Antibiotics

Volume I

Mechanism of Action

Edited by

David Gottlieb and Paul D. Shaw

With 197 Figures

Springer-Verlag Berlin Heidelberg GmbH 1967

David Gottlieb
Professor of Plant Pathology
University of Illinois
Urbana, Illinois

Paul D. Shaw
Associate Professor of Biochemistry
University of Illinois
Urbana, Illinois

ISBN 978-3-662-37649-2 **ISBN 978-3-662-38439-8 (eBook)**
DOI 10.1007/978-3-662-38439-8

Originally published by Springer-Verlag Berlin · Heidelberg in 1967
Softcover reprint of the hardcover 1st edition 1967

Library of Congress Catalog Card Number 67—21462.

Dedication

For most areas of scientific pursuit, there is usually that rare investigator who has the imagination to conceive ideas, who has faith in his visions, and who has the ability to critically test his concepts in the laboratory. Almost invariably, this scientist also inspires younger men to enthusiastically enter into his research program. To him should go the accolades and the recognitions of the esteem in which he is held. As only a small part of this esteem, we wish to dedicate these books to Professor SELMAN A. WAKSMAN in appreciation of his leadership and contributions in all facets of antibiotic research.

Preface

The idea for publishing these books on the mechanism of action and on the biosynthesis of antibiotics was born of frustration in our attempts to keep abreast of the literature. Gone were the years when we were able to keep a bibliography on antibiotics and feel confident that we could find everything that was being published on this subject. These fields of investigation were moving forward so rapidly and were encompassing so wide a range of specialized areas in microbiology and chemistry that it was almost impossible to keep abreast of developments. In our naiveté and enthusiasm, however, we were unaware that we were toying with an idea that might enmesh us, that we were creating an entity with a life of its own, that we were letting loose a Golom who instead of being our servant would be our master.

That we set up ideals for these books is obvious; they would be current guides to developments and information in the areas of mechanism of action and biosynthesis of antibiotics. For almost every subject, we wished to enlist the aid of an investigator who himself had played a part in determining the nature of the phenomena that were being discussed. One concept for the books was that they include only antibiotics for which a definitive, well-documented mechanism of action or biosynthetic pathway was known. Yet, such an approach would not entirely serve the purpose we projected, for it would not encompass all of the information available in these fields of antibiotic investigations and blind searches for the original literature would still have to be made. We therefore chose to include any and all antibiotics about which some pertinent information had been published. It was obvious even at the start that such a compilation, integration, and analysis of information could never be complete unless scientific investigations ceased at the moment the last manuscript was submitted—an end that was neither desirable nor possible. An addendum was therefore included at the end of the volume and left open for the addition of new information until the last pages of the regular articles had been printed.

The original concept has also been further expanded as the authors of several papers found it advisable to elaborate on their subject. Some of the articles included discussions of compounds that were not strictly antibiotics, but were vital in giving a more comprehensive picture of the biosynthesis of an entire series of natural products. In other cases, the antibiotics have served as tools for the elucidation of metabolic pathways and the contributions included clear and current descriptions of various phases of cellular metabolism.

The clinical and industrial aspects of antibiotics have not been emphasized and for most of them only enough information has been given to allow an evaluation of the studies. There is one notable exception, the chapter on the *in vivo* behavior of penicillin. This exposition highlights the important fact that antibiotics have been sought primarily for their use in controlling diseases. The action of antibiotics in a diseased animal are far more complex than in our *in vitro* systems. To understand the mechanism of action of an antibiotic in disease, data from *in vitro* studies must be considered in light of the effects of the compound in the natural, multifaceted system in which it is used.

Though the ideals for this book became clear, their realization proved more difficult. We had to deal with a real world, one in which people are very much involved in their own enterprises. Our colleagues were all busy, with their own research and teaching. There were commitments for lectures, for committee meetings, for surveys of the state of science, and for almost any other concievable phase of scientific activities. We pleaded, we cajoled, we called attention to their debt to science in this matter. We bullied some acquaintances and praised others. We called on their aid for friendship's sake until we finally had commitments to all our topics.

Soon we became aware that editing these books was teaching us more than scientific facts; we were also learning how individualistic our colleagues were. No editor could indicate to them how to write their papers, nor could he dragoon them to a time schedule or insist on a general style of organization. Instead, we were told how the books should be organized, how individual papers should be written, and what topics should be covered. Under such conditions, the best plan was to retreat and allow the authors as much leeway as possible to express their individual approaches and styles of writing. Each retreat was not without resistance from the editors and battle lines were always set beyond which further withdrawal could not go. Many friendships hung in balance during the process, but in the end these relationships persevered.

Finally, there were the many colleagues who helped us and whom we wish to thank. This book would not have existed if it were not for the cooperative effort of our students who gave much time to searching the literature and making certain that our records of antibiotics were complete. We wish to thank them for this aid. Our gratitude goes also to the authors of the papers who were invariably cooperative and understanding during the many trials through which their manuscripts have gone. Finally, we wish to thank Dr. KONRAD F. SPRINGER of Springer-Verlag for his humanistic approach to the project and for his sensitive discernment of the relationship between the publishing media and the sciences which they serve.

Urbana, Illinois, 1967

DAVID GOTTLIEB

PAUL D. SHAW

Contents

Addenda

Contributors

GEORGE ACS, Institute of Muscle Disease, 515 East 71 St., New York, N.Y./USA

B. K. BHUYAN, Biochemical Research, The Upjohn Company, Kalamazoo, Michigan/USA

THOMAS D. BROCK, Department of Bacteriology, Indiana University, Bloomington, Indiana/USA

PAUL G. CALTRIDER, Eli Lilly and Company, Indianapolis, Indiana/USA

A. CERAMI, Rockefeller University, New York, N.Y./USA

F. N. CHANG, Department of Pharmacology, University of Wisconsin, Medica School, Madison, Wisconsin/USA

JOHN M. CLARK, Jr., Biochemistry Division, Department of Chemistry and Chemical Engineering, University of Illinois, Urbana, Illinois/USA

A. DI MARCO, Istituto Nazionale per lo Studio e la Cura dei Tumori, Piazzale Gorini 22, Milano/Italia

JAMES R. FLORINI, Department of Zoology, Syracuse University, Syracuse, New York/USA

EDWIN H. FLYNN, The Lilly Research Laboratories, Eli Lilly and Company, ndianapolis, Indiana/USA

LAURA FRONTALI, Istituto di Fisiologia Generale, Cattedra di Chimica delle Fermentazioni, Universita di Roma, Roma/Italia

G. F. GAUSE, Institute of New Antibiotics, Academy of Medical Sciences of USSR, Bolshaia Pirogovskaia 11, Moscow G 21/USSR

CARL W. GODZESKI, The Lilly Research Laboratories, Eli Lilly and Company, Indianapolis, Indiana/USA

LUIGI C. GORINI, Department of Bacteriology and Immunology, Harvard Medical School, Boston 15, Massachusetts/USA

DAVID GOTTLIEB, Department of Plant Pathology, University of Illinois, Urbana, Illinois/USA

ARMAND J. GUARINO, Department of Biochemistry, Woman's Medical College of Pennsylvania, Philadelphia, Pennsylvania/USA

FRED E. HAHN, Department of Molecular Biology, Walter Reed Army Institute of Research, Washington, D. C./USA

LADISLAV J. HANKA, Department of Microbiology, The Upjohn Company, Kalamazoo, Michigan/USA

C. L. HARVEY, Hoffman-La Roche, Inc., Nutley, New Jersey/USA

I. B. HOLLAND, Department of Genetics, University of Leicester, Leicester/England

FLOYD M. HUBER, Eli Lilly and Company, Indianapolis, Indiana/USA

D. E. HUNT, Kettering-Meyer Laboratories, Southern Research Institute Birmingham, Alabama/USA

F. EDMUND HUNTER, Jr., Department of Pharmacology, Washington University, St. Louis 10, Missouri/USA

V. N. IYER, Microbiology Research Institute, Canada Department of Agriculture, Ottawa/Canada

G. A. JACOBY, Department of Bacteriology and Immunology, Harvard Medical School, Boston 15, Massachusetts/USA

D. C. JORDAN, Microbiology Department, University of Guelph, Ontario/Canada

STEPHEN C. KINSKY, Washington University, School of Medicine, St. Louis, Missouri/USA

S. G. KNIGHT, Department of Bacteriology, University of Wisconsin, Madison, Wisconsin/USA

F. KNÜSEL, Research Laboratories, Pharmaceutical Division, CIBA Ltd., Basel/Switzerland

ALLEN I. LASKIN, The Squibb Institute for Medical Research, New Brunswick, New Jersey/USA

TOMOMASA MISATO, Rikagaku Kenkyusho, The Institute of Physical and Chemica Research, Honkomagome Bunkyo-ku, Tokyo/Japan

DANIEL NATHANS, Department of Microbiology, The John Hopkins University, School of Medicine, Baltimore, Maryland/USA

FRANCIS C. NEUHAUS, Biochemistry Division, Department of Chemistry, Northwestern University, Evanston, Illinois/USA

MASAYASU NOMURA, Laboratory of Genetics, University of Wisconsin, Madison, Wisconsin/USA

JACOB NÜESCH, Research Laboratories, Pharmaceutical Division, CIBA Ltd., Basel/Switzerland

R. F. PITTILLO, Kettering-Meyer Laboratories, Southern Research Institute, Birmingham, Alabama/USA

EDWARD REICH, Rockefeller University, New York, N.Y./USA

F. REUSSER, Department of Microbiology, The Upjohn Company, Kalamazoo, Michigan/USA

P. E. REYNOLDS, Sub-department of Chemical Microbiology, Department of Biochemistry, University of Cambridge, Cambridge/England

JOHN S. RIESKE, Department of Physiological Chemistry, School of Medicine, Ohio State University, Columbus, Ohio/USA

LOIS S. SCHWARTZ, Department of Pharmacology, Washington University, St. Louis, Missouri/USA

OLDRICH K. SEBEK, Department of Microbiology, The Upjohn Company, Kalamazoo, Michigan/USA

PAUL D. SHAW, Department of Plant Pathology, University of Illinois, Urbana Illinois/USA

HAROLD T. SHIGEURA, Merck Sharp & Dohme Research Laboratories, Division of Merck & Company, Inc., Rahway, New Jersey/USA

MALCOLM R. SIEGEL, Department of Plant Pathology, University of Kentucky, Lexington, Kentucky/USA

C. J. SIH, School of Pharmacy, University of Wisconsin, Madison, Wisconsin/USA

JASWANT SINGH, Oregon State College, Corvallis, Oregon/USA

HUGH D. SISLER, University of Maryland, Department of Botany, College Park, Maryland/USA

LIBOR SLECHTA, Research Laboratories, The Upjohn Company, Kalamazoo, Michigan/USA

JACK L. STROMINGER, Department of Pharmacology, The University of Wisconsin Medical Center, Madison, Wisconsin/USA

SHAN-CHING SUNG, Kinsmen Laboratory of Neurological Research, University of British Columbia, Vancouver 8, British Columbia/Canada

WACLAW SZYBALSKI, McArdle Laboratories, University of Wisconsin, Madison, Wisconsin/USA

NOBUO TANAKA, Institute of Applied Microbiology, University of Tokyo, Tokyo/Japan

GIORGIO TECCE, Istituto di Fisiologia Generale, Cattedra di Chimica delle Fermentazioni, Universita di Roma, Roma/Italia

D. VAZQUEZ, Instituto de Biologia Celular, Centro de Investigaciones Biologicas, Madrid/España

D. C. WARD, Rockefeller University, New York, N.Y./USA

EUGENE D. WEINBERG, Department of Microbiology, Indiana University, Bloomington, Indiana/USA

B. WEISBLUM, Department of Pharmacology, University of Wisconsin, Medical School, Madison, Wisconsin/USA

Penicillins and Cephalosporins

I. In Vitro

Edwin H. Flynn and Carl W. Godzeski

Interpretation of the meaning of a term such as "mechanism of action" as applied to antimicrobial substances is certain to be highly variable and dependent to a considerable degree on the background and area of interest of the individual reader. To a classically trained microbiologist, morphological effects may be dominant and of the greatest significance while a biochemically minded individual will wish to know the nature of specific metabolic changes; a clinician interested in infectious diseases wishes to know what events are observable in the host and how these relate to the probable success or failure of his therapy.

It is proposed that this chapter will attempt to present our available knowledge on mechanism of action of penicillins and cephalosporins from two points of view. Observation based on experimental work done under substantially artificial conditions (artificial, if viewed from the standpoint of infectious disease) has led to detailed information about alteration in the life of the "isolated" bacterial cell. This will be presented to supply basic understanding for a discussion of the second area of interest; namely, the effects of penicillins and cephalosporins on the bacterial cell in a host environment. It is hoped that such an approach will clarify for the reader the significance of laboratory observations made with an essentially isolated, three or two compartment system (antibiotic and cell, with or without nutrient medium) and allow use of these data to achieve a more complete understanding of the bacterial invader-host-antibiotic interactions (the "triad of infection").

Discussion here will be restricted to compounds represented by structure (I) (penicillins) and structure (II) (cephalosporins). Other related structures have been described in the chemical literature, but studies of their effects on the bacterial cell have not been published to our knowledge.

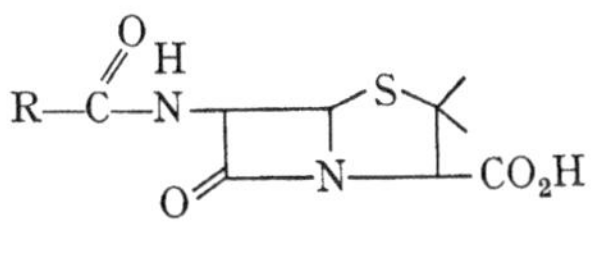

(I)

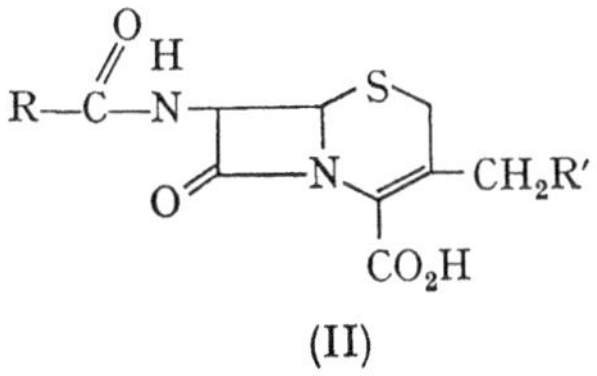

(II)

A brief word about the meaning of the phrase "antibiotic activity" may be appropriate. In a strict sense, to label some substance as having antibiotic activity or not having antibiotic activity is meaningless, since the term depends on a quantitative assessment and there is no fixed value which has been adopted. Our difficulty can be illustrated by pointing out the fact that a β-hemolytic streptococcus may be inhibited by benzylpenicillin at a concentration as low as 0.008 μg/ml while strains of certain "sensitive" Gram-negative organisms may require 25 μg/ml, a 3×10^3 change in magnitude. Yet, in general, investigators would feel that effects observable within this range constitute meaningful activity. Antibiotic substances of many other classes show an activity only at concentrations of 0.5 μg/ml or higher and may be classed as inactive unless they inhibit growth at 25 μg/ml or less, a 50-fold difference in magnitude. It is reasonable to say that the tendency has been to relate activity to potentially achievable blood levels in the therapeutic situation; a consensus would surely place the upper limit of meaningful activity, then, at 25—50 μg/ml. As with most generalized statements, of course, there will be exceptions to this broad rule of thumb.

The Bacterial Cell

Essential to an understanding of the events through which an antibiotic exerts its action is a familiarity with physical and chemical characteristics of the bacterial cell. Since the unique appeal of antibiotic substances is based mainly on their selective toxicity for the microbial as compared to the mammalian cell, differences in these cell types are germane to the discussion.

During the past fifteen years, much has been learned about the structure of the bacterial cell and function of many of the components. It is not possible to consider in detail all of the available information. For comprehensive discussions the reader is referred to a series of volumes edited by GUNSALUS and STANIER (1960—1964). Other pertinent references may be cited (POLLOCK and RICHMOND, 1965; PERKINS, 1963; SALTON, 1962; HUGHES, 1962). Very briefly stated, it can be said the bacterial cell consists of an outer layer called the cell wall (other material may be found on the outer surface of the cell wall, e.g. capsular polysaccharide, etc., with certain organisms), a (cytoplasmic) cell membrane immediately adjacent to the inner wall surface and more or less intimately connected with it, and a protoplasm enclosed by these structures which contains a variety of ultrastructural components. Mitochondria as such are not recognized in the bacterial protoplasm; ribosomes are abundant, together with chromatin bodies. These two components seem to be the essential protein synthesizing materials. Also commonly found in bacterial protoplasm is highly polymerized inorganic phosphate. Other components when found are likely to be less general in their occurrence and restricted to various genera or families.

An experimental approach to studies of the bacterial cell wall became available when MUDD *et al.* (1941) showed that sonic rupture of bacterial cells left a resistant wall structure. DAWSON (1949), following a report by KING and ALEXANDER (1948) on the mechanical killing of bacteria by shaking with glass beads, demonstrated a relatively clean separation of cell walls from protoplasmic material using this technique. A number of workers have since contributed knowledge concerning cell wall preparations; one of the principal investigators in this field, M. R. J. SALTON [see GUNSALUS and STANIER (1960—1964), Vol. I], has written a useful description of such studies.

The bacterial cell wall is a relatively rigid structure capable of retaining much of its original shape even after loss of the cell contents. The wall constitutes from 20 to 40% of the cell, depending on age and conditions for growth of the culture. The high value was obtained with valine as a limiting factor in the medium (SHOCKMAN *et al.*, 1958). Wall thickness may vary two-fold, from 100—200 Å or greater, being generally in the higher range for Gram-positive organisms and the lower range for Gram-negatives. Structural integrity of the wall and its resistance to deformation supply the reason that the bacterial cell may have a solute concentration corresponding to an osmotic pressure of 5—25 atmospheres as shown by MITCHELL and MOYLE (1956) and earlier by WEIBULL (1955). Osmotic fragility is characteristic of most bacteria when the wall structure is removed or damaged, as by the action of lysozyme, for example.

Studies of cell wall composition have shown that, in bacteria, gross differences exist between those organisms which give a Gram-positive stain and those which are classified as Gram-negative. The Gram-negative group have a cell wall composition high in protein and lipid and low in reducing sugar and hexosamine content when compared with Gram-positive bacteria. These differences are given in Table 1 for representatives of each class of organism.

Table 1 [1]

Organism	% Dry weight of cell wall			
	Reducing substances	Hexosamine	Lipid	Total N
Sarcina lutea (G+)	46.5	16.3	1.1	7.6
B. subtilis (G+)	34.0	8.5	2.6	5.1
E. coli (G—)	16.0	3.0	20.8	10.1
S. *pullorum* (G—)	46.0	4.8	19.0	6.4

[1] Abstracted from SALTON (1953).

It is evident, from examination of the figures in Table 1, that response to the Gram staining technique is related to chemical composition of the cell wall. More detailed analysis of amino acid constitution showed that cell wall material from the Gram-negative organisms possessed a large number of naturally occurring amino acids, including the sulfur containing ones, while Gram-positive cell wall substance was essentially free of the aromatic amino acids as well as the sulfur amino acids.

CLARKE and LILLY (1962) have proposed a general structure for cell walls of Gram-negative bacteria. They suggest that the surface layers of these organisms consist of two membranes with a rigid wall structure between them which is composed of mucopeptide and teichoic acid. The inner or "cytoplasmic" membrane would be made up of the layers, protein-lipid-lipid-polysaccharide while the outer membrane would be reversed, i.e. polysaccharide-lipid-lipid-protein; the rigid wall could be linked to either or both of these membranes which it separates.

The foregoing description of gross characteristics of the bacterial cell is sufficient to delineate that marked differences exist between these cells and the mammalian cell. The most striking difference, in a general sense, is the presence of a cell wall which is characterized by its thickness and a high degree of rigidity, this structure being much less prominent in mammalian cells. Again, one must be cautious of exceptions because of the existence of bacterial forms with, probably, nearly all variations in degree of cell wall structure (L-forms, protoplasts, spheroplasts, and mycoplasma).

The gross aspects of cell wall composition have been mentioned in abbreviated form. It is possible to describe more fully the chemistry of certain components of wall structure, especially in the case of a few Gram-positive bacteria. Much less is known with respect to Gram-negative microorganisms.

In the space allotted we are unable to review completely the historical development of our present knowledge of cell wall structure. For those interested, competent coverage has been given in a number of publications (SALTON, 1964; ROGERS, 1965; PERKINS, 1963). Work on this complex structure problem was

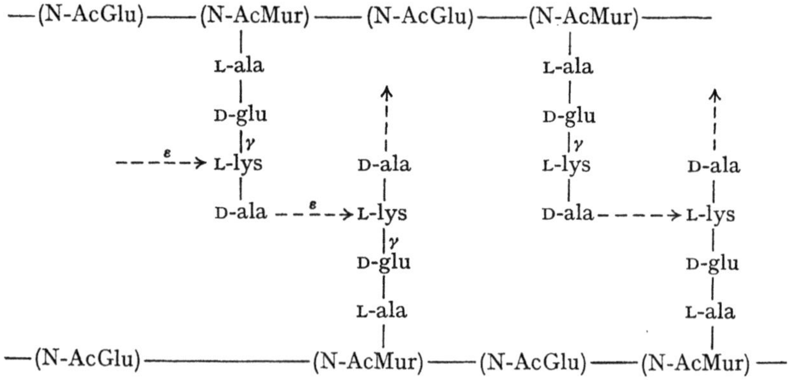

Fig. 1. General structure for cell wall mucopeptide, taken from WISE and PARK (1965). Dotted arrows indicate probable cross links to the epsilon amino groups of lysine. N-AcGlu = N-acetylglucosamine; N-AcMur = N-acetylmuramic acid

only possible after SALTON and HORNE (1951) made available a method for purification of cell walls. It can be said now that all walls of Gram-positive bacteria are composed of a macromolecule called mucopeptide (also glycopeptide), teichoic acids, occasionally teichuronic acids, in many cases polysaccharide, and in certain instances protein (if protein must be made up of a wide variety of amino acids to be so classified). The mucopeptide and teichoic acids seem to be very general in their occurrence, while polysaccharide and protein are probably restricted.

A general structure for cell wall mucopeptide has been proposed by WISE and PARK (1965) as shown in Fig. 1.

Although the foregoing structure gives a generalized conception, variations of it occur among bacterial species. Lysine may be replaced by *meso* or L,L-diaminopimelic acid, α,γ-diaminobutyric acid, or ornithine (WISE and PARK, 1965). D-aspartic acid is also found, notably in lactobacilli (IKAWA and SNELL, 1960), probably linked to lysine. Evidence is available to indicate glutamic acid is present as isoglutamine (TIPPER and STROMINGER, 1965) and that crosslinkage between peptide chains is through polyglycine bridges in, for example, *Staphylococcus aureus*. In another species, *Micrococcus lysodeikticus*, the α-carboxyl group of glutamic acid forms an amide bond with the amino group of a glycine molecule (TIPPER and STROMINGER, 1965). Not shown in the general structure above is the presence of O-acetyl groups which may occur in amounts up to 7% (*Lactobacillus bulgaricus*) (IKAWA and SNELL, 1960). Linkage of the peptide to the aminopolysaccharide "backbone" is through the carboxyl group of the lactic acid component of N-acetylmuramic acid (III). N-Acetylglucosamine (IV) is linked with the N-acetylmuramic acid through a $\beta(1\rightarrow4)$ bond as indicated by the evidence of JEANLOZ, SHARON, and FLOWERS (1963) for the structure of a disaccharide produced when *M. lysodeikticus* is digested with lysozyme. JEANLOZ and OSAWA (1965) have also published an improved synthesis of muramic acid, the D-lactyl ether of D-glucosamine. N-Acetylmuramic acid to N-acetylglucosamine bonding is indicated as $\beta(1\rightarrow4)$ from evidence provided by SALTON and GHUYSEN (1959) in work on *M. lysodeikticus* cell wall components.

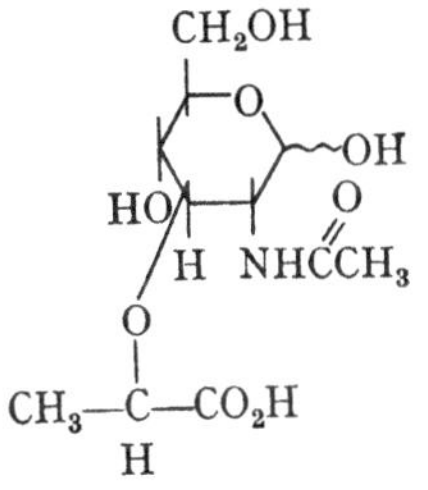

(III)

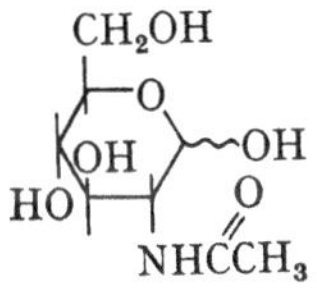

(IV)

As mentioned, dotted arrows in the generalized structure, Fig. 1, indicate crosslinking through pentaglycine bridges such that the terminal glycine carboxyl is attached to the epsilon amino group of lysine; the amino group at the other end of the pentaglycine bridge is attached to the alanine carboxyl of the pentapeptide. Thus, a more detailed representation may be drawn based on present knowledge (WISE and PARK, 1965; TIPPER and STROMINGER, 1965), at least for *S. aureus* mucopeptide, as shown in Fig. 2.

The teichoic acids, which have been mentioned in passing as being cell wall components, undoubtedly serve an important function. Much is known of their chemical structure, although principally where Gram-positive bacteria have been the source. In spite of rather detailed chemical structural information, their role in cell structure is undefined. The subject has been reviewed (SALTON, 1964; BADDILEY, 1964). Detailed chemical studies have shown the teichoic acids to be polymers composed of chains of glycerol or ribitol residues joined by phosphate groups with sugars attached to the glycerol or ribitol. D-Alanine residues have been found in ester linkage with some of the hydroxyl groups. Both the glycerol and ribitol teichoic acids are found in cell wall preparations, principally of Gram-positive bacteria. The glycerol teichoic acids are also found in bacterial preparations which are supposedly free of cell wall (protoplasts) and have been called intracellular teichoic acids when this is the case. However, it appears that these fractions may actually reside at the membrane, perhaps at the surface between membrane and wall. A representative structure is shown in Fig. 3.

Although a structural role for teichoic acids has not been defined, it is known that they are involved in determination of serological groupings of certain

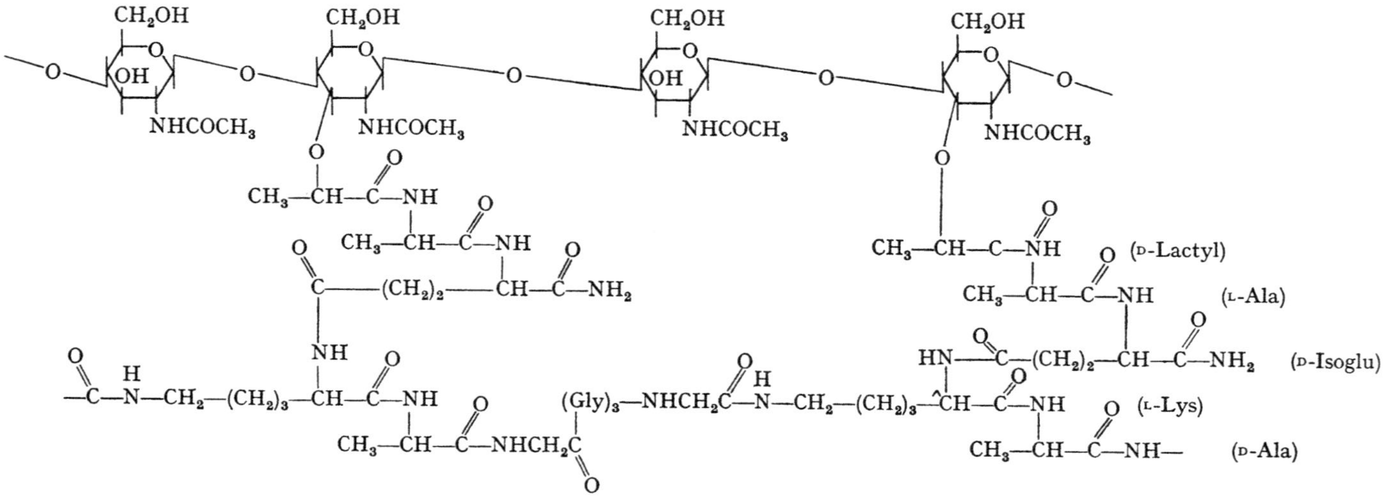

Fig. 2. Detailed structure of cell wall mucopeptide arrived at by incorporating data from SALTON (1964), WISE and PARK (1965), TIPPER and STROMINGER (1965), and JEANLOZ, *et al.* (1963). Still to be placed are O-acetyl groups and inter-chain cross links. This structure may be most representative of *S. aureus* mucopeptide. Other species will vary (see text and Fig. 1). Linear mucopeptide is comparable to the above without the pentaglycine bridge completed

bacteria. This has been shown to be the case for lactobacilli (BADDILEY, 1964; BADDILEY and DAVISON, 1961) and staphylococci (STROMINGER and GHUYSEN, 1963). Moreover, their presence in the wall (or wall-membrane?) as an integral, covalently bonded component seems fairly certain, at least for strains of *S. aureus* (STROMINGER and GHUYSEN, 1963).

A more detailed discussion of bacterial cell membrane is of interest. It is quite likely that, apart from selective permeability functions, it or closely contiguous and included structures carry an active synthetic role. Modern electron microscope studies show that in a healthy Gram-positive bacterium the membrane looks like a sandwich in which the outer layers are thought to be of a lipid character and the filling to be protein, as discussed earlier.

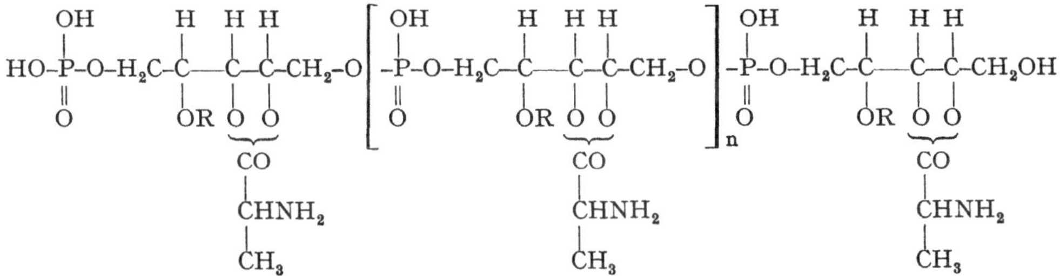

Fig. 3. Ribitol teichoic acid from *S. aureus*. R = α- and β-N-acetylglucosaminyl; n = 6. Taken from BADDILEY (1964). Ribitol may be replaced by glycerol in other cases to form the glycerol teichoic acids. C-2 of the glycerol residues is then substituted by alanine and N-acetylglycosamine in an alternating sequence or with β-glucosyl-[1 → 6]-β-glucosyl

Actual separation of membranes has been achieved at least for Gram-positive bacteria, and was reported first by WEIBULL (1953) following treatment of *B. megaterium* with lysozyme to produce protoplasts which were then lysed by exposure to hypotonic conditions. Differential sedimentation separated the so-called "ghost" fraction which is considered to represent cytoplasmic membrane. Several investigations of the chemical and enzymic make-up of the membrane structure from various bacteria have been published. A recent paper by SALTON and FREER (1965) provides references to pertinent earlier literature. Gram-positive bacteria in several instances have been shown to have cell membrane which constitutes from 10—25% of the dry weight of the cell (SALTON and FREER, 1965). The membrane is mostly protein (50—75%) and lipid (20—30%) with some carbohydrate (10—20%) and does not vary greatly in composition with changes in conditions of growth, although SHOCKMAN *et al.* (1963) have indicated a change in both amount and composition of membrane from *S. fecalis* when grown under different conditions. Little information has appeared concerning isolated cell membranes from Gram-negative bacteria; some studies of membrane-cell wall preparations have been made.

The *Mycoplasma* offer a potential source of relatively pure cell membrane since a primary characteristic of these organisms is the lack of cell wall structure. RAZIN and co-workers (1963) have reported membrane composition from *Mycoplasma laidlawii* to be 37—40% lipid and 50—60% protein with 2—4% carbohydrate and traces of nucleic acids. They have presented evidence (RAZIN *et al.*, 1965) that such membranes appear to be composed of centrifugally homogeneous lipid-protein subunits which are formed from the membrane on treatment with a surfactant. Such subunits can be caused to reaggregate by removal of surfactant and exposure to divalent cations. The reaggregated material bears some resemblance to original membrane as judged by electron micrographs.

Structures called mesosomes are associated with the membrane in certain instances and may be an integral component, occurring as invaginations of the membranous structure. The mesosomes may be one of the sites of enzymic activity since certain reactions have been found to be associated with a membrane preparation (WEIBULL *et al.*, 1959). An important part of these activities are those represented by cytochrome linked electron transport systems and respiratory enzymes. Many other enzymes occur in the membrane or particles closely associated with it. For a helpful discussion, the reader is referred to the paper by HUGHES (1962).

Mechanism of Antibacterial Action of Penicillin

The foregoing discussion of bacterial cell structure is included in this chapter to enable readers to appreciate more fully the implications of what can be said concerning the means by which penicillin may cause death of a bacterial cell. Involvement of the structural integrity of a cell in this killing effect was evident and reported as early as 1940 by GARDNER (1940). He described "grotesque giant forms" from Gram-negative rods, and from staphylococci the occurrence of "spherical enlargement of the cell and imperfect fission". Fleming's original report on penicillin mentioned lysis of staphylococci in the presence of the agent (FLEMING, 1929). The implication, that impairment of structural integrity was an early consequence of exposure to penicillin, was strongly supported by Lederberg's observations (LEDERBERG, 1956) on enteric bacteria which were transformed from their original rod shape into spherical bodies on exposure to penicillin. Carried out in the presence of a hypertonic concentration of sucrose and in the presence of magnesium ion, the protoplasts which were formed remained viable and reverted to rods when penicillin was removed. This was considered to support the hypothesis that the "primary" action of penicillin was on synthesis or maintenance of a component of the cell wall.

A further characteristic of penicillin action is that this substance exerts little killing effect except during an active growth phase (HOBBY *et al.*, 1942; CHAIN and DUTHIE, 1945). Resting cells show no change in oxygen consumption even when large amounts of penicillin are present, but during the early lag and logarithmic phases of growth a strong inhibitory effect is observed.

In addition to the foregoing evidence of an effect of penicillin on cell wall integrity, electron micrographs have been published which indicate defects in cross wall formation may be an early occurrence (SALTON, 1964, p. 212). Furthermore, a highly specific binding of penicillin has been demonstrated for *S. aureus*, using 1-^{14}C labeled penicillin. Moreover, the binding, which is irreversible, seems to involve a definite "penicillin binding component (PBC)" which is intimately associated with cell wall membrane. A thorough discussion has been published by COOPER (1956).

Composition of a picture is emerging, then, which makes reasonable another earlier observation. PARK and JOHNSON (1949) noted, using penicillin concentrations of 0,1—1,0 μg/ml, the accumulation of abnormal amounts of acid-soluble, labile phosphate in *S. aureus* cells. A later paper by PARK (1952) demonstrated the nature of the labile phosphate compounds, showing that one was a uridine pyrophosphate derivative containing an amino sugar, and two others were derived from this by having amino acids attached to the amino sugar component. Studies published in the interim by others, which described some characteristics of bacterial cell wall composition, led PARK and STROMINGER (1957) and STROMINGER *et al.* (1959) to propose that uridine nucleotides were cell wall precursors. These substances were caused to accumulate as a consequence of the intervention of penicillin in biosynthetic steps for wall synthesis. They further speculated that this interference might be as a specific inhibitor of a transglycosidation reaction involving the nucleotide.

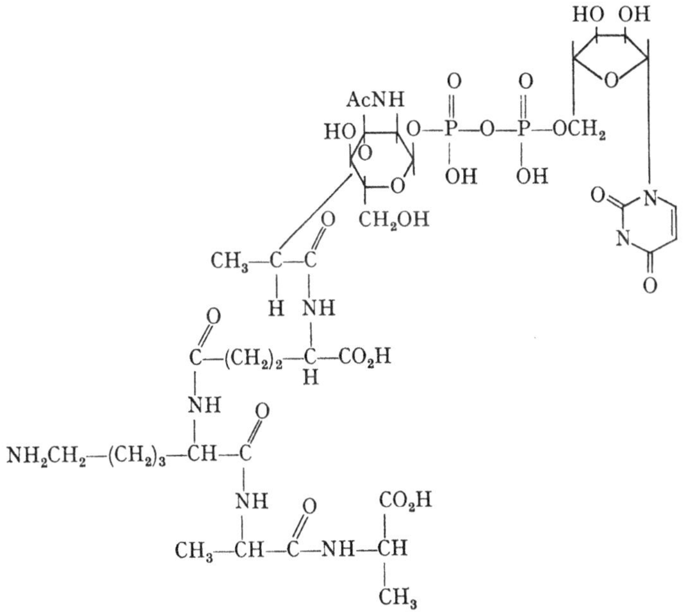

Fig. 4. Uridine nucleotide peptide structure proposed by PARK and STROMINGER (1957). Peptide sequence is ala-D-glu-L-lys-ala-ala

In the period 1956—1959, data from a number of sources (STRANGE and KENT, 1959; STROMINGER, 1959; STROMINGER *et al.*, 1959; STROMINGER, 1962) allowed the logical deduction that uridine nucleotide-peptides were present in varying structural modifications (of the peptide chain) in a number of bacteria, that these structures were as represented, e.g. in Fig. 4, and that penicillin was capable of causing accumulation of the compounds, which appeared to be precursors of bacterial cell wall substance. However, there does not seem to be direct evidence for incorporation of the amino sugar-peptide component of these nucleotides into cell wall as yet (SALTON, 1960, p. 80).

Buildup of the linear glycopeptide polymer (illustrated in Fig. 1 and 2) does not appear to be affected by penicillin (ANDERSON *et al.*, 1965; CHATTERJEE and PARK, 1964; MEADOW *et al.*, 1964), nor does formation of a lipid monomer complex which may be necessary for transport (ANDERSON *et al.*, 1965; MATSUHASHI *et al.*, 1965).

An interesting observation by MEADOW and co-workers (1964) was that formation of the linear glycopeptide polymer required, in addition to enzyme and substrates (UDP-acetylmuramyl-ALA-GLU-LYS-ALA-ALA and UDP-GlcNAc), the presence of filter paper before polymerization proceeded. A later reference (ANDERSON *et al.*, 1965) noted that preparation of enzyme from cells, which was accomplished by grinding with alumina rather than by sonic disintegration, gave an active system requiring no filter paper. These requirements illumine a tantalizing facet of the biosynthetic sequence; polymerization requires a matrix or support of some size before a realistic rate is observed. An effect of

UTP
↓ N-AcGlu-1-P
UDP-N-AcGlu
↓ $CH_3—CH(OPO_3H_2)—CO_2H$
UDP-N-AcMur
↓ 4 steps; addition of amino acids
UDP-N-AcMur pentapeptide
↓ 1. phospholipid 2. UDP-N-AcGlu
Disaccharide-pentapeptide
↓ pentaglycine (activated)
Disaccharide-pentapeptide-pentaglycine
Penicillin block ⟶ ↓ acceptor linear mucopeptide
Cross-linked mucopeptide + D-alanine

Fig. 5. Steps in synthesis of mucopeptide adapted from STROMINGER and TIPPER (1965). UDP = uridine diphosphate; UTP = uridine triphosphate; N-AcGlu = N-acetyl-glucosamine; N-AcMur = N-acetylmuramic acid

penicillin on this matrix requirement does not seem to be the answer since, at least *in vitro*, the antibiotic has no effect at meaningful concentrations. One could speculate, perhaps, that in the growing cell penicillin may interfere with *formation* of the natural matrix but, once formed, has no effect. This would still seem to be a possibility.

The foregoing observations, many of them originating from experiments with cell free systems, have been extended still further by WISE and PARK (1965) and by TIPPER and STROMINGER (1965). WISE and PARK have noted, using *S. aureus* cells exposed to penicillin for twenty minutes in an amino acid medium, that the mucopeptide formed contained a higher amount of alanine than controls and a greater number of free amino groups in terminal glycine residues. Newly synthesized mucopeptide was crosslinked, but the amount of crosslinkage was considered to be less than that found in controls. They suggest that penicillin may act specifically by inhibiting the transpeptidation reaction in which the alanyl-alanine bond is replaced by alanyl-glycyl. The "normal" sequence postulated is outlined in Fig. 5 with the presumed point of attack by penicillin indicated.

From these observations, WISE and PARK (1965) have proposed that penicillin bears a close resemblance to the L-alanyl-γ-D-glutamyl portion of the glycopeptide molecule. Because of this resemblance, it would substitute in that portion of the active site of the presumed transpeptidase in which the L-alanyl-γ-D-glutamyl portion usually fits and the β-lactam would react to form a covalent bond. A part of their hypothesis notes the free carboxyl of the γ-glutamyl moiety in the glycopeptide and suggests that this is matched by the carboxyl group of penicillin. However, TIPPER and STROMINGER (1965) have contributed evidence that the glutamyl carboxyl is present as the primary amide, i.e. that the amino acid is actually isoglutamine. Moreover, benzylpenicillin amide (HOLYSZ and STAVELY, 1950) and the morpholide (BARNDEN *et al.*, 1953) are biologically active; whether the activity is inherent or results from hydrolysis hasn't been proven.

TIPPER and STROMINGER (1965) and STROMINGER and TIPPER (1965) propose a closely analogous explanation to that of WISE and PARK but with some differences. They view penicillin as an analog of the acyl-D-alanyl-D-alanine fragment in the linear glycopeptide instead of the alanyl-glutamyl portion of the molecule. They suggest the penicillin carboxyl mimics the alanine carboxyl. Again, the question of activity of benzylpenicillin amides may be raised.

FITZ-JAMES and HANCOCK (1965) have made a detailed study of morphological changes induced by penicillin acting on *B. megaterium* both in the absence and the presence of an osmotically stabilizing medium. Serial sections were made of the cells at short time intervals after exposure to penicillin, then examined with the electron microscope. Their results clearly show that the first discernible morphologic change occurs at the developing septa in the form of a distortion of the normal wall-membrane relationship. They observed, in addition, the accumulation of fibrous material, thought to be unorganized wall mucopeptide, in pockets between existing wall and membrane. Since earlier studies on nucleotide accumulation induced by penicillin were done using cells without osmotic stabilization, they suggest that uridine-linked mucopeptides found by PARK may represent only a part of the accumulating cell wall precursors; there may be other small molecules and other larger polymers. These authors reason that penicillin action may not only block entry of UDP-linked mucopeptides into wall polymer but also prevent further incorporation of polymer into integral cell wall structure. Could the secondary effect be related to accumulation of precursors for teichoic acids which may be part of a membrane-wall bridging structure? Although the presence of teichoic acids in *B. megaterium* is not established (SALTON, 1964, p. 164), some evidence for their presence has been advanced.

Still unexplained is an observation by SAUKKONEN (1961) that penicillin causes accumulation of large amounts of cytidine-diphosphoribitol in cells of *S. aureus* 209P. It has been shown that penicillin causes a 30—40% inhibition of teichoic acid synthesis by *S. aureus* (Oxford strain) (ROGERS, 1963). As discussed by ROGERS (1963), synthesis of mucopeptide and teichoic acids may be interdependent; it is conceivable that both could be dependent on initial synthesis of a "primer" or ground substance at a specific point on the wall, e.g. the septal region. One is then faced with the problem of defining the *primary* site or consequence of action of penicillin as distinguished from secondary sites or consequences. Is the proposed site of action on the alanine transpeptidase referred to earlier, a primary or a secondary effect?

Structure-Activity Relationships of the Penicillins

It is beyond the scope of this chapter to discuss, in detail, variations in activity of penicillin with variation in structure. It must be said that integrity of the β-lactam is critical to activity. Modification of the carboxyl group is always accompanied by decreased activity; oxidation of the sulfur in the thiazolidine ring diminished inhibitory effect greatly. All gradations of activity are possible by alteration of the acyl group on the 6-amino position. Many changes represent substantial alterations chemically, such as the difference between penicillin N (V) and penicillin V (VI), yet both exhibit antibiotic activity of consequence, its magnitude depending on the test system.

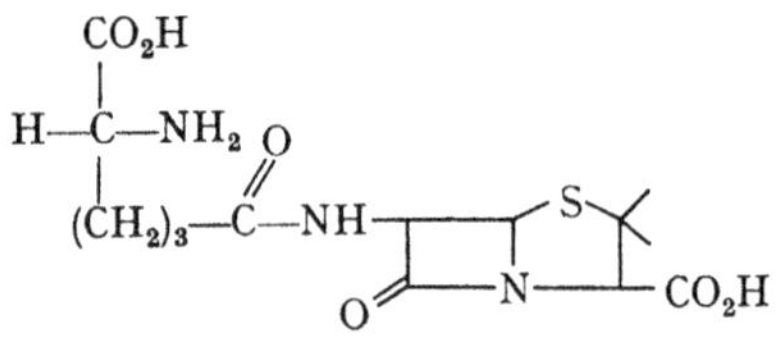

(V)

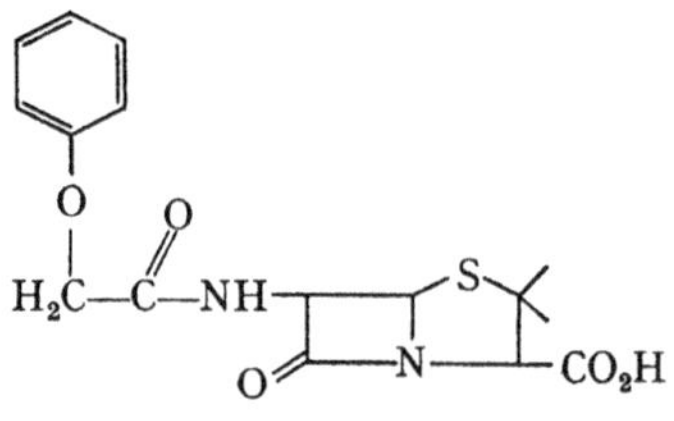

(VI)

Although studies are limited with respect to mechanism of action of penicillins other than benzyl penicillin, little has been published (however, see Part II) to suggest a different mechanism for these compounds.

Many of the quantitative differences in activity might be related to changes in permeability of cells by the compounds. Also certain to be a factor is relative reactivity of the β-lactam ring. Changes may be subtle, such as conversion of one asymmetric center in the acyl side chain to its enantiomorph; this is a change sufficient to alter substantially the antibacterial activity (GOUREVITCH *et al.*, 1961). STEWART (1965) has discussed some of the factors involved in structure-activity relationships, as have DOYLE and NAYLER (1964).

Mechanism of Action of Cephalosporins

The cephalosporins, a family of antibiotics whose evolution has extended over the past fifteen years, bear at least a formal relationship to the penicillins as is evident from their structures. Undoubtedly, cephalosporin C also represents a biogenetic link. Cephalosporin C, progenitor to those compounds which are of medicinal value currently, is produced by a species of *Cephalosporium* which was isolated off the coast of SARDINIA by BROTZU (FLOREY, 1955). The structure (Fig. 6) was obtained as a result of outstanding work by ABRAHAM and NEWTON (1961a). The compound occurs in the fermentation concurrently with penicillin N (V) (cephalosporin N) and cephalosporin P, a steroid antibiotic bearing no structural resemblance to the penicillins and cephalosporins (ABRAHAM, 1957). Although cephalosporin C exhibits antibiotic activity, the magnitude is such as to render it of little practical value. Cleavage of cephalosporin C to produce 7-aminocephalosporanic acid (7-ACA) has not been successful by enzymatic means. A fermentation to produce 7-ACA directly has not been reported.

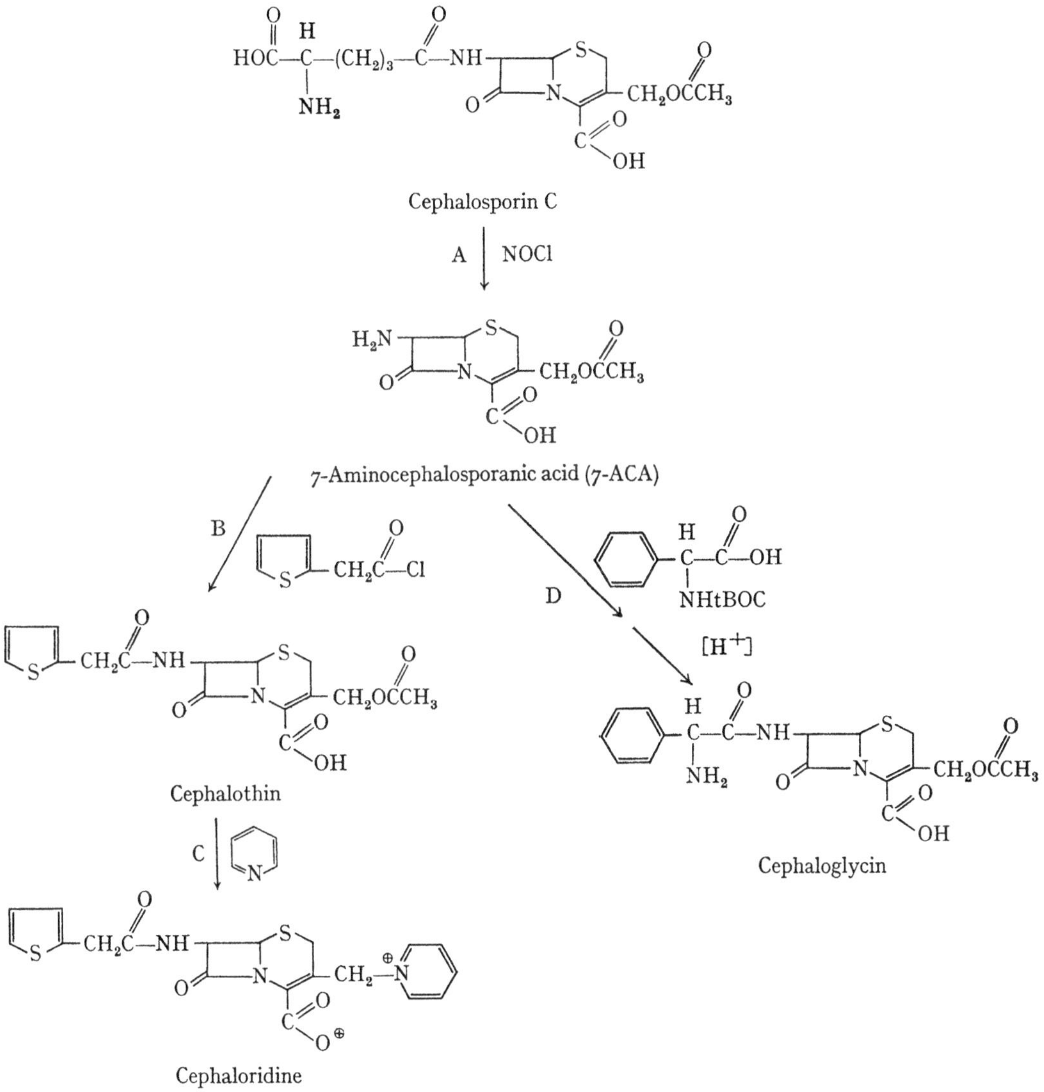

Fig. 6. 7-Aminocephalosporanic acid derivatives. Reactions A and B have been reported (Morin *et al.*, 1962; Chauvette *et al.*, 1962). Procedures C and D, in preparation. t-BOC = tert. butoxycarbonyl

Chemical removal of the aminoadipic acid side chain of cephalosporin C was achieved by Loder *et al.* (1961) and by Morin and co-workers (1962); the latter reaction making available the desired 7-ACA in practical quantities. 7-ACA was readily converted by appropriate reactions to produce those cephalosporins which are of present interest and are depicted in Fig. 6.

Cephalothin, derived by workers at the Lilly Research Laboratories, is stable to penicillinase and exhibits considerable Gram-negative activity (BONIECE *et al.*, 1962). Cephaloridine, a derivative of cephalothin, has been introduced into medical practice in England. It, too, shows considerable Gram-negative activity (WICK and BONIECE, 1965; MUGGLETON *et al.*, 1964). Cephaloglycin, the D-phenylglycine derivative of 7-ACA, is apparently the most active substance against Gram-negative bacteria. Assessment of its activity in the laboratory is complicated by lack of stability; its activity in curing animals with experimental infections is somewhat better than might be predicted from conventional inhibition tests (WICK and BONIECE, 1965).

The only study directed specifically at the question of mechanism of action of cephalosporins is that of CHANG and WEINSTEIN (1964), although ABRAHAM and NEWTON (1961 b) have reported lysis of growing staphylococci and apparent inhibition of synthesis of staphylococcal cell walls by cephalosporin C. CHANG and WEINSTEIN, using methods similar to those employed in penicillin studies, showed a striking decrease in incorporation of lysine into bacterial cell wall mucopeptide in cells incubated with cephalothin. A pronounced accumulation of N-acetyl glucosamine was also evident. Morphologic changes were similar to those observed with penicillin so that circumstantial evidence exists to encourage further work comparing the cephalosporin and penicillin groups.

Whatever the situation, certain of the cephalosporins exhibit a wide range of activity against both Gram-positive and Gram-negative pathogens as evidenced by the antibacterial spectra of cephalothin, cephaloglycin, and cephaloridine (see Tables 2 and 3). It might be surmised that some of this increased Gram-negative activity results from better penetration into the bacterial cell, a better fit at whatever enzyme site is involved, or greater resistance to enzymatic destruction by the bacterial cell if this is a determinant in bacterial resistance. FLEMING *et al.* (1963) have demonstrated existence of a cephalosporinase (β-lactamase) capable of inactivating cephalosporin C and phenylacetamido-cephalosporanic acid. They observed that enzymes which degrade the cephalosporins are widely distributed among the *Enterobacteriaceae*. They comment that the most resistant species are among those which produce these enzymes, while their presence has not been detected among the sensitive species. In any event, it is true that, aside from reactions involving the β-lactam bond as the primary site, chemistry of the β-lactam-dihydrothiazine ring system found in the cephalosporins is radically different from that of the penicillins.

Discussion of *in vitro* testing methods and their inadequacy as a predictor of *in vivo* effectiveness has been published with particular reference to a cephalosporin derivative (GODZESKI *et al.*, 1963). Although it has been notably difficult to develop resistance to cephalothin with staphylococci (GODZESKI *et al.*, 1963), Gram-negative bacteria do become resistant when exposed repeatedly under laboratory conditions. The relation of this observation to the *in vivo* situation has not been explored. The *in vitro* resistance may be related to induction of a cephalosporinase whose existence has been referred to earlier (FLEMING *et al.*, 1963) and confirmed (GODZESKI, unpublished observation).

A brief report from PRESSMAN *et al.* (1964) noted an apparent synergistic reaction between cephalothin and polymyxin against *Pseudomonas aeruginosa.*

Table 2. *Disc-plate sensitivity*[1] *of Gram-negative bacteria to 30 μg discs of six antibiotics*

Organism	Total strains	No. sensitive to					
		Ce-phalo-glycin	Ce-phalo-ridine	Ce-phalo-thin	Tetra-cycline	Chlor-amphe-nicol	Ampi-cillin
Escherichia coli	46	45	45	41	27	40	44
Proteus sp. (indole negative)	21	21	21	21	7	21	21
Proteus sp. (indole positive)	5	0	0	0	1	0	1
Pseudomonas sp.	13	0	1	0	8	2	2
Klebsiella-Aerobacter spp.	25	25	9	10	25	24	12
Salmonella sp.	16	16	16	16	4	16	16
Shigella sp.	11	11	11	11	9	11	10
Paracolobactrum sp.	4	3	0	1	2	4	2
Alcaligenes sp.	2	0	0	0	2	0	1
Haemophilus influenzae	4	4	4	2	4	4	4

[1] The organisms were judged sensitive whenever distinct zones of inhibition were observed. Because of the relative instability of cephaloglycin, these plates were observed more frequently.

Table 3. *Tube-dilution sensitivity of Gram-positive bacteria to three cephalosporin antibiotics*[2]

Organism	Strain	Minimal inhibitory conc. μg/ml		
		Cephalothin	Cephalo-ridine	Cephalo-glycin
Streptococcus sp. (Group A)	C-203	0.1	0.01	0.2
	12385	0.1	0.01	0.2
Streptococcus sp. (Viridans)	9961	0.4	0.02	1.6
	9943	0.4	0.06	1.6
Streptococcus sp. Group D)	Sal.	0.2	0.01	0.2
	9960	>25.0	>2.0	>25.0
S. aureus	3055	0.3	0.02	1.6
	S 112[3]	0.3	0.06	6.3[4]
	H 43[3]	ND	0.06	6.3[4]
	H 114[3]	ND	0.06	6.3[4]
D. pneumoniae	Type I	0.3	0.06	0.4
	Type II	0.3	0.06	0.4
	Type VII	0.3	0.03	0.4
	Type XIV	0.5	0.06	0.4
Cl. tetani	OX	ND	0.6	0.6
	Harvard	0.1	ND	ND
Cl. perfringens	PB6K	0.6	0.6	2.5
C. diphtheriae	mitis	0.6	0.2	1.3
	gravis	0.6	0.2	1.3

[2] 10^5 inoculum in TSB broth except where indicated otherwise. 5% rabbit blood added for streptococci. Abstracted from WICK and BONIECE (1965) and BONIECE *et al.* (1962).

[3] Penicillin-resistant strains.

[4] 12-Hour readings at 10^5 organisms/ml inoculum. Values with 10^3 cells/ml inoculum were 3.1 at 12 hours.

These workers discussed 3 cases of pseudomonas endocarditis that were cured by combination therapy. The high mortality rate common for this form of the disease makes the Pressman results most impressive. There may be underlying factors which are not yet understood in these cases. Confirmation of the *in vivo* results presented is needed.

Table 2 illustrates the nature of Gram-negative antibiotic spectrum activity observed with those cephalosporins for which a place in the treatment of infection would seem to exist. Data are from the work of WICK and BONIECE (1965). Because of a stability problem when in solution, conventional liquid medium tests with cephaloglycin may give misleading data. WICK and BONIECE (1965) have discussed the problem. The data include information on three other widely used compounds, supplied for the purpose of allowing direct comparison since actual figures obtained are so highly dependent on testing prodedures.

Table 3 contains data on the Gram-positive antibiotic spectrum activity of the cephalosporins listed. Results with disc-plate evaluation were comparable to those obtained with the tube-dilution procedure.

See Addendum

References

ABRAHAM, E. P.: Biochemistry of some peptide and steroid antibiotics. In: Ciba lectures in microbial biochemistry. New York: J. Wiley & Sons 1957.

ABRAHAM, E. P., and G. G. F. NEWTON: The structure of cephalosporin C. Biochem. J. **79**, 377 (1961a).

ABRAHAM, E. P., and G. G. F. NEWTON: New penicillins, cephalosporin C, and penicillinase. Endeavour **20**, 92 (1961b).

ANDERSON, J. S., M. MATSUHASHI, M. A. HASKIN, and J L. STROMINGER: Lipid-phosphoacetylmuramyl-pentapeptide and lipid-phosphodisaccharide-pentapeptide: Presumed membrane transport intermediates in cell wall synthesis. Proc. Natl. Acad. Sci. U.S. **53**, 881 (1965).

BADDILEY, J., and A. L. DAVISON: The occurrence and location of teichoic acids in lactobacilli. J. Gen. Microbiol. **24**, 295 (1961).

BADDILEY, J.: Teichoic acids and the bacterial cell wall. Endeavour **23**, 33 (1964).

BARNDEN, R. L., R. M. EVANS, J. C. HAMLET, B. A. HEMS, A. B. A. JANSEN, M. E. TREVETT, and G. B. WEBB: Some preparation uses of benzylpenicillinic ethoxy-formic anhydride. J. Chem. Soc. **1953**, 3733.

BONIECE, W. S., W. E. WICK, D. H. HOLMES, and C. E. REDMAN: *In vitro* and *in vivo* laboratory evaluation of cephalothin, a new broad spectrum antibiotic. J. Bacteriol. **84**, 1292 (1962).

CHAIN, E., and E. S. DUTHIE: Bactericidal and bacteriolytic action of penicillin on the staphylococcus. Lancet **1945**, 652.

CHANG, T., and L. WEINSTEIN: Inhibition of synthesis of the cell wall of *Staphylococcus aureus* by cephalothin. Science **143**, 807 (1964).

CHATTERJEE, A. N., and J. T. PARK: Biosynthesis of cell wall mucopeptide by a particulate fraction from *Staphylococcus aureus*. Proc. Natl. Acad. Sci. U.S. **51**, 9 (1964).

CHAUVETTE, R. R., E. H. FLYNN, B. G. JACKSON, E. R. LAVAGNINO, R. B. MORIN, R. A. MUELLER, R. P. PIOCH, R. W. ROESKE, C. W. RYAN, J. L. SPENCER, and E. VAN HEYNINGEN: Chemistry of cephalosporin antibiotics. II. Preparation of a new class of antibiotics and the relation of structure to activity. J. Am. Chem. Soc. **84**, 3401 (1962).

CLARKE, P. H., and M. D. LILLY: A general structure for cell walls of gram-negative bacteria. Nature **195**, 516 (1962).

COOPER, P. D.: Site of action of radiopenicillin. Bacteriol. Rev. **20**, 28 (1956).

DAWSON, I. M.: Discussion on nature of bacterial surface. Symposium Soc. Gen. Microbiol. **1**, 119 (1949).
DOYLE, F. P., and J. H. C. NAYLER: Penicillins and related structures. Advances in Drug Research **1**, 2 (1964).
FITZ-JAMES, P., and R. HANCOCK: The initial structural lesion of penicillin action in *Bacillus megaterium*. J. Cell Biol. **26**, 657 (1965).
FLEMING, A.: On the antibacterial action of cultures of a penicillium with special reference to their use in the isolation of *B. influenzae*. Brit. J. Exptl. Pathol. **10**, 226 (1929).
FLEMING, P. C., M. GOLDNER, and D. G. GLASS: Observations on the nature, distribution, and significance of cephalosporinase. Lancet **1963**$_{I}$, 1399.
FLOREY, H. W.: Antibiotic products of a versatile fungus. Ann. Internal Med. **43**, 480 (1955).
GARDNER, A. D.: Morphological effects of penicillin on bacteria. Nature **146**, 837 (1940).
GODZESKI, C. W., G. BRIER, and D. E. PAVEY: Cephalothin, a new cephalosporin with a broad antibacterial spectrum. Appl. Microbiol. **11**, 122 (1963).
GOUREVITCH, A., S. WOLFE, and J. LEIN: Effects of side chain on the activity of certain semisynthetic penicillins. Antimicrobial Agents and Chemotherapy, p. 577 (M. FINLAND and G. SAVAGE, eds.). 1961.
GUNSALUS, I. C., and R. Y. STANIER, eds.: The bacteria. A treatise on structure and function (five volumes). New York: Academic Press 1960—1964.
HOBBY, G. L., K. MEYER, and E. CHAFEE: Observations on the mechanism of action of penicillin. Proc. Soc. Exptl. Biol. Med. **50**, 281 (1942).
HOLYSZ, R. P., and H. E. STAVELY: Carboxy derivatives of penicillin. J. Am. Chem. Soc. **72**, 4760 (1950).
HUGHES, D. E.: The bacterial cytoplasmic membrane. J. Gen. Microbiol. **29**, 39 (1962).
IKAWA, M., and E. E. SNELL: Cell wall composition of lactic acid bacteria. J. Biol. Chem. **235**, 1376 (1960).
JEANLOZ, R. W., N. SHARON, and H. M. FLOWERS: The chemical structure of a disaccharide isolated from *Micrococcus lysodeikticus* cell wall. Biochem. Biophys. Research Commun. **13**, 20 (1963).
JEANLOZ, R. W., and T. OSAWA: An improved stereoselective synthesis of 2-amino-3-O-(D-1-carboxyethyl)-2-deoxy-D-glucose (Muramic acid). J. Org. Chem. **30**, 448 (1965).
KING, H. K., and H. ALEXANDER: The mechanical destruction of bacteria. J. Gen. Microbiol. **2**, 315 (1948).
LEDERBERG, J.: Bacterial protoplasts induced by penicillin. Proc. Natl. Acad. Sci. U.S. **42**, 574 (1956).
LODER, B., G. G. F. NEWTON, and E. P. ABRAHAM: The cephalosporin C nucleus (7-aminocephalosporanic acid) and some of its derivatives. Biochem. J. **79**, 408 (1961).
MATSUHASHI, M., C. P. DIETRICH, and J. L. STROMINGER: Incorporation of glycine into the cell wall glycopeptide in *Staphylococcus aureus:* Role of sRNA and lipid intermediates. Proc. Natl. Acad. Sci. U.S. **54**, 587 (1965).
MEADOW, P. M., J. S. ANDERSON, and J. S. STROMINGER: Enzymatic polymerization of UDP-acetylglucosamine by a particulate enzyme from *Staphylococcus aureus* and its inhibition by antibiotics. Biochem. Biophys. Research Commun. **14**, 382 (1964).
MITCHELL, P., and J. MOYLE: Liberation and osmotic properties of the protoplasts of *Micrococcus lysodeikticus* and *Sarcina lutea*. J. Gen. Microbiol. **15**, 512 (1956).
MORIN, R. B., B. G. JACKSON, E. H. FLYNN, and R. W. ROESKE: Chemistry of cephalosporin antibiotics. I. 7-Aminocephalosporanic acid from cephalosporin C. J. Am. Chem. Soc. **84**, 3400 (1962).
MUDD, S., K. POLAVITSKY, T. F. ANDERSON, and L. A. CHAMBERS: Bacterial morphology as shown by the electron microscope. II. The bacterial cell wall in the genus *bacillus*. J. Bacteriol. **42**, 251 (1941).

MUGGLETON, P. W., C. H. O'CALLAGHAN, and W. K. STEVENS: Laboratory evaluations of a new antibiotic — cephaloridine. Brit. Med. J. **1964$_{II}$**, 1234.

PARK, J. T., and M. J. JOHNSON: Accumulation of labile phosphate in *Staphylococcus aureus* grown in the presence of penicillin. J. Biol. Chem. **179**, 585 (1949).

PARK, J. T.: Uridine-5'-pyrophosphate derivatives. III. Amino acid-containing derivatives. J. Biol. Chem. **194**, 897 (1952).

PARK, J. T., and J. L. STROMINGER: Mode of action of penicillin. Science **125**, 99 (1957).

PERKINS, H. R.: Chemical structure and biosynthesis of bacterial cell walls. Bacteriol. Rev. **27**, 18 (1963).

POLLOCK, M. R., and M. H. RICHMOND: Function and Structure in Microorganisms. Cambridge: Cambridge University Press 1965.

PRESSMAN, R. S., V. MARANHAO, and H. GOLDBERG: *Pseudomonas* endocarditis: A therapeutic challenge. Ann. Internal. Med. **61**, 809 (1964).

RAZIN, S., M. ARGAMAN, and J. AVIGAN: Chemical composition of mycoplasma cells and membranes. J. Gen. Microbiol. **33**, 477 (1963).

RAZIN, S., H. J. MOROWITZ, and T. M. TERRY: Membrane subunits of *Mycoplasma laidlawii* and their assembly to membrane-like structures. Proc. Natl. Acad. Sci. U.S. **54**, 219 (1965).

ROGERS, H. J.: The bacterial cell wall. The result of adsorption, structure or selective permeability. J. Gen. Microbiol. **32**, 19 (1963).

ROGERS, H. J.: The outer layers of bacteria: The biosynthesis of structure. Symposium Soc. Gen. Microbiol. **15**, 186 (1965).

SALTON, M. R. J., and R. W. HORNE: Bacterial cell wall. II. Methods of preparation and some properties. Biochim. et Biophys. Acta **7**, 177 (1951).

SALTON, M. R. J.: Studies of the bacterial cell wall. IV. The composition of the cell walls of some gram-positive and gram-negative bacteria. Biochim. et Biophys. Acta **10**, 512 (1953).

SALTON, M. R. J., and J. M. GHUYSEN: The structure of di- and tetrasaccharides released from cell walls by lysozyme and *Streptomyces* F_1 enzyme and the $\beta(1\rightarrow4)$N-acetylhexosaminidase activity of these enzymes. Biochim. et Biophys. Acta **36**, 552 (1959).

SALTON, M. R. J.: Microbial cell walls. In: Ciba Lectures in microbial biochemistry, p. 80—81. NewYork: John Wiley & Sons. 1960.

SALTON, M. R. J.: Cell wall structure synthesis. J. Gen. Microbiol. **29**, 15 (1962).

SALTON, M. R. J.: The bacterial cell wall. Amsterdam: Elsevier Publ. Co. 1964.

SALTON, M. R. J., and J. H. FREER: Composition of the membranes isolated from several gram-positive bacteria. Biochim. et Biophys. Acta **107**, 531 (1965).

SAUKKONEN, J. J.: Acid-soluble nucleotides of *Staphylococcus aureus:* Massive accumulation of a derivative of cytidine diphosphate in the presence of penicillin. Nature **192**, 816 (1961).

SHOCKMAN, G. D., J. J. KOLB, and G. TOENNIES: Relations between bacterial cell wall synthesis, growth phase, and autolysis. J. Biol. Chem. **230**, 961 (1958).

SHOCKMAN, G. D., J. J. KOLB, B. BAKAY, M. J. CONOVER, and G. J. TOENNIES: Protoplast membrane of *Streptococcus faecalis*. J. Bacteriol. **85**, 168 (1963).

STEWART, G. T.: The penicillin group of drugs, p. 98. New York: Elsevier Publ. Co. 1965.

STRANGE, R. E., and L. H. KENT: The isolation, characterization, and chemical synthesis of muramic acid. Biochem. J. **71**, 333 (1959).

STROMINGER, J. L.: The amino acid sequence in the uridine nucleotide-peptide from *Staphylococcus aureus*. Compt. rend. trav. lab. Carlsberg **31**, 181 (1959).

STROMINGER, J. L., J. T. PARK, and R. E. THOMPSON: Composition of the cell wall of *Staphylococcus aureus:* Its relation to the mechanism of action of penicillin. J. Biol. Chem. **234**, 3263 (1959).

STROMINGER, J. L.: Biosynthesis of bacterial cell walls. Federation Proc. **21**, 134 (1962).

STROMINGER, J. L., and J. GHUYSEN: On the linkage between teichoic acid and the glycopeptide in the cell wall of *Staphylococcus aureus*. Biochem. Biophys. Research Commun. **12**, 418 (1963).
STROMINGER, J. L., and D. L. TIPPER: Bacterial cell wall synthesis and structure in relation to the mechanism of action of penicillins and other antibacterial agents. Amer. J. Med. **39**, 708 (1965).
TIPPER, D. J., and J. L. STROMINGER: Mechanism of action of penicillins: A proposal based on their structural similarity to acyl-D-alanyl-D-alanine. Proc. Natl. Acad. Sci. U.S. **54**, 1133 (1965).
WEIBULL, C.: Characterization of the protoplasmic constituents of *Bacillus megaterium*. J. Bacteriol. **66**, 696 (1953).
WEIBULL, C.: Osmotic properties of protoplasts of *Bacillus megaterium*. Exp. Cell Research **9**, 294 (1955).
WEIBULL, C., H. BECKMANN, and L. BERGSTROM: Localization of enzymes in *B. megaterium* strain M. J. Gen. Microbiol. **20**, 519 (1959).
WICK, W. E., and W. S. BONIECE: *In vitro* and *in vivo* laboratory evaluation of cephaloglycin and cephaloridine. Appl. Microbiol. **13**, 248 (1965).
WISE jr., E. M., and J. T. PARK: Penicillin: Its basic site of action as an inhibitor of a peptide cross-linking reaction in cell wall mucopeptide synthesis. Proc. Natl. Acad. Sci. U.S. **54**, 75 (1965).

Penicillins and Cephalosporins

II. In the Host

Carl W. Godzeski and Edwin H. Flynn

Penicillin-Host Interactions

The host environment is so different and complex compared to *in vitro* systems that to expect the mechanism of action of this or any other antibiotic agent to be sequentially identical in both environments is unreasonable. The relative importance of primary, secondary, or later effects as measured in the laboratory test tube may be markedly shifted by interactions of the host polyphasic system. To quote HIRSCH (1965) "... The pathogenesis of infectious disease in many ways illustrates well the infinite complexity of biologic systems, with living things existing in a state of delicate balance under the constant influence of interactions between themselves and their environment." Humoral and cellular mechanisms play varied and complex roles in the host resistance system, changing with such diverse factors as sex, age, hormonal influences, nutrition, intestinal microbial flora and, yes, even the weather (COBURN *et al.*, 1957).

Infectious disease is, then, coexistence or symbiosis which has gotten out of control due to alteration in one or more of the physiological or environmental variables. Infectious disease involves two complex and highly adaptable living systems, host and parasite. As and when host resistance requires supplementation via antibiotic therapy, there arises the triad of infection (disease); host-parasite-drug. This concept is of importance if only to emphasize to the paramedical, iatro- or medical scientist that the three forces interact, one with the other. The manipulation of one always involves alteration of the other two. It is in this extremely plastic environment that chemotherapy should be considered. With this concept in mind, microbiological test results obtained under conditions so far removed from the triad environment as to include distilled water and a simple, standardized synthetic medium seem to lose some of their relevancy. Extrapolation of laboratory results to more complex situations than existed therein may, at times, lead to erroneous or misleading interpretations. This has happened with regularity in the past and will probably continue to happen in the future. We offer here a word of precaution (see GALE, 1959, and MCDERMOTT, 1958) and quote GALE who said, "Things have advanced since that time (1929); now we bomb our way into the house and study the dying spasms of the remains". Let us be aware that the disrupted remains may not have been so disrupted before their organization was "bombed" and that studies on isolated events may not directly relate to the process in the cells or tissues.

In vitro experimental studies on antibiotic mechanism of action cannot include the antibiotic's effect on the subtle and almost unknown nonspecific host resistance factors. These nonspecific factors may be either increased or decreased during therapy and they may profoundly influence the microbe to react to antibiotic stress in a manner that can not be determined *in vitro*. Experimental facts must be related back to the triad of infection before they can be evaluated in the disease state.

The antibiotic age, ushered in via the clinical application of penicillin, has provided the biochemist with powerful tools to ease the study of cellular chemistry but this same age has contributed very little to the understanding of chemotherapeutic mechanisms. The fact that antibiotic therapy may alter many response systems in the host is well known but when this is compounded by alternating or combination antibiotic therapy the effect on host resistance and the complex immunologic system becomes highly unpredictable. Fortunately, antimicrobial effectiveness of the drugs is so great that the patient usually benefits. We say usually, for there are always cases of infectious disease that do not respond as quickly or as completely as might be desired. Thus there are a few patients that carry the infection throughout their lives, sometimes relapsing to overt symptomatic disease states and sometimes not. We have no conclusive evidence on the cause of these clinical problems but the literature is rife with possibilities and speculations (PEASE, 1965; SMADEL, 1963; McDERMOTT, 1958).

As background reading, the essay by McDERMOTT (1958) is an elaborate and provocative piece of writing. He has considered the phenomenon known as "microbial persistence" and it is a recommended reference to anyone interested in the chemotherapy of infectious disease. Microbial plasticity or adaptability allows the cells to survive deleterious environmental influences. As McDERMOTT states, the microbes can "play dead" when menaced by an antibiotic. This is, however, no game to a patient who suffers from the results of a relapsing, persisting infection. To date, clinical research has no sure prevention or cure of this microbial problem. Nor has laboratory research on antibiotic locus of action, as measured in pure cultures or on isolated systems, helped to understand this situation. We must attempt to relate antibiotic action to the cure of disease if we are ever to develop a therapeutic rationale. And we must constantly try to learn more about antibiotic action *in vivo* as well as *in vitro*.

Data so far examined have provided a reasonable and, though still somewhat obscure, rational theory of the mechanism of penicillin's antibacterial action. It is time to emphasize, however, that there are shortcomings in the extrapolation of some of the accumulated information to the *in vivo* situation.

The action of penicillin against bacteria residing within a host is unlikely to be bactericidal without the participation of host resistance factors. Antibiotics used, as penicillin is used, for the cure of disease must exert their effects on organisms adapted to the host environment. The activity of penicillin in the host environment is probably similar to its activity in stabilized media. Blood and tissue fluids have competing stabilizing and lytic effects on microbes and microbial spheroplasts. The influences of antibody, complement, opsonins, phagocytin, lysozyme, miscellaneous proteins, polyamines, amino acids, vitamins and hormones, and other circulating or fixed biochemical substances in host tissues, lymph, and blood are almost totally unknown in regard to penicillin activity. These factors also affect the growth and survival capacity of the invading bacterium, increasing or decreasing the apparent activity of penicillins in a rather indirect manner. The effect of bacterial adaptation to the environment has long been recognized in the laboratory (NEIDHARDT, 1963; BROWN, 1964; MEYNELL, 1961). Research on chemotherapeutic problems seems to have intentionally ignored this information.

The specificity that some organisms have for certain tissues undoubtedly has a biochemical basis. Pneumococcal involvement in lung tissue, streptococcal preference for heart tissue, staphylococcal ubiquity in lesions and generalized infections all have a probable requirement for, or sensitivity to, biochemical tissue components. PEARCE (1962) demonstrated that *Brucella* organisms have an affinity for placental membrane tissue because of a *Brucella* growth stimulating factor, erythritol. The growth stimulatory effect of placental tissue on certain mycoplasma is as yet unexplained (CLARK *et al.*, 1965). A concentrated study of the physiology and biochemistry of the site of bacterial fixation seems to be in order. Very little is known about these propensities.

For symptomatic infectious bacterial disease to occur there must have been bacterial replication in the host. Regrettably, symptoms are not generally recognized until the invading microorganisms are 1. fairly well established in the host, 2. growth has been sufficient to cause a derrangement of the host biochemistry and immunologic mechanisms, and 3. there has been some toxicity from endotoxins, exotoxins, virulence factors (e.g. hemolysins, coagulase, hyaluronidase, leucocidin, etc.). The host reaction to these has either been expressed by this time (via inflammatory processes, fever, phagocytic mobilization, hypersensitive reactions) or is beginning to be expressed. It is quite obvious that this may not be the most propitious time to administer penicillin-type antibiotics which depend upon young rapidly growing cells for their bactericidal properties to be expressed (HOBBY *et al.*, 1942). However, TODD (1945) assumed that the older bacteria would be spontaneously lysing and/or phagocytically cleared more readily than the young cells which would still be actively producing antiphagocytic materials to maintain their virulence and invasive powers.

BIGGER (1944b) proposed alternating therapeutic periods for treatment of more serious disease states with penicillin. His viewpoint was that older bacterial cells and a certain percentage of all the bacteria would not be in a rapidly growing state at the time of exposure to penicillin. These cells would then become "persisters" and survive the initial onslaught of penicillin therapy. A period of non-exposure to antibiotic would allow the resting cells time to revitalize themselves and initiate active growth processes, thereby increasing their susceptibility to delayed penicillin treatment. This therapeutic idea is as sound today as it was in 1944. There have been indications that alternating therapy so modified as to use different antibiotics has some effect on chronic disease states (GUZE and KALMANSON, 1964; FEINSTEIN *et al.*, 1965; MONTGOMERIE *et al.*, 1965). The "persister" problem was discussed by MCDERMOTT (1958), but there remain many aspects of chronic and relapsing infections that have defied analysis.

GARBER (1960) has gone so far as to describe the host as a bacterial growth medium. He states that "pathogenicity ... assumes that the parasite is capable of utilizing the host environment as a growth medium and that it can overcome the total defense mechanisms of the host." These observations led GARBER (1956, 1960) to postulate a nutrition-inhibition hypothesis of pathogenicity that concentrates on the ability of the parasite to propagate and metabolically survive post-host entry. He also felt that organ specificity of many parasites may reflect nutritional requirements. However, it may just as well be due to the absence or reduced concentration of specific parasite inhibitors. Experimental evidence for either view is slim.

Many bacterial products have demonstrated antigenicity in various *in vivo* systems. These may or may not affect the immunologic response of the host (SMITH, 1960). Antigenic factors are found in all non-pathogenic and pathogenic bacteria. The extra factors that increase the virulence of the organism are environmentally responsive, phenotypically determined though genetically controlled. Bacterial genotypes determine a range of phenotypic responses. The phenotypic responses *in vivo* are relatively unknown but some virulence factors may well be produced as a direct reaction to host defenses (SMITH, 1960). Smith's short summary of his very interesting studies on *Brucella abortus*, *Pasteurella pestis*, and *Bacillus anthracis* should be read for background information concerning *in vivo* experimentation. The interplay of penicillin-type antibiotics was not considered in this summary but it points to areas where such studies could be fruitful.

The importance of genetic endowment and the "host factor" was examined by OSBORNE (1961) and the epidemiological factors involved in communicable disease were considered by SCHWEITZER (1961) in a symposium of the New York Academy of Sciences. SCHWEITZER noted that accurate descriptions of disease should not be limited by observations on the sick. He examined the occurrence and spread of rheumatic fever as an infection that may be transferred from person to person with individual recurrences regarded as exacerbations of existing disease. Rheumatic fever organisms have a low degree of infectivity and there exists the possibility of a familial tendency. Why penicillin therapy doesn't cure this disease has not been adequately explained. Is it that the rheumatic fever victim has a peculiar susceptibility to the streptococci involved and is constantly reinfected or are the persisting organisms lodged in sites where penicillin is unable to enter? Is there some peculiarity of the group A streptococcal cell envelope which persists, either directly or indirectly, in host tissues (KAPLAN and MEYESERIAN, 1962; KAPLAN and SVEC, 1964)? The answer to some of the questions concerning rheumatic disease may affect our thinking on host resistance factors.

That there are differences in efficiencies of host resistance factors from individual to individual is well known. JENKIN (1963) reviewed some of these cases and considered recurring, relapsing infections as of particular interest. We hope his stimulating article will lead to increased research activity.

The bacterial or microbial invader of host tissue discovers a battery of defense lines and factors. Fortunately, the invader is usually fought off. After tissue invasion there is a period of ischemia followed by vascular dilatation. Increased blood flow brings leucocytes to the area and stimulates the transport of invading microbes away to other areas more dilute in their bacterial population. This enables liver and spleen tissues to perform their filtration function. There is a simultaneous increase in lymph flow to the area, removing and diluting potentially toxic metabolites. These initial reactions induce overall stimulation of host mechanisms of resistance and the blood soon becomes enriched in gamma globulins, enzymes, and phagocytic cells. The phagocytes, along with some erythrocytes, move through capillary walls to the site of infection. The extent of this inflammatory reaction is generally related to the amount of initial tissue damaged during invasion. Adrenaline flow may affect the process and was studied by Miles *et al.* (1957) in a time course reaction. The effect of the adrenal corticoids on the inflammatory process is well documented and need not be discussed here. Other hormonal effects are relatively unknown.

There are both advantages and disadvantages to the inflammatory reaction. Fibrin clots are formed that may protect bacteria from phagocytes when the phagocytes are present initially in small numbers and are inefficient when so dilute. Hirsch (1965) has recently summarized current views on phagocytosis. He commented that the rate of phagocytosis is influenced by such features as presence of opsonins, pH, temperature, antibody, surface properties of the bacteria, and rate of entry. All these features, and more, determine the eventual outcome of the phagocytic encounter; that the situation is both complex and dynamic has been stated by Suter and Ramseier (1964) and Munoz (1964). Taliaferro (1949) emphasized the central role of phagocytosis in combating infection and noted that living lymphocytes have some protective power of value in nonspecific or innate immunity. Therefore, the host defenses and any antibiotic supplementation are not acting in normal tissue and tissue fluids but in tissue and fluid modified by the invader, by phagocytic and antibiotic products and by materials leaking out of damaged or necrotic tissue (Spector and Willoughby, 1963).

Lymphatic defenses may destroy some of the bacteria within the lymph node as these organs trap and provide a phagocytic base for microbial destruction. Wood and Smith (1956) have studied bacterial flow through the lymph and we shall discuss their studies more completely in a subsequent section.

Systemic defense systems consist entirely of phagocytosis. The liver and spleen trap massive numbers of organisms and the reticuloendothelial system is operative. Taliaferro (1949) has termed the RES the lymphoid-macrophage system, which has all the potential and actual macrophage cells including the non-granular leucocytes but excluding the granular polymorphonuclear leucocytes. Thus the system we call the RES contains both sessile and wandering histiocytes, the most active of which are the endothelial cells of the liver capillaries, spleen, marrow and lymph sinuses, adrenal and pituitary capillaries and the reticular cells of the spleen, thymus and lymphatic nodes. Therefore, the overrun of all these tissues and cells by invading bacteria of microbes would hardly allow survival of the host.

Mere engulfment of the microbe does not necessarily lead to death and lysis of that microbe. Phagocytosis is an active, energy requiring process (Karnovsky, 1962). It requires such serum factors as antibody and various opsonins to proceed (Rowley, 1962; Hirsch, 1965). The nature of the bacterial cell engulfed also affects the phagocytic process as some of them have active antiphagocytic properties (Hirsch and Strauss, 1964). An excellent summary of immunity, nonspecific resistance, phagocytosis, and the reticuloendothelial system action is presented in Topley and Wilson's Principles of Bacteriology and Immunity by Sir Graham S. Wilson and A. A. Miles; Williams and Wilkins publishers.

This is the fifth edition of this monumental work, published in 1964. (See also Ann. N.Y. Acad. Sci., *66*, Natural Resistance to Infections, 1956 and *ibid.*, *88*, Biochemical Aspects of Microbial Pathogenicity, 1960).

The inflammatory response, phagocytosis, and humoral reaction are all required to combat infection. The specific loci of phagocytic action are yet in doubt, but the activity of antibody and various opsonins are coming to light. A most interesting facet of current research interest is the phenomenon called "immune adherence" and its role in phagocytic stimulation and in host resistance to infection (NELSON, 1963). Within this area of opsonin-like effects, penicillin may act as an aid to normal host resistance mechanisms.

It is in this *in vivo* milieu that penicillin must act. There is no evidence for direct tissue stimulation by penicillin. The high degree of selective toxicity that is dependent upon marked cell wall structural differences between bacteria and mammalian tissue cells would seem to preclude a direct tissue cell effect.

Bacteria respond to their environment. Like all living cells, they adapt or die. (Dormancy via spore formation, encystment, etc. may be considered as adaptation for survival.) These bacterial adaptive responses include enzymatic changes due to a variety of causes (among these are penicillin-type antibiotics), changes in flagellation, spore formation and germination, and alterations of radiation sensitivity, chemical composition and genetic recombination. Thus the environment can alter a bacterial population either via genetic or nongenetic mechanisms. Since we know of some areas in microbiology where "cytoplasmic-genes" or "plasmids" or "episomes" have been postulated, it is a little soon to define the fundamental basis for changes we will discuss (DATTA, 1965; HAYES, 1964; RICHMOND, 1965; WATANABE, 1963; WILKIE, 1964; JINKS, 1964).

Bacteria respond to their environment in very unique ways when that environment is another living system, commonly referred to as the host. It is common knowledge that to increase virulence, invasive powers, toxigenicity, etc. of many bacteria, it is wise to try animal passage. When large or loading doses are injected into animals, we may select out of the population those individual cells capable of surviving the host defenses. These cells grow, propagate and can be re-isolated for further passage. A short series of such transfers is all that is required to develop a bacterial population with highly increased lethal powers in the particular host we have selected.

Studies have suggested that amino acid levels in a host may play a role in susceptibility and resistance through their effect on virulence properties (Page *et al.*, 1951). *In vivo* addition of threonine enhanced the virulence of *Salmonella typhimurium* due to selection of a threonine resistant population. Malonate has also been reported to enhance bacterial virulence (BERRY *et al.*, 1954). Under *in vivo* cultural conditions, *Pasteurella pestis* produced an extracellular antiphagocytic factor that was, perhaps, useful in the survival of this organism in host tissue (BURROWS, 1955). Avirulent organisms failed to elaborate this factor. A somewhat different view of phagocytic resistance has been stated by JANSSEN *et al.* (1963).

It has been said that dietary change can lower resistance (SCHNEIDER, 1956; TOPLEY and WILSON p. 393, 1964) yet it is known that in starved animals phagocytosis is increased (KUNA *et al.*, 1951). These results may have been predetermined by the host for there is a difference in reaction dependent upon the species of host as noted by BRAUN (1956). *Brucella suis* inoculated into guinea pigs led to a virulent population whereas infection of chicks yielded the avirulent population.

There is another property of bacterial variation or adaptation that should be considered here and again at a later point. That is the variation associated with changes in growth rate (MEYNELL, 1961). Staining properties (WADE, 1955), surface antigens (BURROWS and BACON, 1956), and antibiotic resistance patterns (BIGGER, 1944a) are examples of growth rate variables. Various phases of the growth cycle thus determine sensitivity to a variety of agents but, oddly, have no effect on the sensitivity of *E. coli* or *Shigella sonnei* to "phagocytin" or on the *E. coli* reaction to histone (HIRSCH, 1956); HIRSCH, 1958).

MEYNELL (1961) states "the numerous kinds of phenotypic variation open to microorganisms suggest that the bacterial population in an infected host is likely to appear extremely heterogeneous, if only because the population is scattered among different sites, each providing a different environment. However, a bacterial population is often heterogeneous even when growing in an environment which appears uniform, such as a stirred, aerated broth culture".

Thus virulence, as a relative degree of pathogenicity, resistance to normal body defense mechanism, metabolism and antibiotic or inhibitor resistance, can be altered via modification of the bacterial environment. The range of phenotypic alteration possible *in vivo* has no known limits.

The Triphasic System

This section is intended to emphasize some of the less well understood effects of penicillin-type antibiotics on bacteria, on the host, and on the outcome of infectious disease situations. The material has been filtered through the prejudiced prism of personal interests.

Evidence that the primary site of penicillin's antibacterial action is on the synthesis of the rigid layer in the cell envelope is overwhelming (see part I of this chapter).

PARK (1963) and STROMINGER and TIPPER (1965) have confirmed DUGUID'S (1946) comment that the lytic action induced by penicillin is due to continued spheroplast growth while the cell wall synthesis has been inhibited so that the wall is ruptured and the spheroplast subjected to osmotic derangement.

It is of historical interest to note that not only did FLEMING discover penicillin and lysozyme, both of which are cell wall destroying materials of continuing scientific interest, but he also observed the apparent stimulation of phagocytosis by penicillin (FLEMING *et al.*, 1943). At the time, he defined penicillin's action as bacteriostatic rather than bactericidal, but his statement did not include the test he used nor the precise environmental conditions upon which his definition was based. The descriptive terms, bactericidal and bacteriostatic, as currently used in the literature have little meaning without defining the experimental test system and the cultural history of the microbe being studied. WOODS and TUCKER (1958) commented on the difficulty of determining bactericidal action and made the important point that successful chemotherapy does not necessarily require bactericidal activity. Inhibition of the invader proliferation is all that is required and this will allow defense mechanisms of the host to operate in the elimination process. They (WOODS and TUCKER, 1958), of course, assumed an undamaged and fully capable host resistance system.

As cited in earlier discussion, the site of initial cellular lesion due to penicillin action was suggested to be the "growing point" or the developing cross wall system by a number of workers. MURRAY and his colleagues (1959) reaffirmed the contentions of SALTON and SHAFA (1958) and BRENNER, *et al.* (1958) that lysozyme-induced "protoplasts" and penicillin-induced "spheroplasts" are not equivalent structures. The MURRAY group noted at this time that the initial lesion was followed by rapid recovery when penicillin-resistant strains were examined. Evidence has since been presented by MURRAY, *et al.* (1965) that the innermost layer of Gram-negative bacteria is the mucopeptide layer and it is only this layer that seems to be involved, along with the cytoplasmic membrane in septum formation. Most, if not all, of the later or secondary antibacterial effects of penicillin are likely due to cytoplasmic membrane distortion incidental to disruption of cell wall integrity. HANCOCK (1958) and others have demonstrated the marked protective effect of osmotic stabilization of the medium in which penicillin acts. When cells are stabilized in this manner, there is no cytoplasmic leakage (FITZ-JAMES and HANCOCK, 1965) and, in fact, in the presence of penicillin these authors suggest that an extra-membranous wall mucopeptide of considerable size appears. This is quite different from the sequence of events that take place in the presence of lysozyme.

RYTER and LANDMAN (1964) demonstrated stabilization of *Bacillus subtilis* L-state cells by mesosome loss. It is interesting to note the rapid mesosome damage that occurred at the points of the membrane where the septum was formed when penicillin was present, even though septum damage occurred before visual changes took place in the mesosome structure (FITZ-JAMES and HANCOCK, 1965). Mesosome structures may be the cellular site of penicillin action for they seem to fit some of the requirements for binding site and cell wall structural associations. FITZ-JAMES (1965) stated that it was doubtful, however, that these structures are involved with the penicillin sensitivity mechanism. His reasoning depends upon structural damage-time relationships of penicillin action.

To summarize, the data discussed in preceding sections indicates:

A. Penicillin blocks a transpeptidation reaction that leads to newly forming polyglycine cross linkages in the cell wall. The evidence for this is good when applied to *S. aureus* but not very definite when the data are examined for application to reactions of Gram-negative bacteria and many Gram-positive types.

B. Penicillin is active only against growing, propagating bacterial cells (HOBBY *et al.*, 1942), but this concept may be modified in view of the proposal by SHOCKMAN *et al.*, (1965) that only the potential for active mucopeptide synthesis is critical.

C. Penicillin action ultimately leads to death of the cell via lysis, or to viable spheroplasts (L-state, L-form, L-phase, transitional forms), depending upon the concentration of antibiotic present and the stabilizing nutrient and protective characteristics of the medium.

D. Reported penicillin effects on amino acid accumulation and transfer, nucleic acid and protein synthesis inhibition may likely be due to secondary effects on the cytoplasmic membrane.

Most of the data so far discussed have been obtained from *in vitro* simple growth medium studies. Many of the secondary effects, including the killing action, of penicillin's antibacterial activity cannot be validly applied to an *in vivo* situation.

In the infected but immunologically normal host, the initial bacterial lesion caused by penicillin action is probably all that is necessary for adequate therapy and host recovery. Once the stage of rapid proliferation of the invading microbe has been stopped or slowed and the cell envelope disorganized, host resistance mechanisms can complete the job.

It is obvious from what has been said that a dominating feature of penicillin action on bacteria is the formation of spheroplasts resulting from disorganization of the cell wall structure. The term spheroplast is used in this discussion as suggested by HURWITZ *et al.* (1958), SALTON and SHAFA (1958), and BRENNER *et al.* (1958). If these spheroplasts are osmotically stabilized and properly handled, they may be propagated as the L-phase or L-form of the bacterium.

We use the term L-phase to designate propagating spheroplasts which are still capable of reversion to the classic parental rigid cell walled organism upon removal of inducing agent. The term L-form is used here to designate non-reverting, stable, propagating spheroplasts. Transitional forms designate the "long forms" and involutionary forms that seem to lie someplace between L's and classic parental forms of bacteria. The term protoplast is used to designate cells existing without a rigid cell wall structure and in which the rigid structural material has been specifically shown to be absent. Protoplasts arise in this discussion when lysozyme has been used as the induction or cell wall destroying agent. WEIBULL (1958) and McQUILLEN (1960) have discussed bacterial protoplasts from a variety of viewpoints. DIENES and WEINBERGER (1951) published a classic review on the L forms of bacteria which has since been supplemented by KLIENEBERGER-NOBEL (1960, 1962). That the L-phase and possible L-form bacteria are formed *in vivo* by either natural (e.g. serum factors, antibody, complement, lysozyme), or unnatural (e.g. antibiotics) inducing agents or both is no longer questioned. A number of laboratories have isolated these forms in association with experimental or accidental disease states (MORTIMER, 1965; GUTMAN *et al.*, 1965; BRAUDE *et al.*, 1961; CAREY *et al.*, 1960; KAGAN, 1961; BRIER *et al.*, 1962; GODZESKI *et al.*, 1965; GUZE *et al.*, 1963; MATTMAN *et al.*, 1960 and WITTLER *et al.*, 1960). There is no incontrovertible evidence that the L-phase is directly the cause of, or the immediate etiological agent in, infectious disease. The possibility that they are involved in the disease state in some as yet unspecified manner is of current interest in many laboratories all over the world.

The occurrence of structural modification of living cells in response to antibiotic stress factors in the environment may extend to the psittacosis-lymphogranuloma venereum-trachoma group of organisms. On the basis of their relationship to the Gram-negative bacteria, MOULDER (1964) reviewed the physiology and metabolic properties of these cells, which he called the bedsoniae. These organisms react to penicillin and cycloserine as do bacteria, via "spheroplast" formation but they are more difficult to observe, since they are induced intracellularly (MOULDER, 1964). It is apparent from this observation that the activity of penicillins on microbial cell wall structures, which results in spheroplast formation, may be a general biological phenomenon.

Studies on specific differences in permeation capabilities between bacterial and other types of cells in regard to antibiotic transport are noticeably absent from the literature. Is there a permease for penicillin-type antibiotics present in bacterial cells as has now been postulated for streptomycin (HURWITZ and ROSANO, 1965)? What is the need for such active transport systems when these substances are metabolic poisons?

In order to establish, to an admittedly minor degree, the possible role of penicillin-type antibiotics in therapy of infectious disease, it is necessary to refer back to the work of EAGLE (1950, 1952). In these studies it was established that the time of initiation of treatment in relation to the onset of disease was most critical and that penicillin was bactericidal only during the early stages of the disease state. The work of WOOD and SMITH (1956) attempted to define the relation of cellular defenses to penicillin's curative actions. In a series of well-performed experiments, WOOD and SMITH confirmed the fact that penicillin is very effective against rapidly dividing cells of pneumococci but much less so when the bacteria are in a stationary phase of growth. In central portions of the pneumococcal lesions, bacterial destruction was more dependent upon the phagocytic process of the host. These authors stated (WOOD and SMITH, 1956), "... penicillin therapy of mature pneumococcal myositis is more effective in unirradiated mice than it is in previously irradiated mice because leucocytes assist the drug in destroying the bacteria." This was essential confirmation of FLEMING'S (1943) notion concerning increased phagocytosis occurring in the presence of penicillin. This should not be construed as a direct effect of penicillin upon the phagocyte but rather a "team operation". WOOD and SMITH (1956) also stated that "when penicillin is employed in the treatment of established bacterial infections, its curative effect is manifestly due to the cellular defenses of the host as well as to the antimicrobial properties of the drug". Their interpretation of the curative effect of penicillin in such diseases as tonsillitis, otitis media, and pneumonia was that penicillin and host combined to rid the body of the bacteria and host defense mechanisms were of equal importance. WOOD and SMITH (1956) point out, however, that their conclusions applied only to penicillin in acute infections caused by penicillin sensitive bacteria, which act in the host as extracellular parasites, and do not necessarily apply to staphylococci which may not be readily phagocytized. ROGERS and TOMSETT (1952) had already pointed out that staphylococci may survive phagocytosis and SKINSNES (1948) had come to the same conclusions as WOOD and SMITH (1956) but in a less elaborate way. All these authors recommended longer than usual penicillin therapy in established infections or in patients having impaired host resistance mechanisms. SKINSNES (1948) also stated that "penicillin does not increase the qualitative efficiency of impaired defense mechanisms as immune sera are known to do". Thus he didn't postulate any direct effect of penicillin on the host.

That there are natural substances in serum which are antagonistic to bacteria and act on a wide variety of bacteria types has been known since the latter part of the last century (MYRVIK and WEISER, 1955; ADLER, 1953a, 1953b). The manifold activities of the bacteriocidins, serum lysins, complement, antibody, nonspecific resistance factors and their interactions with antibiotic substances are still largely undefined. All of the factors in normal non-immune and in immune sera lead to destruction of the bacterium either by unknown mechanisms or via spheroplast (and consequent L-phase cell) induction processes. Quantitative evidence for the previous statement is poor as yet, but the qualitative data are becoming massive.

MUSCHEL *et al.* (1959) reported the finding that the antibody-complement system and lysozyme, operating together, were the factors responsible for protoplast formation by serum. Guinea pig serum was used in their study and even though the characteristic "rabbit ear" effect was not noticed, protoplasts were apparently formed. The "rabbit ear" effect referred to cell aberrations obtained by spheroplast induction with penicillin, as published by HAHN and CIAK (1957) and LEDERBERG (1957). MUSCHEL, *et al.* (1959) postulated a two stage process ".... in which the antibody-complement system paves the way for lysozyme action that results in protoplasts". This result was analogous to those obtained earlier by WARREN, *et al.* (1957) who showed that polymyxin B sulfate paved the way for lysozyme action, leading to lysis. These data also pointed to cell wall structures as the site of serum action. More recently, ALDRICH and SWORD (1964) noted that methicillin pretreatment of a lysozyme-resistant staphylococcus rendered the cell very susceptible to lysozyme lytic action. There seem to be some different properties of methicillin that we shall discuss later. It appears that methicillin may have a site of action which differs from that of the other penicillins. This would be most interesting, if true.

In further experiments with a serum-*Salmonella* system (CAREY and BARON, 1959) it was revealed that serum-induced protoplasts did not carry unique specific antigens. The somatic complex of antigens associated with parental forms was retained by the protoplast membrane; however, this may be characteristic of the particular induction method.

CAREY *et al.* (1960) demonstrated the production of protoplasts *in vivo* with a *loss* of antibody reaction to intact cell anti-serum. Their studies were performed in mice and the protoplast induction occurred in peritoneal fluid and within the the leucocytes, using both *Salmonella* sp. and *Shigella* sp. Immune mice, elevated nonspecific resistance prepared mice, and normal mice gave similar basic effects in which the degree of protoplast induction was correlated with the degree of resistance elevation. CAREY *et al.*, in the same paper, stated that "... the factors responsible for protoplast formation *in vitro* are those which determine the outcome of the host parasite relationship" and "protoplasts may represent a parasite defense mechanism ... persist in the animal body .... possibly multiply as protoplasts or revert to whole cells". CAREY and his colleagues theorized that the animal may thus be saved from death but not chronic infection.

The results of studies like those of CAREY *et al.* (1960) may be combined with those of MICHAEL and BRAUN (1959) who reported serum induction of *Shigella dysenteriae* into the spheroplast phase when the cells were in the post exponential state of growth. Normal human serum was used in the experiments and 20% sucrose was the stabilizing agent. It is conceivable that penicillin (or other antibiotics for that matter) and serum factors form a highly effective team for bactericidal activity. Certainly these aspects deserve a good deal more investigation.

There are mechanisms of protection other than major serum and/or antibiotic systems. MACKANESS (1964) and ERCOLI (1964) have discussed some of the most interesting aspects of non-specific resistance, an area ripe for a major breakthrough of new knowledge. And most assuredly there are bacteria highly resistant to serum factors. At least some organisms appear to be resistant from our present experimental laboratory determinations. There is no serum *per se* in the body of an animal. And, regrettably, citrate and heparin additions to blood create problems due to their own involvement. OSAWA and MUSCHEL (1964) studied two such "serum resistant" organisms, *Paracolobactrum ballerup* and *Salmonella paratyphosa* C and found that these bacteria became sensitive to serum factors when the temperature was elevated. The effect of penicillin on these organisms was also altered as the temperature was varied. The particular strain of bacterium studied may have marked qualitative and quantitative effects upon penicillin action *in vivo* as well as in the *in vitro* tests cited here. It is likely that the organism which we isolate and study in the laboratory is the mutant that has been selected for survival under the imposed environment (BRAUN, 1953).

That penicillin had a definite time of optimal action and that this was related to cell division processes was shown by LARK (1958). Penicillin effectiveness was altered by the time of addition to synchronously dividing *Alkaligenes fecalis* culture. That there is a point in time which is optimal for antibiotic treatment of a microbial infectious process is a reasonable theoretical speculation. Experimental evidence that this is so comes from the work of DINEEN (1961), but more studies are required to evaluate the range of microbes for which time treatment factors are so important. There is a possibility that, during infection, a cycling of lesser and greater microbial susceptibility exists, but we have no knowledge of studies on such events.

Of more than passing interest is a study by A. N. PILIPENKO (1964) on the elimination of hemolytic activity of streptoococci by serial culturing in the presence of sub-bacteriostatic concentrations of penicillin or penicillin-streptomycin combinations. His experimental results were obtained *in vitro*, however, without animal pathogenicity studies during and after this virulence factor diminution.

HIJMANS (1962) noted the loss of group specific antigen of group D streptococci, a supposedly intracellular antigen, while FREEMAN (unpublished private communication) has noted differential antigen retention when glycine and penicillin were used in separate experiments to induce spheroplast formation in smooth strains of *Brucella suis*. Therefore, we cannot join the chorus of "a spheroplast by any other name is just as lytic".

A confusing aspect of penicillin-serum-antigen interaction that remains unexplained is the protection from penicillin offered to staphylococci by Gram-negative bacterial "O" antigen (ZABLOCKI and HOLT, 1961). This protective layering also protected other Gram-positive bacteria and it was highly specific for penicillin. This "O" antigen could partially explain some of the Gram-negative bacteria's ability to resist to a certain degree the antibiotic effect of penicillin. More information is needed concerning Gram-negative wall structures, antigens, and serum-antibiotic interplay.

Immune lysis of *Vibrio cholerae* (FREEMAN *et al.*, 1963) has interesting implications and penicillin interaction in this system should be studied. FREEMAN suggested that "the primary effect of antibody and complement on the cholera vibrio is a breakdown of the cell structure to give an osmotically fragile but viable form".

The possible role of autolytic enzymatic reactions in the mechanism of penicillin action has been considered insufficiently. Spheroplast formation can occur from this action (MOHAN *et al.*, 1965; STOLP and STARR, 1965) and PRESTIDGE and PARDEE (1957) actually postulated the induction of an autolytic enzyme by penicillin. This concept has yet to be disproven. YUDKIN (1963) reported interesting effects of antibiotics on membrane synthesis, but his results using lysozyme induced protoplasts do not negate, as the author implies, the autolytic enzyme concept. That penicillin has an effect on the membrane cannot be questioned unless one assumes that the rigid mucopeptide layer is unattached to the cytoplasmic membrane and the enzymes involved (something less than 30 in number) all operate exterior to the cytoplasm.

Antibiotic Induced Bacterial Phenotypic Variation

MEYNELL (1961) stated that "the range of phenotypic variation open to bacterial pathogens is already known to be so great that it must be considered one of the major factors determining the course of the infection". Obviously, one of these phenotypic variations is the existence and survival *in vivo* of bacterial organisms in the spheroplast state. Stabilization of this state may lead to L-*form* survival while short term conditions may only allow L-*phase* survival with subsequent reversion to parental forms. Either sort of L-type existence is potentially damaging to the host. Studies of bacterial L-variants arose independently from research concerned with antibiotic action (KLIENEBERGER, 1935). It wasn't until 12 years later that DIENES (1947a, 1947b) noted L-phase associated with penicillin action. It is probable that most microbiologists still consider the L-type bacterial cell as being separate and distinct from penicillin-induced aberrant forms when, in actuality, these various spheroplast-protoplast forms are interrelated. The differences in cell envelope structure demonstrated between these related forms of bacteria are dependent upon the degree of mucopeptide alteration involved in their formation (KLIENEBERGER-NOBEL, 1960; STOLP and STARR, 1965).

Increasing interest has been generated during recent years in the relationship of spheroplasts and L-phase organisms to various antibiotic activities (GODZESKI *et al.*, 1963). We would like to note here, however, that almost all of the published information on antibiotic L-phase interaction has been from the viewpoint of the antibiotic mechanism of action *in vitro* and in a medium as simple as could be devised. Also spheroplasts, protoplasts, L-phase and L-form organisms are treated as if they were equivalent creatures. There is no evidence of their equivalence. That they may be related in some way implies nothing concerning their differential reactions to environmental modifications. As pointed out by ROGERS and JELJASZEWICZ (1961) and others, experiments that have used high penicillin levels (HUGO and RUSSELL, 1961) should be viewed with caution. We would like to make the same comment concerning a great many published reports on antibiotic activity data obtained utilizing glycine or lysozyme induced protoplasts. Results derived with cells obtained by these induction methods do not necessarily relate to those obtained with penicillin or other antibiotically induced microbial forms (PULVERTAFT, 1952; HANCOCK and FITZ-JAMES, 1964; SHOCKMAN and LAMPEN, 1962.

The measurable differences between spheroplasts induced by diverse agents may be striking. FREEMAN and RUMACK (1964) had good evidence for differential cytopathogenic effects when comparing glycine and penicillin-induced spheroplasts of *Brucella*. Earlier studies did not find such differences between forms induced by diverse agents (FREIMER *et al.*, 1959).

It is not unreasonable that there should be a difference in the cells propagated, depending upon the manner of induction and subsequent treatment. L-phase induction may result in antigenic variations that would be difficult to explain on any basis other than unique actions on a variety of reacting sites of the cell envelope.

We referred earlier to the work of ALDRICH and SWORD (1964). They reported that methicillin treatment of lysozyme resistant cells rendered them sensitive to the enzyme. Other interesting aspects of methicillin action are appearing. In a study of antibiotic sensitivity of L-forms which were derived from methicillin-resistant staphylococci by exposure to high levels of this agent, KAGAN *et al.* (1962) found them to be very sensitive to non-cell wall inhibiting antibiotics. One of the authors of this discussion (C.W.G.) has studied such a strain through the courtesy of Dr. KAGAN. It was noted that total growth and rate of growth in solid media was markedly influenced by the presence of methicillin. The L-form strain grew much better in the presence of the agent than in its absence. If the actions of other antibiotics are studied using such a culture, what is their effect? Does the second antibiotic negate a growth stimulation requirement for methicillin or does it act on the cell in a more direct manner?

Related to the peculiar or unexpected effect of methicillin on staphylococcal L-forms is the observation that a methicillin-dependent strain of *Pediococcus cerevisiae* can be developed (WHITE, 1962). To the authors' knowledge, methicillin is the only penicillin so far reported which can induce a metabolic dependent state in a bacterium. More studies along this line are indicated before conclusions may be reached.

Methicillin action *in vivo* has been noted to be unexpectedly ineffective in a penicillin-resistant staphylococcal infection (DINEEN and MANNIX, 1962). That the apparent decreased potency may have a rational explanation was commented on by FROST and VALIANT (1964). These authors found that the route of infection and treatment were equally important in determining the outcome of the infection, using penicillinase producing staphylococci. Three days were required before *in vivo* penicillinase production took place.

Resistance Development

Consideration of penicillin resistance development in microorganisms would occupy another chapter. Presently, there seems to be at least two forms of resistance, i.e. inherent, and penicillinase production (POLLOCK, 1964). That there may be a third is suggested by DINEEN and MANNIX (1962) and by some of the data from studies concerned with innate resistance of Gram-negative bacteria (AYLIFF, 1965). PERCIVAL *et al.* (1963) have concluded that the β-lactamase (i.e. the penicillinase) of Gram-negative organisms is more active against penicillin G than against ampicillin, 6-(D-α-aminophenylacetamido) penicillanic acid; penicillinases may also differ.

Identification of the genetic factors in penicillinase mediated resistance to penicillin action has been summarized by DATTA (1965) and DATTA and KONTOMICHALOU (1965) and for further information on penicillinase-cephalosporinase activities, excellent papers by BARBER and WATERWORTH (1964), COLLINS (1964), and STEWART and HOLT (1963) should be consulted.

Penicillin Combination Therapy

There are few conclusive indications of benefit from penicillin combinations with other agents. Synergistic action with penicillinase blocking substances would be expected and has been demonstrated by CRAWFORD and ABRAHAM (1957). Bacitracin apparently competes for the site of penicillin action on Gram-positive cell surfaces so that antagonism may exist, yet not be demonstrated *in vitro* (REYNOLDS, 1962). There is an apparent antagonistic effect between penicillin and a tetracycline that was discussed by JAWETZ and GUNNISON (1953). An unexplained synergistic activity in treatment of experimental endocarditis has been reported by RICHTARIK and SEAGER (1965). A stilbamidine and penicillin combination was used in this study. Erythromycin-penicillin combinations may be of value (HERRELL *et al.*, 1960) and the penicillin-streptomycin team still works well (ROBBINS, 1949).

See Addendum

References

ADLER, F.: Studies on the bactericidal reaction. 1. Bactericidal action of normal sera against a strain of *Salmonella typhosa*. J. Immunol. **70**, 69 (1953a).

ADLER, F.: Studies on the bactericidal reaction. 2. Inhibition by antibody and antibody requirements of the reaction. J. Immunol. **70**, 79 (1953b).

ALDRICH, K. M., and C. P. SWORD: Methicillin-induced lysozyme-sensitive forms of staphylococci. J. Bacteriol. **87**, 690 (1964).

AYLIFF, G. A. J.: Cephalosporinase and penicillinase of gram-negative bacteria. J. Gen. Microbiol. **40**, 119 (1965).

BARBER, M., and P. M. WATERWORTH: Penicillinase-resistant penicillins and cephalosporins. Brit. Med. J. **2**, 344 (1964).

BERRY, L. J., B. MERRITT, and R. B. MITCHELL: The relation of the tricarboxylic acid cycle to bacterial infection. III. J. Infectious Diseases **94**, 144 (1954).

BIGGER, J. W.: The bactericidal action of penicillin on *Staphylococcus pyogenes*. Irish J. Med. Sci. **6**, 553 (1944a).

BIGGER, J. W.: Treatment of staphylococcal infections with penicillin by intermittent sterilization. Lancet **1944II**b, 497.

BRAUDE, A. I., J. SIEMIENSKI, and I. JACOBS: Protoplast formation in human urine. Trans. Assoc. Am. Physicians **74**, 234 (1961).

BRAUN, W.: Bacterial genetics. Philadelphia: W. B. Saunders Co. 1953.

BRAUN, W.: Cellular products affecting the establishment of bacteria of different virulence. Ann. N.Y. Acad. Sci. **66**, 348 (1956).

BRENNER, S., F. A. DARK, P. GERHARDT, M. H. JEYNES, O. KANDLER, E. KELLENBERGER, E. KLIENEBERGER-NOBEL, K. MCQUILLEN, M. RUBIO-HUERTOS, M. R. J. SALTON, R. E. STRANGE, J. TOMCKIS, and C. WEIBULL: Bacterial protoplasts. Nature **181**, 1713 (1958).

BRIER, G., L. ELLIS, and C. W. GODZESKI: Survival *in vivo* (*in ovo*) of L-phase bacteria. Antimicrobiol. Agents and Chemotherapy, 854 (1962).

BROWN, A. D.: Aspects of bacterial response to the ionic environment. Bacteriol. Rev. **28**, 296 (1964).

BURROWS, T. W.: The basis of virulence for mice of *Pasteurella pestis*. In: Mechanisms of microbial pathogenicity, Fifth Symp. Soc. Gen. Microbiol., p. 152—175. Cambridge University Press, 1955.

BURROWS, T. W., and G. A. BACON: The basis of virulence in *Pasteurella pestis:* An antigen determining virulence. Brit. J. Exptl. Pathol. **37**, 481 (1956).

CAREY, W. F., and L. S. BARON: Comparative immunologic studies of cell structures isolated from *Salmonella typhosa*. J. Immunol. **83**, 517 (1959).

CAREY, W. F., L. H. MUSCHEL, and L. S. BARON: The formation of bacterial protoplasts *in vivo*. J. Immunol. **84**, 183 (1960).

CLARK, H. W., J. S. BAILEY, and T. P. MCBROWN: New observations of mycoplasma infectivity and immunity. Abstr. Fifth Intersci. Conf. Antimicrobial Agents and Chemotherapy, p. 3, (1965).

COBURN, A. F., P. F. FRANK, and J. NOLAN: Studies on the pathogenicity of *Streptococcus pyogenes*. IV. The relation between the capacity to induce fatal respiratory infections in mice and epidemic respiratory diseases in man. Brit. J. Exptl. Pathol. **38**, 256 (1957).

COLLINS, J. F.: The distribution and formation of penicillinase in a bacterial population of *Bacillus licheniformis*. J. Gen. Microbiol. **34**, 363 (1964).

CRAWFORD, K., and E. P. ABRAHAM: The synergistic action of cephalosporin C and benzylpenicillin against a penicillinase-producing strain of *S. aureus*. J. Gen. Microbiol. **16**, 604 (1957).

DATTA, N.: Infectious drug resistance. Brit. Med. Bull. **21**, 254 (1965).

DATTA, N., and P. KONTOMICHALOU: Penicillinase synthesis controlled by infectious R factors in Enterobacteriacease. Nature **208**, 239 (1965).

DIENES, L.: Isolation of pleuropneumonia-like organisms from pathological specimens with the aid of penicillin. Proc. Soc. Exptl. Biol. Med. **64**, 165 (1947a).

DIENES, L.: Isolation of pleuropneumonia-like organisms from *H. influenzae* with the aid of penicillin. Proc. Soc. Exptl. Biol. Med. **64**, 166 (1947b).

DIENES, L., and H. J. WEINBERGER: The L-forms of bacteria. Bacteriol. Rev. **15**, 245 (1951).

DINEEN, P.: A period of unusual microbial susceptibility in an experimental staphylococcal infection. J. Infectious Diseases **108**, 174 (1961).

DINEEN, P., and H. MANNIX, jr.: An evaluation of the mechanism of penicillin resistance *in vivo*. J. Surg. Res. **2**, 151 (1962).

DUGUID, J. P.: The sensitivity of bacteria to the action of penicillin. Edinburgh Med. J. **53**, 401 (1946).

EAGLE, H., R. FLEISHMAN, and A. D. MUSSELMAN: The bactericidal action of penicillin *in vivo*. The participation of the host and the slow recovery of the surviving organisms. Ann. Internal Med. **33**, 344 (1950).

EAGLE, H.: Experimental approach to the problem of treatment failure with penicillin. 1. Group A streptococci infection in mice. Am. J. Med. **13**, 389 (1952).

ERCOLI, N.: Nonspecific antibacterial action. In: Experimental chemotherapy, vol. III (R. J. SCHNITZER and F. HAWKING, eds.), p. 387. New York: Academic Press 1964.

FEINSTEIN, A. R., M. SPAGUOLO, S. JONAS, E. TURSKY, E. K. STERN, and M. LEVITT: Prophylaxis of recurrent rheumatic fever. J. Am. Med. Assoc. **191**, 107 (1965).

FITZ-JAMES, P. C.: Discussion. In a symposium on the fine structure and replication of bacteria and their parts. 1. Fine structure and replication of bacterial nucleoids (G. W. FUKS). Bacteriol. Rev. **29**, 293 (1965).

FITZ-JAMES, P., and R. HANCOCK: The initial structural lesion of penicillin action in *Bacillus megaterium*. J. Cell Biol. **26**, 657 (1965).

FLEMING, A., H. W. FLOREY, D. C. BODENHAM, E. C. CUTLER, R. V. HUDSON, R. V. CHRISTIE, J. S. JEFFREY, M. E. FLOREY, and J. N. ROBINSON: Discussion on penicillin. Proc. Roy. Soc. Med. **37**, 101 (1943).

FREEMAN, B. A., G. M. MUSTEIKIS, and W. BURROWS: Protoplast formation as the mechanism for immune lysis of *Vibrio cholera*. Proc. Soc. Exptl. Biol. Med. **113**, 675 (1963).

FREEMAN, B. A., and B. H. RUMACK: Cytopathogenic effect of brucella spheroplasts on monocytes in tissue culture. J. Bacteriol. **88**, 1310 (1964).
FREEMAN, B. A.: Private communication 1965.
FREIMER, E. H., R. M. KRAUSE, and M. MCCARTY: Studies of L-forms and protoplasts of group A streptococci. J. Exptl. Med. **110**, 853 (1959).
FROST, B. M., and M. E. VALIANT: An evaluation of cephalosporin derivates *in vitro* and in experimental infections. J. Pathol. Bacteriol. **88**, 125 (1964).
GALE, E. F.: Synthesis and organization in the bacterial cell. New York: John Wiley and Sons, Inc. 1959.
GARBER, E. D.: A nutrition-inhibition hypothesis of pathogenicity. Am. Naturalist **90**, 183 (1956).
GARBER, E. D.: The host as a growth medium. Ann. N.Y. Acad. Sci. **88**, 1187 (1960).
GODZESKI, C. W., R. M. HISKER, and G. BRIER: Predominant characteristics of the growth of some antibiotic-induced L-phase bacteria. Antimicrobial Agents and Chemotherapy 507 (1963a).
GODZESKI, C. W., G. BRIER, R. S. GRIFFITH, and H. R. BLACK: Association of bacterial L-phase organisms in chronic infections. Nature **205**, 1340 (1965).
GUTMAN, L. T., M. TURCK, R. G. PETERSDORF, and R. J. WEDGWOOD: Significance of bacterial variants in urine of patients with chronic bacteriuria. J. Clin. Invest. **44**, 1945 (1965).
GUZE, L. B., and G. M. KALMANSON: Persistence of bacteria in "protoplast" form after apparent cure of pyelonephritis in rats. Science **143**, 1340 (1963).
GUZE, L. B., and G. M. KALMANSON: Effect of erythromycin on *in vivo* "protoplast" infection. Antimicrobial Agents and Chemotherapy 730 (1964).
HAHN, F. E., and J. CIAK: Penicillin induced lysis of *Escherichia coli*. Science **125**, 119 (1957).
HANCOCK, R.: Protection of *Staphylococcus aureus* from some effects of penicillin by media of high osmotic pressure. Biochem. J. **70**, 15 (1958).
HANCOCK, R., and P. C. FITZ-JAMES: Some differences in the action of penicillin, bacitracin, and vancomycin on *Bacillus megaterium*. J. Bacteriol. **87**, 1044 (1964).
HAYES, W.: The genetics of bacteria and their viruses: Studies in basic genetics and molecular biology. Oxford: Blackwell 1964.
HERRELL, W. E., A. BALLOWS, and J. BECKER: Erythrocillin: A new approach to the problem of antibiotic-resistant staphylococci. Antibiotic Med. & Clin. Therapy **7**, 637 (1960).
HIJMANS, W.: Absence of the group-specific and the cell-wall polysaccharide antigen in L-phase variants of group D streptococci. J. Gen. Microbiol. **28**, 177 (1962).
HIRSCH, J. G.: Phagocytin: A bactericidal substance from polymorphonuclear leucocytes. J. Exptl. Med. **103**, 589 (1956).
HIRSCH, J. G.: Bactericidal action of histone. J. Exptl. Med. **108**, 925 (1958).
HIRSCH, J. G., and B. STRAUSS: Studies on heat-labile opsonin in rabbit serum. J. Immunol. **92**, 145 (1964).
HIRSCH, J. G.: Phagocytosis. Ann. Rev. Microbiol. **19**, 339 (1965).
HOBBY, G. L., K. MEYER, and E. CHAFEE: Observations on the mechanism of action of penicillin. Proc. Soc. Exptl. Biol. Med. **50**, 281 (1942).
HUGO, W. B., and A. D. RUSSELL: Action of penicillin on *Aerobacter cloacae*. J. Bacteriol. **82**, 411 (1961).
HURWITZ, C., J. M. REINER, and J. V. LANDAU: Studies in the physiology and biochemistry of penicillin-induced spheroplasts of *Escherichia coli*. J. Bacteriol. **76**, 612 (1958).
HURWITZ, C., and C. L. ROSANO: Evidence for a streptomycin permease. J. Bacteriol. **90**, 1233 (1965).
JANSSEN, W. A., W. D. LAWTON, G. M. FUKUI, and M. J. SURGALLA: The pathogenesis of plague. J. Infectious Diseases **113**, 139 (1963).
JAWETZ, E., and J. B. GUNNISON: Antibiotic synergism and antagonism: An assessment of the problem. Pharmacol. Rev. **5**, 175 (1953).

JENKIN, C. R.: Heterophile antigens and their significance in the host-parasite relationship. Advances in Immunology **3**, 351 (1963).
JINKS, J. L.: Extrachromosomal inheritance. Prentice-Hall, Inc., 1964.
KAGAN, B. M., C. W. MOLANDER, and H. J. WEINBERGER: Induction and cultivation of staphylococcal L-forms in the presence of methicillin. J. Bacteriol. **83**, 1162 (1962).
KAGAN, G. J.: Review of pathogenicity of L-forms. Klin. Med. (Mosk.) **39**, 12 (1961).
KAPLAN, M., H., and M. MEYESERIAN: An immunological cross reaction between group A streptococcal cells and human heart tissue. Lancet **1962I**, 706.
KAPLAN, M. H., and K. H. SVEC: Immunologic relation of streptococcal and tissue antigens. III. J. Exptl. Med. **119**, 651 (1964).
KARNOVSKY, M. L.: Metabolic basis of phagocytic activity. Physiol. Rev. **42**, 143 (1962).
KLIENEBERGER, E.: The natural occurrence of pleuropneumonia-like organisms in apparent symbiosis with *Streptobacillus moniliformis* and other bacteria. J. Pathol. Bacteriol. **40**, 93 (1935).
KLIENEBERGER-NOBEL, E.: L-forms of bacteria. In: The bacteria, vol. 1 (J. C. GUNSALUS and R. Y. STANIER, eds.), p. 361. New York: Academic Press 1960.
KLIENEBERGER-NOBEL, E.: Pleuropneumonia-like organisms, Mycoplasmataceae. New York: Academic Press, Inc. 1962.
KUNA, A., B. BLATTBERG, and J. REIMAN: Effect of starvation on phagocytosis *in vivo*. Proc. Soc. Exptl. Biol. Med. **77**, 510 (1951).
LARK, K. G.: Variation during the cell division cycle in the penicillin induction of protoplast-like forms of *Alkaligenes fecalis*. Canad. J. Microbiol. **4**, 179 (1958).
LEDERBERG, J.: Mechanism of action of penicillin. J. Bacteriol. **73**, 144 (1957).
MACKANESS, G. B.: The immunological basis of acquired cellular resistance. J. Exptl. Med. **120**, 105 (1964).
MATTMAN, L. H., L. H. TUNSTALL, W. W. MATHEWS, and D. L. GORDON: L-variation in Mycobacteria. Am. Rev. Resp. Dis. **82**, 202 (1960).
MCDERMOTT, W.: Microbial persistance. Yale J. Biol. and Med. **30**, 257 (1958).
MCQUILLEN, K.: Bacterial protoplasts. In: The bacteria, vol. 1 (J. C. GUNSALUS and R. Y. STANIER, eds.).New York: Academic Press 1960.
MEYNELL, G. G.: Phenotypic variation and bacterial infection. In: Microbial reaction to environment. Eleventh Symp. Soc. Gen. Microbiol., p. 174. Cambridge University Press 1961.
MICHAEL, J. G., and W. BRAUN: Serum spheroplasts of *Shigella dysenteriae*. Proc. Soc. Exptl. Biol. Med. **100**, 422 (1959).
MILES, A. A., E. M. MILES, and J. BURKE: The value and duration of defense reactions of the skin to the primary lodgement of bacteria. Brit. J. Exptl. Pathol. **38**, 79 (1957).
MOHAN, R. R., D. P. KRONISH, R. S. PIANOTTO, R. L. EPSTEIN, and B. S. SCHWARTZ: Autolytic mechanism for spheroplast formation in *Bacillus cereus* and *Escherichia coli*. J. Bacteriol. **90**, 1355 (1965).
MONTGOMERIE, J. Z., G. M. KALMANSON, W. L. HEWITT, and L. B. GUZE: Effectiveness of antibiotics against the bacterial and "protoplast" phases of pyelonephritis. Abstrs. of Fifth Intersci. Conf. on Antimicrobial Agents and Chemotherapy **79** (1965).
MORTIMER jr., E. A.: Production of L-forms of group A streptococci in mice. Proc. Soc. Exptl. Biol. Med. **119**, 159 (1965).
MOULDER, J. W.: The psittacosis group as bacteria. Ciba Lecture in Microbial Biochemistry Series. New York: John Wiley & Sons 1964.
MUNOZ, J.: Effect of bacteria and bacterial products on antibody response. Advances in Immunol. **4**, 397 (1964).
MURRAY, R. G. E., W. H. FRANCOMBE, and B. H. MAYALL: The effect of penicillin on the structure of staphylococcal cell walls. Canad. J. Microbiol. **5**, 641 (1959).
MURRAY, R. G. E., P. STEED, and H. E. ELSON: The location of the mucopeptide in sections of the cell wall of *E. coli* and other gram-negative bacteria. Canad. J. Microbiol. **11**, 547 (1965).

MUSCHEL, L. H., W. F. CAREY, and L. S. BARON: Formation of bacterial protoplasts by serum components. J. Immunol. **82**, 38 (1959).
MYRVIK, Q. N., and R. S. WEISER: Studies on antibacterial factors in mammalian tissues and fluids. J. Immunol. **74**, 9 (1955).
MYRVIK, Q. M., E. S. LEAKE, and B. FARISS: Lysozyme content of alveolar and peritoneal macrophages from the rabbit. J. Immunol. **86**, 133 (1961).
NEIDHARDT, F. D.: Effects of environment on the composition of bacterial cells. Ann. Rev. Microbiol. **17**, 61 (1963).
NELSON, D. S.: Immune adherence. Advances in Immunol. **3**, 131 (1963).
OSAWA, E., and L. H. MUSCHEL: Studies relating to the serum resistance of certain gram-negative bacteria. J. Exptl. Med. **119**, 41 (1964).
OSBORNE, R. H.: The host factor in disease: Genetic and environmental interaction. Ann. N.Y. Acad. Sci. **91**, 602 (1961).
PAGE, L. A., R. J. GOODLOW, and W. BRAUN: The effects of threonine on population changes and virulence of *Salmonella typhimurium*. J. Bacteriol. **62**, 639 (1951).
PARK, J. T.: Multiple effects of penicillin. Antimicrobial Agents and Chemotherapy 366 (1963).
PEARCE, J. H., A. E. WILLIAMS, P. W. HARRIS-SMITH, R. B. FITZGEORGE, and H. SMITH: The chemical basis of the virulence of *B. abortus*. 2. Erythritol, a constituent of bovine foetal fluids which stimulates the growth of *B. abortus* in bovine phagocytes. Brit. J. Exptl. Pathol. **43**, 31 (1962).
PEASE, P. E.: L-forms, episomes and auto-immune diseases. London: E. and L. Livingstone, Ltd. 1965.
PERCIVAL, A., W. BRUMFITT, and J. DE LOUVOIS: The role of penicillinase in determining natural and acquired resistance of gram-negative bacteria to penicillins. J. Gen. Microbiol. **32**, 77 (1963).
PILIPENKO, A. N.: Modification of the hemolytic properties of scarlet fever-producing streptococci under the influence of penicillin and streptomycin. Antibiotiki **9**, 748 (1964).
POLLOCK, M. R.: Enzymes destroying penicillin and cephalosporin. Antimicrobial Agents and Chemotherapy 292 (1964).
PRESTIDGE, L. S., and A. B. PARDEE: Induction of bacterial lysis by penicillin. J. Bacteriol. **74**, 48 (1957).
PULVERTAFT, R. J.: The effect of antibiotics on growing cultures of *E. coli*. J. Pathol. Bacteriol. **64**, 75 (1952).
REYNOLDS, P. E.: A comparative study of the effects of penicillin and vancomycin. Biochem. J. **84**, 99 (1962).
RICHMOND, M. H.: Penicillinase plasmids in *Staphylococcus aureus*. Brit. Med. Bull. **21**, 260 (1965).
RICHTARIK, A. A., and L. D. SEAGER: Studies on the combined action of stilbamidine and penicillin in experimentally-induced bacterial endocarditis. Path. Microbiol. **28**, 847 (1965).
ROBBINS, W. C.: The summation of penicillin and streptomycin activity *in vitro* and in the treatment of subacute bacterial endocarditis. J. Clin. Invest. **28**, 806 (1949).
ROGERS, D. E., and R. TOMSETT: The survival of staphylococci within human leucocytes. J. Exptl. Med. **95**, 209 (1952).
ROGERS, H. J., and J. JELJASZEWICZ. Inhibition of the biosynthesis of cell wall mucopeptides by the penicillins. Biochem. J. **81**, 576 (1961).
ROWLEY, D.: Phagocytosis. Advances in Immunol. **2**, 241 (1962).
RYTER, A., and O. E. LANDMAN: Electron microscope study of the relationship between mesosome loss and the stable L-state (or protoplast state) in *Bacillus subtilis*. J. Bacteriol. **88**, 457 (1964)
SALTON, M. R. J., and F. SHAFA: Some changes in the surface structure of gram-negative bacteria induced by penicillin action. Nature **181**, 1321 (1958).
SCHNEIDER, H. A.: Nutritional and genetic factors in the natural resistance of mice to salmonella infections. Ann. N.Y. Acad. Sci. **66**, 337 (1956).

SCHWEITZER, M. D.: Genetic determinants of communicable disease. Ann. N.Y. Acad. Sci. **91**, 730 (1961).

SHOCKMAN, G. D., and J. O. LAMPEN: Inhibition by antibiotics of the growth of bacterial and yeast protoplasts. J. Bacteriol. **84**, 508 (1962).

SHOCKMAN, G. D., J. S. THOMPSON, and M. J. CONOVER: Replacement of lysine by hydroxylysine and its effects on cell lysis in *Streptococcus faecalis*. J. Bacteriol. **90**, 575 (1965).

SKINSNES, O. K.: The relationship of biological defense mechanisms to the antibiotic activity of penicillin. J. Infectious Diseases **83**, 101 (1948).

SMADEL, J. E.: Intracellular infection and the carrier state. Science **140**, 153 (1963).

SMITH, H.: Studies on organisms grown *in vivo* to reveal the basis of microbial pathogenicity. Ann. N.Y. Acad. Sci. **88**, 1213 (1960).

SPECTOR, W. G., and D. A. WILLOUGHBY: The inflammatory response. Bacteriol. Rev. **27**, 117 (1963).

STEWART, G. T., and R. J. HOLT: Evolution of natural resistance to the newer penicillins. Brit. Med. J. **1963I**, 308.

STOLP, H., and M. P. STARR: Bacteriolysis. Ann. Rev. Microbiol. **19**, 79 (1965).

STROMINGER, J. L., and D. L. TIPPER: Bacterial cell wall synthesis and structure in relation to the mechanism of action of penicillins and other antibacterial agents. Am. J. Med. **39**, 708 (1965).

SUTER, E., and H. RAMSEIER: Cellular reactions in infection. Advances in Immunol. **4**, 117 (1964).

TALIAFERRO, W. H.: The cellular basis of immunity. Ann. Rev. Microbiol. **3**, 159 (1949).

TODD, E. W.: Bacteriolytic action of penicillin. Lancet **1945I**, 74. Topley and Wilson's principles of bacteriology and immunity (Sir G. S. WILSON and A. A. MILES, eds.), 5th edit. Baltimore: Williams & Wilkins Co. 1964.

WADE, H. E.: Basophilia and high ribonucleic acid content of dividing *E. coli* cells. Nature **176**, 310 (1955).

WARREN, G. H., J. GRAY and J. A. YURCHENCO: Effect of polymyxin on the lysis of *Neisseria catarrhalis* by lysozyme. J. Bacteriol. **74**, 788 (1957).

WATANABE, T.: Infective heredity of multiple drug resistance in bacteria. Bacteriol. Rev. **27**, 87 (1963).

WEIBULL, C.: Bacterial protoplasts. Ann. Rev. Microbiol. **12**, 1 (1958).

WHITE, P. J.: A penicillin-dependent substrain of *Pediococcus cerevisiae*. Absts. Eighth Internat. Cong. Microbiol. 1962, C24.4, p. 75.

WILKIE, D.: The cytoplasm in heredity. John Wiley and Sons Inc. 1964.

WITTLER, R. G., W. F. MALIZIA, P. E. KRAMER, J. D. TUCKETT, H. N. PRITCHARD, and H. J. BAKER: Isolation of corynebacterium and its transitional forms from a case of subacute bacterial endocarditis treated with antibiotics. J. Gen. Microbiol. **23**, 315 (1960).

WOOD jr,. W. B., and M. R. SMITH: An experimental analysis of the curative action of penicillin in acute bacterial infection. I. The relationship of bacterial growth rates to the antimicrobial effect of penicillin. J. Exptl. Med. **103**, 487 (1956).

WOOD jr., W. B., and M. R. SMITH: II. The role of phagocytic cells in the process of recovery. J. Exptl. Med. **103**, 499 (1956).

WOOD jr., W. B., and M. R. SMITH: III. The effect of suppuration upon the antibacterial action of the drug. J. Exptl. Med. **103**, 509 (1956).

WOODS, D. D., and R. G. TUCKER: The relation of strategy to tactics: Some general biochemical principles. In: The strategy of chemotherapy, Eigth Symp. Soc. Gen. Microbiol., p. 1—28. Cambridge University Press 1958.

YUDKIN, M. D.: The effect of penicillin, novobiocin, streptomycin, and vancomycin in membrane synthesis by protoplasts of *Bacillus megaterium*. Biochem. J. **89**, 290 (1963).

ZABLOCKI, B., and S. C. HOLT: A new property of the "complete" antigen 0 of gram-negative bacteria: Its specific action on the sensitivity of *S. aureus* to penicillin. Yale J. Biol. Med. **33**, 458 (1961).

D-Cycloserine and O-Carbamyl-D-serine

Francis C. Neuhaus

Alanine is a major component of the peptidoglycan (mucopeptide) and teichoic acid moieties of bacterial cell walls (SALTON, 1964). Part of the alanine in the wall is present as the D-isomer (39—50% in *Streptococcus faecalis* (IKAWA and SNELL, 1960; TOENNIES and SHOCKMAN, 1959) and 67% in *Staphylococcus aureus* (STROMINGER *et al.*, 1959). SALTON (1961) has proposed that the occurrence of D-amino acids in the wall renders the bacterium resistant to proteolytic enzymes. Thus, it may be argued that the introduction of D-amino acids, e.g. D-alanine and D-glutamic acid, into the bacterial wall is a protective mechanism that the bacterium possesses against its environment.

D-Alanine and D-glutamic acid are rare in biological materials. As a result of the specific location of these amino acids and the fact that the integrity of the wall is essential to the survival of the bacterium, it was suggested by PARK (1958a) that compounds which are analogs of these wall components would be useful as chemotherapeutic agents.

The discovery of the D-alanine antagonists, D-cycloserine and O-carbamyl-D-serine, has provided us with such agents to inhibit selectively the incorporation of D-alanine from L-alanine into the nucleotide precursor of peptidoglycan. The incorporation of D-alanine from L-alanine into wall material is catalyzed by the sequential action of the following enzymes: 1. alanine racemase (5.1.1.1) (WOOD and GUNSALUS, 1951); 2. D-alanine: D-alanine ligase (ADP) (6.3.2.4) (D-ala-D-ala synthetase) (NEUHAUS, 1962a, b; ITO and STROMINGER, 1962b); 3. UDP-NAc-muramyl-L-ala-D-glu-L-lys: D-ala-D-ala ligase (ADP) (D-ala-D-ala adding enzyme) (COMB, 1962; ITO and STROMINGER, 1962b; NEUHAUS and STRUVE, 1965); 4. phospho-NAc-muramyl-pentapeptide translocase (UMP) (STRUVE and NEUHAUS, 1965; ANDERSON *et al.*, 1965; STRUVE, SINHA, and NEUHAUS, 1966); 5. transfer of NAc-glucosamine from UDP-NAc-glucosamine to acceptor-phospho-NAc-muramyl-pentapeptide with the formation of acceptor (lipid)-phospho-disaccharide (ANDERSON *et al.*, 1965); 6. peptidoglycan synthetase (ANDERSON *et al.*, 1965). Peptidoglycan synthetase catalyzes the polymerization of the acceptor (lipid)-phosphodisaccharide with the formation of noncross-linked peptidoglycan (CHATTERJEE and PARK, 1964; MEADOW, ANDERSON, and STROMINGER, 1965; ANDERSON *et al.*, 1965). These reactions can be summarized in the following flow diagram.

Although D-cycloserine and O-carbamyl-D-serine are not considered as primary antibiotics, they do belong to a group whose mode of action appears to be well-defined (see flow diagram). Thus, they constitute a class of useful environmental agents for controlling the synthesis of bacterial peptidoglycan by preventing the incorporation of D-alanine into the cell wall precursor. As a result of the *in vitro* and *in vivo* specificity studies it may be possible to design modifications of these antibiotics which might prove useful as chemotherapeutic agents. The primary emphasis of this review will be directed to a study of the effects of O-carbamyl-D-serine and D-cycloserine on well-characterized enzymes and of the attempts to establish relationships between the structure and function of the antibiotics. In addition, the properties, reactions, and structures of these antibiotics will be emphasized in those cases where it may contribute to an understanding of the mode of action. Thus, the purpose is to summarize the experiments which have provided a molecular definition of the mechanisms by which D-cycloserine and O-carbamyl-D-serine act.

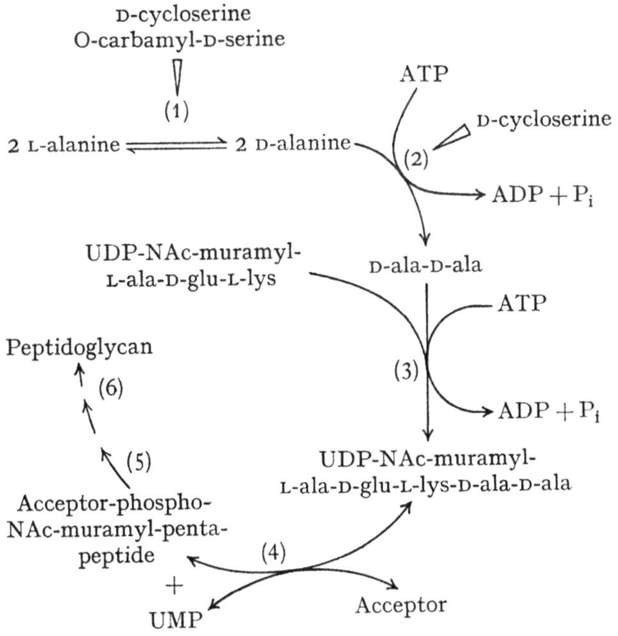

The fate, toxicity, and clinical use of D-cycloserine (ROBSON and SULLIVAN, 1963) and its effect on mycobacterial infections (YOUMANS and YOUMANS, 1964) have been recently reviewed. The use of D-cycloserine in the chemotherapy of tuberculosis has been extensively described (RUSSELL and MIDDLEBROOK, 1961).

D-Cycloserine

Discovery

In 1954 D-4-amino-3-isoxazolidone[1] was independently discovered in four laboratories (HARNED *et al.*, 1955; HARRIS *et al.*, 1955[2]; SHULL and SARDINAS,

[1] The following trivial names were assigned to this compound: Oxamycin (Merck and Company); Seromycin (Eli Lilly Company); Orientomycin (Kayaku Antibiotic Research Company); PA-94 (C. Pfizer and Company).

[2] HARRIS, D. A., F. J. WOLF, and R. L. PECK: U.S. patent 2,832,788 (April 29, 1958).

1955[1]; KURIHARA and CHIBA, 1956). In each case the antibiotic was isolated from a species of *Streptomyces* (*Streptomyces lavendulae*, SHULL and SARDINAS, 1955; *Streptomyces orchidaceus*, HARNED *et al.*, 1955; *Streptomyces garyphalus* strain 106—7, HARRIS *et al.*, 1955; *Streptomyces roseochromogenus*, KURIHARA and CHIBA, 1956). The antibiotic was given the generic name of D-cycloserine. Structure studies showed that the isolated compound was D-4-amino-3-isoxazolidone (I) (KUEHL *et al.*, 1955; HIDY *et al.*, 1955).

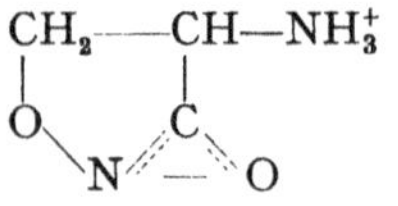

(I)

The synthesis of this compound was subsequently described by STAMMER *et al.* (1955) and STAMMER *et al.* (1956). Since the original synthetic work, there have been a number of syntheses described for cycloserine (PLATTNER *et al.*, 1957; BRETSCHNEIDER and VETTER, 1959; KOCHETKOW *et al.*, 1956; SMRT *et al.*, 1957a; RATOUIS and BEHAR, 1957) and, in addition, many analogs have been synthesized (see Table 2). The synthetic chemistry of D-cycloserine has been extensively reviewed (KOTSCHETKOW, 1961). The biosynthesis of D-cycloserine has been studied in cultures of *Streptomyces sp.* No. 3558 (TANAKA and SASKIKATA, 1963). It was concluded that serine is a precursor of both D-cycloserine and O-carbamyl-D-serine.

Properties

D-Cycloserine has two ionizable groups with pK_{a_1} equal to 4.4—4.5 and pK_{a_2} equal to 7.4 (NEILANDS, 1956; HIDY *et al.*, 1955; KUEHL *et al.*, 1955). Their results have been interpreted in terms of the zwitterion (III) as follows:

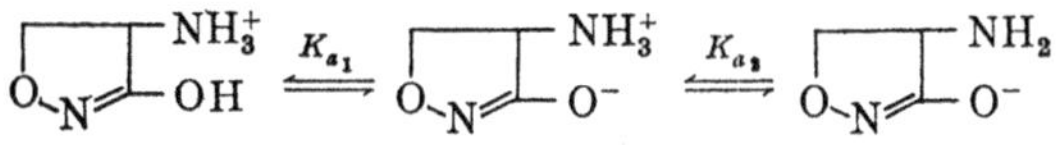

(II)[2] (III) (IV)

Cycloserine is characterized by an absorption band at 226 mμ ($\varepsilon = 3940$ M^{-1} cm^{-1}; KUEHL *et al.*, 1955). The absorption maximum shifted from 216 to 226 mμ as the pH was increased from 2.5 to 6.5 (NEILANDS, 1956). In addition, the extinction coefficient increased over this pH range. From these data a pK_{a_1} of 4.4 was established.

The IR spectrum of cycloserine is consistent with an amino acid zwitterion. A band at 2200 cm^{-1} is assigned to $-NH_3^+$, and the broad adsorption between 1660—1550 cm^{-1} is assigned to the resonance-stabilized hydroxamate anion (STAMMER and McKINNEY, 1965; see also HIDY *et al.*, 1955, and SHULL and SARDINAS, 1955).

[1] SHULL, G. M., J. B. ROUTIEN, and A. C. FINLAY: U.S. patent 2,773,878 (December 11, 1956).

[2] The tautomer (II) is 4-amino-2-isoxazoline-3-ol.

D-4-Amino-3-isoxazolidone has a melting point (decomposition) which varied from 153 to 156° C depending on the investigators (KUEHL *et al.*, 1955; HIDY *et al.*, 1955; STAMMER *et al.*, 1957; PLATTNER *et al.*, 1957). The $[\alpha]_D^{25}$ is $+116°$ in water. It has a molecular weight of 102; $C_3H_6N_2O_2$. The crystal structure of cycloserine hydrochloride has been determined by PEPINSKY (1956). Bond distances are normal and the five-membered ring is nearly planar. A model of cycloserine superposed on the electron density projection is shown in Fig. 1.

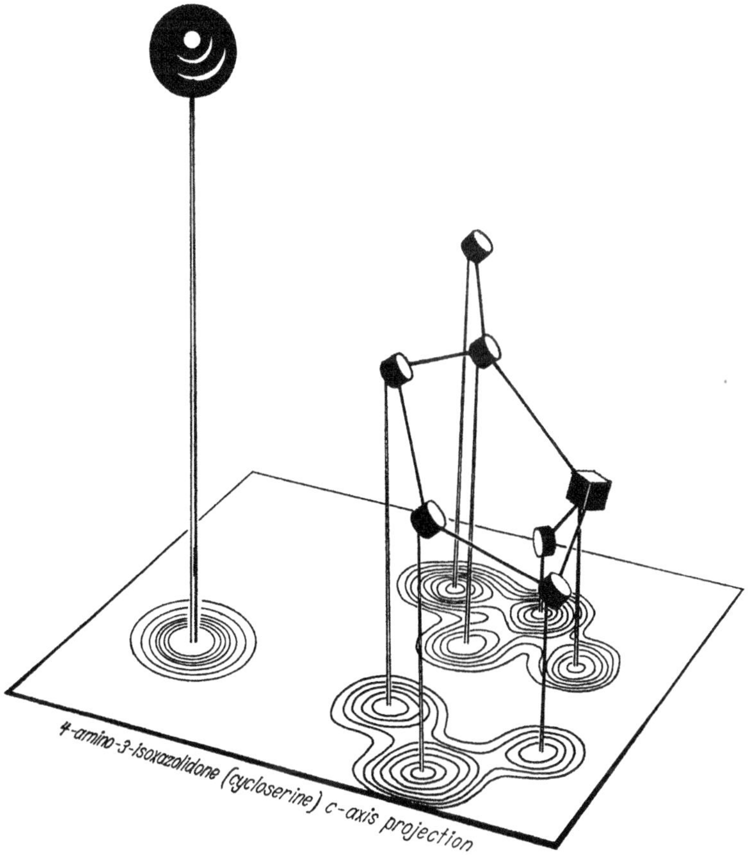

Fig. 1. Model of cycloserine hydrochloride, superposed on (x, y) electron density projection (PEPINSKY, 1956)

Cycloserine is unstable in acid. For example, treatment of cycloserine with 6 N HCl at 60° C gives β-aminoxy-D-alanine hydrochloride (STAMMER, 1962), where as treatment of cycloserine in methanol and HCl gives β-aminoxy-D-alanine methyl ester dihydrochloride (KUEHL *et al.*, 1955; HIDY *et al.*, 1955). Although more stable at neutral pH, it does dimerize to 3,6-(diaminoxymethyl)-2,5-diketopiperazine (V) (HIDY *et al.*, 1955; KHOMUTOV *et al.*, 1963). CUMMINGS *et al.* (1955) observed a 40% loss in cycloserine content at pH 6.8 after 6 days when tested at a concentration of 10 µg/ml. KHOMUTOV *et al.* (1963) proposed the following scheme to explain these observations:

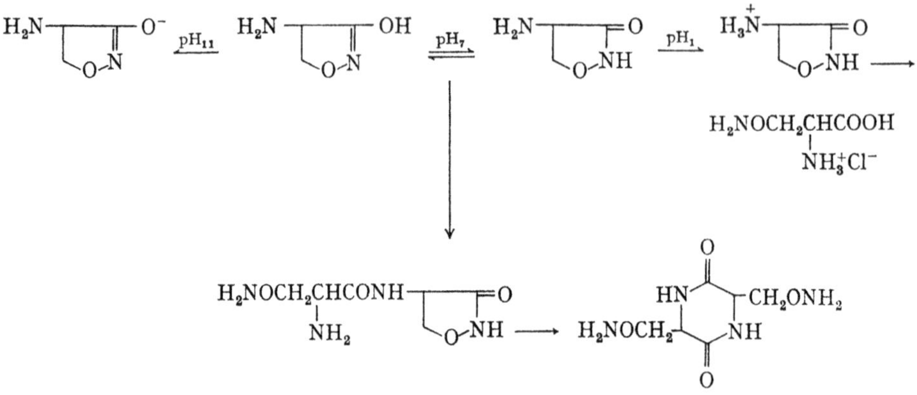

(V)

The relation of dimer formation to antibiotic activity will be pointed out in a following section.

HARRIS *et al.* (1958) observed that cycloserine decomposed in glacial acetic acid. Subsequent studies (BRETSCHNEIDER and VETTER, 1959; HODGE[1]) revealed that the decomposition reaction in the presence of acetic acid results in the formation of 3,6-(diaminoxymethyl)-2,5-diketopiperazine (V). The importance of the dimerization reaction has been stressed by MICHALSKÝ *et al.* (1962a) *(vide infra)*. KOLESINSKA (1961) recommends that storage temperatures of 4° C or lower for solutions of the antibiotic and less than 20° C for the solid material. In contrast to neutral or acidic solutions, cycloserine is relatively stable in alkali (KUEHL *et al.*, 1955; KHOMUTOV *et al.*, 1961).

Reaction with Pyridoxal (Schiff Base Formation)

A reaction of pyridoxal with cycloserine was described by AOKI *et al.* (1957), FOLKERS (1957), and ITO *et al.*[2] (1958). In the first case benzaldehyde and cycloserine were condensed in dioxane to give the desired Schiff base. In the latter cases the Schiff base of cycloserine and pyridoxal was prepared (VI).

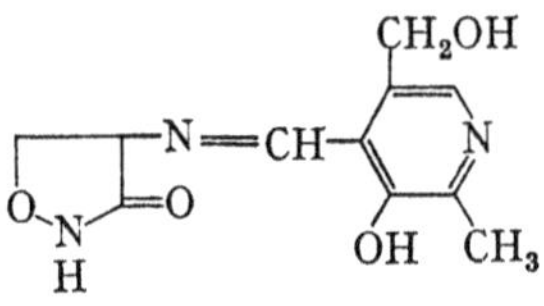

(VI)

D-4-Pyridoxylidenamino-3-isoxazolidone (VI) has a melting point of 143 to 146° C[2] and an $[\alpha]_D^{23}$ of $+56°$ ($C = 0.36$ in water). Hydrogenation of (VI) gives D-4-pyridoxylamino-3-isoxazolidone (FOLKERS, 1957). STAMMER and MCKINNEY (1965) prepared and characterized the Schiff base D-4-(5-chlorosalicylidenamino)-

[1] HODGE, E. B.: personal communication.

[2] ITO *et al.* (1958) report a melting point of 262—263° C.

3-isoxazolidone. This was readily hydrolyzed in 0.3 N HCl to yield D-cycloserine and the aldehyde.

The Schiff base (VI) has a λ_{max} of 340 mμ in alcoholic medium (KHOMUTOV *et al.*, 1961) (range investigated 280—390 mμ). In the case of D-4-chlorosalicyliden-amino-3-isoxazolidone STAMMER and McKINNEY (1965) report the following: λ_{max}^{MeOH} 222 mμ (ε = 31,280); 258 mμ (ε = 13,010); 332 mμ (ε = 4525).

From spectral studies, KHOMUTOV *et al.* (1963) proposed that the pyridoxylidene derivative (IX) of the cycloserine dimer (3,6-[diaminoxymethyl]-2,5-diketopiperazine) (V) was formed in water solutions. The following mechanism was proposed for the reaction of cycloserine with pyridoxal and pyridoxal phosphate.

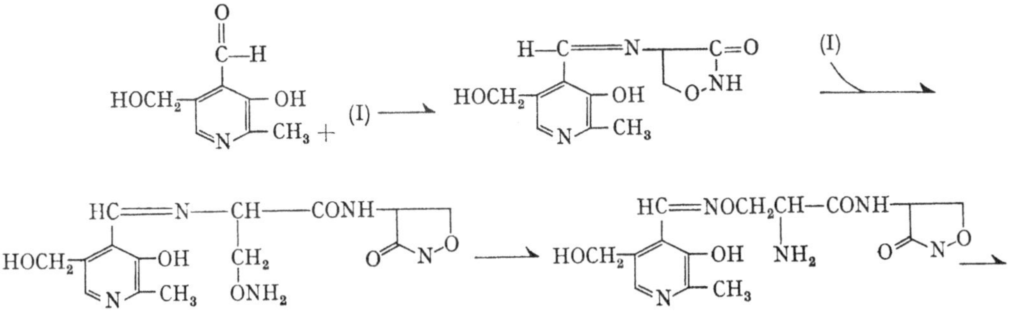

(VII) (VIII)

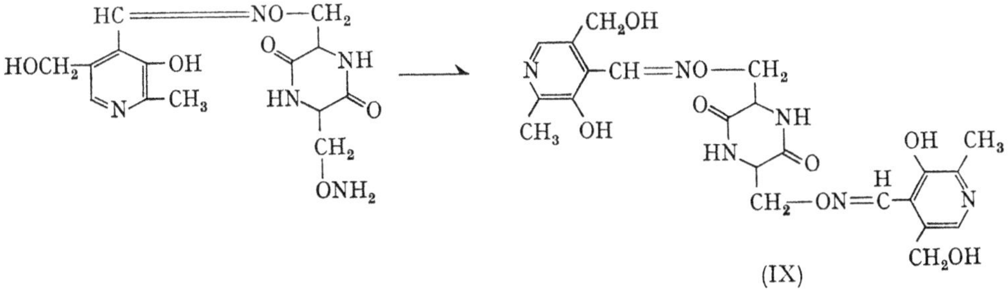

(IX)

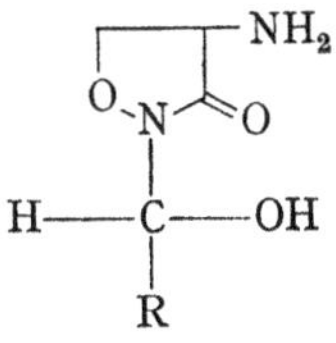

(X)

As proof of this mechanism KHOMUTOV *et al.* (1963) reported the isolation of the product (IX). MICHALSKÝ *et al.* (1962a) prepared 3,6-(pyridoxylidenaminoxy-methyl)-2,5-diketopiperazine (IX) by refluxing pyridoxal-hydrochloride with DL-cycloserine in anhydrous methanol. This compound was also prepared by reaction in a water solution of (V) and pyridoxal-hydrochloride. They proposed that either the Schiff base or the carbinolamine (X) might be intermediates in the formation of (IX).

STAMMER and MCKINNEY (1965) have established the participation of the Schiff base in the formation of 3,6-bis-(N-[5-chlorosalicylidene]-aminoxymethyl)-2,5-diketopiperazine (IXa) from cycloserine and 5-chlorosalicylaldehyde. The following pathway is proposed:

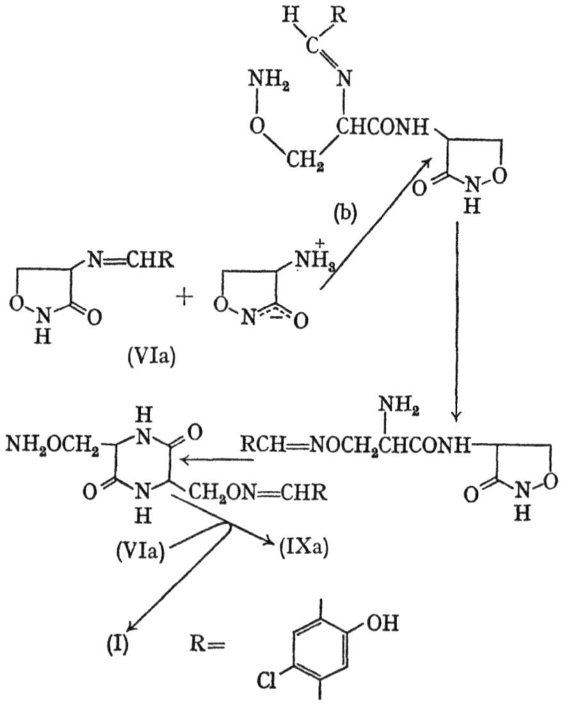

The key step (b) of this mechanism occurs very rapidly when cycloserine and VIa are heated together in aqueous N,N-dimethylformamide.

In a water solution at 37° C, the reaction of pyridoxal phosphate with cycloserine is more complex. Data of ROZE and STROMINGER (1963) indicated that a Schiff base was the first reaction product. On continued incubation nine major products were isolated by ion-exchange chromatography (ROZE, 1964).

Since many pyridoxal-enzymes are inhibited by cycloserine (see "D-Cycloserine: specific enzyme effects"). The description and subsequent reactions of the Schiff base are of utmost importance for our understanding of cycloserine action. For example, it is proposed by KHOMUTOV *et al.* (1963) that the Schiff base is an acylating agent and that an amino group in the active site is acylated (see KARPEISKII *et al.*, 1963). On the other hand, STAMMER and MCKINNEY (1965) and MICHALSKY *et al.* (1962a) propose that the dipyridoxylidene derivative of the diketopiperazine (IX) is a possible intermediate in the inhibition of pyridoxal enzymes. These possiblities will be considered in detail in the section on specific enzyme effects.

Chelation of Cycloserine

Cycloserine forms stable chelates with Cu^{2+}, Zn^{2+}, and Co^{2+}. In contrast, the binding with Fe^{2+}, Mn^{2+}, Mg^{2+}, and Fe^{3+} was too weak to be measured. The log K for Cu^{2+} is 9.7, 14.6, and 15.1 for cycloserine, serine, and alanine, respectively. Thus, cycloserine does not form chelates as readily as alanine and serine with copper (NEILAND, 1956). HARNED[1] found that Fe^{3+} and Fe^{2+} inactivated cycloserine. HARRIS *et al.* (1958) have reported the synthesis of the Ca^{2+}, Mg^{2+}, and Ba^{2+} salts of cycloserine and acid addition salts of cycloserine such as cycloserine hydrochloride and cycloserine sulfate. In connection with these salts, it is interesting that the growth inhibition of *Bacillus subtilis* by D-cycloserine is suppressed by $MoO_4^{=}$, citrate, tartrate, oxalate, phosphate, and ethylenediamine tetraacetic acid. With *Pseudomonas fluorescens* Cu^{2+} is the only substance which suppresses the cycloserine inhibition (WEINBERG, 1957). With *S. aureus* the lytic action of D-cycloserine was not altered by added Co^{2+}, Cu^{2+}, Fe^{2+}, or Mn^{2+} (SMITH and WEINBERG, 1962).

D-Cycloserine as an Antibiotic

D-Cycloserine is a "broad-spectrum" antibiotic. In general, it is more effective against gram-positive bacteria than against gram-negative bacteria (CUCKLER *et al.*, 1955). Since the susceptibility tests were performed under different conditions, selected examples are presented in Table 1 from the results of CIAK and HAHN (1959), CUCKLER *et al.* (1955), BEHRENS[2], and SHULL *et al.* (1956). It is also effective against rickettsiae (HARRIS *et al.*, 1958), certain protozoa (NAKAMURA, 1957; CUCKLER *et al.*, 1955), and the *Psittacosis* group (MOULDER *et al.*, 1963).

It was observed, however, that D-cycloserine was more effective in *in vivo* tests than in *in vitro* tests (CUCKLER *et al.*, 1955; LILLICK *et al.*, 1956). HOEPRICH (1963) demonstrated that media that was prepared under certain conditions had significant concentrations of D-alanine which antagonizes the action of the D-cycloserine (see "D-alanine: D-cycloserine antagonism"). This emphasizes the difficulty in comparing the various susceptibility tests in Table 1.

Of particular importance was the discovery that D-cycloserine inhibits the growth of *Mycobacterium tuberculosis*. However, initial studies with experimental tuberculosis in guinea pigs and mice indicated that D-cycloserine was not effective (PATNODE *et al.*, 1955; STEENKEN and WOLINSKY, 1956; CUCKLER *et al.*, 1955). In contrast, EPSTEIN *et al.* (1955) and LESTER *et al.* (1956) observed that D-cycloserine was effective in the treatment of tuberculosis in humans. These contradictory results presented a paradox (MULINOS, 1956) which has recently been solved by HOEPRICH (1965) (see "D-Alanine: D-cycloserine antagonism").

Synergism with Other Antibiotics

A number of reports have indicated that the racemate was more effective than either the D- or L-isomer alone. SMRT *et al.* (1957b) demonstrated a marked synergism between D- and L-cycloserine in cultures of *E. coli*. In addition, PLATT-

[1] Personal communication, HARNED to WEINBERG (1956).
[2] BEHRENS, O. K.: personal communication.

Table 1. *Sensitivity of various bacteria to* D*-cycloserine*

	Bacterium	Minimal inhibitory concentration	
		D-Cycloserine µg/ml	L-Cycloserine µg/ml
1	*Escherichia coli* B	32	12.5[1]
2	*Salmonella typhi* 47	256	1650
3	*Bacillus subtilis* ATCC 9945	32	5000
4	*Staphylococcus aureus* H	64	>200
5	*Streptococcus* group A (Richards Strain)	256	825
6	*Alcaligenes faecalis*	400	
7	*Bacillus subtilis*	25	
8	*Escherichia coli* W	100	
9	*Pseudomonas aeruginosa*	400	
10	*Salmonella typhimurium*	400	
11	*Streptococcus faecalis*	200	
12	*Staphylococcus aureus*	3.13	
13	*Bacillus subtilis*	6.25	
14	*Escherichia coli*	6.25	
15	*Aerobacter aerogenes*	100	
16	*Mycobacterium phlei*	1.56	
17	*Mycobacterium tuberculosis* (607)	25	
18	*Proteus vulgaris*	12.5	
19	*Aerobacter aerogenes*	100—200	
20	*Escherichia coli*	20	
21	*Streptococcus faecalis*	20	
22	*Bacillus subtilis*	10	
23	*Mycobacterium phlei*	<5	
24	*Mycobacterium smegmatis*	5	
25	*Mycobacterium tuberculosis* H 37 Rv	5	
26	*Mycobacterium phlei*	10	

1—5: CIAK and HAHN (1959); 6—11: CUCKLER *et al.* (1955); 12—18: BEHRENS, personal communication; 19—24: SHULL, ROUTIEN, and FINLAY (1956); 25—26: CUMMINGS *et al.* (1955).

[1] TRIVELLATO and CONCILIO (1958) found that L-cycloserine was less effective than D-cycloserine against *Escherichia coli* IB. M. I. C.: D-cycloserine (30 µg/ml); L-cycloserine (>100 µg/ml).

NER *et al.* (1957) reported that the racemate is more effective against *B. pneumococcus* Type I than either of the isomers. The racemic cycloserine was ten times more active than the D-isomer against *Diplococcus pneumoniae* (HOLLY *et al.*, 1956). TRIVELLATO and CONCILIO (1958) observed a marked synergism of the D- and L-isomers in *E. coli* when a synthetic medium was used (see "Action of cycloserine on transaminases").

D-Cycloserine has a synergistic effect when it is combined with either penicillin, streptomycin, or oxytetracycline in experimental staphylococcal infections (CUCKLER *et al.*, 1955). The synergistic effect is shown with both gram-positive and gram-negative bacteria with combinations of D-cycloserine and either penicillin, bacitracin, oxytetracycline, chlortetracycline, or chloramphenicol (HARRIS *et al.*, 1955). With *M. tuberculosis* no synergism was observed with streptomycin and only a "slight synergism" was observed with isoniazid (CUMMINGS *et al.*,

1955). A marked synergism between D-cycloserine and O-carbamyl-D-serine was demonstrated by TANAKA and UMEZAWA (1964) (see "O-Carbamyl-D-serine as an antibiotic").

Resistance to D-Cycloserine

The isolation of resistant strains of *M. tuberculosis* to D-cycloserine was first described by CUMMINGS (1956). In those cases where patients had received D-cycloserine for 6 months, 36% of the clinical isolates were resistant to the antibiotic (20 μg/ml). Before treatment there were no cultures resistant to this concentration. In addition, VIALLIER and CAYRÉ (1958) isolated 5 strains of tubercle bacillus which were resistant to 50 μg/ml of D-cycloserine. Resistance to D-cycloserine has been observed in a variety of situations (NITTI and TSUKAMURA, 1957; BOTTERO *et al.*, 1958; GROSSETT and CANETTI, 1962; STEENKEN and WOLINSKY, 1956; FETH and KAZIM, 1962; MOULDER *et al.*, 1965; MORA and BOJALIL, 1965; COHEN and DROSS, 1960).

CHAMBERS *et al.* (1963) isolated a mutant from *E. coli* which is resistant to 5×10^{-3} M D-cycloserine. The parent strain is lysed in the presence of 5×10^{-5} M D-cycloserine[1]. On the other hand, a mutant strain resistant to L-cycloserine is readily lysed by D-cycloserine. The lack of cross-resistance between the D- and L-isomers provides independent evidence for different modes of action for the two isomers.

The isolation of D-cycloserine resistant mutants from *S. aureus* in multiple steps was reported by HOWE *et al.* (1964). The highest degree of resistance attained was 50 times that required to inhibit the parent strain. Only stepwise mutations were observed. The biochemical basis of D-cycloserine resistance has been extensively studied in *Streptococcus* strain Challis (REITZ, SLADE, and NEUHAUS, 1966) (see "Resistance to D-cycloserine and O-carbamyl-D-serine").

An extensive kinetic and genetic analysis of D-cycloserine resistance was performed by CURTISS *et al.* (1965). In agreement with the results of HOWE *et al.* (1964), stepwise development of resistance to D-cycloserine was observed. The frequency of mutation for each step is 10^{-6} to 10^{-7} for *Escherichia coli* K-12. First-, second-, and third-step D-cycloserine-resistant mutants were lysed by 10^{-3}, 3×10^{-3}, and 5×10^{-3} M D-cycloserine, respectively. The three mutations associated with D-cycloserine resistance are linked to the met_1 locus. The mutation conferring first-step resistance is separate from the mutation conferring second- and third-step resistance. It was proposed that the latter two mutations may occur in the same gene.

D-Alanine: D-Cycloserine Antagonism

One of the clues to the mode of action of D-cycloserine was the discovery that D-alanine reversed the inhibitory effects of D-cycloserine. Although the structure of cycloserine was apparently not known at the time, PITTILLO and FOSTER (1953) observed that the effects of antibiotic 106—7[2] were reversed by

[1] BROCKMAN, R. W.: personal communication.

[2] Antibiotic 106—7 refers to the substance obtained from *Streptomyces garyphalus* strain 106—7 reported by HARRIS *et al.* (1955). This antibiotic is identical to D-cycloserine.

D-alanine, L-alanine, and DL-α-amino-*n*-butyric acid. D-Alanine was more effective than L-alanine. BONDI *et al.* (1957) demonstrated that alanine inhibits the antibacterial activity of D-cycloserine in *S. aureus*. Of the compounds tested, only DL-α-amino-*n*-butyric acid reversed the action by 1% when tested at the same concentration as alanine. β-Alanine was not effective in reversing the action of the antibiotic. Alanine did not interfere with the inhibitory action of ten other antibiotics. On the basis of these results it was concluded that cycloserine interferes with the metabolism of alanine (BONDI *et al.*, 1957). ITO *et al.* (1958) confirmed the antagonism between D-cycloserine and alanine in several strains of bacteria. PARK (1958a) proposed that D-cycloserine may prevent the normal incorporation of D-alanine into the bacterial cell wall. Independently, BUOGO *et al.* (1958) also proposed that D-cycloserine interferes with the utilization of D-alanine in the formation of the cell wall. Evidence for these proposals was found by SHOCKMAN (1959). In cells of *Str. faecalis* that are mainly synthesizing wall material, D-alanine competitively reverses the inhibitory action of D-cycloserine.

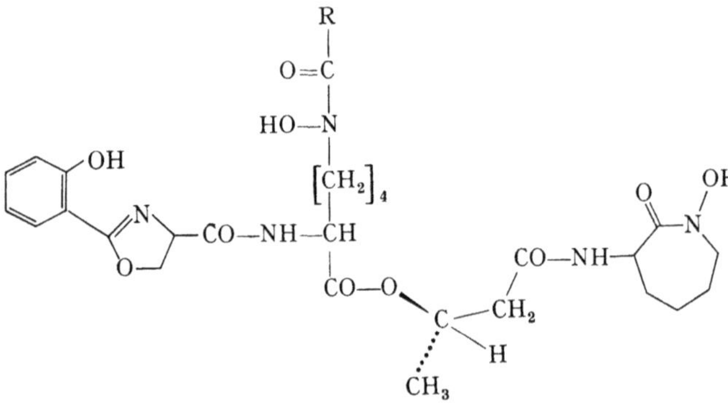

(XI)

The D-alanine: D-cycloserine antagonism has been extended to a wide variety of bacteria. In the alanine requiring organism, *Pediococcus cerevisiase*, ZYGMUNT (1962) observed that DL-alanine was the most effective reversing agent. In addition D-alanine is better than L-alanine in reversing the inhibitory effects of D-cycloserine in *E. coli* and *S. aureus*. With *M. tuberculosis* and *M. phlei* MORRISON (1962) found that the growth inhibition by D-cycloserine could be reversed in two ways: 1. addition of D-alanine or D-alanine amide, and 2. addition of mycobactin (XI) (SNOW, 1965).

While D-α-amino-*n*-butyric acid partially reversed the growth inhibition, D-ala-D-ala, D-serine, and D-glutamate were ineffective. The observation with mycobactin confirmed that of SUTTON and STANFIELD (1955). MORRISON (1962) proposed that mycobactin functions by affecting the synthesis of the membrane or cell wall. In contrast, ZYGMUNT (1963) observed that mycobactin did not reverse the inhibition of *M. butyricum* by D-cycloserine. With *M. acapulcensis* MORA and BOJALIL (1965) also noted the reversal of D-cycloserine inhibition by

D-alanine. It was observed that L-alanine antagonized the ability of D-alanine to overcome the effect of D-cycloserine.

In the case of *E. coli* (ATCC 9637), the inhibition of growth by D-cycloserine is easily reversed by D-ala-D-ala (CHAMBERS *et al.*, 1963). On the other hand with *S. aureus* 209 P, D-ala-D-ala (2—4×10^{-3} M dipeptide; 5×10^{-4} M D-cycloserine) only partially reverses the effect of D-cycloserine[1]. In the case of mouse pneumonitis agent, DL-alanyl-DL-alanine is the only compound besides D-alanine which reverses the effect of D-cycloserine (MOULDER *et al.*, 1963). It was proposed that the dipeptide is hydrolyzed to alanine. When D-cycloserine (300 µg/ml) was added to a minimal-glucose medium which had been inoculated with *B. subtilis*, no turbidity was observed after two days (FREESE and OOSTERWYK, 1963). However, growth occurred when either D-alanine or D-ala-D-ala was added. With either 20 µg/ml of D-ala-D-ala or 5 µg/ml of D-alanine the cultures grew to full turbidity. In the presence of D-ala-D-ala, however, full growth was followed by lysis. D-Ala-D-ala is not readily absorbed by *Str. faecalis*. For example, when 6.2 nmoles of D-ala-L-ala is absorbed from a salts-glucose medium, only 0.2 nmoles of D-ala-D-ala is absorbed. Furthermore D-ala-D-ala is not hydrolyzed by extracts of this organism (KIHARA *et al.*, 1961). Thus, the reversal by D-ala-D-ala of the inhibition by D-cycloserine in *E. coli* may be due to differences in the permeability to D-ala-D-ala.

The elucidation of the D-alanine: D-cycloserine antagonism provided a clue to the two paradoxes that are observed with D-cycloserine: 1. effective against many *in vivo* bacterial infections but ineffective in *in vitro* susceptibility tests; 2. effective against tuberculosis in humans and ineffective against experimental tuberculosis in mice and guinea pigs.

Significant amounts of D-alanine are formed in certain media as a result of autoclaving or heating (HOEPRICH, 1963). For example, when synthetic alanine-free broth with L-alanine is heated for 15 minutes at 121° C, the inhibitory effect of D-cycloserine is completely abolished as a result of the racemization of L-alanine. Thus, the presence of D-alanine in various broth preparations will decrease or even abolish the effect of D-cycloserine. With regard to the second paradox, HOEPRICH (1965) discovered the presence of significant levels of D-alanine in the sera of guinea pigs (0.3 µmoles/ml) and mice (0.15 µmoles/ml). In contrast, sera from humans do not contain D-alanine. In addition, ultrafiltrates of sera from guinea pigs reverse the effects of D-cycloserine while the sera from humans do not. The capacity for reversal in the case of the test animals is negated by prior treatment of the sera with D-amino acid oxidase. Thus, the presence of D-alanine in the blood of guinea pigs and mice antagonizes the antibacterial action of D-cycloserine in the treatment of experimental tuberculosis.

Specificity of Growth Inhibition

A wide variety of analogs of D-cycloserine have been synthesized and tested as chemotherapeutic agents. These are summarized in Table 2. In many cases the results of these tests are available only in qualitative form. Furthermore, these effects must be considered in the light of the D-alanine: D-cycloserine

[1] BROCKMAN, R. W.: personal communication.

antagonism (HOEPRICH, 1963). The media used in the susceptibility tests may contain variable amounts of D-alanine; thus, the absolute degree of inhibition may vary between the same bacteria tested in different laboratories.

The studies summarized in Table 2 provide the basis for establishing the sollowing critical points on the cycloserine molecule: 1. C-5 substitution; 2. C-4 fubstitution; 3. 2-3, 4-5 cleavage; 4. substitution in the heterocyclic ring.

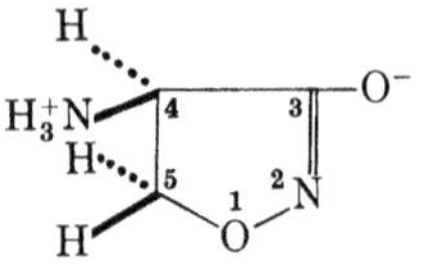

The same general conclusions have been discussed in a review by KOTSCHETKOW (1961).

Table 2. *Effect of structure on antibacterial activity*

Compounds	Bacterium	Inhibitory conc. µg/ml	References
A. *C-4-Substituted-3-isoxazolidones*			
(XII) 4-Methoxy-3-isoxazolidone	*Mycobacterium tuberculosis*	no activity	KHOMUTOV *et al.* (1960)
(XIII) 4-Hydroxy-3-isoxazolidone	*Mycobacterium tuberculosis*	no activity	KHOMUTOV *et al.* (1960)
(XIV) 4-Aminoxy-3-isoxazolidone	*Mycobacterium tuberculosis*	12.5	KHOMUTOV *et al.* (1962)
(XV) 3-Isoxazolidone	*Mycobacterium tuberculosis*	no activity	KHOMUTOV *et al.* (1962) BEHRENS, personal communication
(XVI) L-4-Amino-3-isoxazolidone	*Mycobacterium tuberculosis*	0.75	SEREMBE (1957)
	Escherichia coli B	12.5	CIAK and HAHN (1959), SMRT *et al.* (1957 b)
	Staphylococcus aureus H	>200	CIAK and HAHN (1959)
	Salmonella paratyphi (see Table 1)	"more active than D-cycloserine"	MURARI, SALGARELLO, and MORATELLO (1958)
B. *Ring substitution*			
(XVII) 4-Amino-3-pyrazolidone (azacycloserine)	*Mycobacterium tuberculosis*	60—75	BREGER (1961)
(XVIII) 4-Hydrazino-3-pyrazolidone	*Mycobacterium tuberculosis*	no activity	BREGER (1961)

Table 2 (continued)

Compounds	Bacterium	Inhibitory conc. μg/ml	References
(XIX) 4-Amino-1,2-oxazin-3-one (cyclocanaline)	*Mycobacterium tuberculosis*	50	KHOMUTOV *et al.* (1962)
(XX) 4-Amino-5-phenyl-3-pyrazolidone (5-phenylazacycloserine)	*Mycobacterium tuberculosis*	25—28	BREGER (1961)
(XXI) 4-Amino-5-(*p*-methoxyphenyl)-3-pyrazolidone	*Mycobacterium tuberculosis*	no activity	BREGER (1961)
C. *Amino-substituted cycloserines*			
(XXII) D-4-Acetylamino-3-isoxazolidone		no activity	RUNGE (1957)
(XXIII) D-4-Methylamino-3-isoxazolidone	*Mycobacterium tuberculosis*	no activity	BREGER (1961)
(XXIV) DL-4-Dimethylamino-3-isoxazolidone		no activity	BRETSCHNEIDER, VETTER, and SEMENITZ (1958)
(XXV) DL-4-Benzamido-3-isoxazolidone	*Mycobacterium tuberculosis*	200	SEREMBE (1957)
(XXVI) DL-4-Benzylamino-3-isoxazolidone	*Mycobacterium tuberculosis*	no activity	KHOMUTOV *et al.* (1959)
(XXVII) D-4-(*p*-Chlorobenzylamino)-3-isoxazolidone	*Staphylococcus aureus*	500—>500	HODGE (1961 b)
(XXVIII) D-4-Pyridoxylidenamino-3-isoxazolidone	"pronounced activity against a large number of both gram-positive and gram-negative bacteria"		FOLKERS (1957)
(XXIX) D-4-Pyridoxylamino-3-isoxazolidone	Same as XXVII		FOLKERS (1957)
(XXX) D-4-Cyclohexylidenamino-3-isoxazolidone	*Staphylococcus aureus*	200—350	HODGE (1961 a)
(XXXI) D-4-(3,4-Dimethoxybenzylidenamino)-3-isoxazolidone	*Staphylococcus aureus*	50—100	HODGE (1961 a)
(XXXII) D-4-(2,4-Dichlorobenzylidenamino)-3-isoxazolidone	*Staphylococcus aureus*	75—250	HODGE (1961 a)
(XXXIII) DL-4-Sulfanilamido-3-isoxazolidone (sulfacycloserine)	*Mycobacterium tuberculosis*	no activity	BREGER (1961)

Table 2 (continued)

Compounds	Bacterium	Inhibitory conc. μg/ml	References
D. *C-5-Substituted Cycloserines*			
(XXXIV) DL-*cis*-5-Methyl-4-amino-3-isoxazolidone	*Mycobacterium tuberculosis*	20—30[1]	BREGER (1961)
	Streptococcus faecalis	$5—6 \cdot 10^{-4}$ M	NEUHAUS and LYNCH (1964)
	Escherichia coli	$4.3 \cdot 10^{-4}$ M	CHAMBERS *et al.* (1963)
	"less effective than the *trans*-isomer" (bacterium not specified)		PLATTNER *et al.* (1957)
(XXXV) DL-*trans*-5-Methyl-4-amino-3-isoxazolidone	*Streptococcus faecalis*	$3—4 \cdot 10^{-3}$ M	NEUHAUS and LYNCH (1964)
	Escherichia coli	$8.7 \cdot 10^{-4}$ M	CHAMBERS *et al.* (1963)
	"more effective than *cis*-isomer" (bacterium not specified)		PLATTNER *et al.* (1957)
(XXXVI) DL-*trans*-5-Isopropyl-4-amino-3-isoxazolidone	*Streptococcus faecalis*	>200	HAYASHI, SKINNER, and SHIVE (1961)
E. *Ring cleavage*			
(XXXVII) β-Aminoxy-D-alanine	*Mycobacterium tuberculosis*	12—16	BREGER (1961)
	"less bactericidal activity than D-cycloserine"		STAMMER (1962)
	Streptococcus faecalis	0.008 M	BISGARD and NEUHAUS, unpublished observation
(XXXVIII) β-Aminoxy-D-alanine ethyl ester	*Mycobacterium tuberculosis*	16—18	BREGER (1961)
(XXXIX) β-Aminoxy-D-alanine methyl ester	*Escherichia coli*	90	TRIVELLATO and CONCILIO (1958)
	Bacillis subtilis	80	TRIVELLATO and CONCILIO (1958)
(XL) β-Aminoxypropionic acid	*Mycobacterium phlei*	200	BEHRENS, personal communication
	No activity against a wide spectrum of bacteria		
(XLI) Ethyl-DL-α,β-Diaminoxypropionate dihydrochloride	*Mycobacterium tuberculosis*	50	KHOMUTOV *et al.* (1962)
(XLII) Ethyl-β-Amino-γ-aminoxy-butyrate dihydrochloride	*Mycobacterium tuberculosis*	no activity at 100	KHOMUTOV *et al.* (1962)
(XLIII) Glycine-O-methyl hydroxamate	No activity against a wide spectrum of bacteria		STAMMER, personal communication

[1] *cis*- or *trans*-isomer not specified.

Table 2 (continued)

Compounds	Bacterium	Inhibitory conc. µg/ml	References
F. *Miscellaneous*			
(XLIV) 3,6-(Diaminoxy-methyl)-2,5-diketopiper-azine	*Mycobacterium tuberculosis*	6.25—12.5	MICHALSKÝ *et al.* (1962b)
	Mycobacterium tuberculosis	75	KHOMUTOV *et al.* (1962)
	Streptococcus faecalis	no activity	NEUHAUS and LYNCH (1964)
(XLV) 3-Iminoisoxazoli-dine	"Useful antibac-terial properties against Mycobacteria"		POHLAND (1956)
(XLVI) 2-Phenyl-5-benzyliden-1-imidazolin-3-ol-4-one	Gram-positive and gram-nega-tive bacteria	10—50	KOCHETKOV *et al.* (1959)
(XLVII) α-Benzamido-β-(*p*-dimethylaminophe-nyl) acrylic acid hydrazide[1]	*Mycobacterium tuberculosis*	25—28	BREGER (1961)

[1] In addition to this hydrazide, the susceptibility results of eight other hydrazides are presented (BREGER, 1961).

1. Analogs with substituents in the C-5 position show a decrease in the antibacterial activity. For example, *cis*-5-methyl (XXXIV) and *trans*-5-methyl (XXXV) substitution decreases the activity. In the case of *Str. faecalis* and *E. coli*, the *cis*-isomer is more effective than the *trans*-isomer. The introduction of a *trans*-5-isopropyl group (XXXVI) abolishes the activity.

2. Analogs in which the amino group is alkylated (XXIII, XXIV, XXVI) or acylated (XXII, XXV) are inactive. If the amino group is omitted (XV) or substituted by a 4-methoxy (XII) or 4-hydroxy group (XIII), there is no antibacterial activity. The only exception to this is 4-aminoxy-3-isoxazolidone (XIV). A change in the configuration at the α-carbon results in an effective antibacterial agent (XVI) in the case of several bacteria (see "L-cycloserine"). However, the mode of action is different from that for D-cycloserine.

3. Substitution in the heterocyclic ring results in a decrease of the antibacterial activity. For example, azacycloserine (XVII) is only 10% as active as D-cycloserine when tested with *M. tuberculosis*. In addition, the introduction of a methylene group (XIX) in the heterocyclic ring reduces the activity to 10% of that observed with D-cycloserine.

4. Ring-cleavage results in a decrease of the antibacterial activity. For example, β-aminoxy-D-alanine (XXXVII) has only 25% of the activity observed with D-cycloserine when tested against *M. tuberculosis*. If the amino group of the β-aminoxy-D-alanine is omitted (XL), the antibacterial activity is abolished. Cleavage between positions 4 and 5 (XLIII) also abolishes the activity.

Thus, for antibacterial activity, a free amino group is required. Substitution in the 5-position, substitution in the ring, or cleavage of the ring decreases the activity. It is unfortunate that each of these derivatives has not been tested for reversal by D-alanine. It is possible that some of the compounds could have a site of action different from that observed for D-cycloserine. For example, the mode of action of L-cycloserine has been established to be different from that observed for D-cycloserine.

The antibacterial activity of the Schiff bases (XXVIII, XXX, XXXI, and XXXII) is probably the result of hydrolysis to D-cycloserine.

"Protoplast" (Spheroplast) Formation

Growth in the presence of D-cycloserine and 0.32 M sucrose results in "protoplast" (spheroplast) formation (CIAK and HAHN, 1959). BUOGO *et al.* (1958) observed that the formation of "protoplasts" from *E. coli* occurred only in the presence of D-cycloserine. For example, in the presence of 50 μg/ml of either D-, L-, or DL-cycloserine, 62, 0, and 85% of the cells were converted to "protoplasts," respectively. Only D- and DL-alanine were found to inhibit "protoplast" formation. In *Alcaligenes faecalis* spheroplast induction occurs after a lag of 2—3 minutes when the D-cycloserine concentration is 400 μg/ml (LARK and SCHICHTEL, 1962). The formation of spheroplasts is inhibited if the D-cycloserine treated cells are diluted into growth medium that contains 0.02 M D-alanine. The formation of spheroplasts from *Proteus mirabilis* can also be induced by D-cycloserine (PLAPP and KANDLER, 1965). Protoplast formation in the presence of D-cycloserine is dependent on growing cells (CIAK and HAHN, 1959). Omission of sources of nitrogen or carbon abolish the action of D-cycloserine.

The growth of protoplasts from *Str. faecalis* is not affected by the presence of D-cycloserine (2000 μg/ml). In contrast, the minimal inhibitory concentration for intact *Str. faecalis* is 25 μg/ml (SHOCKMAN and LAMPEN, 1962). HANCOCK and FITZ-JAMES (1964) confirmed these observations in *B. megaterium*. Thus, these results reinforce the conclusion that D-cycloserine is a specific inhibitor of peptidoglycan (mucopeptide) formation (PARK, 1960) (see "Inhibition of peptidoglycan synthesis and accumulation of nucleotides by D-cycloserine").

The spheroplasts formed in the presence of D-cycloserine appear to be different from those formed in the presence of lysozyme (MALAMY and HORECKER, 1964). In the latter case 93% of the alkaline phosphatase was readily released while in the former only 18% was released to the medium. The D-cycloserine spheroplasts contain existing wall structure which prevents the release of the phosphatase.

In an *Erwinia* species, D-cycloserine not only inhibits growth, but at levels which allow some growth, it inhibits cell division. The elongated cells show thickening and swelling. Although low levels of D-alanine overcome the growth inhibition, a 330-fold higher concentration is required to overcome completely the inhibition of division. With this bacterium, L-alanine was almost as effective as D-alanine in reversing the effects of D-cycloserine (GRULA and GRULA, 1965). With *E. coli* the sequence of protoplast formation, vacuolization, and lysis was identical to that observed with penicillin (CIAK and HAHN, 1959; HAHN and CIAK, 1957).

D-Cycloserine is a poor inducer of the L-phase of *Streptobacillus moniliformis*. However, the action of the combination of D-cycloserine and glycine or DL-serine is equal to that obtained with penicillin and the same amino acids (MICHEL and HIJMANS, 1960). Propagation of L-phase organisms was accomplished in the presence of 1% glycine and within a narrow range of D-cycloserine.

Inhibition of Peptidoglycan Synthesis and Accumulation of Nucleotides by D-Cycloserine

PARK (1958b) and CIAK and HAHN (1959) observed a marked accumulation of UDP-NAc-amino sugar when either *S. aureus* or *E. coli* were grown in the presence of D-cycloserine. A direct relationship between the accumulation of UDP-NAc-amino sugar and the inhibition of peptidoglycan synthesis was established by PARK (1958b, 1960) (Table 3). The synthesis of protein is not affected by either D-cycloserine or penicillin. When a species of *Erwinia* is grown in the presence of D-cycloserine, the peptidoglycan content as measured by glucosamine and muramic acid is 40% below that of normal cells (GRULA and GRULA, 1964). In addition to the inhibition of peptidoglycan synthesis, ROGERS and GARRETT (1965) observed that D-cycloserine (100 μg/ml) also inhibits the synthesis of teichoic acid by 78%. Peptidoglycan formation under these conditions was inhibited 78%. In contrast to the results with D-cycloserine, growth of *S. aureus* in the presence of L-cycloserine does not result in the accumulation of UDP-NAc-amino sugar (CIAK and HAHN, 1959). In *E. coli*, BARBIERI *et al.* (1960) demonstrated that D-cycloserine inhibits the incorporation of DL-alanine-1-[^{14}C] into the cell wall and to a lesser extent into the protein fraction.

The structure of the UDP-NAc-amino sugar which accumulates in the presence of D-cycloserine was elucidated by STROMINGER, THRENN, and SCOTT (1959) and found to be:

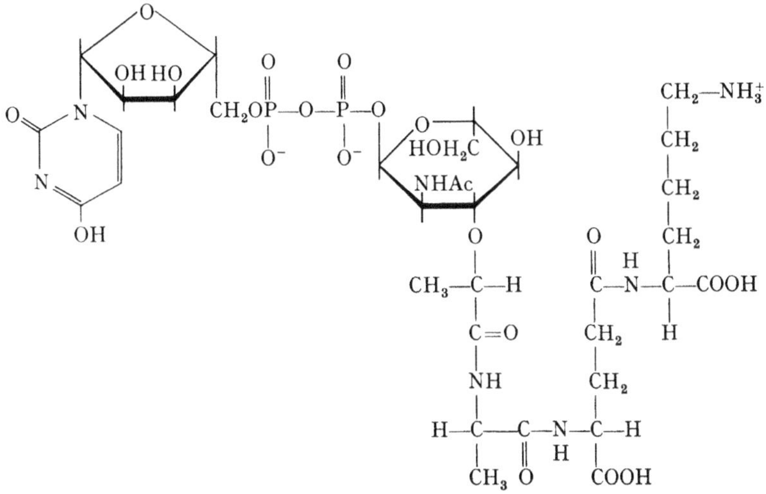

(XLVIII) UDP-NAc-muramyl-L-ala-D-glu-L-lys

In *S. aureus*, the accumulation of this nucleotide was reversed by the addition of D-alanine to the medium. L-Alanine, DL-alanyl-DL-alanine, and D-serine at high concentrations were not effective (STROMINGER, THRENN, and SCOTT, 1959). LYNCH and NEUHAUS[1] observed that high concentrations (6×10^{-3} M) of D-ala-

[1] LYNCH and NEUHAUS: unpublished observation.

Table 3. *Correlation of inhibition of mucopeptide synthesis with accumulation of precursors (UDPX)*[1]

Inhibitor	μg/ml	UDPX formed[2] μmole/g	Lysine incorporation	
			Mucopeptide[2] μmole/g	Protein[2] μmole/g
None		5	25.0	3.2
Penicillin	5	40	5.7	3.7
D-Cycloserine	100	29	9.0	2.9
Chlortetracycline	10	5	25.0	0.5

[1] Park (1961).

[2] Mucopeptide (peptidoglycan), UDP-NAc-amino sugar, and protein were determined by the method of Park and Hancock (1960).

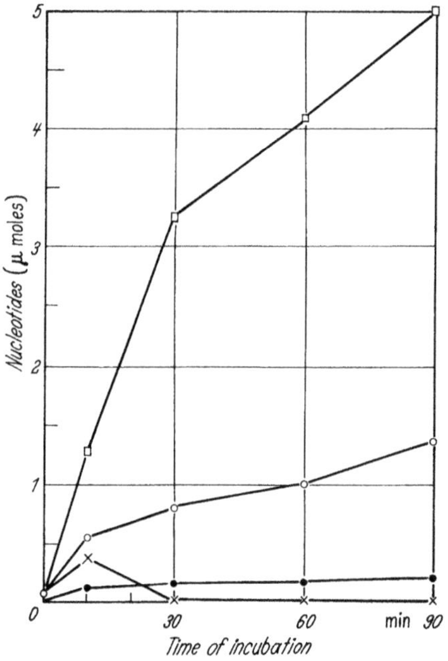

Fig. 2. Time course of accumulation of UDP-N-acetylamino sugar derivatives in cells grown in nutrient broth after the addition of D-cycloserine. D-Cycloserine (2×10^{-3} M) was added to the culture in nutrient broth at the point of half-maximum cell-growth. ×—× UDP-NAc-glucosamine; ○—○ UDP-NAc-muramic acid; ●—● UDP-NAc-muramyl-L-ala; □—□ UDP-NAc-muramyl-L-ala-D-glu-L-lys (Ito and Saito, 1963)

D-ala were effective in reversing the nucleotide accumulation induced by D-cycloserine (3×10^{-4} M) in *S. aureus* Copenhagen. This observation is consistent with the reversal of the growth inhibition by D-ala-D-ala (see "D-Alanine: D-cycloserine antagonism").

The kinetics of UDP-NAc-muramyl-L-ala-D-glu-L-lys accumulation were examined in cultures of *S. aureus* 209 P by Ito and Saito (1963) (Fig. 2). The UDP-NAc-muramyl-L-ala-D-glu-L-lys rapidly accumulated during the 90 minute incubation. To a lesser extent UDP-NAc-muramic acid and UDP-NAc-muramyl-L-ala accumulated. Wishnow *et al.* (1965) also observed that UDP-NAc-muramic acid and UDP-NAc-muramyl-L-ala accumulated when cells of *S. aureus* Copenhagen were grown in the presence of D-cycloserine. When *S. aureus* 209 P was grown in the presence of penicillin, the accumulation of UDP-NAc-muramyl-L-ala-D-glu-L-lys (0.9 μmole per 26 liters) is minor in comparison with UDP-NAc-muramyl-L-ala-D-glu-L-lys-D-ala-D-ala (28.8 μmoles per 26 liters) (Saito, Ishimoto, and Ito, 1963). With *P. mirabilis*, growth in the presence of D-cycloserine resulted in the accumulation of UDP-NAc-muramyl-L-ala-D-glu-mesodiaminopimelic acid (Plapp and Kandler, 1965). The composition of this intermediate reflects the substitution of diaminopimelic acid for L-lysine in the peptidoglycan fraction. In contrast to penicillin, D-cycloserine does not cause the accumulation of CDP-ribitol, a precursor of teichoic acid (SAUKKONEN and VIRKOLA, 1963). In mutants of *E. coli* which are resistant to D-cycloserine there is no accumulation of UDP-NAc-muramyl-L-ala-D-glu-mesodiaminopimelic[1].

D-Cycloserine: Specific Enzyme Effects

Since the accumulation of UDP-NAc-muramyl-L-ala-D-glu-L-lys in the presence of D-cycloserine is reversed by D-alanine, enzymes utilizing D-alanine were examined by STROMINGER and co-workers for inhibition by D-cycloserine. It was observed that the alanine racemase is competitively inhibited by D-cycloserine. Since L-alanine was not effective in the reversal of the D-cycloserine induced accumulation of nucleotide, a second site of action was considered. In addition to the racemase, the D-ala-D-ala synthetase was found to be competitively inhibited by the antibiotic (STORMINGER, ITO, and THRENN, 1960). During the course of this work, the action of D-cycloserine on various transaminases has been extensively investigated. For example, the D-alanine-D-glutamic acid transaminase is effectively inhibited by the antibiotic (PASKHINA, 1964; MARTINEZ-CARRION and JENKINS, 1965). It is difficult, however, to correlate this site with the accumulation of UDP-NAc-muramyl-tripeptide and its reversal by D-alanine.

Inhibition of Alanine Racemase

Alanine racemase occupies a key position in the incorporation of D-alanine from L-alanine into the cell wall precursor UDP-NAc-muramyl-L-ala-D-glu-L-lys-D-ala-D-ala (see "Introduction"). This enzyme was discovered and purified by WOOD and GUNSALUS (1951) and observed to require pyridoxal phosphate as a coenzyme. The racemase is specific for alanine. As shown in Fig. 3, D-cycloserine is an effective competitive inhibitor of the reaction catalyzed by the racemase (STROMINGER, ITO, and THRENN, 1960). The K_i for D-cycloserine is 6×10^{-5} M, and the K_m for D-alanine and L-alanine is 6.1×10^{-3} M and 6.5×10^{-3} M, respectively (cf. LYNCH and NEUHAUS, 1966).

Table 4. *Inhibition of alanine racemase*[2]

Inhibitor	K_i mM	Type of inhibition
NH_2OH	0.012	Competitive
NH_2NH_2	0.10	Competitive
KCN	>10	No inhibition
Semicarbazide	>10	No inhibition
β-Aminoxy-D-alanine	0.04	Competitive
D-Cycloserine	0.05	Competitive
L-Cycloserine	≫10	No inhibition

[2] ROZE and STROMINGER (1965).

ROZE and STROMINGER (1966) have established an inhibitor profile for alanine racemase (Table 4). Of the compounds tested, only hydroxylamine, hydrazine, β-aminoxy-D-alanine, and D-cycloserine inhibit the enzyme. In addition, LYNCH

[1] BROCKMAN, R. W.: personal communication.

and NEUHAUS (1966) observed that O-carbamyl-D-serine is an effective inhibitor of the racemase (see Table 10). Both L-cycloserine and O-carbamyl-L-serine are not effective inhibitors of the racemase. Unfortunately most of the analogs of D-cycloserine presented in Table 2 have not been tested in the reaction catalyzed by the racemase. Although the experiments have not been performed, it is reasonable to assume that D-cycloserine reacts with the enzyme bound pyridoxal phosphate to form a Schiff base. Secondary reactions may then occur which would result in the irreversible inhibition of the enzyme. This proposal is based on the results observed with the transaminases (see "Action of cycloserine on transaminases"). ROZE and STROMINGER (1966) proposed that D-alanine and L-alanine have the same conformation on the enzyme surface, and that this conformation is the one present in D-cycloserine.

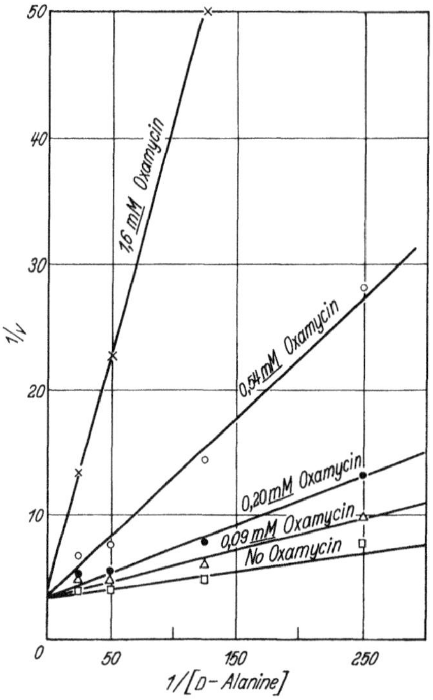

Fig. 3. Competitive inhibition of alanine racemase by D-cycloserine (oxamycin) (STROMINGER, ITO, and THRENN, 1960)

Inhibition of D-ala-D-ala Synthetase

The biosynthesis of D-ala-D-ala is catalyzed by the enzyme D-ala-D-ala synthetase (STROMINGER, 1962; NEUHAUS, 1962), as shown in the reaction:

$$2\ \text{D-alanine} + \text{ATP} \xrightarrow[K^+]{Mg^{2+}} \text{D-ala-D-ala} + \text{ADP} + P_i.$$

This enzyme has been observed in *Str. faecalis* (NEUHAUS, 1962a), *E. coli* (COMB, 1962), and *S. aureus* (ITO and STROMINGER, 1962b). STROMINGER, ITO, and THRENN (1960) observed that D-cycloserine competitively inhibited the synthetase (K_i for D-cycloserine $= 2$—4×10^{-5} M, K_m for D-alanine $= 3$—5×10^{-3} M). The experiments with *S. aureus* were performed with Mn^{2+} while those with *Str. faecalis* were performed with Mg^{2+}.

Specificity studies with analogs of D-cycloserine revealed a high specificity for the antibiotic (NEUHAUS and LYNCH, 1964) (Table 5). The only compounds that were effective at low concentrations were *cis*- (XXXIV) and *trans*-DL-cyclothreonine (XXXV) and β-aminoxy-D-alanine methylester (XXXIX). The inhibition by β-aminoxy-D-alanine methylester was complicated by the cyclization reaction, i.e., the formation of cycloserine via a dimer derivative. 3-Isoxazolidone (XV) and 3-iminoisoxazolidine (XLV) have no apparent inhibitory activity. Analogs of D-cycloserine that have the isoxazolidone ring cleaved (D-serine amide, D-serine methylester, β-aminoxy-D-alanine, and D-serine) have little or no inhibitory activity. In contrast to the results with the transaminases (KARPEISKII

Table 5. *Inhibition of D-ala-D-ala synthetase*[1]

Compound	Inhibition K_i moles/liter	%
D-Cycloserine	0.9×10^{-4}	
cis-DL-Cyclothreonine	1.2×10^{-4} [2]	
trans-DL-Cyclothreonine	4.8×10^{-4} [2]	
β-Aminoxy-D-alanine methyl ester	3.1×10^{-4}	
trans-5-Isopropyl-DL-cycloserine (0.0025 M D-)		0
DL-Serine amide (0.02 M D-)		28
D-Serine methyl ester (0.02 M)		16
D-Serine (0.02 M)		3
3-Isoxazolidone (0.02 M)	(stimulation)	+12
3-Iminoisoxazolidine (0.02 M)		0
β-Aminoxy-propionic acid (0.02 M)		29
L-Cycloserine (0.001 M)		0
β-Aminoxy-D-alanine (0.02 M)		0
3,6-(Diaminoxymethyl)-2,5-diketopiperazine (0.02 M)		0

[1] NEUHAUS and LYNCH (1964).
[2] Molarity on the basis of the D-isomer.

et al., 1963b; BRAUNSTEIN *et al.*, 1961; POLYANOVSKII and TORCHINSKII, 1961; VYSHEPAN *et al.*, 1961), the inhibition is instantaneous and completely reversible.

Kinetic and specificity studies on the D-ala-D-ala synthetase from *Str. faecalis* provided evidence for two D-alanine binding sites which have different specificity patterns and Michaelis constants (NEUHAUS, 1962a, b). The sites are characterized by the following equilibria:

$$\mathrm{E} + \mathrm{A} \rightleftharpoons \mathrm{EA}\ (K_A) \qquad (1)$$
$$\mathrm{EA} + \mathrm{A} \rightleftharpoons \mathrm{EAA}\ (K_{AA}) \qquad (2)$$

where EA and EAA are binary and ternary complexes of enzyme (E) and D-alanine (A), respectively. These reactions are characterized by their respective Michaelis constants, K_A (6.6×10^{-4} M) and K_{AA} (0.01 M).

Inhibitor studies with D-cycloserine (NEUHAUS and LYNCH, 1964) are consistent with the following series of equilibria:

$$\mathrm{E} + \mathrm{I} \rightleftharpoons \mathrm{EI}\ (K_I) \qquad (3)$$
$$\mathrm{EA} + \mathrm{I} \rightleftharpoons \mathrm{EAI}\ (K_{AI}) \qquad (4)$$
$$\mathrm{EI} + \mathrm{I} \rightleftharpoons \mathrm{EII}\ (K_{II}) \qquad (5)$$
$$\mathrm{EI} + \mathrm{A} \rightleftharpoons \mathrm{EIA}\ (K_{IA}) \qquad (6)$$

On the basis of these reactions and those described above (1 and 2), the following rearranged reciprocal equation was obtained by an equilibrium derivation:

$$[A]\left[\frac{1}{v} - \frac{1}{V_{\max}}\right] = \frac{K_{AA}}{V_{\max}}\left[1 + \frac{K_A[I]}{K_I K_{IA}} + \frac{[I]}{K_{AI}}\right] + \frac{K_A K_{AA}}{[A]V_{\max}}\left[1 + \frac{[I]}{K_I} + \frac{[I]^2}{K_I K_{II}}\right].$$

If $[I]=0$, then K_A and K_{AA} can be established (Fig. 4). From the secondary plots of slope and intercept the values for K_I and K_{AI} have been established (assumes $K_{IA}=K_{AA}$). These results are summarized in Table 6. In addition, the results for *cis*- and *trans*-D-cyclothreonine are presented. On the basis of these studies it is concluded that both sites bind D-cycloserine and that the donor site (N-terminal) has a higher affinity for D-cycloserine than the acceptor site (C-terminal) (see Discussion, NEUHAUS and LYNCH, 1964).

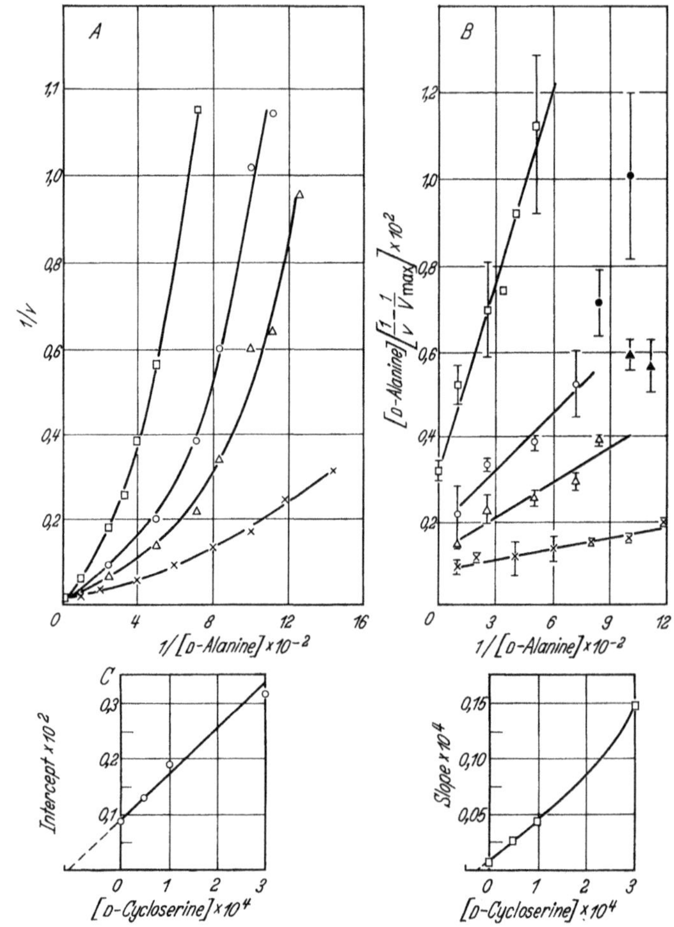

Fig. 4. Analysis of D-cycloserine inhibition. The concentrations are: ×—× 0; △—△ 5×10^{-5} M; ○—○ 1×10^{-4} M; and □—□ 3×10^{-4} M. The Lineweaver-Burk plots (A) and rearranged plots (B) are presented. In C the secondary plots for the evaluation of K_I and K_{AI} are presented (NEUHAUS and LYNCH, 1964)

Table 6. *Summary of inhibitor constants*[1]

Compound	K_I moles/liter	K_{AI} moles/liter	m.i.c.[2] moles/liter
D-Cycloserine	2.2×10^{-5}	1.4×10^{-4}	1.5—2×10^{-4}
cis-DL-Cyclothreonine[3]	1.2×10^{-4}	1.9×10^{-4}	5—6×10^{-4}
trans-DL-Cyclothreonine[3]	5.4×10^{-4}	5.6×10^{-4}	30—40×10^{-4}

[1] NEUHAUS and LYNCH (1964).
[2] Minimal inhibitory concentration.
[3] Molarity on the basis of the D-isomer.

STROMINGER (1962) has proposed that the substrate on the enzyme surface has the conformation of D-cycloserine. The molecular models of D-alanine and D-cycloserine are compared in Fig. 5. Experimental support for this proposal has been found in an independent series of experiments (NEUHAUS and LYNCH, 1964).

If D-alanine and a related amino acid are incubated with the synthetase, a mixed dipeptide can be isolated in addition to D-ala-D-ala, i.e.,

$$\text{ATP} + \text{D-alanine} + \text{D-threonine} \rightarrow \text{D-ala-D-thr} + \text{ADP} + P_i.$$

Substitution of D-allothreonine for D-threonine in the above reaction mixture results in a higher rate of mixed dipeptide formation, i.e., D-allothreonine is a better acceptor than D-threonine. In the hydrophobic environment of the binding site, it is suggested that an intramolecular hydrogen bond between the hydrogen

Oxamycin (D-cycloserine) D-alanine

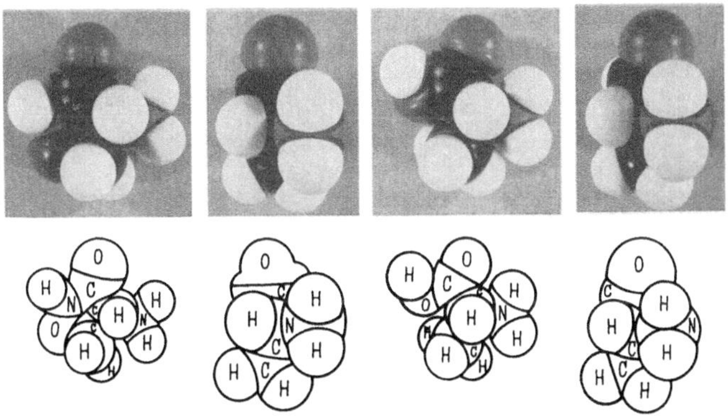

Fig. 5. Molecular models of D-alanine and D-cycloserine (STROMINGER, 1962). In each case on the left, the models are viewed looking down on the hydrogen on the asymmetric carbon atom. On the right, the models are viewed looking at the amino group on this carbon atom. In the latter view the two structures appear to be identical

of the hydroxyl and the carboxyl group stabilizes the amino acid in a single conformation. This is illustrated in Fig. 6. If one compares the fixed conformations of the *cis*-cyclothreonine and the *trans*-cyclothreonine with the conformations of D-allothreonine and D-threonine, there is a striking correlation between *cis*-cyclothreonine and D-allothreonine and between *trans*-cyclothreonine and D-threonine. In the former case a fixed planar conformation exists while in the latter a fixed folded conformation exists. Thus, there is a correlation between the effectiveness of *cis*-D-cyclothreonine as an inhibitor and D-allothreonine as an acceptor and between *trans*-D-cyclothreonine and D-threonine. This correlation lends support to the hypothesis that the substrate on the enzyme surface has a conformation similar (or identical) to that of D-cycloserine. The ratio of K_A/K_I is 30 and the ratio of K_{AA}/K_{AI} is 72. STROMINGER observed a K_m/K_i of 100. These ratios may be interpreted to mean that the effective substrate concentration is equal to the concentration of alanine which has the conformation of D-cycloserine. Additional support for this interpretation is given by the high value for K_i (0.019 M) observed for β-aminoxy-D-alanine. The major difference between this analog and D-cycloserine is the fixed conformation.

In the case of 5-methyl substitution, a good correlation exists between the enzyme-specificity data and the growth inhibitor studies (Table 6). If the primary site of antibiotic action were the acceptor site of the synthetase, one might predict that *cis*-D-cyclothreonine and D-cycloserine would have the same inhibitory activity in bacterial growth experiments. It was observed, however, that a 4-fold greater concentration of *cis*-D-cyclothreonine than D-cycloserine was required to observe lysis. Since these results correlate with the specificity of the donor site rather than the acceptor site, it is proposed that the donor site may be a primary site of antibiotic action.

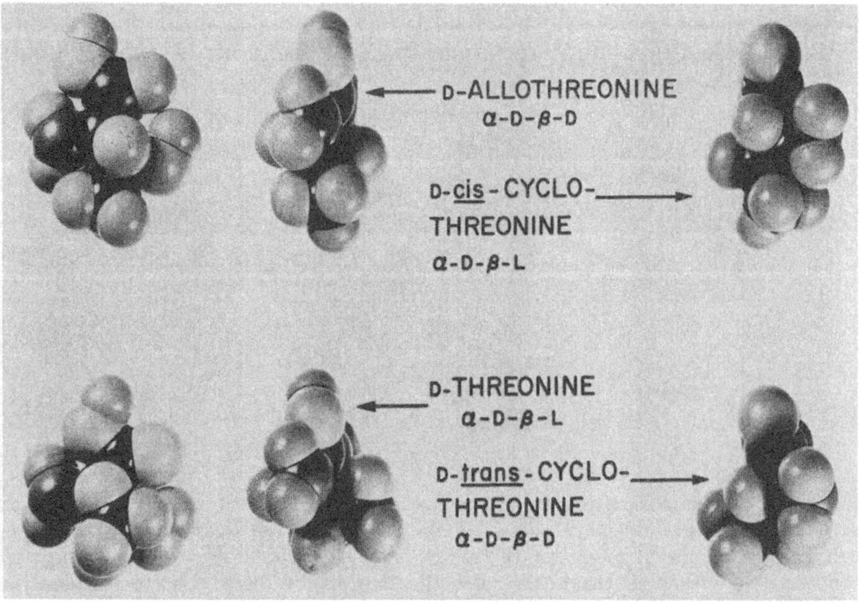

Fig. 6. Molecular models for the comparison of D-allothreonine with *cis*-D-cyclothreonine and D-threonine with *trans*-D-cyclothreonine (NEUHAUS and LYNCH, 1964)

D-Cycloserine and the Permeability of D-Alanine

MORA and SNELL (1963) observed that D-cycloserine inhibits the permease in *Str. faecalis* that is responsible for the transport of L-alanine-^{14}C and D-alanine-^{14}C. The values for K_i of D-cycloserine are 1×10^{-5} M with D-alanine and 1.4×10^{-5} M with L-alanine. L-Cycloserine has no effect at concentrations similar to those of D-cycloserine. Additional experiments with spheroplasts indicated that the permease is associated with the membrane. MORA and BOJALIL (1965) eliminated the permease as a major site of D-cycloserine action in *M. acapulcensis*. Since the antibiotic inhibits in a minimal medium, it was concluded that D-cycloserine must compete with the formation or utilization of D-alanine inside the cell. In *S. aureus* Copenhagen, the permeability of ^{14}C-alanine was not affected by 10^{-3} M D-cycloserine when tested at 10^{-4} M, 10^{-5} M, and 10^{-6} M alanine (STROMINGER, ITO, and THRENN, 1960).

Action of Cycloserine on Transaminases

One of the first sites of action of D-cycloserine that was discovered was the inhibition of the transamination reaction. AOKI (1957) and ITO *et al.* (1958) observed that D-cycloserine (10^{-3} M) inhibited the L-glutamic-L-aspartic transaminase in extracts of *E. coli* K-12 and tubercle bacilli. In addition to this transaminase the L-glutamic-L-alanine transaminase (VYSHEPAN, IVANOVA, and CHERNUKH, 1959; ALIOTO, 1962), the L-glutamic-L-asparagine transaminase (AZARKH *et al.*, 1960; BRAUNSTEIN, AZARKH, and SYUI, 1961), the L-glutamic-γ-aminobutyric acid transaminase (DANN and CARTER, 1964), and D-glutamic-D-alanine transaminase (PASKHINA, 1964; MARTINEZ-CARRION and JENKINS, 1965) are effectively inhibited by either D- or L-cycloserine.

Table 7. *Inhibition of the glutamic-aspartic transaminase by derivatives of hydroxylamine and isoxazolidone-3*[1]

No.	Compound	I_{50} at 5 min of preincubation at pH 5.8 moles/liter
	Hydroxylamine	1.5×10^{-6}
	O-Methylhydroxylamine	1×10^{-6}
(XXXVII)	β-Aminoxy-D-alanine	4×10^{-5}
(XLIV)	3,6-(Diaminoxymethyl)-2,5-diketopiperazine	5×10^{-6}
	α-Aminobutyrolactone	$\gg5\times10^{-3}$
(I)	DL-Cycloserine	1.5×10^{-4}
(XV)	3-Isoxazolidone	3×10^{-4}
(XXIII)	N-Methylcycloserine	5×10^{-3}
(XXXIV)	Cyclothreonine[2]	1×10^{-3} 43% inhibition
(XIX)	Cyclocanaline	6.5×10^{-5}
(XIV)	4-Aminoxy-3-isoxazolidone	6.0×10^{-7}

[1] KARPEISKII *et al.* (1963a).
[2] *cis*- or *trans*-isomer not specified.

With purified L-glutamic-L-aspartic transaminase (2.6.1.1) from human brain, BONAVITA (1959) observed that D-cycloserine inhibits the enzyme with a K_i of approximately 5×10^{-5} M. It was suggested that a reaction between D-cycloserine and pyridoxal phosphate was probable. The specificity of inhibition of a highly purified L-glutamic-L-aspartic transaminase from heart is described in Table 7 (KARPEISKII *et al.*, 1963a). The most effective inhibitor is 4-aminoxy-3-isoxazolidone (XIV). DL-Cycloserine is a poor inhibitor when compared with the dimerization product, 3,6-(diaminoxymethyl)-2,5-diketopiperazine (XLIV).

The inhibition of the L-glutamic-L-alanine transaminase (2.6.1.2) by L-cycloserine has been studied in detail. VYSHEPAN *et al.* (1959, 1961) showed that 2×10^{-5} M DL-cycloserine inhibits the transaminase from rat liver. In addition, the following compounds are inhibitors at 10^{-3} M: β-aminoxy-D-alanine ethyl ester (XXXVIII), β-aminoxy-D-alanine (XXXVII), ethyl γ-aminoxy-butyrate, N-methyl cycloserine (XXIII), and 3-isoxazolidone (XV). BRAUNSTEIN, AZARKH, and SYUI (1961) established the inhibitor constants for D- and L-cycloserine. The K_i for L-cycloserine is 8.0×10^{-6} M while the K_i for D-cycloserine is $\cong10^{-3}$ M.

The L-glutamic-L-asparagine transaminase (2.6.1.14) is very sensitive to the action of L-cycloserine (BRAUNSTEIN, AZARKH, and SYUI, 1961). The K_i for the L-isomer is 5×10^{-7} M while the K_i for the D-isomer is 3×10^{-3} M. BRAUNSTEIN (1962) proposed that the conformation of L-asparagine on the enzyme surface is similar to that of L-cycloserine. An intramolecular hydrogen bond would serve to give a conformation similar to L-cycloserine, i.e.,

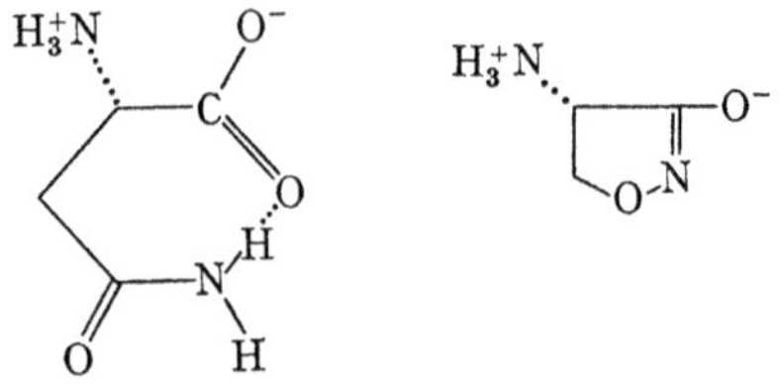

It should be noted that L-cycloserine is a more effective inhibitor of growth in *E. coli* when L-asparagine is the carbon source than when either pyruvate or glucose is the carbon source (TRIVELLATO, 1958).

The D-glutamic-D-alanine transaminase is inhibited by very low concentrations of D-cycloserine (PASKHINA, 1964; MARTINEZ-CARRION and JENKINS, 1965). The K_i for D-cycloserine is 1—5×10^{-7} M, and for L-cycloserine it is 1—5×10^{-4} M (PASKHINA, 1964). MARTINEZ-CARRION and JENKINS (1965) observed that 2.5×10^{-8} M D-cycloserine inhibited the activity 50% while 1×10^{-6} M L-cycloserine inhibited the activity 50%.

BRAUNSTEIN proposed two categories of sensitivity in the inhibition of transaminases by cycloserine (AZARKH *et al.*, 1960). They are:

1. High sensitivity systems: K_i from 5×10^{-7} M to 10^{-5} M. Examples: L-cycloserine and L-glutamic-L-alanine transaminase; L-cycloserine and L-glutamic-L-asparagine transaminase; D-cycloserine and D-alanine-D-glutamic acid transaminase.

2. Low sensitivity systems: K_i around 10^{-3} M. Examples: L-cycloserine and L-glutamic-L-aspartic transaminase; D-cycloserine and L-glutamic-L-alanine transaminase.

The latter category (2) comprises those situations in which there is *nonspecific* binding followed by Schiff base formation with pyridoxal phosphate (see "Reaction with pyridoxal"). The high sensitivity category comprises those cases in which there is *specific* binding followed by Schiff base formation with pyridoxal phosphate.

Incubation of the D-alanine-D-glutamic acid transaminase with 0.1 mM D-cycloserine results in the appearance of a new absorption band at 335 mμ and a small shoulder at 410 mμ associated with the disappearance of the 415 mμ band (MARTINEZ-CARRION and JENKINS, 1965). The interaction of cycloserine at pH 4.5 with the pyridoxylidene form of the L-glutamic-L-aspartic transaminase results in a shift of the absorption maximum from 430 mμ to 335 mμ (KARPEISKII *et al.*, 1963). In addition, a small maximum or a shoulder appears at 380 mμ. The results with the transaminases are similar to the reaction of pyridoxal phosphate and cycloserine to form the Schiff base in alcoholic medium (see "Reaction with pyridoxal").

The inhibition by D-cycloserine of the transaminases increases with time of incubation and requires a preincubation period for maximum effect. Although the inhibition is competitive with respect to L-alanine in the case of the L-glutamic-L-alanine transaminase, it is reactivated to only a slight extent by dialysis or passage over Sephadex G-50 (BRAUNSTEIN *et al.*, 1961). These results are explained on the basis of a biphasic inhibition. The first is reversible and involves the formation of a Schiff base (VI). The second, which is irreversible, involves the acylation of a reactive nucleophile (e.g., the ε-amino group of lysine) in or near the active site to form XLIX (cf. with VII). This is followed by a rearrangement with the formation of an oxime (L).

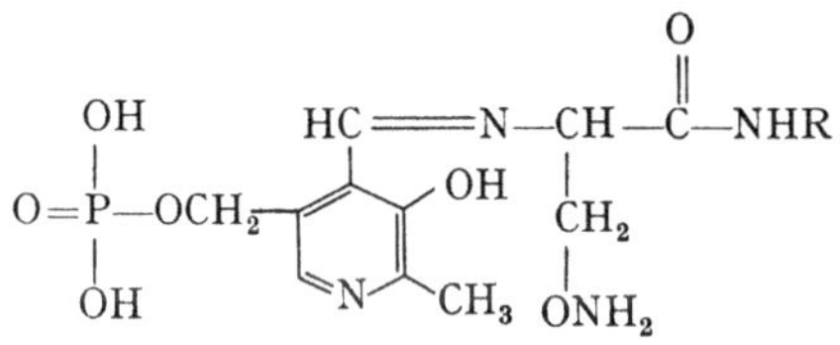

(XLIX, RNH_2=lysine)

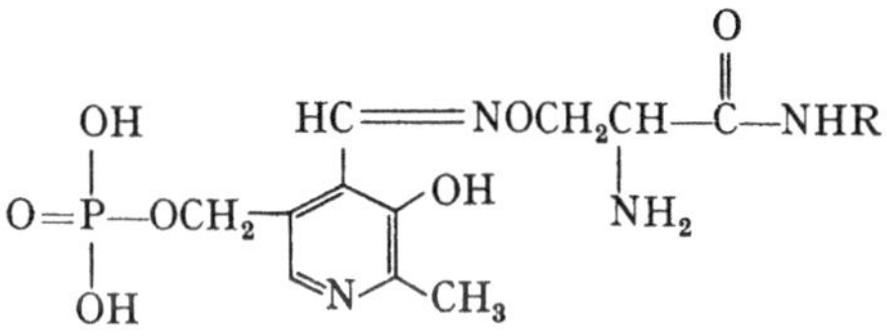

(L)

KARPEISKII and BREUSSOV (1965) treated the L-cycloserine inhibited L-glutamic-L-aspartic transaminase with acid in an ammonium sulfate solution. The cycloserine-pyridoxal phosphate compound was released under conditions in which no denaturation of the apo-enzyme occurred. The structure of this compound was assumed to be LI since $NaBH_4$ treatment of the EI complex followed by acid hydrolysis released α-N-pyridoxyl-β-aminoxyalanine (LII). The formation of oxime (L) in the second stage is a slow reaction and is associated with the absorption at 380 mμ (KARPEISKII *et al.*, 1963).

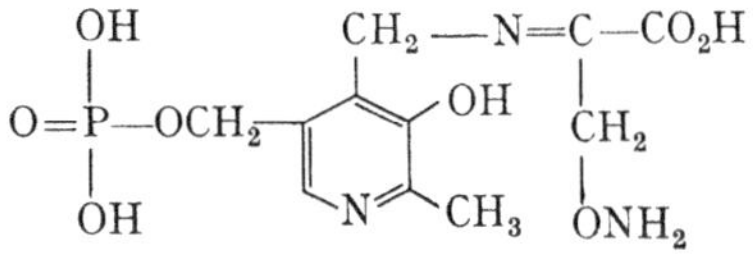

(LI)

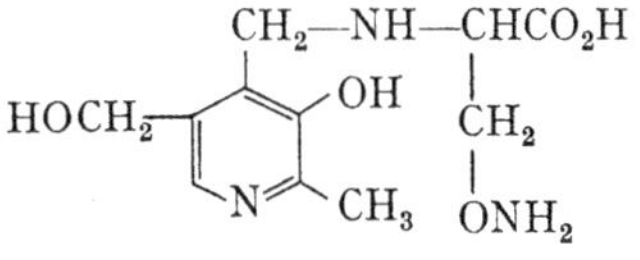

(LII)

The administration of cycloserine to rats and guinea pigs resulted in a marked increase of the γ-aminobutyric acid concentration. DANN and CARTER (1964) observed that DL-cycloserine inhibited the transamination of γ-aminobutyric acid in the following reaction:

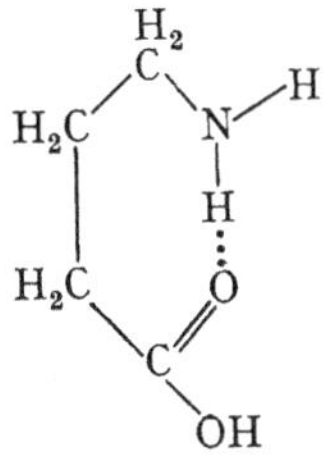

+ α-ketoglutaric acid ⇌ glutamic acid + succinic semialdehyde

The inhibition was characterized by two phases: (1) a rapid, reversible, and competitive stage; (2) followed by a slow, progressive, and irreversible stage. In the initial stage γ-aminobutyric acid reversed the inhibition. The brain transaminase exhibits a K_i of 2.3×10^{-4} M for DL-cycloserine and a K_m of 4.5×10^{-4} M for γ-aminobutyric acid.

Inhibition of Decarboxylases

In addition to the transaminases, the decarboxylation of several amino acids has been shown to be inhibited by cycloserine. For example, glutamic acid decarboxylase (4.1. 1.15) from *E. coli* is inhibited approximately 50% by 10^{-3} M cycloserine (YAMADA, SAWAKI, and HAYAMI, 1957; ITO *et al.*, 1958). PIETRA *et al.* (1963) showed that the treatment of rats with D-cycloserine (500 mg/kg) gave a 66% inhibition of the glutamic acid decarboxylase. In *in vitro* experiments 5×10^{-4} M D-cycloserine gave a 53% inhibition.

The decarboxylation of 3,4-dihydroxyphenylalanine by L-DOPA decarboxylase (4.1. 1.26) is inhibited by L- and D-cycloserine with a K_i of 5.9 and 6.1×10^{-3} M, respectively (DENGLER, 1962). With *cis*- (XXXIV) and *trans*-DL-cyclothreonine (XXXV) the values for K_i are 1.6 and 3.4×10^{-2} M, respectively. The most effective inhibitor is 3,6-(diaminoxymethyl)-2,5-diketopiperazine (XLIV) ($K_i = 2.4 \times 10^{-4}$ M).

On the Mode of Action

The inhibition of alanine racemase and D-ala-D-ala synthetase deprives the bacterium of the D-ala-D-ala necessary for the biosynthesis of the complete wall precursor UDP-NAc-muramyl-L-ala-D-glu-L-lys-D-ala-D-ala. This results in the accumulation of UDP-NAc-muramyl-L-ala-D-glu-L-lys and the inhibition of peptidoglycan synthesis. In growing cells, osmotic fragility results when peptidoglycan synthesis is inhibited. Thus, in many bacteria D-cycloserine at low concentrations is bactericidal. In others, osmotic fragility does not appear to be a major factor even though peptidoglycan synthesis is inhibited. In *E. coli*, D-cycloserine is bactericidal at low concentrations and bacteriostatic at high concentrations (CURTISS *et al.*, 1965). At high concentrations it is reasonable to assume that the antibiotic inhibits transaminases which results in an inhibition of protein synthesis. The effective inhibition of the D-glutamic-D-alanine transaminase by D-cycloserine is difficult to assess. If the major site were this transaminase, the formation of D-glutamic acid from D-alanine and α-ketoglutarate would be inhibited; therefore, an accumulation of UDP-NAc-muramyl-L-ala would occur. As previously described, this is not the case. Thus, the primary sites of D-cycloserine action are concerned with the inhibition of the alanine racemase and the D-ala-D-ala synthetase. These results are consistent with the inhibition of peptidoglycan synthesis and the accumulation of the incomplete wall precursor UDP-NAc-muramyl-L-ala-D-glu-L-lys. The D-ala-D-ala adding enzyme which catalyzes the addition of the dipeptide to the incomplete wall precursor is not inhibited by D-cycloserine (ITO and STROMINGER, 1962b).

There is evidence to indicate that D-alanine has the conformation of D-cycloserine when it is bound to the D-ala-D-ala synthetase. A similar situation may exist with the alanine racemase. It is of interest that the D-alanine activating enzyme

(6.1. 1.8) which catalyzes the activation of D-alanine according to the following reaction (BADDILEY and NEUHAUS, 1959),

$$\text{Enzyme} + \text{ATP} + \text{D-alanine} \xrightarrow{Mg^{2+}} \text{Enzyme-AMP-D-alanine} + \text{PP},$$

is not inhibited by D-cycloserine (NEUHAUS and LYNCH, 1964; ITO and STROMINGER, 1962b). The enzyme catalyzes a [^{32}P]-pyrophosphate-ATP exchange in the presence of D-alanine and Mg^{2+}, and the formation of D-alanine hydroxamate in the presence of ATP, Mg^{2+}, hydroxylamine, and D-alanine. The action of D-cycloserine was measured in the exchange reaction. It may be concluded that the D-alanine is bound to this enzyme in a conformation different from that involved in the alanine racemase and the D-ala-D-ala synthetase.

L-DOPA-decarboxylase and L-glutamic-γ-aminobutyric acid transaminase were investigated because of the toxicity of D-cycloserine. The inhibition of these enzymes in the host may explain its neurophysiological effects.

Other Effects

The competitive inhibition of D-amino acid oxidase has been demonstrated by HOEPRICH (1966). The K_m for D-alanine is 2.8×10^{-3}M and the values for K_i of L- and D-cycloserine are 3.1×10^{-3}M and 6.8×10^{-4}M, respectively. Inhibition of the mammalian D-amino acid oxidase by D-cycloserine could lead to the accumulation of D-alanine in the host, and thus lead to antagonism of the antimicrobial effect of D-cycloserine (see "D-Alanine: D-cycloserine antagonism").

ISHII and SEVAG (1956) observed that D-cycloserine inhibits the accumulation of 5-amino-4-imidazolecarboxamide in a purine dependent strain of *E. coli* in media which contains glucose and either glutamic acid or serine. It is not clear which enzyme is inhibited by the antibiotic in this case. In addition to the pyridoxal phosphate dependent enzymes that have been described, tryptophanase (4.2. 1.20) is also inhibited by D-cycloserine (YAMADA, SAWAKI, and HAYAMI, 1957; ITO *et al.*, 1958).

L-Cycloserine

L-Cycloserine is more effective than D-cycloserine as an inhibitor of growth in *E. coli* (CIAK and HAHN, 1959), *M. tuberculosis* (SEREMBE, 1957; SALGARELLO and TURRI, 1958), and *Salmonella paratyphi* (MURARI, SALGARELLO, and MORATELLO, 1958). The site of action of the L-isomer, however, is readily distinguished from that observed with the D-cycloserine. In contrast to the D-isomer, L-cycloserine does not cause protoplast formation or result in the accumulation of cell wall nucleotides (CIAK and HAHN, 1959) (see "Protoplast" [spheroplast] formation" and "Inhibition of peptidoglycan synthesis and accumulation of nucleotides by D-Cycloserine").

O-Carbamyl-D-Serine

Discovery

O-Carbamyl-D-serine was originally isolated by HAGEMANN *et al.* (1955) from a strain of *Streptomyces*. In 1963 OKAMI *et al.* isolated this antibiotic from *S. fragilis*. In some strains of Streptomycetes, both D-cycloserine and O-carbamyl-D-serine are produced simultaneously (TANAKA and SASHIKATA, 1963). The synthesis of this compound (LIII) was accomplished by SKINNER *et al.* (1955).

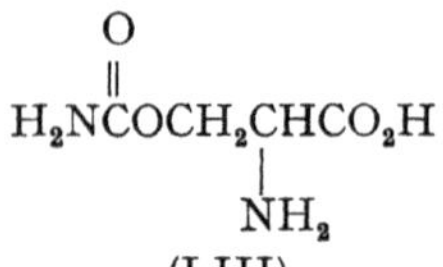

(LIII)

Properties

O-Carbamyl-D-serine has three titratible groups: $pK_{a_1} = 2.25$, and two between 8.00 and 9.10[1] (TANAKA *et al.*, 1963). The following decomposition points were observed: 212—215°C (SKINNER *et al.*, 1955); 226—234°C (HAGEMANN *et al.*, 1955); 198°C (TANAKA *et al.*, 1963). The following specific rotations for O-carbamyl-D-serine were found: $[\alpha]_D = -19.6°$ ($c = 2$ in 1 N HCl) and $+2°$ ($c = 2$ in water) HAGEMANN *et al.*, 1955); $[\alpha]_D = -19.1°$ ($c = 2$ in 1 N HCl) (SKINNER *et al.*, 1955); $[\alpha_D^{20}] = +7.6°$ (c = 2.5 in water) and $-19.6°$ ($c = 2$ in 1 N HCl) (TANAKA *et al.*, 1963). O-Carbamyl-D-serine is readily hydrolyzed to serine by 6 N HCl (100°C) for 3 hours (HAGEMANN *et al.*, 1955).

Reaction with Pyridoxal

The incubation of pyridoxal, a metal (Ga^{3+}), and O-carbamyl-serine results in the rapid formation of pyruvate and NH_3. For example, within 15 minutes at 37°C the following amount of pyruvate (mmoles) was formed from 10 mmoles of starting material: O-phosphoserine, 2.0; O-carbamyl-serine, 3.6; and azaserine, 2.7. In the absence of pyridoxal, no pyruvate was formed; in the absence of metal, only 0.3 mmole of pyruvate was formed from O-carbamyl-serine (LONGENECKER and SNELL, 1957).

O-Carbamyl-D-serine as an Antibiotic

Only limited screening data are available on O-carbamyl-D-serine. In Table 8 the minimal inhibitory concentrations of O-carbamyl-D-serine and D-cycloserine

Table 8. *Sensitivity of various bacteria to O-carbamyl-D-serine*

	Bacterium	Minimal inhibitory concentration	
		O-Carbamyl-D-serine µg/ml	D-Cycloserine µg/ml
1.	*Bacillus subtilis*	100	5
2.	*Staphylococcus aureus*	>2000	80
3.	*Mycobacterium phlei*	800	20
4.	*Mycobacterium tuberculosis*	>2000	80
5.	*Streptococcus faecalis* R	500	20
6.	*Streptococcus* strain Challis	300	50

1—4: TANAKA and UMEZAWA (1964); 5: LYNCH and NEUHAUS (1966); 6: REITZ, SLADE, and NEUHAUS (1966).

[1] A single titratible group was observed with a value of 8.3 in this range (LYNCH and NEUHAUS, unpublished observations).

for six bacteria are compared. In every case it is apparent that D-cycloserine is more effective than O-carbamyl-D-serine. SKINNER *et al.* (1956) reported that the D-isomer of O-carbamyl-serine has no effect on *Str. lactis, Lactobacillus arabinosus,* and *E. coli* at 200µg/ml. Since higher levels of antibiotic are required (Table 8) and their medium contains a significant concentration of D-alanine (2.3×10^{-4} M), the results in Table 8 are also in agreement with those reported by SKINNER *et al.* (1956). O-Carbamyl-L-serine inhibits the growth of *Str. lactis, L. arabinosus* 17-5, and *E. coli* 9723 at concentrations of 4, 2, and 20 µg/ml, respectively. The inhibition by the L-isomer is reversed by glutamine (SKINNER *et al.*, 1956).

TANAKA and UMEZAWA (1964) observed a marked synergism between D-cycloserine and O-carbamyl-D-serine. Optimal synergism was observed in the range 90:10 to 50:50 (D-cycloserine: O-carbamyl-D-serine).

D-Alanine: O-Carbamyl-D-serine Antagonism

TANAKA *et al.* (1963) demonstrated that the antibacterial activity could be reversed by D-alanine. This activity was not reversed by glycine, L-alanine, L-serine, L-glutamic acid, L-lysine, or L-glutamine. With *Str. faecalis*, it was observed that D-alanine (3×10^{-3} M) and L-alanine (3×10^{-2} M) completely reversed the effect of O-carbamyl-D-serine (7.0×10^{-3} M) (LYNCH and NEUHAUS, 1966).

Inhibition of Peptidoglycan Synthesis and Accumulation of Nucleotides by O-Carbamyl-D-serine

As in the case of D-cycloserine (Table 3), O-carbamyl-D-serine also inhibits the synthesis of peptidoglycan (Table 9) (TANAKA, 1963). Incorporation of DL-glutamic acid-^{14}C into the protein fraction was only slightly affected. Identical results were observed with *B. subtilis* PCl 219 and *S. aureus* 209 P. The kinetics of accumulation of N-acyl-amino sugar are shown in Fig. 7 and compared with that of D-cycloserine. These results were confirmed in *Str. faecalis* and the major nucleotide was identified as UDP-NAc-muramyl-L-ala-D-glu-L-lys (XLVIII) (LYNCH and NEUHAUS, 1966). This is identical to the major nucleotide which accumulates in the presence of D-cycloserine (see "Inhibition of peptidoglycan synthesis and accumulation of nucleotides by D-cycloserine"). For example, at 120 minutes the cells grown in the presence of O-carbamyl-D-serine contained

Table 9. *Effects of O-carbamyl-D-serine on incorporation of DL-glutamate-3,4-^{14}C into cell wall or into protein in Bacillus subtilis and in Staphylococcus aureus*[1]

Antibiotics	*B. subtilis*		*S. aureus*	
	Cell wall	Protein	Cell wall	Protein
	705[2]	6780	1020	3270
O-Carbamyl-D-serine 0.4 mg/ml	297 (58)	6030 (11)	660 (35)	2970 (9)
Benzylpenicillin 2 units/ml	324 (54)	5580 (17)	50 (95)	2960 (6)

[1] TANAKA (1963).
[2] The number represents cpm/ml of the culture. The number in the bracket shows % inhibition (TANAKA, 1963).

15.6 nmoles UDP-NAc-muramyl-L-ala-D-glu-L-lys per mg (dry wt.) while the control culture contained 0.55 nmole per mg dry wt.

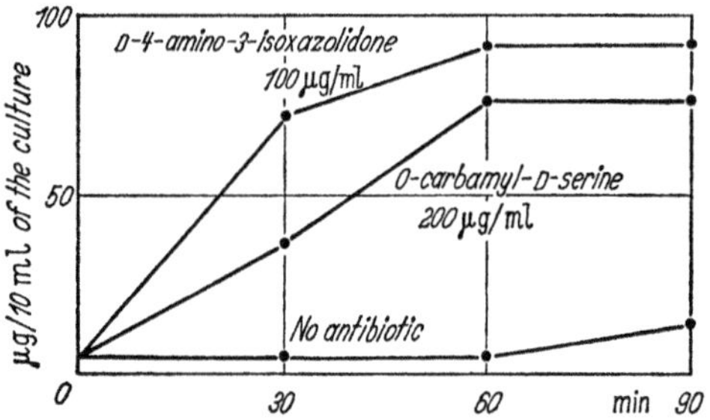

Fig. 7. Intracellular accumulation of N-acylamino sugar in *Bacillus subtilis* (TANAKA, 1963)

O-Carbamyl-D-serine: Specific enzyme Effects

The accumulation of UDP-NAc-muramyl-L-ala-D-glu-L-lys in the presence of the antibiotic suggests that the bacterium is either unable to synthesize adequate amounts of D-ala-D-ala or unable to add the dipeptide to the UDP-NAc-muramyl-tripeptide. Thus, LYNCH and NEUHAUS (1966) have examined the effects of O-carbamyl-D-serine on the alanine racemase, the D-ala-D-ala synthetase, and the D-ala-D-ala adding enzyme.

Alanine Racemase

O-Carbamyl-D-serine is an effective competitive inhibitor of the alanine racemase. The K_m for L-alanine is 6.8×10^{-3} M while the K_i for O-carbamyl-D-serine

Table 10. *Inhibitor specificity of alanine racemase*[1]

Addition[2]	"L-Alanine to D-alanine assay" Inhibition %	"D-Alanine to L-alanine assay" Inhibition %
O-Carbamyl-D-serine	53	38
O-Carbamyl-L-serine	0	0
D-Cycloserine	87	79
L-Cycloserine	8	—[3]
D-Serine	10	9
L-Serine	0	0
D-Threonine	0	0
L-Threonine	0	0
D-α-NH_2-*n*-Butyric acid	12	6
L-α-NH_2-*n*-Butyric acid	0	0
D-Norvaline	0	0
L-Norvaline	0	0
β-Aminoxy-D-alanine	—[4]	84

[1] LYNCH and NEUHAUS (1966).

[2] The concentration of alanine and inhibitor were 5×10^{-3} M and 1×10^{-3} M, respectively.

[3] L-Cycloserine is an effective inhibitor of the glutamic alanine transaminase.

[4] β-Aminoxy-D-alanine inhibits D-amino-acid oxidase.

is 4.8×10^{-4} M. As shown in Table 10, O-carbamyl-L-serine does not inhibit the racemase when tested at 1×10^{-3} M and at a concentration of 5×10^{-3} M L-alanine. Thus, as in the case of cycloserine, the D-isomer is bound more effectively than the L-isomer. In contrast to D-cycloserine and O-carbamyl-D-serine, D-serine and D-α-amino-*n*-butyric acid are poor inhibitors.

D-Ala-D-Ala Synthetase

When O-carbamyl-D-serine was incubated with D-alanine, Mg^{2+}, ATP, and D-ala-D-ala synthetase, D-ala-O-carbamyl-D-ser was formed in addition to D-ala-D-ala, i.e.,

$$\text{D-alanine} + \text{O-carbamyl-D-serine} + \text{ATP} \xrightarrow{Mg^{2+}} \text{D-ala-O-carbamyl-D-ser} + \text{ADP} + P_i$$

The structure of the dipeptide is:

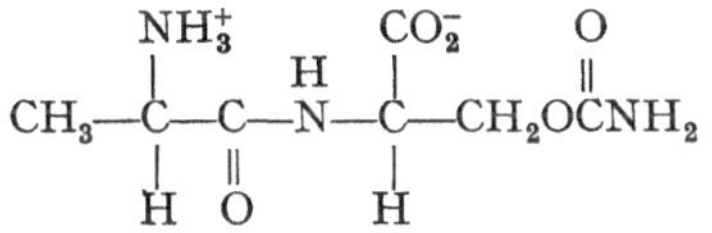

(LIV)

Incubation of D-cycloserine with D-alanine, Mg^{2+}, ATP, and the synthetase did not result in the formation of the corresponding dipeptide D-ala-D-cycloserine. Thus, with the D-ala-D-ala synthetase, we have a clear distinction between the *in vitro* action of O-carbamyl-D-serine and D-cycloserine. However, since high concentrations of O-carbamyl-D-serine are required for mixed dipeptide synthesis, this site appears to be only of secondary importance. For example, at 0.05 M O-carbamyl-D-serine and 0.005 M D-alanine, 0.13 μmole of D-ala-O-carbamyl-D-ser and 0.56 μmole of D-ala-D-ala were formed (LYNCH and NEUHAUS, 1966).

The dipeptide D-ala-D-ala is an effective product inhibitor of the synthetase (NEUHAUS, 1962). If D-ala-O-carbamyl-D-ser should accumulate during growth, the inhibition of the synthetase by the mixed dipeptide (LIV) would be a site of action. Attempts to detect the accumulation of this dipeptide in *Str. faecalis* were not successful. Thus, since D-ala-O-carbamyl-D-ser (LIV) does not accumulate, it would appear that inhibition of the synthetase by the mixed dipeptide does not contribute to the mechanism of O-carbamyl-D-serine action.

D-Ala-D-Ala Adding Enzyme

O-Carbamyl-D-serine (0.05 M) has no effect on the D-ala-D-ala adding enzyme, The dipeptide D-ala-O-carbamyl-D-ser (LIV), however, can be added to UDP-NAc-muramyl-tripeptide (XLVIII) when these components are incubated with the D-ala-D-ala adding enzyme, ATP, and Mg^{2+}. From LINEWEAVER-BURK plots, the Michaelis constants (K_m) for D-ala-O-carbamyl-D-ser (3.6×10^{-3} M) and D-ala-D-ala (1.6×10^{-4} M) were established. Identical V_{max} values for each dipeptide were observed.

On the Mode of Action

From a consideration of the results, it was proposed (LYNCH and NEUHAUS. 1966) that the primary site of action of O-carbamyl-D-serine is the inhibition of the alanine racemase. This conclusion is based on a comparison of the antibiotic effects on the potential enzyme sites, on the observed accumulation of UDP-NAc-muramyl-L-ala-D-glu-L-lys (XLVIII), and on the absence of D-ala-O-carbamyl-D-ser (LIV) accumulation. The inhibition of the racemase deprives the bacterium of the D-alanine necessary for synthesis of D-ala-D-ala; thus, UDP-NAc-muramyl-L-ala-D-glu-L-lys accumulates and peptidoglycan synthesis is inhibited.

Resistance to D-Cycloserine and O-Carbamyl-D-Serine

The emergence of resistance to D-cycloserine has been observed in many situations (see "Resistance to D-cycloserine"). DAVIS and MAAS (1952) proposed and MOYED (1964) has discussed the mechanisms by which a bacterium might acquire resistance to an antibiotic. These are as follows:

a) "Decreased penetration of the drug.
b) Increased destruction of the drug.
c) Increased concentration of a metabolite antagonizing the drug.
d) Increased concentration of an enzyme utilizing this metabolite.
e) Decreased quantitative requirement for a product of the metabolite.
f) Alternative metabolic pathway by-passing the metabolite.
g) Enzyme with decreased relative affinity for the drug compared with the metabolite."

Mutants of *Streptococcus* strain Challis resistant to O-carbamyl-D-serine and D-cycloserine have been analyzed with respect to the enzymes involved in the biosynthesis of UDP-NAc-muramyl-pentapeptide (see "Introduction") (REITZ, SLADE, and NEUHAUS, 1966). In the mutant selected for resistance to D-cycloserine the amounts of alanine racemase and D-ala-D-ala synthetase are elevated by factors of eight and five, respectively (Fig. 8). In the mutant selected for resistance to O-carbamyl-D-serine, only the alanine racemase is increased. These strains were tested for cross-resistance by determining the minimum concentration of antibiotic that was able to inhibit growth 50%. It was observed that the D-cycloserine resistant mutant was completely cross resistant to the O-carbamyl-D-serine while the mutant resistant to O-carbamyl-D-serine was only partially resistant to the action of D-cycloserine. In order to exclude the possibility that the enzymes might have altered sensitivities to the antibiotic or altered Michealis constants, kinetic and inhibitor studies were performed. These results showed no change in either the Michaelis constant or the inhibitor constant (K_i) in the case of alanine racemase (REITZ, SLADE, and NEUHAUS, 1966).

HOWE *et al.* (1964) demonstrated that resistance to D-cycloserine was acquired in discrete steps. In Fig. 9 the levels of four enzymes in three mutants that are resistant to increasing concentrations of O-carbamyl-D-serine are shown (REITZ, SLADE, and NEUHAUS, 1966). The increase in resistance can be correlated with an increase in the alanine racemase.

Perry and Slade[1] showed that resistance to D-cycloserine is a transformable characteristic. With procedures described by Perry and Slade (1964), transformation rates of 1% for D-cycloserine resistance were demonstrated. When the

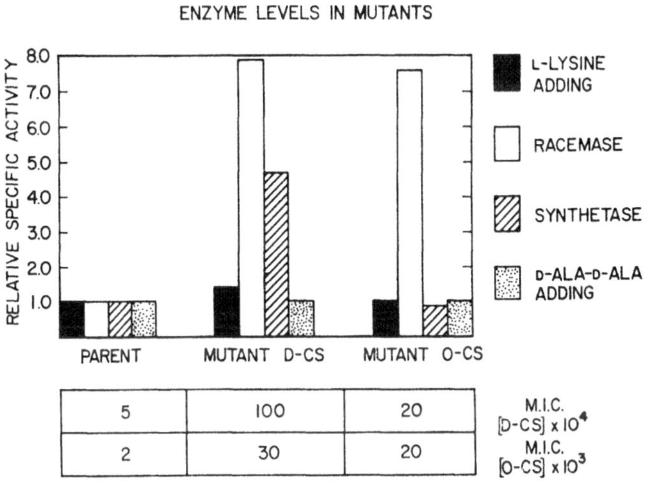

Fig. 8. Enzyme levels in mutants resistant to O-carbamyl-D-serine and D-cycloserine. The specific activities of alanine racemase, L-lysine adding enzyme, D-ala-D-ala synthetase, and the D-ala-D-ala adding enzyme were established in extracts prepared from the mutants. The levels of enzymes in the parent strain were assigned a relative specific activity of one (Reitz, Slade, and Neuhaus, 1966)

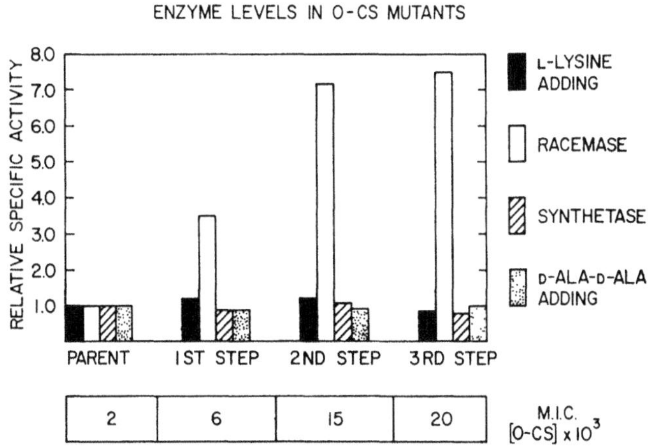

Fig. 9. Enzyme levels in mutants resistant to increasing concentrations of O-carbamyl-D-serine (O-CS). The specific activities are reported in the same manner as in Fig. 8 (Reitz, Slade, and Neuhaus, 1966)

enzyme profiles of the transformants were examined, two general types were found. The first class was characterized by an increase in the racemase while the second class was characterized by an increase in the synthetase (Reitz, Slade,

[1] Perry, D., and H. D. Slade: personal communication.

and NEUHAUS, 1966). These results demonstrated that the acquisition of resistance to D-cycloserine and O-carbamyl-D-serine is a genetic property.

Acknowledgments. The author's research is supported in part by a grant (AI-04615) from the National Institute of Allergy and Infectious Diseases, by a Public Health Service training grant (5 TI GM-626), by a grant (GM 10006) from the Division of General Medical Science, and by a grant-in-aid from the Eli Lilly Company. I am indebted to Dr. O. K. BEHRENS and Dr. M. C. BACHMAN for their interest in this work and for the generous samples of D-cycloserine and O-carbamyl-D-serine; to Drs. P. D. HOEPRICH, J. L. STROMINGER, and C. H. STAMMER for manuscripts that are in press; and to Dr. G. J. LAFFERTY for a bibliography of the cycloserine literature. It is a pleasure to acknowledge the collaboration of Mrs. JUDY LYNCH MILLER and Mr. R. H. REITZ in the work from this laboratory, and Drs. H. D. SLADE, R. W. BROCKMAN, and C. H. STAMMER.

References

ALIOTO, M. R.: In vitro and in vivo action of cycloserine on L-alanine-alpha-ketoglutaric transaminases in rat liver. Biochim. Appl. **9**, 238 (1962).

ANDERSON, J. S., M. MATSUHASHI, M. A. HASKIN, and J. L. STROMINGER: Lipid-phosphodisaccharide-pentapeptide: A presumed membrane transport intermediate in the biosynthesis of bacterial cell walls. Proc. Natl. Acad. Sci. U.S. **53**, 881 (1965).

AOKI, T.: The mode of action of cycloserine. II. The influence on glutamic-aspartic transamination. Kekkaku **32**, 544 (1957); cited from Chem. Abstr. **52**, 7427 (1958).

AZARKH, R. M., A. E. BRAUNSTEIN, T. S. PASKHINA, and T. S. SYUI: The Effect of the optical isomers of cycloserine on the activity of certain transaminases. Biokhimiya **25**, 954 (1960); Biochemistry (U.S.S.R.) **25**, 741 (1961).

BARBIERI, P., A. DI MARCO, I. FUOCO, and A. RUSCONI: Investigations on the mode of action of cycloserine upon protein synthesis in *Escherichia coli*. Biochem. Pharmacol. **3**, 101 (1960).

BONAVITA, V.: Purification and properties of glutamic-oxaloacetic transaminase from human brain. J. Neurochem. **4**, 275 (1959).

BONDI, A., J. KORNBLUM, and C. FORTE: Inhibition of antibacterial activity of cycloserine by alpha-alanine. Proc. Soc. Exptl. Biol. Med. **96**, 270 (1957).

BOTTERO, A., G. PERNA, G. C. COLOMBI, and F. LEIDI: Experimental and clinical studies on cycloserine resistance. Giorn. ital. tuberc. **12**, 10 (1958).

BRAUNSTEIN, A. E.: Studies on the properties, mode of action, and selective inhibition of transaminase, In P. A. E. DESNUELLE (Editor), Proceedings of the Fifth Internat. Congr. of Biochemistry, Moscow, 1962, vol. IV, p. 280. NewYork: Pergamon Press 1963.

BRAUNSTEIN, A. E., R. M. AZARKH, and T. A. SYUI: Kinetics of inhibition of transaminases by cycloserine. Biokhimiya **26**, 882 (1961); Biochemistry (U.S.S.R.) **27**, 760 (1962).

BRETTSCHNEIDER, H., u. W. VETTER: Synthese des DL-4-Amino-3-isoxazolidons sowie seiner D-Form, des natürlichen Cycloserins. Monatsh. Chem. **90**, 799 (1959).

BRETTSCHNEIDER, H., W. VETTER u. E. SEMENITZ: Synthese und antibakterielle Eigenschaften des D,L-N,N-Dimethylcycloserins. Monatsh. Chem. **89**, 627 (1958).

BREGER, M. A.: The biological activity of cycloserine and some of its analogues and homologues. Antibiotiki **6**, 26 (1961).

BUOGO, A., A. DI MARCO, M. GHIONE, A. MIGLIACCI, and A. SANFILIPPO: Antagonism of D- and L-alanine of the enantiomorphic forms of cycloserine. Giorn. microbiol. **6**, 131 (1958); cited from Chem. Abstr. **54**, 17538 (1960).

CHAMBERS, P., J. BING, J. LYNCH, F. C. NEUHAUS, and R. W. BROCKMAN: Effects of cycloserine and related compounds on cell wall synthesis in sensitive and resistant *Escherichia coli*. Bacteriol. Proc. 119 (1963).

CHATTERJEE, A. N., and J. T. PARK: Biosynthesis of cell wall mucopeptide by a particulate fraction from *Staphylococcus aureus*. Proc. Natl. Acad. Sci. U.S. **51**, 9 (1964).

CIAK, J., and F. E. HAHN: Mechanisms of action of antibiotics. II. Studies on the modes of action of cycloserine and its L-stereoisomer. Antibiotics & Chemotherapy 9, 47 (1959).

COHEN, A. C., and I. C. DROSS: High-dosage cycloserine in treatment failures. Transactions of the 19th conference on the chemotherapy of tuberculosis. Veterans Administration-Armed Forces, Washington, D. C., 173 (1960).

COMB, D. G.: The enzymatic addition of D-alanyl-D-alanine to a uridine nucleotide-peptide. J. Biol. Chem. **237**, 1601 (1962).

CUCKLER, A. C., B. M. FROST, L. MCCLELLAND, and M. SOLOTOROVSKY: The antimicrobial evaluation of oxamycin (D-4-amino-3-isoxazolidone), a new broad-spectrum antibiotic. Antibiotics & Chemotherapy **5**, 191 (1955).

CUMMINGS, M. M., R. A. PATNODE, and P. C. HUDGINS: Effects of cycloserine on *Mycobacterium tuberculosis in vitro*. Antibiotics & Chemotherapy **5**, 198 (1955).

CUMMINGS, M. M.: Cycloserine: Resistance data. Transactions of the 15th conference on the chemotherapy of tuberculosis. Veterans Administration-Armed Forces, Washington, D. C., 377 (1956).

CURTISS, R., L. J. CHARAMELLA, C. M. BERG, and P. E. HARRIS: Kinetic and genetic analyses of D-cycloserine inhibition and resistance in *Escherichia coli*. J. Bacteriol. **90**, 1238 (1965).

DANN, O. T., and C. E. CARTER: Cycloserine inhibition of gamma-aminobutyric-alpha-ketoglutaric transaminase. Biochem. Pharmacology **13**, 677 (1964).

DAVIS, B. D., and M. K. MAAS: Analysis of the biochemical mechanism of drug resistance in certain bacterial mutants. Proc. Natl. Acad. Sci. U.S. **38**, 775 (1952).

DEMEREC, M.: Origin of bacterial resistance to antibiotics. J. Bacteriol. **56**, 63 (1948).

DENGLER, H. J.: Zur Hemmung der L-Glutaminsäure- und L-Dopadecarboxylase durch D-Cycloserin und andere Isoxazolidone. Naunyn-Schmiedeberg's Arch. Exptl. Pathol. u. Pharmakol. **243**, 366 (1962).

EPSTEIN, I. G., K. G. S. NAIR, and L. J. BOYD: Cycloserine in the treatment of human pulmonary tuberculosis. Transactions of the 14th conference on the chemotherapy of tuberculosis. Veterans Administration-Armed Forces, Washington, D. C., 326 (1955).

FETH, T., and K. KAZIM: *In vitro* action of cycloserine on *Mycobacterium tuberculosis*. Bacteriol. Proc. **85** (1962).

FOLKERS, K.: 4-Pyridoxylamino-3-isoxazolidone compounds. U.S. Patent 2,776,296 (January 1, 1957).

FRECKING, M. G., and P. D. HOEPRICH: Effect of cycloserines on D-amino acid oxidase. Arch. Biochem. Biophys. **115**, 108 (1966).

FREESE, E., and J. OOSTERWYK: The induction of alanine dehydrogenase. Biochemistry **2**, 1212 (1963).

GROSSET, J., and G. CANETTI: Incidence of resistance to secondary antimicrobials in wild strains of *M. tuberculosis* (PAS, ethionamide, cycloserine, viomycin, and kanamycin). Ann. Inst. Pasteur **103**, 163 (1962).

GRULA, M. M., and E. A. GRULA: Action of cycloserine on a species of *Erwinia* with reference to cell division. Can. J. Microbiol. **11**, 453 (1965).

GRULA, E. A., and M. M. GRULA: Cell division in a species of *Erwinia*. VII. Amino sugar content of dividing and nondividing cells. Biochem. Biophys. Research Commun. **17**, 341 (1964).

HAGEMANN, G., L. PENASSE et J. TEILLON: Sur un derive de la serine, la O-carbamyl-D-serine produit par un streptomyces. Biochim. et Biophys. Acta **17**, 240 (1955).

HAHN, F. E., and J. CIAK: Penicillin-induced lysis of *Escherichia coli*. Science **125**, 119 (1957).

HANCOCK, R., and P. C. FITZ-JAMES: Some differences in the action of penicillin, bacitracin, and vancomycin on *Bacillus megaterium*. J. Bacteriol. **87**, 1044 (1964).

HARNED, R. L., P. H. HIDY, and E. K. LA BAW: Cycloserine. I. A preliminary report. Antibiotics & Chemotherapy **5**, 204 (1955).

HARRIS, D. A., M. RUGER, M. A. REAGAN, F. J. WOLF, R. L. PECK, H. WALLICK, and H. B. WOODRUFF: Discovery, development, and antimicrobial properties of D-4-amino-3-isoxazolidone (oxamycin), a new antibiotic produced by *Streptomyces garyphalus* n. sp. Antibiotics & Chemotherapy **5**, 183 (1955).

HARRIS, D. A., F. J. WOLF, and R. L. PECK: Crystalline alkaline earth metal salts of 4-amino-3-isoxazolidone. U.S. Patent 2,832,788 (April 29, 1958).

HAYASHI, K., C. G. SKINNER, and W. SHIVE: Synthesis and biological properties of 4-amino-5-isopropyl-3-isoxazolidone, a substituted cycloserine. J. Org. Chem. **26**, 1167 (1961).

HIDY, P. H., E. B. HODGE, V. V. YOUNG, R. L. HARNED, G. A. BREWER, W. F. PHILLIPS, W. F. RUNGE, H. E. STAVELEY, A. POHLAND, H. BOAZ, and H. R. SULLIVAN: Structures and reactions of cycloserine. J. Am. Chem. Soc. **77**, 2345 (1955).

HODGE, E. B.: Substituted cycloserines. U.S. Patent 2,971,004 (February 7, 1961 a).

HODGE, E. B.: N-(*p*-Chlorobenzyl)-cycloserine. U.S. Patent 2,967,866 (January 10, 1961 b).

HOEPRICH, P. D.: Alanine: Cycloserine antagonism. III. Quantitative aspects and relations to heating of culture media. J. Lab. Clin. Med. **62**, 657 (1963).

HOEPRICH, P. D.: Alanine: Cycloserine antagonism. VI. Demonstration of D-alanine in the serum of guinea pigs and mice. J. Biol. Chem. **240**, 1654 (1965).

HOLLY, F. W., CRANFORD, and C. H. STAMMER: Synthesis of 4-amino-3-isoxazolidone and its derivatives. U.S. Patent 2, 772, 281 (November 27, 1956).

HOWE, W. B., G. L. MELSON, C. H. MEREDITH, J. R. MORRISON, M. H. PLATT, and J. L. STROMINGER: Stepwise development of resistance to D-cycloserine in *Staphylococcus aureus*. J. Pharmacol. Exptl. Therap. **143**, 282 (1964).

IKAWA, M., and E. E. SNELL: Cell wall composition of lactic acid bacteria. J. Biol. Chem. **235**, 1376 (1960).

ISHII, K., and M. G. SEVAG: Inhibition by cycloserine of the synthesis of 5-amino-4-imidazolecarboxamide by *Escherichia coli*. Antibiotics & Chemotherapy **6**, 500 (1956).

ITO, E., and M. SAITO: Time course of accumulation of UDP-N-acetylamino sugar derivatives in *Staphylococcus aureus*. Biochim. et Biophys. Acta **78**, 237 (1963).

ITO, E., and J. L. STROMINGER: Enzymatic synthesis of the peptide in bacterial uridine nucleotides. I. Enzymatic addition of L-alanine, D-glutamic acid, and L-lysine. J. Biol. Chem. **237**, 2689 (1962a).

ITO, E., and J. L. STROMINGER: Enzymatic synthesis of the peptide in bacterial uridine nucleotides. II. Enzymatic synthesis and addition of D-alanyl-D-alanine. J. Biol. Chem. **237**, 2696 (1962b).

ITO, F., T. AOKI, M. YAMAMOTO, M. YUASA, H. MIZOBATA, and K. TONE: The mode of action of cycloserine (CS). Med. J. Osaka Univ. **9**, 23 (1958).

KARPEISKII, M. YA., R. M. KHOMUTOV, E. S. SEVERIN, and YU. N. BREUSOV: The investigation of the interaction of cycloserine and related compounds with aspartate-glutamate transaminase. In: E. E. SNELL, P. M. FASELLA, A. E. BRAUNSTEIN, and A. ROSSI-FANELLI (editors), Chemical and Biological Aspects of Pyridoxal Catalysis. I.U.B. Symposium Series, vol. 30, p. 323. New York: Pergamon Press 1963a.

KARPEISKII, M. YA., YU. N. BREUSOV, R. M. KHOMUTOV, E. S. SEVERIN, and O. L. POLYANOVSKII: The mechanism of reaction of cycloserine and related compounds with aspartate-glutamate transaminase. Biokhimiya **28**, 345 (1963b); Biochemistry (U.S.S.R.) **28**, 280 (1964).

KARPEISKII, M. YA., and YU. N. BREUSOV: On the structure of the enzyme-inhibitor complex of aspartate-transaminase with L-cycloserine. Biokhimiya **30**, 153 (1965).

KHOMUTOV, R. M., M. YA. KARPEISKII, E. S. SEVERIN, E. I. BUDOVSKII, and N. K. KOCHETKOV: Cycloserine and related compounds. VI. Synthesis of analogs of cycloserine with a substitued amino group. J. gen. Chem. (U.S.S.R.) **29**, 636 (1959).

KHOMUTOV, R. M., M. YA. KARPEISKII, C. CHI-PIN, and N. K. KOCHETKOV: Cycloserine and related compounds. XL. 4-Hydroxy-3-isoxazolidinone and some of its derivatives. Zhur. Obshchei Khim. **30**, 3057 (1960); J. Gen. Chem. (U.S.S.R.) **30**, 3030 (1961).

KHOMUTOV, R. M., M. YA. KARPEISKII, and E. S. SEVERIN: The relationship between biological activity and chemical properties. Biokhimiya **26**, 772 (1961); Biochemistry (U.S.S.R.) **26**, 667 (1962).

KHOMUTOV, R. M., M. YA. KARPEISKII, M. A. BREGER, and E. S. SEVERIN: On some cycloserine derivatives possessing antitubercular activity. Voprosy Med. Khim. **8**, 389 (1962).

KHOMUTOV, R. M., M. YA. KARPEISKII, and E. S. SEVERIN: The predetermined synthesis of inhibitors for pyridoxalic enzymes. In: E. E. SNELL, P. M. FASELLA, A. E. BRAUNSTEIN, and A. ROSSI-FANELLI (editors), Chemical and Biological Aspects of Pyridoxal Catalysis. I.U.B. Symposium Series, vol. 30, p. 323. New York: Pergamon Press 1963.

KIHARA, H., M. IKAWA, and E. E. SNELL: Peptides and bacterial growth. X. Relation of uptake and hydrolysis to utilization of D-alanine peptides for growth of *Streptococcus faecalis*. J. Biol. Chem. **236**, 172 (1961).

KOCHETKOV, N. K., R. M. KHOMUTOV, and M. YA. KARPEISKII: New synthesis of cycloserine. Dokl. Akad. Nauk S.S.S.R. **111**, 831 (1956).

KOCHETKOV, N. K., E. I. BUDOVSKII, R. M. KHOMUTOV, and M. YA. KARPEISKII: Cycloserine and related compounds. V. Cyclization of alpha-benzoylamino-beta-arylacrylohydroxamic acids. J. Gen. Chem. (U.S.S.R.) **29**, 630 (1959).

KOLESINSKA, J.: Cycloserine stability at various temperatures and pH values. Med. Doswiadczalna i. Mikrobiol. **13**, 189 (1961); cited from Chem. Abstr. **55**, 24883 (1961).

KOTSCHETKOW, N. K.: Die Chemie des Antibiotikums Cykloserin. Österr. Chemiker-Ztg. **62**, 276 (1961).

KUEHL, F. A., F. J. WOLF, N. R. TRENNER, R. L. PECK, E. HOWE, B. D. HUNNEWELL, G. DOWNING, E. NEWSTEAD, R. P. BUHS, I. PUTTER, R. ORMOND, J. E. LYONS, L. CHALET, and K. FOLKERS: D-4-Amino-3-isoxazolidone, a new antibiotic. J. Am. Chem. Soc. **77**, 2344 (1955).

KURIHARA, T., and K. CHIBA: Orientomycin, a new antibiotic. Ann. Rept. Tohoku coll. Pharm. **3**, 83 (1956); cited from Chem. Abstr. **51**, 5197 (1957).

LARK, C., and R. SCHICHTEL: Comparison of spheroplast induction in *Alcaligenes faecalis* by three different agents. J. Bacteriol. **84**, 1241 (1962).

LESTER, W., A. SALOMIN, A. F. REIMANN, E. SHULRUFF, and G. S. GERG: Cycloserine therapy in tuberculosis in humans. Am. Rev. Tuberc. **74**, 121 (1956).

LILLICK, L., R. STRANG, L. J. BOYD, M. SCHWIMMER, and M. G. MULINOS: Cycloserine in the treatment of nontuberculosis infections. Antibiotics Ann. **1955/56**, 158.

LONGENECKER, J. B., and E. E. SNELL: Pyridoxal and metal ion catalysis of alpha-beta-elimination reactions of serine-3-phosphate and related compounds. J. Biol. Chem. **225**, 409 (1957).

LYNCH, J. L., and F. C. NEUHAUS: On the mechanism of action of the antibiotic O-carbamyl-D-serine in *Streptococcus faecalis* R. J. Bacteriol. **91**, 449 (1966).

MALAMY, M. H., and B. L. HORECKER: Release of alkaline phosphates from cells of *Escherichia coli* upon lysozyme spheroplast formation. Biochemistry **3**, 1889 (1964).

MARTINEZ-CARRION, M., and W. T. JENKINS: D-Alanine-D-glutamic transaminase. II. Inhibitors and the mechanism of transamination of D-amino acids. J. Biol. Chem. **240**, 3547 (1965).

MEADOW, P. M., J. S. ANDERSON, and J. L. STROMINGER: Enzymatic polymerization of UDP-acetylmuramyl-L-ala-D-glu-L-lys-D-ala-D-ala and UDP-acetylglucosamine by a particulate enzyme from *Staphylococcus aureus* and its inhibition by antibiotics. Biochem. Biophys. Research Commun. **14**, 382 (1964).

MICHALSKÝ, J., J. OPÍCHAL u. J. ČTVRTNIK: Cycloserin und verwandte Verbindungen; Über die Kondensationsprodukte von D,L-4-Amino-3-isoxazolidon und 2,5-Bis-(aminooxymethyl)-3,6-diketopiperazin. Monatsh. Chem. **93**, 618 (1962a).

MICHALSKÝ, J., J. ČTVRTNIK, Z. HORÁKOVÁ u. V. BYDŽOVSKÝ: Über die tuberkulostatische Aktivität von 2,5-Bis-(aminoxymethyl)-3,6-diketopiperazin, eines Umwandlungsproduktes des Cyclo serins Experientia. **18**, 217 (1962b).

MICHEL, M. F., and W. HIJMANS: The additive effect of glycine and other amino acids on the induction of the L-phase of group A beta-haemolytic streptococci by penicillin and D-cycloserine. J. Gen. Microbiol. **23**, 35 (1960).
MORA, J., and L. F. BOJALIL: Antagonism of the D-alanine reversal of D-cycloserine action by L-alanine in *Mycobacterium acapulcensis*. Proc. Soc. Exptl. Biol. Med. **119**, 49 (1965).
MORA, J., and E. E. SNELL: The uptake of amino acids by cells and protoplasts of *Streptococcus faecalis*. Biochemistry **2**, 136 (1963).
MORRISON, N. E.: The reversal of D-cycloserine inhibition of mycobacterial growth. Bacteriol. Proc. 86 (1962).
MOULDER, J. W., D. L. NOVOSEL, and J. E. OFFICER: Inhibition of the growth of agents of the psittacosis group by D-cycloserine and its specific reversal by D-alanine. J. Bacteriol. **85**, 707 (1963).
MOULDER, J. W., D. L. NOVOSEL, and I. I. E. TRIBBY: Changes in mouse pneumonitis agent associated with development of resistance to chlortetracycline. J. Bacteriol. **89**, 17 (1965).
MOYED, H. S.: Biochemical mechanisms of drug resistance. Ann. Rev. Microbiol. **18**, 247 (1964).
MULINOS, M. G.: Cycloserine: An antibiotic paradox. Antibiotics Ann. **1955/56**, 131.
MURARI, G., G. SALGARELLO, and R. MORATELLO: Antibacterial activity of optical isomers of cycloserine and of its synthetic intermediate (isoxazolidone). Action on *Escherichia coli* and *Salmonella*. Boll. soc. ital. biol. sper. **34**, 1534 (1958); cited from Chem. Abstr. **55**, 14583 (1961).
NAKAMURA, M.: Amebacidal action of cycloserine. Experientia **13**, 29 (1957).
NEILANDS, J. B.: Metal and hydrogen-ion binding properties of cycloserine. Arch. Biochem. Biophys. **62**, 151 (1956).
NEUHAUS, F. C., and W. G. STRUVE: Enzymatic synthesis of analogs of the cell-wall precursor. I. Kinetics and specificity of uridine diphospho-N-acetyl-muramyl-L-alanyl-D-glutamyl-L-lysine: D-Alanyl-D-alanine ligase (adenosine diphosphate) from *Streptococcus faecalis* R. Biochemistry **4**, 120 (1965).
NEUHAUS, F. C.: The enzymatic synthesis of D-alanyl-D-alanine. I. Purification and properties of D-alanyl-D-alanine synthetase. J. Biol. Chem. **237**, 778 (1962a).
NEUHAUS, F. C.: The enzymatic synthesis of D-alanyl-D-alanine. II. Kinetic studies of D-alanyl-D-alanine synthetase. J. Biol. Chem. **237**, 3128 (1962b).
NEUHAUS, F. C., and J. L. LYNCH: The enzymatic synthesis of D-alanyl-D-alanine. III. On the inhibition of D-alanyl-D-alanine synthetase by the antibiotic D-cycloserine. Biochemistry **3**, 471 (1964).
NITTI, V., and M. TSUKAMURA: Resistance of tuberculosis mycobacteria to cycloserine *in vitro*. Arch. tisiol. mal. app. respirat. (Naples) **12**, 71 (1957); cited from Chem. Abstr. **51**, 13069 (1957).
OKAMI, Y., K. MAEDA, H. KONDO, T. TANAKA, and H. UMEZAWA: A streptomyces producing O-carbamyl-D-serine. J. Antibiotics (Japan), Ser. A **15**, 147 (1962).
PARK, J. T.: Selective inhibition of bacterial cell-wall synthesis: Its possible applications in chemotherapy. Symp. Soc. Gen. Microbiol. **8**, 49 (1958a).
PARK, J. T.: Inhibition of cell-wall synthesis in *Staphylococcus aureus* by chemicals which cause accumulation of wall precursors. Biochem. J. **70**, 2 P (1958b).
PARK, J. T.: Inhibition of synthesis of bacterial mucopeptide or protein by certain antibiotics and its possible significance for microbiology and medicine. Antimicrobial Agents Ann. 338 (1960).
PARK, J. T., and R. HANCOCK: A fractionation procedure for studies of the synthesis of cell-wall mucopeptide and of other polymers in cells of *Staphylococcus aureus*. J. Gen. Microbiol. **22**, 249 (1960).
PASKHINA, T. S.: Effect of isomers of cycloserine on the activity of D-alanine-D-glutamic transaminase of *Bacillus subtilis*. Voprosy Med. Khim. **10**, 526 (1964); cited from Chem. Abstr. **57**, 2978 (1965).

PATNODE, R. A., P. C. HUDGINS, and M. M. CUMMINGS: Effect of cycloserine on experimental tuberculosis in guinea pigs. Am. Rev. Tuberc. Pulmonary Diseases 72, 117 (1955).
PEPINSKY, R.: X-Rays and the absolute configuration of optically active molecules. Record Chem. Progr. **17**, 145 (1956).
PERRY, D., and H. D. SLADE: Intraspecific and interspecific tranformation in Streptococci. J. Bacteriol. **88**, 595 (1964).
PIETRA, G. D., F. DELORENZO, and G. ILLIANO: Biochim. Appl. **10**, 123 (1963); cited from F. CEDRANGOLO, in E. E. SNELL, P. M. FASELLA, A. E. BRAUNSTEIN, and A. ROSSI-FANELLI (editors), Chemical and Biological Aspects of Pyridoxal Catalysis, p. 343. NewYork: Pergamon Press 1963.
PITTILLO, R. F., and J. W. FOSTER: Potentiation of Inhibitor action through determination of reversing metabolites. J. Bacteriol. **67**, 53 (1953).
PLAPP, R., u. O. KANDLER: Zur Wirkung zellwandhemmender Antibiotica bei gramnegativen Bakterien. II. Die Wirkung von D-Cycloserin auf die Konzentration von Zellwandvorstufen in *Proteus mirabilis* und dessen L-Phase. Arch. Mikrobiol. **50**, 282 (1965).
POHLAND, A.: 3-Isoxazolidones, derivatives and process. U.S. Patent 2,762,815 (September 11, 1956).
POLYANOVSKII, O. L., and Y. M. TORCHINSKII: Effect of cycloserine and of related substances on the activity of pig-heart aspartate-glutamate transaminase and alanine-glutamic transaminase. Doklady Akad. Nauk S.S.S.R. **141**, 488 (1961).
PLATTNER, PL. A., A. BOLLER, H. FRICK, A. FÜRST, B. HEGEDÜS, H. KIRCHENSTEINER, ST. MAJNONI, R. SCHLÄPFER u. H. SPIEGELBERG: Synthesen des 4-Amino-3-isoxazolidinons (Cycloserin) und einiger Analoga. Helv. Chim. Acta **40**, 1531 (1957).
RATOUIS, R., and R. BEHAR: Synthesis of 4-amino-3-isoxazolidinone. Bull. soc. chim. France **1957**, 1255.
REITZ, R., H. D. SLADE, and F. C. NEUHAUS: On the biochemical basis of D-cycloserine resistance. Federation Proc. Abstracts **25**, 344 (1966).
ROBSON, J. M., and F. M. SULLIVAN: Antituberculosis drugs. Pharmacol. Rev. **15**, 195 (1963).
ROGERS, H. J., and A. J. GARRETT: The interrelationship between mucopeptide and ribitol teichoic acid formation as shown by the effect of inhibitors. Biochem. J. **96**, 231 (1965).
ROZE, U.: The non-enzymatic reaction between cycloserine and pyridoxal phosphate. Ph. D. Thesis, submitted to the graduate school of Washington University, St. Louis Missouri 1964.
ROZE, U., and J. L. STROMINGER: The non-enzymatic reaction between D-cycloserine and pyridoxal phosphate. Federation Proc. Abstracts **22**, 423 (1963).
ROZE, U., and J. L. STROMINGER: Alanine racemase from *Staphylococcus aureus:* Conformation of its substrates and its inhibitor; D-cycloserine. J. Mol. Pharmacol. **2**, 92 (1966).
RUNGE, W. F.: Process of producing acetyl cycloserine. U.S. Patent 2,815,348 (December 3, 1957).
RUSSELL, W. F. Jr., and G. MIDDLEBROOK: Chemotherapy of tuberculosis. Springfield (Ill.): Ch. C. Thomas 1961.
SAITO, M., N. ISHIMOTO, and E. ITO: Uridine diphosphate N-acetylamino sugar derivatives in penicillin-treated *Staphylococcus aureus*. J. Biochemistry (Tokyo) **54**, 273 (1963).
SALGARELLO, G., and E. TURRI: Antibacterial activity of optical isomers of cycloserine. Action on *Mycobacterium tuberculosis*. Boll. soc. ital. biol. sper. **34**, 1538 (1958); cited from Chem. Abstr. **55**, 14583 (1961).
SALTON, M. R. J.: The anatomy of the bacterial surface. Bacteriol. Rev. **25**, 77 (1961).
SALTON, M. R. J.: The Bacterial Cell Wall, p. 107. Amsterdam: Elsevier Publ. Co. 1964.
SAUKKONEN, J., and P. VIRKOLA: Acid-soluble nucleotides of *Staphylococcus aureus*. Ann. Med. Exptl. et Biol. Fenniae (Helsinki) **41**, 220 (1963).

SEREMBE, M.: Antituberculous action of levorotatory and dextrorotatory cycloserine and of some synthetic intermediates. Minerva med. **1957**, 3548; cited from Chem. Abstr. **52**, 18837 (1958).

SHOCKMAN, G. D.: Reversal of cycloserine inhibition by D-alanine. Proc. Soc. Exptl. Biol. Med. **101**, 693 (1959).

SHOCKMAN, G. D., and J. O. LAMPEN: Inhibition by antibiotics of the growth of bacterial and yeast protoplasts. J. Bacteriol. **84**, 508 (1962).

SHULL, G. M., and J. L. SARDINAS: PA-94, an antibiotic identical with D-4-amino-3-isoxazolidinone (cycloserine, oxamycin). Antibiotics & Chemotherapy **5**, 398 (1955).

SHULL, G. M., J. B. ROUTIEN, and A. C. FINLAY: Cycloserine and production there of. U.S. Patent 2, 773, 878 (December 11, 1956).

SKINNER, C. G., T. J. MCCORD, J. M. RAVEL, and W. SHIVE: O-Carbamyl-L-serine, an inhibitory analog of L-glutamine. J. Am. Chem. Soc. **78**, 2412 (1955).

SMITH, J. L., and E. D. WEINBERG: Mechanisms of antibacterial action of bacitracin. J. Gen. Microbiol. **28**, 559 (1962).

SMRT, J., J. BERANEK, J. SICHER, and F. SORM: Synthesa 4-amino-3-isoxazolidinonu (cykloserinu). Chem. listy **51**, 112 (1957a).

SMRT, J., J. BERANEK, J. SICHER, J. SKODA, V. F. HESS, and F. SORM: Synthesis of L-4-amino-3-isoxazolidinone, the unnatural stereoisomer of cycloserine and its antibiotic activity. Experientia **13**, 291 (1957b).

SNOW, G. A.: Structure of mycobactin. Biochem. J. **97**, 166 (1965).

STAMMER, C. H.: Beta-Aminoxy-D-alanine. J. Org. Chem. **27**, 2957 (1962).

STAMMER, C. H., and J. D. MCKINNEY: Cycloserine. III. A schiff base and its reactions. J. Org. Chem. **30**, 3436 (1965).

STAMMER, C. H., A. N. WILSON, C. F. SPENCER, F. W. BACHELOR, F. W. HOLLY, and K. FOLKERS: Synthesis of D-4-amino-3-isoxazolidone. J. Am. Chem. Soc. **79**, 3236 (1957).

STAMMER, C. H., A. N. WILSON, F. W. HOLLY, and K. FOLKERS: Synthesis of D-4-amino-3-isoxazolidone. J. Am. Chem. Soc. **77**, 2346 (1955).

STEENKEN, W. JR., and E. WOLINSKY: Cycloserine: Antituberculous activity *in vitro* and in the experimental animal. Am. Rev. Tuberc. Pulmonary Diseases **73**, 539 (1956).

STROMINGER, J. L.: Biosynthesis of bacterial cell walls. Federation Proc. **21**, 134 (1962).

STROMINGER, J. L., R. H. THRENN, and S. S. SCOTT: Oxamycin, a competitive antagonist of the incorporation of D-alanine into a uridine nucleotide in *Staphylococcus aureus*. J. Am. Chem. Soc. **81**, 3803 (1959).

STROMINGER, J. L., E. ITO, and R. H. THRENN: Competitive inhibition of enzymatic reactions by oxamycin. J. Am. Chem. Soc. **82**, 998 (1960).

STROMINGER, J. L., J. T. PARK, and R. E. THOMPSON: Composition of the cell wall of *Staphylococcus aureus*: Its relation to the mechanism of action of penicillin. J. Biol. Chem. **234**, 3263 (1959).

STRUVE, W. G., and F. C. NEUHAUS: Evidence for an initial acceptor of UDP-NAc-muramyl-pentapeptide in the synthesis of bacterial mucopeptide. Biochem. Biophys. Research Commun. **18**, 6 (1965).

STRUVE, W. G., R. K. SINHA, and F. C. NEUHAUS: On the initial stage in peptidoglycan synthesis. Phospho-N-acetyl-muramyl-pentapeptide translocase (uridine monophosphate). Biochemistry **5**, 82 (1966).

SUTTON, W. B., and L. STANFIELD: The reversal of cycloserine inhibition by mycobactin, a growth factor for mycobacteria. Antibiotics & Chemotherapy **5**, 582 (1955).

TANAKA, N.: Mechanism of action of O-carbamyl-D-serine, a new member of cell wall synthesis inhibitors. Biochem. Biophys. Research Commun. **12**, 68 (1963).

TANAKA, N., and K. SASHIKATA: Biogenesis of D-4-amino-3-isoxazolidone and O-carbamyl-D-serine. J. Gen Appl. Microbiol. **9**, 409 (1963).

TANAKA, N., K. SASHIKATA, T. WADA, S. SUGAWARA, and H. UMEZAWA: Mechanism of action of O-carbamyl-D-serine. J. Antibiotics, Ser. A **16**, 217 (1963).

TANAKA, N., and H. UMEZAWA: Synergism of D-4-amino-3-isoxazolidone and O-carbamyl-D-serine. J. Antibiotics, Ser. A **17**, 8 (1964).

TOENNIES, G., and G. D. SHOCKMAN: Growth chemistry of *Streptococcus faecalis*. Proceedings of the fourth internat. Congr. of Biochemistry, vol. 13, p. 365. London: Pergamon Press 1959.

TRIVELLATO, E.: Stereoisomers of cycloserine. II. Activity against *Escherichia coli* in synthetic media. Arch. intern. pharmacodynamie **117**, 317 (1958).

TRIVELLATO, E., and C. CONCILIO: Stereoisomers of cycloserine. I. Bacteriostatic activity towards some microorganisms. Arch. intern. pharmacodynamie **117**, 313 (1958); cited from Chem. Abstr. **53**, 12392 (1959).

VIALLIER, J., and R. M. CAYRÉ: Bacilles tuberculeus résistants à la cyclosérine. Compt. rend. soc. biol. **152**, 776 (1958).

VYSHEPAN, E. D., K. I. IVANOVA, and A. M. CHERNUKH: Inhibition of glutamic-pyruvic transaminase. Byull. Eksptl. Biol. Med. **52**, 76 (1961).

VYSHEPAN, E. D., K. I. IVANOVA, and A. M. CHERNUKH: The effect of D,L-cycloserine on the process of transamination. Byull. Eksptl. Biol. Med. **47**, 52 (1959).

WEINBERG, E. D.: The mutual effects of antimicrobial compounds and metallic cations. Bacteriol. Rev. **21**, 46 (1957).

WISHNOW, R. M., J. L. STROMINGER, C. H. BIRGE, and R. H. THRENN: Biochemical effects of novobiocin on *Staphylococcus aureus*. J. Bacteriol. **89**, 1117 (1965).

WOOD, W. A., and I. C. GUNSALUS: D-Alanine formation: A racemase in *Streptococcus faecalis*. J. Biol. Chem. **190**, 403 (1951).

YAMADA, K., S. SAWAKI, and S. HAYAMI: Inhibitory effect of cycloserine on some enzymic activities related to vitamin B_6. J. Vitaminol. (Osaka) **3**, 68 (1957).

YOUMANS, G. P., and A. S. YOUMANS: Experimental chemotherapy of tuberculosis and other mycobacterial infections. In: R. J. SCHNITZER and F. HAWKING (editors), Experimental Chemotherapy, vol. II, p. 393. New York: Academic Press 1964.

ZYGMUNT, W. A.: Reversal of D-cycloserine inhibition of bacterial growth by alanine. J. Bacteriol. **84**, 154 (1962).

ZYGMUNT, W. A.: Antagonism of D-cycloserine inhibition of mycobacterial growth by D-alanine. J. Bacteriol. **85**, 1217 (1963).

Ristocetin

D. C. Jordan

Ristocetin is a fermentation product of *Nocardia lurida* (GRUNDY *et al.*, 1957). The commercial preparation of this antibiotic, *Spontin*, is a mixture of two closely related components, designated ristocetin A (>90%) and ristocetin B. Although these two ristocetins have the same antimicrobial spectrum and exhibit no major differences in infrared or ultraviolet absorption spectra, optical rotation or elemental analysis, they can be separated by paper strip electrophoresis and paper chromatography. Their isolation, crystallization and chemical properties have been described by PHILIP, SCHENCK and HARGIE (1957). The compounds are amphoteric, can be isolated as free bases and crystallized as sulphates, are soluble in acidic aqueous solutions, are less soluble in neutral aqueous solutions and are generally insoluble in organic solvents. They are very stable in aqueous acidic solutions and although there is no significant alteration in activity over a medium pH of 5.0 to 7.0 there is a rapid loss of activity above a pH of 7.5.

Both ristocetin A and B contain amino and phenolic groups but whereas ristocetin A contains 4 moles of mannose and 2 moles each of glucose, D-arabinose and rhamnose, ristocetin B contains 1 mole of D-arabinose and 2 moles each of mannose, glucose and rhamnose (PHILIP *et al.*, 1961). Measurements of the freezing point depressions of the free bases in aqueous solution suggest a molecular weight of about 2500, although ultracentrifugal studies suggest a value of approximately 5000 (PHILIP, SCHENCK and HARGIE, 1957).

Microbiological assays for ristocetin have been described by GIROLAMI (1963) and ŘEHÁČEK (1961).

Ristocetin is specific for Gram-positive bacteria and mycobacteria (GRUNDY, SINCLAIR *et al.*, 1957) (Table 1). It is inactive against Gram-negative bacteria, yeasts, filamentous fungi and protozoa. Although it is active against streptococci it has little effect against *Leuconostoc mesenteroides* and at least 2 strains of *Lactobacillus*. The tendency of staphylococci to develop resistance to this antibiotic is low (FAIRBROTHER and WILLIAMS, 1958). Ristocetin B is 3 to 4 times more active than ristocetin A on streptococci (PHILIP, SCHENCK and HARGIE, 1957) and about 2 to 3 times more effective in protecting mice infected with *Staphylococcus*, *Streptococcus* and *Diplococcus* (GRUNDY, SINCLAIR *et al.*, 1957). Little or no therapeutic effect of ristocetin has been noted with mouse tuberculosis.

When ristocetin A and B are hydrolyzed with acid the sugars and an amino fragment are split off and the activities against sensitive Gram-positive bacteria are increased up to 30-fold (PHILIP *et al.*, 1961). These degradation products were found not to retain cross-resistance properties with the parent ristocetins against a strain of *Staphylococcus aureus* made resistant to ristocetin A.

In studies on the natural bacterial resistance to ristocetin, GRUNDY, ALFORD and their co-workers (1957) reported that none of 400 clinically-isolated cultures

Table 1. *Sensitivity of various microorganisms to ristocetin*

Culture	Minimum inhibitory concentration (μg/ml)
Actinomyces bovis	2
Bacillus subtilis	0.5
Clostridium perfringens	0.25
Clostridium tetani	0.5
Corynebacterium pseudodiphtheriticum	0.125
Diplococcus pneumoniae	2
Mycobacterium tuberculosis	2
Staphylococcus aureus	4—8
Streptococcus pyogenes	0.5—1

Adapted from GRUNDY, SINCLAIR *et al.* (1957).

of streptococci, staphylococci or pneumococci were resistant. Serial transfer did not readily result in resistance, although two strains of staphylococci were made 100-fold resistant to ristocetin A and a third strain was made 16-fold resistant to ristocetin B. This resistance was acquired in a step-wise fashion with no greater than a 2-fold increase in resistance in any one transfer step. Complete cross resistance was noted between both antibiotics.

Clinically, ristocetin (*Spontin*) has proven successful in the treatment of severe staphylococcal infections, such as sepsis and pneumonia, in children (DRIES and KOCH, 1960). In one such study 7.6% of the 76 patients treated developed severe toxic reactions such as leukopenia and/or neutropenia and these reactions were related to dosage and length of therapy. The commonest change in the peripheral blood count was a mild eosinophilia.

Short-term therapy with ristocetin appears to be a good choice for enterococcal endocarditis (ROMANSKY *et al.*, 1961) and although the side effects include skin rash, drug fever, mild phlebitis and transient leukopenia, the latter two symptoms can be diminished by rapid administration of a daily dose of 25—50 mg in a small volume of solution. The combination of ristocetin and polymyxin B appears excellent for the prevention of peritoneal and wound infections following surgery (SYLVESTER, OLANDER and HUTCHINGS, 1963).

Aside from the possible occurrence of undesirable side effects one other disadvantage to the clinical use of ristocetin is that it must be administered intravenously (FAIRBROTHER and WILLIAM, 1958).

Ristocetin has a pronounced bactericidal activity, the minimum inhibitory concentration (M.I.C.) for staphylococci frequently being the same concentration at which bactericidal activity occurs (GRUNDY, ALFORD *et al.*, 1957). This is not true for all susceptible bacteria, however, for with *M. tuberculosis* the bactericidal concentration is about 4 times the M.I.C. The bactericidal activity is not restricted entirely to the more rapidly dividing cells, as in the case of penicillin and certain other antibiotics.

During an investigation of the mechanism of action of ristocetin WALLAS and STROMINGER (1963) studied the activity of Spontin, pure ristocetin A and B, and partial hydrolysis products of each of these pure substances on uridine nucleotide accumulation and cell wall synthesis in *Staphylococcus aureus*, strain Copenhagen.

They found that accumulation of uridine diphosphate-acetylamino sugar compounds (thought to be cell wall precursors) occurred immediately upon addition of all five ristocetin preparations and reached a maximum in 120 minutes (Fig. 1). The minimum concentration for such accumulation was similar to the minimum growth-inhibiting concentration so that the observed effects appear to represent a primary effect of ristocetin action.

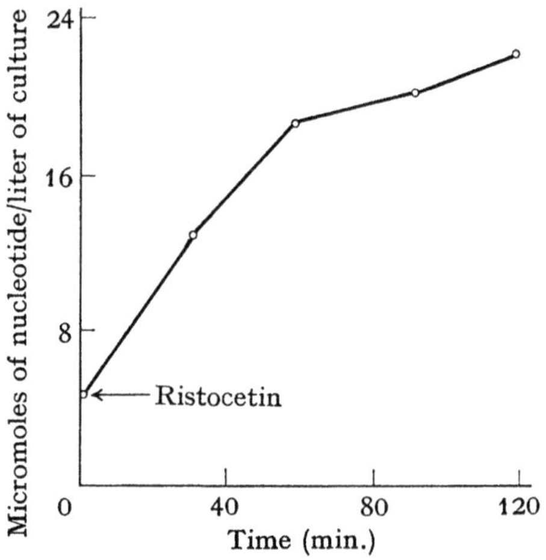

Fig. 1. Rate of nucleotide accumulation in *Staphylococcus aureus* upon the addition of ristocetin (150 μg/ml) at zero time (WALLAS and STROMINGER, 1963)

When the nucleotides were extracted from the cells with trichloroacetic acid and subjected to paper chromatography the pattern of accumulation was similar to that observed when staphylococci were treated with penicillin (STROMINGER, 1962). One prominent compound which accumulated when ristocetin was used was found to be a mixture of uridine diphosphate-N-acetylmuramic acid (UDP-MurNAc) and UDP-MurNAc.L-alanine, while another principal compound was UDP-MurNAc.L-alanine.D-glutamic acid.L-lysine.D-alanine.D-alanine. All three of these nucleotides increase in amount during penicillin treatment of staphylococci (PARK, 1952a—c) and this suggests that ristocetin and penicillin cause inhibition of the synthesis of the cell wall of Gram-positive bacteria. This has been substantiated by the finding that ristocetin causes a 95% inhibition in the incorporation of lysine-^{14}C and inorganic ^{32}P into the staphylococcal cell wall under conditions where little or no inhibition is noted in protein or nucleic acid synthesis (Table 2).

As an inhibitor of cell wall production ristocetin is similar, not only to penicillin, but also to vancomycin, bacitracin, novobiocin and oxamycin. However, because of the extreme complexity of the mechanism of wall synthesis, and because there is no apparent pattern of cross resistance among these antibacterial substances it is unlikely that they act at identical lci. Some support for this view is provided by the work of MEADOW, ANDERSON and STROMINGER (1964) with respect to enzyme systems possibly concerned in wall mucopeptide synthesis. It was reported that ristocetin, like vancomycin, could cause a 50% inhibition in the polymerization of a UDP-MurNAc-peptide and UDP-N-acetylglucosamine (UDP-GlcNAc) by a particulate fraction from *S. aureus*, whereas very large amounts of penicillin

Table 2. *Effect of spontin (ristocetin A and B) on isotope incorporation into several cell fractions of Staphylococcus aureus, var. Copenhagan*

	Cell wall		Trichloroacetic acid precipitates of soluble cell contents (protein and nucleic acids)	
	P^{32}-phosphate	C^{14}-lysine	P^{32}-phosphate	C^{14}-lysine
Control	180,000	16,900	41,600	3,480
+ Spontin, 150 μg/ml	4,180	692	42,200	3,075
% Inhibition	98	97	0	11

Values given are in counts/minutes/mg wall peptide or protein. Adapted from WALLAS and STROMINGER (1963).

and bacitracin were required for the same effect. STRUVE and NEUHAUS (1965), using the same assay procedure, confirmed the result with ristocetin but found, using a different assay system, that this antibiotic (at a level of 50 and 500 μg/ml of reaction mixture) enhanced the incorporation of UDP-MurNAc-pentapeptide-^{14}C into an incompletely defined perchloric acid precipitable fraction. Although vancomycin behaved similarly at the lower concentration it inhibited incorporation at the higher concentration. Although these results have yet to be resolved, of particular interest was the suggestion by these two workers that wall mucopeptide is synthesized in two steps, namely:

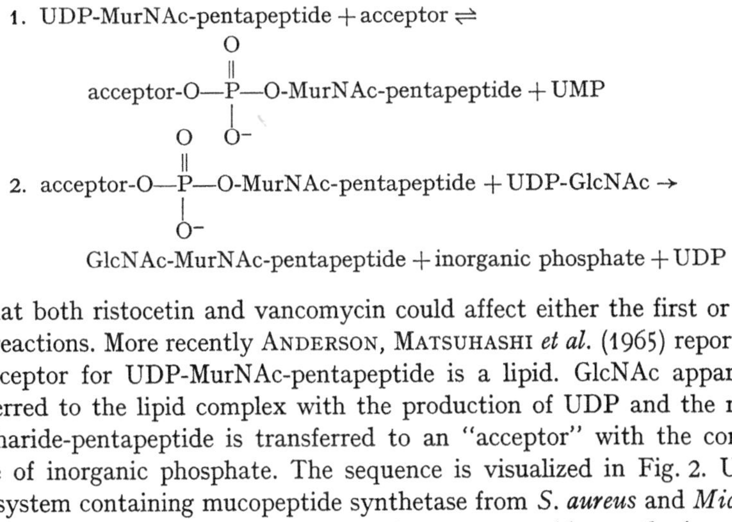

and that both ristocetin and vancomycin could affect either the first or both of these reactions. More recently ANDERSON, MATSUHASHI *et al.* (1965) reported that the acceptor for UDP-MurNAc-pentapeptide is a lipid. GlcNAc apparently is transferred to the lipid complex with the production of UDP and the resulting disaccharide-pentapeptide is transferred to an "acceptor" with the concurrent release of inorganic phosphate. The sequence is visualized in Fig. 2. Using an assay system containing mucopeptide synthetase from *S. aureus* and *Micrococcus lysodeikticus* these investigators found that mucopeptide synthesis was 50% inhibited at a concentration of ristocetin and vancomycin which caused a similar inhibition in the growth of these cells. In addition, at concentrations of these antibiotics which completely prevented growth, there was a rapid accumulation of both types of lipid intermediate (see Fig. 2). Further data revealed that ristocetin (Table 3) and vancomycin specifically prevented the utilization, but not the synthesis, of the second lipid-precursor (lipid-phosphodisaccharide-pentapeptide). Since both of these antibacterial compounds appear to be "glycopeptides" they may, via structural analogue inhibition, block the activity of the

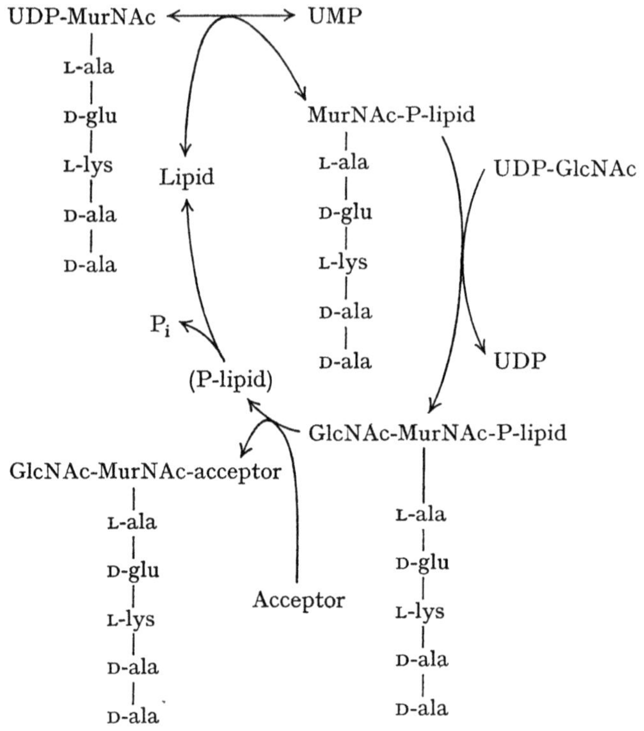

Fig. 2. Scheme for mucopeptide synthesis as proposed by ANDERSON, MATSUHASHI *et al.* (1965), using enzymes from *Staphylococcus aureus* and *Micrococcus lysodeikticus*

natural mucopeptide acceptor (ANDERSON, MATSUHASHI *et al.*, 1965). Nevertheless, since the lipid component may be involved in the passage of the phospho-disaccharide-pentapeptide precursor across the plasma membrane the inhibition by ristocetin and vancomycin of the utilization of this precursor could be manifested in any one of many different ways. Even the binding of these antibiotics near the wall sites where active wall synthesis is occurring might be sufficient to stop

Table 3. *Effect of ristocetin on the utilization of the particle-bound*[1] *intermediate GlcNAc-MurNAc(-pentapeptide)-P-lipid for mucopeptide synthesis*

Additions	Intermediate prepared in			
	Absence of ristocetin		Presence of ristocetin	
	Mucopeptide μμ moles	Δ	Mucopeptide μμ moles	Δ
Zero-time control	41	—	4	—
No Addition	84	43	33	29
UDP-GlcNAc	83	42	32	28
UDP-MurNAc-pentapeptide	87	46	48	44
Ristocetin	48	7	7	3

[1] The particulate enzyme employed was obtained from *Micrococcus lysodeikticus.* See ANDERSON, MATSUHASHI *et al.* (1965) for experimental details.

the utilization of precursors and allow their accumulation. The binding of ristocetin to isolated cell walls of *Bacillus subtilis* has been observed by BEST and DURHAM (1965). However, the exact mechanism by which ristocetin acts is still obscure and will remain so until further details of wall synthesis are unravelled.

References

ANDERSON, J. S., M. MATSUHASHI, M. A. HASKIN, and J. L. STROMINGER: Lipid-phosphoacetylmuramyl-pentapeptide and lipid-phosphodisaccharide-pentapeptide: presumed membrane transport intermediates in cell wall synthesis. Proc. Natl. Acad. Sci. US **53**, 881 (1965).

BEST, G. K., and N. N. DURHAM: Adsorption of the ristocetins to *Bacillus subtilis* cell walls. Abstracts of papers presented at the IVth International Congress of Chemotherapy, Washington, D.C., p. 86, 1965.

DRIES, C. P., and R. KOCH: Clinical evaluation of ristocetin in children. A preliminary report. Amer. J. Diseases Children **99**, 752 (1960).

FAIRBROTHER, R. W., and B. L. WILLIAMS: In vitro activity of ristocetin and framycetin, two new antibiotics. Lancet **1958 II**, 1353.

GIROLAMI, R. L.: Ristocetin: In: F. KAVANAGH (ed.), Analytical microbiology, p. 353. New York: Academic Press, Inc. 1963.

GRUNDY, W. E., E. F. ALFORD, E. J. RDZOK, and J. C. SYLVESTER: Ristocetin, the development of resistance and bactericidal activity. Antibiotics Ann. **1956/57**, 693 (1957).

GRUNDY, W. E., A. C. SINCLAIR, R. J. THERIAULT, A. M. GOLDSTEIN, C. J. RICKLER, H. B. WARREN, JR., T. J. OLIVER, and J. C. SYLVESTER: Ristocetin, microbiological properties. Antibiotics Ann. **1956/57**, 687 (1957).

MEADOW, P. M., J. S. ANDERSON, and J. L. STROMINGER: Enzymatic polymerization of UDP-acetylmuramyl.L-ala.D-glu.L-lys.D-ala.D-ala and UDP-acetylglucosamine by a particulate enzyme from *Staphylococcus aureus* and its inhibition by antibiotics. Biochem. Biophys. Research Commun. **14**, 382 (1964).

PARK, J. T.: Uridine-5-pyrophosphate derivatives. I. Isolation from *Staphylococcus aureus*. J. Biol. Chem. **194**, 877 (1952a).

PARK, J. T.: Uridine-5-pyrophosphate derivatives. II. A structure common to three derivatives. J. Biol. Chem. **194**, 885 (1952b).

PARK, J. T.: Uridine-5-pyrophosphate compounds. III. Amino acid-containing derivatives. J. Biol. Chem. **194**, 897 (1952c).

PHILIP, J. E., J. R. SCHENCK, and M. P. HARGIE: Ristocetins A and B, two new antibiotics. Isolation and properties. Antibiotics Ann. **1956/57**, 699 (1957).

PHILIP, J. E., J. R. SCHENCK, M. P. HARGIE, J. C. HOLDER, and W. E. GRUNDY: The increased activity of ristocetins A and B following acid hydrolysis. Antimicrobial Agents Ann., p. 10 (1961).

ŘEHÁČEK, Z.: Quantitative determination of ristocetin by a microbiological diffusion method. Folia Microbial. **6**, 22 (1961).

ROMANSKY, M. J., C. W. FOULKE, R. A. OLSSON, and J. R. HOLMES: Ristocetin in bacterial endocarditis. An evaluation of short-term therapy. Arch. Internal Med. **107**, 480 (1961).

STROMINGER, J. L.: Biosynthesis of bacterial cell walls. In: I. C. GUNSALUS and R. Y. STANIER (eds.), The bacteria, vol. III, p. 413. New York: Academic Press Inc. 1962.

STRUVE, W. G., and F. C. NEUHAUS: Evidence for an initial acceptor of UDP-NAc-muramyl-pentapeptide in the synthesis of bacterial mucopeptide. Biochem. Biophys. Research Commun. **18**, 6 (1965).

SYLVESTER, J. C., G. A. OLANDER, and V. Z. HUTCHINGS: Intra- and extraperitoneal administration of ristocetin and polymyxin B. Antimicrobial Agents and Chemotherapy 1962, p. 526 (1963).

WALLAS, C. H., and J. L. STROMINGER: Ristocetins, inhibitors of cell wall synthesis in *Staphylococcus aureus*. J. Biol. Chem. **238**, 2264 (1963).

Bacitracin

Eugene D. Weinberg

Bacitracin is produced by strains of *Bacillus licheniformis*. The commercial product contains a main component, bacitracin A (Fig. 1), and at least nine additional closely related polypeptides (REGNA, 1959). In neutral or slightly alkaline solution, bacitracin A is slowly transformed into bacitracin F (Fig. 2) (REGNA, 1959) which has very little antibacterial activity (HICKEY, 1964).

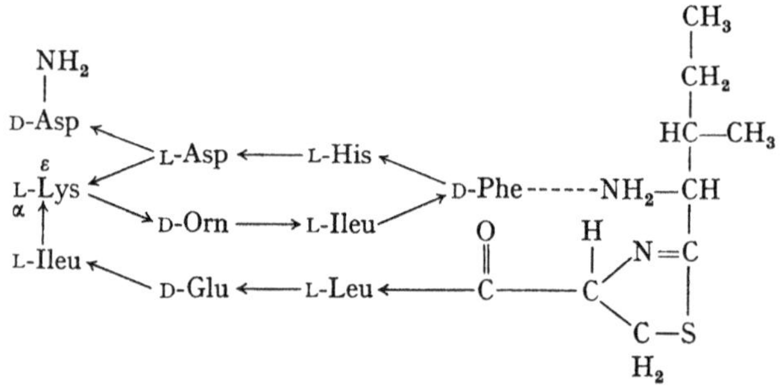

Fig. 1. Probable structural formula of bacitracin A (REGNA, 1959). → Signifies a C—N bond

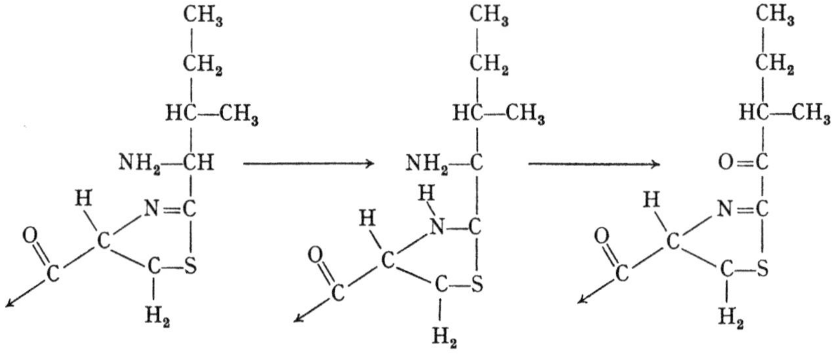

Fig. 2. Transformation of bacitracin A to bacitracin F (REGNA, 1959)

Bacitracin A is highly inhibitory towards growth of many gram positive bacterial genera but, except for *Neisseria*, has little effect on gram negative microorganisms (HICKEY, 1964). Minimal inhibitory concentrations are generally between 0.01 and 2.0 units per ml (JAWETZ, 1961); inasmuch as commercial products contain approximately 55 units per mg; the active concentrations are between 0.18 and 36 μg/ml.

As with other antibiotics, susceptibility of specific microbial strains to bacitracin can be determined only by experimental testing; nevertheless, a generalization that is of considerable diagnostic use is that most strains of group A streptococci are more sensitive to the drug than are strains of all other streptococcal groups. In the original study (MAXTED, 1953) of this phenomenon, 98,3% of 2,386 sensitive strains belonged to group A and, of 851 resistant strains, only 2.5% were members of group A. In subsequent studies, comparable results have been obtained; for example, PETRAN (1961) obtained agreement between sensitivity to discs containing 0.36 μg of bacitracin and group A classification as determined by immunofluorescence in 98% of 439 cultures of hemolytic streptococci.

The development of resistance to bacitracin *in vitro* by serial transfer of bacteria in the presence of sub-inhibitory concentrations of the drug has been studied with *Staphylococcus aureus* (STONE, 1949) and hemolytic streptococci (GEZON *et al.*, 1950). Resistance arose irregularly during approximately 40 transfers and reverted rapidly when the resistant strains were subcultured in the absence of the drug. Resistant bacteria of normally susceptible species are rarely encountered in clinical infections (JAWETZ, 1961); no resistant staphylococci were found in hundreds of cases of burns treated with bacitracin (LOWBURY, 1960). Fortunately, resistance neither emerges readily in infections for which the drug is employed, nor is there cross-resistance between bacitracin and other antimicrobial compounds in either *in vitro* (SZYBALSKI and BRYSON, 1952) or *in vivo* (JAWETZ, 1961) situations.

Bacitracin is well tolerated in topical applications and in instillation directly into joint spaces, pleural cavities, surgical wounds, mucous membranes, ears, eyes, and brain tissue (JAWETZ, 1961; HICKEY, 1964). When administered intramuscularly, however, the drug is excreted via the urinary tract. In the latter case, such nephrotoxic symptoms as proteinuria and hematuria are sometimes observed; if kidney damage does occur, it is not necessarily serious or permanent. However, when the drug is given parenterally for more than three days, continuous laboratory tests for nitrogen retention and the development of uremic poisoning are mandatory. Especially in patients with poor kidney function, bacitracin may accumulate in the excretory organs to cause irreversible damage (JAWETZ, 1961).

Similarly, the principal toxic effect in mice, dogs, and monkeys is associated with damage to kidney tissue (JAWETZ, 1961). The degree, type, and reversibility of the damage varies considerably, not only with individual subjects, but also with the particular sample of bacitracin employed (JAWETZ, 1961). As bacitracin purification procedures have improved and products with more antibacterial potency have become available, reports of satisfactory parenteral use have increased (HICKEY, 1964). Although bacitracin A and F are nearly equally nephrotoxic, if the ratio of A to F could be significantly increased, the improved product would necessarily be less toxic on an activity basis (HICKEY, 1964).

One other possible reason for variation in the amount of nephrotoxicity that develops in various subjects might be a consequence of the considerable fluctuation in content of Cd^{+2} of kidneys. The metallic ion is virtually absent from the human newborn kidney but accumulates in this organ up to the sixth decade of life at which time it begins to decline (SCHROEDER and BALASSA, 1961). The range in adult humans is from 150 to 8000 μg/gm tissue ash (TIPTON and COOK, 1963; TIPTON *et al.*, 1965). Bacitracin forms a fairly stable complex with Cd^{+2}; in fact, the stability constant is approximately 10^4 higher than the constants for the Cd^{+2} complexes of most amino acids (WEINBERG, 1965). It would be of interest to determine if the quantity of bacitracin retained by various kidneys is a function of the content of Cd^{+2} in such tissue.

Mechanisms of Antibacterial Action

Biochemical lesions induced in gram positive bacteria by minimal inhibitory concentrations of bacitracin can result in three distinct manifestations. These consist of interference with protein synthesis, cell wall synthesis, and cell membrane function.

Table. 1. *Suppression by antibiotics of protein synthesis in Staphylococcus aureus*

Test system	Percent suppression	Increase in quantity of drug needed to inhibit test system over that needed to prevent growth	Reference
Synthesis of cell protein	50	penicillin 20,000 X	GALE and FOLKES, 1953
	50	bacitracin 10—20 X	
	50	chloramphenicol 0.2—0.4 X	
Synthesis of induced β-galactosidase	75	penicillin 200 X	GALE and FOLKES, 1955
	80	bacitracin 0.1—0.2 X	
	95	chloramphenicol 1.0—2.0 X	
Synthesis of induced β-galactosidase	73	penicillin 100 X	CREASER, 1955
	100	bacitracin 3.3 X	
	98	chloramphenicol 1.0 X	
Synthesis of induced β-galactosidase	50	penicillin >400 X	SMITH and WEINBERG, 1962
	50	bacitracin 0.9 X	
	50	chloramphenicol 4.0 X	
Synthesis of induced mannitol dehydrogenase	50	penicillin >400 X	SMITH and WEINBERG, 1962
	50	bacitracin 1.8 X	
	50	chloramphenicol 5.5 X	

The type of injury first investigated was that of suppression of protein synthesis (GALE and FOLKES, 1953, 1955; CREASER, 1955; SMITH and WEINBERG, 1962). It may be noted in Table 1 that minimal antibacterial quantities of bacitracin, as well as of chloramphenicol, can inhibit formation of cell protein and of induced enzymes. Penicillin, on the other hand, is active only in amounts far in excess of those needed to prevent cell multiplication. Sub-bacteriostatic concentrations of a group of six antibiotics that inhibit protein synthesis (bacitracin, chloramphenicol, streptomycin, a macrolide, and two tetracyclines) were tested for ability to suppress formation of α-hemolysin by *S. aureus;* of the group, bacitracin is the most effective (HINTON and ORR, 1960). In contrast, bacitracin is the least effective of this group in ability to prevent synthesis of M protein by *Streptococcus pyogenes* (Brock, 1963). Furthermore, it may be seen in Table 2 that, in contrast to tetracycline, bacitracin is unable to suppress incorporation by *S. aureus* of lysine into cell protein. However, in the system summarized in Table 2, chloramphenicol likewise was found to be inactive (Park, 1961).

Table 2. *Suppression by antibiotics of protein and cell wall synthesis in Staphylococcus aureus* (modified from Park, 1961)

Antibiotic	μg/ml	Percent inhibition of lysine incorporation into		Percent change from control in accumulation of uridine-nucleotide-linked precursors of mucopeptide (control = 100)
		protein	mucopeptide	
Penicillin	5.0	0	77.2	800
Bacitracin	50.0	0	94.0	1180
Chloramphenicol	50.0	0	4.0	80
Tetracycline	50.0	87.5	4.0	40

The type of injury next examined was that of suppression of cell wall synthesis. Multiplying cells of *S. aureus* in the early logarithmic phase of growth are induced to lyse by either bacitracin or penicillin but not by chloramphenicol (Abraham and Newton, 1958; Smith and Weinberg, 1962). Like penicillin, bacitracin inhibits incorporation of lysine into mucopeptide whereas both tetracycline and chloramphenicol do not (Mandelstam and Rogers, 1959; Park, 1961). Moreover, penicillin and bacitracin but not tetracycline and chloramphenicol cause uridine nucleotide-linked precursors of mucopeptide to be excreted into the medium. Some of these results are summarized in Table 2. Like tetracycline, however, and in contrast to penicillin, bacitracin is unable to suppress the peptide cross-linking reaction in cell wall mucopeptide synthesis (Wise and Park, 1965). Moreover, bacitracin is not as effective in inhibiting cell wall glycopeptide synthetase as are vancomycin and ristocetin (Anderson *et al.*, 1965).

It soon became apparent that suppression of neither protein synthesis nor cell wall synthesis could be the primary site of antibacterial action of bacitracin (Smith and Weinberg, 1962). As noted above, minimal inhibitory concentrations of the antibiotic are *not always* capable of inhibiting protein synthesis. Moreover, if interference with cell wall synthesis were the primary manifestation of bacitracin action, one would expect the drug to induce the formation of protoplasts and L forms. Of five groups of investigators who have reported attempts to demonstrate this (Ward *et al.*, 1958; Smith and Weinberg, 1962; Williams, 1963; Molander *et al.*, 1964; Rotta *et al.*, 1965), only the last group has been successful. A sixth group (Krawitt and Ward, 1963) obtained protoplasts but not L forms.

Furthermore, protoplasts and L forms obtained either by lysozyme or by penicillin often are as sensitive to the antibacterial action of bacitracin as are the intact parent cells (Ward *et al.*, 1958; Shockman and Lampen, 1962; Williams, 1963; Hancock and Fitz-James, 1964; Snoke and Cornell, 1965). However, in some instances L forms of streptococcal (Ward *et al.*, 1958; Rotta *et al.*, 1965) and of staphylococcal (Williams, 1963; Molander *et al.*, 1964) strains are more resistant than the parent cells. In these cases, the increase in resistance to bacitracin is less than one hundred fold whereas to penicillin the increase is greater than ten thousand fold.

That bacitracin interferes with cell membrane function was first suggested by observations that minimal inhibitory concentrations of the drug, as well as such surfactant germicides as cetyltrimethylammonium bromide (CTAB), stimulate the uptake of tetrazolium dyes (SMITH and WEINBERG, 1962) and the release of ninhydrin-complexing materials (HELMS and WEINBERG, 1963). In these systems, penicillin and chloramphenicol are each inert. Bacitracin is not quite so active as CTAB nor does it possess so much surfactant acitivity. The surface tension of water, for example, is lowered from the normal value at 25 C of 72 dynes per cm to 34,2 dynes per cm by a 0.1 % aqueous solution of CTAB but to only 45.1 dynes per cm by a similar solution of bacitracin (HELMS and WEINBERG, 1963).

Additional evidence that bacitracin alters the permeability function of the cell membrane was provided by HANCOCK and FITZ-JAMES (1964). These investigators observed that concentrations of bacitracin and of penicillin within the range of those needed to inhibit mucopeptide synthesis enhance the efflux of K^{+1} from growing cells of *B. megaterium*. Bacitracin-enhanced leakage of K^{+1} could be either a secondary result of membrane damage subsequent to lesions in the supporting cell wall or a primary result of disruption of the cell membrane by the drug. To differentiate between these two possibilities, chloramphenicol and hypertonic solutions of sucrose were employed in subsequent experiments. Chloramphenicol would be expected to prevent the differential increase of cell protein relative to cell wall, and the sucrose solution would provide osmotic support to replace the mechanical protection provided by the wall. Both the chloramphenicol and sucrose treatments would therefore be expected to prevent penicillin-enhanced K^{+1} efflux; if bacitracin has a primary action on cell membranes, however, neither treatment should alter bacitracin-enhanced leakage and these were the results actually obtained (Table 3). HANCOCK and FITZ-JAMES (1964) noted also that bacitracin causes protoplasts of *B. megaterium* to lyse and this observation has been confirmed by SNOKE and CORNELL (1965) who used protoplasts of *B. licheniformis* and *Micrococcus lysodeikticus*.

Table 3. *Efflux of K^{+1} from Bacillus megaterium exposed to antibiotics* (modified from HANCOCK and FITZ-JAMES, 1964)

Antibiotic	Percent reduction in cellular K^{+1} after 15 minutes		
	Control medium	Medium plus 100 μg/ml chloramphenicol	Medium plus 0.3 M sucrose
None	54	54	65
Penicillin (60 μg/ml)	77	57	65
Bacitracin (30 μg/ml)	84	91	82

The most logical hypothesis, therefore, is that the primary lesion induced in sensitive cells by bacitracin is associated with disruption of the integrity of the cytoplasmic membrane. Effects on the synthesis of proteins and cell walls (in those systems in which such effects have been demonstrated) are undoubtedly sequelae of the loss of membrane functions. It is not at all surprising that bacitracin, a typical member of a large group of polypeptide antibiotics produced by species of *Bacillus*, should have an antibacterial mechanism of action similar to that of polymyxin, tyrocidine, and gramicidin.

Metal Binding Properties of Bacitracin

The majority of the presently known antimicrobial compounds of both synthetic and natural origin possess one or more molecular sites at which metal binding can occur (WEINBERG, 1957). Often, various biological activities of the substances are enhanced by, or may have an absolute requirement for, an appropriate amount of a specific metallic ion (ALBERT, 1958; FOYE, 1961; WEINBERG, 1961, 1964, 1965). That bacitracin forms complexes with metallic ions became apparent in early studies in which the antibiotic was observed to be altered by specific cations in such characteristics as solubility (ANKER *et al.*, 1948), stability to heat and prolonged storage (GROSS, 1954), taste and color (HODGE and LAFFERTY, 1957), and antibacterial activity (WEINBERG, 1959).

Applications of these effects were quickly forthcoming. For example, a method of extraction of the antibiotic from an aqueous concentrate derived from the fermentation medium employs the addition of Zn^{+2} at pH 7.0. The precipitate of Zn^{+2}-bacitracin is then removed and dissolved at pH 4.0 and the Zn^{+2} is exchanged for H^{+1} by means of cation exchange resins (ZINN and CHORNOCK, 1958). Bacitracin, itself, as well as some of its metal complexes, has a very bitter taste. On the other hand, Zn^{+2}-bacitracin is relatively tasteless and is therefore acceptable for use in tablets or troches to be dissolved in the oral cavity (HODGE and LAFFERTY, 1957). Complexes of bacitracin with Zn^{+2} (CHORNOCK, 1957), Ni^{+2} (ZORN, 1959), Mn^{+2} (ZORN *et al.*, 1961), and Co^{+2} (ZORN, 1962), as well as with ZnO and CdO (ZIFFER and CAIRNEY, 1962), are more stable at a variety of temperatures than is the antibiotic itself (Tables 4 and 5). In contrast, at pH 8.4, Cu^{+2} inactivates the antibiotic possibly by catalyzing the oxidation of the sulfur atom (SHARP *et al.*, 1949).

Potentiometric titration showed that bacitracin forms complexes with metallic ions (GARBUTT *et al.*, 1961); the order of ability of the ions to complex with the drug is $Cu^{+2} > Ni^{+2} > (Co^{+2}, Zn^{+2}) > Mn^{+2}$. Each of the first four cations combines with a group in bacitracin that titrates between pH 5.5 and 7.5, and Mn^{+2} combines with the antibiotic above pH 7.2. Histidine forms complexes with Cu^{+2}, Ni^{+2}, Co^{+2}, and Zn^{+2} between pH 5.0 and 7.5; in both bacitracin and histidine, complexes with Cu^{+2} but not Zn^{+2} result in a shift in the ultraviolet absorption maximum to longer wave lengths. Thus, GARBUTT *et al.* (1961) have postulated that the group in bacitracin with which Cu^{+2}, Ni^{+2}, Co^{+2}, and Zn^{+2} combines between pH 5.5 and 7.5 is probably the imidazole ring of histidine, whereas the site at which Mn^{+2} is complexed is possibly a free amino group (Fig. 1).

Attachment to the α-amino group of the terminal isoleucine residue by the metallic ions that stabilize the molecule (i.e., Zn^{+2}, Cd^{+2}, Ni^{+2}, Co^{+2}, Mn^{+2}) might retard conversion of bacitracin A to the inactive 'F' form (GARBUTT *et al.*, 1961).

Table 4. *Stability of bacitracin in feed stored for three months* (modified from CHORNOCK, 1957)

	25 C Relative humidity			40 C Relative humidity		
	30%	60%	80%	30%	60%	80%
Bacitracin	98[1]	71	23	72	27	—
Zn^{+2}-bacitracin	104	92	79	96	66	49

[1] Percent of activity of original sample.

Table 5. *Stability of bacitracin stored at 99 C* (modified from ZORN *et al.*, 1961)

	1 hr	2 hr	3 hr
Bacitracin	19.4[2]	9.4	5.1
Mn^{+2}-bacitracin	84.8	68.9	61.1

[2] Percen t of activity of original sample.

The nitrogen atom of the thiazoline ring could participate with the aforementioned α-amino group in binding the metallic ion (Dr. JOHN N. ARONSON, personal communication) (Fig. 3).

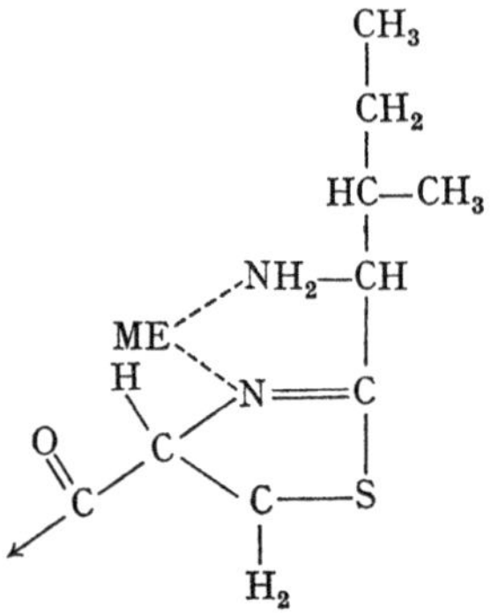

Fig. 3. Possible site of metal-binding by bacitracin (JOHN N. ARONSON, personal communication)

The content of Zn^{+2} in Zn^{+2}-bacitracin varies between 4.3 and 7.0% (GROSS, 1954); the lower limit indicates that one atom of Zn^{+2} combines with one molecule of drug. Additional quantities of Zn^{+2} in preparations containing up to 7.0% would represent one-half atom per molecule and would indicate a second site of attachment in which the metallic ion might link two adjacent molecules. Clearly, additional work is needed to establish the actual sites of binding of the metallic ions to the drug and the alteration in molecular structure that ensues.

Ions of the three elements of group IIB of the Periodic Table (Zn^{+2}, Cd^{+2}, Hg^{+2}) strongly enhance the antibacterial action of bacitracin *in vitro;* 18 other metallic ions were found to be inactive (WEINBERG, 1959). In the absence of added cations, the drug undoubtedly utilizes ions (most probably Zn^{+2}) in the culture media inasmuch as such metal binding agents as ethylene-diaminetetraacetic acid (EDTA) and cyclohexanediaminetetraacetic acid (CDTA) markedly reduce its antibacterial potency (WEINBERG, 1959). The quantity of metallic ion required for significant activation of bacitracin is in the order of 0.5×10^{-5} M; a complex medium such as nutrient agar contains approximately this much Zn^{+2} but less than 15% of this concentration of Mn^{+2} and less than 2% of this quantity of Cd^{+2} (WEINBERG, 1965). There exists a difference of 770 fold in dose of the drug required to inhibit *S. aureus* in nutrient agar (at pH 7.0) that contains added 10^{-4} M Zn^{+2} versus nutrient agar that contains added 10^{-4} M EDTA (Table 6) (WEINBERG, 1959, 1965).

Table 6. *Effect of Zn^{+2} or EDTA on bacitracin activity at different pH reactions against Staphylococcus aureus* (modified from WEINBERG, 1965)

pH of nutrient agar	MIC of bacitracin ($\times 10^{-5}$ M) in nutrient agar enriched with			Difference in activity of drug between Zn^{+2} and EDTA-enriched media
	10^{-4}M Zn^{+2}	neither Zn^{+2} nor EDTA	10^{-4}M EDTA	
6.0	0.14	2.3	100	714-fold
7.0	0.026	1.0	20	770-fold
8.0	0.021	0.7	2.5	124-fold

ADLER and SNOKE (1962) confirmed the observation that EDTA suppresses and that Zn^{+2} and Cd^{+2} enhance the activity of bacitracin; in addition, Mn^{+2} was found to increase the potency of the drug. The latter cation is most active at pH reactions above 7.0 (WEINBERG, 1965) and this finding complements the potentiometric titration data (GARBUTT *et al.*, 1961) in which bacitracin was observed to complex with Mn^{+2} at pH reactions above 7.2. Rapid lysis of protoplasts of *B. licheniformis* and *M. lysodeikticus* by bacitracin requires either Zn^{+2} or Cd^{+2} (SNOKE and CORNELL, 1965); Mn^{+2} was found to be inactive in this system even though the pH of the incubation mixture was 8.5.

Unfortunately, the majority of investigators who have examined the mechanisms of antibacterial action of bacitracin have failed to adjust the concentrations of Zn^{+2}, Cd^{+2}, or Mn^{+2} in their assay systems and, in most cases, did not report the quantities of these cations that might be present. It is probable that in some instances the concentrations of useful cations were insufficient for optimal performance of the antibiotic. In at least one study (BROCK, 1963), the investigator noted that the ability of the drug to inhibit growth was tested in a much more complicated medium than that used for the synthesis of protein; the former would be expected to contain more Zn^{+2} and Mn^{+2} than the latter.

The biological activity of a considerable variety of synthetic and naturally occurring antimicrobial compounds have been reported to be enhanced by Cd^{+2}; of these, more than half are potentiated also by Zn^{+2} (WEINBERG, 1964). In contrast, suppression of many antimicrobial substances is achieved by cations of group IIA of the Periodic Table (especially Mg^{+2} and Ca^{+2}). The ions of group IIB (Zn^{+2} and Cd^{+2}) are often found to be biological antagonists of those of group IIA; it is possible that the former interfere with the ability of the latter to maintain the integrity of cell membranes and other surface structures. Alteration of the integrity of cell membranes could result in increased accessibility of sensitive intracellular sites to antimicrobial compounds. In the case of bacitracin, however, the enhancing metallic ions most probably act simply by stabilizing the drug molecules in a structural configuration that is ideal not only for efficiency of antibacterial action, but also for ability to withstand destruction.

Because bacitracin forms water-insoluble complexes with each of the five cations studied by GARBUTT *et al.* (1961), it is not possible to calculate stability constants from the potentiometric titration data. However, by means of a biological method, the stability constants for Zn^{+2}, Cd^{+2}, and Mn^{+2} have been found to be approximately 14, 12.5, and 11, respectively (WEINBERG, 1965). In this method, the antibacterial activity of the drug is determined at pH 6.0, 7.0, and 8.0 in the presence of each of the three cations both with and without each of 15 metal-binding agents whose stability constants for the three metallic ions are known. The method is based on the assumption that ligands with stability constants greater than those of the antibiotic can depress its antibacterial action whereas those whose constants are below those of bacitracin have no effect on the drug.

Of special interest is ethylenebis (oxyethylenenitrilo) tetraacetic acid (EBONTA; EGTA) whose constant for Zn^{+2} is 12.8 and for Cd^{+2} is 15.6 (normally, the constants for Zn^{+2} are either higher or similar to those for Cd^{+2}). This ligand depresses bacitracin activity when the antibiotic is dependent on Cd^{+2} but not when it is dependent on Zn^{+2} (WEINBERG, 1965). Apparently, EBONTA can compete successfully with bacitracin for Cd^{+2} but not for Zn^{+2}.

The growth-promoting activity of 28 non-antimicrobial ligands for turkey poults on a Zn^{+2}-deficient diet containing soybean protein depends on the Zn^{+2} stability constants of the compounds; those ligands with Zn^{+2} constants close to 14 possess highest activity (VOHRA and KRATZER, 1964). For effectiveness, the chelating agent must have a stronger stability constant than the Zn^{+2}-binding agents in the feed and a weaker constant than the Zn^{+2}-transporting chelating system in the tissues of the birds. Inasmuch as the stability constant of bacitracin for Zn^{+2} is approximately 14, it is possible that the antibiotic stimulates growth in a manner similar to that of the active ligands examined by VOHRA and KRATZER (1964).

The ingestion of a typical low level dose (11 µg/gm) of bacitracin in poultry feed results in concentrations between 32 and 54 µg/ml in the intestine and cecum (BARE *et al.*, 1965). Such low quantities would not be expected to alter the gram negative bacterial flora. Therefore, it is possible that growth stimulation by low level doses of bacitracin would occur in both contaminated and germ-free birds and mammals when diets are employed that are either low in Zn^{+2} and/or high in ligands (e.g., those in soybean protein) that interfere with normal assimilation of Zn^{+2}.

Summary

Bacitracin, a polypeptide synthesized by *Bacillus licheniformis*, is highly active against gram positive bacteria. Inasmuch as resistance does not develop readily, the antibiotic has medicinal usefulness; because of potential renal toxicity, however, bacitracin is generally restricted to non-systemic applications. Three distinct chemical manifestations of the antibacterial action of bacitracin have been observed: a) suppression of protein synthesis, b) suppression of cell wall synthesis, and c) interference with cell membrane function. The first two of these manifestations are considered to be sequels of the third. The known and suspected roles of Zn^{+2}, Cd^{+2}, and Mn^{+2} in stability, antibacterial action, nutritional action, and toxicity of bacitracin are described.

Acknowledgment. This work was supported in part by research grant AI-06268-01 from the National Institute of Allergy and Infectious Diseases, U.S. Public Health Service.

References

ABRAHAM, E. P., and G. G. F. NEWTON: Structure and function of some sulfur containing peptides. In: CIBA foundation symposium on amino acids and peptides with antimetabolic activity, p. 205. London: J. & A. Churchill Ltd. 1958.

ADLER, R. H., and J. E. SNOKE: Requirement of divalent metal ions for bacitracin activity. J. Bacteriol. **83**, 1315 (1962).

ALBERT, A.: Metal-binding agents in chemotherapy: the activation of metals by chelation. In: The strategy of chemotherapy, p. 112. Cambridge: Cambridge University Press 1958.

ANDERSON, J. S., M. MATSUHASHI, M. A. HASKIN, and J. L. STROMINGER: Lipid-phosphoacetylmuramylpentapeptide and lipid-phosphodisaccharide-pentapeptide: presumed membrane transport intermediates in cell wall synthesis. Proc. Natl. Acad. Sci. U.S. **53**, 881 (1965).

ANKER, H. S., B. A. JOHNSON, J. GOLDBERG, and F. L. MELENEY: Bacitracin: methods of production, concentration, and partial purification, with a summary of the chemical properties of crude bacitracin. J. Bacteriol. **55**, 249 (1948).

BARE, L. N., R. F. WISEMAN, and O. J. ABBOTT: Levels of antibiotics in the intestinal tract of chicks fed bacitracin and penicillin. Poultry Sci. **44**, 489 (1965).

BROCK, T. D.: Effect of antibiotics and inhibitors on M protein synthesis. J. Bacteriol. **85**, 527 (1963).

CHORNOCK, F. W.: Zinc bacitracin feed supplement. U.S. Patent 2, 809, 892 (1957).

CREASER, E. H.: The induced (adaptive) biosynthesis of β-galactosidase in *Staphylococcus aureus*. J. Gen. Microbiol. **12**, 288 (1955).

FOYE, W. A.: Role of metal-binding in the biological activities of drugs. J. Pharmaceut. Sci. **50**, 93 (1961).

GALE, E. F., and J. P. FOLKES: The assimilation of amino acids by bacteria. 15. Actions of antibiotics on nucleic acid and protein synthesis in *Staphylococcus aureus*. Biochem. J. **53**, 493 (1953).

GALE, E. F., and J. P. FOLKES: The assimilation of amino acids by bacteria. 21. The effect of nucleic acids on the development of certain enzymatic activities in disrupted staphylococcal cells. Biochem. J. **59**, 675 (1955).

GARBUTT, J. T., A. L. MOREHOUSE, and A. M. HANSON: Metal binding properties of bacitracin. J. Agr. Food Chem. **9**, 285 (1961).

GEZON, H. M., D. M. FASAN, and G. R. COLLINS: Antibiotic studies on beta hemolytic streptococci. VII. Acquired in vitro resistance to bacitracin. Proc. Soc. Exptl. Biol. Med. **74**, 505 (1950).

GROSS, H. M.: Zinc bacitracin in pharmaceutical preparations. Drug & Cosmetic Ind. **75**, 612 (1954).

HANCOCK, R., and P. C. FITZ-JAMES: Some differences in the action of penicillin, bacitracin, and vancomycin on *Bacillus megaterium*. J. Bacteriol. **87**, 1044 (1964).

HELMS, V., and E. D. WEINBERG: Mechanism of antibacterial action of N^1,N^5-di-(3,4-dichlorobenzyl)-biguanide. In: Antimicrobial Agents and Chemotherapy 1962, p. 241. Ann Arbor (Mich.): Amer. Soc. Microbiol. 1963.

HICKEY, R. J.: Bacitracin, its manufacture and uses. Progr. Ind. Microbiol. **5**, 95 (1964).

HINTON, N. A., and J. H. ORR: The effect of antibiotics on the toxin production of *Staphylococcus aureus*. Antibiotics & Chemotherapy **10**, 758 (1960).
HODGE, E. B., and G. J. LAFFERTY: Zinc bacitracin-containing troche. U.S. Patent 2,803,584 (1957).
JAWETZ, E.: Polymyxin, colistin, and bacitracin. Pediat. Clin. North Am. **8**, 1057 (1961).
KRAWITT, E. L., and J. R. WARD: L phase variants related to antibiotic inhibition of cell wall biosynthesis. Proc. Soc. Exptl. Biol. Med. **114**, 629 (1963).
LOWBURY, E. J. L.: Clinical problems of drug-resistant pathogens. Brit. Med. Bull. **16**, 73 (1960).
MANDELSTAM, J., and H. J. ROGERS: The incorporation of amino acids into the cell-wall mucopeptide of staphylococci and the effect of antibiotics on the process. Biochem. J. **72**, 654 (1959).
MAXTED, W. R.: The use of bacitracin for identifying group A haemolytic streptococci. J. Clin. Pathol. **6**, 224 (1953).
MOLANDER, C. W., B. M. KAGAN, H. J. WEINBERGER, E. M. HEIMLICH, and R. J. BUSSER: Induction by antibiotics and comparative sensitivity of L-phase variants of *Staphylococcus aureus*. J. Bacteriol. **88**, 591 (1964).
PARK, J. T.: Inhibition of synthesis of bacterial mucopeptide or protein by certain antibiotics and its possible significance for microbiology and medicine. In: Antimicrobial Agents Ann. 1960, p. 338. New York: Plenum Press 1961.
PETRAN, E. I.: Comparison of the fluorescent antibody and the bacitracin disk methods for identification of group A streptococci. Amer. J. Clin. Pathol. **41**, 224 (1961).
REGNA, P. P.: The chemistry of antibiotics. In: Antibiotics; their chemistry and non-medical uses, p. 58. New York: D. van Nostrand Co., Inc. 1959.
ROTTA, J., W. W. KARAKAWA, and R. M. KRAUSE: Isolation of L forms from group A streptococci exposed to bacitracin. J. Bacteriol. **89**, 1581 (1965).
SCHROEDER, H. A., and J. J. BALASSA: Abnormal trace metals in man: cadmium. J. Chronic Diseases **14**, 236 (1961).
SHARP, V. E., A. ARRIAGADA, G. G. F. NEWTON, and E. P. ABRAHAM: Ayfivin: extraction, purification, and chemical properties. Brit. J. Exptl. Pathol. **30**, 444 (1949).
SHOCKMAN, G. D., and J. O. LAMPEN: Inhibition by antibiotics of the growth of bacterial and yeast protoplasts. J. Bacteriol. **84**, 508 (1962).
SMITH, J. L., and E. D. WEINBERG: Mechanisms of antibacterial action of bacitracin. J. Gen. Microbiol. **28**, 559 (1962).
SNOKE, J. E., and N. CORNELL: Protoplast lysis and inhibition of growth of *Bacillus licheniformis* by bacitracin. J. Bacteriol. **89**, 415 (1965).
STONE, J. L.: Induced resistance to bacitracin in cultures of *Staphylococcus aureus*. J. Infectious Diseases **85**, 91 (1949).
SZYBALSKI, W., and V. BRYSON: Genetic studies on microbial cross resistance to toxic agents. 1. Cross resistance of *Escherichia coli* to fifteen antibiotics. I. Bacteriol. **64**, 489 (1952).
TIPTON, I. H., and M. J. COOK: Trace elements in human tissue. Part II. Adult subjects from the United States. Health Physics **9**, 103 (1963).
TIPTON, I. H., H. A. SCHROEDER, H. M. PERRY jr., and M. J. COOK: Trace elements in human tissue. Part III. Subjects from Africa, the Near and Far East, and Europe. Health Physics **11**, 403 (1965).
VOHRA, P., and F. H. KRATZER: Influence of various chelating agents on the availability of zinc. J. Nutrition **82**, 249 (1964).
WARD, J. R., S. MADOFF, and L. DIENES: In vitro sensitivity of some bacteria, their L forms and pleuropneumonia-like organisms to antibiotics. Proc. Soc. Exptl. Biol. Med. **97**, 132 (1958).
WEINBERG, E. D.: The mutual effects of antimicrobial compounds and metallic cations Bacteriol. Rev. **21**, 46 (1957).

WEINBERG, E. D.: Enhancement of bacitracin by the metallic ions of group IIB. In: Antibiotics Annual 1958/59, 924. New York (N.Y.): Medical Encyclopedia, Inc. 1959.
WEINBERG, E. D.: Known and suspected roles of metal coordination in actions of antimicrobial drugs. Federation Proc. **20** (Suppl. 10), 132 (1961).
WEINBERG, E. D.: Antibacterial action of polyamines in presence of trace metals: enhancement by cadmium. In: Antimicrobial Agents and Chemotherapy 1963, 573. Ann Arbor (Mich.): Amer. Soc. Microbiol. 1964.
WEINBERG, E. D.: Microbiological method for estimation of stability constants of bacitracin complexes of zinc, cadmium, and manganese. In: Antimicrobial Agents and Chemotherapy 1964, 120. Ann Arbor (Mich.): Amer. Soc. Microbiol. 1965.
WILLIAMS, R. E. O.: L forms of *Staphylococcus aureus*. J. Gen. Microbiol. **33**, 325 (1963).
WISE, E. M., and J. T. PARK: Penicillin: its basic site of action as an inhibitor of a peptide cross-linking reaction in cell wall mucopeptide synthesis. Proc. Natl. Acad. Sci. U.S. **54**, 75 (1965).
ZIFFER, J., and T. J. CAIRNEY: Bacitracin composition as feed additive. U.S. Patent 3,025,216 (1962).
ZINN, E., and F. W. CHORNOCK: Production of bacitracin. U.S. Patent 2,834,711 (1958).
ZORN, R. A.: Stabilization of bacitracin. U.S. Patent 2,903,357 (1959).
ZORN, R. A.: Bacitracin product. U.S. Patent 3,021,217 (1962).
ZORN, R. A., R. C. MALZAHN, and A. M. HANSON: Bacitracin. U.S. Patent 2,985,534 (1961).

Vancomycin

D. C. Jordan and P. E. Reynolds

The antibiotic, vancomycin, was isolated in the Eli Lilly Company laboratories from a *Streptomyces* species found in soil obtained in Borneo and India. This organism, which is also found in domestic soils, has been described by PITTENGER and BRIGHAM (1956), who the named it *Streptomyces orientalis*. The hydrochloride of this antibiotic bears the trade name Vancocin.

The chemical properties of vancomycin hydrochloride have been reported by McCORMICK *et al.* (1956), NISHIMURA *et al.* (1957) and HIGGINS *et al.* (1958). It is a white, acid-stable solid, very soluble in water, moderately soluble in aqueous methanol and insoluble in higher alcohols, ether and acetone. It is a complex amphoteric compound, containing about 7% nitrogen and 16—17% carbohydrate, has an apparent molecular weight of 3200—3500 ± 200 and shows an ultraviolet maximum at 282 mμ in acid, shifting to 305 mμ in alkali. It is resistant to a variety of hydrolytic enzymes and although it is reasonably stable in 2% glycine buffers within the pH range 3 to 5 (providing the temperature is kept low, 5° C) it shows marked instability at 37° C.

The chelating properties of vancomycin have been employed in a purification method (MARSHALL, 1965) based on the formation of a copper complex. Analysis of vancomycin regenerated from this complex has yielded a tentative formula of $C_{148}H_{185}Cl_4N_{21}O_{56}$. Removal of a glucose residue leads to the formation of an aglucovancomycin which still retains about 75% of the biological activity of the unaltered antibiotic. Upon mild hydrolysis vancomycin is converted into a crystalline substance (CDP-1) with the tentative formula $C_{83}H_{185}Cl_2N_{10}O_{32-33}$. The yield of CDP-1 corresponds to 93% of the initial weight of the vancomycin molecule although from the molecular weight and chlorine content CDP-1 appears to be slightly more than one half of the vancomycin molecule. This suggests that vancomycin contains two CDP-1 units. Table 1 summarizes the data on the structural components of vancomycin comprising about one half of the molecule, although the nature of most of the N-containing portions are as yet unknown. MARSHALL (1965) suggests that this antibiotic may be made up of repeating units, perhaps linked through the glucose and amino acid units. Of some interest was the finding that acylation of the N-methylleucine residue results in a marked decrease (about 25%) in the antibacterial activity of the vancomycin molecule and suggests that this amino acid plays a role in the antibiotic's mechanism of action.

Vancomycin is a narrow-spectrum antibiotic active against gram-positive bacteria and some spirochetes (McCORMICK *et al.*, 1956; FAIRBROTHER and

Table 1. *Components of part of the vancomycin molecule*

Component	Number of residues	Number of C atoms
Glucose	2	12
Aspartic acid	2	8
N-methylleucine	1	7
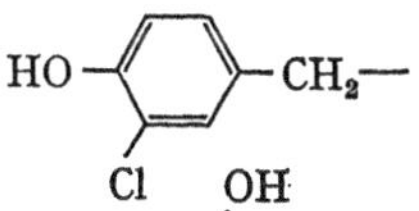	4	28
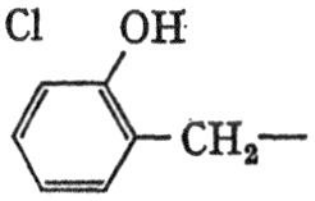	1	7
$C_2H_5COCH(CH_3)—CH_2COOH$[1]	1	7

[1] The 3-methyl-4-ketohexanoic acid is included as a component but may arise during acid treatment, perhaps from an unusual sugar — adapted from MARSHALL (1965).

WILLIAM, 1956; ZIEGLER *et al.*, 1956) and its biological activity is shown in Table 2. The outstanding potency of this antibiotic against staphylococci has been reported by a large number of workers, including WAISBREN and STRELITZER (1958), SCHNEIERSON and AMSTERDAM (1957), KIRBY and DIVELBISS (1957), DAIKOS *et al.* (1960) and JORDAN and INNISS (1962). Of particular significance is the fact that the development of staphylococal resistance and cross-resistance to vancomycin is considerably less than that observed with most other antibiotics (ZIEGLER, WOLFE and MCGUIRE, 1956; GARROD and WATERWORTH, 1956; GRIFFITH and PECK, 1956; GERACI *et al.*, 1957; KIRBY, 1963). Microbiological assays for vancomycin have been described by KAVANAGH (1963).

Table 2. *Biological activity of vancomycin*

Organism	Minimum inhibitory concentration (μg/ml)
Streptococcus pyogenes	0.15—2.5
Staphylococcus aureus[2]	0.15—>10
Diplococcus pneumoniae	0.29
Corynebacterium diphtheriae	0.8
Streptococcus faecalis	0.31—2.5
Sarcina lutea	0.4—1.6
Leptospira pomona	1.0

[2] Strains resistant to penicillin, erythromycin or streptomycin are inhibited by 0.4—1.6 μg/ml.

Microorganisms insensitive to 100 μg/ml include *Mycobacterium tuberculosis, Pseudomonas aeruginosa, Proteus vulgaris, Escherichia coli,* most *Shigella* and *Salmonella* species, filamentous fungi, and yeasts. At a concentration of 50 μg/ml vancomycin does not protect HeLa cells against the effects of vaccinia or herpes simplex virus (GERACI *et al.*, 1957).

Both acute and chronic toxicity tests in mice, rats, guinea pigs, dogs and monkeys show vancomycin to have a low order of toxicity with little or no effect on respiration, blood pressure, electrocardiogram, urinary flow, intestinal motility or the isolated ileum of experimental animals (ANDERSON *et al.*, 1957; LEE and ANDERSON, 1962). Intravenous acute toxicity tests in mice indicate an LD_{50} dose of 400—500 mg/kg while daily oral doses of 1000 mg/kg and subcutaneous doses of 100 mg/kg are tolerated and produce no abnormalities upon necropsy. Tissue culture tests show little toxicity in comparison with other clinically-used antibiotics (McCORMICK *et al.*, 1956).

Since there is little absorption of vancomycin from the gastrointestinal tract (LEE *et al.*, 1957) and since intramuscular injection causes mild to moderate pain, clinical administration of this antibiotic is limited to the intravenous route. In man intravenous doses of 50—100 mg yield serum levels of 0.5—2.0 μg/ml within 2—6 hr with high urine concentrations in 24 hr. Doses of this size, given every 6—8 hr for periods up to 7 days are well tolerated (GRIFFITH and PECK, 1956). However, side effects of vancomycin therapy can occur (KIRBY and DIVELBISS, 1957) and include local tissue irritation, drug fever and renal irritation. In the presence of impaired renal function, unnecessarily high blood levels of vancomycin (about 100 μg/ml) may damage the eight cranial nerve and cause tinnitus or deafness (GERACI *et al.*, 1958) making it necessary to institute a system of serial serum assays to ensure keeping the serum level at a safe therapeutic dose of 10 μg/ml (DUTTON and ELMES, 1959).

Vancomycin is used clinically mainly for severe staphylococcal infections, especially when the responsible organism is resistant to the more commonly used antibiotics or when a bactericidal drug is desirable, as with patients whose normal defense mechanisms are defective. Good clinical responses to vancomycin therapy have been observed in cases of pneumococcal pneumonia, streptococcal pharyngitis and erysipelas (GRIFFITH and PECK, 1956) and it would appear to be the antibiotic of choice in the treatment of staphylococcal ileocolitis, in which case it should be administered orally (GERACI *et al.*, 1957). Further clinical data have been presented by KIRBY, PERRY and LANE (1959), EHRENKRANZ (1959), LOURIA, KAMINSKI and BUCHANAN (1961) and KIRBY (1963).

Non-clinical uses of vancomycin include its employment for the prevention of certain plant diseases (MEHTA *et al.*, 1959; BOYLE and PRICE, 1963) and its incorporation into media for the selective isolation of *Veillonella* (ROGOSA *et al.*, 1958), *Fusobacterium*, and *Leptospira* (McCARTHY and SNYDER, 1963).

Mode of Action

When the concentration of vancomycin is plotted against the growth response of *Staphylococcus aureus* an unusually steep dose-response curve results (McCORMICK *et al.*, 1956) where, after a certain critical point, small increments in antibiotic concentration cause large increases in growth inhibition. The phenomenon was investigated by ZIEGLER *et al.* (1956) who found that the activity of vancomycin against both a beta hemolytic streptococcus and a strain of staphylococcus was characterized by an immediate bactericidal action without any preceding lag phase. It is this rapid bactericidal action of vancomycin (also observed by

GERACI *et al.*, 1957) which probably accounts for the slow development of bacterial resistance toward it.

Vancomycin does not kill resting staphylococci at either 5° C or 37° C and dye reduction studies show that it inhibits neither glucose oxidation by such cells (ZIEGLER *et al.*, 1956) nor the dehydrogenation of ethyl alcohol, sodium lactate and sodium malate (INNISS, 1959). On the other hand, REYNOLDS (1964b) has found that cultures of *S. aureus*, after pretreatment with vancomycin at 0° followed by removal of free vancomycin, are no longer able to grow and divide, or to synthesize the inducible enzyme β-galactosidase; furthermore, they accumulate uridine N-acetylmuramyl-peptides. Recovery of cells that have been treated with vancomycin under these conditions takes a number of hours.

In an initial report, JORDAN and INNISS (1959) indicated that vancomycin caused an inhibition of RNA synthesis in growing cells of *S. aureus* prior to any observed inhibition of DNA or protein synthesis. However, further work demonstrated that, although the synthesis of protein as determined by the Folin-Ciocalteu reagent was unaffected by vancomycin, there was a blockage in the incorporation of certain radioactive amino acids into an internal "bound form" which remained in the cell after removal of the pool constituents and nucleic acid. This suggested that there was an interference in the synthesis of a polypeptide such as the cell-wall mucopeptide, devoid of aromatic amino acids. Using the procedure of PARK and HANCOCK (1960), which yields five cellular fractions, including wall mucopeptide, it was found that vancomycin, at a concentration of 83 μg/mg cell dry weight, had no early effect on the incorporation of glycine-2-^{14}C into either the ethanol soluble "protein" and lipid fraction or the trypsin-soluble protein (JORDAN, 1961; JORDAN and INNISS, 1962). In addition, using the procedure of HANAWALT (1959) it was found that vancomycin did not inhibit the incorporation of ^{32}P into RNA or DNA for 20 and 30 minutes respectively following addition of the antibiotic. There was, however, a marked depression in the rate of incorporation of radioactive glycine into the cell wall mucopeptide (Fig. 1) which was absolute within a few minutes of antibiotic addition. This inhibition, which also occurs when ^{14}C-glutamic acid or ^{14}C-lysine is substituted for ^{14}C-glycine, was found at a vancomycin level as low as 17 μg/mg cell dry weight (MALLORY, 1963). A similar observation with respect to an interference in wall mucopeptide manufacture was made simultaneously by REYNOLDS (1961), and later by BEST and DURHAM (1964) (using *Bacillus subtilis*). The lack of any early effect of vancomycin on protein synthesis was confirmed by REYNOLDS (1961) and BROCK (1963).

In addition to the data concerning the incorporation of radioactive amino acids into the cell wall mucopeptide there were several other early observations which also pointed to wall inhibition as a possible primary site of vancomycin action. First, after the addition of the antibiotic to logarithmically growing staphylococci, the total cell count becomes constant, the culture nephelos (total protoplasm) continues to increase, and the viable count decreases rapidly (JORDAN and INNISS, 1959; REYNOLDS, 1961). This would be the expected result if there was an interference in wall synthesis with a simultaneous inhibition of cell division. Second, there is an immediate accumulation of certain intracellular nucleotides (Fig. 2) when vancomycin, at a concentration very close to the minimum growth inhibitory concentration, is added to growing staphylococcal cells (REYNOLDS, 1961). Anion-exchange chromatography has resolved two hexosamine-containing substances which upon subsequent concentration and desalting were found to contain uracil. The major compound also contained alanine, glutamic acid and lysine in a 3:1:1 ratio, whereas the only amino acid present in the other compound was alanine. These substances appear identical to those compounds ("Park" compounds) which PARK and STROMINGER (1957) believe to be wall precursors,

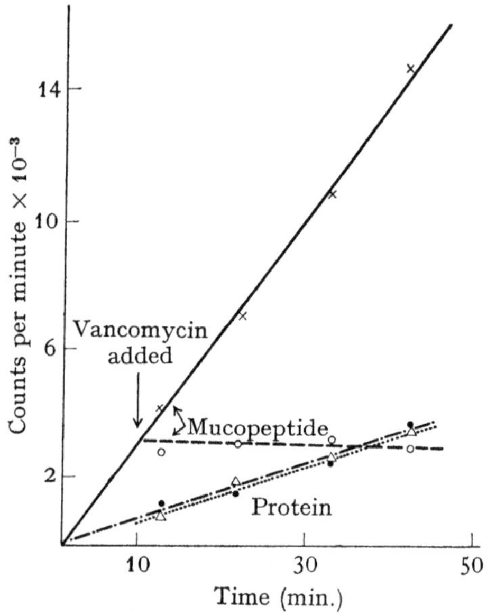

Fig. 1. The effect of vancomycin (83 μg/mg cell dry weight) on the incorporation of glycine-2-^{14}C into the trypsin-solubilized protein and cell-wall mucopeptide of *Staphylococcus aureus* (×—×, mucopeptide control; ○—○, mucopeptide plus vancomycin; △—△, protein control; ●—●, protein plus vancomycin). See JORDAN (1961) for details

and an accumulation of these nucleotides might well signify an inhibition of wall synthesis. Evidence that such nucleotides are actually wall precursors has been provided by REYNOLDS (1964a), who has shown that radioactively-labelled uridine nucleotide-peptides allowed to accumulate in the presence of vancomycin can be reutilized when treated cells are resuspended in a medium devoid of vancomycin, and that more than one half of the radioactivity is transferred to the wall without any concurrent increase in the radioactivity of the cellular protein.

It might be thought that further circumstantial evidence of altered wall synthesis is provided by the finding that in *Pseudomonas* there is a structural weakening of the cell wall formed in the presence of vancomycin, resulting in the formation of filaments and an increased fragility to sonic vibrations (DURHAM, 1963), and by the finding (RUSSELL, 1964) that this antibiotic produces spheroplasts of *Escherichia coli* in the presence of Mg^{++}. However, these are both gram-negative organisms and the concentrations of vancomycin needed to demonstrate the observed effects in each case have been extremely high (160 μg/ml for *Pseudo-*

monas and 500 to 1000 µg/ml for *E. coli*); it is difficult to evaluate such data, especially when these effects cannot be observed with *S. aureus* strains at the minimum inhibitory concentration of 0.1 to 10 µg/ml.

Other evidence for the cell wall as the primary target of vancomycin's activity include the finding (WILLIAMS, 1963; MOLANDER *et al.*, 1964) that L-phase cells of *S. aureus*, which lack the mucopeptide component of the cell wall, are either uninhibited by vancomycin or inhibited at antibiotic levels considerably greater than those necessary to kill normal cells (KAGAN *et al.*, 1964). The situation can be quite complex, and the finding by DAY and COSTILOW (1961) that vancomycin

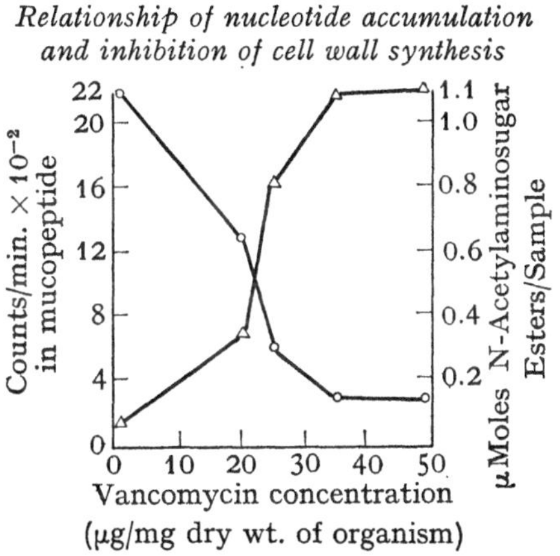

Fig. 2. The effect of vancomycin concentration on the incorporation of ^{14}C amino acids into the wall mucopeptide and on the accumulation of hexosamine-containing nucleotides (*Staphylococcus aureus*). See REYNOLDS (1961) for details. o——o, mucopeptide; Δ——Δ, N-acetylamino sugar esters

inhibits sporulation of *Clostridium botulinum* only after a lag of several hours may be related to a secondary effect of vancomycin on nucleic acid synthesis or to the time period during which a vancomycin-sensitive layer is laid down about the developing spore body.

Although the wall-inhibiting activity of vancomycin appears similar to that of certain other antibiotics such as penicillin, ristocetin, bacitracin and D-cycloserine (oxamycin), there are distinct differences among these antibiotics, which indicate that they act at different sites in the sequence of events leading to wall production. REYNOLDS (1962) found that exponentially-growing cells of *S. aureus* lost the ability to accumulate ^{14}C-labelled amino acids from the medium when treated with either penicillin or vancomycin, but, whereas the penicillin effect was prevented by molar NaCl or molar NH_4Cl, the vancomycin effect was not. With *Bacillus megaterium* KM penicillin caused a 50% conversion of the rods to spheroplasts in the presence of 10% sucrose with a simultaneous reduction in amino acid uptake, but osmotic stabilization did not protect these cells from vancomycin since the inhibition of amino acid uptake was not abolished, and the culture lysed in several hours. In addition, pretreatment of *S. aureus* and *B. megaterium* at 0 C with non-labelled penicillin or bacitracin prevented the subsequent uptake of radioactive penicillin, but similar pretreatment with vancomycin (or novobiocin) did not reduce the secondary penicillin uptake. Consequently it appears that bacitracin can compete with penicillin for a site adjacent to, or identical with, the penicillin binding site, whereas vancomycin has a different attachment point. HANCOCK and FITZ-JAMES (1964) have confirmed this lack of competition between vancomycin and penicillin for cellular binding sites although they reported that bacitracin failed to reduce penicillin binding in *B. megaterium*.

Several workers have suggested that vancomycin may only affect wall synthesis indirectly and that the plasma (cytoplasmic) membrane may represent the primary site of action. SHOCKMAN and LAMPEN (1962) examined the growth of *Streptococcus faecalis* protoplasts by a turbidimetric method and reported that although penicillin had no effect, certain other antibiotics, such as vancomycin, inhibited the growth at concentrations which also inhibited growth of intact cells. HANCOCK and FITZ-JAMES (1964) used both turbidity and ^{14}C-leucine incorporation as a measure of growth and found that vancomycin and bacitracin (in contrast to penicillin and D-cycloserine) inhibited the growth of *B. megaterium* KM protoplasts. A permeability defect was suggested as a possible mechanism of inhibition by vancomycin since, although all the antibiotics tested caused an early efflux of potassium ions from growing cells within 5 minutes of addition, the effect of penicillin was prevented by hypertonic sucrose or chloramphenicol while the effect of vancomycin (and bacitracin) was unaffected by these substances. The addition of chloramphenicol was an attempt to protect the plasma membrane from rupture as a result of a large increase in protein relative to cell wall, while the sucrose was expected to give similar protection by replacing the mechanical support normally provided by the wall.

The implication that the cell wall does not represent the only locus of vancomycin activity also was supported by YUDKIN (1963) who studied the effects of the antibiotic on the incorporation of three ^{14}C-labelled amino acids into the protein fraction, and of ^{14}C-glycerol into the lipid fraction, of plasma membranes of growing protoplasts of *B. megaterium* KM. The amino acids chosen were arginine, histidine and tyrosine since they were unlikely to be converted into other amino acids or to give rise to fatty acids. In this work vancomycin, at a concentration of 2 μg/ml, caused a decreased incorporation of the labelled compounds into the membranes which reached 75% inhibition at the end of 3 hours. However, vancomycin also caused a decrease in the incorporation of ^{14}C from all these labelled substances into the trichloroacetic acid-precipitable fraction of whole protoplasts so that there was no evidence of a selective interference of incorporation into the plasma membrane. However, samples for analysis were removed at hourly intervals, and it is impossible to tell if the rather small inhibition noted after one hr contact with vancomycin could be detected as early as the inhibition of wall mucopeptide synthesis in intact organisms (JORDAN, 1961; JORDAN and MALLORY, 1965).

In an effort to determine which of the two entities, the cell wall or the plasma membrane, was the primary locus of vancomycin action JORDAN (1965) and JORDAN and MALLORY (1965) used protoplasts of *S. aureus* prepared by the use of *Chalaropsis* B enzyme (HASH, 1962). Vancomycin at a concentration of 83 μg/mg cell dry weight caused a rapid inhibition in the incorporation of ^{14}C-amino acids and inorganic ^{32}P into the plasma membranes. The incorporation of ^{14}C-leucine was inhibited strongly within 10 minutes of antibiotic addition, while the inhibition of ^{32}P incorporation, which could not be detected prior to 1.5 minutes after vancomycin addition, was also severe but was not complete for at least 30 minutes. Since this was in contrast with the prevention of glycine uptake into the wall mucopeptide of intact cells, which became absolute in about 0.9 minutes, it seemed that wall inhibition occurred earlier than the membrane inhibition. However, such results cannot constitute conclusive evidence for the cell wall hypothesis since a minute undetected change in plasma membrane composition might result in a major change in wall manufacture.

Additional support for the idea that vancomycin has a primary effect on cell wall synthesis comes from the fact that, for a period of at least 10 minutes, the antibiotic did not prevent the synthesis of a trypsin-insoluble portion of the wall mucopeptide which is believed to be a portion of the plasma membrane. Of even more interest was the observation that when intact cells were pre-exposed to vancomycin their walls become resistant to attack by *Chalaropsis* B enzyme, and this effect was used to show that vancomycin firmly binds to the cell wall within 6—10 sec of its addition. The inability to remove the antibiotic from pre-exposed cells by washing in various buffers and the rapidity of the binding suggest that vancomycin is bound to sites in or on the wall but is not metabolically incorporated into the wall structure, while the finding that ethylenediamine tetra-acetic acid does not prevent vancomycin activity suggests that metallic ions are not essential for this binding process. The amount of antibiotic bound can be considerable since *S. aureus* can remove about 99% of the vancomycin from the growth medium when it is present at the minimum growth inhibitory concentration (REYNOLDS, unpublished data). It would seem, therefore, that vancomycin binds to the wall either at, or near, the potential sites of action of the *Chalaropsis* B enzyme. Such sites, apparently, are the glycosidic linkages between N-acetylmuramic acid or N,O-diacetylmuramic acid and N-acetylglucosamine in the wall mucopeptide (TIPPER, STROMINGER and GHUYSEN, 1964). Consequently, results obtained with protoplasts, where direct contact between antibiotic and cytoplasmic membrane is possible, may not be comparable to results obtained with intact cells where a rigid wall could prevent the influx of antibiotic molecules.

Attempts by several workers (ZIEGLER *et al.*, 1956; JORDAN and INNISS, 1962; JORDAN and MALLORY, 1965) to enhance, minimize or prevent the effect of vancomycin on growing cells of *S. aureus* by the addition of various inorganic ions, amino acids, vitamins, reducing agents and a variety of other compounds to the test medium failed to give any conclusive positive results. DURHAM (1963) found that magnesium ions (and to some extent manganous ions, L-aspartic acid and L- and D-glutamic acid) tended to reverse vancomycin action on growth of *Ps. fluorescens* after 6—12 hr. L-Alanine showed a slight reversal of inhibition at a later period (12—14 hr) but these results are rather atypical since the test organism employed required large amounts of antibiotic (MIC = 144.7 µg/ml) for inhibition. However, in a later study BEST and DURHAM (1964) reported that the inhibition of growth and mucopeptide synthesis in a strain of *B. subtilis* by vancomycin at a level of 1.3 µg/mg cell dry weight could be reduced by the addition of 4 µmoles/ml of magnesium, especially when that ion was added simultaneously with the antibiotic. This inhibition of mucopeptide production by vancomycin was studied only after the excessively long contact period of 90 minutes; nevertheless, although the low ratio of antibiotic to cell mass resulted in only a 43% inhibition, the addition of magnesium returned the level of mucopeptide synthesis to slightly less than 90% of the control level. This activity of magnesium, was not related to an ability to precipitate vancomycin from solution. However, increased magnesium was unable to reduce the leakage of C^{14}-labelled metabolites from the cells at this sublytic vancomycin concentration and was unable to prevent the lysis which occurred when the cells were shaken in the presence of 8.5 μg vancomycin/mg cell dry weight. The observed leakage may have been the result of an alteration in membrane permeability or may represent the efflux of turnover material, but since magnesium was unable to overcome the cellular leakage then this phenomenon cannot represent a primary effect of vancomycin.

Recently BEST and DURHAM (1965) demonstrated that the binding of vancomycin to isolated cell walls of *B. subtilis* during a 90 minutes contact period could be reduced by magnesium, manganese, calcium and ferrous ions (and by the polycationic compounds spermine and polylysine), but not by sodium ions. The effective levels of magnesium were similar to those reducing the vancomycin-induced inhibition of wall mucopeptide synthesis. The unexpected finding that manganese, calcium and ferrous ions appeared unable to prevent growth inhibition by vancomycin is a consequence of these ions being toxic to the test organism when used at the same concentration as magnesium (DURHAM, personal communication). Since esterification of isolated walls with diazomethane under mild conditions completely prevented vancomycin adsorption it was suggested that the antibiotic complexes with the walls by electrostatic binding to anionic groups and that certain cations compete with the antibiotic for these binding sites. However, since the maximum effect of magnesium in decreasing vancomycin adsorption depends upon the presence of such ions in the medium prior to or simultaneous with the addition of the antibiotic, and since these ions are much less effective in eluting previously adsorbed antibiotic, it would appear that after initial vancomycin binding has occurred forces other than ionic bonding may be active. The characteristics of the binding apparently conform to Giles' L2 adsorption isotherms, common for adsorption from dilute solution and often indicative of multiple binding sites. BEST and DURHAM (1965) have calculated that each mg dry weight of isolated *B. subtilis* walls adsorbs more than 750 μg of vancomycin, an amount in excess of that required for growth inhibition of intact cells. The corresponding value for *S. aureus* appears to be about 325 μg/mg dry weight of walls, based on the data of REYNOLDS (1965) that as much as 65 μg can be bound per mg cell dry weight and assuming that the walls of *S. aureus* represent about 20% of the cell dry weight. REYNOLDS (1965) suggests that *S. aureus* cells possess about 10^7 binding sites for vancomycin, in contrast to the 10^3 sites involved in penicillin binding. However, there is no need for all the sites to be occupied by vancomycin for wall synthesis to be inhibited, and in fact only 50% of the sites need to be occupied for nucleotide-peptide accumulation to commence (REYNOLDS, 1964b).

The binding of vancomycin to the cell wall of intact sensitive bacteria, the immediate and marked depression in the incorporation of certain amino acids into the wall mucopeptide and the concurrent accumulation of "Park" compounds strongly suggest that the primary site of vancomycin activity lies in the area of cell wall synthesis. If the wall represents the surface for the collection of enzymes concerned in its own manufacture (ROGERS, 1963) then vancomycin could inhibit these enzymes without any early change in plasma membrane structure. However, if such enzymes are located in or on the plasma membrane then vancomycin could still exert a direct effect on the wall via adsorption, thus preventing the introduction of new structural molecules into the existing wall during growth. The weakening of the cell wall, coupled with the stretching action brought about by the continued synthesis of protein and other protoplasmic constituents would eventually damage the plasma membrane. Another possibility is that by binding to the wall, vancomycin changes the molecular configuration of the wall and consequently that of the underlying layer of the plasma membrane. The resulting change in charge distribution might then cause a generalized loosening of the membrane lipid component which could also interfere with normal membrane synthesis and function. Such membrane damage, representing a secondary effect of vancomycin, would account for the inhibition of glutamic acid transport in *S. aureus*, which occurs about 20 to 30 minutes following addition of the antibiotic, for the complete inhibition of the induction of the membrane-bound enzyme β-galactosidase, and for eventual cellular lysis (REYNOLDS, 1964b).

With intact protoplasts the primary site of vancomycin action seemingly directly involves the plasma membrane and is manifested by an effect on amino acid incorporation in *B. megaterium* protoplasts (YUDKIN, 1963), and on the incorporation of ^{14}C-leucine and inorganic-^{32}P into the membrane structure of *S. aureus* protoplasts (JORDAN and MALLORY, 1965), resulting in inhibition of protoplast growth. Thus the action of vancomycin is of a dual nature, and appears to vary depending on whether the sensitive microorganisms are intact cells or protoplasts. More recently REYNOLDS (unpublished observations) has found that vancomycin has little effect on protoplasts of *B. megaterium* if it is not added until the protoplasts have started to grow. In the particular incubation medium used, the turbidity of protoplast suspensions increases at the same exponential rate as that of whole cells incubated under identical conditions. In these circumstances vancomycin has little effect either on the growth of protoplasts or on the incorporation of ^{14}C-amino acids (Fig. 3). In this respect protoplasts of *B. megaterium* appear to differ from those of *S. aureus* in their susceptibility to vancomycin action.

With respect to a possible direct effect by vancomycin on enzymes concerned in wall manufacture, there have been several studies made on the effect of this antibiotic on the synthesis of wall components in cell-free systems. With respect to teichoic acid synthesis BURGER and GLASER (1964), using a particulate enzyme (polyglycerophosphate synthetase) obtained from the plasma membranes of *B. subtilis* and *B. licheniformis*, noticed that vancomycin, at a level of 150 μg/mg dry weight of enzyme preparation (1.5 mg/ml reaction mixture), caused a 50% inhibition in the synthesis of polyglycerophosphate from ^{14}C-labelled cytidine diphosphate glycerol. In addition GLASER (1964) reported that 250 μg vancomycin/ml reaction mixture inhibited the enzymatic synthesis of polyribitol phosphate from cytidine diphosphate ribitol by a particulate enzyme closely related with the cell wall of *Lactobacillus plantarum*, an organism *not inhibited* by vancomycin. This rather unexpected finding, again coupled with high antibiotic concentrations, even when expressed as a ratio of enzyme dry weight to inhibitor weight, makes the interpretation of these results somewhat uncertain.

In view of the probable direct effect of vancomycin on mucopeptide synthesis it was important that the sensitivity of the different enzymic steps to vancomycin should be determined. Until recently the assembly of the complete mucopeptide was envisaged as the sequential transfer of N-acetylglucosamine and N-acetylmuramylpentapeptide from the corresponding nucleotide-sugar derivatives to

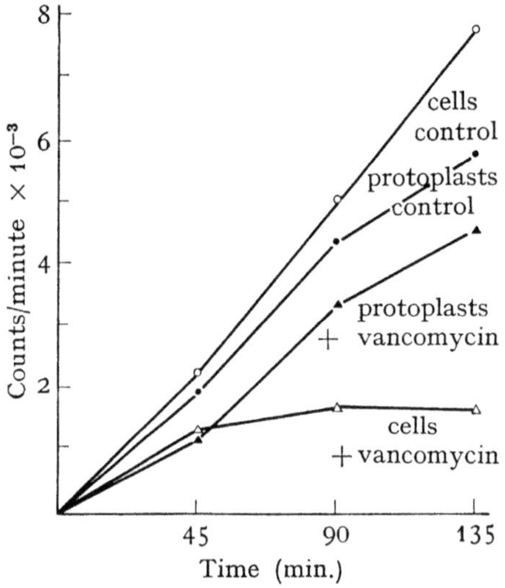

Fig. 3. Effect of vancomycin on the incorporation of ^{14}C-arginine by whole cells and protoplasts of *Bacillus megaterium*. Whole cells or protoplasts were incubated with gentle shaking in a peptone-buffered salts-glucose medium containing 10% sucrose and ^{14}C-arginine (0.01 μC/ml). Incorporation of radioactivity into the cold-acid precipitable fraction was measured

an unfinished mucopeptide backbone. CHATTERJEE and PARK (1964) and MEADOW *et al.* (1964) independently reported the development of particulate enzyme preparations from *S. aureus* which would incorporate radioactivity from lysine-labelled UDP-N-acetylmuramyl-pentapeptide. The cell-free system used by CHATTERJEE and PARK (1964) was insensitive to vancomycin with the exception that the enzyme preparation prepared from cells that had been grown in the presence of the antibiotic was inactive in the assay system. The particulate fraction used by MEADOW *et al.* (1964) contained membranes and ribosomes from sonically-disrupted cells and in this system, incorporation of radioactivity occurred only when the reaction mixture was spread on filter paper. The reaction was inhibited by 200 μg vancomycin/ml.

In a more detailed investigation using milder techniques for preparation of the membrane fraction ANDERSON *et al.* (1965) studied a number of distinct enzymic activities concerned in mucopeptide synthesis and put forward a scheme (Fig. 4) that was consistent with their results: much of their work has been confirmed by CHATTERJEE and PARK (personal communication). It is believed that N-acetylmuramyl-pentapeptide and N-acetylglucosamine are added sequentially to an unidentified lipid acceptor to give rise to a lipid-phospho-disaccharide-pentapeptide. It is the first stage in this reaction that releases UMP and is sensitive to high concentrations of vancomycin (STRUVE and NEUHAUS, 1965). ANDERSON *et al.* (1965) confirmed the sensitivity of this reaction to vancomycin but were unable to detect any inhibition of the formation of the lipid intermediates at the limiting growth inhibitory concentration of the antibiotic;

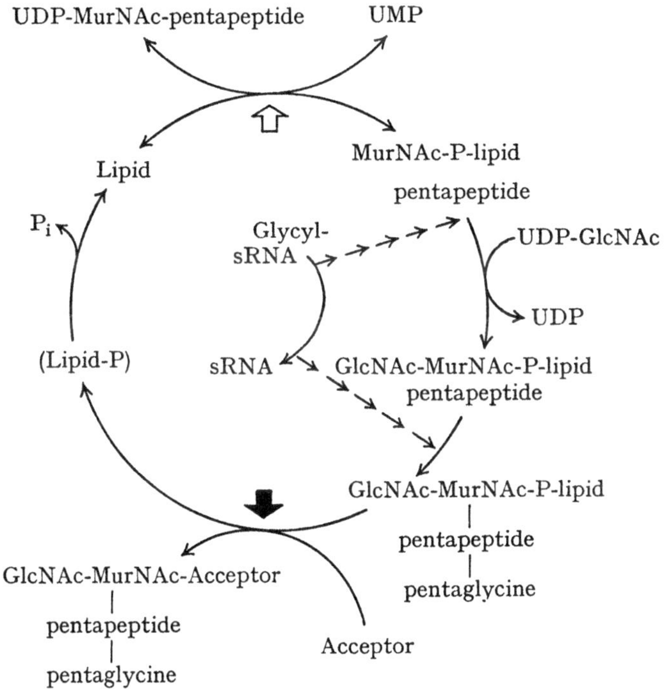

Fig. 4. Scheme for wall-mucopeptide synthesis. *After* MATSUHASHI, DIETRICH and STROMINGER (1965). The broad black arrow indicates the probable site of vancomycin at limiting growth inhibitory concentrations. High concentrations of vancomycin also inhibit the reaction indicated by the broad open arrow. (UDP and UMP = uridine di- and mono-phosphate; MurNAc = N-acetylmuramic acid; GlcNAc = N-acetylglucosamine)

at this concentration, production of the lipid intermediates was stimulated twofold on account of the inhibition of a subsequent reaction. Five glycine residues are then added to the lipid-phospho-disaccharide-pentapeptide from glycyl-s-RNA. The resultant product, N-acetylglucosamine-N-acetylmuramyl-(pentapeptide-pentaglycine)-phospho-lipid, apparently reacts with an acceptor (presumably an unfinished mucopeptide backbone chain) with the release of phospho-lipid and the formation of lysozyme-sensitive glycopeptide material. It is the final polymerisation reaction that is inhibited by vancomycin (and ristocetin and probably bacitracin) at the limiting growth inhibitory concentration of the antibiotic. The inhibition by vancomycin is obtained when the antibiotic is present in the cell-free system or when the enzyme used in the *in vitro* incorporation system is prepared from cells that have been treated with vancomycin *in vivo*. From this result it might be inferred that the *in vivo* mode of action of vancomycin may well be concerned with the final polymerisation reaction referred to above though it is not necessary to postulate an inhibition of the glycopeptide synthetase itself; blockage of the addition sites on the acceptor molecule would have the same effect. In this connection, it should be mentioned that vancomycin is itself a glycopeptide, and hence may act as a structural analogue of the natural glycopeptide. ANDERSON *et al.* (1965) suggest that the lipid derivatives are transport intermediates, and it is of interest that vancomycin does not appear to affect this transport process.

References

ANDERSON, J. S., M. MATSUHASHI, M. A. HASKIN, and J. L. STROMINGER: Lipid-phosphoacetylmuramyl-pentapeptide and lipid-phosphodisaccharide-pentapeptide: presumed membrane transport intermediates in cell wall synthesis. Proc. Natl. Acad. Sci. U.S. **53**, 881 (1965).

ANDERSON, R. C., H. M. WORTH, P. N. HARRIS, and K. K. CHEN: Vancomycin, a new antibiotic. IV. Pharmacologic and toxicologic studies. Antibiotics Ann. **1956/57**, 75 (1957).

BEST, G. K., and N. N. DURHAM: Effect of vancomycin on *Bacillus subtilis*. Arch. Biochem. Biophys. **105**, 120 (1964).

BEST, G. K., and N. N. DURHAM: Vancomycin adsorption to *Bacillus subtilis* cell walls. Arch. Biochem. Biophys. **111**, 685 (1965).

BOYLE, A. M., and R. M. PRICE: Vancomycin prevents crown gall. Phytopathology **53**, 1272 (1963).

BROCK, T. D.: Effect of antibiotics and inhibitors on M protein synthesis. J. Bacteriol. **85**, 527 (1963).

BURGER, M. M., and L. GLASER: The synthesis of teichoic acids. I. Polyglycerophosphate. J. Biol. Chem. **239**, 3168 (1964).

CHATTERJEE, A. N., and J. T. PARK: Biosynthesis of cell wall mucopeptide by a particulate fraction from *Staphylococcus aureus*. Proc. Natl. Acad. Sci. U.S. **51**, 9 (1964).

DAIKOS, G. K., M. ATHANASIADOU u. E. PAPADAKIS: Empfindlichkeit pathogener Staphylokokken und gramnegativer Bakterien gegenüber Vancomycin und anderen Antibiotica. Arch. Mikrobiol. **35**, 248 (1960).

DAY, L. E., and R. N. COSTILOW: Studies on the sporulation of *Clostridium botulinum* 62-A. Bacteriol. Proc. 75 (1961).

DURHAM, N. N.: Inhibition of microbial growth and separation by D-serine, vancomycin and mitomycin C. J. Bacteriol. **86**, 380 (1963).

DUTTON, A. A. C., and P. C. ELMES: Vancomycin: Report on treatment of patients with severe staphylococcal infections. Brit. Med. J. **1959I**, 1144.

EHRENKRANZ, N. J.: The clinical evaluation of vancomycin in treatment of multi-antibiotic refractory staphylococcal infections. Antibiotics Ann. **1958/59**, 587 (1959).

FAIRBROTHER, R. W., and B. L. WILLIAMS: Two new antibiotics. Antibacterial activity of novobiocin and vancomycin. Lancet **1956II**, 1177.

GARROD, L. P., and P. M. WATERWORTH: Behaviour in vitro of some new anti-staphyloccal antibiotics. Brit. Med. J. **1956II**, 61.

GERACI, J. E., F. R. HEILMAN, D. R. NICHOLS, and W. E. WELLMAN: Antibiotic therapy of bacterial endocarditis. VII. Vancomycin for acute micrococcal endocarditis. Proc. Mayo Clinic **33**, 172 (1958).

GERACI, J. E., F. R. HEILMAN, D. R. NICHOLS, W. E. WELLMAN, and G. T. ROSS: Some laboratory and clinical experiences with a new antibiotic, vancomycin. Antibiotics Ann. **1956/57**, 90 (1957).

GLASER, L.: The synthesis of teichoic acids. II. Polyribitol phosphate. J. Biol. Chem. **239**, 3178 (1964).

GRIFFITH, R. A., and F. B. PECK, JR.: Vancomycin, a new antibiotic. III. Preliminary clinical and laboratory studies. Antibiotics Ann. **1955/56**, 619 (1956).

HANAWALT, P.: Use of phosphorus-32 in microassay for nucleic acid synthesis in *Escherichia coli*. Science **130**, 386 (1959).

HANCOCK, R., and P. C. FITZ-JAMES: Some differences in the action of penicillin, bacitracin, and vancomycin on *Bacillus megaterium*. J. Bacteriol. **87**, 1044 (1964).

HASH, J. H.: Formation of *Staphylococcus aureus* protoplasts by enzymes from *Chalaropsis* sp. Federation Proc. **21**, 248 (1962).

HIGGINS, H. M., W. H. HARRISON, G. M. WILD, H. R. BUNGAY, and M. H. MCCORMICK: Vancomycin: A new antibiotic. VI. Purification and properties of vancomycin. Antibiotics Ann. **1957/58**, 906 (1958).

INNIS, W.: Studies on possible modes of action of a new antibiotic (vancomycin) on strains of *Staphylococcus aureus*. M.S.A. Thesis, University of Toronto 1959.

JORDAN, D. C.: Effect of vancomycin on the synthesis of the cell wall mucopeptide of *Staphylococcus aureus*. Biochem. Biophys. Research Commun. **6**, 167 (1961).

JORDAN, D. C.: Effect of vancomycin on the synthesis of the cell wall and cytoplasmic membrane of *Staphylococcus aureus*. Can. J. Microbiol. **11**, 390 (1965).

JORDAN, D. C., and W. INNISS: Selective inhibition of ribonucleic acid synthesis in *Staphylococcus aureus* by vancomycin. Nature **184**, 1894 (1959).

JORDAN, D. C., and W. INNISS: Mode of action of vancomycin on *Staphylococcus aureus*. Antimicrobial Agents and Chemotherapy 1961, p. 218 (1962).

JORDAN, D. C., and H. D. C. MALLORY: Site of action of vancomycin on *Staphylococcus aureus*. Antimicrobial Agents and Chemotherapy 1964, p. 489 (1965).

KAGEN, B. M., C. W. MOLANDER, S. ZOLLA, E. M. HEIMLICH, H. J. WEINBERGER, R. BUSSER, and S. LIEPNIEKS: Antibiotic sensitivity and pathogenicity of L-phase variants of staphylococci. Antimicrobial Agents and Chemotherapy 1963, p. 517 (1964).

KAVANAGH, F.: Vancomycin. In: F. KAVANAGH (ed.), Analytical microbiology, p. 375. New York: Academic Press Inc. 1963.

KIRBY, W. M. M.: Vancomycin therapy of staphylococcal infections. Antibiotics & Chemotherapy **11**, 84 (1963).

KIRBY, W. M. M., and C. L. DIVELBISS: Vancomycin, clinical and laboratory studies. Antibiotics Ann. **1956/57**, 107 (1957).

KIRBY, W. M. M., D. M. PERRY, and J. L. LANE: Present status of vancomycin therapy of staphylococcal and streptococcal infections. Antibiotics Ann. **1958/59**, 580 (1959).

LEE, C. C., and R. C. ANDERSON: Toxicologic studies on vancomycin and polyethylene glycol 200. Toxicol. Appl. Pharmacol. **4**, 206 (1962).

LEE, C. C., R. C. ANDERSON, and K. K. CHEN: Vancomycin, a new antibiotic. V. Distribution, excretion, and renal clearance. Antibiotics Ann. 1956/57, 82 (1957).

LOURIA, D. B., T. KAMINSKI, and J. BUCHANAN: Vancomycin in severe staphylococcal infections. A.M.A. Arch. Internal Med. **107**, 225 (1961).

MCCARTHY, C., and M. L. SNYDER: Selective medium for *Fusobacterium* and *Leptospira*. J. Bacteriol. **86**, 158 (1963).

MCCORMICK, M. H., W. M. STARK, G. E. PITTENGER, R. C. PITTENGER, and J. M. MCGUIRE: Vancomycin, a new antibiotic. I. Chemical and biologic properties. Antibiotics Ann. **1955/56**, 606 (1956).

MALLORY, H. D. C.: Further studies on the effects of vancomycin on *Staphylococcus aureus*. M.S.A. Thesis, University of Toronto 1963.

MARSHALL, F. J.: Structure studies on vancomycin. J. Med. Chem. **8**, 18 (1965).

MATSUHASHI, M., C. P. DIETRICH, and J. L. STROMINGER: Incorporation of glycine into the cell wall glycopeptide in *Staphylococcus aureus:* role of sRNA and lipid intermediates. Proc. Natl. Acad. Sci. U.S. **54**, 587 (1965).

MEADOW, P. M., J. S. ANDERSON, and J. L. STROMINGER: Enzymatic polymerization of UDP-acetylmuramyl. L-ala. D-glu. L-lys. D-ala. D-ala and UDP-acetylglucosamine by a particulate enzyme from *Staphylococcus aureus* and its inhibition by antibiotics. Biochem. Biophys. Research Commun. **14**, 382 (1964).

MEHTA, P. P., D. GOTTLIEB, and D. POWELL: Vancomycin, a potential agent for plant disease prevention. Phytopathology **49**, 177 (1959).

MOLANDER, C. W., B. M. KAGAN, H. J. WEINBERGER, E. M. HEIMLICH, and R. J. BUSSER: Induction by antibiotics and comparative sensitivity of L-phase variants of *Staphylococcus aureus*. J. Bacteriol. **88**, 591 (1964).

NISHIMURA, H., S. OKAMOTO, K. NAKAJIMA, M. SHIMOHIRA, and N. SIMAOKA: Studies on vancomycin. I. Physical, chemical properties and in vitro antibacterial studies. Shionogi's Ann. Rep. **7**, 465 (1957).

PARK, J. T., and R. HANCOCK: A fractionation procedure for studies on the synthesis of cell wall mucopeptide and of other polymers in cells of *Staphylococcus aureus*. J. Gen. Microbiol. **22**, 249 (1960).

PARK, J. T., and J. L. STROMINGER: Mode of action of penicillin. Science **125**, 99 (1957).

PITTENGER, R. C., and R. B. BRIGHAM: *Streptomyces orientalis n. sp.*, the source of vancomycin. Antibiotics & Chemotherapy **6**, 642 (1956).

REYNOLDS, P. E.: Studies on the mode of action of vancomycin. Biochim. et Biophys. Acta **52**, 403 (1961).

REYNOLDS, P. E.: A comparative study of the effects of penicillin and vancomycin. Biochem. J. **84**, 99P (1962).

REYNOLDS, P. E.: Mucopeptide synthesis in *Staphylococcus aureus* after treatment with vancomycin. J. Gen. Microbiol. **35**, v (1964a).

REYNOLDS, P. E.: The mode of action of vancomycin. Ph. D thesis, University of Cambridge 1964b.

REYNOLDS, P. E.: Antibiotics affecting cell wall synthesis. In: Sixteenth Symposium of the Society for General Microbiology 1965 (to be published).

ROGERS, H. J.: The bacterial cell wall. The result of absorption, structure or selective permeability. J. Gen. Microbiol. **32**, 19 (1963).

ROGOSA, M., R. J. FITZGERALD, M. E. MACINTOSH, and A. J. BUCHANAN: Improved medium for selective isolation of *Veillonella*. J. Bacteriol. **76**, 455 (1958).

RUSSELL, A. D.: Mode of action of vancomycin. J. Pharm. and Pharmacol. **16**, 37 (1964).

SCHNEIERSON, S. S., and D. AMSTERDAM: In vitro sensitivity of erythromycin-resistant strains of staphylococci and enterococci to vancomycin and novobiocin. Antibiotics & Chemotherapy **7**, 251 (1957).

SHOCKMAN, G. D., and J. O. LAMPEN: Inhibition by antibiotics of the growth of bacterial and yeast protoplasts. J. Bacteriol. **84**, 508 (1962).

STRUVE, W. G., and F. C. NEUHAUS: Evidence for an initial acceptor of UDP-NAc-muramyl-pentapeptide in the synthesis of bacterial mucopeptide. Biochem. Biophys. Research Commun. **18**, 6 (1965).

TIPPER, D. J., J. L. STROMINGER, and J.-M. GHUYSEN: Staphylolytic enzyme from *Chalaropsis*: mechanism of action. Science **146**, 781 (1964).

WAISBREN, B. A., and C. L. STRELITZER: A five year study of the antibiotic sensitivities and cross resistance of staphylococci in a general hospital. Antibiotics Ann. **1957/58**, 350 (1958).

WILLIAMS, R. E. O.: L forms of *Staphylococcus aureus*. J. Gen. Microbiol. **33**, 325 (1963).

YUDKIN, M. D.: The effect of penicillin, novobiocin, streptomycin and vancomycin on membrane synthesis by protoplasts of *Bacillus megaterium*. Biochem. J. **89**, 290 (1963).

ZIEGLER, D. W., R. N. WOLFE, and J. M. MCGUIRE: Vancomycin, a new antibiotic. II. In vitro antibacterial studies. Antibiotics Ann. **1955/56**, 612 (1956).

Pyocyanine

P. G. Caltrider

Pyocyanine is a blue pigment produced by *Pseudomonas aeruginosa* (formerly *Ps. pyocyanea*). FARBER (1951) reported the isolation of pyocyanine from a bacterium named *Cyanococcus chromospirans*. The antibiotic activity of pyocyanine was observed first by EMMERICH and LOW (1899). They found that old cultures of *Ps. aeruginosa* inhibited the growth of a number of Gram-positive and Gram-negative bacteria. Due to the lytic action of culture broths on suspensions of *Vibrio comma* and *Bacillus anthracis*, they ascribed the inhibition to an enzyme termed pyocyanase. Later investigations, however, showed that several factors were present, none of which had enzymatic activity, and that the major active principle was pyocyanine. The isolation and chemical nature of pyocyanine has been described by SCHOENTAL (1941) and the structure was elucidated by WREDE and STRACK (1924, 1929) and HILLEMAN (1938).

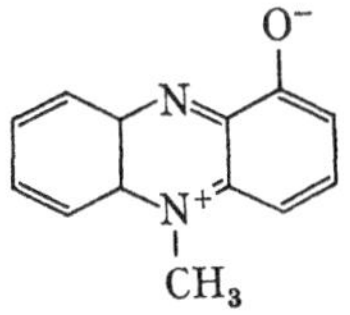

The chemistry and biological properties of pyocyanine and related phenazine compounds have been reviewed by SWAN and FELTON (1957).

Pyocyanine is a broad-spectrum bacteriostatic agent. WAKSMAN and WOODRUFF (1942) found considerable variation in the bacteriostatic effect of pyocyanine tested in different media. Inhibitory concentrations of the antibiotic in nutrient agar for selected bacteria are shown in Table 1.

Table 1. *Collected data on the bacteriostatic effect of pyocyanine on selected organism* (WAKSMAN and WOODRUFF, 1942)

Test Organism	Inhibitory Concentration of Pyocyanine µg/ml
Aerobacter aerogenes	100
Escherichia coli	30
Bacillus subtilis	3
Sarcina lutea	3
Actinomyces sp.	10

Inhibition of growth of pathogenic fungi and yeast *in vitro* by pyocyanine and its α-hydroxy derivatives has been studied (STOKES *et al.*, 1942; STIEB and WALKER, 1957). A dilution of 1/10,000 of pyocyanine inhibited growth of both Gram-positive and Gram-negative bacteria. Hemipyocyanine was less active against yeast and fungi. Growth of amoebae and paramecia was reduced when these organisms were fed cells of *Ps. aeruginosa* but not when they were fed non-pigmented bacteria (IMSHENSTSKII, 1947; GROSCOP and BRENT, 1964). *In vitro* cultures of embryonic chicken tissue treated with the antibiotic increased in cell multiplication (SORESINA, 1939). Generally, respiration is affected by pyocyanine. In cats and dogs, the antibiotic caused an increase in cerebral oxygen utilization which was followed by a decrease. These cerebrial respiratory changes were accompanied by symptoms of disturbed function of the central nervous system (FAZEKAS *et al.*, 1939). Relatively low levels of pyocyanine (0.4 mg/kg) caused respiration to speed up in rabbits; 0.3—0.5 mg caused depression of reflex activity in frogs (KHARCHENKO *et al.*, 1947). Pyocyanine has no therapeutic use because of its general toxicity to animals.

The function first ascribed to pyocyanine in *Ps. aeruginosa* was that of a respiratory catalyst (STHEEMAN, 1927). FRIEDHEIM (1931) reported that pyocyanine increased oxygen consumption several fold in cells grown under conditions not conducive to pigment production. Increased respiratory activity by pyocyanine also has been observed in a number of organisms and animal tissues (FRIEDHEIM, 1932; 1934; EHRISMANN, 1934; YOUNG, 1937; CARLSON and BODINE, 1939; SORESINA, 1939; MOORE *et al.* 1945; LANDAU *et al.*, 1963).

Several lines of evidence indicate that pyocyanine exercises the role of an oxygen transfer catalyst in the place of the cyanide and azide sensitive heme-containing respiratory enzymes. The inhibition of oxygen uptake in both bacteria and animal tissue systems by cyanide or azide could at least partially be overcome by pyocyanine (DE MEIO *et al.*, 1934; LICHSTEIN and SOULE, 1944). Generally, the stimulation of respiratory activity by pyocyanine was dependent upon an oxidizable substrate (WEIL-MALHERBE, 1937a and b; KURACHI, 1960).

DICKENS and MCILWAIN (1938) and ZAWAGG (1964) reported that the oxidation-reduction potential (E_h) of pyocyanine was similar to that of flavin enzymes and thus the antibiotic could substitute for them. WEIL-MALHERBE (1936b) found that oxidation of α-ketoglutarate by animal tissues was enhanced by pyocyanine and by closely related phenazine derivatives with the formation of hydrogen peroxide.

The interference in the terminal electron transport system by pyocyanine affects oxidative phosphorylation. LENNERSTRAND (1938) found that in a system with apoenzyme, cozymase, glucose, NaF, and phosphate buffer, and pyocyanine, more phosphate became organically bound and nonhydrolyzable ester was formed. Pyocyanine caused an increase in oxygen consumption in brain tissue and mitochondria of liver, but phosphorylation decreased (CASE and MCILWAIN, 1951; JUDAH and ASHMAN, 1951). HILL and WALKER (1959) reported that pyocyanine increased phosphorylation by chloroplasts.

There is evidence that catabolic pathways for glucose oxidation are affected by pyocyanine. LANDAU *et al.* (1963) reported that it caused more of the substrates, which were expected to enter the phosphogluconate and Embden-Meyerhof pathway, to be oxidized to carbon dioxide by liver slices. Furthermore, pyocyanine increased the incorporation of labeled substrates into glycogen and fatty acids. CAMPBELL *et al.* (1957) found that pyocyanine stopped oxidation of glucose, 2-ketogluconate, malate and lactate by cells of *Ps. fluorescens* at the keto acid stage. An inhibition of anaerobic oxidation of glucose in an amoeba has been reported by KUN *et al.* (1955).

Diamine oxidase and L-amino acid oxidase were inhibited by pyocyanine in several species of *Mycobacterium* (OWEN *et al.*, 1951). MARCUS and FULY (1962) reported that the inhibition of the latter enzyme by the antibiotic appeared to involve reduction of the amino acid oxidase flavin to a form which reacted poorly with oxygen. Succinic dehydrogenase of rat liver (WEIL-MALHERBE, 1937b) and brain tissue (HARMAN and MACBRINN, 1963) is inhibited by pyocyanine. The data of HARMAN and MACBRINN (1963) suggest that an active site of the enzyme is blocked by pyocyanine. Staphylocoaglulase of *Staphalococcus aureus* was found to be inhibited by pyocyanine by PACHECO and TREJAS (1945).

CAVALLITO *et al.* (1945) and CAVALLITO (1946) demonstrated that pyocyanine was inactivated by sulfhydryl compounds. On the basis of these data, the binding of sulfhydryl groups was suggested as the mechanism of action *in vivo*. Bacteriostasis of *S. aureus* by pyocyanine, however, was not reversed by cysteine (BAILEY and CAVALLITO, 1951).

Experiments with pyocyanine suggest a complex mode of action. It appears evident, however, that its primary site of action evolves around its high affinity for reduced flavoprotein.

References

BAILEY, J. H., and C. J. CAVALLITO: The reversal of antibiotic action. J. Bacteriol. **55**, 175 (1951).

CAMPBELL, J. J. R., A. M. MACQUILLAN, B. A. EAGLES, and R. A. SMITH: The inhibition of keto acid oxidation by pyocyanine. Can. J. Microbiol. **3**, 313 (1957).

CARLSON, L. D., and J. H. BODINE: Action of certain stimulating and inhibiting substances on the respiration of the grasshopper embryo, *Melanoplus differentialis*. J. Cell. Comp. Physiol. **14**, 159 (1939).

CASE, E. M., and H. MCILWAIN: Respiration and phosphorylation in preparations from mammalian. Biochem. J. **48**, 1 (1951).

CAVALLITO, C. J.: Relationships of thiol structures to reaction with antibiotics. J. Biol. Chem. **164**, 29 (1946).

CAVALLITO, C. J., J. H. BAILEY, T. H. HASKELL, J. R. MCCORMICK, and W. F. WARNER: The inactivation of antibacterial agents and their mechanism of action. J. Bacteriol. **50**, 61 (1945).

DEMEIO, R. H., M. KISSIN, and K. S. G. BARRON: Studies on biological oxidations. IV. On the mechanism of the catalytic effect of reversible dyes on cellular respiration. J. Biol. Chem. **107**, 579 (1934).

DICKENS, F., and H. MCILWAIN: Phenazine compounds as carriers in the hexose monophosphate system. Biochem. J. **32**, 1615 (1938).

EHRISMANN, O.: Pyocyanine and bacterial respiration. Z. Hyg. Infektionskrankh. **116**, 209 (1934). Chem. Abstr. **28**, 5489 (1934).

EMMERICH, R., u. O. LOW: Bakteriologische Enzyme als Ursache der erworbenen Immunität und die Heilung von Infektionskrankheiten durch dieselben. Z. Immunitätsforsch. **31**, 1 (1899).

FARBER, G.: New isolated chromogenic microorganism with a high oxidative potency. Sbornik Českoslov. akad. zemědělské **23**, 355 (1951). Chem. Abstr. **45**, 9605 (1951).

FAZEKAS, J. F., H. COLYER, S. NESIN, and H. E. HIMIVICH: Effect of pyocyanine on cerebral metabolism. Proc. Soc. Exptl. Biol. Med. **42**, 446 (1939).

FRIEDHEIM, E. A. H.: Pyocyanine, an accessory respiratory enzyme. J. Exptl. Med. **54**, 207 (1931).

FRIEDHEIM, E. A. H.: The influence of pyocyanine on the respiration of normal tissues and tumors. Naturwissenschaften **20**, 171 (1932). Chem. Abstr. **26**, 3841 (1932).

FRIEDHEIM, E. A. H.: Effect of pyocyanine on the respiration of some normal tissues and tumors. Biochem. J. **28**, 173 (1934).

GROSCOP, J. A., and M. M. BRENT: The effects of selected strains of pigmented microorganisms on small, free living amoeba. Can. J. Microbiol. **10**, 579 (1964).

HARMAN, J. W., and M. C. MACBRINN: The effect of phenazine methosulphate pyocyanine and EDTA on mitochondrial succinic dehydrogenase. Biochem. Pharmacol. **12**, 1265 (1963).

HILL, R., and D. A. WALKER: Pyocyanine and phosphorylation with chloroplasts. Plant Physiol. **34**, 240 (1959).

HILLEMANN, H.: Phenazine. I. Action of dimethyl sulfate on phenazine, l-methoxyphenazine and l-hydroxyphenazine. Ber. deut. chem. Ges. **71**B, 34 (1938). Chem. Abstr. **32**, 21319 (1938).

IMSHENITSKII, A. A.: Ecology of pigmented microorganisms. II. Antibiotic action of pigments. Mikrobiologiya **16**, 3 (1947).

JUDAH, J. D., and H. G. WILLIAMS-ASHMAN: The inhibition of oxidative phosphorylation. Biochem. J. **48**, 33 (1951).

KHARCHENKO, N. S., E. O. RYABUSHKO, and O. I. PETRUKHOVA: Biological activity of a new antibiotic pyocyanine. Vrachebnoe Delo. **27**, 19 (1947). Chem. Abstr. **42**, 4675f (1948).

KUN, E., J. L. BRADIN jr., and J. M. DECHARY: Effect of metabolic inhibitors on production of CO_2 and H_2S by *Endamoeba histolytica*. Proc. Soc. Exptl. Biol. **89**, 604 (1955).

KURACHI, M.: Biosynthesis of pyocyanine. IX. Effect of pyocyanine on respiration of bacterial cells of *Pseudomonas aeruginosa*. Bull. Inst. Chem. Research, Kyoto Univ. **38**, 364 (1960).

LANDAU, B. R., A. B. HASTINGS, and S. ZOTTER: Pyocyanine and metabolic pathways in liver slices in vitro. Biochim. et Biophys. Acta **74**, 629 (1963).

LANNERSTRAND, A.: Über die Konkurrenz zwischen Azetaldehyd und Pyacyanin + mobkularem Sauerstoff im fluoridvergifteten Apozymasesystem. Naturwissenschaften **26**, 45 (1938).

LICHSTEIN, H. C., and M. H. SAULE: Studies on the effect of sodium azide on microbic growth and respiration. III. The effect of sodium azide on the gas metabolism of *Bacillus suvtilis* and *Pseudomonas aeruginosa* and the influence of pyocyanine on the gas exchange of a pyocyanine-free strain of *Pseudomonas aeruginosa* in the presence of sodium azide. J. Bacteriol. **47**, 239 (1944).

MOORE, A. R., H. S. BLISS, and E. H. ANDERSON: Effects of pyocyanine and of lithium on the development and respiration of the eggs of two echinoderms. J. Cell. Comp. Physiol. **25**, 27 (1945).

MARCUS, A., and J. FEELEY: Effect of phenazine methosulfate and pyocyanine on the L-amino acid oxidase reaction. Biochim. et Biophys. Acta **59**, 398 (1962).

OWEN jr., C. A., A. G. KARLSON, and E. A. ZELLER: Enzymology of tubercule bacilli and other mycobacteria. V. Influence of streptomycin and other basic substances on diamine oxidase and various bacteria. J. Bacteriol. **62**, 53 (1951).

PACHECO, G., and A. TREJOS: Influence of pyocyanine on staphylocoagulase with a method for determining pyocyanine. Brasil-med. **59**, 169 (1945). Chem. Abstr. **45**, 693b (1951).

SCHOENTAL, R.: The nature of the antibacterial agents present in *Pseudomonas pyocyanea* cultures. Brit. J. Exptl. Pathol. **22**, 137 (1941).

SORESINA, C.: The effect of pyocyanine on the growth of tissue cultures in vitro. Tumori **12**, 306 (1939).

STHEEMAN, A. A.: Die Rolle des Pyocyanins im Stoffwechsel von *Pseudomonas pyocyanea*. Biochem. Z. **191**, 320 (1927).

STIEB, E. W., and G. C. WALKER: Antagonism exhibited by *Pseudomonas aeruginosa* and *Pseudomonas fluorescens* toward certain fungus pathogens. II. Can. Pharm. J. **90**, 235 (1957).

STOKES, J. L., R. L. PECK, and C. R. WOODWARD jr.: Antimicrobial action of pyocyanine, hemipyocyanine, pyocyanase and tyrothricin. Proc. Soc. Expl. Biol. **51**, 126 (1942).

SWAN, G. A., and D. G. I. FELTON: Phenazines, p. 174. New York: Interscience Publ. Inc. 1957.

WAKSMAN, S. A., and H. B. WOODRUFF: Selective antibiotic action of various substances of microbial origin. J. Bacteriol. **44**, 373 (1942).

WEIL-MALHERBE, H.: Studies on brain metabolism. II. Formation of succinic acid. Biochem. J. **31**, 299 (1937a).

WEIL-MALHERBE, H.: The oxidation of 1(—)a-hydroxyglutaric acid in animal tissues. Biochem. J. **31**, 2080 (1937b).

WREDE, F., and E. STRACK: Pyocyanin, the blue pigment of *Bacillus pyocyaneus*. Z. Physiol. Chem. **140**, 1 (1924). Chem. Abstr. **19**, 302 (1925).

WREDE, F., and E. STRACK: Pyocyanin, the blue pigment of *Bacillus pyocyaneus*. IV. The constitution and synthesis of pyocyanin. Hoppe-Seyler's Z. physiol. Chem. **181**, 58 (1929). Chem. Abstr. **23**, 2717 (1929).

YOUNG, L.: The effect of pyocyanine on the metabolism of cerebral cortex. J. Biol. Chem. **120**, 659 (1937).

ZAUGG, W. S.: Spectroscopic characteristics and some chemical properties of N-methylphenazinium methyl sulfate (phenazine methosulfate) and pyocyanine at the semiquinoid oxidation level. J. Biol. Chem. **239**, 3964 (1964).

Polyene Antibiotics

Stephen C. Kinsky

The early clinical and economic success of antibacterial antibiotics prompted many laboratories to undertake a search for products of natural origin that would be equally effective in the treatment of fungal infections. These endeavors have led to the isolation and characterization of numerous antibiotics, which share certain chemical and biological properties, and are now designated as the polyene antibiotics. Although polyene antibiotics have been known since the discovery of nystatin by HAZEN and BROWN (in 1950), it is only within recent years that sufficient data has accumulated to allow a discussion of their mechanism of action in other than broadly descriptive terms. The polyenes have attracted the attention of numerous investigators because these antibiotics were toxic to fungi, yet had no effect on bacteria. Thus, the polyenes promised to reveal some interesting biochemical differences between bacteria and fungi. Delay in understanding the mechanism of polyene antibiotic action can therefore not be attributed to a lack of interest but, instead, to the gradual realization that very few antibiotics inhibit simple metabolic pathways. Most antibiotics interfere with the formation or function of macromolecules and subcellular structures (DAVIS and FEINGOLD, 1962). Such is the case with the polyenes, and, in this review, we shall present in approximate chronological order the evidence which indicates that:

1. The polyene antibiotics cause permeability alterations in sensitive organisms which lead to the loss of essential cytoplasmic constituents culminating in cell death.

2. The cell membrane is the site of action of the polyene antibiotics and that, as a result of polyene binding, it is no longer able to function as a selective restraining barrier.

3. The selective toxicity of the polyene antibiotics is due to interaction with a unique component present only in the membranes of sensitive organisms and that this component is a sterol.

The final section will consider some current speculations on the molecular basis of polyene action and the use of these antibiotics as specific biochemical tools in problems of membrane structure.

I. Biological Activity and Clinical Application

Extensive discussion of the clinical uses of the polyene antibiotics does not fall within the scope of this review. This material is covered fully in the recent treatise by HILDICK-SMITH, BLANK, and SARKANY (1964). Nystatin and amphotericin B are the polyenes which are mainly used clinically at the present time.

Infections due to Blastomyces, Candida, Cryptococcus, and Histoplasma, among others, have been successfully treated with these antibiotics. The polyenes have also been found effective in the control of certain protozoal infections. Nystatin is employed topically, or given orally in cases of intestinal involvement, whereas amphotericin B is usually administered intravenously for systemic infections. The polyene antibiotics show varying degrees of toxicity; for example, prolonged amphotericin B therapy may produce renal damage and hemolytic anemia.

Non-pathogenic strains of Candida, Saccharomyces, and the mold, Neurospora, have been primarily employed in studies on the mechanism of polyene antibiotic action. Growth of sensitive organisms is inhibited at *in vitro* concentrations of 0.1 to 20 μg/ml, depending on the antibiotic used. The effective minimum inhibitory concentration is also influenced by several factors, particularly, medium composition and size of inoculum. In general, the polyenes are fungicidal at concentrations which inhibit growth completely. Resistance to the antibiotics is rarely developed and does not constitute a serious obstacle to the clinical use of the polyenes.

II. Classification and Chemistry

The present classification of these antibiotics is due to OROSHNIK *et al.* (1955) who characterized them as conjugated polyenes rather than polyenynes on the basis of their ultraviolet absorption spectra. At that time, only 9 antibiotics had been isolated in reasonably pure form and these fell into three distinct groups, each having the same chromophore: tetraenes, hexaenes, and heptaenes which contain 4, 6, and 7 conjugated double bonds, respectively. Since then, pentaenes (5 conjugated double bonds) have also been isolated but, to date, no triene or octaene has been reported. A recent census (WAKSMAN and LECHEVALIER, 1962) lists 51 polyene antifungal antibiotics (17 tetraenes, 12 pentaenes, 5 hexaenes, 17 heptaenes). An earlier tabulation (VINING, 1960) lists 41 polyenes of which 14 are tetraenes, 10 pentaenes, 4 hexaenes, and 13 heptaenes. Undoubtedly, some of the polyenes have been reported more than once but it can nevertheless be safely predicted that more of these antibiotics are awaiting discovery.

A brief description of some of the polyenes is presented in Table 1. The articles by VINING (1960) and WAKSMAN and LECHEVALIER (1962) should be consulted for references to the discovery, isolation and chemical properties of these antibiotics. Approximately 30 polyenes have been crystallized and in this state they are stable for years when kept cold, dry, and dark. The antibiotics are insoluble in water and poorly soluble in low boiling esters, alcohols, ketones, and ethers. They are dissolved by polar organic solvents such as dimethylformamide, dimethylsulfoxide and aqueous mixtures of alcohols. These solutions may be diluted carefully with water; the antibiotics will usually not precipitate out if the final concentration is less than 50 μg/ml. LAMPEN *et al.* (1959) have reported that nystatin is not dialysable under these conditions. Therefore, it seems possible that, even at low concentrations, the antibiotics are not in true solution but exist as micelles in an aqueous environment. The antibiotics may be stored for several weeks in neutral solutions without appreciable loss in activity if they are kept cold and particular care is taken to exclude light and oxygen. ZONDAG *et al.* (1960) and POSTHUMA and BERENDS (1960, 1961) have shown that "photooxidation" of

Table 1. *Some representative polyene antibiotics*

Class and wavelength maxima (mμ)[1]	Antibiotic	Ionizable groups	Mycosamine presence
Tetraenes	Amphotericin A	Amphoteric	? (contains N)
290—292	Antimycoin	?	?
300—305	Etruscomycin	Amphoteric	? (contains N)
317—322	Nystatin	Amphoteric	+
	Pimaricin	Amphoteric	+
	Rimocidin	Amphoteric	? (contains N)
Pentaenes	Filipin[5]	Neutral	—
317—324	Fungichromin[2]	Neutral	—
330—340	Lagosin	Neutral	—
349—358	Pentamycin	?	?
Hexaenes	Endomycin	Amphoteric	?
335—338	Flavicid	Acidic	? (contains N)
355—359			
373—380			
Heptaenes	Amphotericin B	Amphoteric	+
358—366	Ascosin	Amphoteric	?
377—388	Candicidin	Amphoteric	+[3]
399—410	Candidin	Amphoteric	+
	Hamycin	?	?
	Perimycin	Basic	? (contains N[4])
	Trichomycin	Amphoteric	+[3]

[1] Exact position of maxima depends on nature of organic solvent.
[2] Fungichromin may be similar to filipin.
[3] Candicidin and trichomycin also contain a p-amino-acetophenone residue.
[4] Amino sugar present in perimycin but not yet identified; also contains p-amino-phenylacetone residue. No carboxyl group in perimycin.
[5] Filipin is a registered trademark of the Upjohn Co., Kalamazoo, Michigan, USA.

pimaricin in water is stimulated markedly by low concentrations of flavin derivatives. This phenomenon has been developed into a method for determining polyene concentration when high levels of interfering substances preclude the use of direct spectrophotometric analysis (Kinsky, 1962b).

Complete, or nearly complete, structures have been proposed for relatively few polyenes: pimaricin (Patrick *et al.*, 1958); fungichromin (Cope *et al.*, 1962); lagosin (Dhar *et al.*, 1964); filipin (Ceder and Ryhage, 1964); nystatin (Birch *et al.*, 1964). The structure of the pentaene, filipin, is shown in Fig. 1. This formula indicates certain structural features which all polyenes apparently possess in common. They are all characterized by a large macrolide ring containing the conjugated chromophore. It is generally believed that both the lactone group and the conjugated double bond series are necessary for biological activity. The presence of highly polar and non-polar regions within the molecule renders the polyenes amphipathic; this accounts for the peculiar solubility properties described above and may have considerable bearing on their mode of action (see Section VIII). It should be emphasized that filipin is a neutral polyene. The majority of the polyenes are amphoteric substances. The acidity of these polyenes is due to a caboxyl group. The basicity of the amphoteric polyenes is due to mycosamine, a unique amino sugar first isolated from nystatin and amphotericin B and identified as 3-amino-3,6-dideoxy-D-mannose (WALTERS *et al.*, 1957). The site of linkage between mycosamine and the macrolide ring has not yet been determined. Mycosamine has also been isolated from pimaricin, candicidin, candidin, and trichomycin; the sugar may be present in amphotericin A, etruscomycin, rimocidin, flavicid and perimycin since these polyenes contain nitrogen. Candicidin and trichomycin each contain a p-amino-acetopenone residue, and a p-amino-phenylacetone substituent has been detected in perimycin.

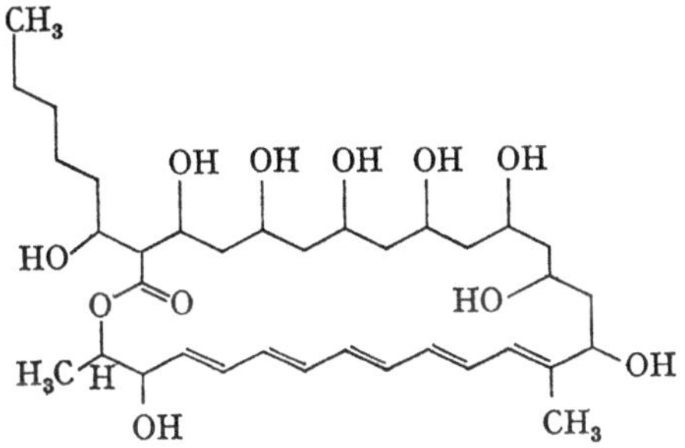

Fig. 1. The structure of filipin. CEDAR and RYHAGE (1964)

N-acetylation of candidin, amphotericin B, candicidin, and trichomycin converts these amphoteric polyenes into acid substances which readily form water soluble salts. The N-acetyl derivatives show significantly less biological activity than the parent compounds (LECHEVALIER *et al.*, 1961). Perimycin is a basic polyene, which possesses no free carboxyl group, and accordingly its N,N-diacetyl derivative is a neutral compound insoluble in water.

In spite of the number of polyene antibiotics, and the diverse types of substituents, the available evidence indicates that they all act by the same general mechanism. There are, however, some significant differences which are discussed in greater detail in Section VI. It is indeed unfortunate that the structures of so few have been determined and that little is known of the geometrical and optical configuration of these antibiotics. Our present knowledge of polyene mechanism at the cellular level has advanced to such a stage that a detailed analysis of structure-activity relationship would undoubtedly contribute greatly to an understanding of polyene action at the molecular level.

III. Mechanism of Action

a) Early Work

Studies on polyene antibiotic mechanism prior to 1960 were reviewed at the Second Conference on Medical Mycology sponsored by the New York Academy of Sciences. The proceedings of this conference, particularly the papers by BRADLEY and JONES (1960) and DROUHET *et al.* (1960), should be consulted for references to the original literature. These studies, as well as those of HARMAN and MASTERSON (1957), LAMPEN *et al.* (1957), SCHOLZ *et al.* (1959), and GALE (1960), revealed that nystatin and amphotericin B influenced a number of processes in sensitive yeasts, including: a) endogenous glycolysis and respiration, b) utilization of exogenous substrates such as sugars and phosphate, c) induced enzyme formation d) nucleic acid synthesis, etc. Both stimulatory and inhibitory effects were recorded; the exact response depended on the particular metabolic parameter under investigation, age of culture, antibiotic concentration, pH, media composition, etc. No clear-cut pattern was apparent and all attempts to demonstrate an effect of the antibiotics on cell free systems were consistently negative. Several investigators interpreted these results to indicate that the polyenes interfered with cell permeability, as suggested also by the phase and electron microscopic observations of HARMAN and MASTERSON (1957) and BLANK (1957), but no direct experiments to test this hypothesis were undertaken. In retrospect, these early studies on polyene mechanism can be best summarized by the statement of DAVIS and FEINGOLD (1962): "Because of the multiple consequences of an outpouring of metabolites from a damaged cell, it is hardly surprising that a multiplicity of metabolic defects have been observed in cells that we now know to have suffered damage to the wall or membrane."

b) Polyene-Induced Permeability Changes

Direct evidence that the polyene antibiotics caused permeability alterations in sensitive organisms was obtained simultaneously in 1961 by several laboratories (GOTTLIEB *et al.*; GHOSH and CHATTERJEE; KINSKY; LAMPEN *et al.*). In this section we shall summarize only the evidence obtained with fungi; the extensive investigations performed with protozoa are reviewed in Section IV. We shall also confine the present discussion to the "major" polyenes. By "major" we mean those antibiotics, particularly nystatin, amphotericin B, and filipin that have been most thoroughly studied, either because they are widely used clinically or because they are the purest and best characterized chemically. The "minor" polyenes are reviewed in Section V.

KINSKY (1961 a, b), studied the action of the polyenes on the mold, *Neurospora crassa*, and observed that all of the polyenes tested caused a marked decrease in the dry weight of mycelial mats when incubated for short periods with low concentrations (ca. 10^{-6} M) of the antibiotics. Mycelial atrophy was accompanied by the appearance of various cytoplasmic constituents in the medium: material absorbing at 260 and 280 mμ, amino acids, free and phosphorylated sugars, peptides, inorganic phosphate, etc. Mycelial atrophy was produced specifically by nystatin, amphotericin B, and filipin, and was not obtained with any other agent (iodoacetamide, azide, p-fluorophenylalanine) or non-polyene antibiotics (cycloheximide, viridin) that also inhibited growth of Neurospora. GOTTLIEB *et al.* (1961), in confirmation of earlier work cited in Section III a, reported that filipin inhibited both aerobic and anaerobic oxidation of glucose, acetate, and endogenous substrate by intact cells of the yeast, *Saccharomyces cerevisiae*. High concentrations of the antibiotic had no effect on the oxidative capabilities of cell-free homogenates. They also observed that filipin caused a decrease in cellular dry weight and the leakage of compounds containing nitrogen and phosphorous from the cell. These observations suggested that the metabolic effects of the polyenes were a consequence of an altered cellular permeability and that ultimate death of the fungal cell was caused by leakage of some essential cytoplasmic component(s).

Experiments from LAMPEN'S laboratory with *S. cerevisiae* led to the same conclusion (MARINI *et al.*, 1961; SUTTON *et al.*, 1961; LAMPEN, 1962). It was found that the glycolytic inhibition caused by low concentrations of nystatin at neutral pH could be reversed by the addition of K^+ and/or NH_4^+ ions to the medium. Since potassium is required for maximal activity of several glycolytic enzymes in yeast, this observation suggested that nystatin had caused the loss of K^+ from the cell. Analysis of yeast cells by flame photometry indicated a significant reduction in K^+ content after antibiotic treatment. When Saccharomyces was treated with higher concentrations of nystatin (> 10 μg/ml) at neutral pH, the intracellular concentration of other essential cofactors apparently fell below a critical level. In this case, reversal of glycolytic inhibition was not obtained with K^+-NH_4^+ alone but also required the addition of ATP, NAD, TPP, Mg^{++} and pyruvate to the medium. At acid pH (< 5.8), inhibition of glycolysis by nystatin could not be reversed or prevented by mixtures of cations, cofactors, and a boiled yeast extract. LAMPEN (1962) has suggested that this may be due to an increased permeability of nystatin treated yeast to H^+ and that acidification of the cell interior results in the activation of lytic enzymes. It should be noted that, even under conditions which led to reversal of glycolytic inhibition, the fungicidal activity of nystatin could not be prevented. Apparently other cytoplasmic constituents needed for survival of the cell, but not necessary for glycolysis, had also leaked out.

Subsequent studies by A. GHOSH and J. J. GHOSH (1963a, b) and STACHIEWICZ and QUASTEL (1963) have corroborated the conclusion that the polyene antibiotics produce permeability alterations in sensitive fungi.

c) The Site of Polyene Antibiotic Action: The Cell Membrane

Because the cell membrane is the structural unit primarily responsible for the maintenance of selective permeability, it seemed likely that this would be the principal site of polyene action. The effect of the antibiotics on Neurospora protoplast morphology support this assumption. The same concentrations of the polyenes, which caused mycelial atrophy, produced rapid shrinkage and crenation of protoplasts stabilized in sucrose (KINSKY, 1962a). This phenomenon could be followed either microscopically or, more conveniently, by the increase in absorbancy of a protoplast suspension. Sucrose can penetrate Neurospora protoplasts slowly, if at all, and these observations indicate that the polyenes induced the loss of cytoplasmic constituents (and, consequently, water) at a rate greater than the rate of entrance of osmotic stabilizer. Conversely, all the polyene antibiotics caused lysis of protoplasts in the presence of osmotic stabilizers, such as NaCl or mannitol, which might be expected to enter the cell at a rate greater than the exit rate of cytoplasmic constituents (KINSKY, 1963).

Polyene induced permeability alterations could conceivably result if the antibiotics interfere with cell membrane synthesis analogous to the way penicillin inhibits the manufacture of certain bacterial cell walls in growing cultures. This possibility was rendered unlikely, however, because conditions conducive to growth were not required for the polyenes to induce a weight loss in Neurospora mycelia. The rate and extent of mycelial atrophy or protoplast shrinkage were neither duplicated nor modified by agents, such as cycloheximide, iodoacetamide, azide, p-fluorophenylalanine, and sucrose deprivation, which inhibited growth and synthetic processes in Neurospora (KINSKY, 1961b, 1962a).

These results suggested as an alternative mechanism, that binding of the polyenes to the fungal cell membrane in some manner interfered with its ability to function as a restraining barrier. This hypothesis was particularly attractive because it implied, as a corollary, that the selective toxicity of these antibiotics was due to a unique binding component present in the membrane of sensitive fungi, but absent in bacteria. Indeed, several years prior to the realization that the polyenes interfered with cellular permeability, LAMPEN and coworkers found that nystatin absorption by cells is a critical factor in determining sensitivity to the antibiotic (LAMPEN *et al.*, 1959; LAMPEN and ARNOW, 1959). They observed that fungal cells (Saccharomyces, Candida, Penicillium) bound significant amounts of nystatin when the antibiotic was present at the minimum growth inhibitory concentration. The bound antibiotic could be recovered by extraction of the yeast cells with isopropanol. Bacteria (e.g. *Escherichia coli*, *Streptococcus faecalis*), whose growth is not inhibited by concentrations of nystatin as high as 100 μg/ml, absorbed negligible amounts of the antibiotic. Uptake of nystatin by Saccharomyces was dependent on the initial antibiotic concentration, did not occur at 4 C, and was more extensive at acid pH than at neutrality. Heated yeast cells also bound nystatin but, in this case, absorption showed less dependence on temperature and pH. Subsequent investigations on the binding of nystatin, amphotericin B, and filipin to Saccharomyces, Candida, and Neurospora have largely confirmed these observations (GOTTLIEB *et al.*, 1961; A. GHOSH and J. J. GHOSH, 1963c, d; KINSKY, 1962b, 1964). The finding that polyene binding by Saccharomyces and Candida was stimulated by the presence of a metabolizable substrate has led to the suggestion that the initial uptake of the antibiotic was an energy requiring process (LAMPEN *et al.*, 1959; A. GHOSH and J. J. GHOSH, 1963c, d). This interesting possibility is somewhat at variance with the results obtained by KINSKY (1961b, 1962a) with Neurospora mycelia and protoplasts, and deserves further attention.

Although only cells of sensitive fungi bind appreciable amounts of the antibiotics, this observation does not *per se* justify the conclusion that the selective toxicity of the polyenes is due to interaction with a unique component present in the fungal cell membrane. It is also possible that bacteria possess the same component but that access of the antibiotics is limited by the complex bacterial cell wall. To decide between these alternatives, the effect of nystatin on lysozyme — prepared protoplasts of *Bacillus megaterium* was examined (KINSKY, 1962b; SHOCKMAN and LAMPEN, 1962). Growth of *B. megaterium* is not affected by any of the polyenes at concentrations of 100 μg/ml. This concentration of nystatin did not promote shrinkage of the bacterial protoplast in sucrose, or lysis in saline, and did not induce leakage of K^+. It was also found that nystatin could be recovered completely from the medium after incubation with *B. megaterium* protoplasts whereas, under identical conditions, Neurospora protoplasts rapidly absorbed the antibiotic. These results are consistent with the contention that the selective toxicity of the polyenes is due to the presence of a specific receptor in the fungal cell membrane and also indicate that the polyene insensitivity of bacteria cannot be attributed to inactivation of the antibiotics.

d) Selective Toxicity of the Polyene Antibiotics: The Role of Sterols in Polyene Binding

In 1958, GOTTLIEB *et al.* reported that addition of several sterols (e.g. cholesterol, ergosterol, stigmasterol, sitosterol) to the medium could antagonize growth inhibition by the polyene antibiotics. GOTTLIEB *et al.* (1958) originally suggested, on the basis of these results, that the polyenes may either inhibit the synthesis of sterols which are necessary for fungal growth, or, replace the sterols as cofactors in an essential metabolic reaction. LAMPEN *et al.* (1960) investigated further the mechanism by which sterols nullified growth inhibition by the antibiotics. They obtained spectrophotometric evidence for complex formation between the antibiotics and sterols. Incubation of the polyenes with numerous sterols in aqueous media had a pronounced effect on the spectra of the antibiotics which was distinguished mainly by a decrease in extinction and, with the possible exception of filipin, no spectral shift or change in the relative peak heights. These observations indicated a decreased solubility of the polyenes in the presence of sterols and, on this basis, the physiological significance of polyene-sterol interaction was originally discounted. It was suggested instead that sterols antagonized the action of the polyenes by a reduction in the effective free antibiotic concentration due to complex formation. Although the latter conclusion is probably valid, more recent evidence, summarized below, leaves little doubt that polyene interaction with sterols *localized in the cell membrane* underlies the basis of action and selective toxicity of these antibiotics. It must be emphasized, however, that the above interpretations were offered before the existence of any direct evidence, as reviewed in Sections IIIb, c, that the polyenes produced permeability alterations by binding to the cell membrane of sensitive fungi. Thus, although subsequent studies have shown that the conclusions of GOTTLIEB and LAMPEN require revision, the significance of these observations for our eventual understanding of polyene mechanism can hardly be exaggerated.

It is generally accepted that sterols are important structural components of cell membranes. The principal *a priori* reason for suspecting that sterols may be involved in binding of the antibiotics to the cell membrane is the conspicuous absence of these compounds from bacteria (FIERTEL and KLEIN, 1959; ASSELINEAU and LEDERER, 1960). Therefore, sterols meet the main requirement of a membrane constituent capable of binding the polyenes and their presence in fungi, but absence in bacteria, can account for the selective toxicity of these antibiotics.

In the past few years convincing evidence has been obtained which indicates that ergosterol, the main sterol in fungi, is involved in binding of the polyenes to the fungal cell membrane. KINSKY (1962b) showed that as much as 80% of Neurospora mycelial binding capacity for nystatin was localized in the "microsomal" fraction of cell free homogenates. Competition experiments between nystatin, amphotericin B, and filipin indicated that these polyenes were bound at the same site. This fraction possessed enzymatic activity (e.g. chitin synthetase) which would be expected in particles derived from the cell membrane. Extraction of the Neurospora membrane particles with a mixture of ethanol-acetone completely abolished their ability to take up nystatin. The capacity to bind the antibiotic could be partially restored by preincubation of the extracted particles with ergosterol (KINSKY, 1962b, 1964). LAMPEN *et al.* (1962) demonstrated a close correlation between the ability of various subcellular fractions from Saccharomyces to bind nystatin and their ergosterol content. They further observed that bound nystatin could be released by subsequent incubation with digitonin, a sterol-specific complexing agent which mimics the effects of the polyenes on fungi. Digitonin has also been shown to inhibit polyene binding to the fungal membrane by A. A. GHOSH and J. GHOSH (1963c, d), who studied the absorption of nystatin and amphotericin B by *Candida albicans*, and by KINSKY (1964).

The above evidence is, of course, circumstantial. All attempts to isolate a polyene-ergosterol complex from the fungal cell membrane have failed. This is undoubtedly due to the fact that, unlike the interaction between digitonin and certain sterols, polyene-sterol complex formation is readily reversed by the presence of organic solvents (LAMPEN *et al.*, 1960). It should also be noted that sterols are not the only conceivable membrane constituents which have been reported to antagonize the polyenes or inhibit binding of the antibiotics. Similar effects have been reported for oleic acid, linoleic acid, and vitamin A (A. A. GHOSH and J. GHOSH, 1963c, d, e) STACHIEWICZ and QUASTEL (1963). These compounds may be competing with the ergosterol present in the cell membrane for the available polyene; this is probably the mechanism by which free sterol added to the growth medium inhibits antibiotic binding. It is more likely, however, that these compounds, like digitonin, are themselves bound to the fungal cell membrane thereby inhibiting access of the polyenes. It is unlikely that direct interaction of the antibiotics with unsaturated fatty acids or carotenoids in the membrane plays a significant role since these compounds, in contrast to sterols, are present in both fungi and bacteria and would not, therefore, provide a basis for the selective toxicity of the polyene antibiotics.

IV. The Polyene Sensitivity of Other Organisms

Although ergosterol is the predominant structural sterol in fungi, several other sterols are also able to prevent fungal growth inhibition by the polyenes: cholesterol, sitosterol, stigmasterol and, to a lesser extent, lanosterol (GOTTLIEB *et al.*, 1958). LAMPEN *et al.* (1960) found that the sterols, which were most effective in nullifying polyene activity, had the greatest effect on the absorption spectra of the polyenes. These results suggest that the ability to interact with the polyenes is shared by numerous sterols. Accordingly, the sterol hypothesis of polyene selective toxicity would predict that other organisms known to contain sterols should also be sensitive to the polyenes. Indeed, one of the strongest arguments in support of the sterol hypothesis is the fact that fungi are not the only organisms affected by these antibiotics. Some of the earlier observations in this area were merely by-products of other investigations. Thus, the finding that some polyene antibiotics are toxic to snails (SENECA and BERGENDAHL, 1955) and planaria (JOHNSON *et al.*, 1962) arose from attempts to maintain cultures of these organisms free of fungal contamination.

Algae

The polyene sensitivity of algae (HUNTER and MCVEIGH, 1961; LAMPEN and ARNOW, 1961) constitutes convincing support of the sterol hypothesis. HUNTER and McVEIGH (1961) observed that the tetraenes, amphotericin A and nystatin, inhibited growth of higher algae but had no effect on blue-green algae. In 1939, CARTER *et al.* reported that, unlike the higher forms, blue-green algae were devoid of sterols; this observation has been recently confirmed with contemporary analytical methods (LEVIN and BLOCH, 1964).

Protozoa

B. K. GHOSH and coworkers have extensively studied the effect of nystatin on the protozoan, *Leishmania donovani*. These investigations, begun around 1960, parallel, confirm, and extend the observations on fungi described in Section III. Nystatin inhibited endogenous and exogenous respiration of the protozoan (GHOSH, HALDER, and CHATTERJEE, 1960), although no effect of the antibiotic on several key enzymes participating in glycolytic or respiratory pathways could be detected (GHOSH and CHATTERJEE, 1962a). Nystatin caused the loss of various intracellular constituents from the cell: 260 mμ absorbing materials, amino acids, phosphate, and small amounts of RNA and protein (GHOSH and CHATTERJEE, 1961). Nystatin induced the lysis of cell suspensions of *L. donovani* (GHOSH and CHATTERJEE, 1963a); the cytological and cytochemical changes which occur within the cell during the lytic process have been described (GHOSH, 1963a). These observations clearly indicate that nystatin alters the selective permeability of this protozoan. Subsequent experiments have shown that the cell membrane is the site of action and implicated a sterol, probably ergosterol, in the binding of the antibiotic to the membrane. *L. donovani* cells rapidly absorbed nystatin; the presence of cholesterol in the incubation medium antagonized antibiotic binding. Digitonin also inhibited nystatin uptake and caused the release of bound nystatin from the cell (GHOSH and CHATTERJEE, 1962b, 1963b). The absorption of nystatin by isolated cell membrane is similarly inhibited by digitonin. Nystatin is preferentially bound by the subcellular fractions which possesses the highest sterol content (GHOSH, 1963b). These valuable studies are discussed further in Section VIII.

Mammalian erythrocytes

The polyene antibiotics are quite toxic to mammals. The principle side effects in humans undergoing amphotericin B therapy are renal damage and hemolytic anemia. The polyenes can cause the lysis of rat and human erythrocytes in isotonic saline (KINSKY *et al.*, 1962; KINSKY, 1963). For this reason, it has been suggested that fungicidal activity and mammalian toxicity may share the same basic cause: nte raction with sterols present in the cell membrane. There is a close correlation between hemolytic potency and human toxicity. Filipin, which may be too toxic for clinical use, is the most potent, and nystatin is the least effective, hemolytic agent; amphotericin B occupies an intermediate position. However, because serum in low concentrations can inhibit hemolysis by the polyenes (KINSKY, 1963), direct action of the antibiotics on the erythrocyte membrane may not be the main cause of hemolytic anemia observed in patients (BUTLER *et al.*, 1965). BANDRISS *et al.* (1964) did not observe any effect of amphotericin B administration on red cell survival time and have suggested that anemia is a consequence of decreased erythrocyte production due to bone marrow suppression. This interesting proposal merits further study since it is possible that the polyenes may interfere with the incorporation of cholesterol into the red blood cell membrane.

Mycoplasma (Pleuropneumonia-like Organisms)

Mycoplasma possess many morphological and biochemical properties in common with bacterial spheroplasts and L-forms. However, in contrast to the polyene-insensitive spheroplasts and L-forms, most mycoplasma (excluding saprophytic species) require sterol for growth. LAMPEN *et al.* (1963) have shown that growth of *M. gallisepticum*, which has an absolute sterol requirement, was inhibited by several polyenes. WEBER and KINSKY (1965) and FEINGOLD (1965) investigated the action of filipin and amphotericin B, respectively, on *M. laidlawii*. *M. laidlawii* is an especially appropriate organism for study of the polyene antibiotics. Neither *M. gallisepticum* nor *M. laidlawii* can synthesis sterols; however, unlike the former, *M. laidlawii* will grow almost equally well in the presence and absence of exogenous sterol, e.g. cholesterol. When grown in the presence of cholesterol, *M. laidlawii* will incorporate the sterol into the cell membrane. It was found (WEBER and KINSKY, 1965) that filipin inhibited growth, and caused lysis, of cells which had been cultured in the presence of cholesterol. The antibiotic had no effect on *M. laidlawii* grown in the absence of sterol. Identical results were obtained with amphotericin B (FEINGOLD, 1965). Both groups observed that cholesterol-grown cells gradually became resistant to the polyenes when incubated in cholesterol-free medium at 37 C; polyene sensitivity was retained when the incubation was carried out at 4 C. Loss of polyene sensitivity was accompanied by a decreased sensitivity to the lytic action of digitonin (WEBER and KINSKY, 1965) and disappearance of a portion of the cholesterol from the cell (FEINGOLD, 1965). Thus, these studies with *M. laidlawii* provide particularly strong evidence for the contention that the presence of sterols in the cell membrane is a prerequisite for polyene sensitivity.

V. The "Minor" Polyene Antibiotics

Although these polyenes have not been investigated as thoroughly as nystatin, amphotericin B, and filipin, the available evidence, summarized below, indicates that all the polyenes act by the same basic mechanism. In spite of a common mode of action, it should be emphasized, however, that the polyenes manifest a wide range of biological potency; this aspect is discussed in greater detail in Section VI.

Pimaricin, Etruscomycin

Growth of *S. cerevisiae* and *C. albicans* by these tetraenes is nullified by several sterols: cholesterol, ergosterol, sitosterol, and stigmasterol (PERRITT *et al.*, 1960; GHIONE *et al.*, 1961). These antibiotics also cause loss of potassium from yeast (LAMPEN, 1962; LAMPEN and ARNOW, 1963) and the lysis of mammalian erythrocytes (KINSKY, 1963).

Candicidin, Candidin, N-acetyl candidin, Hamycin

Growth inhibition by these heptaenes is also antagonized by sterols (GOTTLIEB *et al.*, 1958; RAMACHANDRAN, 1961). Candidin, N-acetyl candicidin, and candicidin induce potassium leakage from *S. cerevisiae*, thereby inhibiting glycolysis (LECHEVALIER *et al.*, 1961; LAMPEN, 1962; HARSCH and LAMPEN, 1963; CIRILLO *et al.*, 1964; LARSEN and DEMIS, 1964). Candidin can promote the lysis of mammalian erythrocytes (KINSKY, 1963). Hamycin causes the leakage of compounds containing nitrogen and phosphorous from *S. cerevisiae* (RAMACHANDRAN, 1961).

Ascosin

HENIS and GROSOWICZ (1960) first studied the influence of this heptaene on yeast metabolism and observed many effects now interpretable as an altered cell permeability. They concluded that the antibiotic interfered with phosphate uptake. Growth inhibition can be antagonized by cholesterol (GOTTLIEB *et al.*, 1958) and ascosin induces the lysis of mammalian erythrocytes (KINSKY, 1963). In spite of the preceeding observations, the mode of action of ascosin has been in dispute for a long time. GOTTLIEB and RAMACHANDRAN (1961) concluded that the prevention of phosphate accumulation was due to an effect of ascosin on mitochondrial respiration resulting in an inhibition of oxidative phosphorylation. They reported that ascosin blocked succinate and pyridine nucleotide-linked cytochrome c reduction catalyzed by cell free extracts, and mitochondrial fractions, obtained from various fungal, plant, and mammalian sources. These results would imply that all of the polyene antibiotics do not act in the same way since previous work by the same laboratory has shown that filipin had no effect on oxidation of citric acid cycle intermediates (GOTTLIEB *et al.*, 1961). KINSKY, GRONAU, and WEBER (1965) have reinvestigated these observations and were able to demonstrate that the ascosin preparation was contaminated by sufficient antimycin A to account for the observed inhibition of electron transport.

VI. Relative Potencies of the Polyene Antibiotics

The extensive studies of LAMPEN and coworkers have revealed that the various polyenes differ in the degree of damage which they produce to the yeast cell membrane. The original papers by LAMPEN (1962), LAMPEN and ARNOW (1963), HARSCH and LAMPEN (1963), and CIRILLO, HARSCH, and LAMPEN (1964) should be consulted for experimental details. As examples, we may consider the permeability changes caused by N-acetylcandidin (NAC), nystatin, and filipin. Each of these polyenes induced the rapid loss of K^+ from the cell. Over a wide range of antibiotic concentrations, the effects of NAC on glycolyssis could be reversed by K^+ and NH_4^+. However, these ions will only antagonize the glycolytic inhibition caused by low concentrations of nystatin; they do not reverse the effects of high levels of the antibiotic unless other essential glycolytic cofactors are added to the medium (see Section IIIb). In the case of filipin, glycolytic inhibition could not be reversed or prevented by mixtures of cations, cofactors, and a boiled yeast extract even at low antibiotic concentrations. These results suggest that filipin causes more extensive damage to the cell membrane than NAC; at low concentrations, nystatin resembles NAC but at high concentrations it behaves like filipin. These experiments also indicate that cation permeability is probably most sensitive to the polyene antibiotics. Thus, leakage of inorganic phosphate or sorbose was not obtained with NAC at any concentration, was marginal with low concentrations of nystatin, and was significant only with high concentrations of nystatin or low concentrations of filipin. A rapid effect of nystatin on cation permeability was also suggested by the experiments of SLAYMAN and SLAYMAN (1962) who demonstrated that nystatin (2.2×10^{-7} M) abolished the membrane potential of Neurospora hyphae within 2 minutes.

On the basis of these studies, LAMPEN has divided the polyenes into two groups. The first group consists of those antibiotics (e.g. NAC, nystatin, candidin, candicidin, and amphotericins A and B) whose effects on glycolysis can be completely or partially reversed under appropriate circumstances. These antibiotics have a more or less specific effect on cation permeability at low concentrations. The second group is represented by the polyenes (e.g. filipin, etruscomycin, pimaricin) which cause more extensive cell membrane damage than members of the first group since their effects cannot be reversed or prevented. This classification is also supported by experiments on Neurospora protoplasts and mammalian erythrocytes (KINSKY, 1962a, 1963) which indicate that the antibiotics cause increasing damage to the membrane in the following order: nystatin, pimaricin, candidin, amphotericin B, etruscomycin, filipin. LAMPEN has emphasized that there is no apparent correlation between the degree of membrane damage and the number of conjugated double bonds, net charge, or presence of —COOH, —NH_2 or aromatic side chains in the antibiotic. There does seem to be a significant relationship between the number of carbon atoms, and presumably the size of the macrolide ring, and the destructive power of the antibiotics. The most damaging polyenes, i.e. those in group 2, are smaller (33—37 carbon atoms) than the antibiotics in group 1 (46—63 carbon atoms). It should also be noted this classification of the polyenes is based on the degree of damage to the membrane and not on the relative potency of the antibiotics in inhibiting growth. In general, the heptaenes inhibit growth at the lowest concentrations although these antibiotics cause the milder type of membrane damage.

VII. Resistance to the Polyene Antibiotics; Effect on Subcellular Membranes

Studies with other antibiotics, e.g. streptomycin, have profited greatly from the characterization of resistant strains. Attempts to isolate strains of yeast resistant to high levels of the polyenes have generally been unsuccessful. Several laboratories have been able to obtain low-level (2—15 fold) resistant strains of Saccharomyces and Candida (STOUT and PAGANO, 1956; LITTMAN *et al.*, 1958; BRADLEY, 1958). The isolation of only low level resistant strains is understandable if one assumes that any major change in membrane composition and structure involving sterols constitutes a letal mutation. Recently, however, HEBEKA and SOLOTOROVSKY (1962, 1965) have reported the isolation of *C. albicans* strains which showed a 4—60 fold resistance to amphotericin B and a 150 fold resistance to candidin. These strains demonstrated cross resistance between candidin and amphotericin B but not with nystatin. The basis of this resistance has not yet been established and may possibly be due to elaboration of an enzyme system which rapidly inactivates the polyenes or a decreased access of the antibiotics to membrane sterols.

Of special interest in this regard is the fact that some subcellular membrane systems seem to be unaffected by the polyenes. B. K. GHOSH (1963a) and GALE

(1963) have published photomicrographs showing that the nucleus and mitochondria remained intact when protozoa and fungi were incubated with extremely high concentrations of several polyenes sufficient to cause a massive leakage of cytoplasmic material into the medium. Studies with isolated Neurospora and rat liver mitochondria have shown that pure polyenes did not have any influence on oxidative phosphorylation, ion accumulation or electron transport (LARDY *et al.*, 1958; PRESSMAN, 1965; KINSKY *et al.*, 1965). An *in vivo* effect of filipin on yeast mitochondrial electron transport has been postulated by SHAW *et al.* (1964), but it seems probable that these results reflect secondary changes occurring as a result of polyene-induced permeability alterations (KINSKY *et al.*, 1965). Although mitochondria function is not disturbed by the polyenes, KINSKY *et al.* (1965) have shown that Neurospora mitochondria contain ergosterol and are able to bind filipin. However, the total steroı content of the mitochondria was significantly less than the sterol content of the microsomes which are presumably derived from the cell membrane. These experiments suggest that, although sterols are *necessary* for interaction with the antibiotics, their presence in a membrane may not be a *sufficient* prerequisite for polyene sensitivity. It has been suggested that the relative proportion of sterols and other lipids, particularly phospholipids, may play an important role in determining whether or not a membrane is sensitive to the polyenes (KINSKY *et al.*, 1965).

Other factors are probably also involved. For example, STACHIEWICZ and QUASTEL (1963) have shown that Ca ions protect the yeast cell from the action of nystatin. They suggest that binding or removal of Ca^{++} from the membrane may lead to the observed permeability alterations. This possibility seems unlikely since it would not account for the selective toxicity of the antibiotics and the action of the non-amphoteric neutral polyenes, such as filipin, which are ineffective Ca^{++} complexing agents. The possibility, however, that the presence of Ca^{++} in the membrane may be an important modifying factor cannot be overlooked especially if one considers that mitochondria are capable of accumulating large amounts of this ion.

VIII. Molecular Basis of Polyene Antibiotic Action

Although the experiments described in the preceeding sections have established the basis for the selective toxicity of the polyenes, very little is yet known of the events, occurring after the antibiotics are bound to membrane sterols, which ultimately produce the observed permeability alterations. This state of affairs reflects our limited knowledge of cell membrane structure, particularly the role of sterols. Further investigation into the molecular basis of polyene action will undoubtedly contribute much to this problem and, just as penicillin has helped unravel bacterial cell wall structure, it seems likely that the polyenes will prove useful biochemical tools for determination of the structure of the cell membrane. However, as pointed out in Section II, efforts along this line are currently hampered by the fact that the geometrical and optical configuration of the polyenes must still be elucidated. Nevertheless, a comparison of the polyenes with other lytic agents, such as vitamin A, ionic detergents, and saponin, provides some useful clues.

The polyenic compound, vitamin A, has been shown by DINGLE and LUCY (1962) to be a powerful hemolytic agent. Since the action of vitamin A can be prevented by certain anti-oxidants, LUCY and DINGLE (1964) have suggested that cell lysis may be due to oxidation of vitamin A within the cell membrane. It has not yet been determined whether anti-oxidants, such as vitamin E, protect sensitive cells from the lytic action of the antibiotics. However, as regards binding to the cell membrane, there is good reason to believe that vitamin A and the polyene antibiotics may not share the same mechanism. KINSKY (1963) has demonstrated that Neurospora protoplasts, which are rapidly lysed in NaCl by low concentrations of the polyenes, are relatively resistant to high concentrations of vitamin A. Conversely, *B. megaterium* protoplasts, which are unaffected by the antibiotics at concentrations as high as 100 μg/ml, are rapidly lysed by low concentrations of vitamin A (10 μg/ml). These results suggest that sterols are not necessary for interaction of the vitamin with the cell membrane. This conclusion is also supported by the monolayer experiments of BANGHAM *et al.* (1964) which indicate that vitamin A interacts more strongly with lecithin than with cholesterol.

An extensive study of the effects of cetyltrimethyl ammonium bromide (CTAB), sodium dodecyl sulfate (SDS), nystatin and amphotericin B on *L. donovani* and *C. albicans* has been carried out by B. K. GHOSH and CHATTERJEE (1963 a), B. K. GHOSH (1963 b), and A. GHOSH and J. J. GHOSH (1963 b). Although the polyenes are surface active agents, these experiments indicate that the antibiotics do not act as the detergents. Maximum effects of nystatin and amphotericin B were observed at concentrations which produced a surface pressure of 12—14 dynes/cm whereas SDS activity was greatest at a detergent concentration having a surface pressure of 30 dynes/cm. It was also observed that CTAB and SDS, but not nystatin, were capable of solubilizing isolated cell membrane fractions. A detergent action of the polyenes has also been excluded by KINSKY (1964) who showed that incubation of Neurospora mycelial mats with high concentrations of the antibiotics did not result in extraction of ergosterol.

On the basis of the available evidence, it appears most probable that saponin and the polyene antibiotics act by an identical mechanism although the structures of these compounds are quite different. In 1937, SCHULMAN and RIDEAL demonstrated that saponin preferentially penetrated cholesterol monolayers and gave only weak interaction with monolayers of lecithin. DEMEL, KINSKY, and VAN DEENEN (1965) have recently performed analogous experiments with the polyenes, filipin and nystatin. They observed that filipin and nystatin readily penetrate monolayers of cholesterol and ergosterol at initial surface pressures greater than the collapse pressure of the antibiotics. With monolayers of either sterol, a greater surface pressure increase was obtained with filipin than with nystatin. Essentially no interaction was obtained with a variety of pure synthetic phospholipids unless sterol was present. Filipin did not penetrate monolayers prepared from lipid extracts of bacteria but did penetrate monolayers of lipids isolated from beef erythrocytes. When the erythrocyte lipid extract was separated into a neutral lipid and a phospholipid fraction, filipin did not penetrate a monolayer of the phospholipids but did interact with the neutral lipids consisting primarily of cholesterol. Thus, these experiments provide an excellent correlation between the ability of the polyenes to penetrate lipid monolayers, the selective toxicity of these antibiotics as revealed by the studies described in Sections III and IV, and the relative potencies of filipin and nystatin as discussed in Section VI.

Further insight into the mechanism of saponin lysis has been obtained from the electron microscopy studies of DOURMASHKIN *et al.* (1962). They observed that membranes from various sources, when treated with saponin and then negatively stained with phosphotungstate, displayed a regular array of hexagonal pits and concluded that saponin acted by *extracting* sterols from the cell membrane. Subsequent experiments by BANGHAM and HORNE (1962), GLAUERT, DINGLE, and LUCY (1962), BANGHAM and HORNE (1964), and LUCY and GLAUERT (1964) indicate, however, that the pits were a consequence of saponin *addition to* the membrane. These studies suggest that the lytic effect of saponin is brought about by a reorientation of the lipids in sensitive cell membranes. As pointed out by LUZZATI and HUSON (1962), phase transistions of a membrane, such as from a lamellar to micellar configuration, would produce marked changes in selective permeability. Some preliminary evidence that the polyenes may also produce a change in the association (spatial arrangement) of sterols was obtained by DEMEL *et al.* (1965). It should however be emphasized that monomolecular layers at best only approximate the lipid architecture of the cell membrane and that reactions occurring at the air/water interface may not be applicable to biological membranes.

Acknowledgements. In the preparation of this review, I have benefited greatly from numerous invaluable discussions with Professor L. L. M. VAN DEENEN, Der Rijksuniversiteit, Utrecht, The Netherlands. I am also indebted to Professor J. O. LAMPEN, Rutgers University, New Brunswick, N. J. for the manuscript of his review on the polyenes which was presented at the 16th Symposium of the Society for General Microbiology, April, 1966.

Work in the author's laboratory has been supported by grants RG-6941 and AI-05114, and Research Career Development award K3-AI-6388, from the United States Public Health Service.

See Addendum

References

ASSELINEAU, J., and E. LEDERER: Bacterial lipids. In: Lipide metabolism (K. BLOCH, ed.). New York: John Wiley & Sons 1960.

BANGHAM, A. D., and R. W. HORNE: Action of saponin on biological cell membranes. Nature **196**, 952—953 (1962).

BANGHAM, A. D., J. T. DINGLE, and J. A. LUCY: Studies on the mode of action of excess vitamin A. 9. Penetration of lipid monolayers by compounds in the vitamin A series. Biochem. J. **90**, 133—140 (1964).

BANGHAM, A. D., and R. W. HORNE: Negative staining of phospholipids and their structural modification by surface active agents as observed in the electron microscope. J. Mol. Biol. **8**, 660—668 (1964).

BIRCH, A. J., C. W. HOLZAPFEL, R. W. RICHARDS, C. DJERASSI, P. C. SEIDEL, M. SUZUKI, J. WESTLEY, and J. D. DUTCHER: Nystatin. Part VI. Chemistry and partial structure of the antibiotic. Tetrahedron Letters **23**, 1491—1497 (1964).

BLANK, H.: Antifungal antibiotics in clinical medicine. Arch. Dermatol. **75**, 184—189 (1957).

BRADLEY, S. G.: Interactions between phosphate and nystatin in *Candida stellatoidea.* Proc. Soc. Exptl. Biol. Med. **98**, 786—789 (1958).

BRADLEY, S. G., and L. A. JONES: Mechanisms of action of antibiotics. Ann. N.Y. Acad. Sci. **89**, 122—133 (1960).

BRANDRISS, M. W., S. M. WOLFF, R. MOORES, and F. STOHLMAN: Anemia induced by amphotericin B. J. Am. Med. Assoc. **189**, 89—92 (1964).

BUTLER, W. F., D. W. ALLING, and E. COTLOVE: Potassium loss from human erythrocytes exposed to amphotericin B. Proc. Soc.Exptl. Biol. Med. **118**, 297—300 (1964).

CARTER, P. W., I. M. HEILBRON, and B. LYTHGOE: The lipochromes and sterols of the algal classes. Proc. Roy. Soc. (London) B **128**, 82—109 (1939).

CEDER, O., and R. RYHAGE: The structure of filipin. Acta Chem. Scand. **18**, 558—560 (1964).

CIRILLO, V. P., M. HARSCH, and J. O. LAMPEN: Action of the polyene antibiotics filipin, nystatin and N-acetylcandidin on the yeast cell membrane. J. Gen. Microbiol. **35**, 249—259 (1964).

COPE, A. C., R. K. BLY, E. P. BURROWS, O. J. CEDER, E. CIGANEK, B. T. GILLIS R. F. PORTER, and H. E. JOHNSON: Fungichromin: Complete structure and absolute configuration at C_{26} and C_{27}. J. Am. Chem. Soc. **84**, 2170—2178 (1962).

DAVIS, B. D., and D. S. FEINGOLD: Antimicrobial agents: mechanisms of action and use in metabolic studies. In: The bacteria, vol. IV, (I. C. GUNSALUS and R. STANIER, eds.). New York: Academic Press 1962.

DEMEL, R. A., L. L. M. VAN DEENEN, and S. C. KINSKY: Penetration of lipid monolayers by polyene antibiotics. Correlation with selective toxicity and mode of action. J. Biol. Chem. **240**, 2749—2753 (1965).

DHAR, M. L., V. THALLER, and M. C. WHITING: Researches on polyenes. Part VIII. The structures of lagosin and filipin. J. Chem. Soc. **1964**, 842.

DINGLE, J. T., and J. A. LUCY: Studies on the mode of action of excess vitamin A. 5. The effect of vitamin A on the stability of the erythrocyte membrane. Biochem. J. **84**, 611—621 (1962).

DOURMASHKIN, R. R., R. R. DOUGHERTY, and R. J. C. HARRIS: Electron microscopic observations on Rous sarcoma virus and cell membranes. Nature **194**, 1116—1119 (1962).

DROUHET, E., L. HIRTH, and G. LEBEURIER: Some aspects of the mode of action of polyene antifungal antibiotics. Ann. N.Y. Acad. Sci. **89**, 134—155 (1960).

FEINGOLD, D. S.: The action of amphotericin B on *Mycoplasma laidlawii*. Biochem. Biophys. Research Comm. **19**, 261—267 (1965).

FIERTEL, A., and H. KLEIN: On sterols in bacteria. J. Bacteriol. **78**, 738—739 (1959).

GALE, G. R.: The effects of amphotericin B on yeast metabolism. J. Pharmacol. Exptl. Therap. **129**, 257—261 (1960).

GALE, G. R.: Cytology of *Candida albicans* as influenced by drugs acting on the cytoplasmic membrane. J. Bacteriol. **80**, 151—157 (1963).

GHIONE, M., A. SANFILIPPO, R. MAZZOLENI e A. MIGLIACCI: Sul meccanismo d'azione della etruscomicina, un nuovo antibiotico polienico. Giorn. microbiol. **9**, 73—82 (1961).

GHOSH, A., and J. J. GHOSH: Changes in the intracellular constituents of *Candida albicans* on nystatin and amphotericin B treatment. Ann. Biochem. and Exptl. Med. (Calcutta) **23**, 113—122 (1963a).

GHOSH, A., and J. J. GHOSH: Release of intracellular constituents of *Candida albicans* in presence of polyene antibiotics. Ann. Biochem. and Exptl. Med. (Calcutta) **23**, 611—626 (1963b).

GHOSH, A., and J. J. GHOSH: Factors affecting the absorption of nystatin by *Candida albicans*. Ann. Biochem. and Exptl. Med. (Calcutta) **23**, 101—112 (1963c).

GHOSH, A., and J. J. GHOSH: Absorption of amphotericin B by *Candida albicans*. Ann. Biochem. and Exptl. Med. **23**, 603—610 (1963d).

GHOSH, A., and J. J. GHOSH: Effect of nystatin and amphotericin B on the growth of *Candida albicans*. Ann. Biochem. and Exptl. Med. (Calcutta) **23**, 29—44 (1963e).

GHOSH, B. K.: Action of an antifungal antibiotic, nystatin, on the protozoa, *Leishmania donovani*. Part IV: Studies on the cytological and cytochemical changes. Ann. Biochem. and Exptl. Med. (Calcutta) **23**, 193—200 (1963a).

GHOSH, B. K.: Action of an antifungal antibiotic, nystatin, on the protozoa, *Leishmania donovani*. Part VI: Studies on the action on isolated membrane and the isolation of antibiotic rich cell particle from *L. donovani*. Ann. Biochem. and Exptl. Med. (Calcutta) **23**, 337—344 (1963b).

GHOSH, B. K., and A. N. CHATTERJEE: Action of an antifungal antibiotic, nystatin, on the protozoa, *Leishmania donovani*. Part II: Studies on the release of intracellular constituents. Ann. Biochem. and Exptl. Med. (Calcutta) **21**, 343—354 (1961).

GHOSH, B. K., and A. N. CHATTERJEE: Leishmanicidal activity of nystatin, a polyene antifungal antibiotic: I. The probable mechanism of action of nystatin on *Leishmania donovani*. Antibiotics & Chemotherapy **12**, 204—206 (1962a).

GHOSH, B. K., and A. N. CHATTERJEE: Leishmanicidal activity of nystatin, a polyene antifungal antibiotic: II. Isolation of bound nystatin from cells of *Leishmania donovani* and its clinical application. Antibiotics & Chemotherapy **12**, 221—224 (1962b).

GHOSH, B. K., and A. N. CHATTERJEE: Action of an antifungal antibiotic, nystatin, on the protozoa, *Leishmania donovani*. Part III. Studies on the lysis of the cells of *L. donovani*. Ann. Biochem. and Exptl. Med. (Calcutta) **23**, 173—186 (1963a).

GHOSH, B. K., and A. N. CHATTERJEE: Action of an antifungal antibiotic, nystatin, on the protozoa, *Leishmania donovani*. Part V: Studies on the absorption of nystatin by *L. donovani*. Ann. Biochem. and Exptl. Med. (Calcutta) **23**, 309—318 (1963b).

GHOSH, B. K., D. HALDAR, and A. N. CHATTERJEE: Effect of nystatin on the metabolism of a protozoal organism, *Leishmania donovani*. Ann. Biochem. and Exptl. Med. (Calcutta) **20**, 55—56 (1960).

GLAUERT, A. M., J. T. DINGLE, and J. A. LUCY: Action of saponin on biological cell membranes. Nature **196**, 953—955 (1962).

GOTTLIEB, D., H. E. CARTER, J. H. SLONEKER, and A. AMMANN: Protection of fungi against polyene antibiotics by sterols. Science **128**, 361 (1958).

GOTTLIEB, D., H. E. CARTER, J. H. SLONEKER, L. C. WU, and E. GAUDY: Mechanisms of inhibition of fungi by filipin. Phytopathology **51**, 321—330 (1961).

GOTTLIEB, D., and S. RAMACHANDRAN: Mode of action of antibiotics. I. Site of action of ascosin. Biochim. et Biophys. Acta **53**, 391—396 (1961).

HARMAN, J. W., and J. G. MASTERSON: The mechanism of nystatin action. Irish J. Med. Sci., Ser. VI, p. 249 (1957).

HARSCH, M., and J. O. LAMPEN: Modification of K^+ transport in yeast by the polyene antifungal antibiotic N-acetylcandidin. Biochem. Pharmacol. **12**, 875—883 (1963).

HEBEKA, E. K., and M. SOLOTOROVSKY: Development of strains of *Candida albicans* resistant to candidin. J. Bacteriol. **84**, 237—241 (1962).

HEBEKA, E. K., and M. SOLOTOROVSKY: Development of resistance to polyene antibiotics in *Candida albicans*. J. Bacteriol. **89**, 1533—1539 (1965).

HENIS, Y., and N. GROSSOWICZ: Studies on the mode of action of antifungal heptaene antibiotics. J. Gen. Microbiol. **23**, 345—355 (1960).

HILDICK-SMITH, G., H. BLANK, and I. SARKANY: Fungus diseases and their treatment. Boston: Little, Brown & Co. 1964.

HUNTER, E. O., JR., and J. MCVEIGH: The effects of selected antibiotics on pure cultures of algae. Am. J. Botany **48**, 179—185 (1961).

JOHNSON, W., C. A. MILLER, and J. H. BRUMBAUGH: Induced loss of pigment in planarians. Physiol. Zoöl. **35**, 18—26 (1962).

KINSKY, S. C.: The effect of polyene antibiotics on permeability in *Neurospora crassa*. Biochem. Biophys. Research Comm. **4**, 353—357 (1961a).

KINSKY, S. C.: Alterations in the permeability of *Neurospora crassa* due to polyene antibiotics. J. Bacteriol. **82**, 889—897 (1961b).

KINSKY, S. C.: Effect of polyene antibiotics on protoplasts of *Neurospora crassa*. J. Bacteriol. **83**, 351—358 (1962a).

KINSKY, S. C.: Nystatin binding by protoplasts and a particulate fraction of *Neurospora crassa*, and a basis for the selective toxicity of polyene antifungal antibiotics. Proc. Natl. Acad. Sci. U.S. **48**, 1049—1056 (1962b).

KINSKY, S. C.: Comparative responses of mammalian erythrocytes and microbial protoplasts to polyene antibiotics and vitamin A. Arch. Biochem. Biophys. **102**, 180—188 (1963).

KINSKY, S. C.: Membrane sterols and the selective toxicity of polyene antifungal antibiotics. Antimicrobial Agents and Chemotherapy—1963, p. 384—394 (1964).
KINSKY, S. C., J. AVRUCH, M. PERMUTT, H. B. ROGERS, and A. A. SCHONDER: The lytic effect of polyene antifungal antibiotics on mammalian erythrocytes. Biochem. Biophys. Research Comm. 9, 503—507 (1962).
KINSKY, S. C., G. R. GRONAU, and M. M. WEBER: Interaction of polyene antibiotics with subcellular membrane systems. I. Mitochondria. Mol. Pharmacol. **1**, 190—201 (1965).
LAMPEN, J. O.: Intermediary metabolism of fungi as revealed by drug reaction. In: Fungi and fungus diseases (G. DALLDORF, ed.). Springfield (Ill.): C. C. Thomas 1962.
LAMPEN, J. O., and P. ARNOW: Significance of nystatin uptake for its antifungal action. Proc. Soc. Exptl. Biol. Med. **101**, 792—797 (1959).
LAMPEN, J. O., and P. ARNOW: Inhibition of algae by nystatin. J. Bacteriol. **82**, 247—251 (1961).
LAMPEN, J. O., and P. M. ARNOW: Differences in action of large and small polyene antifungal antibiotics. Bull. Research Council Israel **11A4**, 286—291 (1963).
LAMPEN, J. O., P. M. ARNOW, Z. BOROWSKA, and A. I. LASKIN: Location and role of sterol at nystatin-binding sites. J. Bacteriol. **84**, 1152—1160 (1962).
LAMPEN, J. O., P. M. ARNOW, and R. S. SAFFERMAN: Mechanism of protection by sterols against polyene antibiotics. J. Bacteriol. **80**, 200—206 (1960).
LAMPEN, J. O., J. W. GILL, P. M. ARNOW, and A. MAGANA-PLAZA: Inhibition of the pleuropneumonia-like organism, *Mycoplasma gallisepticum*, by certain polyene antifungal antibiotics. J. Bacteriol. **86**, 945—949 (1963).
LAMPEN, J. O., E. R. MORGAN, and A. SLOCUM: Effect of nystatin on the utilization of substrates by yeast and other fungi. J. Bacteriol. **74**, 297—302 (1957).
LAMPEN, J. O., E. R. MORGAN, A. SLOCUM, and P. ARNOW: Absorption of nystatin by microorganisms. J. Bacteriol. **78**, 282—289 (1959).
LARDY, H. A., D. JOHNSON, and W. C. MCMURRAY: Antibiotics as tools for metabolic studies. I. A survey of toxic antibiotics in respiratory, phosphorylative and glycolytic systems. Arch. Biochem. Biophys. **78**, 587—597 (1958).
LARSEN, W. G., and D. J. DEMIS: Metabolic studies of the effect of griseofulvin and candicidin on fungi. J. Invest. Dermatol. **41**, 335—342 (1963).
LECHEVALIER, H., E. BOROWSKI, J. O. LAMPEN, and C. P. SCHAFFNER: Water-soluble N-acetyl derivatives of heptaene macrolide antifungal antibiotics: Microbiological studies. Antibiotics & Chemotherapy **11**, 640—647 (1961).
LEVIN, E. Y., and K. BLOCH: Absence of sterols in blue-green algae. Nature **202**, 90—91 (1964).
LITTMAN, M. L., M. A. PISANO, and R. M. LANCHASTER: Induced resistance of Candida species to nystatin and amphotericin B. Antibiotics Ann. **1957/58**, 981—987 (1958).
LUCY, J. A., and J. T. DINGLE: Fat-soluble vitamins and biological membranes. Nature **204**, 156—160 (1964).
LUCY, J. A., and A. M. GLAUERT: Structure and assembly of macromolecular lipid complexes composed of globular micelles. J. Mol. Biol. **8**, 727—748 (1964).
LUZZATI, V., and F. HUSSON: The structure of the liquid-crystalline phases of lipid-water systems. J. Cell Biol. **12**, 207—219 (1962).
MARINI, F., P. ARNOW, and J. O. LAMPEN: The effect of monovalent cations on the inhibition of yeast metabolism by nystatin. J. Gen. Microbiol. **24**, 51—62 (1961).
OROSHNIK, W., L. C. VINING, A. D. MEBANE, and W. A. TABER: Polyene antibiotics. Science **121**, 147—149 (1955).
PATRICK, J. B., R. P. WILLIAMS, and J. S. WEBB: Pimaricin. II. The structure of pimaricin. J. Am. Chem. Soc. **80**, 6688—6689 (1958).
PERRITT, A. M., A. W. PHILLIPS, and T. ROBINSON: Sterol protection against pimaricin in *Saccharomyces cerevisiae*. Biochem. Biophys. Research Comm. **2**, 432—435 (1960).

POSTHUMA, J., and W. BERENDS: Triplet-triplet transfer as a mechanism of a photodynamic reaction. Biochem. et Biophys. Acta **41**, 538—541 (1960).
POSTHUMA, J., and W. BERENDS: Energy transfer in aqueous solutions. Biochem. et Biophys. Acta **51**, 392—394 (1961).
PRESSMAN, B. C.: Induced active transport of ions in mitochondria. Proc. Nat. Acad. Sci. U.S. **53**, 1076—1083 (1965).
RAMACHANDRAN, S.: Studies of the mode of action of antibiotics. I. Hamycin. Hindustan Antibiotics Bull. **4**, 74—79 (1961).
SCHOLZ, R., H. SCHMITZ, TH. BUCHER u. J. O. LAMPEN: Über die Wirkung von Nystatin auf Bäckerhefe. Biochem. Z. **331**, 71—86 (1959).
SCHULMAN, J. H., and E. K. RIDEAL: Molecular interaction in monolayers. I. Complexes between large molecules. Proc. Roy. Soc. (London) B **122**, 29—45 (1937).
SENECA, H., and E. BERGENDAHL: Toxicity of antibiotics to snails. Antibiotics & Chemotherapy **5**, 737—741 (1955).
SHAW, P. D., A. M. ALLAM, and D. GOTTLIEB: Effect of filipin on the terminal electron transport system of *Saccharomyces cerevisiae*. Biochem. et Biophys. Acta **89**, 33—41 (1964).
SHOCKMAN, G., and J. O. LAMPEN: Inhibition by antibiotics of the growth of bacterial and yeast protoplasts. J. Bacteriol. **84**, 508—512 (1962).
SLAYMAN, C. L., and C. W. SLAYMAN: Measurement of membrane potentials in Neurospora. Science **136**, 876—877 (1962).
STACHIEWICZ, E., and J. H. QUASTEL: Amino acid transport in yeast and effects of nystatin. Canad. J. Biochem. and Physiol. **41**, 397—407 (1963).
STOUT, H. A., and J. F. PAGANO: Resistance studies with nystatin. Antibiotics Ann. **1955/56**, 704—710 (1956).
SUTTON, D. D., P. M. ARNOW, and J. O. LAMPEN: Effect of high concentrations of nystatin upon glycolysis and cellular permeability in yeast. Proc. Soc. Exptl. Biol. Med. **108**, 170—175 (1961).
VINING, L. C.: The polyene antifungal antibiotics. Hindustan Antibiotics Bull. **3**, 37—54 (1960).
WAKSMAN, S., and H. LECHEVALIER: The actinomycetes, vol. III. Antibiotics of actinomycetes. Baltimore: Williams & Wilkins Co. 1962.
WALTERS, D. R., J. D. DUTCHER, and O. WINTERSTEINER: The structure of mycosamine. J. Am. Chem. Soc. **79**, 5076—5077 (1957).
WEBER, M. M., and S. C. KINSKY: Effect of cholesterol on the sensitivity of *Mycoplasma laidlawii* to the polyene antibiotic filipin. J. Bacteriol. **89**, 306—312 (1965).
ZONDAG, E., J. POSTHUMA, and W. BERENDS: On the mechanism of a photodynamic reaction. Biochem. et Biophys. Acta **39**, 178—180 (1960).

Polymyxins and Circulin

Oldrich K. Sebek

Polymyxins are peptide antibiotics which have almost identical biological properties and very similar chemical characteristics. Their discovery was announced in 1947 independently in the United States (BENEDICT and LANGLYKKE, 1947; STANSLY *et al.*, 1947), and in England (AINSWORTH *et al.*, 1947). It soon became apparent that all three groups of investigators had discovered closely related substances. At a conference in 1948 which was organized by the New York Academy of Sciences to clarify the relationship among these antibiotics (MINOR, 1949), five major and chemically distinct polymyxins were recognized and designated alphabetically as polymyxins A-E. The original aerosporin of AINSWORTH *et al.* became polymyxin A and the material discovered by STANSLY *et al.* was named polymyxin D. Polymyxin E was found to be identical with colistin[1] (WILKINSON, 1963; WILKINSON and LOWE, 1964). Still another member of this group was described by KHOKHLOV *et al.* (1960) and designated as polymyxin M.

All these antibiotics are produced by bacteria which were identified as *Bacillus polymyxa* (BREED *et al.*, 1948) and have essentially the same antibacterial spectra. They are active in similar concentrations, but exhibit undesirable side-effects to different degrees. Because of their high nephrotoxicity, polymyxins A and D have never been used in medical practice. On the other hand, polymyxins B and E were shown to be the least toxic of the group (BROWNLEE *et al.*, 1952) and are at present the only ones which are manufactured and used, polymyxins B and E as sulfates and polymyxin E as methane sulfonate.

Polymyxins have practically no effect on Gram-positive organisms, pathogenic Gram-negative cocci and mycobacteria. Strains of the *Proteus* group are singularly resistant to them. However, most of the Gram-negative bacteria (*Aerobacter, Brucella, Eberthella, Escherichia, Hemophillus, Klebsiella, Pasteurella, Salmonella, Shigella,* and *Vibrio*) are inhibited by these antibiotics in concentrations of 0.02 to 5.0 μg/ml, and *Trichomonas vaginalis* at 125—250 μg/ml (SENECA and IDES, 1953). Polymyxin B was found active against practically all strains of *Pseudomonas aeruginosa* in <8 μg/ml concentrations (JAWETZ, 1956; see also Table 1). It also inhibited the photosynthesis, respiration, carbon dioxide fixation, and to some extent, growth of *Chlorella pyrenoidosa*. These effects were less pronounced in *Scendesmus obliquus* (GALLOWAY and KRAUSS, 1959a and b; TOMISEK *et al.*,1957).

Polymyxins exhibit an almost complete lack of absorption when administered topically on skin, or orally to the digestive tract, and do not diffuse through the body membranes and body tissues to any significant degree. Because of this property, they are not effective against diffuse systemic or deep-seated infections

[1] Colistin was independently isolated as a product of *B. colistinus* in Japan (KOYAMA *et al.*, 1950).

of tissues and parenchymatous organs. They are, therefore, agents of choice in the treatment of infections limited to surfaces such as wounds, burns, grafts or of mucous membranes of the intestine, pleural cavity or dural space. They are also highly effective in the treatment of meningeal, pulmonary and urinary tract infections, in corneal ulcers and in external otitis caused by *Ps. aeruginosa*, and are, in such cases, the drugs of choice.

Table 1. *Antibacterial spectra of circulin and polymyxin*

Test organism	Inhibitory concentrations (μg/ml)	
	Circulin Sulfate	Polymyxin Hydrochloride
Aerobacter aerogenes	3.1	0.8
Bacillus anthracis	100.0	>100.0
B. subtilis	>100.0	>100.0
Brucella bronchiseptica	0.8	0.1
Escherichia coli	0.8	0.8
Klebsiella pneumoniae	3.1	6.2
Staphylococcus aureus	100.0	>100.0
S. albus	25.0	>100.0
Neisseria catarrhalis	3.1	6.2
Pseudomonas aeruginosa	3.1	3.1
Salmonella sp. group B	1.6	0.4
S. enteritidis	1.6	0.2
S. gallinarum	0.4	0.2
S. paratyphi	6.2	1.6
S. pullorum	0.8	0.4
S. schottmuelleri	6.2	0.8
S. typhimurium	1.6	<0.4
S. typhosa	3.1	<0.4
Shigella dysenteriae	<0.4	<0.4

MURRAY *et al.* (1949).

These antibiotics may also serve as useful diagnostic agents to differentiate the true cholera vibrio (*Vibrio comma*) which is inhibited by polymyxins B and E, from its El Tor type which is resistant to them (HAN and KHIE, 1963; ABE *et al.*, 1966).

Polymyxins are frequently combined with other antibiotics in order to extend antimicrobial spectra and are used for sterilization of the digestive tract. When administered intramuscularly (up to 2.5 mg/kg/day) to persons with normal renal function, they may produce annoying neurotoxic side effects (HOPPER *et al.*, 1953). At higher levels (3 mg or more/kg/day), nitrogen retention and decrease in glomerular filtration rate are common but cease if the therapy is stopped. Chick embryo heart explants were not affected by concentrations of polymyxin B usually attainable in the body fluids (0.1 mg/ml) but were completely inhibited by higher concentrations (2.5 mg/ml; METZGER *et al.*, 1952). Pharmacologically, polymyxin was reported to produce inhibition of impulses at the neuromuscular junction (ADAMSON *et al.*, 1960; LÜLLMANN and REUTER, 1960).

The potency and concentration of polymyxins in biological fluids are determined by conventional microbiological techniques by means of polymyxin-sensitive bacteria (e.g. *Escherichia coli*). Their effectiveness in *vitro* decreases in the presence of serum or blood. Effectiveness appears to be directly proportional to the amount of the inoculum; the larger it is, the larger concentrations of the antibiotic are required to arrest the growth. Resistance to these antibiotics develops only rarely; but naturally resistant strains appear occasionally in susceptible populations. There is complete cross-resistance among all polymyxins. Except for one report by Szybalski and Bryson (1952), the cross-resistance does not extend to any other clinically used antibiotics. A synergistic effect was observed between polymyxins and streptomycin, tetracycline, and chloramphenicol (Jawetz *et al.*, 1954).

Another antibiotic, circulin, was discovered in 1949 in cultures of *Bacillus circulans* (Murray *et al.*, 1949). This material was later separated into circulins A and B. There is a close relationship between polymyxins and circulins as both have almost identical antibacterial spectra (Table 1), strikingly similar structures (Fig. 1) and the cultures which elaborate them are also taxonomically very similar (Table 2).

Table 2. *Characteristics of Bacillus polymyxa and B. circulans* (Breed *et al.*, 1948)

Test	*B. polymyxa*	*B. circulans*
Movement	Motile	
Spores	Ellipsoidal, usually central to terminal	
Sporangia	Swollen and clavate	
Hydrolysis	Starch, gelatin	
C and N utilization	Glucose, sucrose, arabinose, xylose; NH_4^++	
Indole	Not formed	
Citrate	Not utilized	
Reduction	Nitrate to nitrite; methylene blue	
Growth optimum (C)	28—35	
Growth maximum (C)	40 but not at 45	40—45, some strains at 50—55
Gram stain	Variable	Negative
Casein	Hydrolyzed	Not hydrolyzed
Acetoin	Formed	Not formed
Vitamin required for growth	Biotin[1]	Thiamine[2]
Gas from sugar, milk and soybean broth	Formed	Not formed

[1] Katznelson and Lochhead (1944).
[2] Sebek (1964).

Polymyxin and circulin developed an almost reciprocal resistance to each other, and strains of *E. coli* resistant to both antibiotics exhibited a 2—6 fold increase of resistance to streptomycin and neomycin (Szybalski and Bryson, 1952). Both antibiotics are readily soluble in water and are very stable in the physiological range of temperature and pH. Chemically, they are basic peptides with molecular weights of about 1200 and readily form water-soluble salts with mineral acids. They all contain L-threonine, L-α,γ-diaminobutyric acid, and

(+)-6-methyloctanoic (or, as in case of polymyxin B_2, isooctanoic) acid. Although several cyclic structures have been proposed for them, recent investigations show that polymyxins and circulin A are heptapeptides with structures illustrated by examples in Fig. 1.

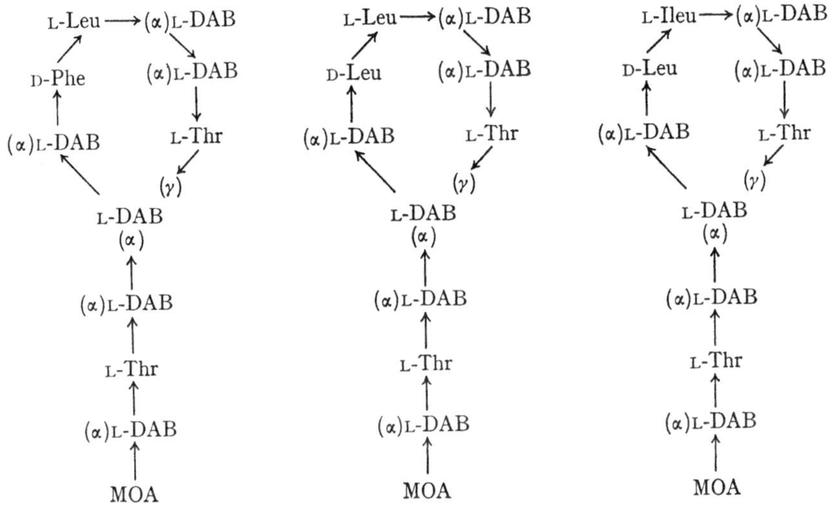

Polymyxin B_1 Colistin A Circulin A

Fig. 1. Structures of polymyxin B_1, Colistin A and Circulin A.
The (α) and (γ) designations indicate that the respective NH_2-groups are involved in the peptide linkages.
DAB = α,γ-Diaminobutyric acid residue;
MOA = (+)-6-Methyloctanoic acid residue.
FUJIKAWA *et al.* (1965), HAYASHI and SUZUKI (1965), SUZUKI *et al.* (1963), SUZUKI and FUJIKAWA (1964), SUZUKI *et al.* (1964)

Action on Cytoplasmic Membrane

All polymyxins contain both hydrophilic and hydrophobic groups in their molecules. Since they are also positively charged at neutral pH values, they can be classified as cationic surface-active compounds. They differ from other such compounds by being more active against Gram-negative than against Gram-positive bacteria. As in the case of cationic detergents, the antibacterial activity of polymyxins decreases in the presence of anionic compounds. Soap, phospholipid extracts of soybean and of bacterial origin, and cephalin also act in this manner (BLISS *et al.*, 1947; FEW, 1955).

Minimum inhibitory concentrations of polymyxins halt the growth of sensitive organisms only temporarily while 2—4 times higher levels become rapidly bactericidal. This bactericidal action does not depend on the growth of the organism as is true in the case of certain other antibiotics, e.g. penicillin. Sensitive bacteria have a high affinity for the antibiotic which was absorbed by them almost completely when added in about 50 μg/ml concentrations. At higher concentrations (310—375 μg polymyxin E/ml), saturation of the organisms occurred and was about four times higher than in the resistant bacteria. With the assumption that

1 mg of polymyxin E occupies an area of 160 A^2/mol, it was calculated that at saturation levels, the amount of polymyxin taken up by *Pseudomonas denitrificans* would cover cell surface area about twelve times, by *E. coli* ten times, and by *Streptococcus faecalis* four times (FEW and SCHULMAN, 1953a, 1953b).

When several sensitive organisms (*Ps. denitrificans, Bacillus subtilis, Micrococcus lysodeikticus, E. coli*) were treated with polymyxin E, a pentose, phosphate and a material absorbing at 260 mμ (corresponding to free purines, pyrimidines and nucleosides), were released from the cells into the medium. At concentrations lower than those required for 99% kill, the amount of this material was proportional to the amount of the cells killed (FEW and SCHULMAN, 1953b; NEWTON, 1953a; cf. also KISHIDA *et al.*, 1965; NAKAJIMA and KAWAMATA, 1965a; SUGANUMA *et al.*, 1965). In most bacteria treated with polymyxin, the release of the 260 mμ absorbing material was rapid and its total quantity corresponded to the purine, pyrimidine and nucleotide content which had been originally present free in the cells. The release of the 260 mμ absorbing material from *Ps. aeruginosa* on the other hand was slow, extended to several hours and was concomitant with the release of equimolar quantities of a pentose and a phosphate. It was correlated with a breakdown of the ribonucleic acid of the cells. The leakage of the material was prevented by low temperature, high concentrations of polymyxin (NEWTON, 1953a; NAKAJIMA and KAWAMATA, 1965c) and by magnesium ions which are known to inhibit ribonuclease. Other divalent cations (calcium, manganese, and ferrous iron) also exhibited such antagonistic activity. The antagonism of these cations was believed to be due to the competitive absorption between them and the antibiotic for specific sites of attachment on the bacterial cell membrane (NEWTON, 1953b).

In addition to the leakage, an ingenious application of N-tolyl-α-naphthylamine-8-sulfonic acid provided still another and more direct evidence of the permeability changes in the polymyxin-treated cells. The compound was also used to investigate the competition between polymyxin and selected cations for sites in the bacterial cells. This dye does not fluoresce when excited by ultraviolet light unless it combines with negatively charged groups of protein. Since the cells of *Ps. aeruginosa* have no groups on their surface that would combine with the dye, they did not fluoresce in its presence. When, however, polymyxin was added to such washed suspensions, it altered the cell permeability, allowed the dye to penetrate through the wall and to react with the proteinaceous parts of the cell. As a result, an immediate fluorescence of the cell suspension resulted. The affinities of the cations for the polymyxin-combining groups of the cell and their ability to reverse the charge on certain colloids suggested that polymyxin reacts with phosphate groups on or near the cell surface (NEWTON, 1954).

Electron micrographs showed that the treatment of sensitive cells with polymyxin resulted in the damage of the cell surface and released most of the electron-dense material from the cells. Nuclear material disappeared from its normal sites and was no longer demonstrable, and the bacterial cytoplasm lost its granular appearance (NEWTON, 1953a; CHAPMAN, 1962a, 1962b). Leptospirae, on the other hand, were reported to be completely lysed by polymyxin (BYSTRICKÝ *et al.*, 1962). Only polymyxin-sensitive bacteria were affected by this antibiotic in this way, since none of these phenomena were observed in polymyxin-resistant microorganisms.

The leakage of soluble constituents from the cells and the rapid loss of viability were also brought about by circulin. As in the case of polymyxin, the amount of the 260 mμ absorbing material released was proportional to the amount of the added antibiotic (COLASITO *et al.*, 1955). Heavy cell suspensions of *Bacillus megaterium* absorbed relatively large amounts of the antibiotic (125-350 μg/mg dry cells). The absorbed material was bound to cytoplasmic membrane. Some was also found in the cell wall fraction, probably due to an incomplete fractionation. None was detected in the cytoplasm (COLASITO *et al.*, 1956).

A similar relationship existed between cetylammonium bromide and the leakage of such material from six Gram-positive and Gram-negative bacteria (SALTON, 1951), as well as between the bactericidal action of tyrocidin and the release of amino acids from the intracellular metabolic pool in *Streptococcus faecalis* (GALE and TAYLOR, 1947). These results supported an hypothesis originally proposed by BAKER *et al.* (1941) which was based on their work with synthetic cationic detergents. They postulated that the rapid effect of these substances on bacterial metabolism and on the viability of the cells was caused by disorganization of the cell membrane and by denaturation of certain proteins essential for metabolism and growth. HOTCHKISS (1946) pointed out that the penetration of surface-active agents would be appreciable only if the cell membrane was damaged.

The site of polymyxin interference was also indicated in other studies. The antibiotic caused only a slight increase in electrophoretic mobility of several strains of *Ps. aeruginosa* thus suggesting that it did not combine with their surface. However, it was calculated that it could combine with structures located about 100 A below the cell surface without affecting the charge at the surface itself. Such structures were also indicated when it was observed that polymyxin affected both electrophoretic mobility and agglutination of the rough form of *Ps. aeruginosa* (MCQUILLEN, 1956). These data agreed with earlier findings which showed that polymyxin agglutinated only the rough forms of *S. aureus* and *E. coli* (LATTERRADE and MACHEBOEUF, 1950). Further studies in which a fluorescent derivative of polymyxin was used, also showed that the antibiotic combined with the protoplasmic membrane. The derivative was prepared by a careful coupling of l-dimethyl-aminonaphthalene-5-sulfonyl chloride with the γ-amino group of the α,γ-diaminobutyric acid residues in the polymyxin B molecule. As with polymyxin itself, this derivative was readily absorbed by sensitive cells and was rapidly bactericidal. An analysis of the cell fractions of three organisms, *Bacillus megaterium, Sarcina lutea* and *Micrococcus lysodeikticus*, obtained by mechanical disintegration and differential centrifugation, showed that 90% of the fluorescent conjugate corresponded to the material derived from the structure underlying the cell wall. Additional evidence for the site of action was obtained by exposing the cells to this polymyxin derivative whereupon the fluorescent material became clearly visible in the peripheral structures of the cells. When the cell walls of these cells were removed by controlled lysozyme treatment, the resulting protoplasts strongly fluoresced while no fluorescent material was detected in the supernatant fluid after centrifugation of the protoplast suspension. After the destruction of the protoplast by sonic vibration and subsequent ultracentrifugation, the fluorescent material was again recovered in the fraction which originated from the cytoplasmic membrane (NEWTON, 1955).

When these findings are taken collectively, they show quite convincingly that polymyxins exert their activity by damaging the bacterial cell membrane. The membrane is a part of the cell envelope and is located between the cell wall and the protoplast which it encloses. It is generally pictured as a three-layer structure consisting of a middle double-layer of oriented phospholipid molecules and enclosed from both sides by two protein layers. The membrane is semi-permeable and acts as an osmotic barrier. It mantains internal osmotic pressure, which may reach as much as 20 atmospheres. Functionally, it is involved in many biochemical processes of the organism. It is credited with the selective transport of substances into the cell (ions and small-molecular nutrients), with the excretion of other materials to the outside (metabolic waste products, exoenzymes) and with the retention of the cellular content within the cell. The membrane contains cytochromes and other respiratory enzyme systems, complexes responsible for oxidative phosphorylation and permeation, the photosynthetic apparatus and is involved in cellular division. It is also postulated as a site of the synthesis of the cell wall, of proteins, capsular components and exoenzymes (see FINEAN, 1966; POLLOCK and RICHMOND, 1965).

Since the cytoplasmic membrane is of such vital importance to the cell, any impairment or modification of its structure inevitably affects the metabolism and viability of the cell. Antibiotics may interfere with any of these functions and it is through such interference that thèir action upon the bacterial cell may be expressed. Polymyxins combine with the cell membrane through their lipophilic and lipophobic groups (phosphatidic acids) whereby they become oriented between the lipid and protein layers of the membrane. Such combination disorients the layers to the extent that the membrane can no longer function normally as an effective osmotic barrier. The osmotic equilibrium of the cell is disturbed, the cellular content is rapidly released and the death of the cell follows. This mechanism is similar to the one postulated for the hemolysis of red blood cells by ionic detergents. This hemolytic action was described to be due to the collapse of a cholesterol-phospho-lipid-lipoprotein complex of the blood cells (PETHICA and SCHULMAN, 1953). In bacterial systems, the cell wall helps to prevent the loss of high molecular constituents from the inside of the cells. Consequently, the damage to such cells caused by polymyxins is less complete than the hemolysis of the erythrocytes.

In view of these profound effects which polymyxins exert on the membranous structure of bacterial cells, other observations that have been made, are of comparatively minor importance for the understanding of the action of these antibiotics. Thus, in experiments with washed cells of *Ps. aeruginosa*, polymyxins inhibited endogenous respiration and oxidation of several intermediates of glucose metabolism (2-ketogluconate, pyruvate, oxalacetate, succinate, and acetate) and of mevalonate; however, the concentrations needed were three times higher than those required for bactericidal effects. On the other hand, glucose oxidation was not inhibited (NEWTON, 1953c; MOHAN *et al.*, 1962). The esterase activity of several mycobacteria but not of pseudomonads was inhibited by the antibiotic (COHEN *et al.*, 1954). The antibiotic was not inactivated by pepsin, trypsin, pancreatin or erepsin (STANSLY and ANANENKO, 1947). Streptokinase and streptodornase increased its action on *Cryptococcus neoformans* (CARTON and LIEBIG,

1953). Polymyxin B was also found to be a potent inhibitor of enzymatic depolymerization of poly-β-hydroxybutyric acid (MERRICK, 1965).

Nucleic acids of the cells were also implicated in the action of polymyxins. It was postulated that polymyxin does not act on Gram-positive bacteria because they possess magnesium ribonucleate coating. Gram-negative bacteria, which have no such structure, are, therefore, vulnerable to the action of this antibiotic (RHODES *et al.*, 1953). Yeast ribonucleic acid and polymyxin formed a complex insoluble in water (LATTERRADE and MACHEBOEUF, 1950), and highly polymerized DNA from various sources, yeast RNA, and *E. coli* ribosomes were precipitated by polymyxin and other basic antibiotics (POTTER *et al.*, 1965; NAKAJIMA and KAWAMATA, 1965b, 1966). MITCHELL and MOYLE (1954) proposed that higher sensitivity of Gram-negative bacteria might be related to their high phosphorus content since it was found that they contain twice as much phosphorus as Gram-positive bacteria.

The antibiotic had no effect on the sporulation of bacilli (WEINBERG, 1955; BROCK, 1962). It induced aberrant bacillary forms to the normally spiral shaped *Rhodospirillum rubrum*, and sequential lysozyme-polymyxin treatment yielded completely transparent spherical bodies sharply delineated by a thin membrane. The addition of polymyxin was also attended by an extensive release of protein (TUTTLE and GEST, 1959).

Little is known about the structural characteristics responsible for the antibacterial action of polymyxins. As shown in experiments with l-dimethylamino-naphthalene-5-sulfonyl chloride, at least one of the available free amino groups of the diaminobutyric acid residues can be substituted without loss of activity, but acetylation of amino acid groups generally results in a complete loss of activity (HOTCHKISS, 1944). The function of the methyloctanoic acid part of the molecule has not been ascertained since it has not been removed without simultaneous destruction of the whole antibiotic molecule. The cyclic structure and the size of polymyxins are undoubtedly important since they impart a higher degree of rigidity to the molecule. Because of these features, the molecule is apt to undergo less kinetic flexing and to absorb more firmly at the intracellular interface than its acyclic form. These properties should give the molecule higher biological activity and specificity (FEW, 1957), and should also render the antibiotic less susceptible to enzymatic attack and destruction. The nature and function of the amino acid components and their particular cyclic arrangements must also be of significance in view of the specific activity of polymyxins against Gram-negative bacteria. Virtually nothing is known, however, about this important aspect of the polymyxin problem[1].

See Addendum

References

ABE, H., S. GOTO, and S. KUWAHARA: Colistin disc — a differential method between *Vibrio cholerae* and *Vibrio eltor*. J. Antibiotics (Japan), Ser. A **19**, 13 (1966).

ADAMSON, R. H., F. N. MARSHALL, and J. P. LONG: Neuromuscular blocking properties of various polypeptide antibiotics. Proc. Soc. Exptl. Biol. Med. **105**, 494 (1960).

[1] Other discusions and reviews on polymyxins are by BRUNNER and MACHEK (1965), NEWTON (1956), and by GALE (1963). The action of surface-active bactericides as chemotherapeutic agents are discussed by NEWTON (1958).

AINSWORTH, G. C., A. M. BROWN, and G. BROWNLEE: "Aerosporin", an antibiotic produced by *Bacillus aerosporus* Greer. Nature **160**, 263 (1947).
BAKER, Z., R. W. HARRISON, and B. F. MILLER: The bactericidal action of synthetic detergents. J. Exptl. Med. **74**, 611 (1941).
BENEDICT, R. G., and A. F. LANGLYKKE: Antibiotic activity of *Bacillus polymyxa*. J. Bacteriol. **54**, 24 (1947).
BLISS, E. A., C. A. CHANDLER, and E. B. SCHOENBACH: *In vitro* studies of polymyxin. Ann. N.Y. Acad. Sci. **51**, 944 (1949).
BREED, R. S., E. G. D. MURRAY, and N. R. SMITH: Bergey's manual of determinative bacteriology, 6th ed., pp. 720, 722. Williams & Wilkins Co. 1948.
BROCK, T. D.: Inhibition of endotrophic sporulation by antibiotics. Nature **195**, 309 (1962).
BROWNLEE, G., S. R. M. BUSHBY, and E. I. SHORT: The chemotherapy and pharmacology of the polymyxins. Brit. J. Pharmacol. **7**, 170 (1952).
BRUNNER, R., u. G. MACHEK, Hrsg.: Die Antibiotica, Bd. 2, S. 214, 235. Nürnberg: H. Carl 1965.
BYSTRICKÝ, V., K. LADZIANSKA, and M. HALAŠA: Electron microscopy of the action of polymyxin on Leptospirae. J. Bacteriol. **84**, 864 (1962).
CARTON, C. A., and C. S. LIEBIG: Treatment of central nervous system cryptococcosis. A.M.A. Arch. Internal. Med. **91**, 773 (1953).
CHAPMAN, G. B.: Cytological aspects of antimicrobial antibiosis. I. Cytological changes associated with the exposure of *Escherichia coli* to colistin sulfate. J. Bacteriol. **84**, 169 (1962a). II. Cytological changes associated with the exposure of *Pseudomonas aeruginosa* and *Bacillus megaterium* to colistin sulfate. J. Bacteriol. **84**, 180 (1962b).
COHEN, S., C. V. PURDY, and J. B. KUSHNICK: Inhibition of mycobacterial esterases by polymyxin B. Antibiotics & Chemotherapy **4**, 18 (1954).
COLASITO, D. J., H. KOFFLER, H. C. REITZ, and P. A. TETRAULT: The probable site of action of circulin. Bacteriol. Proc. **1956**, 72.
COLASITO, D. J., H. KOFFLER, P. A. TETRAULT, and H. C. REITZ: Assay for circulin based on the release of cellular constituents. Canad. J. Microbiol. **1**, 685 (1955).
FEW, A. V.: The interaction of polymyxin E with bacterial and other lipids. Biochim. et Biophys. Acta **16**, 137 (1955).
FEW, A. V.: Structure in relation to surface and biological properties of cyclic decapeptide antibiotics. Proc. 2nd Internatl. Congr. Surface Activity, vol. 4, p. 288. London: Butterworth & Co. 1957.
FEW, A. V., and J. H. SCHULMAN: Absorption of polymyxin by bacteria. Nature **171**, 644 (1953a).
FEW, A. V., and J. H. SCHULMAN: The absorption of polymyxin E by bacteria and bacterial cell walls and its bactericidal action. J. Gen. Microbiol. **9**, 454 (1953b).
FINEAN, J. B.: The molecular organization of cell membranes. Progress in Biophysics and Molecular Biology **38**, 145 (1966). Pergamon Press, J. A. V. BUTLER, and H. E. HUXLEY, eds.
FUJIKAWA, K., Y. SUKETA, K. HAYASHI, and T. SUZUKI: Chemical structure of circulin A. Experientia **21**, 307 (1965).
GALE, E. F.: Mechanisms of antibiotic action. Pharmacol. Revs. **15**, 481 (1963).
GALE, E. F., and E. S. TAYLOR: The assimilation of amino acids by bacteria. 2. The action of tyrocidin and some detergent substances in releasing amino acids from the internal environment of *Streptococcus faecalis*. J. Gen. Microbiol. **1**, 77 (1947).
GALLOWAY, R. A., and R. W. KRAUSS: Differential action of chemical agents, especially polymyxin B, on certain algae, bacteria and fungi. Amer. J. Botany **28**, 40 (1959b).
GALLOWAY, R. A., and R. W. KRAUSS: Mechanism of action of polymyxin B on Chlorella and Scenedesmus. Plant Physiol. **92**, 380 (1959a).
HAN, GAN KOEN, and TJIA SOE KHIE: A new method for the differentiation of *Vibrio comma* and *Vibrio El Tor*. Amer. J. Hyg. **77**, 184 (1963).
HAYASHI, K., and T. SUZUKI: Chemical structures of polymyxin series antibiotics. Bull. Inst. Chem. Res., Kyoto Univ. **43**, 259 (1965).

HOPPER, J., E. JAWETZ, and F. HINMAN: Polymyxin B in chronic pyelonephritis: observations on the safety of the drug and on its influence on the renal infection. Amer. J. Med. Sci. **225**, 402 (1953).
HOTCHKISS, R. D.: Gramicidin, tyrocidine and tyrothricin. Advances in Enzymol. **4**, 153 (1944).
HOTCHKISS, R. D.: The nature of the bactericidal action of surface active agents. Ann. N.Y. Acad. Sci. **46**, 479 (1946).
JAWETZ, E.: Polymyxin, neomycin, bacitracin, p. 11—35. New York: Medical Encyclopedia, Inc. 1956.
JAWETZ, E., V. COLEMAN, and J. B. GUNNISON: The participation of polymyxin B in combined antibiotic action. Ann. Internal Med. **41**, 79 (1954).
KATZNELSON, H., and A. G. LOCHHEAD: Studies with *Bacillus polymyxa*. III. Nutritional requirements. Canad. J. Research C **22**, 273 (1944).
KHOKHLOV, A. S. (and fourteen coauthors): A new type of polymyxin — polymyxin M. Antibiotiki **5** (1), 3 (1960).
KISHIDA, T., SUGANUMA, W. HARA and Y. FUJITA: The mode of action of colistin. J. Kyoto Prefect. Med. Univ. (in press) (1965).
KOYAMA, Y., A. KUROSASA, A. TSUCHIYA, and K. TAKAKUTA: A new antibiotic, 'colistin', produced by spore-forming soil bacteria. J. Antibiotics (Japan), Ser. B **3**, 457 (1950).
LATTERRADE, C., et M. MACHEBOEUF: Recherches biochimiques sur le mode d'action de la polymyxine. Ann. Inst. Pasteur **78**, 751 (1950).
LÜLLMANN, H., u. H. REUTER: Über die Hemmung der neuromuskulären Übertragung durch einige Antibiotika. Chemotherapia **1**, 375 (1960).
McQUILLEN, K.: Unpublished data quoted by B. A. NEWTON 1956.
MERRICK, J. M.: Effect of polymyxin B, tyrocidine, gramicidin D and other antibiotics on the enzymatic hydrolysis of poly-β-hydroxybutyrate. J. Bacteriol. **90**, 965 (1965).
METZGER, J. F., M. H. FUSILLO, and D. M. KUHNS: Effect of polymyxin and viomycin on embryonic cells in tissue cultures. Antibiotics & Chemotherapy **2**, 227 (1952).
MINOR, R. W., ed.: Antibiotics derived from *Bacillus polymyxa*. Ann. N.Y. Acad. Sci. **51**, 853 (1949).
MITCHELL, P., and J. MOYLE: The Gram reaction and cell composition: nucleic acids and other phosphate fractions. J. Gen. Microbiol. **10**, 533 (1954).
MOHAN, R. R., R. S. PIANOTTI, R. LEVERETT, and B. S. SCHWARTZ: Effect of colistin on the metabolism of *Pseudomonas aeruginosa*. Antimicrobial Agents and Chemotherapy **1962**, 801.
MURRAY, F. J., P. A. TETRAULT, O. W. KAUFMANN, H. KOFFLER, D. H. PETERSON, and D. R. COLINGSWORTH: Circulin, an antibiotic from an organism resembling *Bacillus circulans*. J. Bacteriol. **57**, 305 (1949).
NAKAJIMA, K., and J. KAWAMATA: Effect of colistin and actinomycin sensitivity on *Escherichia coli*. Biken J. **8**, 115 (1965a).
NAKAJIMA, K., and J. KAWAMATA: Studies on the mechanism of action of colistin. I. Formation of an insoluble complex with nucleic acids. Biken J. **8**, 225 (1965b).
NAKAJIMA, K., and J. KAWAMATA: Studies on the mechanism of action of colistin. II. Alteration of permeability of *Escherichia coli* by colistin. Biken J. **8**, 233 (1965c).
NAKAJIMA, K., and J. KAWAMATA: Studies on the mechanism of action of colistin. III. Precipitation of *Escherichia coli* ribosomes with colistin. Biken J. **9**, 45 (1966).
NEWTON, B. A.: The release of soluble constituents from washed cells of *Pseudomonas aeruginosa* by the action of polymyxin. J. Gen. Microbiol. **9**, 54 (1953a).
NEWTON, B. A.: Reversal of antibacterial activity of polymyxin by divalent cations. Nature **172**, 160 (1953b).
NEWTON, B. A.: The action of polymyxin on *Pseudomonas pyocyanea*. J. Gen. Microbiol. **8**, vi (1953c).
NEWTON, B. A.: Site of action of polymyxin on *Pseudomonas aeruginosa*: Antagonism by cations. J. Gen. Microbiol. **10**, 491 (1954).

NEWTON, B. A.: A fluorescent derivative of polymyxin: its preparation and use in studying the site of action of the antibiotic. J. Gen. Microbiol. **12**, 226 (1955).
NEWTON, B. A.: The properties and mode of action of the polymyxins. Bacteriol. Rev. **20**, 14 (1956).
NEWTON, B. A.: Surface-active bactericides. Strategy of Chemotherapy Symp. Soc. Gen. Microbiol., vol. 8, p. 62. Cambridge: Cambridge University Press 1958.
PETHICA, B. A., and J. H. SCHULMAN: The physical chemistry of hemolysis by surface-active agents. Biochem. J. **53**, 177 (1953).
POLLOCK, M. R., and M. H. RICHMOND, eds.: Function and structure in microorganisms. 15th Symp. Soc. Gen. Microbiol. Cambridge: Cambridge University Press 1965, p. 405.
POTTER, J. L., L. W. MATTHEWS, S. SPECTOR, and J. LEMM: Complex formation between basics antibiotics and deoxyribonucleic acid in human pulmonary secretions. Pediatrics **36**, 714 (1965).
RHODES, R. E., O. A. VILA, and R. J. FERLAUTO: The nature of polymyxin activity against a Gram-positive organism. Antibiotics & Chemotherapy **3**, 509 (1953).
SALTON, M. R. J.: The adsorption of cetyltrimethylammonium bromide by bacteria, its action in releasing cellular constituents and its bactericidal effects. J. Gen. Microbiol. **5**, 391 (1951).
SEBEK, O. K.: Requirements for growth and antibiotic synthesis in *Bacillus circulans*. Unpublished data 1964.
SENECA, H., and D. IDES: The *in vitro* effect of various antibiotics on *Trichomonas vaginalis*. Amer. J. Trop. Med. Hyg. **2**, 1045 (1953).
STANSLY, P. G., and N. H. ANANENKO: Resistance of polymyxin to some proteolytic enzymes. Arch. Biochem. **15**, 473 (1947).
STANSLY, P. G., R. G. SHEPHERD, and H. J. WHITE: Polymyxin: a new chemotherapeutic agent. Bull. Johns Hopkins Hosp. **81**, 43 (1947).
SUGANUMA, A., T. KISHIDA, T. ASANO, T. OTANI, M. TOMITA, M. SUZUKI, and T. SUZUKI: Morphological changes of *E. coli* by colistin sulfate (colimycin). J. Kyoto Prefect. Med. Univ. (in Press) (1965).
SUZUKI, T., and K. FUJIKAWA: Studies on the chemical structure of colistin. IV. Chemical structure of colistin B. J. Biochem. (Japan) **56**, 182 (1964).
SUZUKI, T., K. HAYASHI, K. FUJIKAWA, and K. TSUKAMOTO: Contribution to the elucidation of the chemical structure of polymyxin B. J. Biochem. (Japan) **56**, 335 (1964).
SUZUKI, T., H. INOUYE, K. FUJIKAWA, and Y. SUKETA: Studies on the chemical structure of colistin. I. Fractionation, molecular weight determination, amino acid and fatty acid composition. J. Biochem. (Japan) **54**, 25 (1963).
SZYBALSKI, W., and V. BRYSON: Genetic studies on microbial cross resistance to toxic agents. I. Cross resistance of *Escherichia coli* to fifteen antibiotics. J. Bacteriol. **64**, 489 (1952).
TOMISEK, A. J., M. R. REID, W. A. SHORT, and H. E. SKIPPER: The photosynthetic reaction. III. The effects of various inhibitors upon growth and carbonate fixation in *Chlorella pyrenoidosa*. Plant Physiol. **32**, 7 (1957).
TUTTLE, A. L., and H. GEST: Subcellular particulate systems and the photochemical apparatus of *Rhodospirillum rubrum*. Proc. Natl. Acad. Sci. U.S. **45**, 1261 (1959).
WEINBERG, E. D.: The effect of Mn^{++} and antimicrobial drugs on sporulation of *Bacillus subtilis* in nutrient broth. J. Bacteriol. **70**, 289 (1955).
WILKINSON, S.: Identity of colistin and polymyxin E. Lancet **1963**, 922.
WILKINSON, S., and L. A. LOWE: The identities of the antibiotics colistin and polymyxin E. J. Chem. Soc. **1964**, 4107.

Albomycin

B. K. Bhuyan

Albomycin is a cyclic iron-containing peptide produced by *Actinomyces subtropicus* (GAUSE and BRAZHNIKOVA, 1951). Most of the chemical and biological properties of albomycin have been reviewed by GAUSE (1955). Some of the properties of the antibiotic are listed in Table 1. Albomycin inhibits the growth of gram-positive cocci, chiefly pneumococcus and staphylococcus, and is also effective against several gram-negative bacteria, e.g., the coli-dysentery group. In view of

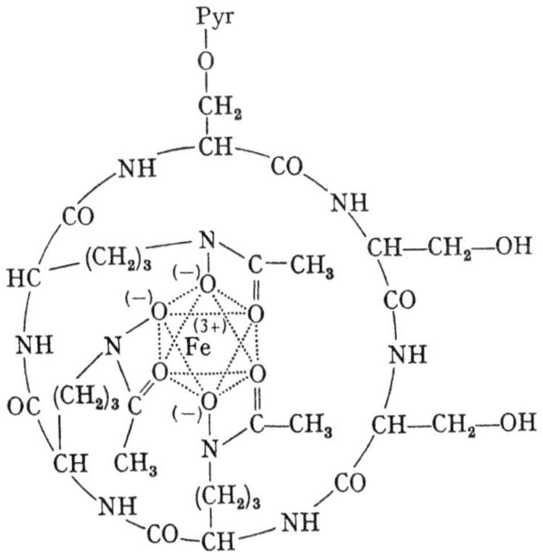

Fig. 1. Partial structure of Albomycin

its marked activity, particularly against penicillin resistant staphylococcus, and lack of toxicity, albomycin has undergone clinical trial in the U.S.S.R. (GAUSE, 1955). In clinical practice albomycin is used mainly in the treatment of infections caused by pathogenic cocci and in various septic conditions caused by penicillin resistant cocci. Albomycin binds partially and reversibly to serum. However, the albomycin-serum complex possesses chemotherapeutic activity, indicating dissociation of the complex *in vivo* (GAUSE, 1955).

The structure of albomycin has been partially determined. It is a basic, cyclic peptide containing three molecules of serine and three of acetylated-N^5-hydroxy ornithine. The iron atom is bound as the trivalent ion by three ionic bonds to the hydroxamate residues of ornithine and by three minor bonds to the carboxyl group of the three acetyl residues (TURKOVÁ *et al.*, 1964). The proposed structure is shown in Fig. 1. Further studies on the nature of the pyrimidine bound to the cyclic peptide has been reported (TURKOVÁ *et al.*, 1965). The iron is necessary for the antibacterial activity of the antibiotic. Removal of iron with 8-hydroxyquinoline results in loss of 90% of the activity. Addition of iron reestablishes the activity (GAUSE, 1955). Ferrichrome reversed the antibacterial activity of albomycin with *B. subtilis* (ŘIČICOVÁ, 1963).

Table 1

Empirical formula	$C_{39}H_{79}FeN_{12}O_{13}S$ (M.W. 1140)
Solubility	Soluble in water, slightly soluble in methanol
Toxicity (I.V., mice)	Nontoxic at 100 mg/kg
Structure	see Figure 1

SHORIN and SAZYKIN (1954) showed that albomycin inhibits growth of *S. aureus* and *E. coli* only in the presence of oxygen O_2. Since albomycin contains iron and is active only in an aerobic system, GAUSE (1955) suggested that albomycin inhibits the respiratory function of the cell by virtue of its similarity to the iron-containing respiratory system of bacteria.

However, GRUNBERGER *et al.* (1957) showed that albomycin does not affect the endogenous respiration of the oxidation of glucose by *E. coli* and *S. aureus*. Albomycin (1 µg/ml), added to *S. aureus* during a logarithmically growing phase, caused accumulation in the cell of acid soluble nucleosides and nucleotides (24% increase) and decreased the content of both RNA and DNA about 30%. SAZYKIN and BORISOVA (1962) reported that in bacteriostasis of *S. aureus* caused by albomycin, RNA and protein synthesis stopped immediately. Albomycin inhibited the uptake of radioactive precursors of proteins and of nucleic acids into the acid soluble pool of cells. This was followed by the inhibition of RNA, DNA and protein synthesis. The antibiotic did not inhibit the activity of RNA-polymerase or polynucleotide phosphorylase *in vitro*. Albomycin did not inhibit incorporation of amino acids into proteins in cell-free systems (VOŘÍŠEK, GRUNBERGER, 1966). The authors suggest that albomycin interferes with the transport of metabolic precursors through bacterial membranes.

References

GAUSE, G. F., i M. G. BRAZHNIKOVA: Nov. Med. (Mosk.) **23**, 3 (1951).

GAUSE, G. F.: Recent studies on albomycin, a new antibiotic. Brit. Med. J. **2**, p. 1177 (1955).

GRUNBERGER, D., Z. ŠHORMORÁ, and F. ŠORM: The effect of albomycin on oxidative processes and nucleic acid metabolism in *S. aureus* and *E. coli*. Biokhimiya **22**, 141 (1957).

ŘIČICOVÁ, A.: Antagonism of ferrichrome towards albomycin. Collection Czechoslov. Chem. Commun. **28**, 1761 (1963).

SAZYKIN, Y. O., i G. N. BORISOVA: Antibiotiki **7**, 975 (1962).

SHORIN, V. A., i Y. O. SAZYKIN: Compt. rend. acad. sci. U.R.S.S. **96**, 645 (1954).

TURKOVÁ, J., O. MIKES, and F. ŠORM: Chemical composition of the antibiotic albomycin. VI. Determination of the structure of the peptide moiety of the antibiotic albomycin. Collection Czechoslov. Chem. Commun. **29**, 280 (1964).

TURKOVÁ, J., O. MIKEŠ, and F. ŠORM: Chemical composition of the antibiotic albomycin. VII. Determination of S atom bond in the molecule of the antibiotic albomycin. Collection Czechoslov. Chem. Commun. **30**, 118 (1965).

VOŘÍŠEK, J., and D. GRUNBERGER: Study of the mechanism of the effect of albomycin with regard to the origin of resistance. IX. Int. Cong. Microbiol. Moscow July, 1966. Collection Czechoslov. Commun. (in press).

Sarkomycin

Shan-ching Sung

Isolation and Chemical Structure of Sarkomycin

Sarkomycin (sarcomycin) is an antitumor agent with weak antibacterial activities that is produced by *Streptomyces erythrochromogenes*. It was discovered during a search for antitumor agents by screening against the Yoshida sarcoma by UMEZAWA *et al.* (1953b). Sarkomycin was later found to be very effective against Ehrlich ascites carcinoma (UMEZAWA *et al.*, 1953a, 1953b; OKAMI *et al.*, 1953; UMEZAWA *et al.*, 1954).

HOOPER *et al.* (1955) described various methods of purification of sarkomycin and their evidence indicated that the active principle of sarkomycin is 2-methylene-3-oxocyclopentanecarboxylic acid.

2-methylene-3-oxocyclopentanecarboxylic acid

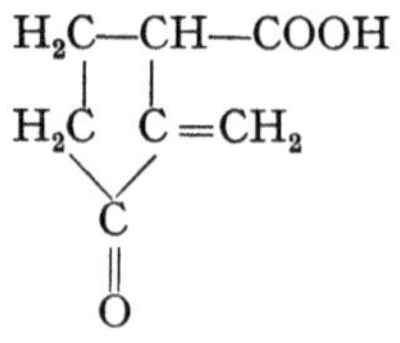

The chemical synthesis of sarkomycin has been described by TOKI *et al.* (1957) and its chemistry has been studied by MAEDA and KONDO (1958). An excellent review by KONDO (1963) appeared in Japanese. The free acid of sarkomycin is colorless and oily (MAEDA and KONDO, 1958). Both the sodium and calcium salts are white, amorphous, hygroscopic powders (TAKEUCHI, 1954). The free acid is soluble in water and many organic solvents, but is insoluble in petroleum ether. The sodium and calcium salts are soluble in water, but only the sodium salt is readily soluble in lower alcohols (UMEZAWA *et al.*, 1954; TAKEUCHI, 1954; MAEDA and KONDO 1958). Hydrogenation of sarkomycin destroys the antibacterial activity (HOOPER *et al.*, 1955). The hydrogenation product is an optically active 2-methyl-3-oxocyclopentanecarboxylic acid which is an active antitumor agent without antibacterial activity.

Some of the isomers or derivatives of sarkomycin which were either isolated from natural sources or synthesized chemically are:

1. Sodium and calcium salt (TAKEUCHI, 1954).
2. β-Sarkomycin (HOOPER *et al.*, 1955).
3. Sarkomycin A, A′ and B (MAEDA and KONDO, 1958).

4. 5-Methylenecyclopentanone-3-carboxylic acid (UMEZAWA and KINOSHITA, 1956).

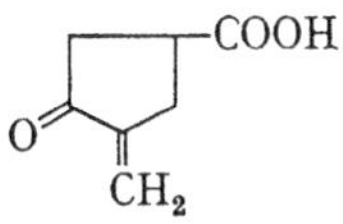

5. 2-Methyl-3-oxocyclopentanecarboxylic acid (Dihydrosarkomycin) (HOOPER *et al.*, 1955).

2-methyl-3-oxocyclopentanecarboxylic acid

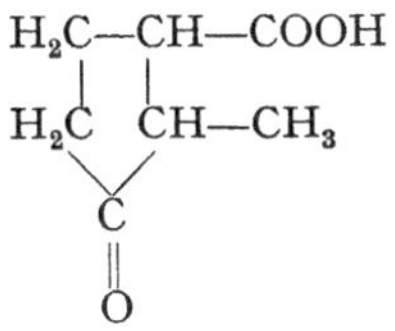

6. Sarkomycin-isonicotinic acid hydrazide (HARA *et al.*, 1957; TAKEUCHI *et al.*, 1958).

7. Sarkomycin S_1 or Di-(2-carboxy-5-oxocyclopentylmethyl) disulfide (TATSUOKA *et al.*, 1958).

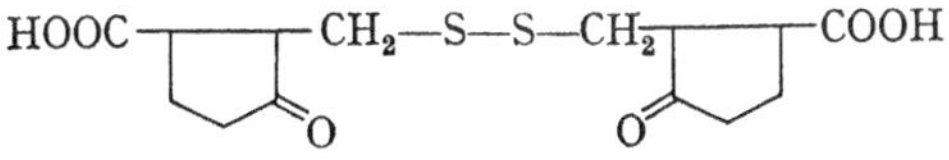

8. Sarkomycin S_2 or Di-(2-carboxy-5-oxocyclopentylmethyl) sulfide (TATSUOKA *et al.*, 1958).

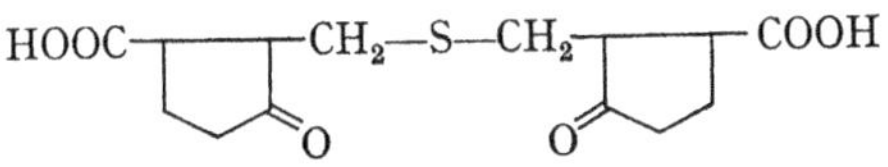

9. Various compounds structurally related to sarkomycin have been synthesized (TAKEUCHI *et al.*, 1961; CAPUTO *et al.*, 1961, 1964).

Effect of Sarkomycin on Ehrlich Ascites Carcinoma and other Tumors

UMEZAWA *et al.* (1954) reported that the development of Ehrlich carcinoma of mice was inhibited either by daily intravenous injection of 1 mg per mouse, or daily intraperitoneal injection of 2.5 mg per mouse, or daily oral administration of 5 mg per mouse. Four out of the 16 sarkomycin-treated ascitic mice died in 20—28 days whilst the other 12 mice survived 35 days or longer after inoculation of tumor cells. TAKEUCHI *et al.* (1955) found the minimum effective daily dose of sarkomycin against Ehrlich ascites carcinoma to fluctuate only between 1.25 mg and 2.5 mg.

The *in vivo* and *in vitro* cytostatic effects of sarkomycin on Ehrlich ascites carcinoma cells have been studied by ISHIYAMA *et al.* (1955). They observed that the antibiotic added *in vitro*, in concentrations over 0.75 mg/ml inhibited the subsequent transplantability of Ehrlich ascites and also morphological changes (or degeneration) of the tumor cells in mice treated with sarkomycin. OBOSHI *et al.* (1955a, 1955b) reported that sarkomycin is not a mitotic poison, but is a specific destroyer of the tumor cells. They also studied the inhibitory effects of sarkomycin on various other ascites tumors. They noted that daily administration of the maximum tolerated doses of sarkomycin resulted in the inhibition of proliferation of the tumor cells in the ascites and the prolongation of survival time of the tumor-bearing animals in a wide spectrum of the tumors, except Hirosaki sarcoma and its nitromin-resistant line. The inhibitory effect of sarkomycin on various mouse, rat and hamster tumors has been studied thoroughly by SUGIURA (1959); some were completely destroyed or inhibited, some partially or slightly inhibited and others were not affected.

ROBERTS *et al.* (1956) investigated the effect of sarkomycin on the Yoshida ascites tumor. In tissues examined 30 minutes after the intraperitoneal injection (on the 5th day after inoculation) they found that most of the tumor cells showed cytoplasmic blebbing. They also noted chromosomal abnormalities such as clumping and irregular scattering at metaphase in cells undergoing mitosis. The cellular damage increased with time, and at 60 minutes the cells showed severe cytoplasmic distortion as a result of blebbing, with irregular processes or atypical amoeboid protrusions. Mitotic arrest occurred at metaphase in increasing numbers of cells and nuclear abnormalities took place in resting cells and at early prophase. Moreover, nuclei began to exhibit a coarse ultrastructure and despiralized or broken down chromonemata, and the number of cells undergoing normal mitosis decreased in number. At 120 and 300 minutes, more marked degenerative changes in the tumor cells had occurred and more than 50% of the tumor cells showed pyknotic aggregations of chromatin following inhibition at metaphase.

These investigators also observed alterations in the Ehrlich ascites tumor cells after the administration of sarkomycin. Five minutes after the administration of sarkomycin, a large number of cells show small blisters on their cytoplasmic surfaces. Some of the mitotic cells, especially those at metaphase, showed marked nuclear abnormalities characterized by clumped or sticky chromosomes. At 40 minutes, there was extensive cytoplasmic damage as well as prominent karyorrhexis in both resting and dividing states. Disintegration of nucleus and cytoplasm appeared to take place simultaneously in many instances. Between 60 and 120 minutes after the injection of the sarkomycin all the damaged cells had disappeared from the ascitic fluid and only a relatively small number of normal-appearing tumor cells could be found.

Antibacterial Activity

In addition to its strong antitumor activity, sarkomycin is slightly inhibitory to bacteria (UMEZAWA *et al.*, 1954). Antibacterial and antifungal spectra have been studied extensively by TAKEUCHI (1954) and TATSUOKA *et al.* (1956). Minimal inhibitory concentrations for bacteria and fungi are listed below (TAKEUCHI, 1954). The antibiotic, however was not pure at that time and the concentration would be lower for pure sarkomycin.

Bacillus anthracis	25 µg/ml
Bacillus subtilis NRRL-B 558	500 µg/ml
Bacillus subtilis PCI 219	1,000 µg/ml
Staphylococcus aureus 209 P	50 µg/ml
Escherichia coli	500 µg/ml
Shigella dysenteriae	100 µg/ml
Salmonella typhosa 63	500 µg/ml
Salmonella paratyphi	100 µg/ml
Proteus vulgaris OX 19	1,000 µg/ml
Pseudomonas aeruginosa	>1,000 µg/ml
Mycobacterium 607	>1,000 µg/ml
Nocardia asteroides	63 µg/ml
Candida albicans	>1,000 µg/ml
Torula utilis	1,000 µg/ml
Trichophyton mentagrophyte	500 µg/ml
Histoplasma capsulatum	63 µg/ml
Penicillium chrysogenum	>1,000 µg/ml
Aspergillus niger	>1,000 µg/ml

The bacteriostatic effect was influenced by cysteine and serum; however, sarkomycin could be extracted from serum mixture with ethyl acetate and hence had not been destroyed by serum (TAKEUCHI, 1954; UMEZAWA *et al.*, 1954). A component of serum influences the bacteriostatic effect, but it does not lower the antitumor effect.

Toxicity

No delayed toxicity was noted by UMEZAWA *et al.* (1954). However they found that sarkomycin was more toxic by subcutaneous injection than by intravenous route. By intravenous injection, no toxic reaction occurred in mice with 800 mg/kg, but all died at a dose of 1,600 mg/kg. Subcutaneous injection caused the death of almost all the mice at 800 mg/kg, but all survived at 400 mg/kg. Subcutaneous injection of not less than 200 mg/kg induced necrosis in the locus of injection. Mice tolerated the oral administration of 4,800 mg/kg. However, all the mice died following the administration of 6,400 mg/kg.

UMEZAWA *et al.* also injected sarkomycin intravenously into a monkey for 20 days. Daily injection of 100 mg/kg produced no evidence of toxicity; when 200 mg/kg was injected, the monkey showed signs of nausea, but survived, and tolerated further daily injection of 100—150 mg/kg. The injection of 100 mg/kg repeated 20 times caused no change in the white or red blood cells count.

The addition of cysteine, glutathione or serum to sarkomycin decreases its toxicity (UMEZAWA *et al.*, 1954; TAKEUCHI, 1954; TAKEUCHI *et al.*, 1955).

Activity of Compounds Structurally Related to Sarkomycin

Of the compounds derived from sarkomycin, dihydrosarkomycin (HOOPER *et al.*, 1955) and disulfide of di-sarkomycin (TATSUOKA *et al.* 1956) have antitumor activity against Ehrlich ascites carcinoma, though their activities are weaker than that of sarkomycin itself. TAKEUCHI *et al.* (1958) prepared sarkomycin-INH, derived from two moles of sarkomycin and one mole of isonicotinic acid hydrazide, and studied its antitumor effect. Sarkomycin-INH which is more stable than sarkomycin was found to be more active on YOSHIDA rat sarcoma than sarkomycin itself, although Ehrlich carcinoma cells are equally sensitive to both sarkomycin-INH and sarkomycin. Various other sarkomycin derivatives have been synthesized and their antitumor activities have been studied (TAKEUCHI *et al.*, 1961; CAPUTO *et al.*, 1961 a, b, 1962, 1964).

CAPUTO, BRUNORI and GIULIANO (1961) synthesized 70 new sarkomycin derivatives and tested the effects of these compounds on the inhibition of tumor growth. The most effective were SB_5, SB_6, SB_7, SB_8, SB_{15}, SB_{19}, SB_{21} and SB_{22} (see CAPUTO *et al.*, 1961 a; for the structures). These compounds were found to be more effective than the original sarkomycin for the prolongation of survival rate and for diminishing the increase in the body weight. They also observed that some compounds, such as SB_{21}, which restrain the growth of tumor cells, produced at least early morphological changes indicating nuclear injuries, diminution in mitotic activity or nuclear enlargement. The data of CAPUTO, BRUNORI and GIULIANO (1961 a) show that some modifications of the sarkomycin molecule modify the antiblastic activity of sarkomycin. Their observations also indicate that the increased antitumor activity of sarkomycin derivatives is probably dependent on the concomitant presence in the molecule of both an ethyl and one or two sustituted methylene groups.

Biochemical Effects of Sarkomycin

Sarkomycin up to concentrations of 500 μg/ml has no effect on the rate of oxygen uptake of Ehrlich ascites cells, either in the presence or absence of glucose (BICKIS *et al.*, 1957; CAPUTO *et al.*, 1961 a; SUNG and QUASTEL, 1963). However, some of the more effective sarkomycin derivatives, such as SB_{21} (CAPUTO *et al.*, 1961 a), markedly inhibit the respiration of Ehrlich ascites tumor cells. The effects on glycolysis resemble those on aerobic respiration. Sarkomycin at a concentration of 200 μg/ml (BICKIS *et al.*, 1957), 400 μg/ml (SUNG and QUASTEL, 1963) or even at a concentration of 1000 μg/ml (CAPUTO *et al.*, 1961 a) does not affect the rate of anaerobic glycolysis. However, BICKIS *et al.* (1957) noted that when the concentration of sarkomycin was increased to 600 μg/ml, a relatively large inhibition of the rates of respiration and glycolysis took place. A marked inhibition of the rate of glycolysis by some of the sarkomycin derivatives, SB_{21} and SB_{22}, has also been reported (CAPUTO *et al.*, 1951 a).

Very low levels of free or easily extractable glutamine are normally observed in tumors (KIT and AWAPARA, 1953; ROBERTS and BORGES, 1955; SHRIVASTAVA and QUASTEL, 1962). A greatly elevated content of glutamine in extracts of Yoshida ascites tumor cells and also in the ascitic fluid was observed by ROBERTS *et al.* (1956) after an intraperitoneal injection of 50 mg sarkomycin per rat. They also showed that treatment with sarkomycin *in vivo* did not destroy the ability of Yoshida tumor cells to take up labeled glutamine *in vitro* rapidly and to convert it to glutamic acid. An elevated level of glutamine also was found in the Ehrlich acites tumors after sarkomycin treatment. They suggested that the glutamine, which was not observed in the control cells, may have come from some intracellular source.

ROBERTS *et al.* (1956) also noticed a marked decrease in glutathione and an increase of valine and leucine in the ascites after sarkomycin treatment. Decreased formation *in vitro* of ^{14}C-glutathione from ^{14}C-glucose in intestine by sarkomycin has been observed by SAHAGIAN and SUNG (unpublished data, 1963). ROBERTS *et al.* (1956) suggested the possibility that one action of sarkomycin might be an interference with some phase of glutamine metabolism by the tumor cells, because of a close resemblance between the rigid structure of sarkomycin and one of the possible configurations of glutamine.

Sarkomycin, at 200 μg/ml, brings about marked diminution in the rates of incorporation of glycine into the tumor proteins, but its uptake into tumor cells is only slightly affected (BICKIS *et al.*, 1957). The inhibition of protein synthesis by sarkomycin, at 200 μg/ml, is about 70%. However, higher concentrations of sarkomycin, e.g. 670 μg/ml, causes more than 90% inhibition of the rate of incorporation of glycine into Ehrlich ascites tumor protein. Incorporation of glycine into the proteins of chick embryo (four days old) or rat spleen slices is also affected by the high sarkomycin concentration (670 μg/ml), but the inhibition (ca. 70%), is not as great as those found with Ehrlich ascites tumor cells (BICKIS *et al.*, 1957).

The mechanism of inhibition of protein synthesis in Ehrlich ascites cells by sarkomycin is obscure. The possibility that sarkomycin depletes the necessary energy supply, presumably the supply of adenosine triphosphate, has been suggested by BICKIS *et al.* (1957). It is not clear whether the inhibition of protein synthesis by sarkomycin is due to a direct affect on the protein synthesizing system or to a secondary action.

ROBERTS *et al.* (1956) suggested that the antitumor activity of sarkomycin might be caused by its interference with an aspect of glutamine metabolism. However, the inhibition by sarkomycin of the incorporation of glycine-1-^{14}C into Ehrlich ascites carcinoma proteins was not reversed by the addition of L-glutamine (BICKIS *et al.*, 1957).

Sarkomycin, 200 μg/ml, greatly reduces the incorporation of phosphate-^{32}P into adenosine mono-, di-, and tri-phosphate and into the ribonucleic and deoxyribonucleic acid fractions (BICKIS *et al.*, 1957; CREASER and SCHOLEFIELD, 1960). The incorporation of adenine-8-^{14}C into ATP or that of thymidine-2-^{14}C into thymidine triphosphate in Ehrlich ascites cells is however, not inhibited by sarkomycin (SUNG and QUASTEL, 1963). The mechanism by which sarkomycin affects the phosphate-^{32}P incorporation into ATP resembles the uncoupling action of dinitrophenol, but a notable difference exists (BICKIS *et al.*, 1957). Sarkomycin does not stimulate the rate of oxygen consumption of ascites whereas such stimulation is a characteristic feature of dinitrophenol activity. Another feature is that sarkomycin, as reported by BICKIS *et al.*, inhibits the anaerobic incorporation of glycine-1-^{14}C into protein in the presence of glucose, whereas there is only feeble, or lack of, inhibition by dinitrophenol under the same conditions (RABINOVITZ *et al.*, 1955).

Deoxyribonucleic Acid Synthesis

At a concentration of 100 μg/ml or higher, the antibiotic inhibits the rate of incorporation of adenine-8-^{14}C, guanine-8-^{14}C, or thymidine-2-^{14}C into deoxyribonucleic acid (DNA) in intact Ehrlich ascites cells more than 90% (SUNG and

QUASTEL, 1963). At the same concentration ribonucleic acid (RNA) synthesis is inhibited only 20%. Below 200 µg/ml antibiotic, no inhibition of the incorporation of adenine-8-^{14}C into acid soluble nucleotides takes place. The incorporation of thymidine-2-^{14}C into thymidine nucleotides is not inhibited by sarkomycin but, on the contrary, increases. This increase might be due to the inhibition of the DNA polymerase step by sarkomycin, or to the smaller pool size of thymidine nucleotides compared with that of adenosine nucleotides. As shown clearly by SUNG and QUASTEL (1963), the inhibition of DNA synthesis by sarkomycin can be prevented by reduced glutathione or cysteine. The following compounds all fail to prevent the sarkomycin inhibition. L-glutamine, D-ribose, D-deoxyribose, nicotinamide, nicotinamide dinucleotide phosphate, reduced nicotinamide dinucleotide phosphate, ascorbic acid, adenine, adenosine, d-AMP, d-GMP, d-CMP, calf thymus DNA, and yeast RNA. The inhibition of DNA synthesis by sarkomycin may be observed not only in the intact Ehrlich ascites cells but also in a cell-free extract prepared from ascites cells. The site of inhibition of DNA synthesis by sarkomycin seems to be DNA polymerase, possibly at a thiol group.

Recently, KEIR and SHEPHERD (1965) have partially purified DNA polymerase (DNA nucleotidyltransferase) from Landschutz ascites tumor cells and shown the inhibitory activity of sarkomycin on this enzyme. Their data also showed that the inhibition by sarkomycin could be partially prevented by glutathione or 2-mercaptoethanol.

Pyridine Nucleotides Synthesis

Both the synthesis of pyridine nucleotides and of nucleic acids involve nucleoside (or deoxynucleoside) triphosphates and the formation of pyrophosphate. At a concentration of 200 µg/ml, sarkomycin inhibits by 60% the incorporation of nicotinamide-7-^{14}C into pyridine nucleotides in Ehrlich ascites cells (SUNG and QUASTEL, 1963). The extent of inhibition of nicotinamide-7-^{14}C incorporation lies between that of DNA synthesis and that of RNA synthesis. Further study of the mechanism involved in the sarkomycin inhibition of pyridine nucleotides synthesis is necessary.

Conclusions

Sarkomycin is an antitumor substance with weak antibacterial activity. The antibiotic is produced by *Streptomyces erythromogenes*. It is active against Ehrlich ascites carcinoma and some other experimental animal tumors. Cytological effects of sarkomycin on tumors, particularly Ehrlich ascites carcinoma cells, have been observed. Although clinical trials by MAGILL et al. (1956) failed to show any appreciable therapeutic value in disseminated cancer, some favorable effects have been reported by Japanese investigators.

Sarkomycin appears to interfere with the adenylic acid system, either by inhibition of the rate of formation of ATP or by an increased rate of the breakdown of ATP. This disturbance of the adenylic acid reaction resembles, in some ways, the uncoupling action of dinitrophenol. However, there is a lack of stimulation of the rate of oxygen consumption of ascites cells and marked inhibition of glycine-1-^{14}C incorporation anaerobically in the presence of glucose. Protein synthesis is also inhibited though the nature of the interference with this system is not known.

A similarity of certain aspects of the molecular models of sarkomycin and glutamine led to the suggestion that sarkomycin might be interfering with some phase of utilization of glutamine in the susceptible cells. Since glutamine plays important roles in the *de novo* synthesis of nucleic acids and proteins, the increase in the amount of free or easily extractable glutamine in tumors after sarkomycin treatment could be due to the accumulation of glutamine caused by any one of a number of ways of inhibiting the biosynthesis of proteins and nucleic acids in cells. However, the inhibitions of both DNA and protein synthesis caused by sarkomycin can not be prevented by the addition of L-glutamine.

Sarkomycin apparently shows multiple effects on the metabolism of ascites cells. These include effects on glycine-1-^{14}C incorporation into protein, changes in free and easily extractable amino acids patterns in ascites cells, pyridine nucleotide synthesis, phosphate-^{32}P incorporation into nucleotides, nucleic acids fractions, etc. The most sensitive reaction affected seems to be that of DNA synthesis at the DNA polymerase step, probably at a thiol group. KEIR and SHEPHERD (1965) have suggested that with sarkomycin, electron displacement induced by the 3-oxo group gives rise to a partial positive charge on the 2-methylene carbon, thus promoting reactivity towards thiol groups.

Acknowledgement. I wish to thank Professor J. H. QUASTEL for his interest and many valuable comments.

See Addendum

Bibliography

BICKIS, I. J., E. H. CREASER, J. H. QUASTEL, and P. G. SCHOLEFIELD: Effects of sarcomycin on the metabolism of Ehrlich ascites carcinoma cells. Nature **180**, 1109 (1957).

CAPUTO, A., M. BRUNORI, and R. GIULIANO: Antitumoral action of new sarcomycin derivatives. I. Importance of ethyl radical and substituted methylene groups. Cancer Research **21**, 1499 (1961 a).

CAPUTO, A., B. GIOVANELLA, and R. GIULIANO: Antitumoral action of new sarcomycin derivatives. Nature **190**, 819 (1961 b)

CAPUTO, A., M. BRUNORI, and R. GIULIANO: Effect of sarcomycin derivatives on solid tumors. Gann **53**, 371 (1962).

CAPUTO, A., M. BRUNORI, and R. GIULIANO: Studies on the action of new sarcomycin derivatives. Acta Unio Intern. contra Cancrum **20**, 309 (1964).

CREASER, E. H., and P. G. SCHOLEFIELD: The influence of dinitrophenol and fatty acids on the P^{32} metabolism of Ehrlich ascites carcinoma cells. Cancer Research **20**, 257 (1960).

HARA, T., Y. YAMADA, and E. AKITA: Studies on sarkomycin. IV. Preparation of sarkomycin-INAH derivative and stability. II. J. Antibiotics (Japan), Ser. A **10**, 62 (1957).

HOOPER, I. R., L. C. CHENEY, M. J. CRON, O. B. FARDIG, D. A. JOHNSON, D. L. JOHNSON, F. M. PALERMITI, H. SCHMITZ, and W. B. WHEATLEY: Studies on sarkomycin. Antibiotics & Chemotherapy **5**, 585 (1955).

ISHIYAMA, S.: Clinical observations of some malignant tumors treated with sarkomycin, a new antitumor antibiotic. J. Antibiotics (Japan), Ser. A **7**, 82 (1954).

ISHIYAMA, S., H. HIRAYAMA, M. TAKAMURA, and T. OHASHI: Further observations upon the cytostatic effects of sarkomycin: An experimental study on the Ehrlich ascites carcinoma in mice. J. Antibiotics (Japan), Ser. A **8**, 57 (1955).

KEIR, H. M., and J. B. SHEPHERD: Thiol groups in deoxyribonucleic acid nucleotidyltransferase. Biochem. J. **95**, 483 (1965).

KIT, S., and J. AWAPARA: Free amino acid content and transaminase activity of lymphatic tissues and lymphosarcoma. Cancer Research **13**, 694 (1953).

KONDO, S.: Sarkomycin [in Japanese]. J. Antibiotics (Japan), Ser. B **16**, 210 (1963).

MAEDA, K., and S. KONDO: Chemistry on sarkomycin. Chemical studies on antibiotics of *Streptomyces*. VI. J. Antibiotics (Japan), Ser. A **11**, 37 (1958).

MAGILL, G. B., R. B. GOLBEY, D. A. KARNOFSKY, J. H. BURCHENAL, C. C. STOCK, C. P. RHOADS, C. E. CRANDALL, S. N. YORUKOGLU, and A. GELLHORN: Clinical experiences with sarkomycin in neoplastic diseases. Cancer Research **16**, 960 (1956).

OBOSHI, S., K. AOKI, and T. SAKURABA: Experimental studies on chemotherapy of malignant tumors. II. Influence of sarkomycin on the tumor cells, especially upon the cell division. J. Antibiotics (Japan), Ser. A **8**, 153 (1955a).

OBOSHI, S., K. AOKI, T. SAKURABA, T. ISHIKURA, T. YOSHIDA, M. SATO, and K. SEKI: Experimental studies on chemotherapy of malignant tumors. III. Inhibitory effects of sarkomycin in a spectrum of ascites tumors in rats and mice. J. Antibiotics (Japan), Ser. A **8**, 156 (1955b).

OKAMI, Y., T. OKUDA, T. TAKEUCHI, K. NITTA, and H. UMEZAWA: Studies on antitumor substances produced by microorganisms. IV. Sarkomycin-producing *Streptomyces* and other two *Streptomyces* producing the anti-tumor substance No. 289 and caryomycin. J. Antibiotics (Japan), Ser. A **6**, 153 (1953).

RABINOVITZ, M., M. E. OLSON, and D. M. GREENBERG: Relation of energy processes to the incorporation of amino acids into proteins of the Ehrlich ascites carcinoma. J. Biol. Chem. **213**, 1 (1955).

ROBERTS, E., and P. R. F. BORGES: Patterns of free amino acids in growing and regressing tumors. Cancer Research **15**, 697 (1955).

ROBERTS, E., K. KANO TANAKA, T. TANAKA, and D. G. SIMONSEN: Free amino acids in growing and regressing ascites cell tumors: Host resistance and chemical agents. Cancer Research **16**, 970 (1956).

SHRIVASTAVA, G. C., and J. H. QUASTEL: Malignancy and tissue metabolism. Nature **196**, 876 (1962).

SUGIURA, K.: Studies in a tumor spectrum. VIII. The effect of mitomycin C on the growth of a variety of mouse, rat, and hamster tumors. Cancer Research **19**, 438 (1959).

SUNG, S. C., and J. H. QUASTEL: Sarcomycin inhibition of deoxyribonucleic acid synthesis in Ehrlich ascites carcinoma cells. Cancer Research. **23**, 1549 (1963).

TAKEUCHI, T.: Bacteriological studies on actinomycetes products exhibiting antitumor activity. II. The bacteriostatic effect of sarkomycin and its relation to sulfhydryl group. J. Antibiotics (Japan), Ser. A **7**, 37 (1954).

TAKEUCHI, T., T. HIKIJI, K. NITTA, Y. MORIKUBO, and H. UMEZAWA: On antitumor effect of sarkomycin-INH. J. Antibiotics (Japan), Ser. A **11**, 212 (1958).

TAKEUCHI, T., K. NITTA, T. HIKIJI, M. KINOSHITA, and H. UMEZAWA: Antitumor activities of synthetic compounds structurally related to sarkomycin. J. Antibiotics (Japan), Ser. A **14**, 54 (1961).

TAKEUCHI, T., K. NITTA, T. YAMAMOTO, and H. UMEZAWA: Effect of sarkomycin on experimental animal tumors. J. Antibiotics (Japan), Ser. A **8**, 110 (1955).

TATSUOKA, S., A. MIYAKE, S. WADA, M. INOUE, E. IWASAKI, and K. OGATA: Studies on sarkomycin. II. Isolation of sarkomycin sulfur compound [in Japanese]. J. Antibiotics (Japan), Ser. B **9**, 107 (1956).

TATSUOKA, S., A. MIYAKE, S. WADA, and E. IWASAKI: Studies on antibiotics. VII. Structure of S_1 and S_2 [in Japanese]. J. Antibiotics (Japan), Ser. B **11**, 275 (1958).

TOKI, K., H. WADA, Y. SUZUKI, and C. SAITO: Synthesis of sarkomycin. J. Antibiotics (Japan), Ser. A **10**, 35 (1957).

UMEZAWA, S., and M. KINOSHITA: Synthesis of 5-methylenecyclopentanone-3-carboxylic acid, an antitumor isomer of sarkomycin. J. Antibiotics (Japan), Ser. A **9**, 194 (1956).

UMEZAWA, H., T. TAKEUCHI, K. NITTA, Y. OKAMI, T. YAMAMOTO, and S. YAMAOKA: Studies on anti-tumor substances produced by microorganisms. III. On sarkomycin produced by a strain resembling to *Streptomyces erythrochromogene*. J. Antibiotics (Japan), Ser. A **6**, 147 (1953a).
UMEZAWA, H., T. TAKEUCHI, K. NITTA, T. YAMAMOTO, and S. YAMAOKA: Sarkomycin, an anti-tumor substance produced by *Streptomyces*. J. Antibiotics (Japan), Ser. A **6**, 101 (1953b).
UMEZAWA, H., T. YAMAMOTO, T. TAKEUCHI, T. OSATO, Y. OKAMI, S. YAMAOKA, T. OKUDA, K. NITTA, K. YAGISHITA, R. UTAHARA, and S. UMEZAWA: Sarkomycin, an anti-cancer substance produced by *Streptomyces*. Antibiotics & Chemotherapy **4**, 514 (1954).

Pluramycin

Nobuo Tanaka

Pluramycin A, obtained from the culture broth of *Streptomyces pluricolorescens* by MAEDA *et al.* (1956), is a basic antibiotic. It forms orange needle crystals which are yellow in acid and purple in alkali. The molecular formula, $C_{20}H_{25}O_5N$, was suggested and confirmed by S. NAKAMURA (personal communications). Another antibiotic, designated pluramycin B, was isolated from the same culture filtrate in a crude form. Both pluramycins A and B inhibit growth of bacteria and tumor cells. OGAWARA *et al.* (1966) observed that a macromolecular antitumor substance (molecular weight 30,000—60,000) is also produced by the same organism. It consists of a pluramycin-like prosthetic group and a glycoprotein, and is designated plurallin.

The antibacterial and antitumor activity of pluramycin A was reported by TAKEUCHI *et al.* (1957) and by NISHIBORI (1957). The minimal inhibitory concentrations, tested by agar dilution method, were 6.25 μg/ml for *Staphylococcus aureus, Bacillus subtilis* and *Mycobacterium phlei;* 25.0 μg/ml for *Salmonella typhosa, Shigella dysenteriae* and *Escherichia coli;* and 100 μg/ml for *Pseudomonas aeruginosa.* However, it inhibited growth of *S. aureus* at the concentrations of 0.02 to 0.1 μg/ml by the broth dilution technique. They considered that the difference in the minimal inhibitory concentrations observed by the two methods may be due to the slow diffusion and lability of the antibiotic in agar. TANAKA *et al.* (unpublished data) observed that the minimal inhibitory concentration for *E. coli* was 1.0 μg/ml by the broth dilution technique.

Pluramycin A exhibited antitumor effects on Ehrlich carcinoma, sarcoma 180 and Yoshida sarcoma. Ehrlich mouse carcinoma was most sensitive and Yoshida rat sarcoma was most resistant. The activity against these tumors was stronger than that of actinomycin J. Pluramycin A significantly inhibited the ascites increase and prolonged the survival period of mice bearing ascitic form of Ehrlich carcinoma. Intraperitoneal or subcutaneous injections of 0.5—2 μg/mouse were effective, even when the treatment started 5 or 7 days after the inoculation of the tumor cells. The intraperitoneal injection of more than 1 μg/mouse inhibited growth of the subcutaneous solid tumor of Ehrlich carcinoma. It exhibited destructive effects on HeLa cells in the tissue culture at 0.06—0.15 μg/ml.

LD_{50} of pluramycin A ascorbate to mice was 1.0 mg/kg by the intravenous injection and 6.6 mg/kg by the intraperitoneal injection.

LEIN *et al.* (1962) observed phage induction of lysogenic bacteria by pluramycin. MATSUMAE and HATA (1964) reported that pluramycin caused elongation and produced filamentous forms of *E. coli* B.

TANAKA *et al.* (1965) investigated the activity of pluramycin A on macromolecular syntheses, and observed that the antibiotic inhibits both protein and nucleic acids syntheses in the intact cells of bacteria. They demonstrated that protein synthesis was not significantly affected in bacterial cell-free systems, but RNA and DNA polymerase reactions were markedly inhibited by the antibiotic.

As illustrated in Fig. 1, RNA polymerase reaction, using salmon sperm DNA as a primer, was markedly inhibited by pluramycin A. Approximately 50% inhibition was observed at the concentration of 2 μg/ml of the antibiotic with native DNA. DNA polymerase reaction, using salmon sperm DNA as a primer, was significantly inhibited by pluramycin A. About 50% inhibition was demonstrated at 2 μg/ml (see Table 1). The source of both enzymes was *E. coli*.

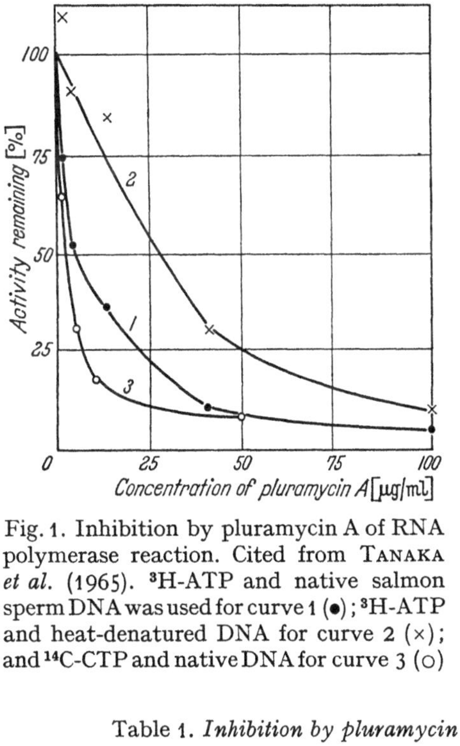

Fig. 1. Inhibition by pluramycin A of RNA polymerase reaction. Cited from TANAKA *et al.* (1965). ^{3}H-ATP and native salmon sperm DNA was used for curve 1 (•); ^{3}H-ATP and heat-denatured DNA for curve 2 (×); and ^{14}C-CTP and native DNA for curve 3 (○)

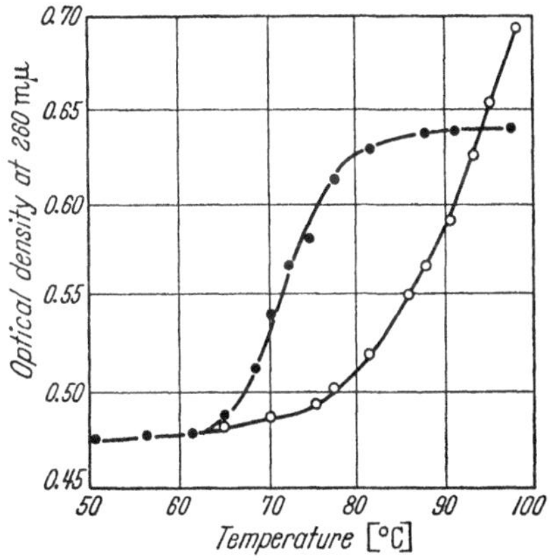

Fig. 2. Transition of melting temperature of salmon sperm DNA in the presence of pluramycin A. Cited from TANAKA *et al.* (1965). The reaction mixture contained 25 μg/ml of salmon sperm DNA with (—○—) and without (—•—) 10 μg/ml of pluramycin A in 0.01 M NaCl, 0.01 M Tris-HCl pH 7.4

Table 1. *Inhibition by pluramycin A of DNA polymerase reaction*

Series	Primer DNA			
	Native		Heat-denatured	
	Incorp. of dATP		Incorp. of dATP	
	cpm	%	cpm	%
Control	885	100	315	100
0 time	22	0	27	0
—DNA	81	6.8	93	22.0
+Pluramycin A 50 μg/ml	25	0.3	40	4.3
25	39	2.0	46	6.4
10	142	14.0	133	36.0
5	289	31.0	207	60.0
2	398	44.0	234	73.0
1	619	69.0	267	84.0

Cited from TANAKA *et al.* (1965)

As illustrated in Fig. 2, the thermal transition curve of salmon sperm DNA was markedly shifted in the presence of pluramycin A. The difference in Tm in the absence and presence of the antibiotic was approximately 15°. It indicated that pluramycin A binds with and stabilizes the double strand structure of DNA to the denaturing effect of heat.

Tanaka *et al.* (1965) concluded that pluramycin A may complex with DNA and consequently inhibit DNA and RNA polymerase reactions. The inhibition of protein synthesis in the intact cells may be the secondary effect of the inhibition of DNA and RNA syntheses.

References

Lein, J., B. Heinemann, and A. Gourevitch: Induction of lysogenic bacteria as a method of detecting potential antitumor agents. Nature **196**, 783 (1962).

Maeda, K., T. Takeuchi, K. Nitta, K. Yagishita, R. Utahara, T. Osato, M. Ueda, S. Kondo, Y. Okami, and H. Umezawa: A new antitumor substance, pluramycin. Studies on antitumor substances produced by actinomycetes. XI. J. Antibiotics (Japan), Ser. A **9**, 75 (1956).

Matsumae, A., and T. Hata: Morphological changes of bacteria induced by chemotherapeutic agents. I. A classification of chemotherapeutic agents based on their activities to induce morphological changes of *Escherichia coli* strain B. J. Antibiotics (Japan), Ser. A **17**, 164 (1964).

Nishibori, A.: Antitumor effect of pluramycin A on experimental animal tumors. Studies on antitumor products of streptomyces. II. J. Antibiotics (Japan), Ser. A **10**, 213 (1957).

Ogawara, H., K. Maeda, K. Nitta, Y. Okami, T. Takeuchi, and H. Umezawa: An antibiotic, plurallin, consisting of a pluramycin-like prosthetic group and a glycoprotein. J. Antibiotics (Japan), Ser. A **19**, 1 (1966).

Takeuchi, T., K. Nitta, and H. Umezawa: Antitumor effect of pluramycin crude powder on Ehrlich carcinoma of mice. Studies on antitumor substances produced by microorganisms. X. J. Antibiotics (Japan), Ser. A **9**, 22 (1956).

Takeuchi, T., T. Hikiji, K. Nitta, and H. Umezawa: Effect of pluramycin A on Ehrlich carcinoma of mice. Studies on antitumor substances produced by actinomycetes. XIII. J. Antibiotics (Japan), Ser. A **10**, 143 (1957).

Tanaka, N., K. Nagai, H. Yamaguchi, and H. Umezawa: Inhibition of RNA and DNA polymerase reactions by pluramycin A. Biochem. Biophys. Research Commun. **21**, 328 (1965).

Edeine and Pactamycin

B. K. Bhuyan

Edeine

Edeine is a basic polypeptide antibiotic produced by *Bacillus brevis* (Kurylo-Borowska, 1959). It inhibits gram-positive and gram-negative bacteria at 10 µg/ml, some fungi and yeasts and mammalian neoplastic cells in tissue culture. Some of its chemical and biological properties are listed in Table 1.

Table 1. *Chemical and biological properties of edeine*

Structure	Basic polypeptide of unknown structure; hydrolysate contains glycine, diaminopropionic acid, spermidine, and tyrosine and two unidentified amino acids (Rancori *et al.*)
Molecular weight	1400 (approx.) (Kurylo-Borowska, 1962)
Solubility	Water soluble, insoluble in organic solvents
Other activities	Inhibits yeasts, molds and replication of DNA and RNA bacteriophages

Edeine selectively inhibited DNA synthesis at concentrations at which protein or RNA synthesis were not affected (Kurylo-Borowska, 1962). Thus DNA synthesis by *E. coli* B growing on synthetic medium was inhibited 60% by 3.3 µg/ml of edeine in two hours with no inhibition of protein synthesis and about a two-fold stimulation of RNA synthesis. Removal of edeine from the cell suspension resulted in normal cell growth. This indicates that incubation of *E. coli* B with sub-inhibitory concentration of edeine induced "unbalanced growth" of cells characterized by prevention of DNA synthesis and accumulation of synthesized RNA in cells which were unable to divide.

In *E. coli*, edeine (10 µg/ml) also inhibited ^{3}H-thymidine uptake into DNA without inhibiting incorporation of ^{14}C-uracil into RNA (Kurylo-Borowska, 1964). Edeine unlike mitomycin C did not induce ^{3}H-thymidine release from pre-labelled DNA. Edeine did not bind to DNA on the basis of the following evidence. There was no change in the absorption spectrum of either edeine or DNA when they were mixed in solution. DNA heat denatured and rapidly cooled in presence of edeine formed a band in CsCl density gradient characteristic of normal denatured DNA. However, mitomycin C under the same conditions formed two bands indicating a thermostable linking of the complementary strains of DNA (Iyer and Szybalski, 1963). DNA isolated from *B. subtilis* cells exposed to edeine had the same banding pattern on CsCl density gradient centrifugation and about the same specific transforming activity as DNA from control cells. *In vitro*, edeine inhibits DNA synthesis apparently by affecting the activity of DNA polymerase (KURYLO-BOROWSKA, 1965a).

In subsequent studies KURYLO-BOROWSKA (KURYLO-BOROWSKA, 1965 a and b) reported the inhibitory action of edeine on polypeptide synthesis in a cell-free system from *E. coli*. Edeine affects protein synthesis by inhibiting the binding of aminoacyl s-RNA to ribosomes. Edeine (0.7 μg/ml), when added at zero time to the cell-free preparation, inhibited by 96% the incorporation of ^{14}C-phenylalanine directed by poly U. However when the cell-free preparation was incubated with poly U and ^{14}C-phenylalanine prior to the addition of edeine, no inhibition was observed on the addition of edeine. Also, the ternary complex of ribosome-poly U, ^{14}C-phenylalanyl-s-RNA was isolated. Edeine did not affect the polymerization of phenylalanine when the ternary complex was incubated with polymerizing enzyme. Therefore, when the ternary functional complex of ribosome, poly U and phenylalanyl s-RNA is formed prior to the addition of edeine, the antibiotic had no effect on polypeptide synthesis. Sucrose density gradient centrifugation of a mixture of ribosome, poly U, ^{14}C-phenylalanyl s-RNA, Tris-HCl, $MgCl_2$ and NH_4Cl showed a radioactivity peak coinciding with the ribosomal peak. Presence of edeine in the above mixture prevented the binding of ^{14}C-phenylalanyl s-RNA to ribosome resulting in a ribosomal peak devoid of ^{14}C-phenylalanine.

Edeine did not affect the transfer of ^{14}C-phenylalanine to s-RNA or the binding of poly U to ribosomes.

Since edeine affected the binding of phenylalanyl-s-RNA to ribosomes, the binding of ^{14}C-edeine to ribosomes was studied. Approximately 1—2 molecules of edeine was bound per 70S ribosome at 1 mM $MgCl_2$. Although edeine binding to ribosomes did not affect poly U-ribosome binding, it completely inhibited the nonenzymic formation of the ternary complex of poly U-ribosome-aminoacyl-s-RNA. The 30S and 50S ribosomal sub-units reassociated in the presence of edeine even at 0.1 mM $MgCl_2$. This concentration of $MgCl_2$ causes dissociation of 70S ribosomes. Edeine, unlike streptomycin, did not alter the coding properties of poly U.

When edeine action is compared *in vivo* and *in vitro*, certain differences become apparent (KURYLO-BOROWSKA, 1965a). *In vivo* edeine selectively inhibits DNA synthesis by *E. coli* with no effect on protein synthesis. DNA synthesis *in vitro* is inhibited only 50% at an edeine concentration which completely inhibits DNA synthesis *in vivo*. RNA synthesis *in vitro* is unaffected at this edeine concentration. However, this concentration of edeine is ten times higher than that required for complete inhibition of polyphenylalanine synthesis *in vitro*.

Pactamycin

Pactamycin is an antitumor antibiotic produced by *Streptomyces pactum* var. *pactum* (BHUYAN *et al.*, 1961). It is active *in vitro* against a variety of gram-positive and gram-negative bacteria. It is also active *in vivo* against many tumors in mice and hamsters. On the basis of its antitumor activity, it has undergone clinical trial under the auspices of the Cancer Chemotherapy National Service Center (CCNSC) (EVANS *et al.*, 1965). Some of the chemical and biological properties of pactamycin are listed in Table 2.

Table 2. *Chemical and biological properties of pactamycin*

Empirical formula	$C_{28}H_{40}N_4O_8$ (ARGOUDELIS, 1961)
Solubility	Soluble in methanol, ethanol, ethyl acetate and chloroform
Stability	Relatively unstable in solution
Cytotoxicity (ID_{50})	KB cell = 0.01 μg/ml
Minimum inhibitory concentration (μg/ml)	*B. subtilis*, 0.8; *S. aureus*, 0.2; *E. coli*, 6.5; *K. pneumoniae*, 0.8; *P. vulgaris*, 110
Acute toxicity (LD_{50} mice, I.V.)	15.6 mg/kg

Pactamycin caused 50% inhibition of KB (human epidermoid carcinoma) cells in tissue culture at 0.01 μg/ml. Growth inhibition was not reversed by the addition of mixtures of purines or pyrimidine bases, nucleosides and nucleotides, or amino acids or vitamin mixtures (BHUYAN, 1965a).

Pactamycin (0.1 μg/ml) inhibited protein synthesis 94% (in KB cells in suspension) compared to 39% and 18% inhibition of DNA and RNA synthesis respectively (BHUYAN, 1965a). Also pactamycin (0.04 μg/ml) caused 40% inhibition of protein synthesis within five minutes, but no inhibition of DNA or RNA synthesis. Inhibition of protein synthesis was also observed by YOUNG *et al.* (1965) in cells in tissue culture, by COLOMBO *et al.* (1965) in reticulocyte cells and cell-free system, and by BHUYAN (1965a) in rat liver when pactamycin was injected intravenously. These results indicated that the primary locus of pactamycin action is the inhibition of protein synthesis.

Pactamycin did not affect the activation of amino acids by ATP in a cell-free system (BHUYAN, 1965b), nor did it inhibit the formation of amino acyl-s-RNA in a cell-free system (COLOMBO *et al.*, 1965). These observations suggested that protein synthesis is inhibited at some later step.

FELICETTI *et al.* (1965) showed that pactamycin acts by inactivating some function of the ribosomes which is essential to protein synthesis. Thus ribosomal and supernatant fractions were obtained from reticulocyte cells preincubated with and without pactamycin. Ribosomes (from cells preincubated with pactamycin) and control supernatant (S-100) showed little amino acid incorporation. However when control ribosomes were incubated with supernatant fraction (S-100) from cells preincubated with pactamycin, amino acid incorporation was equal to that in the system consisting of control ribosomes and control supernatant. Similar results were also obtained (BHUYAN, 1965b) when the activity of ribosomes and supernatant fractions isolated from the livers of rats injected with pactamycin where compared with those from control rats. Pactamycin also degraded polysomes to single ribosomes (FELICETTI, 1965).

References

ARGOUDELIS, A. D., H. K. JAHNKE, and J. F. FOX: Pactamycin, a new antitumor antibiotic. II. Isolation and characterization. Antimicrobial Agents and Chemotherapy, p. 191 (1961).

BHUYAN, B. K., A. DIETZ, and C. G. SMITH: Pactamycin, a new antitumor antibiotic. I. Discovery and biological properties. Antimicrobial Agents and Chemotherapy, p. 184 (1961).

BHUYAN, B. K.: Studies on the mode of action of pactamycin on mammalian cells. Tissue Culture Association 1965a.

BHUYAN, B. K.: Unpublished observations 1965b.

COLOMBO, B., L. FELICETTI, and C. BAGLIONI: Inhibition of protein synthesis in reticulocytes by antibiotics. I. Effects on polysomes. Biochim. et Biophys. Acta **119**, 109 (1966).

EVANS, A. M., B. H. DESSEL, W. M. FOWLER, A. PISCIOTTA, P. S. HAGEN, and J. LOUIS: To be published.

FELICETTI, L., B. COLOMBO, and C. BAGLIONI: Inhibition of protein synthesis in reticulocytes by antibiotics. II. The site of action of cycloheximide, streptovitacin A and pactamycin. Biochim. et Biophys. Acta **119**, 120 (1966).

IYER, V. N., and W. SZYBALSKI: Mitomycins and porfiromycins. Chemical mechanism of activation and cross-linking of DNA. Science **145**, 55 (1964).

KURYLO-BOROWSKA, Z.: Bull. State Inst. Marine and Trop. Med. Gdansk, Poland **10**, 83 (1959).

KURYLO-BOROWSKA, Z.: On the mode of action of edeine. Biochim. et Biophys. Acta **61**, 897 (1962).

KURYLO-BOROWSKA, Z.: On the mode of action of edeine. Effect of edeine on bacterial DNA. Biochim. et Biophys. Acta **87**, 305 (1964).

KURYLO-BOROWSKA, Z.: On the mode of action of edeine. I. Effect of edeine on the synthesis of polyphenylalanine in a cell-free system. Biochim. et Biophys. Acta **95**, 578 (1965).

KURYLO-BOROWSKA, Z.: On the mode of action of edeine. II. Studies on the binding of edeine to *E. coli* ribosomes. Biochim. et Biophys. Acta **95**, 590 (1965).

RANCORI, G., Z. KURYLO-BOROWSKA, and L. C. CRAIG: Unpublished data.

YOUNG, C. W.: Inhibitory effects of acetoxycycloheximide, puromycin and pactamycin upon synthesis of protein and DNA in asynchronous populations of HeLa cells. Mol. Pharm. **2**, 50 (1966).

Phleomycin, Xanthomycin, Streptonigrin, Nogalamycin, and Aurantin

B. K. Bhuyan

Phleomycin

Phleomycin was isolated from a culture of *Streptomyces verticillius* by MAEDA *et al.* (1956). It is a water-soluble copper containing antibiotic complex and is effective against a variety of bacteria. The antibiotic can be freed of its copper by treatment with 8-hydroxy-quinoline and can regain its copper on addition of $CuSO_4$. The copper-free phleomycin had almost the same antibacterial activity as the copper containing antibiotic except against mycobacteria, where the former was less active (TAKITA, 1959). Some of the chemical and biological properties of phleomycin are listed in Table 1.

Table 1. *Chemical and biological properties of phleomycin*

Molecular formula	$C_{53}H_{91}N_{17}O_{32}Cu$
Solubility	Soluble in H_2O, methanol, insoluble in acetone, ether
Structure	Unknown
Minimum inhibitory concentration (μg/ml) (TAKITA, 1959)	*B. subtilis*, 0.26; *M. pyogenes* var. *aureus*, 0.52; *E. coli*, 0.26; *M. phlei*, 0.05
Antitumor activity (BRADNER *et al.*, 1962)	Active against Ehrlich carcinoma, sarcoma 180 and carcinoma 755
Acute toxicity (LD_{50}, I.V., mice) (TAKITA, 1959)	Copper-containing phleomycin = 40—60 mg/kg, copper-free phleomycin = 150 mg/kg

TANAKA *et al.* (1963) showed that phleomycin inhibited total DNA synthesis to a much greater extent than either RNA or protein synthesis by *E. coli* K-12. Cells growing logarithmically were exposed to 2 μg/ml phleomycin for 60 minutes. During this period the turbidity and total protein and RNA content of the cell suspension increased about 1.6 fold but no increase in DNA was observed. Phleomycin at 10 μg/ml also caused 58% inhibition of ^{3}H-thymidine incorporation into *E. coli* DNA. At this level, uptake of ^{14}C-labelled amino acids or ^{32}Phosphate into RNA was not inhibited. When HeLa cells were processed for autoradiography, TANAKA *et al.* (1963) observed 54% inhibition of ^{3}H-thymidine incorporation into cell nuclei at 1 μg/ml phleomycin.

Subsequent to this FALASCHI and KORNBERG (1964) showed that phleomycin inhibited DNA polymerase at concentrations at which negligible inhibition of RNA polymerase was observed. Thus with poly dAT as primer 0.33 μg/ml phleomycin caused 11% and 90% inhibition of RNA and DNA polymerase respectively. TANAKA (1965) also observed inhibition of DNA polymerase by phleomycin.

Several lines of evidence indicate that phleomycin inhibits DNA polymerase by binding to primer DNA (FALASCHI *et al.*, 1964). First, under the ionic conditions used for DNA polymerase assay phleomycin affects the thermal melting behavior of DNA. Second, variation in primer DNA level affected the degree of inhibition of DNA polymerase indicating either a competitive relationship between phleomycin and the primer in binding to the polymerase or a direct binding between phleomycin and primer DNA. Finally, the inhibition of DNA polymerase depended on the A-T content of primer DNA. Thus, with increasing A-T content of primer DNA, the per cent inhibition of polymerase increased, indicating that phleomycin interacts with either A or T or both in primer DNA. Phleomycin also inhibited exonuclease-I (an enzyme which like DNA polymerase acts sequentially from the 3'-OH end of the chain) but had no significant effect on the action of endonuclease I. These results indicate that the inhibition of DNA synthesis by phleomycin is due to a binding of DNA which in turn inhibits its replication by DNA polymerase. However in extending these *in vitro* data to the effect of phleomycin on *E. coli*, it is found that 50% inhibition of DNA polymerase with *E. coli* DNA as primer requires 470 μg/ml of phleomycin as compared to 10 μg/ml needed for suppression of DNA synthesis in a culture of *E. coli*. This discrepancy may be due to a concentration of the agent in the bacterial cell, or to a more effective binding of DNA and inhibition of DNA polymerase under the ionic conditions of the nuclear region of the cell. These results point out the difficulty of extending *in vitro* data to the action of the antibiotic *in vivo*.

Phleomycin did not have any effect on the oxidation of glucose and lactose by *E. coli*. It did not cause marked breakdown of HeLa DNA, in contrast to mitomycin C (TANAKA *et al.*, 1963).

Recent studies of KAJIWARA *et al.* (1966) indicate that phleomycin acts primarily by inhibiting mitosis. Thus, addition of 5 μg/ml phleomycin to synchronously growing HeLa cells caused marginal inhibition of DNA synthesis but almost completely blocked cell division. The phleomycin sensitive step followed completion of DNA synthesis; and microscopic evidence suggested that it prevented the cells from entering prophase. Therefore, phleomycin must inhibit some process concerned with the induction of mitosis other than DNA replication.

Xanthomycin

Xanthomycin is a mixture of three antibiotics, xanthomycin A, B and C. The antibiotics are produced by a streptomyces sp. (THORNE *et al.*, 1948) in the proportion of A = 70%, B = 25% and C = 5% of the total activity. Most of the discussion will pertain to xanthomycin A; its biological and chemical properties are given in Table 2. Xanthomycin is a basic quinonoidal antibiotic with marked activity against gram-positive bacteria, much less activity against gram-negative bacteria, and highly cytotoxic against mammalian cells in tissue culture. Xanthomycin A tends to convert to xanthomycins B and C.

To study the mode of action of the antibiotic, *E. coli* K_{12} cells growing logarithmically were exposed to 0.6 μg/ml of xanthomycin for ten minutes. DNA synthesis was inhibited more than RNA synthesis while no inhibition of protein synthesis was observed by HORVATH *et al.* (1964). They found that xanthomycin caused accumulation of uridine nucleotides by *Staphylococcus aureus* cells, in a manner similar to penicillin.

Table 2. *Chemical and biological properties of xanthomycin A*

Molecular formula	$C_{23}H_{29-31}N_3O_7$ (free base) (RAO *et al.*, 1954)
Solubility	Soluble in H_2O, CH_3OH, $CHCl_3$ and butanol
Stability	Stable in acid solution — unstable above pH 6
UV absorption maxima	265 mμ ($\varepsilon^{1\%}_{1\,cm} = 185$) and 345 mμ at acid pH
Minimum inhibitory concentration (μg/ml)	*B. subtilis*, 0.006; *S. aureus*, 0.8; *Mycobacterium phlei*, 20; *P. vulgaris*, 4
Cytotoxic activity (ID_{50}, μg/ml)	0.005 (SMITH *et al.*, 1959)
Toxicity (LD_{50}, IV, mice, mg/kg)	0.16
Toxicity (LD_{10}, IV, mice, mg/kg)	0.08

Streptonigrin

Streptonigrin is a broad spectrum antibiotic produced by *Streptomyces flocculus* (RAO *et al.*, 1959). It is a weak acid with quinonoid properties whose structure was reported by RAO *et al.* (1963). Some of its chemical and biological properties are listed in Table 3. Though the chemical nature of streptonigrin has been well defined, its biochemical action has remained confusing.

Streptonigrin inhibited total DNA synthesis by *Salmonella typhimurium* cells (LEVINE *et al.*, 1963) at 10 μg/ml (2×10^{-5} M). Ninety minutes exposure to the antibiotic caused 47 and 57% inhibition of RNA and protein synthesis, compared to 97% inhibition of DNA synthesis. Like many other antibiotics that affect DNA synthesis, such as mitomycin C, short exposures to streptonigrin, induced phage (P_{22}) production in inducible lysogenic *Salmonella typhimurium* (LEVINE *et al.*, 1963). The mechanism of such induction is, however, unknown. Like mitomycin C, streptonigrin also causes degradation of bacterial DNA (RADDING *et al.*, 1963).

Table 3. *Chemical and biological properties of streptonigrin*

Empirical formula	$C_{25}H_{22}N_4O_8$ (506.5 MW)
Solubility	Soluble in dioxane, pyridine or dimethylformamide Slightly soluble in H_2O, alcohol and $CHCl_3$
Stability	Stable at acid pH, unstable and photosensitive at pH 7.8
Minimum inhibitory concentration (μg/ml)	*B. subtilis*, 0.07; *S. aureus*, 0.39; *E. coli*, 0.25; *P. vulgaris*, 6.25; *Candida albicans*, 25; *S. cerevisiae*, 50
Toxicity (LD_{50}, mice, IV, mg/kg)	0.5—2.0
Structure	see Fig. 1, RAO *et al.* (1963)

In common with its effect on DNA synthesis, streptonigrin caused marked inhibition of the mitotic rate and extensive chromosomal damage in cultured human leucocytes (COHEN *et al.*, 1963). The chromosomal breaks were nonrandom in the sense that it was not related to unit chromosomal length. Thus chromosomes 19—20, 21—22 and 7 had significantly fewer breaks while significantly larger number of breaks were found in chromosomes 1, 2 and 3 (COHEN, 1963). Thus, like 5-bromouracil deoxyriboside and hydroxylamine, chromosome damage following streptonigrin treatment appears to be aggregated into specific chromosomal segments. However, it would be premature to postulate a biochemical relationship due to the lack of information regarding its mode of action. The antibiotic also caused genetic recombination in phage (LEVINE *et al.*, 1964).

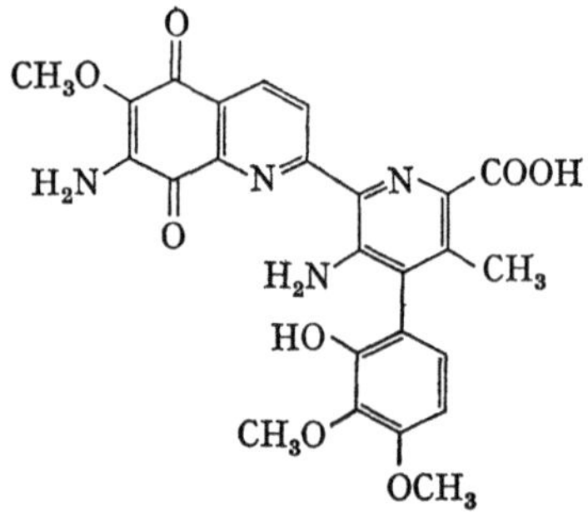

Fig. 1. Structure of Streptonigrin

Streptonigrin catalyzed a non-phosphorylating oxidation of intra- and extramitochondrial DPNH and extra-mitochondrial TPNH (HOCHSTEIN *et al.*, 1965). Since the oxidation was sensitive to dicoumarol, it was presumably mediated by DT diaphorase. The same results were obtained when purified DT diaphorase was used. This oxidation was insensitive to antimycin A_3 and cyanide and was not coupled to phosphorylation, leading instead to the production of H_2O_2. The authors visualize toxicity to result from the (1) depletion of cellular DPNH or TPNH, (2) uncoupling of phosphorylation and depletion of ATP, and (3) formation of H_2O_2.

WHITE and WHITE (1964) reported that the bactericidal action of streptonigrin, like mitomycin C, was affected by the intracellular redox environment of the *E. coli*. Agents which made the intracellular environment reducing (such as cyanide) increased the bactericidal action of the antibiotic. Phenazine methosulfate, on the other hand, completely reversed streptonigrin action, presumably by preempting electrons, which in the absence of phenazine methosulfate would be available for reducing the antibiotic. These results therefore indicate that streptonigrin, like mitomycin C, is bactericidal in its reduced form. However, the synergistic effect of cyanide on the bactericidal effect of the antibiotic is contradictory to the lack of effect of cyanide on the streptonigrin catalyzed oxidation of DPNH or TPNH. Further work is needed to coordinate into an integrated unit the effect of the antibiotic on DNA synthesis and its catalytic effect on oxidation of DPNH or TPNH.

Nogalamycin

Nogalamycin, a cytotoxic antibiotic, produced by *Streptomyces nogalater* var *nogalater* (Bhuyan, Dietz, 1965) has a varied spectrum of biological effects. Some of its chemical and biological properties are listed in Table 4.

Table 4. *Chemical and biological properties of nogalamycin*

Empirical formula and molecular weight	$C_{38}H_{51}NO_{17}$ (M.W. 793.8)
Solubility	Soluble in chloroform, ethyl acetate, and acetone, insoluble in water and alcohol
Absorption spectra and molar absorption coefficient (in neutral ethanol)	237 mμ ($\varepsilon^{1\%}_{1\,cm} = 630$); 258 mμ, 293 mμ, 480 mμ ($\varepsilon^{1\%}_{1\,cm} = 180$)
Minimum inhibitory concentration (μg/ml)	*B. subtilis*, 50; *S. aureus*, 0.4; *S. fecalis*, 0.4; *P. vulgaris* and *E. coli*, > 100
Toxicity (LD_{50}; I.V., rats)	4.6 mg/kg

KB (human epidermoid carcinoma) cell growth in tissue culture was completely inhibited for three days at 0.05 μg/ml (Bhuyan *et al.*, 1965a). Growth inhibition was not reversed by the addition of a mixture of purine and pyrimidine bases, nucleosides, deoxynucleosides, amino acids or vitamins. DNA added to the medium in high concentration partially reversed the cytotoxicity of nogalamycin.

Nogalamycin (0.6 μg/ml) caused much greater inhibition of RNA synthesis (74%) in KB cells than of DNA (31%) or protein (2%) synthesis. The antibiotic was shown (Bhuyan *et al.*, 1965a) to bind to DNA on the basis of: a) change in nogalamycin absorption spectra on mixing with DNA; b) inability to extract with ethyl acetate all the nogalamycin from a nogalamycin-DNA mixture; and c) change in the melting temperature (Tm) of DNA. When excess nogalamycin was mixed with different amounts of calf thymus DNA (in 0.1 M potassium phosphate buffer, pH 7), 173 μg of the antibiotic were irreversibly bound per mg DNA. Nogalamycin increased the Tm of DNA; the increase (ΔTm) being proportional to the ratio of nogalamycin to DNA. When DNA from different sources were compared, the ΔTm at constant nogalamycin: DNA ratio corresponded to the per cent adenine (A) and thymine (T) in the DNA. Furthermore, nogalamycin markedly increased the Tm of poly dAT in contrast to that with poly dGdC. These results indicated that nogalamycin binds to the adenine or thymine or both in DNA (Bhuyan *et al.*, 1965a).

This hypothesis was confirmed when it was found that nogalamycin (10 μg/ml) caused 99% inhibition of RNA synthesis, by *E. coli* RNA polymerase, when poly dAT was used as the primer. Only 3% inhibition was obtained when poly dGdC was used as the primer (Bhuyan *et al.*, 1965a). This was in contrast to the results with actinomycin which forms a hydrogen bond with the deoxyguanosine moiety of DNA.

Nogalamycin, like actinomycin D, inhibited DNA polymerase from KB cells much less than RNA polymerase. It also inhibited DNA viruses and did not inhibit RNA viruses (where RNA synthesis is RNA directed). Nogalamycin also did not inhibit RNA synthesis by RNA polymerase when poly A, C, U, I or UG were used as primers (WARD *et al.*, 1965). These results indicated that nogalamycin, like actinomycin D, inhibits DNA directed RNA synthesis by binding to DNA (BHUYAN *et al.*, 1965 a). However, nogalamycin binds to the dA or dT or both moieties of DNA, whereas actinomycin binds specifically to the dG moiety. The finding that nogalamycin profoundly affected both the heat stability and template function of poly dAT (whose base sequence is a perfectly alternating one) but not of poly dAdT (which consists of a mixture of homopolymers of dA and dT) suggested that base sequence may determine the binding of nogalamycin to DNA.

In vivo (rat liver), nogalamycin also inhibited RNA synthesis to a greater extent than DNA synthesis with marginal inhibition of protein synthesis (GRAY *et al.*, 1966). Like actinomycin, nogalamycin inhibited the induction of tryptophan pyrollase with hydrocortisone as the inducer. Induction of tryptophan pyrollase by hydrocortisone involves the synthesis of messenger RNA. No inhibition of tryptophan induced tryptophan pyrollase was seen either with nogalamycin or actinomycin (GRAY *et al.*, 1966).

With bacteria (*S. aureus*) nogalamycin (1.2 μg/ml) inhibited nucleic acid synthesis (84%) more than protein (68%) synthesis (BHUYAN, DIETZ, 1965). The marked inhibition of protein synthesis observed in bacteria was in contrast to the marginal inhibition (4% after two hours incubation with drug) seen in mammalian cells.

Preliminary data suggest that the nogalamycin, like proflavin, probably intercalates with DNA (BHUYAN, 1965 a). Difference spectra measurements indicated that nogalamycin-DNA binding was inhibited 94% by 1 M NaCl compared to 45% inhibition for proflavin. Nogalamycin binding to DNA also increased DNA viscosity as has been observed with proflavin (LERMAN, 1961). The actinomycin-DNA complex was completely dissociated at high levels of urea. This level of urea had marginal effects on both the DNA-nogalamycin and DNA-proflavin complexes.

Aurantin

Aurantin (Au), produced by *Actinomycete citriofluorescens* (BITTEVA, 1963), is a mixture of five actinomycins; three of which have been characterized (Fig. 2) (PLANELLES *et al.*, 1964). Au-1 makes up 79% of the total composition of aurantin, Au-2 accounts for 21% while the others account for a fraction of a per cent. Some of the chemical and biological properties of aurantin are listed in Table 5.

Table 5. *Chemical and biological properties of aurantin*

Absorption spectrum	Max. at 443—444 mμ
Minimum inhibitory concentration (μg/ml)	*B. subtilis*, 0.4; *S. aureus*, 0.4; *Streptococcus sp.*, 0.04
Mammalian cell inhibition	HeLa in tissue culture, 0.5 μg/ml
Toxicity (LD_{50}, I.V., mg/kg)	Mice, 1.6; rabbits, 0.15
Structure	see Fig. 2

Clinically, aurantin was most effective against Hodgkin's disease with objective improvement in 26 of 40 patients. Various degrees of improvement were noted in treatment of many forms of leukemia (PLANELLES *et al.*, 1964).

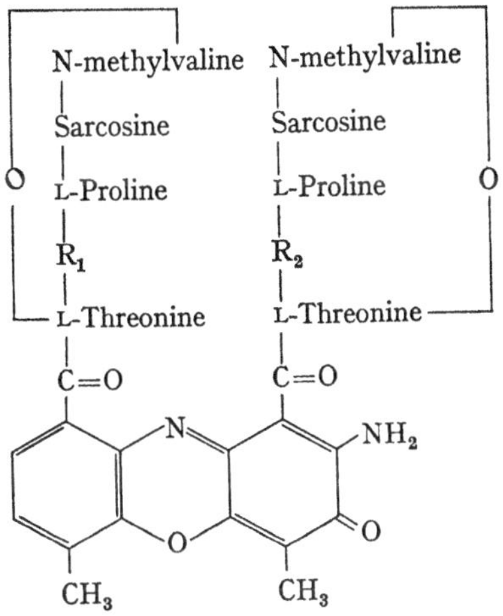

Aurantin-1 — R_1, R_2 = D-alloisoleucine
Aurantin-2 — R_1 = D-alloisoleucine
R_2 = D-valine
Aurantin-3 — R_1, R_2 = D-valine

Fig. 2. Structure of Aurantins

Aurantin (SAZYKIN *et al.*, 1964; GEORGIEN *et al.*, 1963) inhibits RNA synthesis by binding to the primer DNA. This renders the primer unavailable for directing RNA synthesis by RNA polymerase.

References

BHUYAN, B. K., and A. D. DIETZ: Nogalamycin: Fermentation, taxonomic and biological studies, Antimicrobial Agents and Chemotherapy, p. 836 (1965).

BHUYAN, B. K., and C. G. SMITH: Differential interaction of nogalamycin with DNA of varying base composition. Proc. Natl Acad. Sci. U.S. **54**, 566 (1965a).

BITTEVA, M. B.: The taxonomic position of the actinomycete producing aurantin. Mikrobiologiya (Transl.) **31**, 492 (1963).

BRADNER, W. T., and M. H. PINDELL: Antitumor properties of phleomycin. Nature **196**, 682 (1962).

COHEN, M. M.: Specific effects of streptonigrin activity on human chromosomes in culture. Cytogenetics **2**, 271 (1963).

COHEN, M. M., M. W. SHAW, and A. P. CRAIG: Effects of streptonigrin on cultured human leucocytes. Proc. Natl Acad. Sci. U.S. **50**, 16 (1963).

FALASCHI, A., and A. KORNBERG: Phleomycin, an inhibitor of DNA polymerase. Federation Proc. **23**, 940 (1964).

GEORGIEN, G. P., O. P. SAMARINA, M. I. LERMAN, M. N. SMIRNOV, and A. N. SEVERTZOR: Biosynthesis of messenger and ribosomal RNA in the nucleochromosomal apparatus of animal cells. Nature **200**, 1291 (1963).

GRAY, G. D., G. W. CAMIENER, and B. K. BHUYAN: Nogalamycin effects in rat liver: Inhibition of tryptophan pyrolase induction and nucleic acid and protein biosynthesis. Cancer Research **26**, 249 (1966).

Hochstein, P., J. Laozlo, and D. Miller: A unique dicoumarol-sensitive, non-phosphorylating oxidation of DPNH and TPNH catalyzed by streptonigrin. Biochem. Biophys. Research Commun. **19**, 289 (1965).

Horvath, J., I. Gado, O. Kilian, and T. Sik: The action of xanthomycin. Biochem. Pharmacol. **13**, 938 (1964).

Kajiwara, K., U. H. Kim, and G. C. Mueller: Phleomycin, an inhibitor of replication of HeLa cells. Cancer Res. **26**, 233 (1966).

Lerman, L. S.: Structural considerations in the interaction of DNA and acridines. J. Mol. Biol. **3**, 18 (1961).

Levine, M., and M. Bothwick: Action of streptonigrin on bacterial DNA metabolism and on induction of phage production in lysogenic bacteria. Virology **21**, 568 (1963).

Levine, M., and M. Bothwick: Action of streptonigrin on genetic recombinations between bacteriophages. Proc. XI Int. Congr. Genet., The Hague, Netherlands 1963.

Maeda, K., H. Kosaka, K. Yagishita, and H. Umezawa: A new antibiotic phleomycin. J. Antibiotics (Japan), Ser. A **9**, 82 (1956).

Planelles, J. J., Y. V. Soloryeva, Z. N. Belova, A. B. Silaer, M. K. Ebert, N. P. Grachera, A. M. Kharitonora, A. E. Gosheva, and S. S. Akopyants: Aurantin — a complex antibiotic substance of the actinomycin group; its properties and results of clinical trials on various types of neoplasms. Acta Unio Intern. contra Cancrum **20**, 297 (1964).

Radding, C. M.: Uptake of tritiated thymidine by K_{12} (λ) induced by streptonigrin. Proc. XI Intern. Congr. Genet., The Hague, Netherlands 1963.

Rao, K. V., K. Biemann, and R. B. Woodward: The structure of streptonigrin. J. Am. Chem. Soc. **85**, 2533 (1963).

Rao, K. V., and W. P. Cullen: Streptonigrin, an antitumor substance. I. Isolation and characterization. Antibiotics Ann., p. 953 (1960).

Rao, K. V., and W. H. Peterson: Xanthomycin A: production, isolation and properties. J. Am. Chem. Soc. **76**, 1335 (1954).

Sazykin, Y. O., and G. N. Barisova: Effect of specific inhibitors on RNA synthesis dissociated from protein synthesis by bacteriostatic antibiotics. Federation Proc. (Transl. Suppl.) **23**, 380 (1964).

Smith, C. G., W. Lummis, and J. E. Grady: An improved tissue culture assay. II. Cytotoxicity studies with antibiotics, chemicals and solvent. Cancer Research **19**, 847 (1959).

Takita, T.: Studies on purification and properties of phleomycin. J. Antibiotics (Japan), Ser. A **12**, 285 (1959).

Tanaka, N.: Effect of phleomycin on DNA of tumor origin. J. Antibiotics (Japan), Ser. A **18**, 111 (1965).

Tanaka, N., H. Yamagnchi, and H. Umezawa: Mechanism of action of phleomycin, a tumor-inhibitory antibiotic. Biochem. Biophys. Research Commun. **10**, 171 (1963).

Thorne, C. B., and W. H. Peterson: Xanthomycins A and B, new antibiotics produced by a species of streptomyces. J. Biol. Chem. **176**, 413 (1948).

Ward, D. C., E. Reich, and I. H. Goldberg: Base specificity in the interaction of polynucleotides with antibiotic drugs. Science **149**, 1259 (1965).

White, J. R., and H. White: Effect of intercellular redox environment on bactericidal action of mitomycin C and streptonigrin. Antimicrobial Agents and Chemotherapy, p. 495 (1964).

Griseofulvin

Floyd M. Huber

Griseofulvin ($C_{17}H_{17}O_6Cl$) was first isolated from *Penicillium griseofulvum* DIECK by OXFORD, RAISTRICK, and SIMONART (1939). In 1946 BRIAN, CURTIS and HEMMING isolated a "curling factor" from cultures of *P. janczewskii* ZAL., which caused abnormal development of fungal hyphae. The chemical and physical properties of the antibiotic were reported by MCGOWAN (1946). The identity of "curling factor" with griseofulvin was determined chemically by GROVE and MCGOWAN (1947), and biologically by BRIAN *et al.* (1949). Subsequent studies have demonstrated that *P. patulum* and *P. raistrickii* also produce the antibiotic (BRIAN *et al.*, 1949, 1955). The griseofulvin analogs, bromogriseofulvin and dechlorogriseofulvin have also been isolated from fungi (MACMILLAN, 1951, 1954).

Table 1. *Griseofulvin sensitivity of fungi*

Organism	Percent[3] inhibition	Griseofulvin µg/ml	Reference
Alternaria tenuis	39[1]	10	EL-NAKEEB *et al.*, 1965c
Aspergillus niger	ins	—	EL-NAKEEB *et al.*, 1965c
Candida albicans	ins	—	EL-NAKEEB *et al.*, 1965c
Fusarium nivale	ins	—	EL-NAKEEB *et al.*, 1965c
Glomerella cingulata	65[1]	10	EL-NAKEEB *et al.*, 1965c
Microsporum gypseum	97[1]	5	EL-NAKEEB *et al.*, 1965c
Neurospora crassa	ins	—	EL-NAKEEB *et al.*, 1965c
Saccharomyces cerevisiae	ins	—	EL-NAKEEB *et al.*, 1965c
Trichophyton interdigitalis	95[1]	10	EL-NAKEEB *et al.*, 1965c
Trichophyton mentagrophytes	95[1]	5	EL-NAKEEB *et al.*, 1965c
Armillaris mellea	50[2]	1	BRIAN, 1949
Botrytis allii	50[2]	1	BRIAN, 1949
Diaporthe perniciosa	50[2]	1	BRIAN, 1949
Phoma betae	50[2]	1	BRIAN, 1949
Botrytis cinerea	90[1]	20	HUBER and GOTTLIEB
Cryptococcus nigricans	ins	—	ROTH *et al.*, 1959b
Curvularia geniculata	ins	—	ROTH *et al.*, 1959b
Fusarium oxysporum	ins	—	ROTH *et al.*, 1959b
Penicillium chrysogenum	ins	—	ROTH *et al.*, 1959b
Saccharomyces cerevisiae (protoplasts)	ins	—	SHOCKMAN and LAMPEN, 1962

[1] Based on dry weight.
[2] Based on radial growth.
[3] ins — insensitive to griseofulvin.

The structure of griseofulvin (Fig. 1) was proposed by GROVE (1952). Recently, CROSSE *et al.* (1964) reported a large number of griseofulvin relatives with enhanced *in vitro* activity. Other reviews on griseofulvin have been published by BRIAN (1960), GROVE (1963), and ROTH (1960a).

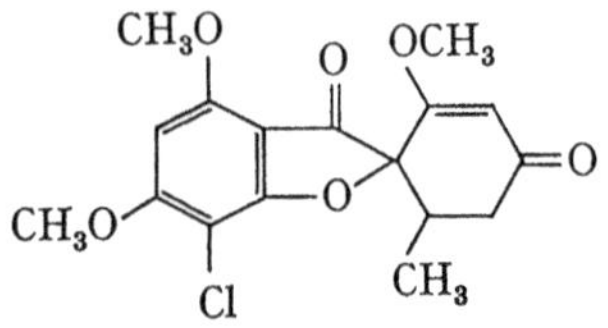

Fig. 1. Griseofulvin

Griseofulvin inhibits the growth of mycelial fungi, but has no effect on bacteria or yeasts (Table 1). The antibiotic does not affect the growth of fungi with cellulose cell walls, but does inhibit fungi that contain chitin (BRIAN, 1949). Griseofulvin resistance in fungi has been developed in vitro (AYTOUN *et al.*, 1960; BRIAN, 1960). However, the resistance was rapidly lost when the organisms were subcultured on griseofulvin-free media.

At 25 μg/ml, griseofulvin inhibited germination and root growth of mustard seeds 39 and 77%, respectively, (BRIAN, 1949). At the same concentration, germination of clover and wheat seeds was not inhibited, but root growth was retarded 48 and 88% respectively. Similar results have been reported by WRIGHT (1951). When lettuce and oat plants were subjected to the antibiotic, both roots and shoots were stunted (BRIAN, 1951). At 5 μg/ml, griseofulvin caused the roots of wheat seedlings to become stunted and swollen just behind the tip (STOKES, 1954).

Griseofulvin administered orally to humans produced essentially no side effects (ROTH and BLANK, 1960b; ROTH *et al.*, 1959b; BURGOON *et al.*, 1960). GOLDMAN *et al.* (1960) observed that the antibiotic had no effect on skin tumors. Large doses of griseofulvin have been reported to cause inhibition of spermatogenisis in mice and necrosis of the seminiferous epithelium in rats (SCHWARZ *et al.*, 1960; PAGET and WALPOLE, 1960). BARICH *et al.* (1960) demonstrated that simultaneous treatment of mice with griseofulvin and methyl cholanthrene caused the production of tumors. However, PAGET and ALCOCK (1960) have shown that the antibiotic was not carcinogenic to rats.

At 100 μg/ml griseofulvin inhibited the growth of both HeLa and skin cell lines (DEMIS *et al.*, 1960). A concentration of 1 mg/ml caused complete destruction of such cells. The antibiotic has also been reported to cause budding of human amnion and monkey kidney cells (MUNTONI and LODDO, 1964).

Reversal of Griseofulvin Inhibition

MCNALL (1960a, b) has shown that adenylic acid, cytidylic acid, guanylic acid, thymine, and uracil partially reversed the inhibition of *M. canis*. With *T. mentagrophytes*, adenylic and guanylic acids reversed the inhibition of growth from 56 to 19% (EL-NAKEEB *et al.*, 1965c). When each compound was used alone, no reversal occurred and pyrimidine derivatives were without effect. The same investigators reported that twelve nucleotides and nucleosides would not reverse the inhibition of *M. gypseum*. The inhibition of *B. cinerea* has also been reported not to be reversed by nucleic acids, nucleotides, purines, and pyrimidines (HUBER and GOTTLIEB, 1966).

Morphological Effects

A paste containing griseofulvin applied to the growing zone of *Phycomyces blakesleeanus* sporangiophores caused the structure to bend in the direction opposite the point of application (BANBURY, 1952). AYTOUN *et al.* (1960) reported that griseofulvin only affects fungal cells in immediate contact with it; thus, aerial hyphae were not affected. However, when aerial hyphae touched the substrate, growth of the contact cells ceased, and the end result was a stolon type of growth.

Although the germination of *B. allii* spores was not inhibited nor the time required for germination altered, the germtubes were greatly distorted (BRIAN *et al.*, 1946). Low concentrations of griseofulvin caused hyphae to curl, to have shortened internodes, form excessive branching and unusual swellings (BRIAN, 1944; BRIAN *et al.*, 1946; SRIVASTAVA and VORA, 1961). At high concentrations of the antibiotic, hyphae lost direction of growth, became larger in diameter and finally ruptured (AYTOUN, 1956; LARPENT, 1963; BRIAN, 1949). NAPIER *et al.* (1956) classified the morphologic responses of fungi exposed to griseofulvin into four groups.

The treatment of *Trichophyton tonsurous*, caused the organism to produce rectangular arthrospores instead of round endospores (REISS *et al.*, 1960). Drawings and photographs of the morphologic abnormalities have been published by BRIAN *et al.* (1946) and ROTH *et al.* (1956b).

Cytological Effects

Intravenous injections of griseofulvin into rats arrested mitosis in metaphase (PAGET and WALPOLE, 1958, 1960). Cells arrested in metaphase exhibited disorientation and scattering of the chromosomes throughout the cytoplasm. Bean roots treated with griseofulvin showed a delay in mitosis at metaphase (PAGET and WALPOLE, 1960). In such cells, spindle formation was not completely inhibited, but multipolar mitosis and nuclei of varying size were observed. DEYSON (1946a, b) has reported the inhibition of mitosis in both allium and rat cells.

THYAGARAJAN (1963) studied dermatophytes exposed to griseofulvin and observed abnormalities only in the growing region of the fungi. Although more nuclei were present in the hyphal tips, they were of abnormal size or shape. Extremely large nuclei were found, suggesting that these structures did not separate after or during division. Electron micrographs of *T. rubrum* revealed that exposure of hyphae to the antibiotic caused swelling, disappearance of cytoplasm, and contraction of cytoplasmic membranes (BLANK *et al.*, 1960).

Respiratory Effects

Griseofulvin has been reported to have no effect on the respiration of *B. allii*, *B. cinerea*, *T. mentagrophytes*, and *T. rubrum* (BRIAN, 1949; HUBER, 1965; LARSEN and DEMIS, 1963; ROTH *et al.*, 1959b).

Effect on Cell Walls

EVELEIGH and KNIGHT (1965) isolated and chemically analyzed cell wall fractions from *T. mentagrophytes*. In preparations from both griseofulvin treated and untreated cells, the content of total carbohydrate, amino sugars, protein, and phosphate were similar. No change was observed in the ratio of glucose to glucosamine.

High magnification electron micrographs of cell walls revealed that the microfibril structure of treated cells was like that of control cells (EVANS, 1964). Lower magnifications have shown that the walls of cells exposed to griseofulvin lose their integrity and become thickened (BLANK *et al.*, 1960).

Effect on Chemical Composition

EL-NAKEEB *et al.* (1965c) incubated *M. gypseum* with griseofulvin (10 μg/ml) for various periods of time and then analyzed the mycelium. When cell composition in griseofulvin treated mycelia are compared to controls on a culture volume basis, the data indicate a marked decrease in protein, RNA, and DNA at various time intervals between 0 and 24 hr. At 72 hr the culture showed significant increased growth, and the RNA and DNA had increased over the controls; protein was still lower than in controls.

Analysis of *B. cinerea* mycelium exposed to griseofulvin (20 μg/ml) for 24 hours indicated that the chitin, protein and total lipid content was the same as that of control mycelium (HUBER and GOTTLIEB, 1966). Total carbohydrate, and in some instances ergosterol, decreased in cells exposed to the antibiotic. Very small decreases were observed in the RNA content of treated cells compared to control cells. Griseofulvin caused an increase in DNA which related directly to antibiotic concentration. The differences in the data obtained from *M. gypseum* and *B. cinerea* can be eliminated if the data of EL-NAKEEB *et al.* (1965c) are recalculated on a dry weight basis. Then the composition of a 24 hr culture of *M. gypseum* showed that protein, RNA, and DNA had increased. No nucleotides have been shown to accumulate in *T. mentagrophytes* exposed to griseofulvin (EVELEIGH and KNIGHT, 1965).

Effect of Griseofulvin on the Uptake of Labeled Substrates

The isotope incorporation date of EL-NAKEEB *et al.* (1965c) have been recalculated as shown in Table 2. When radioactive uridine was used to study the rate of RNA synthesis in *M. gypseum*, the specific activity of the nucleic acid fraction was almost 50% less in cells exposed to griseofulvin. The incorporation of thymidine into griseofulvin treated cells was twice that found in the controls. Radioactive amino acids were rapidly incorporated into both control and treated mycelia during the first six hours of the experiment, but later the specific activity decreased. The amount of labeling in the protein fraction of treated cells was higher at 24 hr than that of control cells.

The synthesis of RNA in *B. cinera*, as measured by the incorporation of labeled glucose and glycine into a RNA fraction, was not inhibited by the antibiotic (HUBER and GOTTLIEB, 1966). When the incorporation of aspartic acid-U-^{14}C into the RNA fraction was measured, the final radioactivity was 50% less

Table 2. *Synthesis by M. gypseum of protein, RNA and DNA from radioactive precursors*[1]

Substrate	Griseofulvin	Incorporation of radioactive precursor			
		hr of incubation			
		0	6	12	24
Uridine	−	167[3]	14.4[2]	25.6[2]	26.2[2]
	+	—	5.7[2]	14.7[2]	14.5[2]
Thymidine	−	3.3[3]	42.5[3]	48.4[3]	118[3]
	+	—	40.0[3]	60.0[3]	230[3]
Leucine	−	133[3]	35.5[2]	21.8[2]	9.85[2]
	+	—	54.9[2]	43.0[2]	29.5[2]
Valine	−	0	24.0[2]	—	2.85[2]
	+	—	32.7[2]	—	8.1[2]

[1] Collation of data in Tables 3 and 4 of El-Nakeeb *et al.* (1965c).
[2] Values represent cpm $\times$ 10^{-3} mg dry weight.
[3] Values represent cpm/mg dry weight.

in mycelia that had been exposed to griseofulvin. The data from radioactive precursors, especially from glycine, revealed an increase in DNA caused by griseofulvin. This was similar to the increases in DNA that were found by direct chemical analyses. The specific activity of the DNA fraction increased with time during the entire period of the experiment when glucose or glycine were used as substrates. On the other hand, the control mycelium rapidly incorporated radioactivity into the DNA fraction for only 12 hr; then the specific activity of the fraction remained constant. With aspartic acid the total incorporation into the DNA fraction was lower, and the pattern was the same as control cells. The difference in incorporation of glycine-U-^{14}C and aspartic acid-U-^{14}C could indicate that the increase in DNA is primarily one of pyrimidines. The rate of incorporation of labeled substrates into the protein fraction of *B. cinerea* was not inhibited by griseofulvin.

Binding of Griseofulvin to Cellular Components

Freedman *et al.* (1962) reported that griseofulvin binds to keratin. Removal of lipids from the protein hindered subsequent sorption of the antibiotic.

RNA isolated from *M. gypseum* has been reported to form complexes with griseofulvin that are stable to dialysis, molecular seive chromatography, and density gradient centrifugation (El-Nakeeb and Lampen, 1964a). The griseofulvin to nucleotide ratio was 1:50. Similar nucleic acid preparations from *A. niger* and *S. cerevisiae* had a low affinity for the antibiotic, and the complexes which formed were unstable. Huber and Gottlieb (1966) also were unable to demonstrate the binding of griseofulvin to yeast RNA.

Ribosomes, isolated from *M. gypseum*, bound griseofulvin at 4 C (El-Nakeeb and Lampen, 1964b). Although the effect was stimulated by small volumes of a 105,000 × g supernatant fraction, large volumes were inhibitory. Incubation of the ribosomes and griseofulvin at 30 C caused the release of nucleotides and griseofulvin.

Approximately 75% of the carbon-14 labeled griseofulvin bound by cell free extracts of *B. cinerea* was associated with a 500 × g pellet (Huber and Gottlieb, 1966). Radioactivity was also found in mitochondrial and ribosomal fractions.

The Uptake of Griseofulvin from Culture Media

The uptake of griseofulvin, as measured by loss from culture media, occurred into *B. allii* and *Mucor ramannianus*, but not *Phycomyces blakesleeanus* (ABBOTT and GROVE, 1959).

EL-NAKEEB and LAMPEN (1965 a, b) found that the uptake of tritiated griseofulvin by *M. gypseum* was dependent on the concentration of antibiotic in the medium, temperature, pH, and an energy source such as glucose. Sodium azide (10^{-2} M), 2,4-dinitrophenol (10^{-3} M) and p-fluorophenylalanine (10 μg/ml) inhibited the uptake with the exception of a small residual uptake. Approximately 50% of the griseofulvin which accumulated in the mycelium was extracted with hot water. The remaining antibiotic was distributed equally between a hot trichloroacetic acid (TCA) extract (nucleic acids) and a hot sodium hydroxide extract (protein). Hot water and hot TCA had little effect on the antibiotic. When griseofulvin-^{3}H was heated at 90° C for 30 minutes in 1 N sodium hydroxide, less than 40% of the radioactivity could be recovered as unchanged griseofulvin. EL-NAKEEB and LAMPEN (1965 d) also found that insensitive yeasts and bacteria did not bind appreciable amounts of griseofulvin. *Aspergillus niger* and *N. crassa*, which are only moderately sensitive to griseofulvin, accumulated some of the antibiotic into a water soluble pool.

In contrast to these results, approximately 40% of the carbon-14 labeled griseofulvin bound by *B. cinerea* was removed by chloroform: methanol extraction (HUBER and GOTTLIEB, 1966). Twenty-one percent of the radioactivity was extracted with 80% ethanol. The remaining radioactivity was distributed between cold TCA, RNA, DNA, protein, and chitin fraction. A total of 0.23 μg griseofulvin were taken up per mg dry weight of mycelium.

Absorption and Translocation of Griseofulvin in Higher Plants

Griseofulvin was absorbed and has been reported to be taken up by plants and translocated unchanged (CROWDY *et al.*, 1955; BRIAN *et al.*, 1951). The initial uptake in broad bean was reduced by azide and 2,4-dinitrophenol (CROWDY *et al.*, 1956). In wheat seedlings the uptake and translocation of the antibiotic was inhibited by azide at 10^{-6} M (STOKES, 1954). CROWDY *et al.* (1959a, b), studying griseofulvin analogues, reported that compounds active *in vitro* and as systemic fungicides were closely related to griseofulvin in structure. Such analogs were translocated unchanged, and they acted directly against the pathogen.

The Metabolism of Griseofulvin

Large amounts of 6-demethylgriseofulvin were found in the urine of humans, rabbits, and rats after these subjects received doses of griseofulvin (BARNES and BOOTHROYD, 1961). The same product was isolated from rat liver slices incubated with the antibiotic. BOOTHROYD *et al.* (1961) incubated griseofulvin with various fungi; *B. allii*, *Cercospora melonis*, and *M. canis* produced griseofulvic acid, 6-demethylgriseofulvin, and 4-demethylgriseofulvin respectively. Recently, EL-NAKEEB and LAMPEN (1965 d) have shown that griseofulvin sensitive fungi also degrade the antibiotic.

Miscellaneous Effects of Griseofulvin

The phosphorus uptake of *M. canis exposed* to griseofulvin has been reported to be interrupted for a short period (ZIEGLER, 1963). The antibiotic did not reduce the proteolytic activity of the culture until 15 days had elapsed.

Summary

The mode of action of griseofulvin is not completely understood. The antibiotic does not inhibit the synthesis of protein, chitin, and total lipid. Furthermore, respiration and glycolysis of fungal cells is not altered by griseofulvin and the ability of fungal protoplasts to synthesize new cell walls is not inhibited. Conflicting data indicate that RNA and DNA synthesis may either be stimulated or reduced by the antibiotic. However, if RNA synthesis was the site of action, it is doubtful that protein synthesis would continue at a normal or accelerated rate.

Since griseofulvin appears to stimulate DNA synthesis and causes the formation of abnormal cells, it is likely that the site of action is in the replicatory system of the fungal cell. Other data supporting this view are the cytological studies showing that griseofulvin inhibits mitosis in the metaphase, causes multipolar mitosis, and produces abnormal nuclei.

References

ABBOTT, M. T. J., and J. F. GROVE: Uptake and translocation of organic compounds by fungi. II. Griseofulvin. Exptl. Cell Research **17**, 105 (1959).

AYTOUN, R. S. C.: The effects of griseofulvin on certain phytopathogenic fungi. Ann. Botany (London) **20**, 297 (1956).

AYTOUN, R. S. C., A. H. CAMPBELL, E. J. NAPIER, and D. A. L. SEILER: Mycological aspects of the action of griseofulvin against dermatophytes. A.M.A. Arch. Dermatol. **81**, 650 (1960).

BANBURY, G. H.: Physiological studies in the mucorales. Part II. Some observations on growth regulation in the sporongiophore of Phycomyces. J. Exptl. Botany **3**, 86 (1952).

BARICH, L. L., T. NAKAI, J. SCHWARZ, and D. J. BARICH: Tumour promoting effect of excessively large doses of oral griseofulvin on tumours induced in mice by methylcholanthrene. Nature **187**, 335 (1960).

BARNES, M. J., and B. BOOTHROYD: The metabolism of griseofulvin in mammals. Biochem. J. **78**, 41 (1961).

BLANK, H., and F. J. ROTH: Systemic control of cutaneous fungus infections. Am. J. Med. Sci. **240**, 104/466 (1960b).

BLANK, H., D. TAPLIN, and F. J. ROTH: Electron microscopic observations of the effects of griseofulvin on dermatophytes. A.M.A. Arch. Dermatol. **81**, 667 (1960).

BOOTHROYD, B., E. J. NAPIER, and G. A. SOMERFIELD: The demethylation of griseofulvin by fungi. Biochem. J. **80**, 34 (1961).

BRIAN, P. W.: Studies on the biological activity of griseofulvin. Ann. Botany (London) **13**, 59 (1949).

BRIAN, P. W.: Griseofulvin. Trans. Brit. Myco. Soc. **43**, 1 (1960).

BRIAN, P. W., P. J. CURTIS, and H. G. HEMMING: A substance causing abnormal development of fungal hyphae produced by *Penicillium janczewskii* ZAL. I. Biological assay, production, and isolation of "curling factor". Trans. Brit. Myco. Soc. **29**, 173 (1946).

BRIAN, P. W., P. J. CURTIS, and H. G. HEMMING: A substance causing abnormal development of fungal hyphae produced by *Penicillium janczewskii* ZAL. III. Identity of "curling factor" with griseofulvin. Trans. Brit. Myco. Soc. **32**, 20 (1949).

BRIAN, P. W., P. J. CURTIS, and H. G. HEMMING: Production of griseofulvin by *Penicillium raistrichii*. Trans. Brit. Myco. Soc. **38**, 305 (1955).
BRIAN, P. W., J. M. WRIGHT, J. STUBBS, and A. M. WAY: Uptake of antibiotic metabolites of soil microorganisms by plants. Nature **167**, 347 (1951).
BURGOON, C. F., J. H. GRAHAM, R. J. KEIPER, F. URBACH, J. S. BURGOON, and E. B. HELWIG: Histopathologic evaluation of griseofulvin in *Microsporum andovini* infections. A.M.A. Arch. Dermatol. **81**, 724 (1960).
CROSSE, R., R. MCWILLIAM, and A. RHODES: Some relations between chemical structure and antifungal effects of griseofulvin analogues. J. Gen. Microbiol. **34**, 51 (1964).
CROWDY, S. H., D. GARDNER, J. F. GROVE, and D. PRAMER: The translocation of antibiotics in higher plants. I. Isolation of griseofulvin and chloramphenicol from plant tissue. J. Exptl. Botany **6**, 371 (1955).
CROWDY, S. H., A. P. GREEN, J. F. GROVE, P. MCCLOSKEY, and A. MORRISON: The translocation of antibiotics in higher plants. 3. The estimation of griseofulvin relatives in plant tissue. Biochem. J. **72**, 230 (1959a).
CROWDY, S. H., J. F. GROVE, H. G. HEMMING, and K. C. ROBINSON: The translocation of antibiotics in higher plants. II. The movement of griseofulvin in broad bean and tomato. J. Exptl. Botany **7**, 42 (1956).
CROWDY, S. H., J. F. GROVE, and P. MCCLOSKEY: The translocation of antibiotics in higher plants. 4. Systemic fungicidal activity and chemical structure in griseofulvin relatives. Biochem. J. **72**, 241 (1959b).
DENNIS, D. J., M. J. DAVIS, and J. C. CAMPBELL: The effects of griseofulvin on epithelial cells in tissue culture. J. Invest. Dermatol. **34**, 99 (1960).
DEYSON, G.: Antimitotic properties of griseofulvin. Ann. pharm. franç. **22**, 17 (1964a).
DEYSON, G.: The influence of griseofulvin on the antimitotic properties of colchicine. Ann. pharm. franç. **22**, 89 (1964b).
EL-NAKEEB, M. A., and J. O. LAMPEN: Formation of complexes of griseofulvin and nucleic acids of fungi and its relation to griseofulvin sensitivity. Biochem. J. **92**, 59p (1964a).
EL-NAKEEB, M. A., and J. O. LAMPEN: Binding of tritiated-griseofulvin by ribosomes and RNA of *Microsporum gypseum*. Bacteriol. Proc. **1964**, P60 (1964b).
EL-NAKEEB, M. A., and J. O. LAMPEN: Uptake of griseofulvin by the sensitive dermatophyte, *Microsporum gypseum*. J. Bacteriol. **89**, 564 (1965a).
EL-NAKEEB, M. A., and J. O. LAMPEN: Distribution of griseofulvin taken up by *Microsporum gypseum:* Complexes of the antibiotic with cell constituents. J. Bacteriol. **89**, 1075 (1965b).
EL-NAKEEB, M. A., W. L. MCLELLAN, and J. O. LAMPEN: Antibiotic action of griseofulvin on dermatophytes. J. Bacteriol. **89**, 557 (1965c).
EL-NAKEEB, M. A., and J. O. LAMPEN: Uptake of H^3-griseofulvin by microorganisms and its correlation with sensitivity to griseofulvin. J. Gen. Microbiol. **39**, 285 (1965d).
EVANS, G.: The antibiotic activity of *Cylindrocarpon radicicola*. Ph. D. Thesis, University of Sydney 1964.
EVELIGH, D. E., and S. G. KNIGHT: The effect of griseofulvin on the cell wall composition of *Trichophyton mentagrophytes*. Bacteriol. Proc. **1965**, G82, p. 27 (1965).
FOLEY, E. J., and G. A. GRECO: Studies on the mode of action of griseofulvin. Antibiotics Ann. **1959/60**, 670 (1960).
FREEDMAN, M. H., R. M. BAXTER, and G. C. WALKER: In vitro sorption of griseofulvin by keratin substrates. J. Invest. Dermatol. **38**, 199 (1962).
GOLDMAN, L., A. BEYER, and J. SCHWARZ: Absence of local cytotoxic change in man from griseofulvin. Nature **187**, 335 (1960).
GROVE, J. F.: Griseofulvin. Quart. Revs. (London) **17**, 1 (1963).
GROVE, J. F., J. MACMILLAN, T. P. C. MULHOLLAND, and M. A. T. ROGERS: Griseofulvin. Part IV. Structure. J. Chem. Soc. **1952**, 3977 (1952).
GROVE, J. F., and J. C. MCGOWAN: Identity of griseofulvin and "curling factor". Nature **160**, 574 (1947).

HUBER, F. M., and D. GOTTLIEB: The mode of action of the antifungal antibiotic griseofulvin (1966). (In Preparation.)
LARPENT, J. P.: Comparative action of griseofulvin and colchicine on growth and branching of the young thallus of *Saprolegnia monoica*. Compt. rend. **157**, 2219 (Chem. Abstr. **61**, 2407f) (1963).
LARSEN, W. G., and D. J. DEMIS: Metabolic studies of the effect of griseofulvin and candicidin on fungi. J. Invest. Dermatol. **41**, 335 (1963).
MACMILLAN, J.: Griseofulvin. Part 9. Isolation of the bromoanalogue from *Penicillium griseofulvum* and *Penicillium nigricans*. J. Chem. Soc. 2585 (1954).
MACMILLAN, J.: Dechlorogriseofulvin — a metabolic product of *Penicillium griseofulvum* DIERCKX and *Penicillium janczewskii* ZAL. Chem. & Ind. (London) 179 (1951).
MCGOWAN, J. C.: A substance causing abnormal development of fungal hyphae produced by *Penicillium janczewskii* ZAL. II. Preliminary notes on the chemical and physical properties of "curling factor". Trans. Brit. Myco. Soc. **29**, 188 (1946).
MCNALL, E. G.: Biochemical studies on the metabolism of griseofulvin. A.M.A. Arch. Dermatol. **81**, 657 (1960a).
MCNALL, E. G.: Metabolic studies on griseofulvin and its mechanism of action. Antibiotics Ann. **1959/60**, 674 (1960b).
MUNTONI, S., and B. LODDO: Griseofulvin — induced budding in cell cultures. Arch. intern. pharmacodynamie **151**, 365 (Chem. Abstr. **62**, 5755g) (1964).
NAPIER, E. J., D. I. TURNER, and A. RHODES: The in vitro action of griseofulvin against pathogenic fungi of plants. Ann. Botany (London) **20**, 461 (1956).
OXFORD, A. E., H. RAISTRICK, and P. SIMONART: Studies on the biochemistry of microorganisms. 60. Griseofulvin, $C_{17}H_{17}O_6Cl$, a metabolic product of *Penicillium griseofulvum* DIECK. Biochem. J. **33**, 240 (1939).
PAGET, G. E., and S. J. ALCOCK: Griseofulvin and colchicine: lack of carcinogenic action. Nature **188**, 867 (1960).
PAGET, G. E., and A. L. WALPOLE: Some cytological effects of griseofulvin. Nature **182**, 1320 (1958).
PAGET, G. E., and A. L. WALPOLE: The experimental toxicology of griseofulvin. A.M.A. Arch. Dermatol. **81**, 750 (1960).
REISS, F., L. KORNBLEE, and B. GORDON: Griseofulvin (fulvicin) in the treatment of fungus infections of the hair, skin, and nails with special reference to mycologic changes produced during therapy. J. Invest. Dermatol. **34**, 263 (1960).
ROTH, F. J.: Griseofulvin. Ann. N.Y. Acad. Sci. **89**, 81, 750 (1960).
ROTH, F. J., B. SALLMAN, and H. BLANK: In vitro studies of the antifungal antibiotic griseofulvin. J. Invest. Dermatol. **33**, 403 (1959b).
SCHWARZ, J., and J. K. LOUTZENHISER: Laboratory experiences with griseofulvin. J. Invest. Dermatol. **34**, 295 (1960).
SHOCKMAN, G. D., and J. O. LAMPEN: Inhibition by antibiotics of the growth of bacterial and yeast protoplasts. J. Bacteriol. **84**, 508 (1962).
SRIVASTAVA, O. P., and V. C. VORA: Effect of griseofulvin on dermatophytes including locally isolated strains of *Trichophyton rubrum* and on *Microsporum canis* grown in keratin. J. Sci. Ind. Research (India) **20C**, 163 (1961).
STOKES, A.: Uptake and translocation of griseofulvin by wheat seedlings. Plant and Soil **5**, 132 (1954).
THYAGARAJAN, T. R., O. P. SRIVASTAVA, and V. V. VORA: Some cytological observations on the effect of griseofulvin on dermatophytes. Naturwissenschaften **50**, 524 (1963).
WRIGHT, J. M.: Phytotoxic effects of some antibiotics. Ann. Botany (London) **15**, 493 (1951).
ZIEGLER, H.: Effect of griseofulvin on *Microsporum canis*. IV. Z. allgem. Mikrobiol. **3**, 211 (1963).

Daunomycin and Related Antibiotics

A. Di Marco

Daunomycin (Da) is a metabolite of *Streptomyces peucetius* (GREIN *et al.*, 1963) which strongly inhibits a variety of experimental tumors (DI MARCO *et al.*, 1964b). The antibiotic substance is a glycoside (Hydrochloride: $C_{27}H_{29}NO_{10} \cdot HCl$) which by acid hydrolysis yields an aglycone, daunomycinone (ARCAMONE *et al.*, 1964b) and a new aminosugar, daunosamine (ARCAMONE *et al.*, 1964a). DUBOST *et al.* (1963) have also described an antibiotic, rubidomycin, whose physico-chemical characteristics correspond to those of daunomycin. Daunomycin is closely related to the anthracyclines. Following BROCKMANN'S suggestion (1963), those antibiotics that contained a tetrahydrotetracenquinone chromophore linked to a sugar should all be included in the anthracycline group. The chromophores of such antibiotics have different substituents on the nucleus (Fig. 1 and Table 1).

Antimicrobial Activity

The antimicrobial activities of daunomycin, cinerubin and aklavin are summarized in Table 2. Gram-positive bacteria and the fungi show a relatively high degree of susceptibility to these antibiotics, but gram-negative bacteria are generally resistant. Different strains of the same organism may have different susceptibilities, e.g. *E. coli* K12 and *E. coli* B.

Antiviral Activity

In *E. coli* K12 a selective interference of Da with the multiplication of bacteriophage of the series T was observed (Table 3). The antibiotic does not, however, inactivate the phages nor does it inhibit the absorption of the virus particles on the cell (SANFILIPPO and MAZZOLENI, 1964; PARISI and SOLLER, 1964).

The protection against the lysis resulting from phage multiplication occurs only if Da is present in the first few minutes after infection (Fig. 2). DNA from fish sperm partially antagonizes the protective effect of Da for the bacteria. In contrast with the observations on T phages (whose genetic material consists of DNA) no protective effect was exerted by Da against infection of *E. coli* K12 by μ2 phages containing only RNA (PARISI and SOLLER, 1964). This lack of activity could be accounted for by the poor ability of Da to bind to RNA. If the Da action on T phage multiplication prevents the release of viral messenger RNA, the lack of protection on bacterial cells infected with μ2 phages might be explained by assuming that the RNA μ2 phage genome itself were the messenger.

Table 1. *Constituents of anthracycline antibiotics*

Antibiotic	Chromophore	Sugar	Reference
Pyrromycin	ε-Pyrromicinone	1 mol. rhodosamine	BROCKMANN, 1959
Rutilantin	ε-Pyrromicinone	?	OLLIS, 1961; OLLIS, 1959
Cinerubin A	ε-Pyrromicinone	1 mol. rhodosamine 1 mol. 2-deoxy-L-fucose 1 mol. dideoxyaldohexose	ETTLINGER, 1959
Cinerubin B	ε-Pyrromicinone	1 mol. rhodosamine	
Cinerubin B	ε-Pyrromicinone	1 mol. rhodosamine 1 mol. 2-deoxy-L-fucose 1 mol. dideoxyaldohexose	ETTLINGER, 1959
Aklavin	Aclavinone	?	STRELITZ, 1956
Rhodomycin A	β-Rhodomycinone	2 mol. rhodosamine	BROCKMANN and SPOLLER, 1961; BROCKMANN and WACHNELDT, 1961; BROCKMANN, 1963
Rhodomycin B	β-Rhodomycinone	rhodosamine	BROCKMANN and SPOLLER, 1961; BROCKMANN and WACHNELDT, 1961; BROCKMANN, 1963
γ-Rhodomycin 1	γ-Rhodomycinone	rhodosamine	BROCKMANN and SPOLLER, 1961; BROCKMANN and WACHNELDT, 1961; BROCKMANN, 1963
γ-Rhodomycin 2	γ-Rhodomycinone	2 mol. rhodosamine	BROCKMANN and SPOLLER, 1961; BROCKMANN and WACHNELDT, 1961; BROCKMANN, 1963
γ-Rhodomycin 3	γ-Rhodomycinone	2 mol. rhodosamine + 1 mol. 2-deoxy-L-fucose	BROCKMANN and SPOLLER, 1961; BROCKMANN and WACHNELDT, 1961; BROCKMANN, 1963
γ-Rhodomycin 4	γ-Rhodomycinone	2 mol. rhodosamine + 1 mol. 2-deoxy-L-fucose + 1 mol. rhodinose	BROCKMANN and SPOLLER, 1961; BROCKMANN and WACHNELDT, 1961; BROCKMANN, 1963
Isorhodomycin A	β-Isorhodomycinone	2 mol. rhodosamine	
Ruticulomycin A	5-Deoxy-pyrromicinone	?	MITSCHER, L. A.,
Ruticulomycin B	5-Deoxy-pyrromicinone	?	MCCRAE, W., W. W. ANDRES, LOVERY, J. A., N. BOHONOS, 1964
Isoquinocycline A	Isoquinocycline	methileptose	TULINSKY, 1964

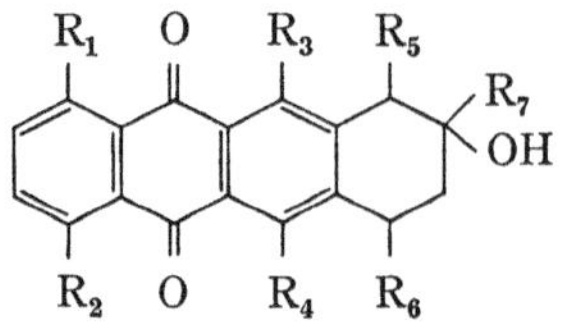

Chromophore group

	R_1	R_2	R_3	R_4	R_5	R_6	R_7
ε-Pyrromycinone	OH	OH	H	OH	$COOCH_3$	OH	C_2H_5
Aclavinone	H	OH	H	OH	$COOCH_3$	OH	C_2H_5
β-Rhodomycinone	H (or OH)	OH (or H)	OH	OH	OH	OH	C_2H_5
γ-Rhodomycinone	H (or OH)	OH (or H)	OH	OH	OH	H	C_2H_5
β-Isorhodomycinone							
5-Desoxy-pyrromycinone	OH	OH	H	H	$COOCH_3$	OH	C_2H_5
Daunomycinone	H (or OCH_3)	OCH_3 (or H)	OH	OH	H	OH	$COCH_3$

Sugars components

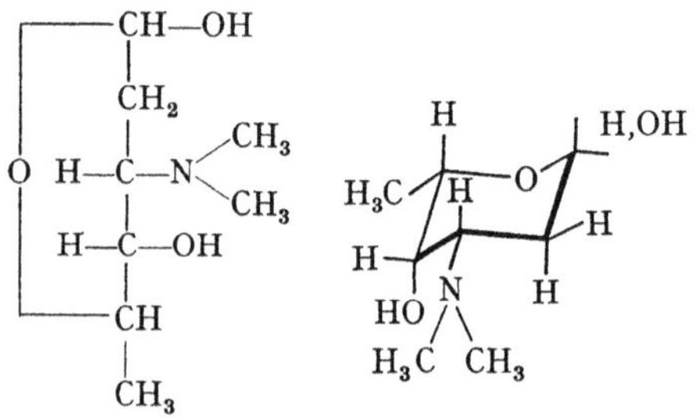

Rhodosamine

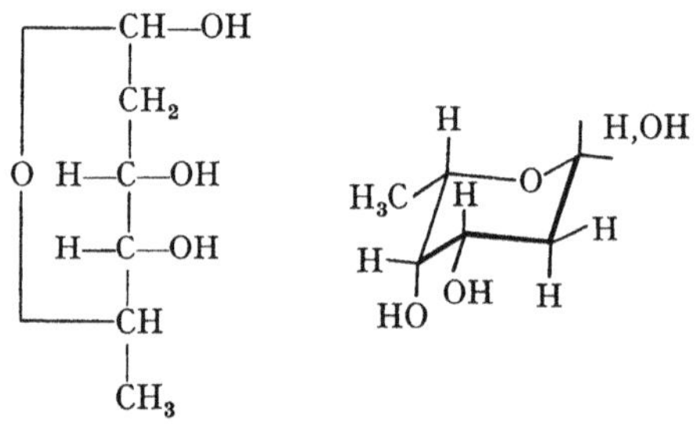

2-Desoxy-L-fucose

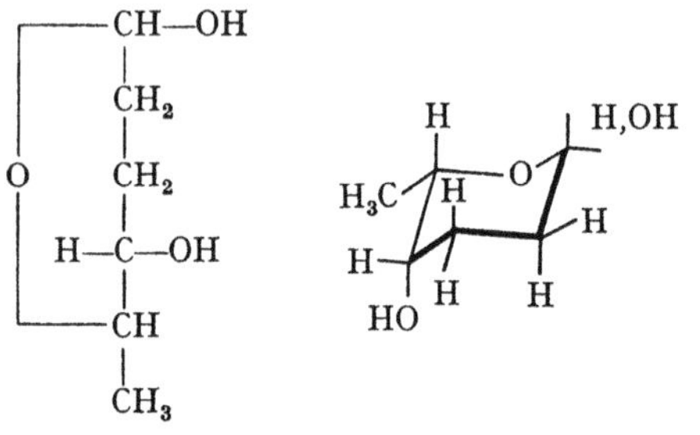

Rhodinose

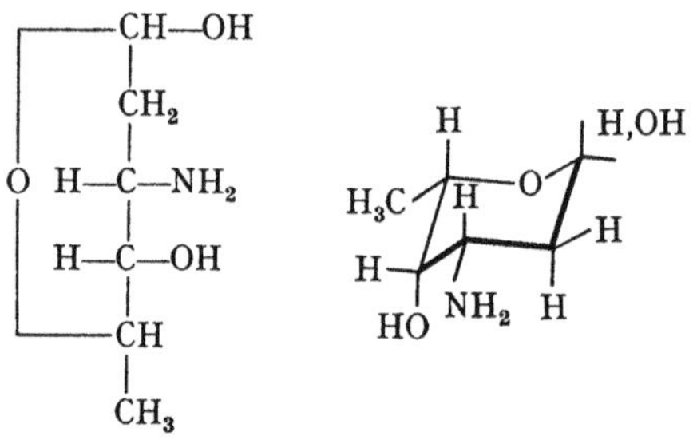

Daunosamine

Fig. 1. Structures of Anthracyclines

Other members of the anthracyclines group also have antiviral activity; an inhibitory effect of aklavin on the reproductive ability of a number of bacterial phages was observed by Strelitz and coworkers (1956). The inhibiting concentration for *B. megaterium* phage was 0.013 µg/ml; for staphylophage 15.0 µg/ml and for *E. coli* phage T-2 50 µg/ml. To attain a phagocidal effect on free phages, a much higher aklavin concentration is needed than to prevent cell lysis; this suggests an action on the host-parasite relationship. Aklavin also inactivated

Table 2. *Antimicrobial spectrum of daunomycin, cinerubin and aklavin*

Microorganism	Antibiotic		
	Daunomycin (LD^{50}) µg/ml (SANFILIPPO e MAZZOLENI, 1964)	Cinerubin (End Inhibiting Dose) µg/ml (ETTLINGER *et al.*, 1959)	Aklavin (Minimum Inhibitory Concentration Dose) µg/ml (STRELITZ *et al.*, 1955)
Bacteria Gram positive			
Micrococcus pyogenes aureus	3.0	10	2—8
Streptococcus faecalis A	—	1	—
Streptococcus faecalis B	—	10	—
Streptococcus mitis A	—	0.01	—
Streptococcus mitis B	—	0.01	—
Streptococcus pyogenes A	—	0.1	—
Streptococcus pyogenes B	—	1	—
Sarcina lutea	2.0	—	—
Mycobacterium Tbc A	—	1	—
Mycobacterium Tbc B	—	10	—
Mycobacterium smegmatis (ATCC 10143)	—	—	1.6
B. *subtilis* (ATCC 6633)	—	—	4.0
Bacteria Gram negative			
Escherichia coli K 12	100	(>100)	—
Escherichia coli B	2.0	—	16.0
Escherichia strain (ATCC 9637 *et al.*)			125.0—250.0
Salmonella tiphosa	2	(>100)	—
Pasteurella pestis	—	(>100)	—
Klebsiella pneumoniae (ATCC 9577)	—	—	16.0
Pseudomonas aeruginosa (ATCC 10145)	—	—	250.0
Fungi			
Endomyces albicans A	—	0.1	—
Endomyces albicans B	—	1	—
Candida vulgaris A	—	0.1	—
Candida vulgaris B	—	1	—
Saccharomyces carlbersgensis	6	—	—
Saccharomyces pasteurianus	—	—	50.0
Ceratostornella fimbriata	—	—	6.25
Trichophyton interdigitale	—	—	25.0
Protozoa			
Entamoeba histolitica	50	100	—

animal viruses; an hour incubation of equine *encephalomyelitis* virus with 0.01 µg of the antibiotic was enough to protect mice from the viral infection. ASHESHOV and GORDON (1961) showed an inhibiting activity of rutilantin on the multiplication of *V. cholerae* phage up to a dilution $1:5\times10^6$. Since the growth of microorganism was inhibited by $1:10^4$—$1:10^5$ dilutions of this antibiotic, there seems to be present a fairly high degree of selective antiphage activity.

Table 3. *Antiphagic activity of daunomycin*

Phage	Daunomycin µg/ml				
	0	0.1	1	10	100
T1 Phage	18	24	41	59	81
T2 Phage	0	8	18	54	77
T4 Phage	17	24	49	58	84

Density of bacterial cultures were measured at 600 mµ after 45 minutes from the infection with bacteriophages T1, T2, and T4. The incubation was at 37°C in presence of different concentrations of daunomycin. From A. SANFILIPPO and R. MAZZOLENI: "Attività antifagica dell' antibiotico Daunomicina", Giorn. di Microbiol., *12*, 83 1964.

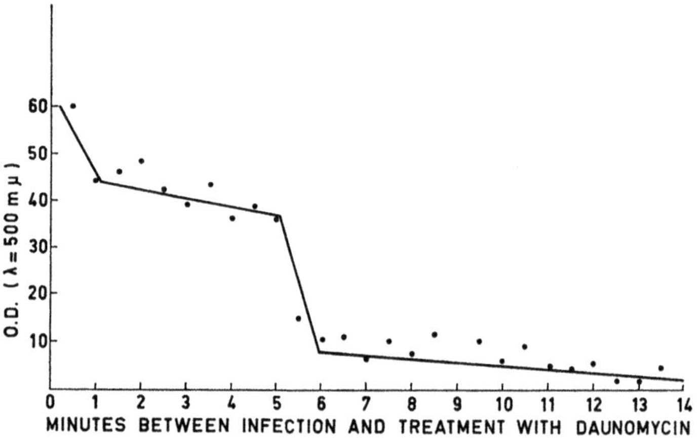

Fig. 2. Action of daunomycin on phage lysis. The antibiotic (10 µg/ml) was added to the cultural medium at different time intervals after the phage infection. Ordinate: density of bacterial population as percent value in comparison with the unifected control. The density of bacterial population was made up after 45 minutes incubation at 37°C (from: SANFILIPPO and MAZZOLENI, 1964)

Activity on *in vitro* Grown Normal and Neoplastic Mammalian cells

Da has a strong inhibiting effect on the *in vitro* growth of mammalian cells; a 0.1 µg/ml dose reduced the mitotic activity of a number of different test cells. An example of the antimitotic effect on slide cultures of rat fibroblasts and HeLa cells is reported in Fig. 3 (DI MARCO *et al.*, 1963b). Comparable activity was shown on cultures of cells originally isolated from carcinoma of the larynx (Helius Lettrè strain) and from human epidermoid carcinoma (KB strain). In *in vitro* mouse and rat bone marrow, both in rotating tubes and hanging drop cultures to which was added 0.1 µg/ml of Da, the absence of mitoses and severe cytological damages was observed after 24 hours (DI MARCO *et al.*, 1963b). At a concentration of 1.0µg/ml to 3µg/ml, Da was found to inhibit the proliferation of stem cells from human lymphocytes, following phyto-hemagglutinin stimulation (COSTA and ASTALDI, 1964).

Cell damage induced by Da is mainly nuclear. In resting cells, a finely granular appearance of the chromatin and marked alterations in the shape and size of the nucleolus have been observed. Cytoplasmic changes, such as vacuolation, are moderate, appear later and only after prolonged treatment by high doses of antibiotic. In mitotic cells, chromosomal damage such as fragmentation and mitotic aberrations, mainly anaphasic bridges, were observed (Di Marco *et al.*, 1963b). The reduction in mitotic index appears rather abruptly after addition of Da. When a sufficient amount of the antibiotic was added to a rat fibroblast culture, phase contrast microscopy reveals a cessation of the mitotic process and an anomalous scattering of the chromosomes within the cell (Di Marco *et al.*, 1963b). The damage induced by Da on the reproductive equipment of the cell seems to be

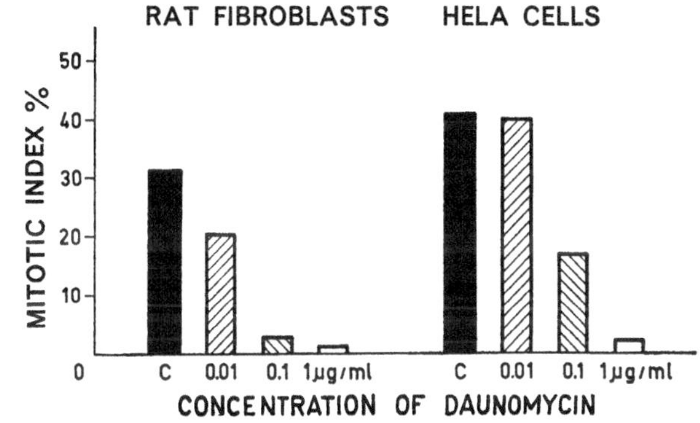

Fig. 3. Action of daunomycin on mitotic index of *in vitro* culture of rat fibroblasts and HeLa cells in solid form. Values of mitotic index found 24 hours after treatment with daunomycin at a dose of 1.0, 0.1 and 0.01 μg/ml. *C* control. Ordinate: mitotic index (from: Di Marco *et al.*, 1963)

a permanent one. HeLa cells exposed for one hour to 0.1 μg/ml of Da, then washed and observed 24 to 48 hours later show chromosomal breaks and bridges in a large percentage of the cells (Silvestrini *et al.*, 1963). The antimitotic effect of Da on HeLa cells cultured in monolayer was much more rapid than actinomycin D at comparable doses (Di Marco *et al.*, 1965b).

Cinerubin also impaired the multiplication of *in vitro* cultured chick embryo fibroblasts and caused morphological alterations of nucleoli (Ettlinger, 1959). Similar cytological effects on the nucleolus and on the process of cellular division were reported by Brindle and coworkers (1961) for the action of cinerubin on *in vitro* cultures of Ehrlich ascites cells and strain L cells.

Activity on Experimental Tumors

The inhibiting effect of different doses of Da (administered i.p. for 5 consecutive days following tumor implantation) on the growth of Ehrlich ascites tumor in albino mice is reported in Fig. 4 (Di Marco *et al.*, 1963a; Di Marco *et al.*, 1964a; Di Marco *et al.*, 1964c). A single dose of 2 mg/kg produced a rapid drop in the number of mitotic cells for 24 hours (Fig. 5). After 48 hours nearly all mitoses showed aberrations, such as anaphasic bridges, anomalous dispersion of chromosomes in the cytoplasm and chromosomal fragmentation. The nucleolus, appeared considerably enlarged from the 48th hour after treatment.

Da also inhibited to various degrees other ascites tumors of mice and rats. A comparative evaluation of the effectiveness of daunomycin, mitomycin and actinomycin C on mice bearing Ehrlich ascites tumor is shown in Fig. 6 (Gaetani, 1965). Da treatment of animals with different solid tumors resulted in various

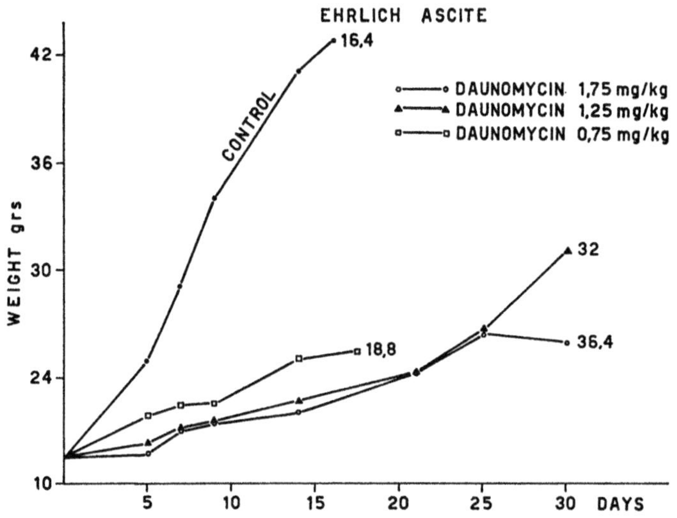

Fig. 4. Effect of daunomycin on growth of Ehrlich ascites tumor. Numbers at end of each curve represent values of average survival of animals in each lot (from: Di Marco *et al.*, 1964b)

amounts of inhibition (Table 4). These tumors show a lower susceptibility to Da compared to the ascite forms, probably because of an impaired penetration of the drug into the tissue. Fig. 7 shows the dose-effect of Da against Walker car-

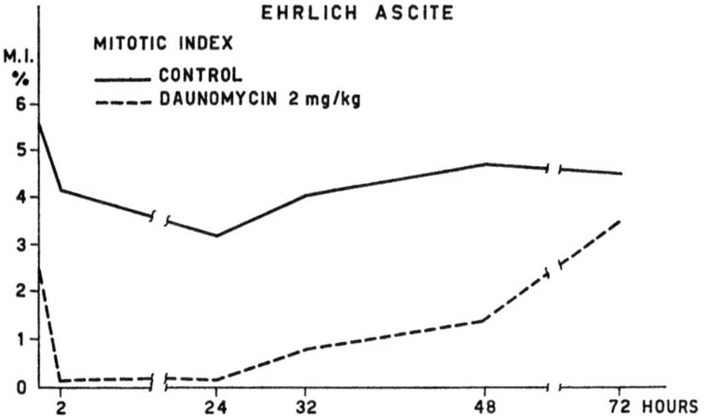

Fig. 5. Variations in mitotic index of Ehrlich ascites carcinoma after treatment with daunomycin (from: Di Marco *et al.*, 1964b)

cinoma, recorded according to the method of Litchfield and Wilcoxon (1949). The average effective dose (ED 50) is about 1.5 mg/kg with 8 i. v. injections.

In experimental leukemia, a therapeutic effect of Da on L 121 was reported (Goldin, 1965); whereas, no significant results were obtained on transplantable

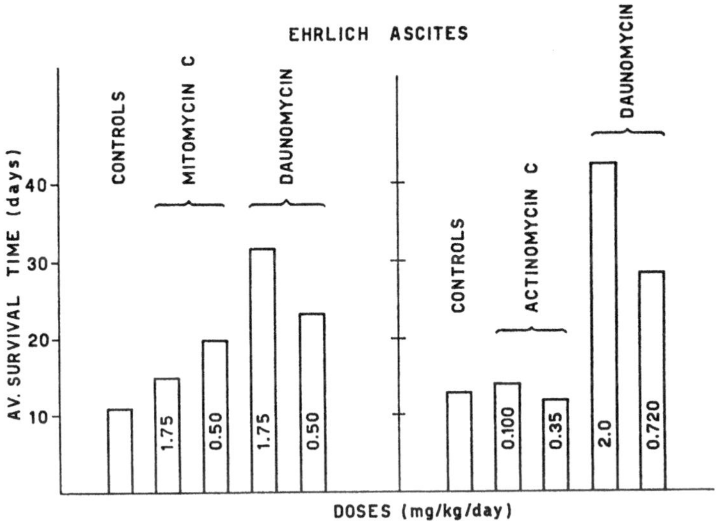

Fig. 6. Comparative evaluation of effectiveness of daunomycin, mitomycin and actinomycin C on mice bearing Ehrlich ascites tumour (from: GAETANI, 1965)

eukemia of C3H mice (Moloney leukemia 10) and a lymphoblastic acute leukemia of the CFW mouse (DI MARCO, DORIGOTTI and GAETANI, 1965c).

A study of the antineoplastic selectivity of Da was made on rats bearing the Walker carcinoma, or O. G. G. myeloma and the foreign-body granuloma, as

Table 4. Effect of daunomycin on solid tumors

Tumor	Dose (mg/kg/day)	% of inhibition	Mortality (treated/ controls)
Ehrlich carcinoma	6×6 s.c.	41.1	0/0
Ehrlich carcinoma	3×6 s.c.	12.—	0/0
SA 180	2×7 i.p.	42.1	0/0
SA 180	2×7 os	24.4	0/0
SA 180	5×8 s.c.	68.4	0/0
SA 180	2.5×8 s.c.	36.5	0/0
Methylcolantrene	1×10 e.v.	22.6	1/0
sarcoma	2×10 e.v.	67.6	1/0
Walker carcinoma	1×8 e.v.	30.8	0/0
Walker carcinoma	1.25×8 e.v.	36.—	0/0
Walker carcinoma	2×8 e.v.	65.27	1/0
Walker carcinoma	2.5×8 e.v.	61.10	1/0
O.G.G. myeloma	1.25×8 e.v.	37.2	0/2
O.G.G. myeloma	2×8 e.v.	70.8	1/2
O.G.G. myeloma	2.5×8 e.v.	82.6	3/2
O.G.G. myeloma	4×4 e.v.	85.2	1/1

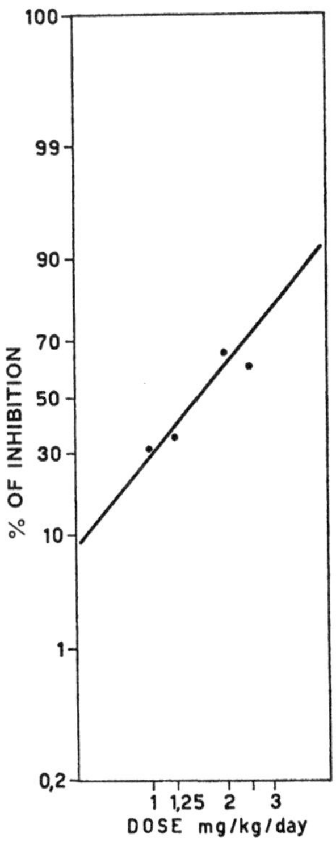

Fig. 7. Dose-response curve of daunomycin for Walker carcinoma after i.v. treatment for 8 days (from: DI MARCO *et al.*, 1964b)

nonmalignant, rapidly growing tissue (Gaetani, 1965). The results, evaluated according to Loustalot *et al.* (1958), are illustrated in Fig. 8. Daunomycin exerted a significant inhibiting effect on tumor growth and a lower one on granuloma growth.

Cinerubin inhibits the growth of some experimental tumors such as transplantable Crocker sarcoma 180, Ehrlich carcinoma in solid form, adeno-carcinoma EO-771, Walker carcinosarcoma 256 (Ettlinger, 1959). Cinerubin A is more active than B and in addition it inhibits Guerin's Epithelioma T8 and the Flexner-Jobling carcinoma. This antibiotic is also partially tumor-inhibiting specific (Loustalot *et al.*, 1958).

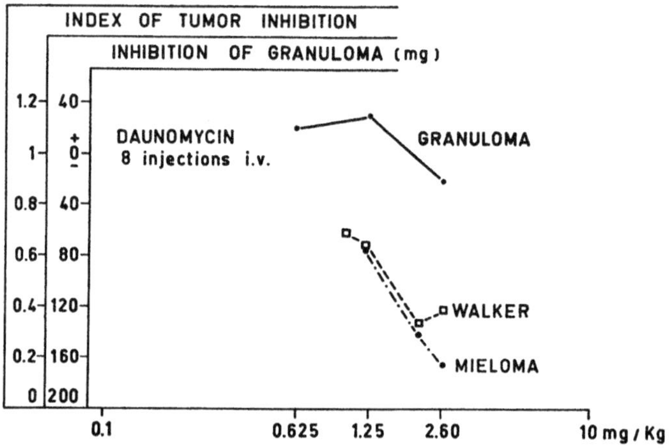

Fig. 8. Growth inhibition, by daunomycin, of cotton pellets granuloma, Walker carcinoma and solid myeloma (from: Gaetani, 1965)

Toxicity

The comparison of the acute LD_{50} values of daunomycin, actinomycin and mitomycin is reported in Table 5 (Bertazzoli and Chieli, 1964). Daily intravenous administration of 1.25 mg/kg for 8—10 days in the mouse did not cause mortality and caused no reduction of body weight. Daily intravenous injection of 2—2.5 mg/kg for 8 days caused a mortality rate of about 10% as well as a slight decrease in the body weight and in the number of circulating lymphomonocytes. A decrease in number of hematopoietic cells, mainly the erythroblastic line, was observed in the bone marrow immediately after treatment. Moreover, the lymphoid follicles of spleen, thymus and lymph nodes were reduced in size. All these lesions were transient and followed by complete recovery within 10—15 days. Daily intravenous administration of 3 mg/kg for 8 days caused a 60—80% mortality, a decrease in the body weight, severe anemia and leukopenia, bone marrow aplasia, marked reduction in spleen and lymph node size. Histological examinations showed a slight hydropic and albuminous degeneration in the kidney and liver. In the dog, daily intravenous injection of 0.25 mg/kg for 30 days was well tolerated; daily intravenous injection of 1 mg/kg caused a severe bone marrow aplasia followed by the death of the animals. Intravenous administration of 0.5 mg/kg three times a week for 30 days was well tolerated without signs of hematological, hepatic and renal toxicity.

Table 5. *Acute toxicity in LD_{50} values (mg/kg)*

Animal	Route or Administration	Daunomycin	Actinomycin D	Mitomycin C
Mouse	i.v.	20	0.67	5—7.5
Mouse	i.p.	5	0.76	5.2—8.5
Rat	i.v.	13—15	0.46	
Rat	i.p.	8	0.40	1—2.5

Complex Formation with DNA

The ability of daunomycin and cinerubin to react with DNA to form complexes can be demonstrated by physico-chemical methods. Daunomycin shows a

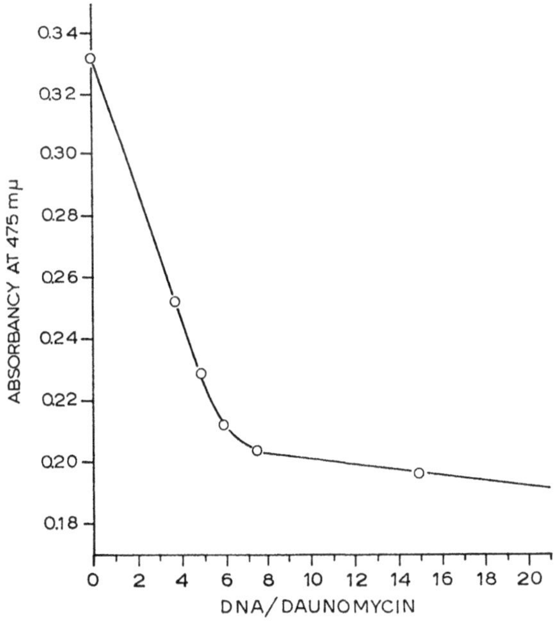

Fig. 9. Absorbancy at 475 mμ of daunomycin (35.6×10^{-6}M) plotted against increasing DNA/daunomycin molar ratios (from: Calendi *et al.*, 1965)

peak extinction at 475 mμ. On addition of DNA, the optical density is reduced proportionally to the added DNA. No further variations appear after a DNA/Da nucleotide molar ratio of about 8.7/1 is attained (Fig. 9). At the same time, the maximum absorption value shifts to a wavelenght of 505 mμ. The reaction between Da and DNA is also revealed by the reduction of daunomycin fluorescence (emission at 580 mμ when excited at 485 mμ) that disappears when a DNA/Da nucleotide ration of 8.7/1 is attained (Fig. 10) (Calendi *et al.*, 1965). Similar changes in the U.V. and visible spectra on addition of DNA are shown by cinerubin (Kersten and Kersten, 1965b). A change in their fluorescence spectra also occurs with rhodomycins and cinerubins (which are excited at 490 mμ and have a light emission at 570 mμ) in the presence of DNA (Calendi *et al.*, 1965). Further evidence of the binding of Da to DNA is given by disappearance of the wave of polarographic reduction, characteristic of anthraquinones (Fig. 11) for the same ratio of the two substances (Calendi *et al.*, 1965).

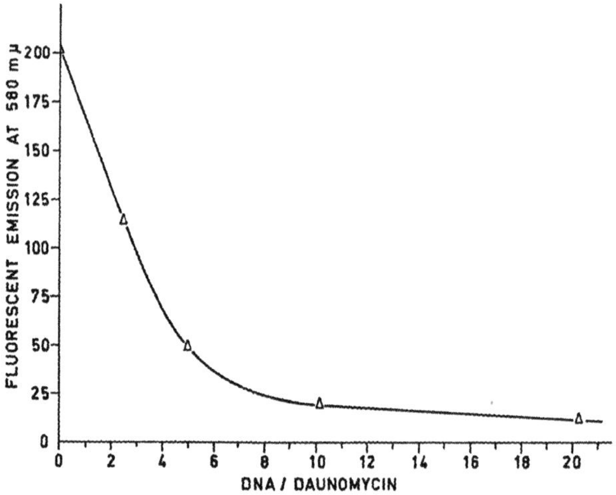

Fig. 10. Fluorescent emission of daunomycin (3.6×10^{-6}M) plotted against increasing DNA/daunomycin molar ratios (from: Calendi *et al.*, 1965)

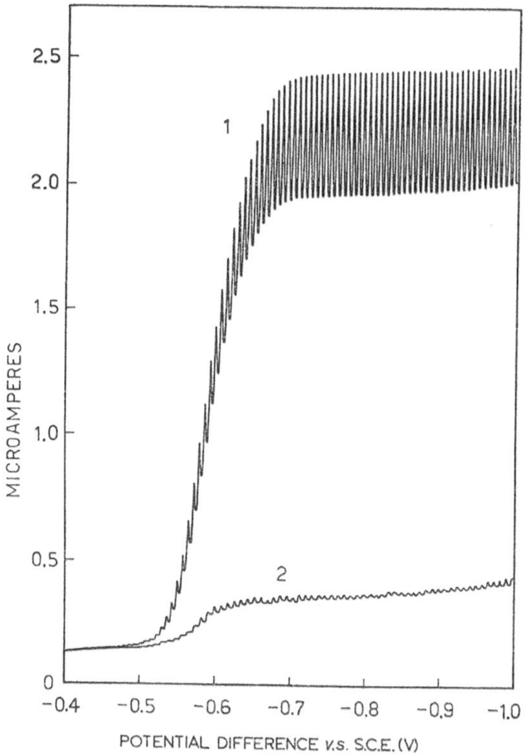

Fig. 11. Polarographic pattern of: 1. daunomycin, 2. daunomycin+DNA (molar ratio DNA: Da=8.7:1). S.C.E. = standard calomel electrode (from Calendi *et al.*, 1965)

Spectral changes, as well as disappearance of the ability to take part in oxido-reductions indicate a binding of the aromatic hydroxyls of the chromophore of the antibiotic to DNA. On the other hand, there is evidence for a linkage of Da to DNA through the amino group of the sugar for the capacity of Da N-acetyl-derivative to bind to DNA was decreased. In fact, dialysis against tap water is sufficient to completely break the bond between the N-acetyl daunomycin and DNA (CALENDI *et al.*, 1965).

The increase in ionic strength and, particularly, the presence in the medium of bivalent metal salts, such as magnesium, affects complex formation between Da and DNA; at sufficiently high concentrations of this cation, a return to the

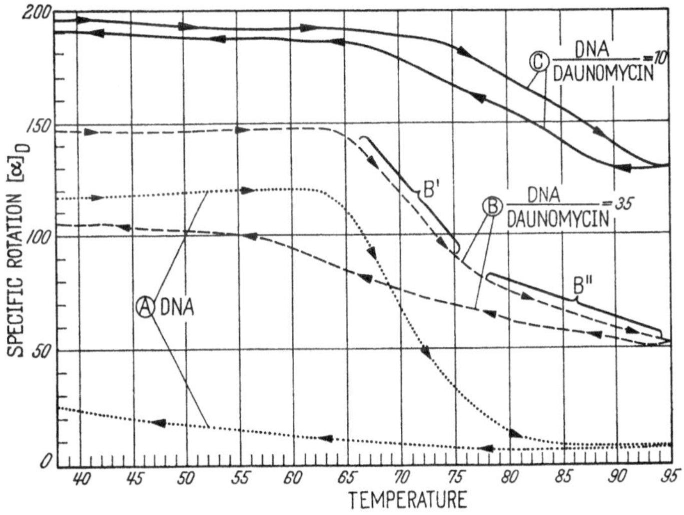

Fig. 12. Thermal denaturation of DNA in the presence of daunomycin. Medium: 0.01 M NaCl. *A* DNA (3100×10^{-6}M); *B* DNA (3100.0×10^{-6}M) + daunomycin (89.0×10^{-6}M); *C* DNA (3100.0×10^{-6}M) + daunomycin (293.7×10^{-6}M) (from CALENDI *et al.*, 1965)

characteristic Da absorbance spectrum is observed, even in the presence of DNA. If substances able to split hydrogen bonds, such as formamide, are present, a complete splitting of the linkage between Da acetyl-derivative and DNA is observed, whereas that between Da and DNA is only partially broken. However, under these conditions, the antibiotic is still partially bound to DNA, as indicated by its sedimentation in ultracentrifuge (CALENDI *et al.*, 1965).

Da also forms spectrophotometrically detectable complexes with RNA; they are, however, not very stable and are easily dissociated by salts even at relatively low concentrations (CALENDI *et al.*, 1965). Some evidence of a binding to RNA was also obtained by sedimentation in the ultracentrifuge (KERSTEN and KERSTEN, 1965 b). REICH (WARD, 1964), moreover, observed a precipitation by Da of purine nucleotide polymers. Purine mononucleotides, but not pyrimidine mononucleotides, caused slight spectral alterations in Da solution. Precipitation does not occur in the presence of manganous ions. Under such conditions difference spectra can be observed.

As the temperature increases, DNA solutions undergo a change of optical absorption which is evidence for the breaking of the hydrogen bonds between the strands of the DNA double helix (thermal transition or melting of DNA). Anthracyclines have a stabilizing effect on DNA structure and raise the temperature required for the hyperchromic shift. This was observed by measuring the optical density of solutions containing both DNA and Da, or DNA and cinerubin (Kersten and Kersten, 1965b). The protecting effect of Da against thermal denaturation of DNA was demonstrable also by following the changes of optical rotation (Fig. 12), (Calendi *et al.*, 1965). In the presence of these antibiotics, an easier renaturation of DNA occurred. This observation indicates a bond between antibiotic and DNA which prevents the detachment of the two helices and promotes their binding after cooling.

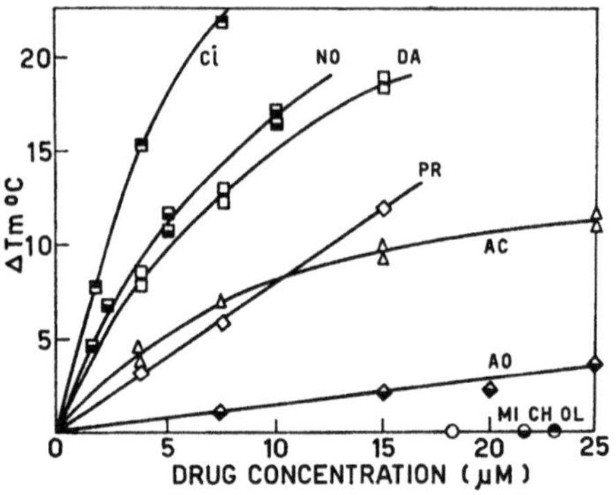

Fig. 13. Effect of antibiotics and acridine dyes on the shift in the melting temperature (ΔT^{m}) of C. Johnsonii DNA (40 μg DNA/ml PE solvent). The following symbols, abbreviations of drug names and their molecular weights were used for calculating the molar concentrations or ratios: Actinomycin D (C_1): AC (△) M.W. = 1200 (Brockmann, 1963); Chromomycin A_3: CH (◓) M. W. = 1052 (Miyamoto *et al.*, 1964); Mithramycin: MI (◒) M.W. = 1100 (Rao *et al.*, 1962; Rao, K.V. pers. comm.); Olivomycin: OL (○) M.W. = 960 (Brazhnikova *et al.* 1964); Cinerubin: CI (⬓) M.W. = 875 (Ettlinger *et al.*, 1959); Daunomycin: DA (□) M.W. = 560 (Arcamone *et al.*, 1964); Nogalomycin: NO (⬒) M.W. = 793 (Wiley, personal comm.) Acridine Orange: AO (⬙) M.W. = 207; Proflavine sulfate (.H_2O) PR (◇) M.W. = 325 (from Kersten W., Kersten, H., and Szybalski, 1965a)

In a comparative evaluation of the different anthracyclines (Fig. 13), cinerubin showed the highest effect on the melting temperature, followed by nogalamycin and daunomycin (Kersten *et al.*, 1965a).

The strong depression of the buoyant density of DNA from *S. lutea* observed in cesium salt gradients was also interpreted to be a consequence of complex formation between anthracyclines and DNA (Kersten, Kersten and Szybalski, 1965a). On a molar basis nogalamycin was the most effective in depressing the buoyant density followed by cinerubin, chromomycin, and daunomycin.

Further evidence for the binding of anthracyclines to DNA is revealed by the sedimentation of these substances with DNA in the ultracentrifuge (Kersten and Kersten, 1965b). The apparent sedimentation coefficients of the complexes with DNA tend to decrease proportionally to the increase in relative viscosity of DNA solutions caused by these antibiotics (Kersten and Kersten, 1965b; Calendi *et al.*, 1965). The effect of different anthracyclines on specific viscosity and sedimentation coefficient of DNA is shown in Table 6 (Kersten *et al.*, 1965a).

This effect on DNA viscosity, indicates a stiffening and elongation of the DNA molecules that are quite specific for anthracyclines. Actinomycin is somewhat different, for the raising of DNA viscosity occurs only at very high concentrations, whereas low concentrations of this antibiotic cause a slight decrease of viscosity and an increase of sedimentation coefficient.

The increased viscosity of DNA caused by anthracyclines, and the consequent decrease of the sedimentation coefficient, recall the analogous changes induced in DNA by Acridine dyes (LERMAN, 1961). The effect of ionic strength on the stability of the Daunomycin-DNA complex (CALENDI *et al.*, 1965) is comparable to its effect on the increase of the dissociation velocity of the complex proflavin-DNA (LIERSCH and HARTMANN, 1964). However at the high ionic strength required for making density gradients, the binding of anthracyclines to DNA is little, whereas the acridine dyes are not bound at these high ionic strengths (KERSTEN *et al.*, 1965a).

Table 6. *Effect of antibiotics on sedimentation coefficient* ($S_{25,w}$) *and on viscosity* (η) *of S. lutea DNA*[1]

	Control	Daunomycin	Cinerubin	Nogalomycin	Chromomycin A_3
Antibiotic concentration (mμM/ml)	—	5	5	6.2	5
$S_{25,w}$[2]	31.0	28.8	28.0	26.5	31.1
η (dl/g)[3]	140	165	190	225	140

[1] 20 μg DNA (60 mμM nucleotide) per ml SSC.
[2] 35.600 rpm, 25°C, 30 mm cell, sedimented in SSC corrected for water.
[3] Reduced specific viscosity measured at 25°C and at 0.01—0.05 sec^{-1} shear rate.
From KERSTEN, W., KERSTEN, H., and SZYBALSKI, W., 1965.

The planarity of the anthracene-like structure of the anthracycline chromophore should have considerable influence on the complex formation with DNA. It would favor hydrophobic interactions of the ring system with the base pairs. In strict analogy with the hypothesis of an intercalation of acridine dyes between adjacent base pairs (LERMAN, 1964), an intercalation of daunomycin between adjacent base pairs of DNA was suggested (WARD *et al.*, 1965). X-ray diffraction studies indicated that in fibres of the complex daunomycin-DNA centrifuged out of solution, one molecule of the drug is intercalated every 4 or 5 base-pairs (W. FULLER — Personal Comm. 1965).

An increase of viscosity and lowering of the sedimentation constant were not observed after binding of anthracyclines to heat denaturated DNA (CALENDI *et al.*, 1965). Since spectral changes of the chromophore are the same with denatured as with native DNA, one can deduce that a more strict structural and chemical relationship is required to change the hydrodynamic properties of DNA. Because of the slight effect of N-acetyl-derivative of daunomycin on DNA viscosity (CALENDI *et al.*, 1965), the amine group present in the sugar residue should be considered responsible for the very tenacious binding that causes the viscosity increase of DNA.

In view of the great importance of the presence of guanine in DNA for the binding of actinomycin (GOLDBERG *et al.*, 1962; HURWITZ *et al.*, 1962), attention should be paid to the effect of base composition of DNA on the ability to bind anthracyclines. Density measurements in cesium chloride gradients indicate a binding of anthracyclines also to poly AT; the binding, however, increases with rising the G+C content of DNA (Kersten *et al.*, 1965a).

Biochemical Effects — RNA-Synthesis

The investigations of Kersten and Kersten (1965b) on the activity of cinerubin and daunomycin on *B. subtilis* show that there is a) a reduction of the RNA content per mg protein with drug concentrations (0.9—1.4) that have little

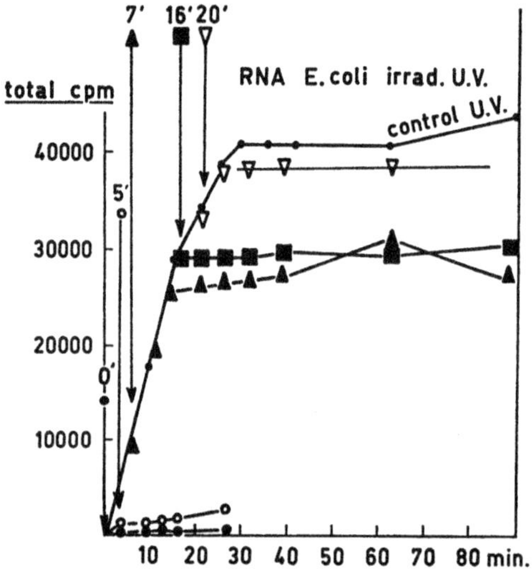

Fig. 14. Incorporation of ^{32}P orthophosphate into RNA of *E. coli* B irradiated with a total dose of 2.200 ergs/mm², without (·—·—·) and with daunomycin, 10 μg/ml, added at 0 minutes (•—•—•), 5 minutes (○—○—○), 7 minutes (▲—▲—▲), 16 minutes (■—■—■) and 20 minutes (▽—▽—▽—▽) after ^{32}P addition in the cultural medium. (From Barbieri *et al.*, 1964)

effect on the growth of the test organism or only delay the onset of growth; and b) an increase in the DNA content per mg protein up to 1.5 to 2 times that of the control organism. From these data the authors conclude that there is primary inhibition of RNA synthesis by these two antibiotics. Confirmatory evidence are available from tracer experiences carried out on the sensitive strain, *E. coli* B (Barbieri, 1964). Da prevents ^{32}P incorporation into RNA in growing cultures (Barbieri *et al.*, 1964). In cultures heavily irradiated with U.V. rays (to stop bacterial multiplication) an inhibition by Da on a high turnover RNA occurred (Barbieri *et al.*, 1964) (Fig. 14). The inhibition of the production of the adaptative enzyme, β-galactosidase (Fig. 15) could be ascribed to the inhibited synthesis of a high-turnover RNA.

In cultures of mammalian cells both Da and actinomycin strongly inhibit adenine-8-^{14}C incorporation into RNA (Rusconi, 1965). Autoradiographic research carried out on *in vitro* cultures of HeLa cells (Di Marco *et al.*, 1965a) showed a different degree of susceptibility to Da of uridine-^{3}H incorporation into RNA in the nucleolar and extranucleolar RNA (Fig. 16).

These observations confirm the previous studies of PERRY (1963) on the higher susceptibility to actinomycin D of the uridine-^{3}H incorporation in the nucleolar area as compared to that occurring in the extranucleolar "chromosomal" area. Therefore, attempts were made to identify by physico-chemical procedures the

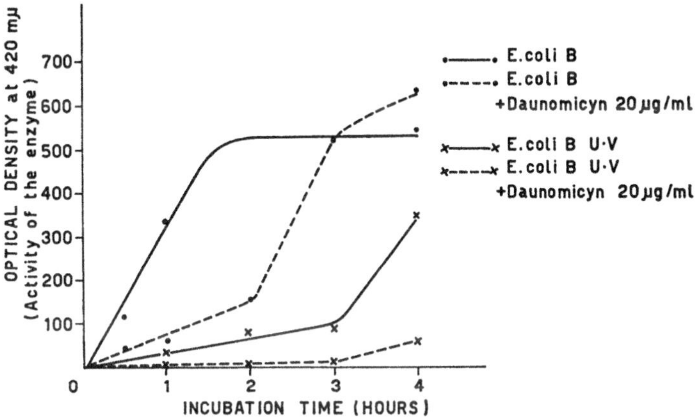

Fig. 15. Action of daunomycin on the induction of β-galactosidase in normally grown and U.V. irradiated cells of *E. coli* B. Galactosidase was measured spectrophotometrically by production of o-nitrophenol from o-nitrophenyl-galactoside (from SANFILIPPO and MAZZOLENI, 1963)

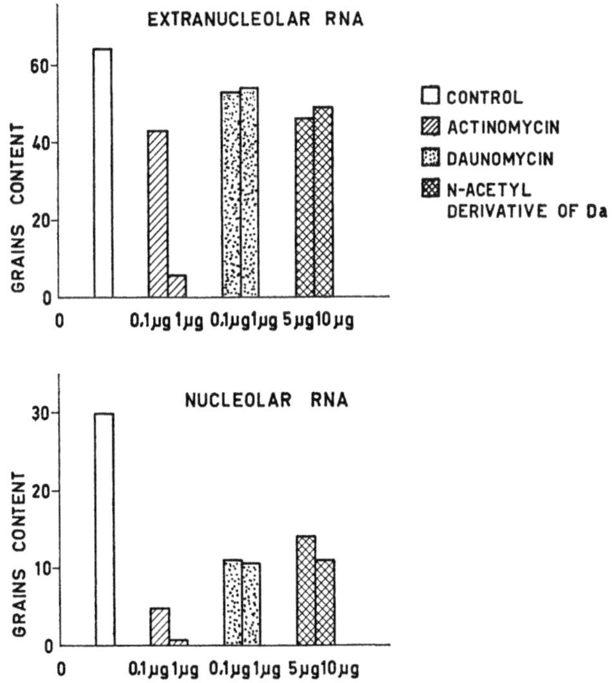

Fig. 16. ^{3}H-uridine incorporation into extranucleolar and nucleolar RNA in cells treated with different antibiotics after a 45 minutes treatment and a 30 minutes contact with the precursor (from DI MARCO *et al.*, 1965a)

RNA fractions whose syntheses are differentially inhibited by these antibiotics. Experiments carried out on HeLa cells demonstrated that Da or actinomycin D exert a comparable degree of inhibition on newly synthesized RNA (extracted by phenol-sodium-dodecyl-sulphate method according to HIATT (1962). This RNA sediments in a sucrose gradient in the 30 S and 20 S zone (RUSCONI and CALENDI, 1965). In contrast, an RNA aliquote not extracted by the Hiatt procedure appeared less sensitive to the action of Da and actinomycin. The base ratio, G+C/A+U, was lower in this fraction than in phenol extracted RNA, 1.08:1.39. At the present stage of research it would be premature to identify this RNA fraction with "chromosomal RNA". The reports of PERRY (1963) and GEORGIEV (1963) refer also to an RNA with DNA-like base composition which is less sensitive to actinomycin.

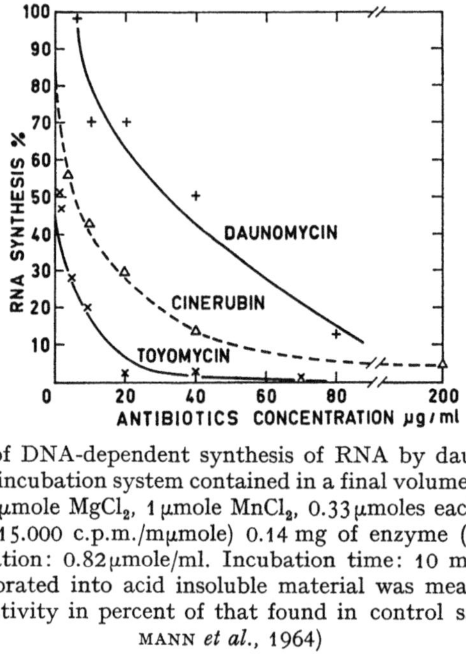

Fig. 17. Inhibition of DNA-dependent synthesis of RNA by daunomycin, cinerubin and toyomycin. The incubation system contained in a final volume of 0.5 ml: 100 µmole Tris-HCl pH 7.8, 10 µmole $MgCl_2$, 1 µmole $MnCl_2$, 0.33 µmoles each GTP, CTP, UTP; 0.06 µmoles $AT^{32}P$ (15.000 c.p.m./mµmole) 0.14 mg of enzyme (from *E. coli*). DNA nucleotide concentration: 0.82 µmole/ml. Incubation time: 10 minutes at 30 C. The radioactivity incorporated into acid insoluble material was measured. Results were expressed as radioactivity in percent of that found in control sample (from HARTMANN *et al.*, 1964)

The interference on the incorporation of labeled precursors into RNA should be related to the inhibition exerted by daunomycin on the activity of DNA-dependent RNA polymerase (HARTMANN *et al.*, 1964; WARD *et al.*, 1965). As observed for actinomycin, the degree of enzyme inhibition increases with the concentration of daunomycin, cinerubin and toyomycin (Fig. 17) and the action of daunomycin can be antagonized by DNA. According to Reich, the effect of daunomycin occurs when the enzymatic polymerization reaction is primed by Crab dAT, dGdC or dIdC. It seems, therefore, that the linkage of daunomycin to DNA involves some groups which are present in all these pairs of bases. If the polymerization is primed by ribopolymers, daunomycin inhibits the template activity of poly A and poly I but not that of poly U or poly C. This effect of the antibiotic on RNA-primed RNA synthesis can be accounted for by the reaction of daunomycin with the purine nucleotide polymers (WARD *et al.*, 1965).

DNA Synthesis

Da inhibits ^{32}P incorporation into DNA of the susceptible strain *E. coli* B. In growing cultures there is a short lag from the moment of the antibiotic addition to the appearance of the block. Sublethal concentrations of this antibiotic on *B. subtilis* allows DNA synthesis to proceed at concentrations which considerably reduce the RNA/protein ratio. The DNA content per mg protein of the treated cultures can attain values 1.5 to 2.0 times higher than in the control (KERSTEN and KERSTEN, 1965b).

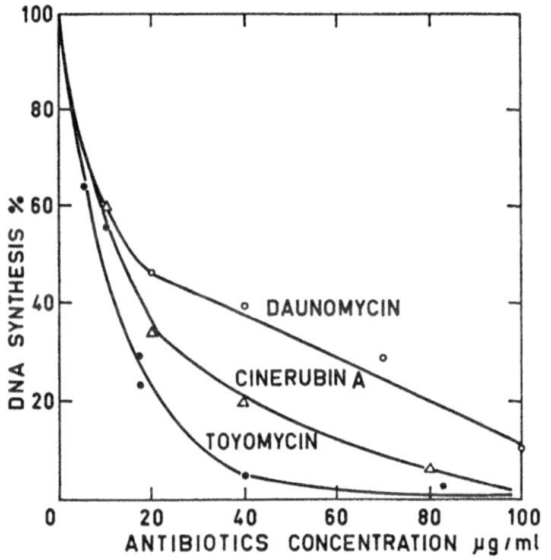

Fig. 18. Inhibition of DNA-dependent synthesis of DNA by daunomycin, cinerubin and toyomycin. The incubation system contained 0.15 μmole of activated thymus DNA/ml and 50 μg of enzymatic protein (purified up to stage IV). The concentration of the antibiotics is reported in the abscissa. Results are expressed in percent of control value (from: HARTMANN et al., 1964)

Interference with DNA synthesis was also observed following the incorporation of adenine-8-^{14}C into nucleic acids of cell suspension of YOSHIDA'S ascites hepatoma (RUSCONI and CALENDI, 1964) and on *in vitro* cultured HeLa cells (RUSCONI, 1965). The inhibiting effect of daunomycin, cinerubin and toyomycin on the incorporation of nucleic acid precursors into DNA is related to the interference exerted by this substance on the activity of DNA-dependent DNA polymerase (Fig. 18) (HARTMANN *et al.*, 1964). The effect exerted by daunomycin is, on a quantitative basis, less than that of cinerubin and toyomycin. With all these substances the inhibition is strongly dependent on the DNA concentration in the medium. From the competitive effect between daunomycin and DNA present, during the inhibition of DNA synthesis, one can hypothesize this inhibition is caused by the formation of a complex between antibiotic and DNA. This assumption is strengthened by the observation that Da N-acetyl-derivative, which has less capacity to bind to DNA (CALENDI *et al.*, 1965) also has a reduced capacity to inhibit the incorporation of different precursors into DNA (DI MARCO *et al.*, 1965).

In postulating a molecular mechanism for the interference of anthracyclines with DNA replication, two different possibilities should be considered. One is that the binding of the antibiotic to DNA causes a steric hindrance to the formation of the hypothetical DNA-DNA polymerase complex. Another is based on the idea that strand separation is a necessary requirement to the function of the catalytic system (BOLLUM, 1963). In this case the observed tendency of these antibiotics to tie together the two strands of DNA molecule should inhibit the very beginning of the polymerization reaction. The observation that the degree of DNA-synthesis inhibition is higher with cinerubin, the antibiotic that is endowed with the stronger binding capacity, is in agreement with the second concept.

Autoradiographic research showed a marked interference of daunomycin with the incorporation of thymidine-^{3}H into nuclear DNA of HeLa cells cultured *in vitro* (DI MARCO *et al.*, 1963b). DNA synthesis decreases proportionally to the dose used. In contrast to results from experiments carried out with Actinomycin treated cells, daunomycin inhibition of DNA synthesis is not complete even with doses which rapidly stop mitotic activity (DI MARCO *et al.*, 1965b).

The question whether the antimitotic activity of Da is correlated with its metabolic effects must be examined in light of the data previously cited:

1. The reduction of the mitotic index appears one hour after the beginning of the treatment; thus, the effect of daunomycin is also exerted on cells which have already completed the DNA synthesis and are in G_2 phase or in mitosis.

2. Marked inhibition of the mitotic index can also take place with concentrations of Da that are inactive or only slightly active on DNA synthesis.

3. In cultures of HeLa cells treated with an amount of Da-N-acetyl-derivative sufficient to considerably reduce the mitotic activity, DNA synthesis can proceed.

That the antimitotic effect is correlated with a metabolic effect on RNA synthesis can also be excluded. A dissociation of the two phenomena is evident when cells are treated with low concentrations of the N-acetyl-derivative (5 and 10μg/ml); marked inhibition of RNA synthesis occurs while the mitotic activity is not affected (DI MARCO *et al.*, 1965b). It is therefore possible that the blockage of mitosis and the serious chromosomal damage which is caused by Da are due to the physico-chemical changes in DNA structures which follow its linkage with the antibiotic.

There is very little experimental evidence on the nature of the changes in the chromosomal molecular structure and one can only speculate on its character. However, it is perhaps useful to consider the stiffening of the chromosomal structure, produced by the complex formation, as preventing the coiling and folding of the DNA strands. This stiffening might also cause the breaking of chromosomes when they are subjected to the forces normally operating in the mitotic process.

References

ARCAMONE, F., G. CASSINELLI, P. OREZZI, G. FRANCESCHI, and R. MONDELLI: Daunomycin. II. The structure and stereochemistry of daunosamine. J. Am. Chem. Soc. **86**, 5335 (1964a).

ARCAMONE, F., G. FRANCESCHI, P. OREZZI, G. CASSINELLI, W. BARBIERI, and R. MONDELLI: Daunomycin. The structure of daunomycinone. J. Am. Chem. Soc. **86**, 5334 (1964b).

ASHESHOV, I. N., and J. J. GORDON: Rutilantin: an Antibiotic substance with antiphage activity. Biochem. J. **81**, 101 (1961).

BARBIERI, P., A. DI MARCO, R. MAZZOLENI, M. MENOZZI e A. SANFILIPPO: Azione della Daunomicina sul metabolismo degli acidi nucleici nell' *E. coli* B. Giorn. Microbiol. **19**, 71 (1964).

BERTAZZOLI, C., e T. CHIELI: Studio tossifarmacologico della Daunomicina. Personal communication 1964.

BOLLUM, F. I.: Primers in DNA polymerase reaction. In: Progress in Nucleic Acid Research (J. H. DAVIDSON and W. E. COHEN, ed.). Academic Press 1963.

BRINDLE, S. A., N. A. GIUFFRE, B. J. AMREIN, R. C. MILLONIG, and D. PERLMAN: Antibiotic sensitivity of Ehrlich ascites cells grown in tissue culture. In: M. FINLAND and G. M. SAVAGE, Antimicrobial agents and chemotherapy, p. 159. Am. Soc. Microbiol. 1961.

BROCKMANN, H., and W. LENK: Pyrromycin. Chem. Ber. **93**, 1904 (1959).

BROCKMANN, H.: Die Actinomycine Jerstchritte. Chem. Org. Naturvt. **18**, 1 (1960).

BROCKMANN, H., u. E. SPOLLER: Zur Konstitution des Rhodomycins A. Naturwissenschaften **48**, 716 (1961).

BROCKMANN, H., u. T. WACHNELDT: Eine neue Gruppe von Rhodomycinen. Naturwissenschaften **48**, 717 (1961).

BROCKMANN, H., P. BOLDT u. J. NIEMEYER: Beta-Rhodomycinon und Gamma-Rhodomycinon. Chem. Ber. **96**, 1356 (1963).

CALENDI, E., A. DI MARCO, M. REGGIANI, B. SCARPINATO, and L. VALENTINI: On physico-chemical interactions between daunomycin and nucleic acids. Biochim. et Biophys. Acta **103**, 25 (1965).

CALENDI, E., and B. SCARPINATO: Personal communication 1965.

COSTA, G., e G. ASTALDI: Effetto della Daunomicina sulla attività proliferativa di cellule staminali ottenute in coltura da sangue umano normale. Tumori **50**, 477 (1964).

DAVIS, B. D., and E. S. MINGIOLI: Mutants of *Escherichia coli* requiring methionine or vitamin B12. J. Bacteriol. **60**, 17 (1950).

DI MARCO, A., M. GAETANI, L. DORIGOTTI, M. SOLDATI e O. BELLINI: Studi sperimentali sull'attività antineoplastica del nuovo antibiotico Daunomicina. Tumori **49**, 203 (1963a).

DI MARCO, A., M. SOLDATI, A. FIORETTI e T. DASDIA: Ricerche sull'attività della Daunomicina su cellule normali e neoplastiche coltivate *in vitro*. Tumori **49**, 235 (1963b).

DI MARCO, A., M. GAETANI, L. DORIGOTTI, M. SOLDATI, and O. BELLINI: Daunomycin: a new antibiotic with antitumor activity. Cancer Chemoth. Rep. **38**, 31 (1964a).

DI MARCO, A., M. GAETANI, P. OREZZI, B. SCARPINATO, R. SILVESTRINI, M. SOLDATI, T. DASDIA, and L. VALENTINI: Daunomycin, a new antibiotic of the rhodomycin group. Nature **201**, 706 (1964b).

DI MARCO, A., M. SOLDATI, A. FIORETTI, and T. DASDIA: Activity of daunomycin, a new antitumor antibiotic, on normal and neoplastic cells grown *in vitro*. Cancer Chemoth. Rep. **38**, 39 (1964c).

DI MARCO, A., R. SILVESTRINI, T. DASDIA, and S. DI MARCO: Nucleolar and chromosomal origin of nuclear RNA and its passage to cytoplasm. Riv. ital. istochimica (in press) (1965a).

DI MARCO, A., R. SILVESTRINI, S. DI MARCO, and T. DASDIA: Inhibiting effect of the new cytotoxic antibiotic daunomycin on nucleic acids and mitotic activity of HeLa cells. J. Cell Biol. **27**, 545 (1965b).

DI MARCO, A., L. DORIGOTTI, and M. GAETANI: Unpublished data (1965c).

DUBOST, M., P. GANTER, R. MARAL, L. NINET, S. PINNERT, J. PREUD-HOMME et G. H. WERNER: Un nouvel antibiotique à propriétés antitumorales. Compt. Rend. **257**, 1813 (1963).

ETTLINGER, L., E. GAUMANN, R. HUTTER, W. KELLER-SCHLIEREIN, F. KRADOLFER, L. NEIPP, V. PRELOG, P. REUSSER, and H. ZARNER: Cinerubine. Chem. Ber. **92**, 1867 (1959).

FULLER, W.: Personal communication 1965.

GAETANI, M.: Personal communication 1965.

GEORGIEV, G. P., O. P. SAMARINA, M. I. LERMAN, M. N. SMIRNOV, and A. N. SEVERTZOV: Biosynthesis of messenger and ribosomal nucleic acids in the nucleolochromosomal apparatus of animal cells. Nature **200**, 1291 (1963).

Goldberg, I. H., M. Rabinowitz, and E. Reich: Basis of actinomycin action. I DNA binding and inhibition of RNA polymerase synthetic reactions by actinomycin. Proc. Natl. Acad. Sci. U.S. **48**, 2094 (1962).

Goldin, A.: Personal communication 1965.

Grein, A., C. Spalla, A. di Marco e G. Canevazzi: Descrizione e classificazione di un attinomicete (*Streptomyces peucetius sp. nova*) produttore di una sostanza ad attività antitumorale: la daunomicina. Giorn. Microbiol. **11**, 109 (1963).

Hartmann, G., H. Goller, K. Koschel, W. Kersten u. H. Kersten: Hemmung der DNA-abhängigen RNA- und DNA-Synthese durch Antibiotica. Biochem. Z. **341**, 126 (1964).

Hiatt, H. H.: A rapidly labeled RNA in rat liver nuclei. J. Mol. Biol. **5**, 217 (1962).

Hurwitz, J., J. J. Furth, M. Malamy, and M. Alexander: The role of deoxyribonucleic acid synthesis. III. The inhibition of enzymatic synthesis of ribonucleic acid and deoxyribonucleic acid by actinomycin D and proflavin. Proc. Natl. Acad. Sci. U.S. **48**, 1222 (1962).

Kersten, W., H. Kersten, and W. Szybalski: Physico-chemical properties of complexes between DNA and antibiotics which affect RNA synthesis. Biochemistry (in press) (1965a).

Kersten, W., and H. Kersten: Die Bindung von Daunomycin, Cinerubin und Chromomycin A_3 an Nucleinsäuren. Biochem. Z. **341**, 174 (1965b).

Lerman, L.: Structural considerations in the interaction of DNA and acridines. J. Mol. Biol. **3**, 18 (1961).

Lerman, L.: Acridine mutagen and DNA structure. J. Cellular Comp. Physiol. **64**, Suppl. **1**, 1 (1964).

Liersch, M., u. G. Hartmann: Die Bindung von Proflavin und Actinomycin und Desoxyribonnucleinsäure. Biochem. Z. **340**, 390 (1964).

Lichtfield, J. T., and F. Wilcoxon: A semplified method of evaluating dose-effect experiments. J. Pharmacol. Exptl. Therap. **96**, 99 (1949).

Loustalot, P., P. A. Desaulles, and R. Meier: Characterization of the specificity of action of tumor-inhibiting compounds. Ann. N.Y. Acad. Sci. **76**, 838 (1958).

Mitscher, L. A., W. McCrae, W. W. Andres, J. A. Larry, and N. Boleanos: Ruticulomycins, new anthracycline antibiotics. J. Pharm. Sci. **53**, 1139 (1964).

Ollis, W. D., I. O. Sutherland, and J. J. Gordon: Rutilantinone. Tetrahedron Letters **16**, 17 (1959).

Ollis, W. D., and I. O. Sutherland: A new family of antibiotics. In: W. D. Ollis, Chemistry of natural phenolic compounds, p. 212. Oxford: Pergamon Press 1961.

Parisi, B., and A. Soller: Studies on the antiphage activity of daunomycin. Giorn. Microbiol. **12**, 183 (1964).

Perry, R. R.: Selective effects of actinomycin D in the intracellular distribution of RNA synthesis in tissue culture cells. Exptl. Cell Research **29**, 400 (1963).

Reich, E.: In: D. Ward, E. Reich. and I. H. Goldberg, Characterization of polynucleotides with drugs. New York (1965).

Rusconi, A.: Personal communication 1965.

Rusconi, A., e E. Calendi: Azione della Daunomicina sulla sintesi nucleica in cellule di epatoma. Tumori **50**, 261 (1964).

Rusconi, A., e E. Calendi: Personal Communication 1965.

Sanfilippo, A., e R. Mazzoleni: Attività antifagica dell'antibiotico Daunomicina. Giorn. Microbiol. **12**, 83 (1964).

Scarpinato, B.: Personal communication 1964.

Silvestrini, R., A. di Marco, S. di Marco e T. Dasdia: Azione della Daunomicina sul metabolismo degli acidi nucleici di cellule normali e neoplastiche coltivate *in vitro*. Tumori **49**, 399 (1963).

Strelitz, F., H. Flon, U. Weiss, and I. N. Asheshou: Aklavin, an antibiotic substance with antiphage activity. J. Bacteriol **72**, 90 (1956).

Tulinsky, A.: The structure of isoquinocycline A. An X-ray crystallographic determination. J. Am. Chem. Soc. **86**, 5368 (1964).

Ward, D., E. Reich, and I. H. Goldberg: Base specificity in the interaction of polynucleotides with antibiotic drugs. Science **149**, 1259 (1965).

The Mitomycins and Porfiromycins

W. Szybalski and V. N. Iyer

Origin and Chemical Structure

The mitomycins and porfiromycins form a group of closely related bactericidal and cytotoxic antibiotics produced by several Streptomyces species. They all can be derived from a common structure, the trivial name of which is mitosane

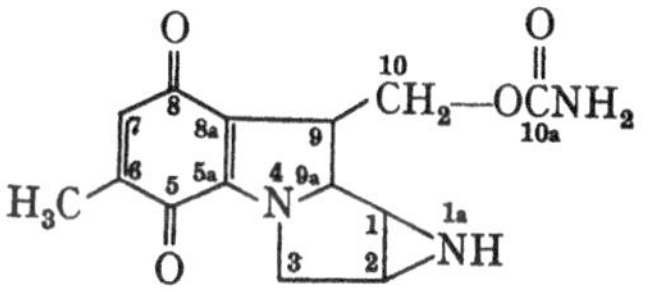

Fig. 1. Structure of mitosane (WEBB *et al.*, 1962)

(I, Fig. 1), as first recognized and named by WEBB *et al.* (1962). This rather unusual compound contains several reactive groups, including *1.* the highly

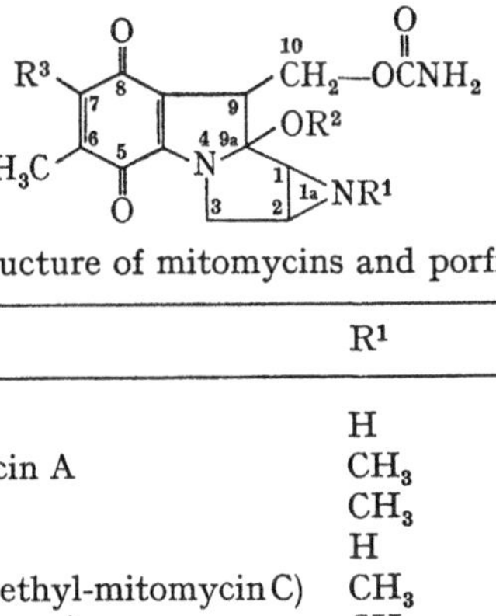

Fig. 2. Structure of mitomycins and porfiromycins

	R^1	R^2	R^3
Mitomycin A	H	CH_3	H_3CO
N-Methyl-mitomycin A	CH_3	CH_3	H_3CO
Mitomycin B	CH_3	H	H_3CO
Mitomycin C	H	CH_3	H_2N
Porfiromycin (N-methyl-mitomycin C)	CH_3	CH_3	H_2N
7-Hydroxy-porfiromycin	CH_3	CH_3	HO

(GARRET, 1963; GARRETT and SCHROEDER, 1964; STEVENS *et al.*, 1965; WEBB *et al.*, 1962)

strained aziridine ring (1-1a-2), *2.* amino- or methoxybenzoquinone (5a-5-6-7-8-8a), *3.* the pyrrolizidine configuration (1-2-3-4-5a-8a-9-9a), and *4.* a methylurethane side chain (10-10a). The various natural mitomycins and porfiromycins vary in the nature of the ring substitutions in positions 1a (hydrogen or methyl), 7 (amino, or methoxy) and 9a (methoxy of hydroxyl). It is not clear whether the nature of the substituents in positions 1a and 7 determines only quantitatively or also qualitatively the biological activity (Tables 1 and 2); substituent 9a should be a good leaving group, because of the aromatization afforded by loss of the 9a substituents, which promotes their elimination, as will become evident in the discussion on the mechanism of mitomycin action. The structures of the mitomycins and porfiromycins (WEBB *et al.*, 1962; TULINSKY, 1962; HERR *et al.*, 1961; WAKAKI, 1961; STEVENS *et al.*, 1965) are shown in Fig. 2. The structures of two other mitomycin-associated antibiotics A_1 and A_2 (mitiromycin) are unknown (LEFEMINE *et al.*, 1962). Three more compounds, which are synthetic products but can be regarded as partially rearranged or degraded mitomycins, and which were shown to possess bactericidal activity, include 7-hydroxyporfiromycin

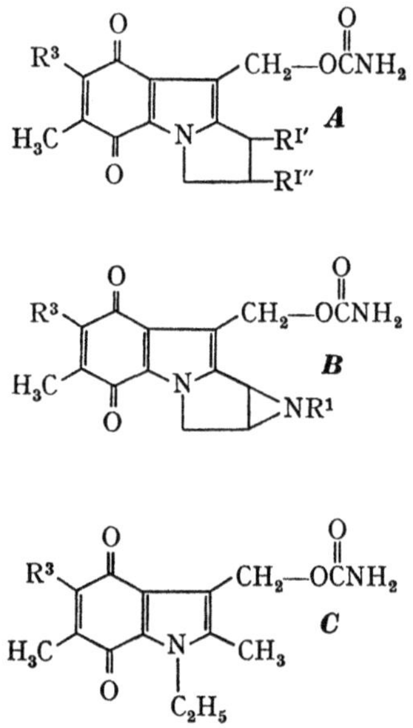

Fig. 3. Structure of (A) mitosenes, (B) 1,2-aziridino-mitosenes, and (C) 1,2-dialkylindoloquinones. mitosene: A, $R^3 = R^{I'} = R^{I''} = H$; 7-methoxymitosene: A, $R^{I'} = R^{I''} = H$, $R^3 = CH_3$; 7-methoxy-1,2-(N-methylaziridino)mitosene: B, $R^1 = CH_3$, $R^3 = CH_3$. (ALLEN *et al.*, 1964a and b; PATRICK *et al.*, 1964; WEBB *et al.*, 1962)

(Fig. 2; GARRETT and SCHROEDER, 1964), 7-methoxymitosene (Fig. 3 A; ALLEN *et al.*, 1964a, 1965) and 7-methoxy-1,2-(N-methylaziridino)mitosene (Fig. 3 B, PATRICK *et al.*, 1964). 7-Methoxymitosene, which is only very remotely related to mitomycins, can be regarded as a monofunctional agent, whereas the other two compounds are bifunctional alkylating agents. A group of antibacterial indoloquinones related in structure and action to 7-methoxymitosene was described by ALLEN *et al.* (1964b), REMERS and WEISS (1966) and ROTH *et al.* (1966). Other more recent papers discussing the chemistry of the mitomycins include those of ALLEN *et al.* (1965, 1966), ALLEN and WEISS (1965), REMERS *et al.* (1963, 1964, 1965), REMERS and WEISS (1965), and STEVENS *et al.* (1965).

The first mitomycins were isolated and described by HATA *et al.* (1956). Two chromatographically separable compounds A and B were produced by a strain of *Streptomyces caespitosus* described by SUGAWARA and HATA (1956). Isolation of mitomycin C, which was also produced by *S. caespitosus*, was described by WAKAKI *et al.* (1958). Porfiromycin produced by *Streptomyces ardus* was reported by DEBOER *et al.* (1961). All these antibiotics and in addition the unidentified bactericidal fractions A_1 and A_2 (mitiromycin A) were found among the fermentation products of *Streptomyces verticillatus* by LEFEMINE *et al.* (1962).

Since all these closely related compounds were found to be similar in structure and biological activity, as related to mode of action, they will be referred to under the general name of *mitomycins*, unless there is specific reference to a particular antibiotic within this group.

Several books and reviews published within the recent period and discussing the chemistry and mode of action of the mitomycins include those of UMEZAWA (1964), NEWTON (1965), and WARING (1966). A complete list of literature pertaining to mitomycin C and covering the period up to June, 1962 was published by the Kyowa Hakko Kogyo Co. (ANONYMOUS, 1962).

Inhibitory Effects

Depending on the concentration, the mitomycins exhibit a variety of inhibitory effects. At very low noninhibitory concentrations they suppress the ability of recipient *Diplococcus pneumoniae* cells to integrate transforming DNA (BALASSA,

Table 1. *Inhibitory concentrations (µg/ml nutrient agar) of mitomycins and porfiromycins for a variety of bacterial strains, as determined by the gradient-plate technique* (SZYBALSKI, 1952)

Bacteria*	mol-% G+C**	Mitomycin A	Mitomycin B	Mitomycin C	Porfiromycin	7-Hydroxy-porfiromycin
Cytophaga johnsonii	34	1	4	0.02	0.5	10
Bacillus subtilis W23	43	0.01	0.3	0.04	0.06	0.3
Bacillus subtilis 168+	43	0.3	>1	0.03	0.03	4
Bacillus subtilis 168 uvr−	43	0.1	>1	0.02	0.02	3
Bacillus subtilis 168mms−	43	0.1	>1	0.02	0.02	4
Escherichia coli B	50	1	4	0.05***	2	2
Escherichia coli K12+	50	2	7	0.5 †	5	4
Escherichia coli K12uvr−	50	0.5	>1	0.06	2	2
Escherichia coli K12rec−	50	0.5	>1	0.06	2	2
Sarcina lutea	71	0.01	0.6	0.3	0.1	8

* uvr−, UV sensitive; mms−, methylmethane sulfonate sensitive; rec−, recombination impaired.

** Guanine + cytosine content of bacterial DNA.

*** Large proportion of mutants resistant up to 0.5 µg mitomycin C/ml.

† Approximately half of bacterial population sensitive to 0.05 µg mitomycin C/ml.

Incubation temperature 37 C, except 28 C for *Cytophaga johnsonii.* Assays performed in the author's laboratory by Mrs. CAROL HOOPER. Mitiromycin, the aziridinomitosenes, mitosenes, and indoloquinones were not included in this study, since these compounds could not be obtained from the Lederle Laboratories. The reported inhibitory concentrations of mitiromycin are over 500 µg/ml for *E. coli* (LEFEMINE *et al.*, 1962), and of 7-methoxymitosene 8 µg/ml for *M. pyrogenes* var. *aureus*, 0.5 µg/ml for *B. subtilis*, and over 150 µg/ml for *E. coli* (ALLEN *et al.*, 1964a). The inhibitory concentrations of the aziridinomitosenes (PATRICK *et al.*, 1964) and indoloquinones (ALLEN *et al.*, 1964b) have not been released by the manufacturer (Dr. G. R. ALLEN JR., personal communication).

1962). Slightly higher, but still noncidal concentrations, inhibit cell division of several bacterial species with formation of long filamentous bacterial forms REILLY *et al.* (1958) GRULA and GRULA (1962a and b); REICH *et al.* (1961). This inhibitory effect can be reversed by pantoyl lactone and several divalent cations, with restoration of normal cell viability (GRULA and GRULA, 1962b; DURHAM, 1963). Still higher mitomycin concentrations result in more complete bacteriostasis and in rapid cidal effects. With some microorganisms there is a 2 to 7 fold difference between the static and cidal concentrations, but with other bacteria as e.g.

Table 2. *Bactericidal concentrations (heart infusion agar) and LD_{50} (mouse) of various mitomycin derivatives*
(abbreviated from the data of MIYAMURA *et al.*, 1967)

Mitomycin derivatives			Inhibitory concentrations		(μg/ml)		LD_{50} mg/kg
R^1	R^2	R^3 *	Gram + †	Gram − †	Vibrio comma	Mycobacterium tuberculosis	
H	CH_3	H_2N	0.2	0.4	2	0.05	9
C_2H_5	CH_3	H_2N	0.3	10	0.02	2	6
C_3H_7	CH_3	H_2N	0.4	20	0.8	0.4	50
C_4H_9	CH_3	H_2N	0.4	30	3	0.4	80
CH_3CO	CH_3	H_2N	0.4	3	6	0.8	20
CH_3SO_2	CH_3	H_2N	10	40	50	4	100
$CH_3 \cdot C_4H_6 \cdot SO_2$	CH_3	H_2N	10	500	800	2	100
H	CH_3	CH_3HNH	0.2	10	0.1	2	30
H	CH_3	$(CH_2)_2N$	0.3	7	0.02	0.1	9
H	CH_3	▷N	0.04	0.2	0.02	0.02	2
H	CH_3	HO	9	10	50	6	100
H	CH_3	CH_3O	0.03	0.5	0.0001	0.6	2
CH_3	H	H_2N	2	20	0.4	0.4	100
CH_3	H	CH_3HN	10	50	30	6	200
CH_3	H	▷N	0.2	4	0.02	0.04	7
CH_3	H	CH_3O	3	50	—	—	3
CH_3	—**	CH_3O	0.01	2	0.01	0.8	9
—OH *** / —$NHCH_3$	—***	CH_3O	1	30	0.8	30	9

* mitosanes (c.f., Fig. 2).
** aziridinomitosene derivative (c.f., Fig. 3B).
*** mitosene derivative (c.f., Fig. 3A; $R^{I\prime}$ = —OH, $R^{I\prime\prime}$ = —$NHCH_3$).
† average for six strains (MIYAMURA *et al.*, 1967).

Escherichia coli there is no difference between the cidal and static levels (LEWIS *et al.*, 1961). The mitomycins are thus principally bactericidal or cytocidal agents. They affect not only bacteria but several other organisms, and their importance is based on their antineoplastic activity (WAKAKI *et al.*, 1958; SUGIURA, 1961). In clinical practice they have proved to be rather toxic, but substantiation of their antineoplastic efficacy can be found in the literature (EVANS, 1961; EVANS *et al.*, 1961).

The minimal inhibitory concentrations of various mitomycins and related compounds against a spectrum of organisms is summarized in Tables 1 and 2.

Inhibition of cell growth and bactericidal or cytotoxic effects are obviously only the final manifestations of action of the mitomycins on several cell components. As discussed in detail in later sections, the mitomycins upon metabolic activation become transformed into very reactive bifunctional "alkylating" agents (IYER and SZYBALSKI, 1964), which can react with many active centers on any cell component. The irreversible cidal effects can be accounted for by crosslinking of the complementary DNA strands (IYER and SZYBALSKI, 1963). Reversible growth inhibition and filament formation might be related either to reaction between activated mitomycins and some cell wall components or to repairable DNA damage due mainly to monofunctional attack by the antibiotic.

Several side effects of mitomycin attack on DNA were reported in earlier papers. 1. Selective inhibition of DNA synthesis, first described in 1958/59 (SHIBA *et al.*, 1958, 1959; SEKIGUCHI and TAKAGI, 1959), is most probably the result of steric hindrance to the replication process imposed by crosslinks between the complementary DNA strands (IYER and SZYBALSKI, 1963). 2. Breakdown of DNA, observed first by REICH *et al.* (1960, 1961) and KERSTEN and RAUEN (1961), is most probably related to the excision phenomenon connected with the repair of mitomycin-alkylated DNA (BOYCE and HOWARD-FLANDERS, 1964) and to nucleases induced during activation of lysogenic phages. 3. The mutagenic effects reported by SZYBALSKI (1958), IIJIMA and HAGAWARA (1960) and TSUKAMURA and TSUKAMURA (1962) are obviously the result of alkylation of DNA. 4. Induction of lysogenic phages (DUDNIK, 1965; KORN and WEISSBACH, 1962; LEIN *et al.*, 1962; LEVINE, 1961; OTSUJI, 1961, 1962; OTSUJI *et al.*, 1959; SUTTON and QUADLING, 1963; WEISSBACH and KORN, 1962) and of colicins (IIJIMA, 1962) is related to the inhibition of DNA synthesis. Lysogenic bacteria are more sensitive to mitomycin (MUSCHEL and SCHMOKER, 1966). 5. Fragmentation of chromosomes is in turn the result of DNA breakdown.

Other processes inhibited by mitomycin include synthesis of induced enzymes (CHEER and TCHEN, 1962, 1963; CUMMINGS, 1965; KIT *et al.*, 1963; SHIBA *et al.*, 1958; TAKAGI, 1963; COLES and GROSS, 1965), repression of alkaline phosphatase (HIRAGA, 1966), cell capacity to serve as phage (HERCIK, 1963) or viral hosts (BEN-PORAT *et al.*, 1961), and DNA-mediated transformation, both by treatment of the recipient cells (BALASSA, 1962) as already mentioned and by inactivation of the DNA donor cells at high mitomycin concentrations (IYER and SZYBALSKI, 1963; NAKATA *et al.*, 1962; TERAWAKI and GREENBERG, 1966a). SUZUKI *et al.* (1965) claimed that mitomycin inhibits early phenotypic expression in half of the potential transformants by interfering with replication of the inactive complementary DNA strand.

Selective inhibition of DNA synthesis by the mitomycins, without or with concomitant effects on RNA (including rapidly labeled mRNA, and its capacity to hybridize with DNAs, SMITH-KIELLAND, 1964, 1966) or protein synthesis, has been the subject of a number of studies (KERSTEN, 1962a; KIRSCH and KORSHALLA, 1964; MAGEE and MILLER, 1962; SEKIGUCHI and TAKAGI, 1959, 1960a; SHIBA *et al.*, 1958, 1959; KONTANI, 1964, in addition to the reports already mentioned). The mitomycins are considered as standard, rapidly acting and selective inhibitors of DNA synthesis.

Depolymerization of Nucleic Acids

Since it is difficult to measure inhibition of DNA synthesis in the presence of DNA depolymerization, the role of the mitomycins as selective inhibitors of DNA synthesis has been questioned (KERSTEN and RAUEN, 1961; REICH *et al.*, 1961; SHATKIN *et al.*, 1962). This problem can be readily resolved by using conditions under which mitomycin-induced DNA breakdown is not observed. Although in two mammalian cell lines a concurrent depolymerization and synthesis of DNA was observed, as measured by release and incorporation of radioactive DNA precursors (SHATKIN *et al.*, 1962), little if any mitomycin-induced DNA breakdown was noted in some other mammalian and bacterial cultures (IYER and SZYBALSKI, 1963; MAGEE and MILLER, 1962; SCHWARTZ *et al.*, 1963b; SMITH-KIELLAND, 1966a; BOYCE and HOWARD-FLANDERS, 1964). Similarly, no DNA breakdown was observed in HeLa cells which showed an elevated DNase content as the result of mitomycin treatment (STUDIZINSKI and COHEN, 1966). Some of these studies and those of HOWARD-FLANDERS *et al.* (1966), BOYCE (1966), and TERAWAKI and GREENBERG (1966b) provide convincing evidence that DNA breakdown bears no direct relationship to lethal mitomycin effects, since there is little DNA depolymerization in the radiosensitive *E. coli* uvr$^-$ mutants hypersensitive to the mitomycins, whereas the radiation and mitomycin-resistant uvr$^+$ mutants show considerable breakdown of DNA at cidal concentrations of the antibiotic. This relationship is to be expected in the light of present concepts of the repair mechanisms for damaged DNA. As expected, 5-bromouracil-labeled DNA shows enhanced enzymic breakdown after UV irradiation but not after mitomycin inactivation of the cells (BOYCE, 1966), since 5-bromouracil presents a site of preferential photochemical damage but is not a substrate for mitomycin alkylation. The relationship, however, between UV, mitomycin and thymine-less deaths is not altogether clear, since some *E. coli* strains (B, B_s) are hyper-sensitive to UV, mitomycin and thymine-less death whereas other strains (K12 uvr$^-$ and rec$^-$) exhibit hypersensitivity only to UV and mitomycin but not to thymine-less death. It was concluded that a single defect in DNA repair connot satisfactorily account for both hypersensitivity to thymine-less death (single-strand breaks in DNA; MENNIGMANN and SZYBALSKI, 1962) and ultrasensitivity to either UV or mitomycin (CUMMINGS and TAYLOR, 1966).

Breakdown of DNA in mitomycin-exposed cells depends on the presence of magnesium ions, is temperature-dependent, and leads to the formation of mononucleotides and free bases (REICH *et al.*, 1961; SHIIO *et al.*, 1962). Synthesis of new nucleases observed during mitomycin-effected induction of λ phages reflects the activity of the induced phage genome, since in the nonlysogenic host no new λ-specific nucleases are induced (WEISSBACH and KORN, 1962; KORN and WEISSBACH, 1964) and since the nuclease-deficient λ_{sus} mutants fail to show an increase in nuclease activity at inducing doses of mitomycin (RADDING, 1964). DNA depolymerization in the absence of any obvious phage induction (KERSTEN, 1962a and b; KERSTEN and KERSTEN, 1963; NAKATA *et al.*, 1962; REICH *et al.*, 1960, 1961) has been postulated to depend on mitomycin-effected damage to the s-RNA and ribosomes and consequent release of ribosome-bound nucleases (KERSTEN, and KERSTEN, 1963; KERSTEN *et al.*, 1964; LEHMAN, 1963; LEOPOLD *et al.*, 1965). Preferential damage by mitomycin to 50s ribosomal subunits and reduction in the incorporation of uracil-2-C^{14} into ribosomal RNA was reported by SUZUKI and KILGORE (1964). An initial increase followed by a decrease in the rate of s-RNA synthesis and a degradation of total RNA in mitomycin-treated *E. coli* cells was reported by SMITH-KIELLAND (1966b). Respiration mutants were reported to be very susceptible to mitomycin-induced DNA breakdown (GAUSE *et al.*, 1963). Streptomycin inhibits this DNA breakdown (REICH *et al.*, 1961), whereas inhibition of protein synthesis by chloramphenicol or 5-methyl tryptophane (but not by several other protein synthesis inhibitors, including puromycin, ethionine or norleucine) does not modify the DNA depolymerization process (CONSTANTOPOULOS and TCHEN 1964). Low concentrations of chloramphenicol or 5-methyltryptophane stimulated mitomycin-induced DNA degradation, whereas at higher levels this effect was not observed. Inhibition of RNA synthesis by 6-azauracil, actinomycin, or by the omission of uracil in uracil-dependent cells, depresses the breakdown of DNA, whereas phenethyl alcohol completely eliminates the mitomycin-induced DNA degradation (MATSUMOTO and TAKAGI, 1966). No change (REICH *et al.*, 1961) or an 80% increase in the activity of DNase (NAKATA *et al.*, 1962) and acid phosphatase (NIITANI *et al.*, 1964) was observed during cell exposure to mitomycin. Mitomycin has no effect on the *in vitro* activity of DNases or on their formation in cell-free systems (KERSTEN, 1962a; KERSTEN *et al.*, 1965; LEHMAN, 1963; NAKATA *et al.*, 1962). Detailed studies on the optimal condition for DNA degradation and on the increase in endodeoxyribonuclease activity during mitomycin treatment were presented by KERSTEN *et al.* (1965). Mitomycin-alkylated DNA (and also UV-irradiated DNA) is degraded at a slower rate than the control native DNA by three *E. coli* exonucleases (λ, Exo I, Exo II), but at an unimpaired rate by RNA-inhibitable *E. coli* endonuclease and pancreatic endo-DNase (PRICER and WEISSBACH, 1965).

Other Biological Effects of Mitomycins

Several other interesting biological effects have been attributed to the mitomycins. A summary of these findings is made available in this section, although little detailed information is available about the mechanisms by which such effects are brought about. As will be clear from later sections of this review, it would appear that all such effects can eventually be described on the basis that the mitomycins first become activated by reduction in the *in vivo* environment and that the reduced molecule, being highly reactive, will attach to and modify one or more cellular sites.

The mitomycins are mutagenic both for bacteria (SZYBALSKI, 1958; IIJIMA and HAGAWARA, 1960; TSUKAMURA and TSUKAMURA, 1962) and for Drosophila (SUZUKI, personal communication) in which such induced mutations appear to be non-randomly distributed. The mitomycins also are instrumental in the stimulation of chromosomal exchanges and crossing-over (SHAW and COHEN, 1965; SUZUKI, 1965) and for genetic recombination (IIJIMA and HAGAWARA, 1960; YUKI, 1962; HOLLIDAY, 1964), and in its inhibition (REICH *et al.*, 1961). They cause fragmentation of chromosomes and other cell structures (BACH and MAGEE, 1962; BIELIAVSKY, 1963; COHEN and SHAW, 1964; KERSTEN and THEMANN, 1962;

KIMURA, 1963; KOSAKA, 1964; KURODA and FURUYAMA, 1963; LAPIS and BERNHARD, 1965; MERZ, 1961; SHATKIN *et al.*, 1962; TRUHAUT and DEYSSON, 1960) resulting in inhibition of the development of pleurodele embryos blocked in the morula stage (BIELIAVSKY, 1963), giant cell formation (SHATKIN *et al.*, 1962), and other abnormal growth as *e.g.*, filament formation, an effect already mentioned. Mitomycin was also found to inhibit postirradiation repair of fragmented chromosomes (MATSUURA *et al.*, 1962, 1963; IWABUCHI *et al.*, 1966).

The mitomycins were found to influence the action of the polymerases, including stimulation of DNA polymerase activity in mammalian cells (BACH and MAGEE, 1962; MAGEE and MILLER, 1962) but not in bacteria (NAKATA *et al.*, 1962; SEKIGUCHI and TAKAGI, 1960a) and 60 to 75% impairment (PRICER and WEISSBACH, 1964, 1965) or little impairment (TAKAGI, 1963; KONTANI, 1964) of the *in vitro* priming capacity of DNA for the DNA polymerase but not for the DNA-dependent RNA polymerase. No changes in RNA base composition were detected in mitomycin-treated Ehrlich ascites cell (AKAMATSU *et al.*, 1963). Inhibition of RNA synthesis by mitomycin C and for the cellular transfer of delayed-type hypersensitivity in guinea pigs was reported by BLOOM *et al.* (1964). From their kinetic studies on the inhibition of DNA, RNA and protein (penicillinase) synthesis, COLES and GROSS (1965) concluded that mitomycin's primary attack is directed toward DNA, with inhibition of mRNA and induced enzyme synthesis as secondary phenomena.

Differential Sensitivity of Viral or Episomal Versus Host DNA

The mitomycins exhibit some selectivity in the cross-linking of DNA, and the resulting depolymerization and inhibition of DNA synthesis, even within the cytoplasm or nucleus of the same cell. Thus, the *E. coli* sex factor F seemed not to be degraded at all or to a lesser extent than the nuclear DNA, although the synthesis of both types of DNA was inhibited by mitomycin C (DRISKELL-ZAMENHOF and ADELBERG, 1963). Mitomycin, like acridine orange, was able to eliminate the F^+ factor from the treated cells, unless F^+ was associated with the colicin factor (MAYNE, 1965). Accumulation of episomal DNA after mitomycin induction was proportional to the rate of the production of colicin E (DE WITT and HELINSKI, 1965).

The inductive effect of mitomycin on lysogenic bacteria was discussed in Section 2. The induction of phage λ by mitomycin follows nearly the same kinetics at 37 and 20° C, and in this respect it differs from thymine-less induction, which is effective at 37° C but little at 20° C (GEISSLER, 1966).

In the case of several bacteriophages (OTSUJI, 1962; SEKIGUCHI and TAKAGI, 1959, 1960a) and other viruses (BEN-PORAT *et al.*, 1961; MAGEE and MILLER, 1962; MUNK and SAUER, 1965) mitomycin seemed to preferentially inhibit the synthesis of host DNA, permitting the synthesis of viral DNA, although the progeny virus was often not viable (BEN-PORAT *et al.*, 1961; COOPER and ZINDER, 1962; OKUBO, 1962; SEKIGUCHI and TAKAGI, 1960b). The genetic material of this inactive phage could be partially rescued by multiplicity reactivation, cross reactivation and host reactivation (OKUBO, 1962; BOYCE and HOWARD-FLANDERS, 1964). Only comparatively high concentrations of mitomycin inhibit viral DNA synthesis (MAGEE and MILLER, 1962; REICH and FRANKLIN, 1961; SEKIGUCHI and TAKAGI, 1960a). On the other hand, some viral DNA's are more effectively cross-linked by mitomycin than the chromosomal host DNA, even if both types of DNA are present in the same nucleus (SZYBALSKI *et al.*, 1964; SZYBALSKI, 1964). As could be predicted, in the absence of the reductive activation, the mitomycins have no lethal effect on free extracellular viral particles (OKUBO, 1962; REICH and FRANKLIN, 1961; SEKIGUCHI and TAKAGI, 1960a; SZYBALSKI and IYER, 1964a; WINKLER, 1962a and b). Production of viruses containing single-stranded RNA is little, if at all affected by moderate concentrations of mitomycin (COOPER and ZINDER, 1962; REICH and FRANKLIN, 1961; KNOLLE and KAUDEWITZ, 1964), with the exception of fowl plague myxovirus (ROTT *et al.*, 1965) and Rous sarcoma virus (VIGIER and GOLDE, 1964a and b) synthesis, which seem to be sensitive to mitomycin. Very selective suppression of the host DNA synthesis without affecting the synthesis of viral DNA was obtained with ΦX174 phage grown in mitomycin treated repair-deficient hcr$^-$ *E.coli* mutants (LINDQVIST and SINSHEIMER, 1966).

In Vivo Effects of Mitomycins on Intracellular DNA

The mitomycins are rapidly acting bactericidal and cytotoxic agents. Exposure to these antibiotics for only short periods of time results in irreversible cell death, unless certain special measures for cell rescue are applied (SZYBALSKI and ARNESON, 1965). The inhibitory concentrations of mitomycins for the wild-type strains of *Cytophaga johnsonii*, *B. subtilis*, *E. coli*, and *Sarcina lutea* used in this laboratory are in the range of 0.01—10 µg/ml (Table 1). The human cell line D98S (SZYBALSKI and SMITH, 1959) is inactivated at 0.02 µg/ml (SZYBALSKI *et al.*, 1964; SZYBALSKI and ARNESON, 1965), while free phage, several strains of *Streptomyces*, and *Neurospora crassa* are unaffected even at concentrations as high as 100 µg/ml. Resistant as well as more sensitive strains of *E. coli* have been described: strain B_{ms} and some radiosensitive B and K12 strains sensitive to 0.01—0.04 µg mitomycin/ml and strains resistant to over 20 µg mitomycin/ml (BOYCE and HOWARD-FLANDERS, 1964 and in press; GREENBERG and WOODY-KARRER, 1963; IYER, 1966; IYER and SZYBALSKI, 1963; SEKIGUCHI and TAKAGI, 1960; SHIBA *et al.*, 1958). A strain of *B. subtilis*, hypersensitive to mitomycin C and to ultraviolet irradiation, has been studied by OKUBO and ROMIG (1966), who from the behaviour of this strain on transformation and infection with ultraviolet-irradiated phages interpret it to be similar to the recombination-deficient mutants of *E. coli* (CLARK and MARGULIES, 1965; HOWARD-FLANDERS, 1965). Mutations that determine resistance to the mitomycins are chromosomally-localizable in *B. subtilis* and clustered in the early-replicating segment of the genome, which bears genetic loci for streptomycin and erythromycin resistance, and for ribosomal and transfer RNAs (IYER, 1966). Although the biochemical basis of mitomycin resistance is not known at present, the above results together with the known pleiotropic effects of mitomycin resistance (GREENBERG *et al.*, 1961; IYER, 1966), and mitomycin effects on ribosomal function (SUZUKI and KILGORE, 1964), suggest that mitomycin resistance might be related to the latter function (IYER, 1966) or to some general permeability barriers. It might be of interest to mention a report by YOSHIOKA and KUNII

(1966), who observed that mitomycin-resistant streptococcus mutants produced a mitomycin-inactivating factor.

The lethal effects of the mitomycins are associated with concomitant dramatic changes in the structure of the DNA. DNA isolated from cells which were exposed for as little as 1 min to this antibiotic is characterized by covalent links between its complementary strands, as demonstrated by the spontaneous reversibility of the denaturation process (IYER and SZYBALSKI, 1963). The schematic comparison of the behavior of normal and mitomycin cross-linked DNA upon thermal denaturation followed by rapid cooling is outlined in Fig. 4. The denaturation of control

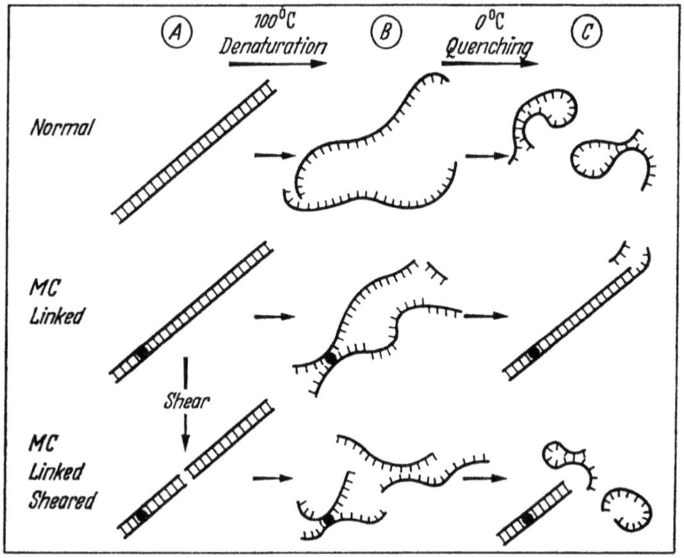

Fig. 4. Schematic presentation of molecular events following denaturation (A to B) and rapid cooling (B to C) of DNA. *Top row:* normal DNA extracted from control cells. *Middle row:* cross-linked DNA extracted from mitomycin C(MC)-inactivated cells. The possibility of hydrolytic cleavage of the phosphate ester bonds and its consequences are illustrated for denatured (B) and spontaneously renatured, quenched form (C). *Bottom row:* cross-linked DNA extracted from mitomycin-inactivated cells and subsequently exposed to shearing forces with resulting double-strand break. Upon heating and rapid cooling only the cross-link-bearing fragment renatures spontaneously. (From IYER and SZYBALSKI, 1963)

DNA (Fig. 4, *top row*) is an irreversible process under the conditions of rapid cooling, since the sorting out and proper alignment of the separated complementary strands is a slow and temperature-dependent process. In cross-linked DNA (Fig. 4, *middle row*) the complementary strands cannot separate completely and remain in original alignment; the "zippering-up" process (for terminology see KOHN *et al.*, 1966) is apparently a rapid one, even under conditions of rapid cooling.

Spontaneously renatured, ("zippered-up"), cross-linked DNA has many properties in common with native helical DNA and can be distinguished from the disordered denatured DNA by several criteria.

a) In cesium chloride or cesium sulfate density gradients, renatured cross-linked DNA (*B. subtilis*) bands at a density very close to that of native DNA, usually 0.015 (cesium chloride) or 0.024 g/cm³ (cesium sulfate) lower than the density of denatured DNA. Thus, analytical (Fig. 5) or preparative equilibrium density gradient centrifugation separates the cross-linked from the non-cross-linked DNA molecules after their subjection to denaturation and low-temperature quenching.

b) Control DNA which was previously denatured and rapidly cooled does not exhibit a sharp thermal transition at its characteristic melting temperature when its optical density (OD_{260}) is measured as a function of temperature (Fig. 6; control *thin dotted line*). Under the same conditions the denatured cross-linked DNA shows a melting behavior similar to that of native DNA (Fig. 6; mitomycin, *thin solid line*). A low degree of such spontaneous renaturation was observed in DNA extracted from mitomycin-treated bacteria by MATSUMOTO and LARK (1963) and interpreted as formation of stable bonds between the two strands of the DNA helix.

c) During thermal denaturation normal DNA loses over 90% of its transforming activity, while the transforming activity of mitomycin cross-linked DNA is not critically and abruptly destroyed under the same conditions (Fig. 7).

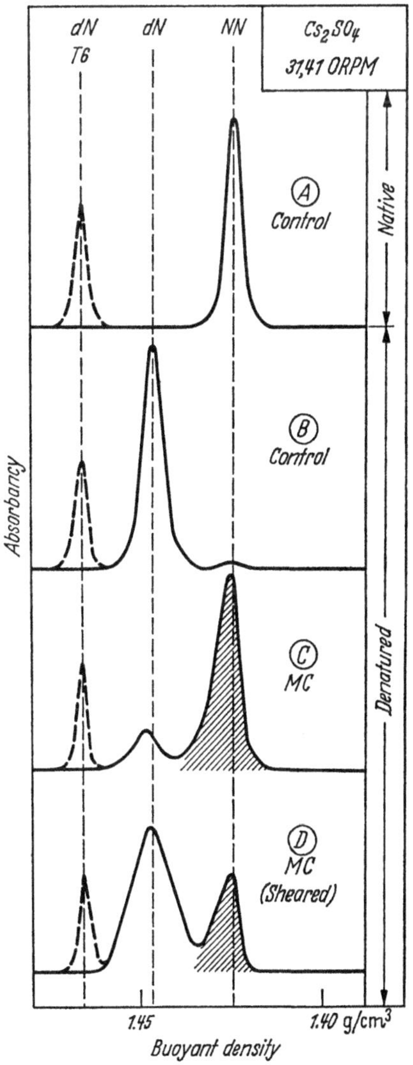

Fig. 5. Microdensitometric tracings of photographs taken after 40 hr of Cs_2SO_4 equilibrium density gradient centrifugation (31,410 rpm, 25 C) of DNA extracted from *B. subtilis* cells never exposed to mitomycin (A, B) or grown for 15 minutes in the presence of 12.5 μg mitomycin C/ml of nutrient broth (C, D). The DNA was either native (A) or denatured (B, C, D) by 6 minutes exposure to 100 C in 0.02 M Na_3·citrate buffer at pH = 7.8 followed by rapid chilling at 0 C. The DNA used in experiment D was mechanically sheared prior to denaturation by forcing a solution of 15 μg DNA/ml three times through a 25-gage needle (I. D. = 0.254 mm) with a spring-loaded, constant-rate syringe CR 700 (Hamilton Co., Whittier, Calif.). The shaded areas correspond roughly to mitomycin cross-linked DNA. The broken lines (dN T6) represent denatured T6 coliphage DNA added as a density marker. The buoyant densities of native (A) and denatured (B) *B. subtilis* DNA correspond to 1.424 (NN) and 1.446 (dN) g/cm³, respectively. The proportion of denatured, non-cross-linked DNA, determined by comparing the areas under the peaks, increases upon shearing from 23% (C) to 73% (D). (From SZYBALSKI and IYER, 1964a)

d) Spontaneously renatured cross-linked DNA can also be separated from denatured DNA by a variety of other procedures, including filtration on cellulose nitrate filters (Nygaard and Hall, 1963), chromatography on methyl-esterified albumin-kieselguhr columns (Mandell and Hershey, 1960), countercurrent paritition (Albertsson, 1962), and other techniques used or reviewed by Summers and Szybalski (1967a) and Szybalski (1967).

Many other features of the *in vivo* cross-linking reaction and the properties of cross-linked DNA were described earlier (Iyer and Szybalski, 1963). These can be summarized as follows. The degree of cross-linking by mitomycin C depends on the concentration of the antibiotic, on the duration of its contact with the cells, and on the temperature. The physiological state of the bacteria has little effect on

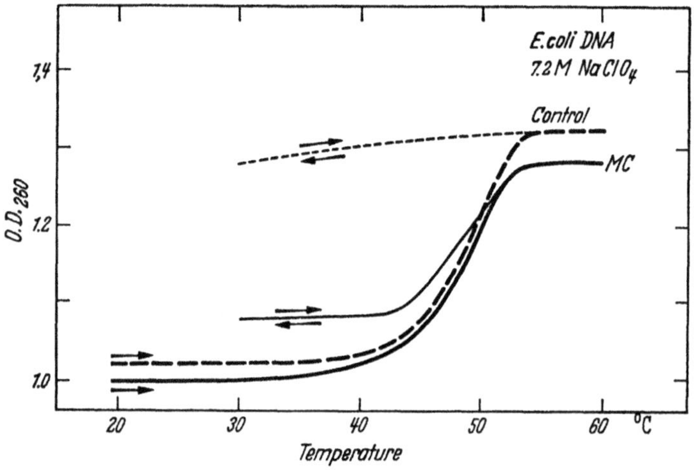

Fig. 6. Thermal denaturation profiles in 7.2 M $NaClO_4$ for DNA's isolated from *E. coli* cells grown in nutrient broth and exposed for 15 minutes to 0 (control, dotted lines) or 10 (MC, solid lines) μg mitomycin C/ml. The first heating (0.5 C/minutes) is indicated by the thicker lines. The absorbance changes (OD_{260}) during subsequent cooling (5 C/minutes) and heating (0.5 C/minutes) cycles, which were carried out in the thermospectrophotometer cuvette compartment, are represented by the thinner lines. The midpoint transition values, Tm (melting temperature), correspond to 48.5 C (control) and 48.0 C (mitomycin-linked DNA). (From Iyer and Szybalski, 1963)

the susceptibility of the DNA to cross-linking. Once formed, the cross-links are quite stable. The loss of the cross-linked fraction observed in some cases is most probably related to the "repair" or nucleolytic breakdown of the DNA with resulting separation of the linked from the nonlinked fragments (Fig. 4, *middle row*). Similar loss of the spontaneously renaturing crosslinked fragments can be observed during hydrodynamic shearing of mitomycin-cross-linked native DNA prior to denaturation and low temperature quenching, according to the scheme presented in Fig. 4 (*bottom row*) and determined by cesium sulfate density gradient centrifugation. The proportion of cross-linked material (*shaded area* under *peaks*) decreases upon shearing from approximately 77% (Fig. 5C) to 28% (Fig. 5D).

The rate of cell death is well correlated with the degree of DNA cross-linking, with mitomycin-resistant *E. coli* mutants showing a parallel decrease in susceptibility to cross-linking and to the lethal effects of mitomycin. Rough calculations indicate that 10 minutes exposure (37 C) to 0.1, 1, and 10 μg mitomycin C/ml results in 90%, 5% and 5×10^{-4}% cell survival (*B. subtilis*) and 1, 10, and 100 cross-links/10^9 daltons of DNA, i.e., per one cell genome respectively (SZYBALSKI and IYER, 1964a). Taking into account that the *B. subtilis* cell has on the average 2—4 nuclei with a partially duplicated genome, these figures indicate that inactivation of all nuclei by one cross-link per genome should result in cell death. It is rather easy to imagine that replication of the DNA would abruptly stop as soon as it reached the mitomycin cross-link, unless some repair phenomenon intervened.

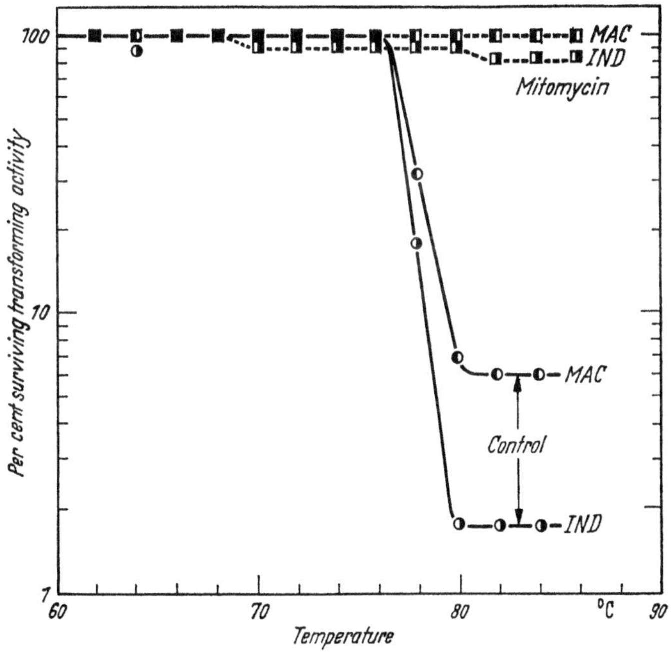

Fig. 7. Thermal inactivation of transforming DNA extracted from *B. subtilis* cells grown in nutrient broth and exposed for 15 minutes (37 C) to 0 (solid lines) or to 12 (dotted lines) μg of mitomycin C/ml. Each point corresponds to an assay performed on an 0.03 ml sample of DNA, dissolved in DSC (0.015 M NaCl, 0.0015 M Na_3·citrate, pH = 7.8) at 10 μg DNA/ml, sealed in a glass capillary, heated for 10 minutes at the indicated temperature, and rapidly chilled in ice water (0° C). The transforming activity was assayed for indole independence (IND) (minimal agar) and for resistance to the macrolide group of antibiotics (MAC) (0.5 μg erythromycin/ml), by plating 0.05 ml of a transforming mixture containing 0.002 μg DNA and approximately 2×10^7 recipient cells. (From IYER and SZYBALSKI, 1963)

The transforming activity of *B. subtilis* DNA is not greatly affected by mitomycin cross-linking. DNA extracted from mitomycin-treated cells exhibiting less than 10^{-4}% survival still has a specific transforming activity only 2—3 times lower than that of DNA extracted from control cells. Since such a DNA would have approximately one cross-link per 10^6 daltons and since much smaller DNA fragments seem to be integrated into the recipient genome during the transformation process, it is not surprising that cross-links distant from the actual genetically integrated fragments would have little effect on their function in the recipient cell. The numerical data quoted here and the experiments and calculations leading to the determination of the frequency of cross-links were outlined earlier (IYER and SZYBALSKI, 1963).

In Vitro Effects of Mitomycins on DNA

As mentioned earlier, the mitomycins do not react *in vitro* with purified DNA or with free phage. On the other hand, it was possible to obtain *in vitro* cross-linking of purified DNA if the reaction mixture composed of DNA and mitomycin was supplemented with a cell-free lysate derived from any of several mitomycin-sensitive species of bacteria (IYER and SZYBALSKI, 1963, 1964). These observations indicated clearly that the mitomycins must be activated prior to cross-linking of the DNA, but at the same time raised the following questions: a) what is the chemical nature of this metabolic activation of the mitomycins; b) can the activation process be duplicated in a purely chemical way; and c) what are the reactive groups on the mitomycin and DNA molecules which participate in the cross-linking reaction? The answers to some of these questions are outlined in this review.

Metabolic Activation of Mitomycins

The cross-linking of purified native DNA by the mitomycins in the presence of cell lysates was studied in some detail (IYER and SZYBALSKI, 1963, 1964). Activation of the mitomycins was observed when a cell lysate of *Bacillus subtilis*, of *Sarcina lutea*, or of *Cytophaga johnsonii*, prepared by exposing approximately 10^9 cells/ml for 10 minutes to 100 μg lysozyme/ml of SSC (0.15 M sodium chloride + 0.02 M sodium citrate; pH = 7.6), was diluted two-fold to eight-fold into the reaction mixture containing per ml 10—100 μg mitomycin and 100—200 μg purified DNA of any of the above-mentioned bacteria or of other species, including T-even and T-odd coliphages, *E. coli*, and human cells. Mitomycins activated in this way cross-linked the purified DNA present in the reaction mixture. Heating (10 minutes at 70 C), aging, aeration, or dialysis against SSC destroyed the mitomycin-activating capacity of the cell lysate. However, the activity of the dialyzed lysate can be almost completely restored by the addition of TPNH (100—200 μg/ml) or of the TPNH-generating system, whereas TPNH in the absence of the lysate is ineffective as a mitomycin-activating agent. These results indicate that the activation process can most probably be equated to TPNH-dependent enzymatic reduction of mitomycin to its hydroquinone derivative by one of the enzymes belonging to the group of quinone reductases, often referred to as diaphorases (MARTIUS, 1963). The commercial preparation of the *Clostridium kluyveri* diaphorase (Nutritional Biochemicals, Cleveland, Ohio) was found to activate mitomycin in the presence of TPNH with concomitant cross-linking of added DNA. Unfortunately this diaphorase preparation also had a nucleolytic activity directed toward DNA. The reductase activity of the cell lysates was associated mainly (90%) with the fraction sedimenting at 198,000 × g (90 minutes) and was not affected by dicumarol, a reported inhibitor (MARTIUS, 1963) of some quinone reductases.

Enzymatic reduction of mitomycin C and its metabolic inactivation by liver homogenates was reported by SCHWARTZ *et al.* (1963a). These authors have also postulated that some reductive steps might be associated with the metabolic activation of mitomycin, although in their experimental system it was possible to measure only the metabolic inactivation of this antibiotic (SCHWARTZ, 1962; SCHWARTZ and PHILIPS, 1961).

Chemical Activation of Mitomycins

Since metabolic experiments clearly indicated that a reductive step seems to be prerequisite to the mitomycin activation and cross-linking reaction, a chemical reduction was also attempted (IYER and SZYBALSKI, 1964). Several reducing agents were tested, but only three were found readily suitable on account of the ease of reduction of mitomycin and the absence of untoward effects on DNA. Sodium borohydride ($NaBH_4$), sodium hydrosulfite ($Na_2S_2O_4$), both at concentrations of 100—200 μg/ml, and hydrogen at atmospheric pressure in the presence of a palladium catalyst (5% palladium-on-charcoal moistened with ethanol) were found to rapidly reduce mitomycin dissolved in 0.15 M phosphate buffer (pH = 7.8; room temperature), as determined by the color change of the solution from purple to yellow and by loss of the absorption peak at 363 mμ (SCHWARTZ, 1962). DNA present in this reaction mixture, or added within seconds after the chemical reduction of the mitomycin, is cross-linked. The active form of mitomycin obtained by chemical reduction must be quite unstable, since for cross-linking to take place the DNA must be added within seconds after completion of the reduction reaction. Reduced and reoxidized mitomycin has no cross-linking activity, and its spectrum is similar to that of the inactive acid-degradation product of mitomycin with open aziridine ring (GARRETT, 1963; WEBB *et al.*, 1962) (Fig. 12D).

The results of two typical experiments which illustrate *in vitro* cross-linking of various DNA's by chemically reduced mitomycin C are presented in Figs. 8 and 9. The reaction mixture was composed of the indicated concentrations of mitomycin (10—100 μg/ml), various DNA's (200 μg/ml), and sodium hydrosulfite (dithionite) (100 μg/ml). The addition of the latter component initiated the reaction, usually carried out under anaerobic conditions with nitrogen bubbling. The reaction was terminated after 1—2 minutes by alcohol (1.5 vol.) precipitation of the DNA, followed by collection on a glass rod, immediate dissolution of the still gelatinous precipitate in DSC, denaturation, and ultracentrifugal examination for cross-links. As can be seen in Figs. 8 and 9, the DNA becomes cross-linked under these conditions, and the proportion of cross-linked DNA (*shadowed area* under *peaks*) depends on the mitomycin concentration and on the type of DNA.

Activated (reduced) mitomycins inactivate also free extracellular viruses and phage (SZYBALSKI and IYER, 1964a), cross-linking their DNA. This result was confirmed by BORENFREUND *et al.* (1965) with the polyoma virus.

Reactive Sites on Mitomycin Molecules

The examination of the structure of all the mitomycins (Fig. 2) reveals an abundance of reactive groups, including the aziridine ring (1-2-1a), a methyl-urethane side chain starting with C-10, a tertiary methoxy or hydroxyl group at C-9a, and the 7-amino-(methoxy-, or hydroxyl-)quinone configuration. Many highly reactive synthetic compounds containing the aziridine ring(s) are known, but the mitomycins are the only known naturally occurring compounds with this configuration. In synthetic compounds the aziridine ring is quite reactive, readily providing an alkylating function as easily determined with γ-(4-nitrobenzyl-) pyridine (EPSTEIN *et al.*, 1955), a specific color reagent for the assay of alkylating centers, or by titration with sodium thiosulfate (ALLEN and SEAMAN, 1955). On the other hand, the aziridine component of the mitomycins in their natural oxidized form was found to be very unreactive, as assayed with two previously discussed reagents (SCHWARTZ *et al.*, 1963a; A. LOVELESS, personal communication). This lack of reactivity might be caused by heavy substitution on the two carbon atoms in the aziridine ring, in analogy with the reported decrease in reactivity of the diepoxides with increasing substitution on the carbon atoms (ROSS, 1962, and personal communication). Cyclohexenimine, an ethylenimine fused to the cyclohexane ring, appears to be a rather stable compound on the basis of the published report (PARIS and FANTA, 1952). While nonreactive under neutral and alkaline conditions, this aziridine ring is readily opened under acid conditions, with simultaneous loss of the tertiary methoxy group (GARRETT, 1963; WEBB *et al.*, 1962). Actually, the aziridine ring in the mitomycins is much more sensitive to low pH (half-life of 0.1 hr in 0.01 N HCl at 30 C) (GARRETT, 1963) than the same ring in many synthetic aziridine derivatives (interpolated half-life c. 10 hr in 1 M HCl at a temperature of 30 C) (SCHATZ and CLAPP, 1955).

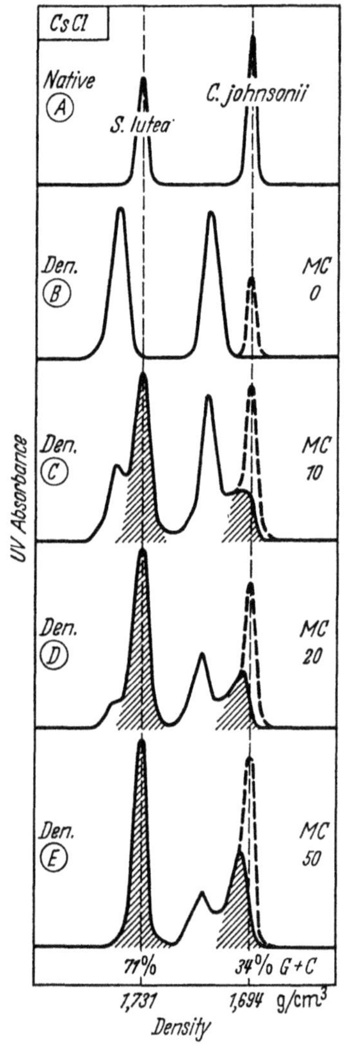

Fig. 8. Microdensitometric tracings of photographs taken after 22 hr of CsCl equilibrium density gradient centrifugation (44,770 rev/minutes, 25 C) of a mixture of deproteinized and RNase-treated DNA's extracted from *C. johnsonii* and *S. lutea* cells, native (A), or denatured (heated for 6 minutes at 100 C in DSC and quenched at 0 C) after *in vitro* exposure to 0 (B), 10 (C), 20 (D), and 50 (E) μg mitomycin C/ml DSC under reducing conditions (200 μg DNA + 100 μg $Na_2S_2O_4$/ml, 1 minute, 20 C, followed by alcohol precipitation and dissolving the precipitate in DSC). The shaded areas roughly correspond to spontaneously renaturable (cross-linked) DNA. The per cent cross-linked DNA, determined by integration of the tracings and correction for hypochromicity, amounted to 0% (B), 79% and 36% (C), 91% and 49% (D), 100% and 62% (E), for *S. lutea* and *C. johnsonii* DNA's, respectively. The dotted peaks correspond to native *C. johnsonii* DNA and were obtained by repeating the centrifugation after addition of c. 1 μg of this density-marker DNA directly to the centrifuge cells. (From IYER and SZYBALSKI, 1964)

The stability of the mitomycins is related to the resonance between forms A and B (Fig. 10), which results in partial withdrawal of electrons from the N_{-4} into the quinone ring and a stabilization of the tertiary methoxy (or hydroxyl) group at C_{-9a} (SZYBALSKI and IYER, 1964a).

Since the quinone ring when reduced to hydroquinone would lose the capacity to withdraw electrons from N_{-4}, the regaining of an electron pair and increase in the basicity of N_{-4} would start the chain of events illustrated in Fig. 10. Thus, reduction of mitomycin to form C would result in loss of the 9a methoxy (hydroxyl) group (Fig. 10D) together with the formation of the fully aromatic indole system (Fig. 10E) (IYER and SZYBALSKI, 1964). No elimination of the 9a group was observed upon electrolytic reduction of mitomycin B to a semiquinone stage (PATRICK *et al.*, 1964). The spontaneous elimination of the 9a methoxy group, which was previously observed during acid solvolysis of mitomycins (GARRETT, 1963; GARRETT and SCHROEDER, 1964; WEBB *et al.*, 1962), was determined analytically. The release of methanol during chemical reduction of mitomycin C was practically quantitative, as determined by the microdiffusion technique (IYER and SZYBALSKI, 1964).

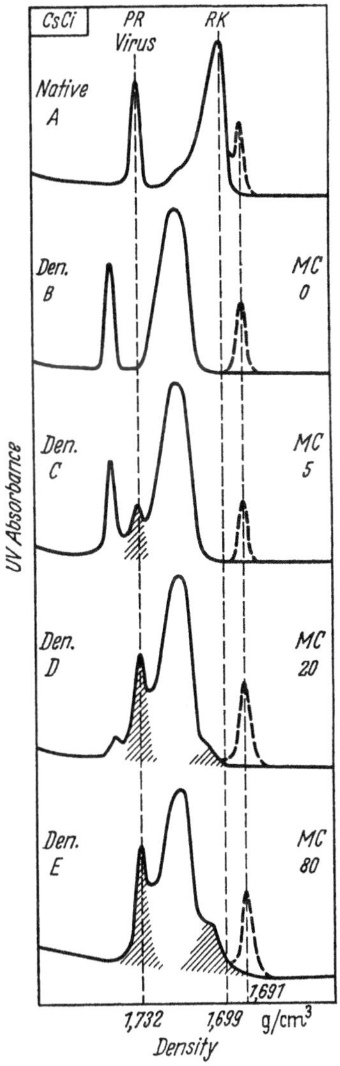

Fig. 9. Microdensitomertric tracings of photographs taken after 23 hr of CsCl equilibrium density gradient centrifugation (44,770 rev/minutes, 25 C) of a once deproteinized (chloroform + butanol) mixture of nucleic acids extracted from rabbit kidney cells (RK) infected with pseudorabies virus (PR), native (A) or denatured (cf. Fig. 7) after *in vitro* exposure to 0 (B), 5 (C), 20 (D), and 80 (E) µg mitomycin C/ml DSC, under reducing conditions (cf. Fig. 7). The shaded areas roughly correspond to spontaneously renaturable (cross-linked) DNA. The dotted peaks correspond to the native *Clostridium perfringens* DNA used as a density marker (1.691 g/cm³). (From SZYBALSKI, 1964)

As pointed out earlier, the reduced (activated) form of mitomycin (Fig. 10E) is very unstable and rapidly loses its capacity to cross-link purified DNA. The cross-linking reaction requires at least two reactive sites on the mitomycin molecule. The reactions leading to the formation of such sites are illustrated in Fig. 11, starting with the protonated form of reduced mitomycin (A). The aromatic indole system would now facilitate the rapid fission of the aziridine ring (A → B, C), because of the stabilization of the positive charge by the indole ring in the transition state of the reaction (B→C). This resonant system would in turn stabilize the carbonium ion at C_{-1}, the most probable reactive site, thus providing the first alkylating center at position "1" (Fig. 12C), forming a covalent link with DNA. Furthermore, one might predict activation of a second alkylating center at C_{-10}, also most probably a carbonium ion, since here again a positive charge in the transition state would be stabilized by the indole nitrogen (Fig. 11 D → E) and

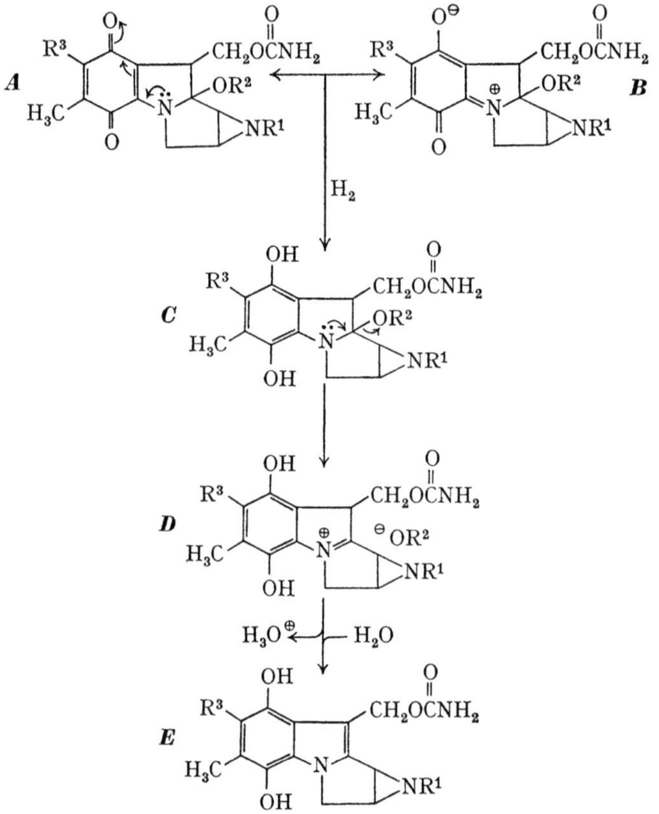

Fig. 10. The resonant structure of the mitomycins in their natural oxidized form (A ↔ B), indicating partial withdrawal of electrons from N_{-4} into the quinone ring (after IYER and SZYBALSKI, 1964) and rearrangement following the reductive step (A, B → C), and including elimination of the tertiary 9a methoxy (hydroxyl) group (C → D) and formation of the fully aromatic indole system (D → E)

since the carbon (C_{-10})-oxygen fission would be similar to that reported for pyrrolizidine alkaloids containing an acyloxymethyldehydropyrrolizidine configuration (CULVENOR *et al.*, 1963) analogous to that in reduced mitomycin. Esters of amino allylic alcohol (N_{-4}-C_{-9a} = C_{-9}-O-R) are known to undergo such a carbon-oxygen fission (CULVENOR *et al.*, 1963).

Reactions leading to activation and inactivation of the mitomycins are summarized in Fig. 12. Although two reactive sites "1" and "2" are sufficient to explain their necessarily bifunctional cross-linking activity, it is difficult at present to exclude the possibility of a third reactive site "3" at the C-7 position. It was suggested by RAO *et al.* (1963) that the presence of the o-aminoquinone moiety not only in mitomycin but also in the antibiotics streptonigrin and actinomycin might indicate similarities in their mechanism of action. However, these similarities might be spurious on account of more then one reason: a) neither streptonigrin nor actinomycin cross-links DNA (IYER and SZYBALSKI, 1964;

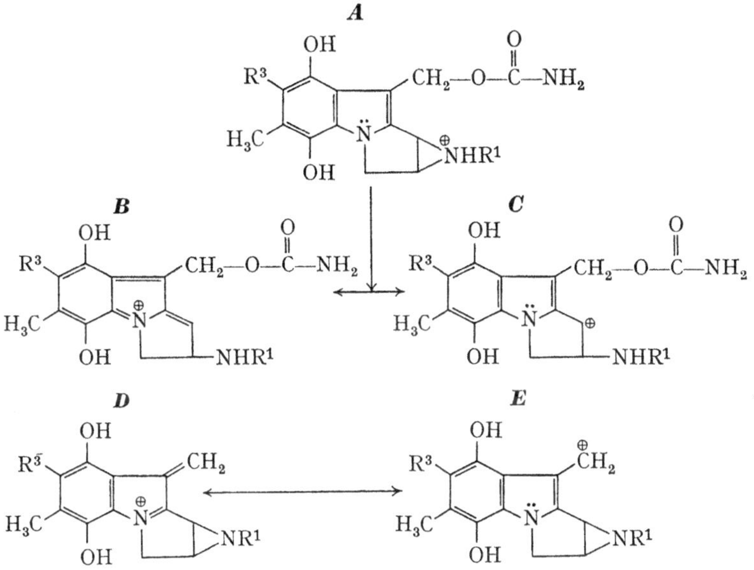

Fig. 11. The resonant forms of the reduced mitomycins after elimination of the 9a methoxy or hydroxyl group and formation of the aromatic indole configuration. (From IYER and SZYBALSKI, 1964)

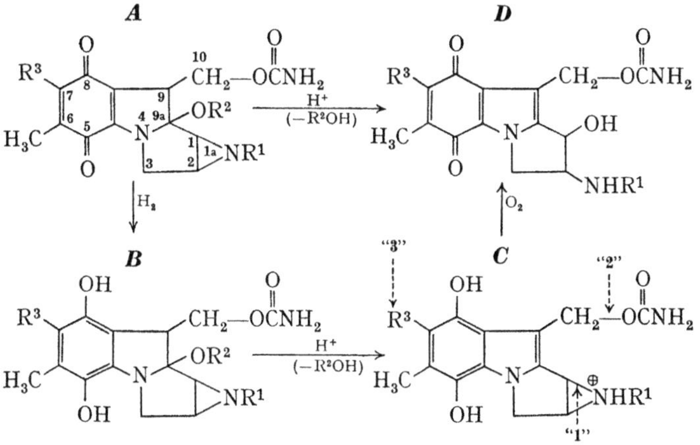

Fig. 12. Structure of the mitomycins and porfiromycins and some of their reduction, protonation, reoxidation, and acid degradation products. A: The natural oxidized form of the mitomycins (cf. Fig. 2). B: The primary reduction product (cf. Fig. 10). C: The postulated structure after secondary rearrangements following the reductive step and protonation in the aziridine ring (cf. Fig. 11 A). The arrows ("1", "2", "3") point to the reactive sites and to points of possible cleavage. D: The product of acid solvolysis (GARRATT, 1963; GARRETT and SCHROEDER, 1964; KIRSCH and KORSHALLA, 1964; WEBB *et al.*, 1962) and the possible products of reduction and late reoxidation of the mitomycins. (From IYER and SZYBALSKI, 1964)

KERSTEN *et al.*, 1966); b) actinomycin does not seem to form stable covalent links with DNA (REICH, 1964); c) chemical reduction of tritiated streptonigrin does not affect its *in vitro* reactivity with DNA (IYER and SZYBALSKI, 1964), and d) on theoretical grounds, site "3" should be more reactive in the oxidized than in the reduced form of mitomycin as pointed out by Dr. J. S. WEBB (personal comm.). The possibility should be considered that the amino-(methoxy-)quinone configuration is responsible for the proper alignment of mitomycin in respect to the DNA molecule prior to the actual cross-linking reaction. Complete removal or inactivation of the 7-amino group would have helped to elucidate the role of site "3" (Fig. 12C), but such derivatives were not available. Replacement of the amino group at C^{-7} by the methoxy (mitomycins A and B) or hydroxyl group (7-hydroxyporfiromycin) did not affect greatly their lethal and DNA cross-linking activities; mitomycin A was actually a somewhat more efficient cross-linking agent, whereas 7-hydroxyporfiromycin was less active than mitomycin C, when tested with the *B. subtilis* W23 strain. With other strains of *B. subtilis*, 7-hydroxyporfiromycin was 100 times less active than porfiromycin, which, however, was not the case for *E. coli* strains (Table 1). On the average 7 hydroxyl substitution results in lower activity than N-pyridine or tertiary amino substitution, with 7-methoxyl, 7-aziridino and 7-amino compounds being most active (Table 2). The nature of the C^{-7} substituent might modify the redox potential of the mitomycins and in this manner affect the biological activity (UZU *et al.*, 1966).

Replacement of the tertiary methoxy group at position 9a by a hydroxyl group (mitomycin B) has little effect on the cross-linking, but, on average, resulted in reduced bactericidal (Tables 1 and 2) and antineoplastic activity (OBOSHI *et al.*, 1967). Methylation at N_{-1_a} affects neither the stability of the aziridine ring in the natural oxidized form of the porfiromycins nor the cross-linking activity of the activated (reduced) form. Since N_{-1_a} has to be protonated prior to expressing its "alkylating" function, substitution of an acyl group (or especially sulfonyl derivatives which cannot be enzymatically removed), which interferes with the protonation, will predictably decrease the biological activity (Table 2) (MIYAMURA *et al.*, 1967). There is little doubt that the aziridine moiety participates in the formation of one covalent link with DNA. Irreversible loss of cross-linking activity upon opening of the aziridine ring (Fig. 12D) attests to its role. The nature of the second covalent link with DNA is less clear, since the formation of a bond from C_{-10} to DNA is based only on analogies with alkylation by the pyrrolizidine alkaloids (CULVENOR *et al.*, 1962); direct chemical proof of the structure of the product is required. The biological activity (Table 2) of the mitosenes (Fig. 3A) and 1,2-dialkylindoloquinones (Fig. 3C), both devoid of aziridine rings, suggests an alkylating role for the C_{-10} carbonium ion. Isolation of a diguanylated mitomycin as a product of *in vitro* reaction between sRNA and reduced mitomycin supports the notion that mitomycin is a *bi*functional "alkylating" agent (LIPSETT and WEISSBACH, 1965). Some degree of cross resistance was observed between mitomycin and nitrogen mustard, a typical alkylating agent, when using Yoshida sarcoma cells made resistant to mitomycin (SAKURAI, 1964).

The methoxy or hydroxyl group in position 9a cannot be directly involved in the formation of the covalent bond with DNA, since an intermediate prepared by catalytic hydrogenation of mitomycin in dimethylformamide followed by its reoxidation, most probably the aziridinomitosene (Fig. 3 B), is still a biologically active DNA cross-linking agent, although it lacks any substituent in position 9a (SZYBALSKI and IYER, 1964a). The yield of aziridinomitosene prepared by reduction and reoxidation was very low, attesting to the instability of the aziridine ring in its intermediary reduced form (Figs. 10E and 12C), and required chromatographic purification of the product. Ultraviolet spectra similar to those of compound D (Fig. 12), together with preservation of the biological activity, were considered as indicative of its structure. Since cross-linking of purified DNA *in vitro* by the aziridinomitosene is more efficient in the presence of reducing agents, the reduced form of this compound (Figs. 10E and 12C) is most probably the biologically active form of mitomycin (SZYBALSKI and IYER, 1964a). 7-Methoxy-1,2-(N-methylaziridino) mitosene (Fig. 3 B) was prepared in 40% yield by reduction and reoxidation of mitomycin B and reported to have bactericidal activity (PATRICK *et al.*, 1964). Unfortunately, however, it was not made available for testing of its *in vitro* DNA cross-linking activity. No quantitative data were published on the antibiotic activities of three aziridinomitosenes derived from mitomycins A, B, and porfiromycin, but it was stated that surprisingly the activity of the latter compound is much lower than that of the derivatives of mitomycins A and B (PATRICK *et al.*, 1964).

After this review was completed, a theoretical paper of MURAKAMI (1966) was published outlining the possible electronic mechanisms of mitomycin activation and DNA cross-linking. The author postulates that the intermediary semiquinoid form of mitomycin is the active intermediate and that the cross-link includes O_{-6} of guanine, N_{-4} and O_{-5} of mitomycin, and N_{-4} of cytosine. The promoting effect of cytosine on DNA cross-linking by mitomycin in a reductive medium, as described by IYER and SZYBALSKI (1964), is interpreted as transformation of the hydroquinone form of mitomycin into the reactive semiquinoid form by transference of its hydrogen atom to the carbonyl oxygen atom of the cystosine. The postulated intermediary role of the semiquinoid form of mitomycin is not confirmed by the data of PATRICK *et al.* (1964), who did not observe any secondary rearrangements upon reduction of mitomycin B to a semiquinone stage.

The relationship between the structure of the mitomycins and their antineoplastic activity is rather complicated (USUBUCHI *et al.*, 1967; OBOSHI *et al.*, 1967). These authors have reported that approximately one third of mitomycin derivatives, most of those listed in Table 2, was more effective than mitomycin C. Many substituents at positions R^{I} and R^{II} (Figs. 2 and 3) had little effect on antineoplastic activity. Most of the heavily substituted primary amines (3 to 6 carbons) at position 7 were more effective than mitomycin C; Secondary amines were less effective. 7-Hydroxyl derivatives were inactive, indicating an important role for the aminoquinone structure. When compared with mitomycin C, the rupture of the aziridine ring (1-hydroxy, 2,7-diamino mitosene) did not reduce the antineoplastic activity on some tumors (USUBUCHI *et al.*, 1967), but decreased the activity against sarcoma 180 (OBOSHI *et al.*, 1967). Since permeability, active transport, inactivation, activation, and toxicity phenomena play great roles in any type of animal experiments, it is difficult to draw any clear-cut conclusion about the primary mode of action of the mitomycins.

Reactive Sites on DNA (and RNA) Molecules

Information about the sites of mitomycin attachment on the DNA molecule is still far from complete. Earlier evidence of indirect nature suggested that the guanine, cytosine, or both moieties of DNA might preferentially react with the mitomycins, since the degree of cross-linking increases with increasing guanine and cytosine (G + C) content. Thus, a higher degree of cross-linking was observed with *S. lutea* DNA (71% G + C) than with *C. johnsonii* (33% G + C), when both were treated simultaneously with reduced mitomycin (Fig. 8). Similar observations have been made with other DNA's of various G + C contents, of mammalian, bacterial, and viral origin (SZYBALSKI and IYER, 1964a).

To obtain more insight into the nature of the reactive sites on the DNA molecule, several types of exotic DNA's were evaluated (SZYBALSKI and IYER, 1964a). The DNA's extracted from T-even coliphages containing glucosylated 5-hydroxymethylcytosine in place of cytosine, and from *B. subtilis* phages PBS-2 containing uracil and SP8 containing 5-hydroxymethyluracil in place of thymine were all found to be cross-linked by mitomycin, demonstrating that these base substitutions have no profound effect on the cross-linking reaction. More surprising, at least on first sight, was that mono- and diglucosylation of 5-hydroxymethylcytosine (HMC) residues had no effect whatsoever on the efficiency of cross-linking, although the bulky glucose molecules fill almost completely the large groove of the DNA double helix; an identical degree of cross-linking under identical *in vitro* conditions was observed with DNA isolated from phage T6 containing 76% diglucosylated HMC residues, phage T4 containing 100% monoglucosylated HMC residues, and phage T6 (o) grown in a UDPG$^-$ host (ERIKSON and SZYBALSKI, 1964) and thus containing less than 7% glucosylated HMC. Inspection of the space-filling DNA model, however, indicates that some types of cross-links would not be sterically hindered by the glucose residues (SZYBALSKI and IYER, 1964a).

The experiments of IYER and SZYBALSKI (1964), demonstrating the possibility of *in vitro* reaction between nucleic acids and activated (reduced) mitomycin, have prompted several attempts to measure directly the binding of radioactive mitomycins to DNA. SZYBALSKI and IYER (1964a and b) have prepared N-methylmitomycin-1a-^{14}C (porfiromycin-^{14}C) by exposing mitomycin C to ^{14}C-methyl iodide for 2 days at 37° C and purifying the product by chromatography on phosphate-buffer (pH = 7)-impregnated Whatman No. 1 paper, using a methanol solvent.

When purified *Bacillus subtilis* DNA (200 μg) was exposed for 3 minutes to 20 μg of N-methylmitomycin-^{14}C per 0.27 ml of 0.15 M NaCl + 0.02 M Na_3·citrate with subsequent addition of 0.03 ml of a freshly prepared aqueous solution of sodium borohydride (1000 μg/ml), which reaction was shown to result in cross-linking of the complementary strands of native DNA (one cross-link per molecular weight of 10^7), the radioactive counts became associated with the DNA. The amount of radioactivity in DNA purified by alcohol precipitation and by cesium chloride-gradient fractionation corresponded to one mitomycin molecule per 2,500 nucleotide pairs, i.e., per molecular weight of 1.5×10^6. The amount of bound mitomycin depended on its concentration during the reaction with DNA.

In control experiments carried out in the absence of the "activating" (reducing) agent only negligible amounts of radioactivity (1 to 2%) remained associated with the repurified DNA.

In similarly designed experiments the extent of mitomycin binding to denatured DNA or to total *B. subtilis* RNA was only slightly lower, whereas binding to bacterial protein was lower by at least one order of magnitude.

These results show directly that mitomycin could be covalently bound to DNA, with only one out of 5 to 10 antibiotic molecules participating in the cross-link and the others reacting with one strand only. Exposure of *B. subtilis* cells to N-methylmitomycin-^{14}C results in similar binding of the antibiotic to intracellular DNA. Similar results were reported by WEISSBACH and LISSIO (1965), LIPSETT and WEISSBACH (1965) and by WHITE and WHITE (1965a), further confirming the notion that mitomycin cross-links DNA by actual chemical binding to DNA. The study of LIPSETT and WEISSBACH (1965) has shown further that reduced porfiromycin reacts preferentially with guanine, although the reaction with other bases is not negligible. The number of porfiromycin molecules bound per 1000 molecules of bases amounted to 10 for guanine, 3.3 for adenine or cytosine and 2 for uracil. The secondary structure and sequence seem to affect the extent of porfiromycin alkylation, since poly GU is alkylated to a level of 1.3% whereas poly G alkylation approaches only 1%. The homopolymers are alkylated to a much greater extent than sRNA. The latter reaction yielded monoalkylated guanine and diguanyl porfiromycin, but no similar attempts were reported on the direct demonstration of the bases involved in the DNA cross-links.

By experimenting with space-filling models of DNA and of mitomycin, it was attempted to fit the mitomycin molecule as a cross-link between the complementary DNA strands (SZYBALSKI and IYER, 1964a). The short span between sites "1" and "2" on the mitomycin molecule (Fig. 12C), corresponding to only four carbon atoms, limited the choice of the hypothetical linking sites on the DNA molecule compatible with preservation of the largely undistorted double-helical configuration of the native DNA. Cross-links between the N_{-7} positions of the guanines on the opposite DNA strands, similar to those postulated for nitrogen or sulfur mustards (LAWLEY and BROOKES, 1963), are probable, but only when one accepts very gross distortion of the DNA. Even with the mustards, in which the alkylating sites are connected through a five-atom chain (four carbons and one nitrogen or sulfur), a major distortion of the DNA structure is necessary to effect the N_{-7} to N_{-7} links between the nearest guanines on the opposite strands, as ascertained by means of the models. The best fit with the models was obtained by postulating links between the O_{-6} groups of guanines. Alkylation of the latter groups was reported to take place during interaction between guanine and diazomethane (FRIEDMAN *et al.*, 1963, 1965). Since experiments designed to determine indirectly the identity of the cross-linked bases, evaluating the competition for mitomycin between the free nucleotides and DNA, were not interpretable (IYER and SZYBALSKI, 1964), the exact localization of the cross-links must be based on systematic study of the reactions between radioactive mitomycin and DNA or synthetic polydeoxyribonucleotides in single and various double-stranded combinations. Up to this time the participation of diguanyl mitomycin in the interstrand cross-link is a suggestive but far from proven notion. No evidence for formation of dicytidyl or cytidyl-guanyl porfiromycin was found by LIPSETT and WEISSBACH (1965) during treatment of sRNA with reduced porfiromycin. The latter paper was not considered by MURAKAMI (1966), who suggested that mitomycin links the O_{-6} of guanine to the N_{-4} of cytosine by its N_{-4}-C_{-5a}-C_{-5}-O_{-5} configuration (Fig. 1).

Since the mitomycin-induced cross-links are relatively rare, not exceeding 1 per 10^3 nucleotide pairs (IYER and SZYBALSKI, 1963), their localization and determination of the exact chemical structure might prove to be a rather difficult task.

Properties and Applications of Cross-Linked DNA

The stability of the cross-links was evaluated in some detail, since sulfur mustard cross-links involving the N_{-7} position of guanine have been reported to be thermally unstable (LAWLEY and BROOKES, 1963), because of the simultaneous labilization of the N_{-9} to sugar bond; the cleavage of the latter bond would destroy the integrity of the cross-link between the complementary strands. In a comparative study it was found that sulfur mustard cross-links are completely destroyed during thermal denaturation of DNA under conditions innocuous to mitomycin cross-links (BROOKES and SZYBALSKI, unpublished), and that mitomycin cross-links seem to be equally stable to the three different modes of DNA denaturation: a) thermal treatment (6—10 minutes exposure to 98 C in 0.02 M sodium citrate at pH = 7.6 followed by rapid cooling at 0 C); b) exposure to high pH (0.7 g disodium phosphate + 5 ml 1 M sodium hydroxide + water up to 100 ml) for 1 minute at 25 C followed by rapid neutralization with NaH_2PO_4 buffer or hydrochloric acid; or c) exposure to formamide in 0.01 N trisodium·citrate at 37 C. A similar ratio of denatured to spontaneously renatured (cross-linked) DNA was found in all the cases, when multiply cross-linked, non-fractionated DNA was employed as a substrate (SZYBALSKI and IYER, 1964a). Prolonged heating (up to 40 minutes) at 100 C resulted in a somewhat decreased proportion of cross-linked material. Such loss, however, is accountable for by a secondary thermal degradation of the DNA, which in parallel experiments was found to affect to a similar degree both the control and the mitomycin cross-linked DNA. As illustrated in Fig. 4, such scissions would free DNA fragments from their association with covalent cross-links. These results strengthen the previously discussed results, indicating low probability of participation of the N_{-7} position of guanine in the mitomycin cross-links. Using a fractionated population of DNA molecules, each cross-linked with only one mitomycin bridge, permitted more sensitive assessment of the stability of the cross-linked DNA. With this substrate (which was principally used for a sensitive assay of radiation-induced single-strand breaks in DNA; SUMMERS and SZYBALSKI, 1965, 1967a and b) it was found that thermal denaturation could result in the loss of a variable proportion of the cross-linked molecules (SUMMERS and SZYBALSKI (1967a). These losses were less severe when alkali denaturation was employed. Using a still different technique based on measuring the amount of DNA-bound radioactive porfiromycin, WEISSBACH and LISIO (1965) observed some instability of the porfiromycin-alkylated DNA.

When employing adequately high mitomycin concentrations (100 µg/ml or higher), it is possible to cross-link all the bacterial DNA fragments (molecules) of molecular weight 10^7 or higher, both *in vitro* (+ 100 µg sodium hydrosulfite/ml) and *in vivo* (in intact cells). On the other hand, it is not possible to cross-link *in vivo* more than 30—40% of the DNA molecules of similar molecular size in mammalian cells exposed to the mitomycins (SZYBALSKI, 1964). This was not caused by the low G + C content of the DNA, which corresponded to approximately 38—40% for the human cell line D98 S and the rabbit kidney cells employed in this study, since under similar conditions it was possible to cross-link 100% of the *C. johnsonii* DNA, which contains only 33% G + C. Incomplete cross-linking of the mammalian chromosomal DNA might reflect either poor penetration of mitomycin into the cell nucleus or the protection of the mammalian DNA within the chromosomal structure. The latter interpretation is more plausible, since viral DNA placed in the nucleus of mammalian cells is easily cross-linked by mitomycin whereas chromosomal DNA is only partially cross-linked under the same conditions (SZYBALSKI, 1964).

As discussed earlier the activation of mitomycin is closely related to the enzymatic inactivation of mitomycin. Inactivation of mitomycin was reported with extracts from the liver and other organs (SCHWARTZ, 1962; SCHWARTZ and PHILIPS, 1961) and with actinomycetes mycelium (GOUREVITCH *et al.*, 1961). The latter case is interesting, since actinomycetes are resistant to the lethal effects of mitomycin, while its destruction suggests the presence of activating enzymes. Lack of permeability to mitomycin cannot be easily invoked in the case of the mitomycin-producing actinomycetes. Although it is difficult to interpret these data until detailed studies of mitomycin effects on resistant organisms are performed, one might postulate that under prevalent, highly aerobic conditions mitomycin cannot be activated (reduced), whereas under anaerobic conditions it is reduced and inactivated. In the case of mitomycin-resistant *E. coli*, a lower degree of *in vivo* cross-linking was observed than in the corresponding sensitive mutant strains (IYER and SZYBALSKI, 1963). As discussed earlier, the cross resistance between mitomycin and radiation observed with some resistant strains (GREENBERG *et al.*, 1961; GREENBERG and WOODY-KARRER, 1963) is most probably related to the similar repair mechanisms observed for UV or mitomycin damaged DNA (BOYCE and HOWARD-FLANDERS, 1964; HOWARD-FLANDERS *et al.*, 1966). The temperature reactivation of mitomycin-exposed cells (WINKLER, 1962a and b) could also be interpreted by involving the differential effect on the repair mechanism: temporary inhibition of DNA synthesis at high temperature permits the effective elimination of mitomycin-modified bases. Alternatively, the temperature reactivation could be ascribed to differential inactivation of the residual activated form of mitomycin at the increased temperatures, before irreversible DNA cross-linking could be accomplished. Similarly, reaction between residual mitomycin and some components of yeast extract could account for the reactivating effect of yeast extract (SHIBA *et al.*, 1958).

Since reduction of mitomycin is related to both its activation and inactivation process, it was attempted to determine whether the addition of a reducing agent to the medium would have any effect on the lethality of this antibiotic. It was found that sodium borohydride at noninhibitory concentrations (50 µg/ml) reverses almost completely the lethal effects of mitomycin when added within 5 minutes (mammalian cell cultures), or 10 seconds (bacteria), after cell exposure to the antibiotic (SZYBALSKI and ARNESON, 1965). On the other hand, sodium cyanide, 2,4-dinitrophenol and carbonyl cyanide phenylhydrazone, which effect electron transport, strongly synergize the bactericidal action of mitomycin, as does the withdrawal of glucose and inhibition of DNA synthesis by phenethyl alcohol (WHITE and WHITE, 1964, 1965b). These compounds had no such effects on mitomycin toxicity as directed toward mammalian cell cultures (SZYBALSKI and ARNESON, 1965). Thus the redox potential of the medium seems to have a profound effect on the lethal activity of the mitomycins. Cytosine arabinoside (EVANS *et al.*, 1964), 4,6-dinitroquinoline-1-oxide (OKAMOTO *et al.*, 1965), 1,4-naphthoquinone derivatives (MIYAKI, 1963), 6-thioguanine and 5-fluorouracil (SARTORELLI and BOOTH, 1965) were reported to synergize the antineoplastic activity of the mitomycins.

Summary

The antibiotics of the mitomycin group, including the porfiromycins, are rather stable compounds in their natural oxidized state, but upon chemical or enzymatic reduction become converted to highly reactive, bifunctional alkylating agents which form covalent bonds with nucleic acids, proteins and any other suitable molecules in the target cell. It appears, however, that in most cases the true lethal reaction is (I) the formation of mitomycin cross-links between the complementary DNA strands, although it cannot be excluded that (II) monofunctional attack on DNA might be lethal, especially in organisms with deficient repair (excision) mechanisms. The phenomenon of reversible filament formation by some bacteria exposed to sublethal mitomycin concentrations might either be related to DNA cross-linking and repair or indicate a reaction between reduced mitomycins and some cell wall components leading to inhibition of cross-wall formation.

Alkylation of DNA by reduced mitomycin, the chemical mechanism of which seems to be fairly well understood, results in a chain of ancillary events. Inhibition of DNA replication is the result of steric hindrance imposed by covalent cross-links. Breakdown of DNA in some but not in all types of cells is most probably associated either with excision and repair of alkylated DNA or with appearance of new nucleases associated with the mitomycin induction of lysogenic (normal or defective) phages. Inhibition of the synthesis of RNA and of induced enzyme becomes evident only a long time after the suppression of DNA synthesis and is probably related to the loss of DNA integrity and template function for the DNA transcription and RNA translation processes. The changes in morphology and in many cell functions could all be related to this chain of sublethal or lethal events initiated by mono- and bifunctional alkylation of DNA by the mitomycins.

Acknowledgments. We gratefully acknowledge helpful discussions with colleagues at the University of Wisconsin, and especially with Drs. J. A. MILLER, J. D. SCRIBNER, C. HEIDELBERGER, P. BROOKES, W. C. SUMMERS, and H. H. MUXFELDT. Our ideas about the mechanism of *in vitro* activation of mitomycin were a direct outcome of consultations with Drs. J. A. MILLER and J. D. SCRIBNER. Drs. W. A. REMERS and J. S. WEBB of the Lederle Laboratories, and W. C. SUMMERS of this laboratory read the manuscript and contributed many helpful suggestions. We are also thankful to Dr. REMERS for pointing out to us that Dr. J. B. PATRICK independently proposed at a Gordon Research Conference a scheme of mitomycin action similar to that outlined in Fig. 11. Dr. S. WAKAKI of Kyowa Hakko Kogyo Co., Tokyo generously supplied us with mitomycins and sent us translations of the papers of MIYAMURA *et al.* (1966), which permitted us to prepare Table 2 listing the activities of a great variety of mitomycin derivatives, and of OBOSHI *et al.* (1966) and USUBUCHI *et al.* (1966).

Drs. G. R. ALLEN JR., and N. BOHONOS of the Lederle Laboratories, Dr. C. C. CULVENOR of the C.S.I.R.O., Melbourne, Australia, Dr. L. B. CLAPP of Brown University, Dr. P. E. FANTA of the Illinois Institute of Technology, Dr. O. M. FRIEDMAN of Brandeis University, Dr. E. R. GARRETT of the University of Florida, Dr. T. HATA of the Kitasato Institute, Tokyo, Drs. H. and W. KERSTEN of the University of Muenster, Drs. A. LOVELESS, W. C. J. ROSS and G. P. WARWICK of the Chester Beatty Research Institute, London, Drs. C. B. REESE and M. J. WARRING of Cambridge University, Drs. W. SCHROEDER and G. M. SAVAGE of the Upjohn Co., Drs. H. S. SCHWARTZ and F. S. PHILIPS of the Sloan-Kettering Institute, New York, Dr. C. L. STEVENS of Wayne University, Dr. A. WEISSBACH of the N.I.H., Bethesda, and Dr. R. B. WOODWARD of Harvard University contributed information for this chapter which is gratefully acknowledged.

We are also indebted to Dr. ELIZABETH H. SZYBALSKA for editorial help.

The original work included in this chapter was supported in part by Grants G-18165 and B-14976 from the National Science Foundation, Grant-CA-07175 from the National Cancer Institute and the Alexander and Margaret Stewart Trust Fund.

Contribution No. 603 from the Microbiology Research Institute, Canada Department of Agriculture.

References

AKAMATSU, N., H. KAJI, and T. ARAI: On the mechanism of action of mitomycin C. Ann. Rep. Inst. Food Microbiology, Chiba University **15**, 74 (1963).

ALBERTSSON, P.-A.: Partition of double-stranded and single-stranded deoxy-ribonucleic acid. Arch. Biochem. Biophys., Suppl. **1**, 264 (1962).

ALLEN, E., and W. SEAMAN: Method of assay for ethylenimine derivatives. Anal. Chem. **27**, 540 (1955).

ALLEN, JR., G. R., J. F. POLETTO, and M. J. WEISS: The mitomycin antibiotics. Synthetic studies. II. The synthesis of 7-methoxymitosene an antibacterial agent. J. Am. Chem. Soc. **86**, 3877 (1964a).

ALLEN, JR., G. R., J. F. POLETTO, and M. J. WEISS: The mitomycin antibiotics. Synthetic studies. III. Related indoloquinones, active antibacterial agents. J. Am. Chem. Soc. **86**, 3878 (1964b).

ALLEN, JR., G. R., J. F. POLETTO, and M. J. WEISS: The mitomycin antibiotics. Synthetic studies. V. Preparation of 7-methoxymitosene. J. Org. Chem. **30**, 2897 (1965).

ALLEN, JR., G. R., C. PIDACKS, and M. J. WEISS: The mitomycin antibiotics. Synthetic studies. XIV. The Nenitzescu indole synthesis. Formation of isomeric indoles and reaction mechanism. J. Am. Chem. Soc. **88**, 2536 (1966).

ALLEN, JR., G. R., and M. J. WEISS: The mitomycin antibiotics. Synthetic studies. VI. Transformation in the 2,3-dihydro-1H-pyrrolo[1,2-*a*]indole system. J. Org. Chem. **30**, 2904 (1965).

ANONYMOUS: Bibliography of mitomycin C, p. 1—49. Tokyo: Kyowa Hakko Kogyo Co., Lt. 1962.

BACH, M. K., and W. E. MAGEE: Interrelationships between the synthesis of host- and vaccinia-DNA. Federation Proc. **21**, 463 (1962).

BALASSA, G.: Action de la mitomycine C sur la transformation du Pneumocoque. Ann. Inst. Pasteur **102**, 547 (1962).

BEN-PORAT, T., M. REISSIG, and A. S. KAPLAN: Effect of mitomycin C on the synthesis of infective virus and deoxyribonucleic acid in pseudorabies virus-infected rabbit kidney cells. Nature **190**, 33 (1961).

BIELIAVSKY, N.: Effects de la mitomycine sur l'incorporation de la thymidine tritiée dans les embryons d'amphibiens au stade morula. Exptl. Cell Research **32**, 342 (1963).

BLOOM, B. R., L. D. HAMILTON, and M. W. CHASE: Effects of mitomycin C on the cellular transfer of delayed-type hypersensitivity in the guinea pig. Nature **201**, 689 (1964).

BORENFREUND, E., M. KRIM, and A. BENDICH: Effects of mitomycin C on the infection of cells by polyoma virus and its DNA. Virology **25**, 393 (1965).

BOYCE, R. P.: Production of additional sites of deoxyribonucleic acid breakdown in bromouracil containing *Escherichia coli* exposed to ultra-violet light. Nature **209**, 688 (1966).

BOYCE, R. P., and P. HOWARD-FLANDERS: Genetic control of DNA breakdown and repair in *E. coli* K-12 treated with mitomycin C or ultraviolet light. Z. Vererbungsl. **95**, 345 (1964).

CHEER, S., and T. T. TCHEN: Effect of mitomycin C on the synthesis of induced β-galactosidase in *E. coli*. Biochem. Biophys. Research Commun. **9**, 271 (1962).

CHEER, S., and T. T. TCHEN: Effect of mitomycin C on induced enzyme synthesis in *Escherichia coli*. Bacteriol. Proc. 38 (1963).

CLARK, A. J., and A. D. MARGULIES: Isolation and characterization of recombination-deficient mutants of *Escherichia coli* K 12. Proc. Natl. Acad. Sci. U.S. **53**, 451 (1965).

COHEN, M. M., and M. W. SHAW: Effects of mitomycin C on human chromosomes. J. Cell Biol. **23**, 386 (1964).

COLES, N. W., and R. GROSS: The effect of mitomycin C on the induced synthesis of penicillinase in *Staphylococcus aureus*. Biochem. Biophys. Research Commun. **20**, 366 (1965).

CONSTANTOPOULOS, G., and T. T. TCHEN: Enhancement of mitomycin C-induced breakdown of DNA by inhibitors of protein synthesis. Biochim. et Biophys. Acta **80**, 456 (1964).

COOPER, S., and N. D. ZINDER: The growth of an RNA bacteriophage: The role of DNA synthesis. Virology **18**, 405 (1962).

CULVENOR, C. C. J., A. T. DANN, and A. T. DICK: Alkylation as the mechanism by which the hepatotoxic pyrrolozidine alkaloids act on cell nuclei. Nature **195**, 570 (1962).

CUMMINGS, D. J.: Macromolecular synthesis during synchronous growth of *Escherichia coli* B/r. Biochim. et Biophys. Acta **85**, 341 (1965).

CUMMINGS, D. J., and A. L. TAYLOR: Thymineless death and its relation to UV sensitivity in *Escherichia coli*. Proc. Natl. Acad. Sci. U.S. **56**, 171 (1966).

DE BOER, D., A. DIETZ, N. E. LUMMIS, and G. M. SAVAGE: Porfiromycin, a new antibiotic. I. Discovery and biological activities. In: Antimicrobial Agents Annual 1960, p. 17—22. New York: Plenum Press 1961.

DE WITT, W., and D. R. HELINSKI: Characterization of colicinogenic factor E, from a non-induced and mitomycin C-induced *Proteus* strain. J. Mol. Biol. **13**, 692 (1965).

DRISKELL-ZAMENHOF, P. J., and E. A. ADELBERG: Studies on the chemical nature and size of sex factors of *Escherichia coli* K 12. J. Mol. Biol. **6**, 483 (1963).

DUDNIK, J. V.: Induction of lysogenic *Micrococcus lysodeikticus* by antibiotics with ability to affect DNA synthesis. Antibiotiki **2**, 112 (1965).

DURHAM, N. N.: Inhibition of microbial growth and separation by D-serine, vancomycin, and mitomycin C. Bacteriol. J. **86**, 380 (1963).

EPSTEIN, J., R. W. ROSENTHAL, and R. J. ESS: Use of γ-(4-nitrobenzyl) pyridine as analytical reagent for ethylenimines and alkylating agents. Anal. Chem. **27**, 1435 (1955).

ERIKSON, R. L., and W. SZYBALSKI: The Cs_2SO_4 equilibrium density gradient and its application for the study of T-even phage DNA: Glucosylation and replication. Virology **22**, 111 (1964).

EVANS, A. E.: Mitomycin C. Cancer Chemoth. Rep. No. 14, 1 (1961).

EVANS, J. S., E. A. MUSSER, and J. E. GRAY: Porfiromycin antitumor and toxicopathologic studies. Antibiotics & Chemotherapy **11**, 445 (1961).

EVANS, J. S., L. BOSTWICK, and G. D. MENGEL: Synergism of the antineoplastic activity of cytosine arabinoside by porfiromycin. Biochem. Pharmacol. **13**, 983 (1964).

FRIEDMAN, O. M., G. N. MAHAPATRA, and R. STEVENSON: The methylation of deoxyribonucleosides by diazomethane. Biochim. et Biophys. Acta **68**, 144 (1963).

FRIEDMAN, O. M., G. N. MAHAPATRA, B. DASH, and R. STEVENSON: Studies on the action of diazomethane on deoxyribonucleic acid. The action of diazomethane on ribonucleosides. Biochim. et Biophys. Acta **103**, 286 (1965).

GARRETT, E. R.: The physical chemical characterization of the products, equilibrium, and kinetics of the complex transformations of the antibiotic porfiromycin. J. Med. Chem. **6**, 488 (1963).

GARRETT, E. R., and W. SCHROEDER: Prediction of stability in pharmaceutical preparations. XIII. Stability, spectrophotometric, and biological assay of the antibiotic porfiromycin in pharmaceutically useful pH ranges. J. Pharm. Sci. **53**, 917 (1964).

GAUSE, G. F., G. V. KOCHETKOVA, and G. B. VLADIMIROVA: Mutants with impaired respiration in *Staphylococcus afermentans*. J. Gen. Microbiol. **30**, 29 (1963).

GEISSLER, E.: Untersuchungen über den Mechanismus der Induktion lysogener Bakterien. IX. Die Temperaturabhängigkeit der Induktion durch Thymin-Mangel und Mitomycin C. Biochim. et Biophys. Acta **114**, 116 (1966).

GOUREVITCH, A., T. A. PURSIANO, and J. LEIN: Destruction of mitomycin by *Streptomyces caespitosus* mycelia. Arch. Biochem. Biophys. **93**, 283 (1961).

GREENBERG, J., J. D. MANDELL, and P. L. WOODY: Resistance and cross-resistance of *Escherichia coli* mutants to antitumour agent mitomycin C. J. Gen. Microbiol. **26**, 509 (1961).

GREENBERG, J., and P. WOODY-KARRER: Radiosensitivity in *Escherichia coli*. J. Gen. Microbiol. **33**, 283 (1963).

GRULA, E. A., and M. M. GRULA: Cell division in a species of *Erwinia*. V. Effect of metabolic inhibitors on terminal division and composition of a "division" medium. J. Bacteriol. **84**, 492 (1962a).

GRULA, M. M., and E. A. GRULA: Reversal of mitomycin C-induced growth and division inhibition in a species of *Erwinia*. Nature **195**, 1126 (1962b).

HATA, T., Y. SANO, R. SUGAWARA, A. MATSUMAE, K. KANAMORI, T. SHIMA, and T. HOSHI: Mitomycin, a new antibiotic from Streptomyces. I. J. Antibiotics (Japan), Ser. A **9**, 141 (1956).

HERCIK, F.: Effects of mitomycin and alpha-rays on the capacity of *Escherichia coli* B for phage T3. Folia Biol. (Prague) **9**, 42 (1963).

HERR, R. R., M. E. BERGY, T. E. EBLE, and H. K. JAHNKE. Porfiromycin, a new antibiotic. In: Antimicrobial Agents Annual 1960, p. 23. New York: Plenum Press 1961.

HIRAGA, S.: Regulation of synthesis of alkaline phosphatase by deoxyribonucleic acid synthesis in a constitutive mutant of *Bacillus subtilis*. J. Bacteriol. **91**, 2192 (1966).

HOLLIDAY, R.: The induction of mitotic recombination by mitomycin C in Ustilago and Saccharomyces. Genetics **50**, 323 (1964).

HOWARD-FLANDERS, P., R. P. BOYCE, and L. THERIOT: Three loci in *Escherichia coli* K-12 that control the excission of pyrimidine dimers and certain other mutagen products from DNA. Genetics **53**, 1119 (1966).

IIJIMA, T.: Studies on the colicinogenic factor in *Escherichia coli* K12. Induction of colicin production by mitomycin C. Biken's J. **5**, 1 (1962).

IIJIMA, T., and A. HAGAWARA: Mutagenic action of mitomycin C on *Escherichia coli*. Nature **185**, 395 (1960).

IWABUCHI, M., T. SAHO, and S. TANIFUJI: Studies on the factors affecting the rejoining of chromosome breaks produced by X-rays. I. Effects of mitomycin C, chloramphenicol, adenosine triphosphate and nucleosides on the yield of X-ray induced chromosome aberations. Japan. J. Genetics **41**, 379 (1966).

IYER, V. N.: Mutations determining mitomycin resistance in *Bacillus subtilis*. J. Bacteriol. **92**, 1663 (1966).

IYER, V. N., and W. SZYBALSKI: A molecular mechanism of mitomycin action: Linking of complementary DNA strands. Proc. Natl. Acad. Sci. U.S. **50**, 355 (1963).

IYER, V. N., and W. SZYBALSKI: Mitomycins and porfiromycin: Chemical mechanism of activation and cross-linking of DNA. Science **145**, 55 (1964).

KERSTEN, H.: Action of mitomycin C on nucleic acid metabolism in tumor and bacterial cells. Biochim. et Biophys. Acta **55**, 558 (1962a).

KERSTEN, H.: Zur Wirkungsweise von Mitomycin C, I. Einfluß von Mitomycin C auf den Desoxyribonucleinsäure-Abbau in ruhenden Bakterien. Hoppe-Seylers Z. physiol. Chem. **329**, 31 (1962b).

KERSTEN, H., and W. KERSTEN: Zur Wirkungsweise von Mitomycin C. II. Einfluß von Mitomycin C, Chloramphenicol und Mg^{2+} auf den RNA- und DNA-Stoffwechsel in Bakterien. Hoppe-Seyler's Z. physiol. Chem. **334**, 141 (1963).

KERSTEN, H., W. KERSTEN, G. LEOPOLD, and B. SCHNIEDERS: Effect of mitomycin C on DNAase and RNA in *Escherichia coli*. Biochim. et Biophys. Acta **80**, 521 (1964).

KERSTEN, W., H. KERSTEN, and W. SZYBALSKI: Physicochemical properties of complexes between DNA and antibiotics which affect RNA synthesis (actinomycin, daunomycin, cinerubin, nogalamycin, chromomycin, mithramycin, and olivomycin). Biochemistry **5**, 236 (1966).

KERSTEN, H., B. SCHNIEDERS, G. LEOPOLD, and W. KERSTEN: Die Deoxyribonucleasen von *Escherichia coli* und die Wirkung von Mitomycin C. Biochim. et Biophys. Acta **108**, 619 (1965).

KERSTEN, H., and H. M. RAUEN: Degradation of deoxyribonucleic acid in *Escherichia coli* cells treated with mitomycin C. Nature **190**, 1195 (1961).

KERSTEN, H., and H. THEMANN: Morphologische und biochemische Veränderungen an Ascites-Tumorzellen der Maus nach Einwirkung von Mitomycin C. Z. ges. exptl. Med. **136**, 209 (1962).

KIMURA, Y.: Cytological effect of chemicals on tumors. XVII. Effect of mitomycin-C and carzinophilin on HeLa cells. Gann **54**, 163 (1963).

KIRSCH, E. J., and J. D. KORSHALLA: Influence of biological methylation on the biosynthesis of mitomycin A. J. Bacteriol. **87**, 247 (1964).

KIT, S., L. J. PIEKARSKI, and D. R. DUBBS: Effects of 5-fluorouracil, actinomycin D and mitomycin C on the induction of thymidine kinase by vaccinia-infected L-cells. J. Mol. Biol. **7**, 497 (1963).

KNOLLE, P., and F. KAUDEWITZ: Degree of host control on RNA production of an RNA phage. Abstracts, Sixth Int. Congr. Biochem. **3**, 234 (1964).

KOHN, K. W., C. L. SPEARS, and P. DOTY: Inter-strand cross-linking of DNA by nitrogen mustard. Appendix. Terminology of configurational changes of DNA in solution. J. Mol. Biol. **19**, 266 (1966).

KONTANI, H.: Effect of mitomycin C on nucleic acid biosynthesis in Ehrlich ascites tumor cells. Biken's J. **7**, 9 (1964).

KORN, D., and A. WEISSBACH: Thymineless induction in *Escherichia coli* K12(λ). Biochim. et Biophys. Acta **61**, 775 (1962).

KORN, D., and A. WEISSBACH: The effect of lysogenic induction of the deoxyribonucleases of *Escherichia coli* K12(λ). II. The kinetics of formation of a new exonuclease and its relation to phage development. Virology **22**, 91 (1964).

KOSAKA, Y.: A cytological study on abnormal mitosis induced by mitomycin C in cultures of HeLa cell. Mie Med. J. **13**, 51 (1964).

KURODA, Y., and J. FURUYAMA. Physiological and biochemical studies of effects of mitomycin C on strain HeLa cells in cell culture. Cancer Research **23**, 682 (1963).

LAPIS, K., and W. BERNHARD: The effect of mitomycin C on the nucleolar fine structure of KB cells in cell culture. Cancer Research **25**, 628 (1965).

LAWLEY, P. D., and P. BROOKES: Further studies on the alkylation of nucleic acids and their constituent nucleotides. Biochem. J. **89**, 127 (1963).

LEFEMINE, D. V., M. DANN, F. BARBATSCHI, W. K. HAUSMANN, V. ZBINOVSKY, P. MONNIKENDAM, J. ADAM, and N. BOHONOS: Isolation and characterization of mitiromycin and other antibiotics produced by *Streptomyces verticillatus*. J. Am. Chem. Soc. **84**, 3184 (1962).

LEHMAN, I. R.: The nucleases of *Escherichia coli*. Progr. Nucleic Acid Research **2**, 83 (1963).

LEIN, J., B. HEINEMANN, and A. GOUREVITCH: Induction of lysogenic bacteria as a method of detecting potential antitumour agent. Nature **196**, 783 (1962).

LEOPOLD, G., B. SCHNIEDERS, H. KERSTEN, and W. KERSTEN: The effect of mitomycin C on ribosomes and soluble ribonucleic acid in *Escherichia coli*. Biochem. Z. **343**, 423 (1965).

LEVINE, M.: Effect mitomycin C on interactions between temperate phages and bacteria. Virology **13**, 493 (1961).

LEWIS, C., H. W. CLAPP, and H. R. REAMES: Porfiromycin, a new antibiotic. III. In vitro and in vivo evaluation. In: Antimicrobial Agents Annual 1960, p. 27. New York: Plenum Press 1961.

LINDQVIST, B., and R. L. SINSHEIMER: The use of mitomycin C als a selective inhibitor of host DNA synthesis in ΦX174-infected, hcr^- cells. Federation Proc. **25**, 651 (1966).

LIPSETT, M. N., and A. WEISSBACH: The site of alkylation of nucleic acids by mitomycin. Biochemistry **4**, 206 (1965).

MAGEE, W. E., and O. V. MILLER: Dissociation of the synthesis of host and viral deoxyribonucleic acid. Biochim. et Biophys. Acta **55**, 818 (1962).

MANDELL, J. D., and A. D. HERSHEY: A fractionating column for analysis of nucleic acids. Anal. Biochem. **1**, 66 (1960).

MARTIUS, C.: Quinone reductases. In: Enzymes (P. D. BOYER, H. LARDY and K. MYRBÄCK, eds.), vol. 7, p. 517. New York: Academic Press 1963.

MATSUMOTO, I., and K. G. LARK: Altered DNA isolated from cells treated with mitomycin C. Exptl. Cell Research **32**, 192 (1963).

MATSUMOTO, I., and Y. TAKAGI: Action mechanism of mitomycin C. Abstracts of Papers, Ninth Intern. Cancer Congress, Tokyo, 1966, p. 353.

MATSUURA, H., S. TANIFUJI, T. SATO, and M. IWABUCHI: Chromosome studies on *Trillium kamtschaticum* Pall. and its Allies. XXVI. The effect of mitomycin C on the frequency of X-ray-induced chromosome aberations. J. Fac. Sci. Hokkaido Univ., Ser. V, **8**, 75 (1962).

MATSUURA, H., S. TANIFUJI, T. SATO, and M. IWABUCHI: Effect of mitomycin-C on the frequency of chromosome aberrations produced by X-rays. Am. Naturalist **97**, 191 (1963).

MAYNE, E.: Essais d'élimination par l'acridine orange ou la mitomycine d'un facteur colicinogène lié a un facteur de fertilité chez *Escherichia coli*. Ann. Inst. Pasteur **109**, 154 (1965).

MENNIGMANN, H.-D., and W. SZYBALSKI: Molecular mechanism of thymine-less death. Biochem. Biophys. Research Commun. **9**, 398 (1962).

MERZ, T.: Effect of mitomycin C on lateral root-tip chromosomes on *Vicia faba*. Science **133**, 329 (1961).

MIYAKI, K.: Inhibitory effects on the growth of Ehrlich ascites tumor of mitomycin C combined with 1,4-naphthoquinone derivatives. Ann. Rep. Inst. Food Microbiol., Chiba Univ. **15**, 49 (1963), abstracted by Cancer Chemother. Abstr. **5**, 484 (1964).

MIYAMURA, S., N. SHIGENO, M. MATSUI, S. WAKAKI, and K. UZU: The antibacterial studies on mitomycin derivatives. I. Antibacterial activities of mitomycin derivatives. J. Antibiotics (Japan), Ser. A (in press) (1967).

MUNK, K., and G. SAUER: Vermehrung und DNS-Synthese des Herpes-simplex-Virus nach Mitomycin C-Behandlung. Z. Naturforsch. **20**b, 671 (1965).

MURAKAMI, H.: Electron aspects of the mode of action of the mitomycin molecule. J. Theoret. Biol. **10**, 236 (1966).

MUSCHEL, L. H., and K. SCHMOKER: Activity of mitomycin C, other antibiotics, and serum against lysogenic bacteria. J. Bacteriol. **92**, 967 (1966).

NAKATA, Y., K. NAKATA, and Y. SAKAMOTO: On the action mechanism of mitomycin C. Biochem. Biophys. Research Commun. **6**, 339 (1962).

NEWTON, B. A.: Mechanism of antibiotic action. Ann. Rev. Microbiol. **19**, 209 (1965).

NIITANI, H., A. SUZUKI, M. SHIMOYAMA, and K. KIMURA: Effect of mitomycin C injection on lysosomal enzymic activities of Yoshida ascites sarcoma. Gann **55**, 447 (1964).

NYGAARD, A. P., and B. D. HALL: A method for the detection of RNA-DNA complexes. Biochem. Biophys. Research Commun. **12**, 98 (1963).
OBOSHI, S., M. MATSUI, S. ISHII, N. MASAGO, S. WAKAKI, and K. UZU: Antitumor studies on mitomycin derivatives. II. Effect on solid tumor of sarcoma 180. Manuscript to be published (1967).
OKAMOTO, T., Y. HASEGAWA, T. KINOSHITA, M. ISHIGURO, and D. MIZUNO: The anti tumor activity of 4,6-dinitroquinoline 1-oxide. Yakugaku Zasshi **85**, 720 (1965).
OKUBO, S.: Genetic studies on the non-infectious phage produced in the presence of mitomycin C. Biken's J. **5**, 51 (1962).
OKUBO, S., and W. R. ROMIG: Impaired transformability of *Bacillus subtilis* mutant sensitive to mitomycin C and ultraviolet radiation. J. Mol. Biol. **15**, 440 (1966).
OTSUJI, N.: The effect of glucose on the induction of lambda phage formation by mitomycin C. Biken's **4**, 235 (1961).
OTSUJI, N.: DNA synthesis and lambda phage development in a lysogenic strain of *Escherichia coli* K12. Biken's J. **5**, 9 (1962).
OTSUJI, N., M. SEKIGUCHI, T. IIJIMA, and T. TAKAGI: Induction of phage formation in the lysogenic *Escherichia coli* K 12 by mitomycin C. Nature **184**, 1079 (1959).
PARIS, O. E., and P. E. FANTA: Cyclohexenimine (7-azabicyclo[4.1.0]heptane) and the stereochemistry of ethylenimine ring-closure and opening. J. Am. Chem. Soc. **74**, 3007 (1952).
PATRICK, J. B., R. P. WILLIAMS, W. E. MEYER, W. FULMOR, D. B. COSULICH, R. W. BROSCHARD, and J. S. WEBB: Aziridinomitosenes: A new class of antibiotics related to the mitomycins. J. Am. Chem. Soc. **86**, 1889 (1964).
PRICER, JR., W. E., and W. WEISSBACH: The effect of lysogenic induction with mitomycin C on the DNA and DNA polymerase of *Escherichia coli* K12λ. Biochem. Biophys. Research Commun. **14**, 91 (1964).
PRICER, JR., W. E., and A. WEISSBACH: Enzymatic utilization and degradation of DNA treated with mitomycin C or ultraviolet light. Biochemistry **4**, 200 (1965).
RADDING, C. M.: Nuclease activity in defective lysogens of phage λ. Biochem. Biophys. Research Commun. **15**, 8 (1964).
RAO, K. V., K. BIEMANN, and R. B. WOODWARD: The structure of streptonigrin. J. Am. Chem. Soc. **85**, 2532 (1963).
REICH, E.: Actinomycin: correlation of structure and function of its complexes with purines and DNA. Science **143**, 684 (1964).
REICH, E., and R. M. FRANKLIN: Effect of mitomycin C on the growth of some animal viruses. Proc. Natl. Acad. Sci. U.S. **47**, 1212 (1961).
REICH, E., A. J. SHATKIN, and E. L. TATUM: Bacteriocidal action of mitomycin C. Biochim. et Biophys. Acta **45**, 608 (1960).
REICH, E., A. J. SHATKIN, and E. L. TATUM: Bacteriocidal action of mitomycin C. Biochim. et Biophys. Acta **53**, 132 (1961).
REILLY, H. C., J. C. CAPPUCCINO, and D. M. HARRISON: Studies on mitomycin X, a tumor-inhibiting antibiotic. Proc. Am. Assoc. Cancer Research **2**, 338 (1958).
REMERS, W. A., P. N. JAMES, and M. J. WEISS: The mitomycin antibiotics. Synthetic studies. I. Synthesis of model quinones. J. Org. Chem. **28**, 1169 (1963).
REMERS, W. A., R. H. ROTH, and M. J. WEISS: The mitomycin antibiotics. Synthetic studies. IV. Introduction of the 9-hydroxymethyl group into the 1-ketopyrrolo [1,2-*a*]indole system. J. Am. Chem. Soc. **86**, 4612 (1964).
REMERS, W. A., R. H. ROTH, and M. J. WEISS: The mitomycin antibiotics. Synthetic studies. VII. An exploration of pyrrolo[1,2-*a*]indole A-ring chemistry directed toward the introduction of the aziridine function. J. Org. Chem. **30**, 2910 (1965).
REMERS, W. A., and M. J. WEISS: The mitomycin antibiotics. Synthetic studies. IX. A versatile new method of indole synthesis. J. Am. Chem. Soc. **87**, 5262 (1965).
REMERS, W. A., and M. J. WEISS: The mitomycin antibiotics. Synthetic studies. XII. Indoloquinone analogs with variations at positions 5 and 6. J. Am. Chem. Soc. **88**, 804 (1966).
ROSS, W. C. J.: Biological alkylating agents, p. 107. London: Butterworth & Co. 1962.

ROTH, R. H., W. A. REMERS, and M. J. WEISS: The mitomycin antibiotics. Synthetic studies. XIII. Indoloquinone analogs with variation at C-5. J. Org. Chem. **31**, 1012 (1966).
ROTT, R., S. SABER, and C. SCHOLTISSEK: Effect on myxovirus of mitomycin C, actinomycin D, and pretreatment of the host cell with ultra-violet light. Nature **205**, 1187 (1965).
SAKURAI, Y.: *In vitro* culture of Yoshida sarcoma cells: methods for determining acquired resistance to drugs. Natl. Cancer Inst. Monograph No. 16, 207 (1964).
SARTORELLI, A. C., and B. A. BOOTH: The synergistic-anti-neoplastic activity of combinations of mitomycins with either 6-thioguanine or 5-fluorouracil. Cancer Research **25**, 1393 (1965).
SCHATZ, V. B., and L. B. CLAPP: Reactions of ethylenimines. V. Hydrolysis. J. Am. Chem. Soc. **77**, 5113 (1955).
SCHWARTZ, H. S.: Pharmacology of mitomycin C: III. *In vitro* metabolism by rat liver. J. Pharmacol. Exptl. Therap. **136**, 250 (1962).
SCHWARTZ, H. S., and F. S. PHILIPS: Pharmacology of mitomycin C. II. Renal excretion and metabolism by tissue homogenates. J. Pharmacol. Exptl. Therap. **133**, 335 (1961).
SCHWARTZ, H. S., J. E. SODERGREN, and F. S. PHILIPS: Mitomycin C: Chemical and biological studies on alkylation. Science **142**, 1181 (1963a).
SCHWARTZ, H. S., S. S. STERNBERG, and F. S. PHILIPS: Pharmacology of mitomycin C. IV. Effects *in vivo* on nucleic acid synthesis; comparison with actinomycin D. Cancer Research **23**, 1125 (1963b).
SEKIGUCHI, M., and Y. TAKAGI: Synthesis of deoxyribonucleic acid by phage-infected *Escherichia coli* in the presence of mitomycin C. Nature **183**, 1134 (1959).
SEKIGUCHI, M., and Y. TAKAGI: Effect of mitomycin C on the synthesis of bacterial and viral deoxyribonucleic acid. Biochim. et Biophys. Acta **41**, 434 (1960a).
SEKIGUCHI, M., and Y. TAKAGI: Noninfectious bacteriophage produced by the action of mitomycin C. Virology **10**, 160 (1960b).
SHATKIN, A. J., E. REICH, R. M. FRANKLIN, and E. L. TATUM: Effect of mitomycin C on mammalian cells in culture. Biochim. et Biophys. Acta **55**, 277 (1962).
SHAW, M. W., and M. M. COHEN: Chromosome exchanges in human leukocytes induced by mitomycin C. Genetics **51**, 181 (1965).
SHIBA, S., A. TERAWAKI, T. TAGUCHI, and J. KAWAMATA: Studies on the effect of mitomycin C on nucleic acid metabolism in *Escherichia coli* strain B. Biken's J. **1**, 179 (1958).
SHIBA, S., A. TERAWAKI, T. TAGUCHI, and J. KAWAMATA: Selective inhibition of formation of deoxyribonucleic acid in *Escherichia coli* by mitomycin C. Nature **183**, 1056 (1959).
SHIIO, T., G. WEINBAUM, H. TAKAHASHI, and B. MARUO: Chromatographic analysis of nucleotidic compounds in *Bacillus subtilis*. J. Gen. Appl. Microbiol. **8**, 178 (1962).
SMITH-KIELLAND, I.: Effect of mitomycin C on the synthesis of messenger RNA in *Escherichia coli*. Biochim. et Biophys. Acta **91**, 360 (1964).
SMITH-KIELLAND, I.: The effect of mitomycin C on deoxyribonucleic acid and messenger ribonucleic acid in *Escherichia coli*. Biochim. et Biophys. Acta **114**, 254 (1966a).
SMITH-KIELLAND, I.: The effect of mitomycin C on ribonucleic acid synthesis in growing cultures of *Escherichia coli*. Biochim. et Biophys. Acta **119**, 486 (1966b).
STEVENS, C. L., K. G. TAYLOR, M. E. MUNK, W. S. MARSHALL, K. NOLL, G. D. SHAH, L. G. SHAH, and K. UZU: Chemistry and structure of mitomycin C. J. Med. Chem. **8**, 1 (1965).
STUDZINSKI, G. P., and L. S. COHEN: Mitomycin C induced increases in the activities of the deoxyribonucleases of HeLa cells. Biochem. Biophys. Research Commun. **23**, 506 (1966).
SUGAWARA, R., and T. HATA: Mitomycin, a new antibiotic from streptomyces. II. Description of the strain. J. Antibiotics (Japan), Ser. A **9**, 147 (1956).

SUGIURA, K.: Antitumor activity of mitomycin C. Cancer Chemoth. Rep. No. 13, 51 (1961).

SUMMERS, W. C., and W. SZYBALSKI: A sensitive assay for single-strand breaks in DNA molecules. Radiation Research 25, 246 (1965).

SUMMERS, W. C., and W. SZYBALSKI: γ-Irradiation of DNA in dilute solutions. I. A sensitive method for detection of single strand breaks in polydisperse DNA samples. J. Mol. Biol. (in press) (1967a).

SUMMERS, W. C., and W. SZYBALSKI: γ-Irradiation of DNA in dilute solutions. II. Molecular mechanisms responsible for inactivation of phage, its transfecting DNA and of bacterial transforming activity. J. Mol. Biol. (in press) (1967b).

SUTTON, M. D., and C. QUADLING: Lysogeny in a strain of *Xanthomonas campestris*. Can. J. Microbiol. 9, 821 (1963).

SUZUKI, D. T.: Effects of mitomycin C on crossing over in *Drosophila melanogaster*. Genetics **51**, 635 (1965).

SUZUKI, H., and W. W. KILGORE: Mitomycin C: effect on ribosomes of *Escherichia coli*. Science **146**, 1585 (1964).

SUZUKI, K., H. YAMAGAMI, and Y. SHIMAZU: Effect of mitomycin C on early phenotypic expression in the transformation of *Diplococcus pneumoniae*. Nature **205**, 929 (1965).

SZYBALSKI, W.: Special microbiological systems. II. Observations on chemical mutagenesis in microorganisms. Ann. N.Y. Acad. Sci. **76**, 475 (1958).

SZYBALSKI, W.: Gradient plate technique for study of bacterial resistance. Science **116**, 46 (1962).

SZYBALSKI, W.: Chemical reactivity of chromosomal DNA as related to mutagenicity: Studies with human cell lines. Cold Spring Harbor Symposia Quant. Biol. **29**, 151 (1964).

SZYBALSKI, W.: Effect of elevated temperatures on DNA and some polynucleotides: Denaturation, renaturation and cleavage of glycosidic and phosphate ester bands. In: Thermobiology (A. H. ROSE, Ed.), Chapter 4. London: Academic Press (in press) 1967.

SZYBALSKI, W., and V. G. ARNESON: Reductive activation and inactivation of mitomycin as studied with human and bacterial cell cultures. Molecul. Pharmacol. **1**, 202 (1965).

SZYBALSKI, W., and V. N. IYER: Cross-linking of DNA by enzymatically or chemically activated mitomycins and porfiromycins, bifunctionally "alkylating" antibiotics. Federation Proc. **23**, 946 (1964a).

SZYBALSKI, W., and V. N. IYER: Binding of C^{14}-labeled mitomycin or porfiromycin to nucleic acids. Microbial Genetics Bull. No. 21, 16 (1964b).

SZYBALSKI, W., G. RAGNI, and N. K. COHN: Mutagenic response of human somatic cell lines. In: Cytogenetics of cells in culture. Symp. Int. Soc. Cell Biol. **3**, 209 (1964); New York: Academic Press.

SZYBALSKI, W., and M. J. SMITH: Genetics of human cell lines. I. 8-Azaguanine resistance, a selective "single-step" marker. Proc. Soc. Exptl. Biol. Med. **101**, 662 (1959).

TAKAGI, Y.: Action of mitomycin C. Japan J. Med. Sci. Biol. **16**, 246 (1963).

TERAWAKI, A., and GREENBERG: Inactivation of transforming deoxyribonucleic acid by carcinophillin and mitomycin C. Biochim. et Biophys. Acta **119**, 59 (1966a).

TERAWAKI, A., and J. GREENBERG: Post-treatment breakage of mitomycin C induced cross-links in deoxyribonucleic acid of *Escherichia coli*. Biochim. et Biophys. Acta **119**, 540 (1966b).

TRUHAUT, R., and G. DEYSSON: Etude des propriétés antimitotiques de la mitomycine C sur les cellules méristématiques d'*Allium sativum* L. Compt. rend. soc. biol. **154**, 718 (1960).

TSUKAMURA, M., and S. TSUKAMURA: Mutagenic effect of mitomycin C on Mycobacterium and its combined effect with ultraviolet irradiation. Japan J. Microbiol. **6**, 53 (1962).

TULINSKY, A.: The structure of mitomycin A. J. Am. Chem. Soc. **84**, 3188 (1962).

UMEZAWA, H.: Recent advances in chemistry and biochemistry of antibiotics, 266 p. Microb. Chem. Res. Found., Tokyo 1964.
USUBUCHI, I., Y. SOBAJIMA, T. HONGO, T. KAWAGUCHI, M. SUGAWARA, M. MATSUI, S. WAKAKI, and K. UZU: Antitumor studies on mitomycin derivatives. I. Effect on ascites Hirosaki sarcoma. Manuscript to be published (1967).
UZU, K., M. SHIMIZU, R. KOJIMA, T. OGAMI, S. WAKAKI, H. ENDO, and M. MATSUI: Mechanism of mitomycin derivatives. Abstracts of Papers, Ninth Intern. Cancer Congress, Tokyo, 1966, p. 354, and personal communication.
VIGIER, P., et A. GOLDE: Action de l'actinomycine D et de la mitomycine C sur le développement du virus de Rous. Compt. rend. **258**, 389 (1964a).
VIGIER, P., and A. GOLDE: Effects of actinomycin D and mitomycin C on development of Rous sarcoma virus. Virology **23**, 511 (1964b).
WAKAKI, S.: Recent advance in research on antitumor mitomycins. Cancer Chemoth. Rep. No. 13, 79 (1961).
WAKAKI, S., H. MARUMO, K. TOMIOKA, G. SHIMIZU, E. KATO, H. KAMADA, S. KUDO, and Y. FUJIMOTO: Isolation of new fractions of antitumor mitomycins. Antibiotics and Chemotherapy **8**, 228 (1958).
WARING, M. J.: Cross-linking and intercalation in nucleic acids. 16th Symp. Soc. Gen. Microbiol. 1966, p. 235—265.
WEBB, J. S., D. B. COSULICH, J. H. MOWAT, J. B. PATRICK, R. W. BROSCHARD, W. E. MEYER, R. P. WILLIAMS, C. F. WOLF, W. FULMOR, C. PIDACKS, and J. E. LANCASTER: The structures of mitomycins A, B and C and porfiromycin — Part I. J. Am. Chem. Soc. **84**, 3185 (1962).
WEISSBACH, A., and D. KORN: The effect of lysogenic induction on the deoxyribonucleases of *Escherichia coli* K12λ. J. Biol. Chem. **234**, PC 3312 (1962).
WEISSBACH, A., and A. LISIO: Alkylation of nucleic acids by mitomycin C and porfiromycin. Biochemistry **4**, 196 (1965).
WHITE, J. R., and H. L. WHITE: Phenethyl alcohol synergism with mitomycin C, porfiromycin, and streptonigrin. Science **145**, 1312 (1964).
WHITE, H. A., and J. R. WHITE: The binding of porfiromycin to deoxyribonucleic acid. J. Elisha Mitchell Sci. Soc. **81**, 37 (1965a).
WHITE, J. R., and H. L. WHITE: Effect of intracellular redox environment on bactericidal action of mitomycin C and streptonigrin. In: Antimicrobial Agents and Chemotherapy — 1964, 495 (1965b).
WINKLER, U.: Über die Inaktivierung UV-sensibler, UV-resistenter und Mitomycin C-resistenter Mutanten von *E. coli* B mit UV und Mitomycin C. Naturwissenschaften **49**, 91 (1962a).
WINKLER, U.: Über die Abhängigkeit der bakteriziden Wirkung von Mitomycin C auf *E. coli* B und B/MC von der Temperatur und dem Nährmedium. Z. Naturforsch. **17b**, 670 (1962b).
YOSHIOKA, M., and T. KUNII: Antibiotic resistant group A streptococci. III. Penicillin resistance and mitomycin C inactivation of mutants which lose soluble hemolysis production. Japan J. Microbiol. **10**, 43 (1966).
YUKI, S.: The effect of mitomycin C on the recombination in *Escherichia coli* K 12. Biken's J. **5**, 47 (1962).

Chromomycin, Olivomycin and Mithramycin

G. F. Gause

Three chemically related cancerostatic antibiotics — chromomycin (toyomycin), olivomycin and mithramycin — have been studied in some detail in recent years. Chromomycin was isolated in Japan, olivomycin in the U.S.S.R. and mithramycin in the United States. The structure of molecules in these antibiotics is similar, but not identical; there are also some differences in the toxicity and pharmacology of these products, which have been compared in a recent review (GAUSE, 1965). Biochemical mechanisms of action of these antibiotics have much in common.

Chromomycin

Chromomycin is produced by *Streptomyces griseus* strain 7 as a complex of closely related variants (TATSUOKA *et al.*, 1958). The main variant was named chromomycin A_3, and the chemical structure of this compound was studied in detail (MIZUNO, 1963; TATSUOKA *et al.*, 1964; MIYAMOTO *et al.*, 1964a, b, c).

It was observed that chromomycin A_3 can be hydrolyzed with 50% acetic acid to give lipid-soluble and water-soluble fractions. From the lipid-soluble fraction a yellow crystalline substance, chromomycinone, containing a saturated carbonyl group, was isolated; the elementary analysis of this substance and the molecular weight measured by the osmotic pressure method were in agreement with the empirical formula $C_{21}H_{24}O_9$. It was also shown that chromomycinone retains the original chromophore of chromomycin A_3.

By repeated chromatography of the water-soluble fraction, four new sugars were isolated in crystalline form. These were named chromose A, B, C, and D, and their structures have been established (MIYAMOTO *et al.*, 1963, 1964c):

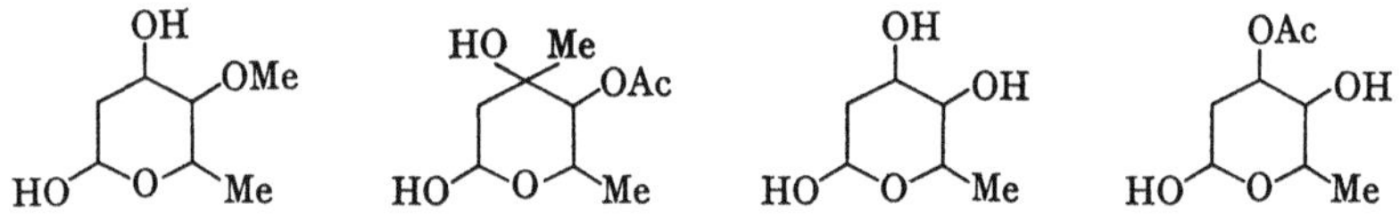

Chromose A   Chromose B   Chromose C   Chromose D

The structure of the chromomycinone, the aglycone of chromomycin A_3, has also been published (MIYAMOTO *et al.*, 1964a). The structural formula for chromomycin A_3 proposed by TATSUOKA *et al.* (Fig. 1) shows that this antibiotic consists of chromophore (chromomycinone), to which four sugars (chromoses A, B, C, D) are attached in the sequence indicated. However, final agreement on the structure of chromomycin A_3 has not yet been reached. Another possible structural formula for this antibiotic is shown in Fig. 2. It has a slightly different configuration of the chromophore, and chromose B and chromose C are attached to the chromophore at a position different from that of chromose A and chromose D (MIYAMOTO *et al.*, 1966).

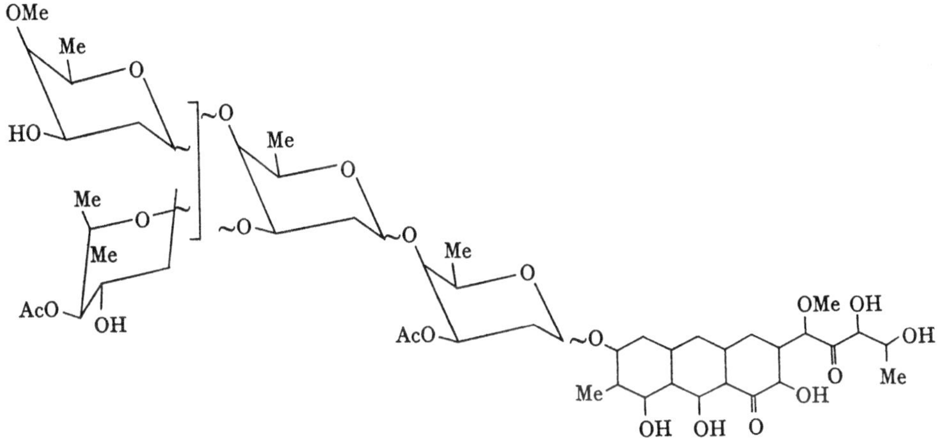

Fig. 1. The structure of chromomycin A_3 from TATSUOKA *et al.* (1964)

Chromomycin A_3 inhibits the growth of *Staphylococcus aureus* and *Bacillus subtilis* at minimum inhibitory concentrations of 0.10 and 0.15 μg/ml, respectively (KAZIWARA *et al.*, 1960, 1961). It also inhibits growth of *Mycobacterium smegmatis*, the minimal bacteriostatic concentration attains 5 μg/ml (TSUKAMURA *et al.*, 1964; TSUKAMURA, 1965). Chromomycin A_3 is inactive against Gram-negative bacteria and fungi.

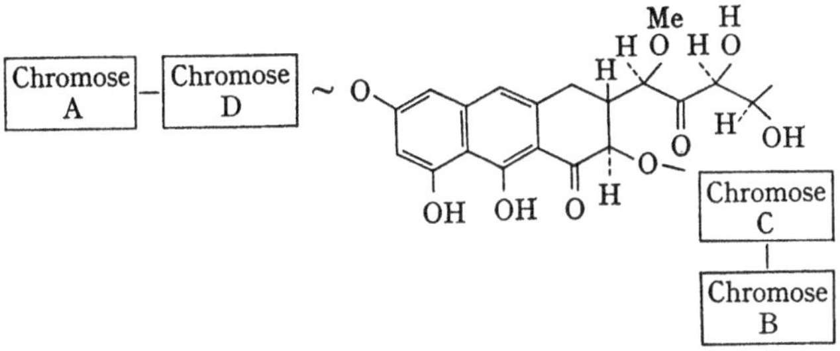

Fig. 2. Probable structure of chromomycin A_3 according to MIYAMOTO *et al.* (1966)

Chromomycin A_3 strongly inhibits multiplication of HeLa cells in tissue culture at the lowest concentration of 0.01 μg/ml (TAKAKI *et al.*, 1960). SATO *et al.* (1960) reported similar results for various other strains of tumor cells grown in vitro.

The study of acute toxicity of chromomycin A_3 has shown that the LD_{50} in mice is 2.1 mg/kg (intraperitoneal; KAZIWARA *et al.*, 1961) and 1.21 mg/kg (intravenous; CHORIN and ROSSOLIMO, 1965).

Some morphological effects of chromomycin A_3 have been observed by BRAHMACHARY and REVERBERI (1964). They studied the action of solutions of chromomycin on eggs and embryos of *Ciona intestinalis* and observed marked effect on the late gastrula stage, with the appearance of abnormal larvae.

The biochemical mechanism of the inhibitory action of chromomycin A_3 was studied by WAKISAKA *et al.* (1963). Chromomycin selectively inhibits the biosynthesis of ribonucleic acid (RNA) in cultures of mammalian cells (rabbit bone marrow cells and leukemic human leucocytes), whereas the formation of deoxyribonucleic acid (DNA) is not affected, as can be seen from the data shown in Table 1.

Table 1. *Effects of chromomycin A_3 on incorporation of adenine-^{14}C into nucleic acids of leukemic human leucocytes*[1]

Concentration of chromomycin A_3 (μg/ml)	Specific activities (cpm/μmole P)	
	RNA	DNA
0	8.970	101
10	5.970	102
100	4.850	109

[1] From WAKISAKA *et al.* (1963).

It was reported that chromomycin A_3 selectively inhibits DNA dependent RNA synthesis as a result of binding of this antibiotic to cellular DNA (HARTMANN *et al.*, 1964; KERSTEN and KERSTEN, 1965). The capacity of chromomycin to form complexes with native DNA can be recognized by decreased buoyant density in cesium chloride gradient. For example, the density of *Sarcina lutea* DNA (1.731 gm/cm^3) changes in the presence of chromomycin (0.4 μM) to 1.670 to 1.710 gm/cm^3 (KERSTEN, KERSTEN and SZYBALSKI, 1965). DNA binding can be followed also by cosedimentation of the DNA-antibiotic complexes and by the spectral shifts. Two other related antibiotics, olivomycin and mithramycin, are in this respect similar to chromomycin. On the other hand, these antibiotics have no effect on the melting temperature of DNA or on its hydrodynamic properties, including viscosity and sedimentation coefficient, properties which are strongly affected by the other DNA-complexing antibiotics, such as actinomycins and anthracyclines (daunomycin, cinerubin, nogalamycin, and others).

WARD, REICH and GOLDBERG (1965) have shown that chromomycin A_3 inhibits RNA synthesis, but only when the governing template is a DNA preparation which contains guanine. Spectrophotometric analysis of the chromomycin-polynucleotide interaction has revealed the following features (WARD, REICH and GOLDBERG, 1965):

1. The spectrum of chromomycin A_3 is altered by Mg^{++} (and by Ca^{++}, Cu^{++}, Mn^{++}, Co^{++}, and Zn^{++}), and by polyamines, but not by Na^+, Li^+, K^+, or Cs^+ ions. The spectral changes evoked by the divalent cations differ somewhat, qualitatively and quantitatively. In the case of the closely related antibiotic olivomycin, these spectral changes were previously reported by BRAZHNIKOVA *et al.* (1964) and related to the capacity of this antibiotic to form complexes with metals. This material will be discussed in more detail in the section of this review dealing with olivomycin.

2. The spectrum of chromomycin A_3 is not altered by polynucleotides in the absence of bivalent cations (Fig. 3). Of the cations tested only Mg^{++}, Mn^{++}, Zn^{++} and, to a lesser extent, Co^{++}, can promote the DNA-chromomycin interaction.

3. The magnitude of the spectral alterations of chromomycin A_3 produced by DNA is a function of Mg^{++} concentration. The amount of Mg^{++} required to promote maximum DNA-antibiotic interaction corresponds to a 1:1 molar equivalence with antibiotic concentration. It follows that the metal probably exerts its effect primarily through a prior interaction with chromomycin A_3 (not by altering the structure of DNA), and that it is the antibiotic-Mg^{++} complex which binds to DNA. The Mg^{++} requirement for chromomycin binding to DNA is also observed if DNA is precipitated by alcohol from chromomycin solutions — the precipitate is yellow in the presence and white in the absence of Mg^{++}.

4. Heat denatured DNA is quantitatively much less effective than native DNA in producing spectral shifts of chromomycin A_3 (Fig. 3).

5. No spectral changes of chromomycin A_3 are produced by RNA, even in the presence of Mg^{++}, nor by any of the normal ribo- or deoxyribonucleosides or nucleotides. This is in contrast with actinomycin which has been shown to react indiscriminately with purine nucleosides and analogues.

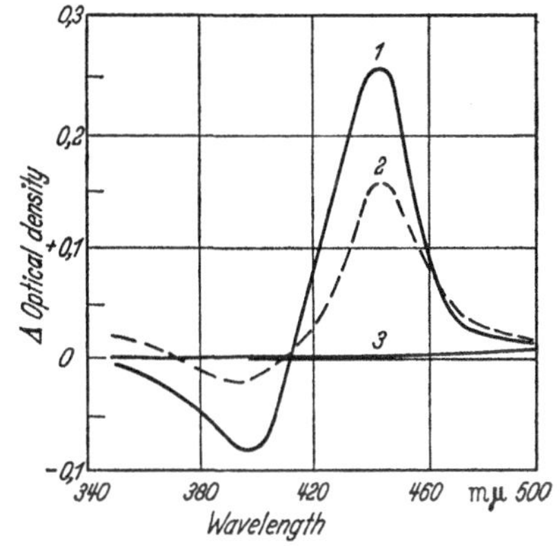

Fig. 3. Effect of Mg^{++} on the interaction of chromomycin A_3 with DNA. Difference spectra of chromomycin solutions (100 mμ moles/ml) read against the same solutions containing DNA (425 mμ moles/ml). Curve 1, native calf thymus (C.T.) DNA, and curve 2, heat denatured C.T. DNA in 0.01 M Tris-HCl, pH 7.4, 0.01 M NaCl containing 0.05 M $MgCl_2$. Curve 3, same as curve 1, but without $MgCl_2$. (From WARD, REICH and GOLDBERG, 1965)

6. The maximum binding capacity for chromomycin A_3 of DNA preparations (per unit phosphorus) increases slightly as their guanine content increases.

7. The interaction between chromomycin A_3 and DNA is unaffected by elevated ionic strengths (1 M NaCl and 5 M CsCl) but is reduced by urea.

8. The behavior of mithramycin and olivomycin is qualitatively indistinguishable from that of chromomycin A_3 in all spectral tests. In addition, neither mithramycin nor olivomycin inhibit RNA synthesis directed by synthetic DNA polymers containing deoxyadenine and deoxythymine at concentrations which completely inhibit the same reaction directed by calf thymus DNA.

The reaction between chromomycin A_3 and Mg^{++}, and the requirement of the latter for the chromomycin-DNA interaction are of considerable interest. Since Mg^{++} alters the visible and UV spectrum of chromomycin A_3, the metal must complex in some way directly either with atoms forming part of, or with functional groups which can be conjugated with, the chromophore. One or more of the numerous available oxygen-containing groups attached to the chromophore seems likely to mediate Mg^{++} binding. Because the spectral alterations produced by DNA appear to accentuate those produced by Mg^{++}, the structural definition of the antibiotic-Mg^{++} complex may provide insight into the nature of the complex subsequently formed with DNA.

Olivomycin

Olivomycin is produced by *Streptomyces olivoreticuli* strain 16,749 (GAUSE, UKHOLINA and SVESHNIKOVA, 1962). The antibiotic can be isolated in the form of crystalline acid from the culture fluid of this organism. The study of crystalline preparations of olivomycin by the counter-current distribution method showed that this substance represents a complex of closely related variants, and the principal component of the complex was named olivomycin I (BRAZHNIKOVA *et al.*, 1962, 1964a). The elementary composition of olivomycin I is similar to that of chromomycin A_3 and mithramycin, as it is shown in Table 2.

Table 2.
Elementary composition of acid forms of olivomycin, chromomycin and mithramycin

Antibiotic	C	H	O	Author
Olivomycin I	57.23	7.36	35.41	BRAZHNIKOVA *et al.* (1962, 1964a)
Chromomycin A_3	56.50	7.23	36.27	MIZUNO (1963)
Mithramycin	55.98	7.39	36.63	RAO *et al.* (1962)

The three antibiotics are similar in certain chemical and physical properties and color reactions. However, each is different and can be separated from the others. Four solvent systems were developed for the paper chromatography of olivomycin and related substances (KRUGLYAK *et al.*, 1963):

1. Benzene-acetic acid-water (20:25:5).
2. Benzene-butanol-water (18:2:20).
3. Chloroform-carbon tetrachloride (saturated with water)-methanol (5:4:1).
4. Diisoamyl ether (saturated with water)-butanol (20:10).

It is possible to separate olivomycin from chromomycin A_3 and mithramycin using these solvent systems.

Olivomycin readily undergoes acid hydrolysis and alcoholysis. Methanolysis under mild conditions for 2 hours at 75—80° in 0.1 N methanolic HCl (BRAZHNIKOVA *et al.*, 1964b), or for 3 hours in 0.1 N methanolic H_2SO_4 (BERLIN *et al.*, 1964a), smoothly cleaved the antibiotic to an aglycone and several carbohydrate components.

The crystalline aglycone, called olivin, has the empirical formula $C_{23}H_{26}O_{11}$ (BRAZHNIKOVA *et al.*, 1964b; MESENTSEV *et al.*, 1966). The chromatography of aglycones of olivomycin (olivin), chromomycin A_3 (chromomycinone), and mithramycin (mithramycinone), as well as of their methyl ethers in five systems of solvents, the study by the counter-current distribution method, the infra-red spectra and the investigation of derivatives clearly demonstrate the identity of chromomycinone with mithramycinone and their difference from olivin (MESENTSEV *et al.*, 1966). According to BERLIN *et al.* (1966) the empirical formula of olivin is $C_{20}H_{22}O_9$ and it has the following structure:

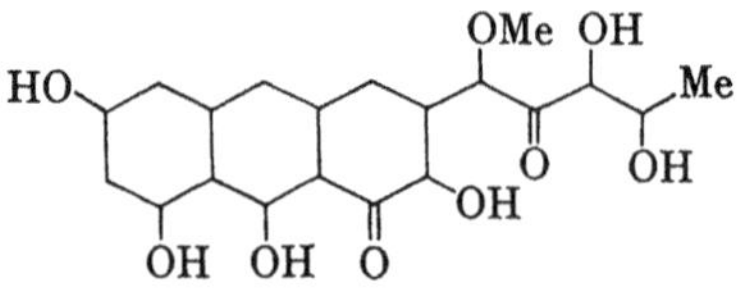

Several components were isolated by chromatography on Al_2O_3 from the mixture of carbohydrate derivatives obtained in the methanolysis of olivomycin, the most important of them being derivatives of three sugars called *olivomycose*, *olivomose*, and *olivose* (BERLIN *et al.*, 1964a). These sugars are different from the chromoses in the chromomycin molecule. As reported by BERLIN *et al.* (1964b), olivomycose is 3-C-methyl-2,6-dideoxy-L-*arabo*-hexose; olivomose is 4-C-methyl-2,6-dideoxy-D-*lyxo*-hexose; and olivose is 2,6-dideoxy-D-*arabo*-hexose. It is evident that olivomycin and chromomycin are two closely related natural products, which nevertheless differ chemically in the structural details of both the aglycone and the sugars attached to it.

The structural formula for olivomycin proposed by BERLIN *et al.* (1966) has the following appearance:

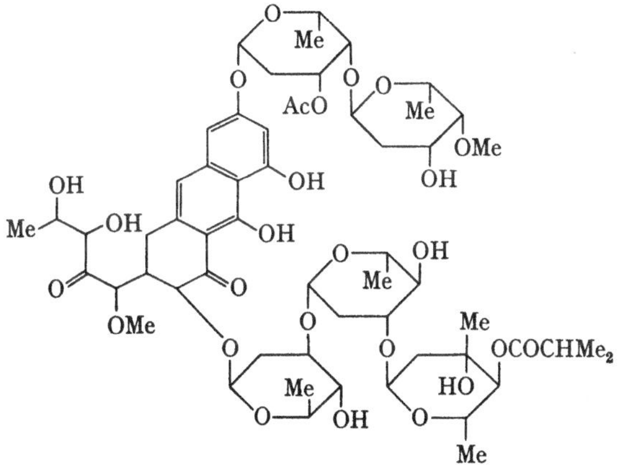

The capacity of the molecule of olivomycin to form complexes with metals is very important for its biochemical mechanism of action, and it has been studied in detail. Olivomycin easily form complex with Fe^{+++}; this antibiotic is yellow in the absence and green in the presence of Fe^{+++}. Olivomycin forms ferric chelate complex in the culture fluid. By treating green preparations of olivomycin by solutions of 8-oxiquinoline, one can isolate yellow olivomycin free of Fe^{+++}. The latter binds to oxiquinoline (BRAZHNIKOVA *et al.*, 1962). Another method using sodium hydrosulfite was found useful for isolating olivomycin from the ferric chelate complex (GRINEV *et al.*, 1964).

Olivomycin is an active "complexon", binding ions of some metals. BRAZHNIKOVA *et al.* (1964a) used solutions of pure olivomycin I in 50% aqueous methanol and added to it various cations (1 part per 5 parts of antibiotic). They observed spectral changes evoked by Al^{+++}, Fe^{+++}, Ni^{++}, Co^{++}, Mg^{++}, and measured bathochromic shifts of the absorption maxima induced by these cations. By adding EDTA to the solutions under investigation, as well as by adding acids or alkalies, the absorption maxima of olivomycin were returned to original positions. The ions of Na^+ and K^+ produced no spectral changes. The results of these measurements are shown in Table 3. It is clear that the capacity to complex with metals is an important feature of the molecule of olivomycin.

Olivomycin inhibits the growth of *S. aureus* and *B. subtilis* at minimum inhibitory concentrations of 0.5 µg/ml (GAUSE *et al.*, 1962). Mutant culture of

S. aureus strain uv-2 is inhibited at 0.004 μg/ml. It also inhibits growth of *B. mycoides*, at a minimal bacteriostatic concentration of 0.05 μg/ml. Olivomycin is inactive against Gram-negative bacteria and fungi.

Table 3. *Effect of various cations upon the position of absorption maxima of olivomycin in ultraviolet* (λ_{max})[1]

	50% methanol in water	50% methanol in water plus 0.01 M EDTA	Formation of complex
Olivomycin (O)	275; 405—410	275; 405—410	
O + $CoCl_2$	281—282; 420—425	275; 405—410	+
O + $FeCl_3$	279; 410—415	274; 400—405	+
O + $AlCl_3$	280—282; 425—430	275; 410	+
O + $MgSO_4$	280; 415		+
O + NaCl	275; 405		—
O + KCl	275; 405		—

[1] From BRAZHNIKOVA *et al.* (1964a).

TOROPOVA (1962) reported that olivomycin strongly inhibits multiplication of tumor cells in vitro; ascitic lympholioma of mice, strain NK/Ly, was used in these experiments. Olivomycin also inhibits multiplication of human amnion cells, strain FL, in tissue cultures at the concentration of 1 μg/ml (ZALMANSON *et al.*, 1965).

The study of acute toxicity of olivomycin has shown that the LD_{50} in mice is 12.7 mg/kg (intraperitoneal), and 13.7 mg/kg (intravenous), as observed by GOLDBERG and KREMER (1962).

It has been clearly shown by a number of investigators that olivomycin selectively inhibits RNA synthesis in bacterial and animal cells. LAIKO (1962) reported that olivomycin at the concentration of 0.3 μg/ml completely stops the synthesis of RNA in cells of staphylococci, whereas the formation of DNA and of protein are not affected to the same extent. These data are shown on Table 4.

Table 4. *Effect of olivomycin (0.3 μg/ml) on the synthesis of RNA, DNA and protein by Staphylococcus aureus*[1]

	Time (hours)	Controls	Treated
RNA	0	0.623	0.623
	1	0.795	0.615
	2	0.958	0.609
DNA	0	0.112	0.112
	1	0.168	0.146
	2	0.224	0.156
Protein	0	0.339	0.339
	1	0.554	0.438
	2	0.827	0.547

[1] From LAIKO (1962). Data are expressed in units of optical density.

G. G. GAUSE, LOSHKAREVA and DUDNIK (1965) observed that in cultures of *B. megaterium* olivomycin in the concentration of 0.8 μg/ml inhibits the synthesis of RNA by 70% in 64 minutes, the synthesis of DNA by 10%, whereas the synthesis of protein is not inhibited at all. It was also concluded that the resistance of Gram-negative bacteria to the action of olivomycin may be related to the impermeability of their cell walls for the antibiotic. In fact, these investigators prepared protoplasts of Escherichia coli and observed that olivomycin in the concentration of 1 μg/ml strongly inhibits incorporation of uracil-^{14}C into RNA of protoplasts, as it is shown on Fig. 4. At the same time both growth and synthesis of RNA in the intact cells of E. coli was resistant to the action of olivomycin in the concentration of 500 μg/ml.

ZALMANSON *et al.* (1965, 1966) reported that olivomycin selectively inhibits the synthesis of RNA of human amnion cells, strain FL, in tissue cultures. They used the method of radioautography, and investigated the incorporation of uridine-^{3}H (for synthesis of RNA), of thymidine-^{3}H (for synthesis of DNA), and of methionine-^{35}S (for synthesis of protein).

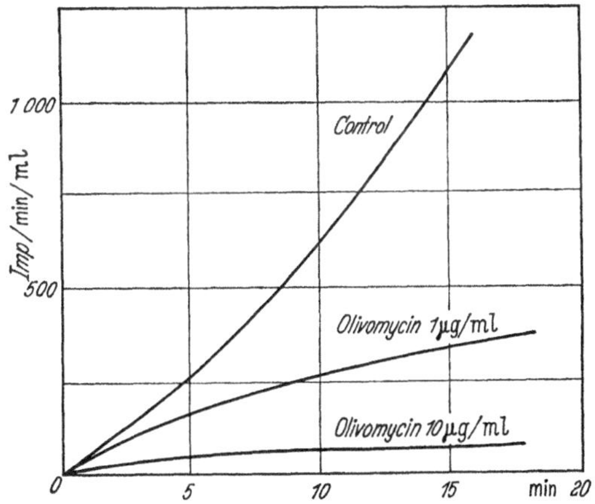

Fig. 4. Effect of olivomycin on the incorporation of C^{14}-uracil into RNA of protoplasts in *Escherichia coli*. (From G. G. GAUSE, LOSHKAREVA and DUDNIK, 1965)

G. G. GAUSE and LOSHKAREVA (1965) studied the action of olivomycin on the cells of Ehrlich ascites carcinoma of mice. They measured the incorporation of ^{32}P into DNA and RNA, as well as the incorporation of valine-^{14}C into the protein fraction of these cells suspended in solutions of olivomycin. The results of their observations are shown on Fig. 5. It is clear that olivomycin selectively inhibits the synthesis of RNA; the synthesis of DNA is affected in much smaller degree, and the synthesis of protein is practically not affected at all by concentrations of olivomycin ranging from 10 to 250 μg/ml. G. G. GAUSE and LOSHKAREVA (1965) reported also that rapidly labelled RNA, which was formed by

Table 5. *Effect of olivomycin upon nucleotide composition of the rapidly labelled RNA of Ehrlich ascites tumor cells of mice*[1]

	Specific activity of RNA (imp/min)	G	A	C	U	$\frac{G+C}{A+U}$
Control	10,200	26.4	22.5	26.6	24.5	1.13
Olivomycin, 250 μg/ml	4,280	27.8	22.1	26.0	24.1	1.17

[1] From G. G. GAUSE and LOSHKAREVA (1965).

tumor cells exposed to olivomycin in the concentration 250 μg/ml, possessed the same nucleotide composition as rapidly labelled RNA of the control cells. Table 5 shows the contents of guanilic, adenylic, cytidylic and uridylic acid in the rapidly labelled RNA of control cells as well as of those treated with olivomycin.

G. G. GAUSE (1965) reported that olivomycin in the concentration of 1 μg/ml inhibited the synthesis of RNA from ribonucleoside triphosphates in the RNA polymerase system prepared from the nuclei of Ehrlich ascites tumor cells. It was concluded that the inhibition of RNA synthesis by olivomycin in tumor cells was due to interference with the RNA polymerase reaction.

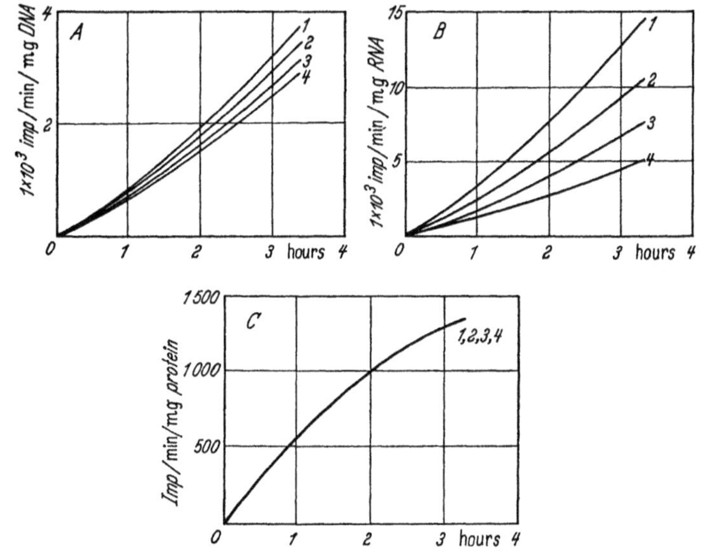

Fig. 5. Effect of olivomycin on the incorporation of P^{32} into DNA (A), RNA (B), and of C^{14}-valine into protein (C) of Ehrlich ascites carcinoma cells. Curves indicate control (1), as well as olivomycin in the increasing concentrations of 10 μg/ml (2), 50 μg/ml (3), and 250 μg/ml (4). (From G. G. GAUSE and LOSHKAREVA, 1965)

G. G. GAUSE, LOSHKAREVA and DUDNIK (1965) observed the capacity of olivomycin to form complexes with DNA, but not with RNA. The binding of olivomycin to DNA strongly reduces the antibacterial activity of the antibiotic, whereas in the presence of RNA the antibacterial activity of olivomycin is not

Table 6. *Effect of DNA and RNA upon the inhibitory action of olivomycin on growth of Staphylococcus aureus*[1]

	Optical density[2]		Optical density[2]
Nutritive broth (NB)	0.337	NB + RNA (300 μg/ml)	0.310
NB + DNA (300 μg/ml)	0.300	NB + olivomycin + DNA	0.230
NB + olivomycin (5 μg/ml)	0.085	NB + olivomycin + RNA	0.080

[1] From G. G. GAUSE, LOSHKAREVA and DUDNIK (1965).

[2] Optical density of bacterial suspension after 2 hours of growth at 37°. Initial optical density attained 0.060.

impaired, as it is shown on Table 6. It was therefore suggested that olivomycin may inhibit DNA dependent RNA synthesis as a result of binding of this antibiotic to cellular DNA. Experiments made by G. G. GAUSE, LOSHKAREVA and DUDNIK (1965) have indeed shown that olivomycin in the concentration of 0.1 μg/ml strongly inhibits DNA-dependent RNA synthesis from ribonucleoside triphosphates. This inhibition is due to a complex formation between olivomycin and DNA. In these experiments DNA preparations from phage T2, as well as from *S. aureus*, *E. coli* and *Micrococcus lysodeikticus*, were used as the governing templates for RNA synthesis.

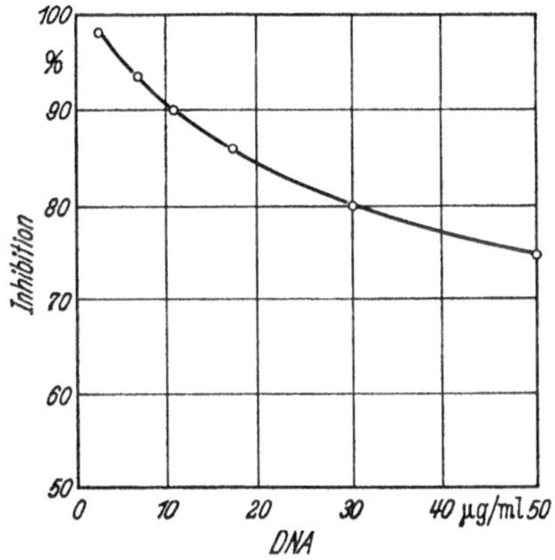

Fig. 6. Effect of increasing concentrations of DNA upon the inhibition by olivomycin of DNA-dependent RNA synthesis from ribonucleoside triphosphates (RNA polymerase reaction). Abscissae: concentrations of DNA (μg/ml) from phage T2. Ordinates: inhibition of incorporation of C^{14}-uracil into RNA, in per cents. Olivomycin 0.1 μg/ml. (From G. G. GAUSE, LOSHKAREVA and DUDNIK, 1965)

It is of interest that the degree of inhibition by olivomycin of DNA-dependent RNA synthesis is decreased with the increase in the concentration of DNA (Fig. 6). This observation also demonstrates that olivomycin complexes directly with DNA.

Mithramycin

Mithramycin is produced by a Streptomyces sp. (RAO *et al.*, 1962), and the empirical formula of this antibiotic (Table 2), is very similar to that for chromomycin and olivomycin. It has been shown that mithramycin can be separated by paper chromatography from olivomycin and chromomycin A_3 (KRUGLYAK *et al.*, 1963). At the same time chromophore of mithramycin molecule (mithramycinone) is identical with chromomycinone, but differs from olivin (MESENTSEV *et al.*, 1966).

Mithramycin inhibits the growth of Staphylococcus aureus and Bacillus subtilis at minimum inhibitory concentrations of 0.039 μg/ml (RAO *et al.*, 1962). It is inactive against Gram-positive bacteria. Mithramycin kills HeLa cells in tissue culture at the concentration of 0.1 μg/ml (RAO *et al.*, 1962). Data on the acute toxicity of this antibiotic for laboratory animals are not available, but the dosage of its clinical application (25 μg/kg) indicates that it is more toxic than olivomycin, which is used clinically in the dose 300 μg/kg (GAUSE, 1965).

YARBRO, KENNEDY and BARNUM (1965, 1966) studied the mechanism of action of mithramycin by measuring the inhibition of DNA and RNA synthesis in a mouse ascites tumor as indicated by incorporation of P^{32} in vitro and in vivo. Mithramycin was found to inhibit the synthesis of RNA to a marked degree with little or no effect on DNA synthesis.

It has been reported by KERSTEN, KERSTEN and SZYBALSKI (1965) as well as by WARD, REICH and GOLDBERG (1965) that the biochemical mechanism of action of mithramycin is qualitatively indistinguishable from that of chromomycin A_3 and olivomycin. Further comparative investigation of this group of closely related antibiotics would be of great interest.

Conclusions

It is abundantly clear that chromomycin, olivomycin and mithramycin are three closely related cancerostatic antibiotics of similar chemical structure, although differing in details of chemical composition. They are also similar in the spectrum of antibacterial action and in the capacity to inhibit the growth of cells in tissue cultures. However, these substances are different in toxicity to animals, and olivomycin is the least toxic member of this group.

All three antibiotics preferentially inhibit the synthesis of RNA in bacterial and animal cells. This effect depends upon the inhibition of DNA-dependent RNA synthesis due to a complex formation between antibiotic and DNA. It is also clear that Mg^{++} is required for interaction of these antibiotics with DNA, and that it is the antibiotic-Mg^{++} complex which binds to DNA. It appears that the structural definition of the antibiotic-Mg^{++} complex may provide insight into the nature of the complex subsequently formed with DNA. One or more of the numerous available oxygen-containing groups attached to the chromophore in the molecules of these antibiotics seems likely to mediate Mg^{++} binding. As far as chromophore of olivomycin differs from those of chromomycin and mithramycin, further comparative study of the effects of these antibiotics may be helpful for understanding of their interaction with DNA.

References

BERLIN, Y. A., S. E. ESIPOV, M. N. KOLOSOV, M. M. SHEMYAKIN, and M. G. BRAZHNIKOVA: Olivomycin. I. Methanolysis. Tetrahedron Letters 1323 (1964a).

BERLIN, Y. A., S. E. ESIPOV, M. N. KOLOSOV, M. M. SHEMYAKIN, and M. G. BRAZHNIKOVA: Olivomycin. II. Structure of the carbohydrate components. Tetrahedron Letters 3513 (1964b).

BERLIN, Y. A., I. V. VASINA, B. A. KLYASHCHITSKII, M. N. KOLOSOV, G. Y. PECK, L. A. PIOTROVICH, O. A. CHUPRUNOVA, and M. M. SHEMYAKIN: Structure of olivin. Doklady Acad. Sci. U.S.S.R. **167**, 1054 (1966).

BERLIN, Y. A., O. A. CHUPRUNOVA, B. A. KLYASHCHITSKII, M. N. KOLOSOV, G. Y. PECK, L. A. PIOTROVICH, M. M. SHEMYAKIN, and I. V. VASINA: Olivomycin. III. The structure of olivin. Tetrahedron Letters 1425 (1966).

BERLIN, Y. A., S. E. ESIPOV, and M. N. KOLOSOV: Olivomycin. IV. The structure of olivomycin. Tetrahedron Letters 1431 (1966).

BRAHMACHARY, R., and G. REVERBERY: On the action of chromomycin on the eggs and embryos of Ciona intestinalis. Experientia **20**, 621 (1964).

BRAZHNIKOVA, M. G., E. B. KRUGLYAK, I. N. KOVSHAROVA, N. V. KONSTANTINOVA, and V. V. PROSHLYAKOVA: Isolation, purification and study of certain physical chemical properties of new antibiotic olivomycin. Antibiotiki **7**, 39 (1962).

BRAZHNIKOVA, M. G., E. B. KRUGLYAK, V. N. BORISOVA, and G. B. FEDOROVA: A study of homogeneity of olivomycin. Antibiotiki **9**, 141 (1964a).

BRAZHNIKOVA, M. G., E. B. KRUGLYAK, A. S. MESENTSEV, and G. B. FEDOROVA: Products of acid hydrolysis of olivomycin. Antibiotiki **9**, 552 (1964b).

CHORIN, V. A., and O. K. ROSSOLIMO: An experimental study of antitumor action of six antibiotics related to olivomycin. Antibiotiki **10**, 48 (1965).

GAUSE, G. F., R. S. UCHOLINA, and M. A. SVESHNIKOVA: Olivomycin — a new antibiotic producd by *Actinomyces olivoreticuli*. Antibiotiki **7**, 34 (1962).

GAUSE, G. F.: Olivomycin, mithramycin, chromomycin: Three related cancerostatic antibiotics. Advances in Chemotherapy **2**, 179 (1965).

GAUSE, G. G.: Effect of olivomycin on the synthesis of RNA. Transactions of the 2nd Conference on Nucleic Acids, Moscow 1965.

GAUSE, G. G., and N. P. LOSHKAREVA: Effect of olivomycin on the cells of Ehrlich ascites carcinoma. Voprosy Med. Chem. (Moscow) **11**, 79 (1965).

GAUSE, G. G., N. P. LOSHKAREVA, and Y. V. DUDNIK: Mechanism of action of olivomycin. Antibiotiki **10**, 307 (1965).

GOLDBERG, L. E., and V. E. KREMER: A pharmacological study of antibiotic olivomycin. Antibiotiki **7**, 53 (1962).

GRINEV, A. N., L. A. KOZLOVA, and A. S. MESENTSEV: A study of chemical properties of olivomycin. Antibiotiki **9**, 138 (1964).

HARTMANN, G., H. GOLLER, K. KOSCHEL, W. KERSTEN u. H. KERSTEN: Hemmung der DNA-abhängigen RNA- und DNA-Synthese durch Antibiotika. Biochem. Z. **341**, 126 (1964).

KAZIWARA, K., J. WATANABE, T. KOMEDA, and T. USUI: Growth inhibiting activities of chromomycin A_3 on transplantable tumors. Ann. Repts. Takeda Research Lab. **19**, 68 (1960).

KAZIWARA, K., J. WATANABE, T. KOMEDA, and T. USUI: Further observations on the inhibiting effect of chromomycin A_3 on transplantable tumors. Cancer Chemoth. Rep. **13**, 99 (1961).

KERSTEN, W., u. H. KERSTEN: Die Bindung von Daunomycin, Cinerubin und Chromomycin A_3 an Nucleinsäuren. Biochem. Z. **341**, 174 (1965).

KERSTEN, W., H. KERSTEN, and W. SZYBALSKI: Physico-chemical properties of complexes between DNA and antibiotics which affect RNA synthesis. Biochemistry **5**, 236 (1965).

KRUGLYAK, E. B., V. N. BORISOVA, and M. G. BRAZHNIKOVA: A chromatographic comparison of olivomycin with some related antibiotics. Antibiotiki **8**, 1064 (1963).

LAIKO, A. V.: The action of certain antitumor antibiotics on the synthesis of nucleic acids in cells of staphylococci. Antibiotiki **7**, 601 (1962).

MESENTSEV, A. S., E. B. KRUGLYAK, V. A. TUTUKOVA, and M. G. BRAZHNIKOVA: The comparative investigation of olivin and of aglycones from chromomycin A_3, mithramycin and antibiotic 3014. Doklady Acad. Sci. U.S.S.R. **168**, 207 (1966).

MIYAMOTO, M., Y. KAWAMATSU, M. SHINOHARA, Y. ASAHI, Y. NAKADAIRA, M. KAKISAWA, K. NAKANISHI, and N. BHACCA: Chromomycin A_3, isolation of chromose A. Tetrahedron Letters 693 (1963).

MIYAMOTO, M., K. MORITA, Y. KAWAMATSU, S. NOGUCHI, R. MARUMOTO, K. TANAKA, S. TATSUOKA, K. NAKANISHI, Y. NAKADAIRA, and N. BHACCA: Chromomycinone, the aglycone of chromomycin A_3. Tetrahedron Letters 2355 (1964a).

MIYAMOTO, M., K. MORITA, Y. KAWAMATSU, M. SASAI, A. NOHARA, K. TANAKA, S. TATSUOKA, K. NAKANISHI, Y. NAKADAIRA, and N. BHACCA: The structure of chromomycin A_3. Tetrahedron Letters 2367 (1964b).

MIYAMOTO, M., Y. KAWAMATSU, M. SHINIHARA, K. NAKANISHI, Y. NAKADAIRA, and N. BHACCA: The four chromoses from chromomycin A_3. Tetrahedron Letters 2371 (1964c).

MIYAMOTO, M., Y. KAWAMATSU, K. KAWASHIMA, M. SHINOHARA, and K. NAKANISHI: The full structures of three chromomycins, A_2, A_3, and A_4. Tetrahedron Letters 545 (1966).

MIZUNO, K.: Chromomycin A_3 and its derivatives. J. Antibiot. (Japan), Ser. A **16**, 22 (1963).

NAKANISHI, K.: The chemistry of chromomycin. Special Organic Seminar, The University of Wisconsin 1965.

RAO, K. V., W. P. CULLEN, and B. A. SOBIN: A new antibiotic with antitumor properties. Antibiotics & Chemotherapy **12**, 182 (1962).

SATO, K., N. OKAMURA, K. UTAGAWA, Y. ITO, and M. WATANABE: Studies on the antitumor activity of chromomycin A_3. Sci. Repts. Research Insts. Tohoku Univ. Ser. C **9**, 224 (1960).

TAKAKI, R., K. SUGI, K. KATSUTA, T. KAMIYA, and T. TAKAHASHI: Effect of chromomycin on the cells in tissue culture. Kyushu J. Med. Sci. **11**, 225 (1960).

TATSUOKA, S., K. NAKAZAWA, A. MIYAKE, K. KAZIWARA, Y. ARAMAKI, M. SHIBATA, K. TANABE, Y. HAMADA, H. HITOMI, M. MIYAMOTO, K. MIZUNO, J. WATANABE, M. ISHIDATE, H. YOKOTANI, and I. USHIKAWA: Isolation, anticancer activity and pharmacology of a new antibiotic chromomycin A_3. Gann **49**, (Suppl.) 23 (1958).

TATSUOKA, S., K. TANAKA, M. MIYAMOTO, K. MORITA, Y. KAWAMATSU, K. NAKANISHI, Y. NAKADAIRA, and N. BHACCA: The structure of chromomycin A_3, a cancerostatic antibiotic. Proc. Japan Acad. **40**, 236 (1964).

TOROPOVA, E. G.: The method of cultivating of tumor cells in vitro and its use in the screening for antitumor antibiotics. Antibiotiki **7**, 598 (1962).

TSUKAMURA, M., S. TSUKAMURA, and S. MIZUNO: Mode of action of chromomycin A_3 on a mycobacterium. J. Antibiot. (Japan), Ser. A **17**, 246 (1964).

TSUKAMURA, M.: Combined effect of chromomycin A_3 on mycobacterium smegmatis with 8-azaguanine or dihydrostreptomycin. J. Antibiotics (Japan), Ser. A **18**, 137 (1965).

WAKISAKA, G., H. UCHINO, T. NAKAMURA, H. SOTOBAYASHI, S. SHIRAKAWA, A. ADACHI, and M. SAKURAI: Selective inhibition of biosynthesis of ribonucleic acid in mammalian cells by chromomycin A_3. Nature **198**, 385 (1963).

WARD, D., E. REICH, and I. H. GOLDBERG: Characterization of base specificity in the interaction of polynucleotides with drugs: echinomycin, daunomycin, ethidium, nogalamycin, chromomycin, mithramycin, and olivomycin. Science **149**, 1259 (1965).

YARBRO, J. W., B. J. KENNEDY, and C. P. BARNUM: Mithramycin inhibition of RNA synthesis in mouse ascites tumor. Proc. Am. Assoc. Cancer Research **6**, 70 (1965).

YARBRO, J. W., B. J. KENNEDY, and C. P. BARNUM: Mithramycin inhibition of ribonucleic acid synthesis. Cancer Research **26**, 36 (1966).

ZALMANZON, E. S., A. V. ZELENIN, K. A. KAFIANI, L. S. LOBAREVA, E. A. LYAPUNOVA, and M. Y. TIMOFEEVA: Effect of some antitumor antibiotics on nucleic acid synthesis and virus reproduction in human amnion cell cultures (strain FL). Antibiotiki **10**, 613 (1965).

ZALMANZON, E. S., A. V. ZELENIN, K. A. KAFIANI, L. S. LOBAREVA, E. A. LYAPUNOVA, and M. Y. TIMOFEEVA: On the mechanism of action of olivomycin. Voprosy Med. Chem. (Moscow) **13**, 58 (1966).

Puromycin*

Daniel Nathans

Puromycin[1], an antibiotic isolated from culture filtrates of *Streptomyces alboniger* (PORTER *et al.*, 1952), is well-characterized chemically and biologically. Its structure, shown in Fig. 1, has been established both by degradative studies and total synthesis as 6-dimethylamino-9-(3'-deoxy-3'-p-methoxy-L-phenylalaninamido-β-D-ribofuranosyl)-purine (WALLER *et al.*, 1953; BAKER *et al.*, 1955a, 1955b). Compared with many other antibiotics, puromycin has an unusually broad range of growth-inhibitory activity. The structural features of the molecule required for activity are known, and its principal mode of action is understood in molecular terms. As will become evident in later sections of this review, puromycin is a notable example of the structural analogue concept of antimetabolite action. By virtue of its structural analogy to aminoacyl-sRNA, an obligatory intermediate in a vital cellular function, protein synthesis, puromycin terminates the growth of polypeptide chains, thereby inhibiting cell growth.

Chemical Properties

Puromycin is a substituted aminonucleoside, made up of three components (Fig. 1): 6-dimethylaminopurine (dimethyladenine), 3-deoxy-3-amino-D-ribose, and p-methoxy-L-phenylalanine. As in natural nucleosides, the glycosidic bond

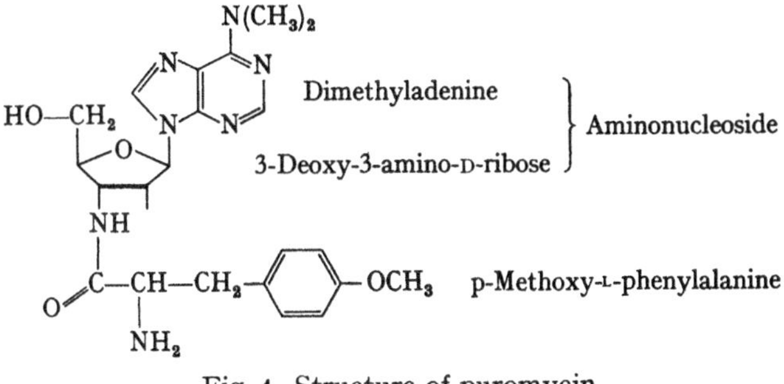

Fig. 1. Structure of puromycin

is of β configuration (BAKER *et al.*, 1955a). The pk_a of the unsubstituted amino group is 7.3, and that of the purine is 3.7. It is stable at pH's near neutrality, and neutral solutions can be stored frozen for long periods. Absorption maxima occur

* The author's research reported in this paper was supported by a grant from the United States Public Health Service.

[1] When originally isolated, puromycin was called "achromycin" and later given the trademark name "stylomycin".

at 275 mμ in 0.1 N NaOH (E 20,300) and at 267.5 mμ in 0.1 N HCl (E 19,500) (WALLER *et al.*, 1953). The glycosidic bond is cleaved quantitatively by strong acids (e.g. 1 N HCl at 100° for 10 minutes) under which conditions the amide linkage of the amino acid is stable (WALLER *et al.*, 1953). The amino acid side chain has been removed by treatment of the phenylthiourea derivative of puromycin with sodium methoxide in methanol, giving the aminonucleoside in 75% yield (BAKER *et al.*, 1955c). By condensing the aminonucleoside with carbobenzoxy amino acids, BAKER *et al.* (1955c) have prepared various analogues of puromycin with different side chain amino acids; radioactive puromycin has been synthesized by this same technique (ALLEN and ZAMECNIK, 1962; NATHANS, 1964).

Inhibition of Growth

Since puromycin is an inhibitor of protein synthesis at a step probably shared by all living cells, it inhibits the growth of many different kinds of organisms, ranging from bacteria and protozoa to complex plants and animals. Table 1

Table 1. *Sensitivity of various organisms or cells to puromycin*

	Conc. for complete inhibition (mMolar)
Bacteria[1]	
Escherichia coli	0.4
Salmonella typhosa	0.5
Klebsiella pneumoniae	0.01
Bacillus subtilus	0.015
Staphylococcus aureus	0.015
Sarcina lutea	0.004
Mycobacterium No. 607	0.08
Protozoa	
Tetrahymena pyriformis[2]	0.01
Mammals	
Mouse	1.1 mMole/kg[3]
HeLa cells	0.1 mMolar[4]

[1] PORTER *et al.* (1952).
[2] BORTLE and OLESON (1954/55).
[3] LD_{50} by intraperitoneal route (SHERMAN *et al.*, 1954/55).
[4] Concentration for complete inhibition of protein synthesis (WHEELOCK, 1962).

illustrates the sensitivities of selected organisms. Among the bacteria, gram positive organisms are generally more sensitive than gram negative organisms (although *Klebsiella pneumoniae* is an exception). The greater resistance of the gram negative group may be related to poor uptake of puromycin, since in cell-free extracts protein synthesis is markedly inhibited at a concentration of puromycin much lower than that required to inhibit growth and sensitivity to puromycin is enhanced by growth in media with low Mg^{++} concentrations (TAKEDA *et al.*, 1960). Although it is not clear that this Mg^{++} effect is related to uptake of drug, the effects of EDTA on bacterial permeability described by LEIVE (1965), suggest that this is the case.

Puromycin is bacteriostatic rather than bacteriocidal, except possibly under unusual conditions. For example, *Escherichia coli*, when treated with puromycin at a concentration of 500 μg/ml, ceased to multiply, but there was no fall in viable count for 2 hrs. (WHITE and WHITE, 1964). On the other hand, KAMMEN *et al.* (1965) have reported that *B. subtilis* was killed by low (30 μg/ml), but not by high (100 μg/ml) concentrations of puromycin, as measured by viable counts. This paradoxical observation may well be explainable by the possible lethality of accumulated long, non-functional peptides expected at low concentrations, but not at high concentrations of the antibiotic. Another interesting observation is the effect of puromycin on the bactericidal potency of aminoglycoside antibiotics (WHITE and WHITE, 1964). When puromycin was added together with such an agent to growing *E. coli*, the rate of loss of viable cells was greater than with the aminoglycoside alone, whereas pretreatment with puromycin decreased the bactericidal effect of the aminoglycoside. These effects were attributed to possible changes in susceptibility of ribosomes to the aminoglycoside, but the actual mechanism is still unknown.

Biosynthesis of Macromolecules

The effects of puromycin on the synthesis of macromolecules has been studied in intact bacteria, mammalian cells and whole animals. CREASER (1955), in a survey of several antibiotics, first observed the inhibition by puromycin of induced enzyme synthesis in bacteria. The specific susceptibility of bacterial protein synthesis to puromycin was shown by measurements of total protein, RNA and DNA synthesis, Fig. 2 (TAKEDA *et al.*, 1960). As shown in the figure, protein synthesis is immediately inhibited, while DNA and RNA synthesis continue for a time at normal or near-normal rates. This pattern of macromolecular synthesis has come to be recognized as characteristic of inhibition of protein synthesis at a step subsequent to formation of aminoacyl-sRNA (NEIDHARDT, 1964). One striking consequence of this imbalance in RNA and protein synthesis is the accumulation of abnormal, RNA-rich ribonucleoprotein particles (NAKADA, 1965).

The sensitivity to puromycin of induced enzyme synthesis by bacteria is considerably greater than the overall synthesis of protein, as measured by amino acid incorporation into an acid-insoluble product (SELLS, 1965). Although this has been attributed to a special effect of puromycin on some aspect of enzyme induction other than at the level of polypeptide formation, it seems likely that this effect is related to the underlying mechanism of puromycin action, whereby incomplete proteins are prematurely released from ribosomes. At low concentrations of puromycin much of the incomplete "protein" would be large enough to be acid-precipitable, but no longer enzymatically or biologically active; for example, see PIECHOWSKI and SUSSMAN (1965).

Studies in mammalian cells have confirmed the rapid, reversible inhibition of protein synthesis by puromycin. For example, WHEELOCK (1962) found complete inhibition of protein synthesis by HeLa cells at 10^{-4} M puromycin, and restoration 30 minutes after removal of the drug. In addition, it has been reported that the synthesis of cellular RNA by HeLa cells is also diminished (HOLLAND, 1963; TAMAOKI and MUELLER, 1963). This effect was gradual compared to the time required for inhibition of protein synthesis, and this effect was restricted to ribosomal RNA. Whether the decrease in RNA synthesis is a primary effect of puromycin or a consequence of the shut-down of protein synthesis is not clear. An interesting, but as yet untested, possibility is that puromycin is hydrolytically cleaved in the cell, liberating the aminonucleoside (see Fig. 1), which is known to inhibit the synthesis of RNA (and preferentially ribosomal RNA) in animal cells (FARNHAM, 1965; FARNHAM and DUBIN, 1965; STUDZINSKI *et al.*, 1965). This explanation also fits in with the relative potency of the aminonucleoside and puromycin analogues in the treatment of neoplasms (BENNETT *et al.*, 1954/55)

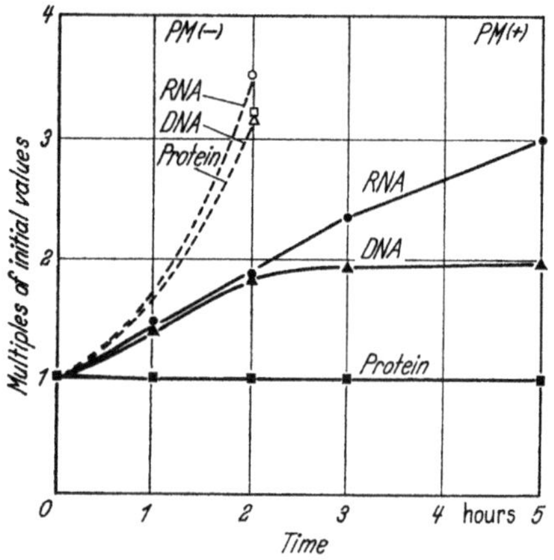

Fig. 2. The effect of puromycin on DNA, RNA and protein synthesis in *Pseudomonas fluorescens*. - - -, PM (—), no puromycin; —, PM (+), 50 μg/ml puromycin. (From TAKEDA *et al.*, 1960)

and trypanosomiasis (HUTCHINGS, 1957) and in the production of nephrosis (BOROWSKY *et al.*, 1958). In contrast with the structural requirements for inhibition of protein synthesis and bacterial growth, the pattern of analogue activity against neoplasms and trypanosomes, as well as in producing nephrotoxicity, strongly suggests that the aminonucleoside fragment of puromycin is formed in these situations and is the most active molecule.

DNA synthesis by HeLa cells is also affected by puromycin (MUELLER *et al.*, 1962). In the presence of the antibiotic, DNA synthesis continues at its prior rate but fails to accelerate. In view of the dependence of initiation of bacterial DNA synthesis on protein synthesis (MAALØE, 1961), it is likely that the puromycin effect on DNA formation is secondary to inhibition of protein synthesis.

The acute effects of puromycin on the biosynthesis of protein, RNA and phospholipid in various tissues of the rat was studied by GORSKI *et al.* (1961). Four hourly injections of 55 mg/kg of puromycin intraperitoneally reduced the incorporation of glycine into protein from 50 to 90% in various tissues during the four hours after the first dose of puromycin. In contrast, RNA synthesis was not inhibited during this same time period, except in the thymus (40% decrease), and phospholipid synthesis in the uterus and liver was stimulated. The slight effect on RNA synthesis *in vivo* compared with the effect on mammalian cells in culture, described above, may be related to dosage, or to differences in metabolism of the types of cells studied. In view of the widespread use of puromycin at various dosages and for varying times to block protein syntheses *in vivo*, it would be worthwhile to extend this kind of study to ensure that under given conditions the effect of puromycin is on protein synthesis specifically. Since puromycin may be broken down in animal tissues to the aminonucleoside, strict specificity in inhibiting protein synthesis cannot be assumed.

Nucleotide Metabolism

Since puromycin is an analogue of adenosine, the possibility that it or the aminonucleoside portion of the molecule directly interferes with nucleotide metabolism has been investigated. Many of these studies have been carried out with intact cells, and it is often difficult to distinguish between direct and indirect effects. For example, in *Tetrahymena piriformis* W., a protozoan which has an absolute requirement for guanine, guanosine or guanylic acid, inhibition by low levels of puromycin is overcome by guanylic acid (BORTLE and OLESON, 1954/55), but whether this reversal is due to a direct effect of puromycin on guanylic acid synthesis or is secondary to inhibition of protein synthesis is not clear. Nor is it clear that the inhibition by puromycin (but not by aminonucleoside) of C^{14}-glycine incorporation into guanine by ascites tumor cells (FRANZ *et al.*, 1964) is a primary effect of the agent, since BUCHANAN (1957) has reported that puromycin does not inhibit any of the enzymes concerned with purine biosynthesis *de novo*. On the other hand, studies with the aminonucleoside of puromycin do point to a direct effect on nucleotide metabolism. For example, the stimulation by adenosine of adenosine triphosphate synthesis by toluenized yeast was blocked by aminonucleoside (KESSNER *et al.*, 1958). The striking glycogenolytic effect of puromycin, aminonucleoside and 6-dimethyladenine observed by HOFERT and his colleagues (HOFERT *et al.*, 1962; HOFERT and BOUTWELL, 1963) might also be due to a direct effect on nucleotide metabolism. These authors clearly showed that the abrupt fall in liver glycogen of mice after a single dose of puromycin or analogue was not correlated with inhibition of protein synthesis, and they suggested that the effect might be due to inhibition of breakdown of adenosine-3′, 5′-phosphoric acid (cyclic AMP), thereby stimulating glycogen phosphorylase activity. Such an effect on cyclic AMP degradation could also explain the action of puromycin and its aminonucleoside on hormone regulation of fatty acid release by fat tissue (KORNER and RABEN, 1964). Further investigation of this phenomenon, particularly at the enzyme level, would be most interesting.

Toxicity for Mammalian Hosts

From what has been noted already, puromycin would be expected to have considerable toxicity in higher animals, and in fact its toxicity, particularly nephrotoxicity, has all but precluded its use in the treatment of human or animal infectious diseases or neoplasms. Toxic manifestations, in addition to signs and symptoms of renal disease, include headache, nausea, vomiting and diarrhea (WRIGHT *et al.*, 1955; SHERMAN *et al.*, 1954/55). The 50% lethal dose for mice by the intraperitoneal route is 580 mg/kg (SHERMAN *et al.*, 1954/55).

The renal lesion in rats is of particular interest as a model for the nephrotic syndrome of humans, which it resembles pathologically and clinically (FRENK *et al.*, 1955; DUBACH, 1964). Although this lesion results from puromycin administration, the aminonucleoside of puromycin is an even more potent agent (BOROWSKY *et al.*, 1958), as already noted. Since the aminonucleoside does not inhibit protein synthesis (NATHANS and NEIDLE, 1963; DECKER *et al.*, 1964), it is likely that this specific renal defect is due not to inhibition of protein synthesis, but to changes in RNA or nucleotide metabolism. Presumably, puromycin is active solely by yielding the aminonucleoside *in vivo*.

Protein Synthesis

After studies with intact cells showed that inhibition of protein synthesis was the principal mode of action of puromycin, extensive investigation of its effect in the protein biosynthetic pathway was carried out with cell extracts. Before presenting these results, however, it is necessary to review briefly what is now known about the way proteins are synthesized.

The biosynthesis of proteins begins with activation of amino acids by ATP and enzymes specific for each amino acid (aminoacyl-sRNA synthetases). The immediate product of this reaction is an enzyme-bound acid anhydride, aminoacyl-adenylate (Fig. 3, reaction 1a). The same enzymes have binding sites for specific sRNA's, to which the activated aminoacyl residue is transferred, resulting in aminoacyl-sRNA in which the amino acid is esterified to the 2′ or 3′ hydroxyl of the terminal adenosine of sRNA (reaction 1b). Aminoacyl-sRNA retains the activated aminoacyl group and serves as the adaptor for positioning the amino acid in the polypeptide chain in accordance with the sequence of codons in messenger RNA.

The next stage of protein synthesis, in which the aminoacyl residue is inserted into peptide linkage, is more complex and is not as well understood as the synthesis of aminoacyl-sRNA. For this reason the following description should be taken as a summary of present knowledge, likely to be correct in general outline, but in need of more detailed verification and amplification. As shown diagrammatically in Fig. 3 (reaction 2a), a molecule of aminoacyl-sRNA becomes bound to a ribosome-messenger RNA complex by hydrogen bonding with the appropriate codon and attaching to a site on the ribosome (site 1, the acceptor site), adjacent to the sRNA to which the growing peptide chain is attached (site 2, the donor site). The carboxyl-activated peptide is then transferred to the amino group of the aminoacyl-sRNA, with displacement of the sRNA from the peptide (reaction 2b). As a result of this reaction the polypeptide is lengthened by one residue and the peptidyl-sRNA now occupies the acceptor site. Movement of the ribosome with respect to the peptidyl-sRNA-messenger RNA unit returns the peptidyl-sRNA to the donor site (reaction 2c) in preparation for the next incoming aminoacyl-sRNA and repetition of the reaction sequence. At least two enzymes are involved in the overall reaction, one of which probably catalyses peptide-bond formation (reaction 2b) and the other, the movement of the ribosome (reaction 2c). In addition, GTP is required, and it has been suggested that this nucleoside triphosphate is needed for movement of the ribosome, in analogy with the role of

Reaction 1

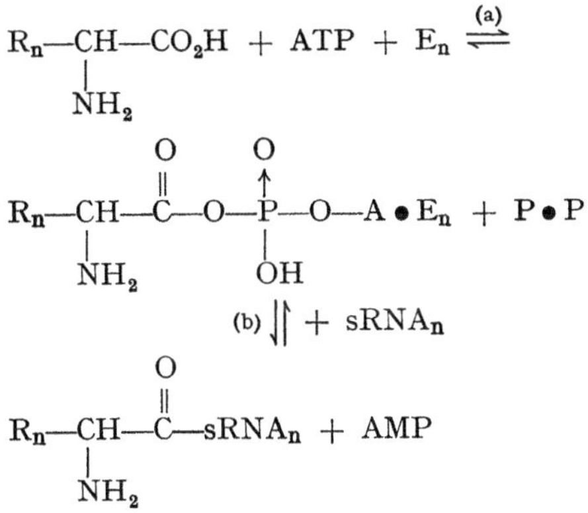

Reaction 2

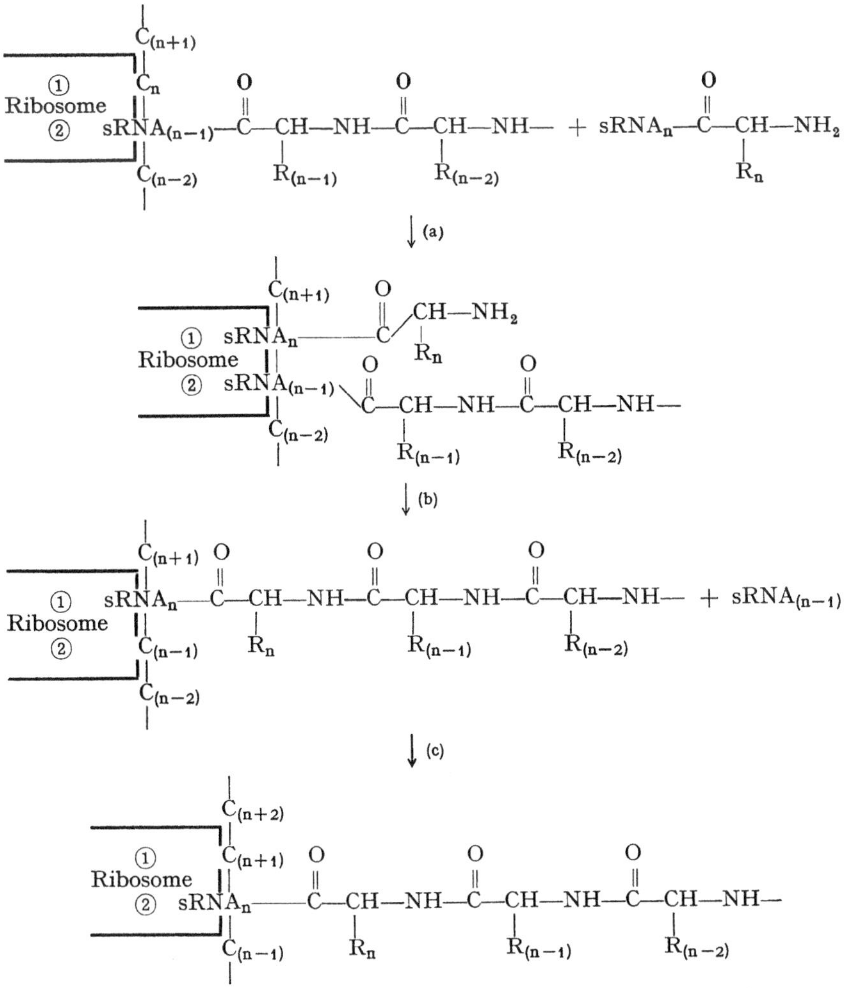

Fig. 3. A diagram of the reactions of protein synthesis. -C-C-C represents the sequence of codons in messenger RNA; (1) and (2), the acceptor and donor sites respectively, on the ribosome

ATP in the contraction of muscle. Although in Fig. 3 only the ribosome is shown attached to messenger RNA, in the cell many ribosomes function simultaneously with the same messenger molecule, the aggregate being termed a polysome.

Two special features of protein synthesis are not included in the above description, viz., chain initiation and chain termination. Presumably initiation is related to ribosome attachment at the beginning of the RNA message and possibly to special aminoacyl-sRNA's; and termination, to ribosome release at the end of the message. In addition, a distinct reaction leading to cleavage of the peptide-sRNA bond is required for chain termination.

Structural Requirements for Inhibition

On examining the structures of the various molecules involved in the protein biosynthetic pathway, YARMOLINSKY and DE LA HABA (1959) were struck with the similarity between the 3′ end of aminoacyl-sRNA and puromycin (Fig. 4).

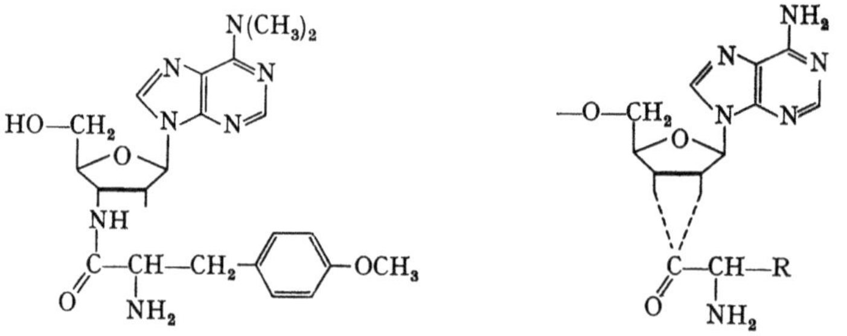

Fig. 4. Comparison of puromycin (left) and the aminoacyl-adenosine end of sRNA (right)

In each case there is a D-ribosyl (or aminoribosyl) group glycosidically linked in the β configuration to position 9 of adenine (or adenine derivative) and substituded in the 2′ or 3′ position with an amino acid. Puromycin has a 3′ amino acid substitutent, whereas aminoacyl-sRNA is thought to be an equilibrium mixture of the 2′ and 3′ aminoacyl esters (WOLFENDEN *et al.*, 1964; MCLAUGHLIN and INGRAM, 1965 a, b). The nature of the amino acid linkage to the nucleoside is thus different in the two cases. In aminoacyl-sRNA the linkage is an ester bond of special lability owing to the vicinal hydroxyl, whereas in puromycin the amino acid is linked by the more stable amide bond to the 3′ amino group of the aminoribose moiety. On the basis of this similarity in structure, YARMOLINSKY and DE LA HABA (1959) proposed that puromycin acts as an analogue of aminoacyl-sRNA, and this has been the guiding hypothesis for most subsequent studies of its mode of action.

The structural requirements for puromycin inhibition of bacterial growth have been extensively studied in an effort to develop more potent and less toxic antimicrobial compounds (HUTCHINGS, 1957). Many analogues of puromycin have also been tested for inhibition of protein synthesis in cell extracts (Table 2; NATHANS and NEIDLE, 1962). The results of these studies, which are in close agreement, can be summarized as follows: 1. both the amino acid side chain and the aminonucleoside are required; 2. the amino acid must be of L-configuration; 3. the amino group of the amino acid must be unsubstituted; 4. the nucleoside amino group must be at the 3′ position; 5. the nature of the amino acid side chain is of considerable importance — compounds with phenylalanine or O-alkyl-tyrosine are most active, whereas compounds with glycine or proline are inactive.

Table 2. *Inhibition of leucine transfer from sRNA to protein by puromycin analogues*[1]

Compound	Conc., M	% Inhibition
puromycin	10^{-4}	83
	10^{-3}	93
2′-puromycin isomer	10^{-3}	0
5′-puromycin isomer	10^{-3}	0
3′-aminonucleoside	10^{-3}	0
L-phenylalanyl analogue	10^{-5}	49
	10^{-4}	79
	10^{-3}	90
D-phenylalanyl analogue	10^{-4}	17
	10^{-3}	35
L-leucyl analogue	10^{-4}	10
	10^{-3}	35
L-prolyl analogue	10^{-4}	10
	10^{-3}	9
glycyl analogue	10^{-3}	7
glycyl-p-methoxy-L-phenylalanyl analogue	10^{-4}	10

[1] From NATHANS and NEIDLE (1963).

A comparison of these structural requirements for acitivity with the structure of aminoacyl-sRNA (Fig. 4) in general supports the analogue concept of puromycin action. It is worth pointing out, however, that the amino acid specificity for activity is unexpected and not explained. In contrast with this specificity of puromycin analogues, TAKANAMI (1964) has found that fragments of aminoacyl-sRNA containing the esterified adenosine terminus of the molecule act like puromycin but have no such amino acid specificity. Also of note is the need for the 3′ rather than the 2′ substituted aminonucleoside. Due to rapid acyl migration, it has not been possible to determine directly whether the active form of aminoacyl-sRNA is a 2′ or 3′ aminoacyl ester (WOLFENDEN et al., 1963; MCLAUGHLIN and INGRAM, 1965; but see SONNENBLICHER *et al.*, 1965). The fact that puromycin is the 3′ amide and that the 2′ isomer is inactive suggests that the active form of aminoacyl-sRNA in protein synthesis is the 3′ ester. Finally, in view of the inhibition of polylysine synthesis by puromycin (GARDNER *et al.*, 1962), and the inhibition of polyphenylalanine synthesis by the tyrosine analogue of puromycin (NATHANS and NEIDLE, 1962), it is clear that the inhibition is not amino acid-specific. This is not unexpected, since there is no amino acid-discriminating step at the stage of protein synthesis inhibited by puromycin (CHAPEVILLE *et al.*, 1962; NATHANS *et al.*, 1963).

Site of Action

At least two enzymes must recognize the aminoacyl-adenosine end of each sRNA: aminoacyl-sRNA synthetase (reaction 1b, Fig. 3) and the peptide-bond forming enzyme (reaction 2b, Fig. 3). It was therefore thought likely that puromycin interfered at one or another, or perhaps both of these steps. Although no thorough study of the effect of puromycin on aminoacyl-sRNA synthesis has been published, in those instances in which this reaction has been tested (formation of leucyl-, phenylalanyl-, tyrosyl-, lysyl- and threonyl-sRNA) no effect of puromycin was detected (YARMOLINSKY and DE LA HABA, 1959; NATHANS, unpublished results). In contrast, as already indicated in Table 2, the incorporation into protein of amino acids from aminoacyl-sRNA is markedly inhibited by puromycin, Table 3 (YARMOLINSKY and DE LA HABA, 1959). This observation localizes the effect to the "ribosome stage" of protein synthesis. Three steps are experimentally distinguishable in this phase of protein synthesis: messenger RNA binding to ribosomes, aminoacyl-sRNA binding to the ribosome-messenger RNA complex, and peptide-bond formation (see Fig. 3, reaction 2). Puromycin does not effect m-RNA or aminoacyl-sRNA binding to ribosomes (SPYRIDES, 1964) but does interfere with normal peptide bond formation (see below).

Table 3. *Effect of puromycin on incorporation of C^{14}-leucine into protein by rat liver extracts*[1]

	Form of C^{14}-leucine	Puromycin (Molarity)	% Inhibition
Exp. 1	free leucine	2×10^{-5}	65
	leucyl-sRNA	2×10^{-5}	64
Exp. 2	leucyl-sRNA	5×10^{-6}	15
	leucyl-sRNA	2×10^{-5}	44
	leucyl-sRNA	2×10^{-4}	87

[1] From YARMOLINSKY and DE LA HABA (1959).

Several observations with whole cells or cell extracts from different sources have indicated that puromycin leads to the release of incomplete protein chains from the ribosome. In ascites tumor cells treated with low concentrations of puromycin, amino acid incorporation into protein associated with ribosomes was diminished, whereas incorporation into soluble protein was enhanced (RABINOVITZ and FISHER, 1960). When reticulocyte ribosomes with which hemoglobin peptide chains are associated were incubated with puromycin, globin peptides were released into the high speed supernatant fraction of the incubate (MORRIS *et al.*, 1963; ALLEN and ZAMECNIK, 1962). In the coliphage RNA-directed synthesis of phage coat protein with *E. coli* extracts, puromycin leads to a series of coat protein fragments of varying length, identifiable by their tryptic peptides, indicating the release of peptide chains at many different points during the stepwise growth of the chain (Fig. 5). Similarly, in the polyuridylate-dependent transfer of phenylalanine from sRNA into polyphenylalanine (NIRENBERG *et al.*, 1962) puromycin inhibits the formation of long (acid-precipitable) peptides but induces the formation of shorter (acid- and alcohol-soluble) phenylalanine peptides (NATHANS *et al.*, 1963).

The point of cleavage of the growing peptide chain which results in its release from the ribosome was identified by GILBERT in his studies on the nature of the polypeptide intermediate in protein synthesis (GILBERT, 1963). Using the polyuridylate-directed synthesis of polyphenylalanine in *E. coli* extracts, GILBERT observed the accumulation of polyphenylalanyl-sRNA attached to 50S ribosomes. In the presence of puromycin and a soluble cell fraction, polypenylalanine chains no longer linked to sRNA were released from ribosomes (Fig. 6). This finding indicates that puromycin leads to cleavage of the peptidyl-sRNA intermediate of protein synthesis, thus releasing incomplete protein chains.

The results detailed in the preceeding paragraph suggest that puromycin releases growing polypeptides from the ribosome-messenger RNA complex by causing a split of the ester linkage between the carboxyl group of the peptide and the hydroxyl group of adenosine at the end of sRNA. Further investigation of this reaction has shown that this bond is not cleaved hydrolytically, but rather that the peptide is transferred from sRNA to puromycin.

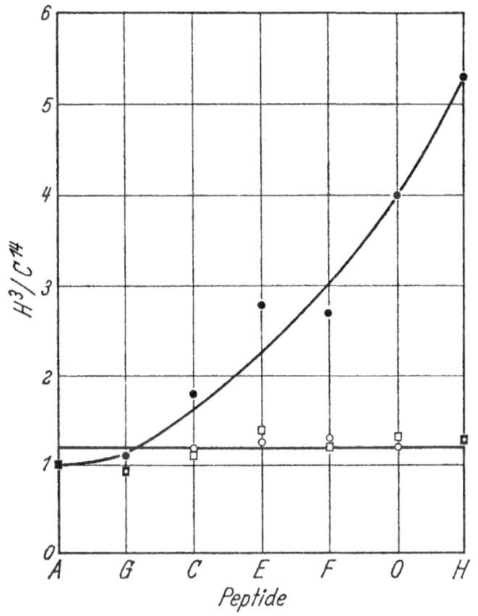

Fig. 5. Analysis of the fragments of coat protein of coliphage MS2 synthesized in the presence of puromycin. Coat protein labeled with H^3-alanine was synthesized in the presence of 1.5×10^{-6} M puromycin (70% inhibition), and in a second tube coat protein labeled with C^{14}-alanine was synthesized in the absence of puromycin. These products were mixed, digested with trypsin and the tryptic peptides separated and counted. The H^3/C^{14} ratio of a peptide, plotted on the ordinate, is a measure of the relative amount made in the presence of puromycin. On the abscissa the individual peptides are plotted in the order of their position in the coat protein molecule (*A* = carboxyl terminal peptide), as determined by pulse-labeling. As controls, similar experiments were carried out with chloramphenical (▫) and tetracycline (∘); (•) puromycin. Note that in the presence of puromycin the relative amount of each peptide is directly related to its proximity to the amino end of the protein, where protein synthesis begins. (From NATHANS, 1965)

The first indication that puromycin acts as an acceptor of the activated peptide came from observations of ALLEN and ZAMECNIK (1962) that rabbit reticulocyte ribosomes, which contain incomplete globin peptides, when incubated with puromycin radioactively labelled in the amino acid, release peptides which are radioactive (Fig. 7). On analysis of the released peptides it was found that for each N-terminal valine (valine is the N-terminal residue of rabbit globin) approximately one molecule of radioactive puromycin is present. Furthermore, the amino group of the amino acid portion of the incorporated puromycin was no longer free. These results indicate that all or part of a puromycin molecule is linked to released peptides via the amino group of the side chain.

The incorporation of puromycin into polypeptide chains has been studied also in intact bacterial cells (NATHANS, 1964). Growing *E. coli* incorporated radioactive puromycin into peptides, from which part of the puromycin could be released by means of trypsin and chymotrypsin. That the entire molecule of puromycin was present in these peptides was shown by chromatographic, electrophoretic, and chemical characterization of the released putative puromycin. By use of a model aminoacyl-puromycin (phenylalanyl-puromycin) in which an aromatic amino acid is bound in peptide linkage to

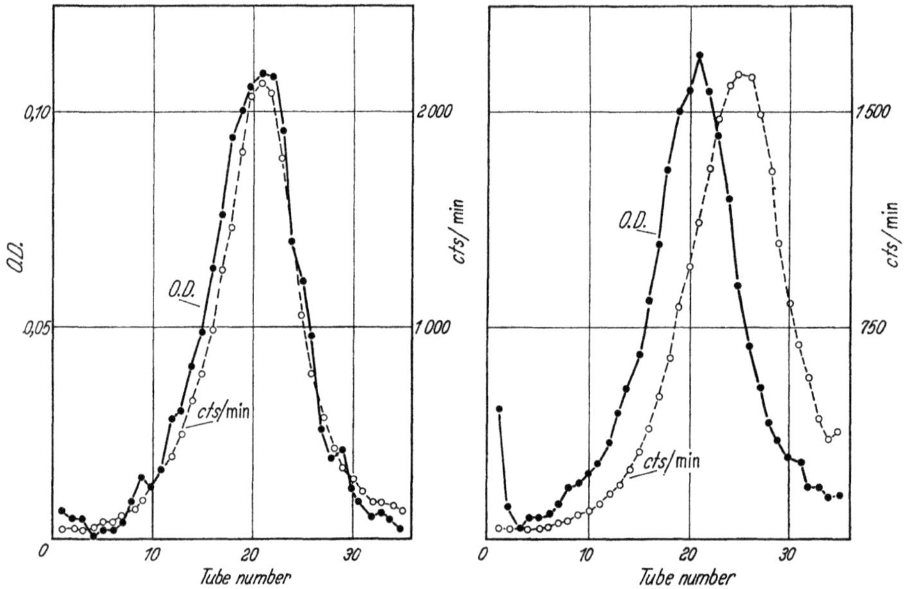

Fig. 6. The release of polyphenylalanine from polyphenylalanyl-sRNA by puromycin. The figure on the left is a sucrose gradient of C^{14}-polyphenylalanyl-sRNA isolated from *E. coli* extracts after polyuridylate-directed incorporation of C^{14}-phenylalanine. Carrier sRNA has been added (O.D.). On the right is a similar sucrose gradient of material isolated from a reaction mixture incubated with puromycin after incorporation of C^{14}-phenylalanine. Note that the O.D. (sRNA) and radioactivity (C^{14}-polyphenylalanine) peaks no longer correspond after incubation with puromycin. (From GILBERT, 1963)

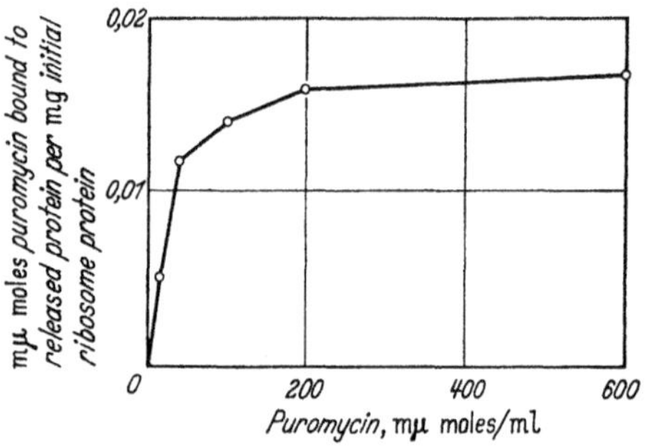

Fig. 7. The binding of C^{14}-puromycin by globin peptides released from reticulocyte ribosomes. Ribosomes were incubated with varying concentrations of C^{14}-puromycin and the released polypeptide precipitated at pH 5.1 and counted. The maximum level of incorporation of puromycin corresponds to about 1 molecule per peptide chain released. (From ALLEN and ZAMECNIK, 1962)

the free amino group of puromycin, it was shown that chymotrypsin liberates free puromycin from such a compound as it does from the peptidyl-puromycins isolated from whole cells. It was therefore concluded that puromycin becomes linked via a peptide bond at the C-terminal end of polypeptides in a reaction analogous to the transfer of peptide from peptidyl-sRNA to the next aminoacyl-sRNA (Fig. 8; compare with reaction 2b, Fig. 3).

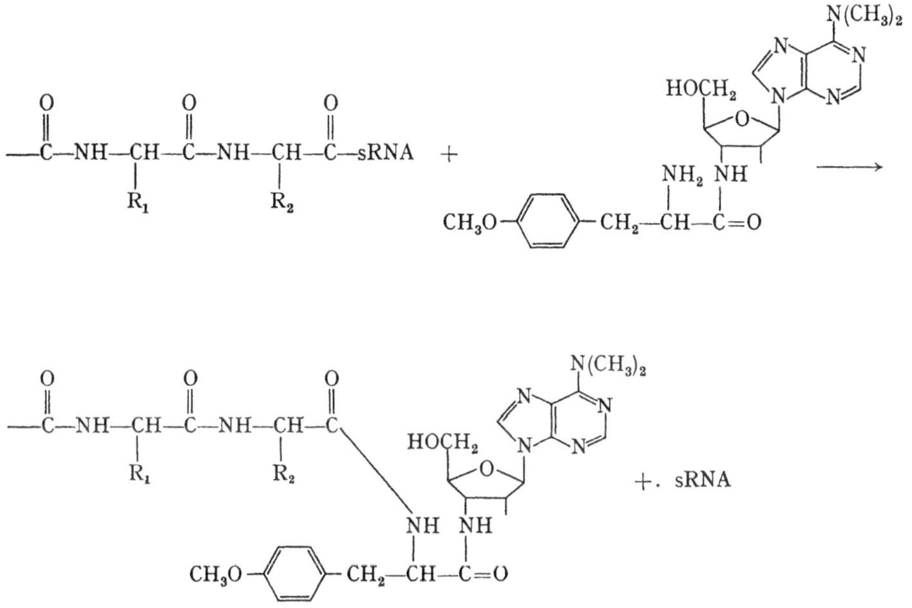

Fig. 8. The transfer of peptide chains from sRNA to puromycin. (From NATHANS, 1964)

The use of polyadenylate-directed synthesis of lysine peptides in the presence of puromycin has permitted more precise characterization of the resulting peptidyl-puromycins (SMITH *et al.*, 1965). SMITH *et al.* prepared an active, radiolabelled analogue of puromycin by reacting puromycin with P^{32} β-cyanoethyl phosphate under anhydrous conditions in the presence of dicyclohexylcarbodiimide, followed by purification of the cyanoethyl phosphate derivative. When this compound was added to *E. coli* extracts synthesizing lysine peptides in the presence of polyadenylate and H^3-lysine, a series of lysine peptides was isolated by column chromatography each of which contained a single molecule of the puromycin analogue (Fig. 9). On treatment of dilysyl-puromycin with trypsin, dilysine was formed, again indicating that puromycin is bound at the carboxyl end of the peptide by a peptide bond. The finding that essentially all released lysine peptides were linked to puromycin is in agreement with the results of ALLEN and ZAMECNIK (1962) that the amount of puromycin attached to globin peptides released from reticulocyte ribosomes is equivalent to the number of released peptide chains. Hence puromycin appears to effect peptide release from sRNA solely by accepting the carboxyl-activated peptide. One further finding of interest was reported in this system: although dilysyl-, trilysyl- and tetralysyl-puromycins were clearly identified, no lysyl-puromycin was found. This points to an unusual feature in the formation of the first peptide bond of the growing polylysine chain.

Although the mode of action of puromycin described above adequately accounts for inhibition of protein synthesis by this agent, a secondary effect on the polysome complex is of considerable interest, viz., the breakdown of polysomes by release of single ribosomes. For example, when intact reticulocytes were incubated with puromycin and the size distribution of isolated polysomes measured, there was a marked fall in the number of large polysomes and concomitant increase in the number of 80 S monosomes (HARDESTY *et al.*, 1963;

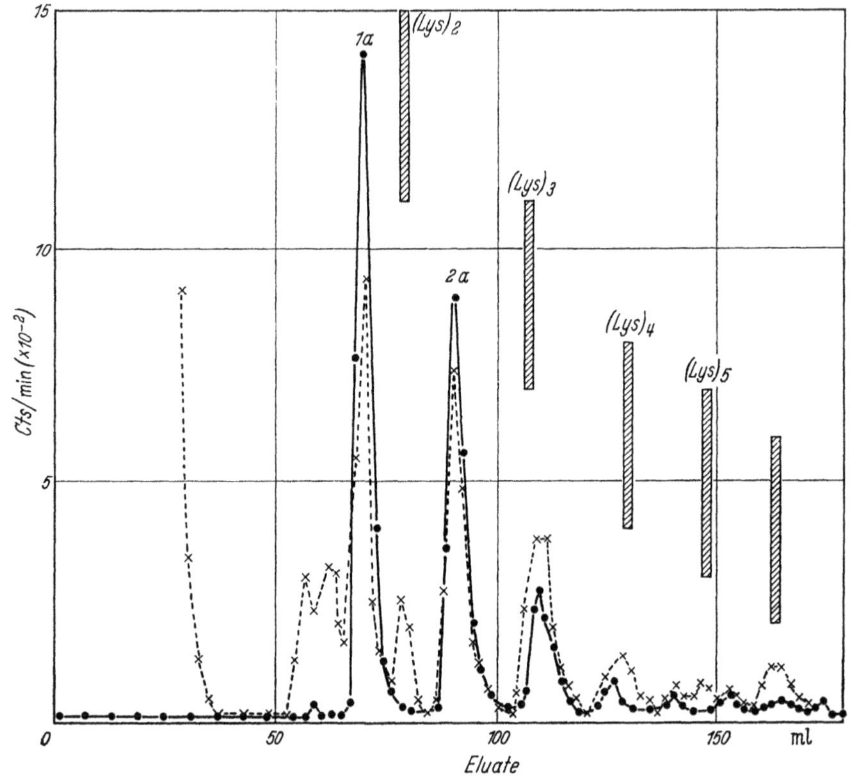

Fig. 9. Separation on cellulose phosphate of released H^3-lysine peptides formed in the presence of polyadenylate and P^{32}-puromycin-5′-β-cyanoethylphosphate. Vertical lines indicate positions of lysine peptides formed in the absence of puromycin analogue. Peaks 1a and 2a were identified as dilysyl-puromycin analogue and trilysylpuromycin analogue, respectively, (• • •) represents P^{32}, and (× × ×) represents H^3. (From SMITH *et al.*, 1965)

BURKA and MARKS, 1964). Similar observations have been made on liver polysomes of rats treated with puromycin (VILLA-TREVINO *et al.*, 1964) and in cell-free preparations of reticulocytes and rat liver (NOLL *et al.*, 1963; WILLIAMSON and SCHWEET, 1965; BURKA and MARKS, 1964) (see Fig. 10). Puromycin-induced polysome breakdown is, however, dissociable from puromycin-induced release of polypeptide chains; for example, in the absence of an energy source (as shown in Fig. 10) or in the presence of another inhibitor of protein synthesis, cyclohexamide, puromycin causes the release of ribosome-bound polypeptide, but fails to cause appreciable release of ribosomes from the polysome (COLOMBO *et al.*, 1965; WILLIAMSON and SCHWEET, 1965). Therefore, polysomal breakdown is not due to instability caused by removal of the peptide chains *per se*. Rather the release of ribosomes appears to be due at least in part, to resumption of protein synthesis from the point of peptidyl-sRNA cleavage, leading to continued movement of ribosomes along the messenger RNA (WILLIAMSON and SCHWEET, 1965). If the rate-limiting-step in extension of peptide chains (and hence in ribosome movement) is the binding of specific aminoacyl-sRNA's to the ribosome-messenger complex, puromycin might accelerate the progression of ribosomes by bypassing the binding step. As a consequence the polysomes would decrease in size (WILLIAMSON and SCHWEET, 1965; VILLA-TREVINO *et al.*, 1965). However, in view of the orderly variation in the relative amounts of MS2 phage coat peptides synthesized in cell extracts in the presence of puromycin (see Fig. 5), it is likely that some of the ribosomes fail to function beyond the point of peptide release. A similar conclusion has been reached by NOLL (1965).

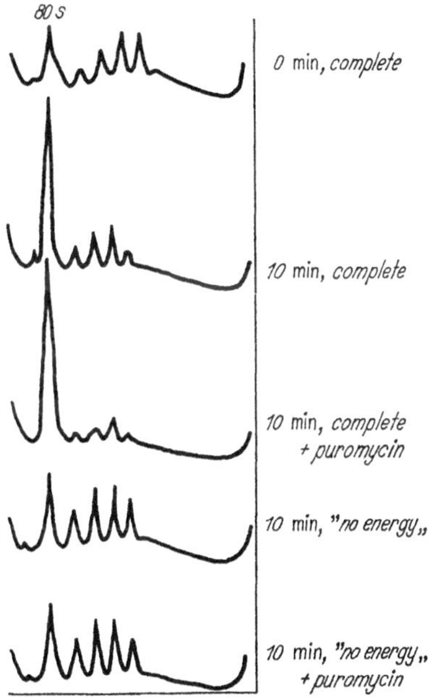

Fig. 10. Sedimentation patterns of rabbit reticulocyte ribosomes incubated with puromycin. The peaks to the right of 80 S are polysomes. "Complete" refers to an incubation in which all components required for protein synthesis are present; "no energy" indicates omission of ATP, GTP and generating system and soluble enzymes. In a separate experiment, puromycin released the growing peptides in the presence or absence of "energy". (From WILLIAMSON and SCHWEET, 1965)

The Puromycin Reaction as a Model for Peptide Bond Formation

The demonstration that puromycin becomes linked to the carboxyl group of peptide chains by means of a peptide bond suggested that this reaction might serve as a model for specifically studying peptide bond formation in protein synthesis (GILBERT, 1963; NATHANS, 1964; TRAUT and MONRO, 1964). Using the puromycin-dependent release of polyphenylalanine from the ribosome-bound peptidyl-sRNA as a measure of peptide-bond formation, TRAUT and MONRO (1965) observed a partial dependence of this reaction on the soluble cell fraction (presumably one or both "transfer enzymes") and GTP. In view of the extent of peptide release in the absence of enzyme and GTP (about 40% of the total polyphenylalanine released), it was suggested that puromycin can accept the peptide chain from peptidyl sRNA only when the latter occupies the "donor" binding site on the ribosome (see Fig. 3 and earlier discussion of protein synthesis), and that GTP and enzyme(s) lead to a shift of peptidyl-sRNA from the "acceptor" site to the "donor" site. Recent evidence obtained in the reticulocyte system supports this notion (SCHWEET *et al.*, 1965). Further studies along these lines should help identify the peptide-bond forming enzyme with certainty and elucidate the mechanism of the reaction which it catalyses.

Conclusion

The principal mode of action of puromycin as an inhibitor of protein synthesis has been clearly defined as a result of investigations on the mechanism of protein biosynthesis. As a structural analogue of aminoacyl-sRNA, puromycin accepts growing polypeptide chains intended for transfer to the next aminoacyl-sRNA, thus terminating further extension of the polypeptide. Presumably puromycin binds to the acceptor site of the peptide bond-forming enzyme, and it remains for future studies to clarify this interaction.

In contrast with this precise localization of puromycin action in the protein biosynthetic pathway are the more complicated effects on animal cells and intact animals. In addition to inhibition of protein synthesis there is evidence for an effect on nucleotide metabolism and RNA synthesis, which may be due in part to breakdown of the molecule to the aminonucleoside. For this reason, the conclusion that any puromycin-sensitive phenomenon is therefore dependent on protein synthesis is unwarranted in the absence of evidence pointing to inhibition of protein synthesis as the relevant site of puromycin action.

References

ALLEN, D., and P. C. ZAMECNIK: The effect of puromycin on rabbit reticulocyte ribosomes. Biochim. et Biophys. Acta **55**, 865 (1962).

BAKER, B. R., R. E. SCHAUB, and J. H. WILLIAMS: Puromycin. Synthetic studies. VIII. Synthesis of 3-amino-3-deoxy-D-ribofuranoside derivatives. A second synthesis of 3-amino-3-deoxy-D-ribose. J. Am. Chem. Soc. **77**, 7 (1955a).

BAKER, B. R., R. E. SCHAUB, J. P. JOSEPH, and J. H. WILLIAMS: Puromycin. Synthetic studies. IX. Total synthesis. J. Am. Chem. Soc. **77**, 12 (1955b).

BAKER, B. R., J. P. JOSEPH, and J. H. WILLIAMS: Puromycin. Synthetic studies. VII. Partial synthesis of amino acid analogs. J. Am. Chem. Soc. **77**, 1 (1955c).

BENNETT, F. L., S. L. HALLIDAY, J. J. OLESON, and J. H. WILLIAMS: The effect of amino acid analogs of puromycin on mouse mammary tumors. Antibiotics Ann. **1954/55**, 766.

BOROWSKY, B. A., D. M. KISSNER, and L. RECANT: Structural analogues of puromycin in production of experimental nephrosis in rats. Proc. Soc. Exptl. Biol. Med. **97**, 857 (1958).

BORTLE, L., and J. J. OLESON: Effect of puromycin on *Tetrahymena pyriformis* nutrition. Antibiotics Ann. **1954/55**, 770.

BUCHANAN, J. M.: Discussion of B. L. HUTCHINGS (1957).

BURKA, E. R., and P. A. MARKS: Protein synthesis in erythroid cells. II. Polyribosome function in intact reticulocytes. J. Mol. Biol. **9**, 439 (1964).

CHAPEVILLE, F., F. LIPMANN, G. V. EHRENSTEIN, B. WEISBLUM, W. J. RAY, JR., and S. BENZER: On the role of soluble RNA in coding for amino acids. Proc. Natl. Acad. Sci. U.S. **48**, 1086 (1962).

COLOMBO, B., L. FELICETTI, and C. BAGLIONI: Inhibition of protein synthesis by cyclohexamide in rabbit reticulocytes. Biochem. Biophys. Research Comm. **18**, 389 (1965).

CREASER, E. H.: The induced (adaptive) biosythesis of β-galactosidase in *Staphylococcus aureus*. J. Gen. Microbiol. **12**, 288 (1955).

DARKEN, M. A.: Puromycin inhibition of protein synthesis. Pharm. Rev. **16**, 223 (1964).

DECKER, K., H. E. FRANZ u. M. FRANZ: Vergleichende Untersuchungen über die Wirkung von Puromycin und Aminonucleosid auf die Proteinsynthese. Klin. Wschr. **42**, 583 (1964).

DUBACH, U. C.: Aminonucleosid-Nephrose. Fortschr. Arzneimittel-Forsch. **7**, 341 (1964).

FARNHAM, A. E.: Effect of aminonucleoside (of puromycin) on normal and encephalomyocarditis (EMC) virus-infected L cells. Virology **27**, 73 (1965).

FARNHAM, A. E., and D. T. DUBIN: Effect of puromycin aminonucleoside on RNA synthesis in L cells. J. Mol. Biol. **14**, 55 (1965).

FRANZ, H. E., M. FRANZ u. K. DECKER: Wirkung von Puromycin und Aminonucleosid auf die Purinbiosynthese. Hoppe-Seyler's Z. physiol. Chem. **336**, 127 (1964).

FRENK, S., I. ANTONOWICZ, J. M. CRAIG, and J. METCAFF: Experimental nephrotic syndrome induced in rats by aminonucleoside. Renal lesions and body electrolyte composition. Proc. Soc. Exptl. Biol. Med. **89**, 424 (1955).

GARDNER, R. S., A. J. WALBA, C. BASILIO, R. S. MILLER, P. LENGYEL, and J. F. SPEYER: Synthetic polynucleotides and the amino acid code. VII. Proc. Natl. Acad. Sci. U.S. **48**, 2087 (1962).

GILBERT, W.: Polypeptide synthesis in *Escherichia coli*. II. The polypeptide chain and sRNA. J. Mol. Biol. **6**, 389 (1963).

GORSKI, J., Y. AIZAWA, and G. C. MUELLER: Effect of puromycin *in vivo* on the synthesis of protein, RNA and phospholipids in rat tissues. Arch. Biochem. Biophys. **95**, 508 (1961).

HARDESTY, B., R. MILLER, and R. SCHWEET: Polyribosome breakdown and hemoglobin synthesis. Proc. Natl. Acad. Sci. U.S. **50**, 924 (1963).

HOFERT, J. S., J. GORSKI, G. C. MUELLER, and R. K. BOUTWELL: The depletion of liver glycogen in puromycin-treated animals. Arch. Biochem. Biophys. **97**, 134 (1962).

HOFERT, J. F., and F. K. BOUTWELL: Puromycin-induced glycogenolysis as an event independent from inhibited protein synthesis in mouse liver; effects of puromycin analogs. Arch. Biochem. Biophys. **103**, 338 (1963).

HOLLAND, J. J.: Effects of puromycin on RNA synthesis in mammalian cells. Proc. Natl. Acad. Sci. U.S. **50**, 436 (1963).

HUTCHINGS, B. L.: Puromycin. In: Chemistry and biology of purines (G. E. W. WOLSTENHOLME and C. M. O'CONNOR, eds.). Boston: Little, Brown & Co. 1957.

KAMMEN, H., R. BELOFF, and E. CANELLAKIS: Transformation in *Bacillus Subtilis*. I. Role of amino acids in stabilization of transformants. (In press.)

KESSNER, D. M., B. A. BOROWSKY, and L. RECANT: Effect of 6-dimethylaminopurine-3'-amino-D-ribose on adenosine triphosphate formation in yeast. Proc. Soc. Exptl. Biol. Med. **98**, 766 (1958).

KORNER, A., and M. S. RABEN: Effect of aminonucleoside and puromycin on insulin and epinephrine control of fatty acid release from adipose tissue. Nature **203**, 1287 (1964).

LEIVE, L.: A nonspecific increase in permeability in *Escherichia coli* produced by EDTA. Proc. Natl. Acad. Sci. U.S. **53**, 745 (1965).

MAALØE, O.: The control of normal DNA replication in bacteria. Cold Spring Harbor Symposia Quant. Biol. **26**, 45 (1961).

MCLAUGHLIN, C. S., and V. M. INGRAM: Chemical studies on amino acid acceptor ribonucleic acids. IV. Position of the amino acid residue in aminoacyl-sRNA: Chemical Approach. Biochemistry **4**, 1442 (1965a).

MCLAUGHLIN, C. S., and V. M. INGRAM: Chemical studies on amino acid acceptor ribonucleic acids. V. Position of the amino acid residue in aminoacyl-sRNA: Chromatographic approach. Biochemistry **4**, 1448 (1965b).

MORRIS, A., R. ARLINGHAUS, S. FLAVELUKES, and R. SCHWEET: Inhibition of hemoglobin synthesis by puromycin. Biochemistry **2**, 1084 (1963).

MUELLER, G. C., K. KAJIWARA, E. STUBBLEFIELD, and R. R. RUECKERT: Molecular events in the reproduction of animal cells. I. The effect of puromycin on the duplication of DNA. Cancer Research **22**, 1084 (1962).

NAKADA, D.: Ribosome formation by puromycin-treated *Bacillus Subtilis*. Biochim. et Biophys. Acta **103**, 455 (1965).

NATHANS, D., J. E. ALLENDE, T. W. CONWAY, G. I. SPYRIDES, and F. LIPMANN: Protein synthesis from aminoacyl-sRNA's. In: Symposium on Information Macromolecules (H. J. VOGEL, V. BRYSON and J. O. LAMPEN, eds.). New York: Academic Press 1963.

NATHANS, D., and A. NEIDLE: Structural requirements for puromycin inhibition of protein synthesis. Nature **197**, 1076 (1963).

NATHANS, D.: Puromycin inhibition of protein synthesis: The incorporation of puromycin into peptide chains. Proc. Natl. Acad. Sci. U.S. **51**, 585 (1964).

NATHANS, D.: Cell-free protein synthesis directed by coliphage MS2 RNA. J. Mol. Biol. **13**, 521 (1965).

NEIDHARDT, F. C.: The regulation of RNA synthesis in bacteria. Prog. in Nucleic Acid. Res. and Mol. Biol. **3**, 145 (1964).

NIRENBERG, M. W., J. H. MATTHAEI, and O. W. JONES: An intermediate in the biosynthesis of polyphenylalanine directed by synthetic template RNA. Proc. Natl. Acad. Sci. U.S. **48**, 104 (1962).

NOLL, H., T. STAEHELIN, and F. O. WETTSTEIN: Ribosomal aggregates engaged in protein synthesis: Ergosome breakdown and messenger RNA transport. Nature **198**, 632 (1963).

NOLL, H.: Polysome organization as a control element. (In press.)

PIECHOWSKI, M. M., and M. SUSSMAN: Studies on phage development. II. The maturation of T4 phage in the presence of puromycin. (In press.)

PORTER, J. N., R. I. HEWITT, C. W. HESSELTINE, G. KRUPKA, J. A. LOWERY, W. S. WALLACE, N. BOHONOS, and J. H. WILLIAMS: Achromycin: A new antibiotic having trypanocidal properties. Antibiot. & Chemotherapy **2**, 409 (1952).

RABINOVITZ, M., and J. M. FISHER: A dissociative effect of puromycin on the pathway of protein synthesis by Ehrlich ascites tumor cells. J. Biol. Chem. **237**, 477 (1962).

SCHWEET, R., R. ARLINGHAUS, R. HEINTZ, and J. SHAEFFER: Mechanism of peptide bond formation in protein synthesis. (In press.)

SELLS, B. H.: Puromycin. Effect on messenger RNA synthesis and β-galactosidase formation in *Escherichia coli* 15 T^-. Science **148**, 371 (1965).

SHERMAN, J. F., D. J. TAYLOR, and H. W. BOND: Puromycin. III. Toxicology and pharmacology. Antibiotics Ann. **1954/55**, 757.

SMITH, J. D., R. R. TRAUT, G. M. BLACKBURN, and R. E. MONRO: Action of puromycin in polyadenylic acid-directed polylysine synthesis. J. Mol. Biol. **13**, 617 (1965).

SONNENBLICHER, J., H. FELDMANN u. H. G. ZACHAU: Kernmagnetische Resonanz-Messungen an Aminoacyl-adenosin aus Aminoacyl-sRNA und an Modellsubstanzen. Hoppe-Seyler's Z. physiol. Chem. **341**, 249 (1965).

SPYRIDES, G. J.: The effect of univalent cations on the binding of sRNA to the template-ribosome complex. Proc. Natl. Acad. Sci. U.S. **51**, 1220 (1964).

STUDZINSKI, G. P., R. D. WOODRUFF, and R. LOVE: Relation between nucleolar morphology and RNA production. Federation Proc. **24**, 239 (1965).

TAKANAMI, M.: The effect of ribonuclease digests of aminoacyl-sRNA on a protein synthesis system. Proc. Natl. Acad. Sci. U.S. **52**, 1271 (1964).

TAKEDA, Y., S. HAYASHI, H. NAKAGAWA, and F. SUZUKI: The effect of puromycin on ribonucleic acid and protein synthesis. J. Biochem. (Tokyo) **48**, 169 (1960).

TAMAOKI, T., and G. C. MUELLER: Effect on puromycin on RNA synthesis in HeLa cells. Biochem. Biophys. Res. Comm. **11**, 404 (1963).

TRAUT, R., and R. E. MONRO: The puromycin reaction and its relation to protein synthesis. J. Mol. Biol. **10**, 63 (1964).

VILLA-TREVINO, S., E. FARBER, T. STAEHELIN, F. O. WETTSTEIN, and H. NOLL: Breakdown and reassembly of rat liver ergosomes after administration of ethionine or puromycin. J. Biol. Chem. **239**, 3826 (1964).

WALLER, C. W., P. W. FRYTH, B. L. HUTCHINGS, and J. H. WILLIAMS: Achromycin. The structure of the antibiotic puromycin. I. J. Am. Chem. Soc. **75**, 2025 (1953).

WHEELOCK, E. F.: The role of protein synthesis in the eclipse period of newcastle disease virus multiplication in HeLa cells as studied with puromycin. Proc. Natl. Acad. Sci. U.S. **48**, 1358 (1962).

WHITE, J. R., and H. L. WHITE: Streptomycinoid antibiotics: Synergism by puromycin. Science **146**, 772 (1964).

WILLIAMSON, A. R., and R. SCHWEET: Role of the genetic message in polyribosome function. J. Mol. Biol. **11**, 358 (1965).

WOLFENDEN, R., D. H. RAMMLER, and F. LIPMANN: On the site of esterification of amino acids to soluble RNA. Biochemistry **3**, 329 (1964).

WRIGHT, J. C., V. B. DOLGOPOL, M. LOGAN, A. PRIGOT, and L. T. WRIGHT: Clinical evaluation of puromycin in human neoplastic disease. Arch. intern. Med. **96**, 61 (1955).

YARMOLINSKY, M. B., and G. L. DE LA HABA: Inhibition of puromycin of amino acid incorporation into protein. Proc. Natl. Acad. Sci. U.S. **45**, 1721 (1959).

Gougerotin*

John M. Clark, Jr.

Gougerotin was first isolated as a water soluble, basic antibiotic from culture filtrates of *Streptomyces gougerotii, No. 21544* by workers at Takeda Chemical Industries, Ltd., Osaka, Japan (KANZAKI *et al.*, 1962). Gougerotin was found to be a broad spectrum antibiotic of only limited commercial value due to its weak antibiotic activity and toxicity to mammalian systems (Table 1). The I.V. LD_{50} in mice is 57 mg/kg.

Table 1. *Inhibitory levels of gougerotin* (KANZAKI *et al.*, 1962)

Organism	Detection limit (µg/ml) using agar streak method
E. coli	200
Prot. vulgaris	800
Staph. aureus 209 P	400
B. subtilis PCI 219	400
B. cereus	>800
Microc. flavus	40
Sarcina lutea	800
Ps. aeruginosa	800
B. brevis	200
Mycobacterium avium	800
M. avium streptomycin-fast	800
Mycobacterium 607	800
Mycobacterium smegmatis	>800
Mycobacterium phlei	800
M. tuberculosis H 37 Rv	100[1]
Pen. chrysogenum Q 176	>500
Sacc. cerevisiae	>500
Candida albicans	>500
Piricularia oryzae	>500
Gib. fujikuroi	>500
Phytophythora infestans	>500
Colleto. lagernarium	>500
Glomerella cingulata	>500
Alternaria kikuchiana	>500

[1] Serial broth dilution method.

* Supported in part by United States Public Health Service Grant, GM 08647.

In spite of the low commercial potential for gougerotin, Dr. IWASAKI of Takeda Chemical Industries, Ltd., carried out initial structural studies on gougerotin. These studies combined with gougerotin's empirical formula ($C_{16}H_{25}N_7O_8$), chemical and spectral properties, and ease of hydrolysis into ammonia, sarcosine, D-serine, and an amino sugar derivative led IWASAKI to propose N^4-sarcosyl-1-(3'-deoxy-3'-D-serylamido-β-D-allopyranosyl-uronamide)-cytosine (Fig. 1) as the structure for gougerotin (IWASAKI, 1962). Yet gougerotin demonstrates pKs at 3.7 and 8.5. IWASAKI's structure for gougerotin did not present a ready explanation for the pK value at 3.7. Accordingly, J. J. FOX and coworkers reexamined the structure of gougerotin. These workers showed that the D-serine in gougerotin exists in a dipeptide (i.e., it does not have free α amino group). Further, they characterized gougerotin's amino sugar as a 4-deoxy-4-amino-D-galactopyranuronamide. This led to the currently accepted gougerotin structure (FOX *et al.*, 1964) of 1-(cytosinyl)-4-sarcosyl-D-serylamino-1,4-dideoxy β-D-galactopyranuronamide (Fig. 2).

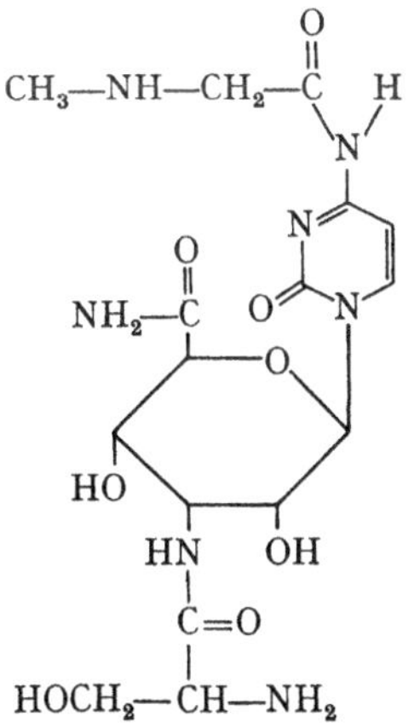

Fig. 1. Structure first proposed for gougerotin

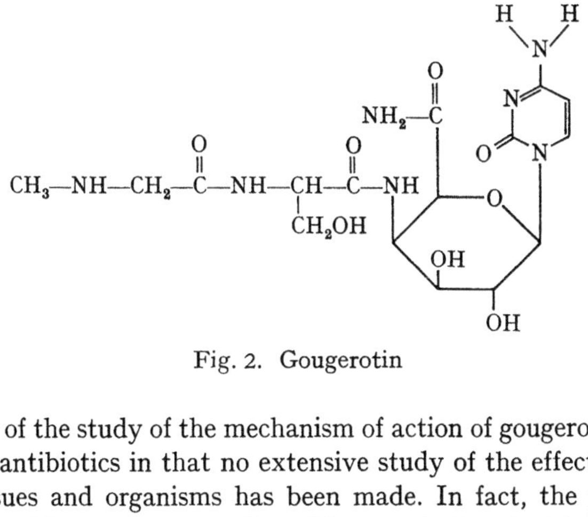

Fig. 2. Gougerotin

The history of the study of the mechanism of action of gougerotin is somewhat unique among antibiotics in that no extensive study of the effects of gougerotin on various tissues and organisms has been made. In fact, the primary site of action was derived from an examination of IWASAKI's theorized (and subsequently incorrect) structure of the antibiotic rather than from any physiological observation. J. M. CLARK, JR., and J. K. GUNTHER, at the University of Illinois, were intrigued with the similarities between IWASAKI's initial structure for gougerotin (Fig. 1) and the known protein synthesis inhibitor, puromycin (Fig. 3). Accordingly they investigated the effect of gougerotin on a cell free protein synthesizing system of *E. coli* (CLARK and GUNTHER, 1963). Their results clearly demonstrate that gougerotin is an inhibitor of protein synthesis in the *E. coli* system. They further demonstrated that gougerotin inhibits protein synthesis by inhibiting the transfer of amino acids from aminoacyl-S-RNA to protein (the "transfer reaction") rather than inhibiting aminoacyl-S-RNA synthesis. Gougerotin has subsequently been shown to be an inhibitor of the "transfer reaction" of protein synthesis in cell free systems obtained from mouse liver (SINOHARA and SKY-PECK, 1965) and rabbit reticulocytes (CLARK and CHANG, 1965; CASJENS and MORRIS, 1965). One can therefore probably safely conclude that gougerotin acts as an inhibitor of the "transfer reaction" in all tissues and organisms.

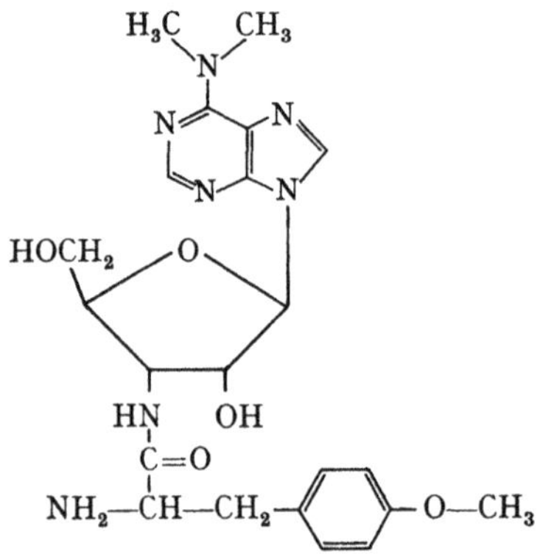

Fig. 3 Puromycin

Two separate laboratories have investigated the mechanism by which gougerotin inhibits the "transfer reaction" of protein synthesis (CLARK and CHANG, 1965 and CASJENS and MORRIS, 1965). Both of these groups independently arrived at the same general conclusions. Their reasoning followed the general pattern illustrated below.

An obvious hypothesis for the specific mechanism by which gougerotin inhibits protein synthesis arises from the structural similarities between gougerotin and puromycin (Fig. 3). Puromycin is known to inhibit protein synthesis by acting as an analog of aminoacyl-S-RNA and thereby catalyzing the release of incomplete protein chains (peptides) that terminate (C terminal) with puromycin (see review by NATHANS). This action of puromycin is conveniently assayed by measuring the release of acid soluble ^{14}C-materials (^{14}C-peptidyl puromycin forms) from ^{14}C-peptidyl-S-RNA, messenger-RNA, ribosome complexes (MORRIS *et al.*, 1963). Therefore, if gougerotin acts analogously to puromycin, then gougerotin should catalyze the release of acid soluble ^{14}C-materials from ribosomes prelabeled with ^{14}C-amino acids. Both groups (CLARK and CHANG, 1965 and CASJENS and MORRIS, 1965) found that gougerotin was incapable of catalyzing the release of peptidyl materials from prelabeled ribosomes capable of reacting with puromycin. Gougerotin therefore inhibits the "transfer reaction" of protein synthesis in a manner different from that of puromycin.

The structural similarities between gougerotin and puromycin suggest a second mechanism of action for gougerotin. The release of peptides containing puromycin at the C terminal end establishes that puromycin acts as a functional analog of aminoacyl-S-RNA. Thus the enzyme(s) involved in peptide bond formation during protein synthesis both recognizes puromycin as an analog of aminoacyl-S-RNA and transfers the growing peptide chain from peptidyl-S-RNA to puromycin. The structural differences between gougerotin and puromycin or aminoacyl-S-RNA suggest that the enzyme(s) involved in peptide bond formation also recognizes gougerotin as an analog of aminoacyl-S-RNA but is incapable of transferring the growing peptide chain from peptidyl-S-RNA to gougerotin. This would result in gougerotin acting as a nonfunctional analog of aminoacyl-S-RNA; i.e., a competitive inhibitor of either aminoacyl-S-RNA or puromycin in the peptidyl transfer mechanism ("peptide synthetase").

There is considerable evidence to support this concept that gougerotin acts as a competitive nonfunctional analog of aminoacyl-S-RNA and puromycin. Gougerotin does inhibit the puromycin dependent release of peptidyl materials from prelabeled ribosomes (CLARK and CHANG, 1965). In this inhibition, gougerotin acts as a strict competitive inhibitor relative to puromycin (CASJENS and MORRIS, 1965). Thus both puromycin and gougerotin act at the same site. Further, gougerotin does inhibit ribosomal motion along messenger-RNA as expressed by its inhibition of the release of free ribosomes from peptidyl-RNA, messenger-RNA, ribosome complexes (CASJENS and MORRIS, 1965). Finally, it has been shown (CLARK and CHANG, 1965) that gougerotin does not inhibit the other steps in the "transfer reaction". For example, gougerotin does not inhibit the binding of aminoacyl-S-RNA into initial aminoacyl-S-RNA, messenger-RNA, ribosome complexes (CLARK and CHANG, 1965) or the final GTP dependent release of completed globin chains from prelabeled rabbit reticulocyte ribosomes (CASJENS and MORRIS, 1965). Thus it can be concluded that gougerotin acts as a nonfunctional or competitive analog of aminoacyl-S-RNA (and puromycin) in the peptidyl transfer step of the "transfer reaction" in protein biosynthesis.

At this writing (1966), the exact mechanism involved in the peptidyl transfer step of the "transfer reaction" of protein synthesis is not defined. Therefore, the specific process or enzyme inhibited by gougerotin cannot be specified. The answer to this question must await further characterization of mechanisms involved in protein biosynthesis.

References

CASJENS, S. R., and A. J. MORRIS: The selective inhibition of protein assembly by gougerotin. Biochim. et Biophys. Acta **108**, 677 (1965).

CLARK, JR., J. M., and J. K. GUNTHER: Gougerotin, a specific inhibitor of protein synthesis. Biochim. et Biophys. Acta **76**, 636 (1963).

CLARK, JR., J. M., and A. Y. CHANG: Inhibitors of the transfer of amino acids from aminoacyl soluble ribonucleic acid to proteins. J. Biol. Chem. **240**, 4734 (1965).

FOX, J. J., Y. KUWADA, K. A. WATANABE, T. UEDA, and E. B. WHIPPLE: Nucleosides. XXV. Chemistry of gougerotin. Antimicrobial agents and chemotherapy (ed. J. C. SYLVESTER), p. 519. Am. Soc. Microbiol., 1964.

IWASAKI, H.: Studies on the structure of gougerotin, 11 structure of gougerotin. Yakagaku Zasshi **82**, 1393 (1962).

KANZAKI, T., E. HIGASHIDE, H. YAMAMOTO, M. SHIBATA, K. NAKAZAWA, H. IWASAKI, T. TAKEWAKA, and A. MIYAKE: Gougerotin, a new antibacterial antibiotic. J. Antibiotics (Japan), Ser. A **15**, 93 (1962).

MORRIS, A., R. ARLINGHAUS, S. FAVELUKES, and R. SCHWEET: Inhibition of hemoglobin synthesis by puromycin. Biochemistry **2**, 1084 (1963).

SINOHARA, H., and H. H. SKY-PECK: Effect of gougerotin on the protein synthesis in the mouse liver. Biochem. Biophys. Research. Commun. **18**, 98 (1965).

Cycloheximide and Other Glutarimide Antibiotics

Hugh D. Sisler and Malcolm R. Siegel

I. Introduction

A number of biologically active glutarimide derivatives have been isolated from various streptomycetes. The derivatives for which chemical structures have been determined include cycloheximide, naramycin B, isocycloheximide, streptimidone, acetoxycycloheximide, inactone and the streptovitacins. All have in common the β (2-hydroxyethyl) glutarimide moiety attached to a cyclic or acyclic ketone. Although the antibiotics are noted particularly for their antifungal properties, they are toxic to a broad spectrum of organisms. Yet, a highly interesting characteristic of these antibiotics is the marked difference in their activity toward closely related organisms.

Cycloheximide has been investigated far more extensively than any other member of this group and, therefore, much of the information in this chapter on mechanism of action is derived from studies of this derivative. However, where comparative studies have been made, the evidence indicates that other glutarimide derivatives act in the same manner as cycloheximide.

This chapter will deal mainly with structure activity relationships and mechanism of action of the antibiotics. Much of the literature on the chemical synthesis of these compounds, their use in control of fungal diseases of plants, and their antitumor properties will not be considered.

II. Structure and Biological Activity

A. Cycloheximide and Stereoisomers

1. Cycloheximide (l-Cycloheximide, Actidione, Naramycin A)

Cycloheximide was first isolated in crystalline form from culture filtrates of *Streptomyces griseus* by LEACH *et al.* (1947), and the chemical structure, β-[2 (3,5-dimethyl-2-oxocyclohexyl)-2-hydroxyethyl]-glutarimide, was determined by KORNFELD *et al.* (1949). Since there are 4 asymmetric centers in such a structure, a number of stereoisomers are possible and, therefore, much additional study was required to determine the stereochemical configuration of cycloheximide and that of certain of its stereoisomers (see JOHNSON *et al.*, 1965; for literature review). On the basis of optical rotatory dispersion analysis, OKUDA and SUZUKI (1961) concluded that the 3 substituents on the cyclohexanone ring of cycloheximide are oriented 2-equatorial, 4-axial, 6-equatorial[1] and that the antibiotic has the structure shown in Fig. 1. These conclusions have since been confirmed by chemical methods and nuclear magnetic resonance spectroscopy measurements (JOHNSON *et al.*, 1965). Clarification of the stereochemistry has made possible the total organic synthesis of *dl*- and *l*-cycloheximide (JOHNSON *et al.*, 1964).

Cycloheximide is toxic to a wide spectrum of organisms. These include fungi, higher plants, and mammals (WHIFFEN, 1948, 1950; FORD *et al.*, 1958; FORD and KLOMPARENS, 1960), algae (PALMER and MALONEY, 1955), and protozoa (LOEFER and MATNEY, 1952). It is not effective against bacteria, however (WHIFFEN, 1948). The antibiotic has antitumor activity, but it is apparently too toxic for practical use (FORD and KLOMPARENS, 1960). Cycloheximide was the most active of 233 chemicals tested as inhibitors of tobacco mosaic virus multiplication (LINDNER *et al.*, 1959). It is used to control certain fungal diseases of plants, although phytotoxicity tends to limit its usefulness for this purpose (FORD *et al.*, 1958). The antibiotic is also a highly effective rat repellent (WELCH, 1954).

Even though cycloheximide is toxic to diverse types of organisms, it displays marked specificity for closely related organisms. For example, growth of some species of yeasts is completely inhibited by concentrations less than 0.2 μg/ml whereas other species grow readily in the presence of 1000 μg/ml (WHIFFEN, 1948). Concentrations of the antibiotic required to prevent growth of 33 species of plant pathogenic fungi ranged from 0.125—100 μg/ml (WHIFFEN, 1950). The LD_{50} administered intravenously is 190 μg/kg in mice and 2.5 μg/kg in rats (FORD and KLOMPARENS, 1960).

2. *Isocycloheximide (d-Isocycloheximide)*

This stereoisomer of cycloheximide was found together with cycloheximide in aged filtrates from cultures of *S. griseus* (LEMIN and FORD, 1960). It has also been produced by isomerization of cycloheximide with acid deactivated alumina (LEMIN and FORD, 1960) and by chemical synthesis (SUZUKI *et al.*, 1963). The antibiotic (Fig. 1) differs from cycloheximide only in absolute configuration of the cyclohexanone ring and in orientation of the methyl group at position 4 in the ring (OKUDA and SUZUKI, 1961; JOHNSON *et al.*, 1965). Isocycloheximide was reported to be 30% as toxic to *Saccharomyces pastorianus* as cycloheximide (LEMIN and FORD, 1960), but SIEGEL *et al.* (1966) found a carefully purified sample to be only 13—14% as toxic to this organism as the latter antibiotic (Table 1).

3. *Naramycin B (d-Naramycin B)*

This antibiotic is a stereoisomer of cycloheximide which is produced together with cycloheximide by *Streptomyces naraensis novo* (OKUDA *et al.*, 1959). It has also been synthesized by hydrogenation of inactone (JOHNSON *et al.*, 1965). The absolute configuration of the cyclohexanone ring as well as the orientation of the methyl groups at both the 2 and 4 positions in the ring differ from those of cyclo-

[1] For the purposes of stereochemical discussions the numbering of the cyclohexanone ring begins at the carbonyl carbon atom, but in chemical designation of the antibiotic the numbering of the ring begins at the carbon attached to the hydroxyethylglutarimide moiety.

heximide (OKUDA and SUZUKI, 1961; OKUDA *et al.*, 1963; JOHNSON *et al.*, 1965). The antibiotic is only 32% as toxic to *Saccharomyces saki* as cycloheximide and relative toxicity of the 2 antibiotics to several other species of fungi (OKUDA *et al.*, 1959) and to *S. pastorianus* (Table 1) is similar to that observed with *S. saki*. However, the best samples of naramycin B prepared thus far apparently contain 25—33% cycloheximide (JOHNSON *et al.*, 1965; SIEGEL *et al.*, 1966). When this is taken into consideration it appears that naramycin B has little if any fungitoxic activity. On the other hand, a naramycin B sample which apparently contained some contaminating cycloheximide was reported to be 5 times as toxic to *Alternaria kikuchiana* as cycloheximide (OKUDA *et al.*, 1959). This implies that naramycin B is peculiarly more toxic to some fungal species than cycloheximide, even though it is almost without toxicity to other species.

4. Neocycloheximide

Neocycloheximide is a stereoisomer of cycloheximide synthesized by JOHNSON *et al.* (1962) which has the substituents on the cyclohexanone ring oriented 2-equatorial, 4-equatorial, 6-axial (JOHNSON *et al.*, 1965). Since the product synthesized is a racemic mixture, both the cycloheximide ring configuration and its mirror image are represented. It is not known, however, which ring configuration is associated with a hydroxyethylglutarimide side chain having the hydroxyl group oriented as in cycloheximide. *dl*-Neocycloheximide is essentially inactive against *S. pastorianus* (Table 1).

5. α-Epi-isocycloheximide (dl-α-Epi-isocycloheximide)

This isomer is apparently not produced by streptomycetes but it has been synthesized by purely chemical procedures (SUZUKI *et al.*, 1963; JOHNSON and CARLSON, 1965). *α-epi*-Isocycloheximide is identical with isocycloheximide except for the orientation of the hydroxyl group in the hydroxyethylglutarimide side chain. The *l* form of the isomer, therefore, differs from *l*-cycloheximide only in orientation of the methyl group at position 4 in the cyclohexanone ring (Fig. 1).

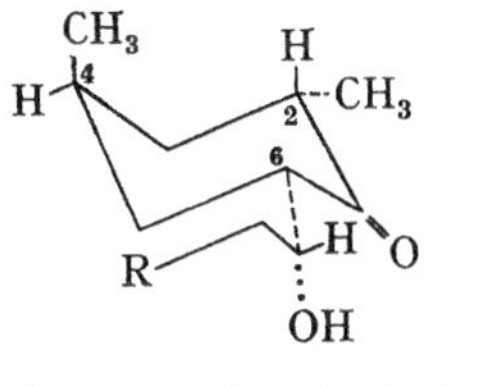
l-Cycloheximide (2e, 4a, 6e)

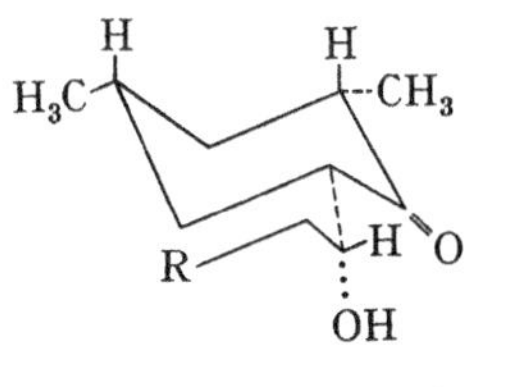
l-α epi Isocycloheximide (2e, 4e, 6e)

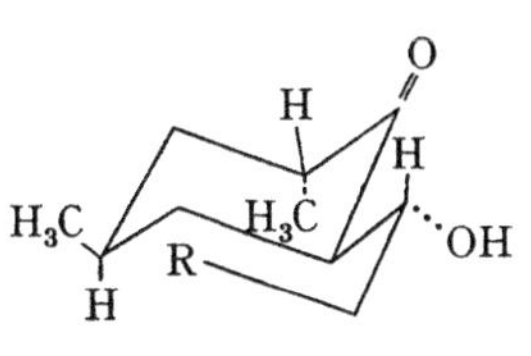
d-Naramycin B (2e, 4e, 6e)

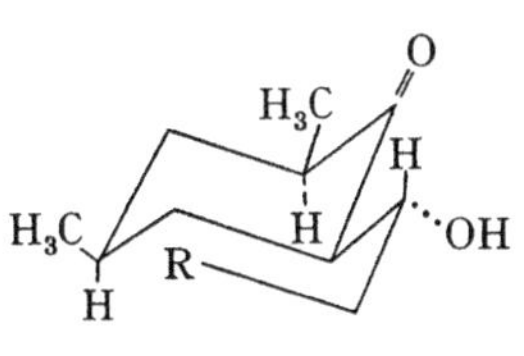
d-Isocycloheximide (2e, 4e, 6e)

Fig. 1. Conformational structures of *l*-cycloheximide and 3 of its stereoisomers. (R = glutarimide)

A racemic mixture of the antibiotic is $^1/_4$ as toxic to *S. pastorianus* as cycloheximide (Table 1). Assuming all activity in the mixture is due to the *l* form, its activity is $^1/_2$ that of cycloheximide.

B. Acetoxycycloheximide (E-73)

This glutarimide derivative (Fig. 3) was isolated from culture filtrates of *Streptomyces albulus* by RAO and CULLEN (1960), and its structure was determined by RAO (1960b). The stereochemistry of the antibiotic has not been fully elucidated. Acetoxycycloheximide is less toxic to *S. pastorianus* than cycloheximide (Table 1), but it is much more effective than the latter antibiotic against tumors (RAO, 1962) or protein synthesis in cell-free systems (see Section VII B).

C. Streptovitacins

Streptovitacins A, B, C_2 and D are a group of closely related antibiotics isolated from culture filtrates of a cycloheximide producing strain of *S. griseus* (EBLE *et al.*, 1959; SOKOLSKI *et al.*, 1959; HERR, 1959a, b). The antibiotics have the gross structure of cycloheximide, but with a single hydroxyl substituent on the cyclohexanone ring. The hydroxyl substituent in streptovitacin A (Fig. 3), B, and C_2 is at position 5, 4 and 3 respectively. Position of substitution in streptovitacin D is unknown (HERR, 1959b). The stereochemistry of these compounds has not been fully elucidated.

Antitumor activity of streptovitacin A is 70—100 times that of B or C_2. Streptovitacin A and D are equally effective against Walker 256 tumor, but the former antibiotic is almost 10 times as effective as the latter against Ehrlich carcinoma (EVANS *et al.*, 1960). The dose of antibiotic producing 50% inhibition of growth of the KB strain of human epidermoid cells in tissue culture is 0.035, 0.48, 90, 0.06 and 0.1 μg/ml respectively for streptovitacin A, B, C_2, D and cycloheximide (SMITH *et al.*, 1959). Streptovitacin A and B are only about 1% as toxic to cells of *S. pastorianus* as cycloheximide (SOKOLSKI *et al.*, 1959). Relative toxicity of the three antibiotics to the protozoan, *Trichomonas vaginalis*, follows the general pattern of their toxicity to KB cells in tissue culture. The 50% inhibitory dose for this organism in μg/ml is 0.04, 0.4 and 0.1 respectively for streptovitacin A, B and cycloheximide (SOKOLSKI *et al.*, 1959).

D. Streptimidone

This glutarimide derivative (Fig. 2) is produced by *Streptomyces rimosus* forma *paramomycinus* (FROHARDT *et al.*, 1959). The ketone in streptimidone is not cyclic as in most other glutarimide antibiotics (FROHARDT *et al.*, 1959; VAN TAMELEN and HAARSTAD, 1960; WOO *et al.*, 1961). The biological activity of streptimidone was investigated by KOHBERGER *et al.* (1960). It is highly toxic to certain species of yeast and filamentous fungi, but many of the latter are not highly sensitive to the antibiotic. The LD_{50} for mice is 192 mg/kg when the antibiotic is administered intravenously. Unlike cycloheximide and streptovitacin A and B, it is not highly toxic to *T. vaginalis*. It is lethal to *Entamoeba histolytica* at 8 μg/ml. Although streptimidone is not markedly toxic to many species of bacteria, 25 μg/ml completely inhibits growth of *Brucella suis*, *Staphylococcus aureus* and *Streptococcus pyogenes*.

E. Inactone

This glutarimide derivative was isolated from culture filtrates of a cycloheximide producing strain of *S. griseus* and the structure (Fig. 2) was determined by PAUL and TCHELITCHEFF (1955). It is only 2—8% as toxic to cells of *S. pastorianus* as cycloheximide (PAUL and TCHELITCHEFF, 1955) (Table 1). Inactone has been reduced over a rhodium-on-alumina catalyst to a product consisting of about 30% cycloheximide and 70% naramycin B (JOHNSON *et al.*, 1965).

F. Actiphenol (C-73)

HIGHET and PRELOG (1959) isolated this glutarimide derivative from culture filtrates of a cycloheximide producing streptomycete and determined its structure (Fig. 2). Independently the compound was isolated by RAO (1960a), who gave it the trivial designation, C-73. The derivative has been produced by aromatization of the cyclohexane ring of cycloheximide with N-bromosuccinimide (HIGHET and PRELOG, 1959), and more recently, JOHNSON (1962) has accomplished total organic synthesis of the compound. The derivative is not toxic to cells of *S. pastorianus* (Table 1).

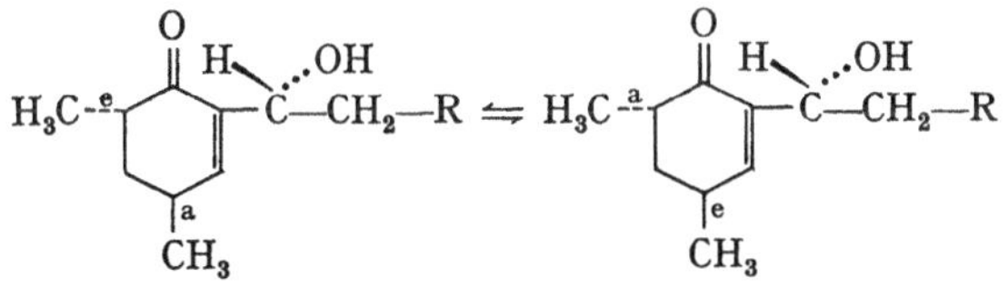

Inactone

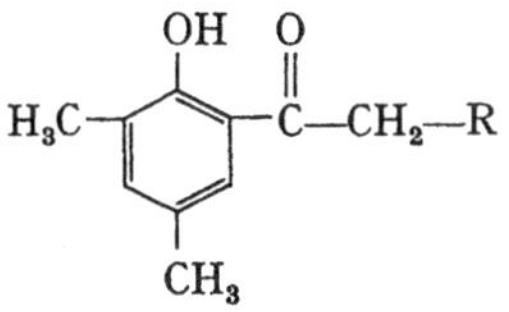

Actiphenol

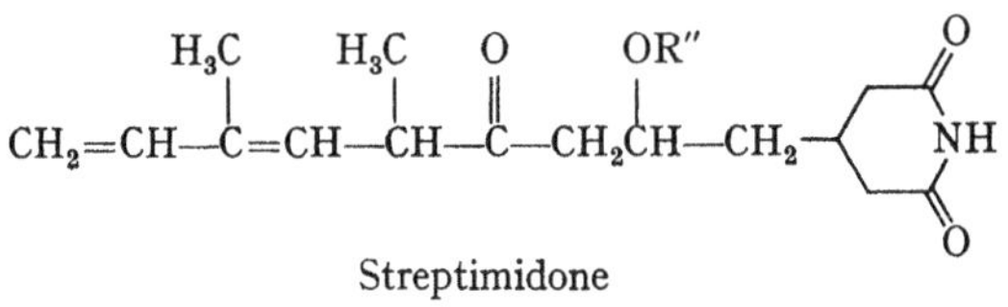

Streptimidone

Glutarimide (R)
Streptimidone (R''=H)
Streptimidone acetate ($R'' = -\overset{O}{\overset{\|}{C}}-CH_3$)

Fig. 2. Structures of inactone, actiphenol, and streptimidone

G. Protomycin, Fermicidin and Niromycins

These are incompletely characterized glutarimide antibiotics.

Protomycin was isolated from culture filtrates of *Streptomyces reticuli*, var. *protomycicus* by HIRABAYASHI (1959). Characteristics of the antibiotic suggest that it is closely related to streptimidone (SUGAWARA, 1963b). It is highly toxic to *Saccharomyces cerevisiae*, *S. saki*, *Aspergillus fumigatus*, *Piricularia oryzae* and *E. histolytica*, but shows little activity toward bacteria (SUGAWARA, 1963a).

Fermicidin is produced by *Streptomyces griseolus* and is toxic to certain yeasts and fungi (IGARASHI and WADA, 1954).

Niromycin A and B are produced by *Streptomyces albus* (OSATO *et al.*, 1960a). Although they have not been completely characterized, they resemble the streptovitacins in some respects (OSATO *et al.*, 1960b). The antibiotics are active against viruses, certain yeasts and filamentous fungi.

H. Derivatives of Glutarimide Antibiotics

A number of derivatives of glutarimide antibiotics have been synthesized which are of interest from the point of view of structure-activity relationships.

Esters of cycloheximide which have been tested for toxicity include the acetate (Fig. 3) (LEMIN and MAGEE, 1957) benzoate, 3,4-dichlorobenzoate, tosylate and mesylate (SUZUKI, 1960). The acetate ester is completely ineffective against *S. pastorianus* (Table 1), but it is toxic to tomato plants (LEMIN and MAGEE, 1957). It is $^{1}/_{32}$ as toxic to *P. oryzae* as cycloheximide, but the remaining 4 esters are either non-toxic or are only $^{1}/_{64}$ as toxic as cycloheximide to this organism or to

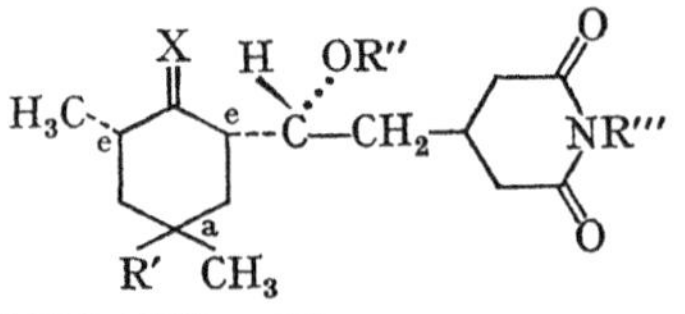

Cycloheximide (X = O, R′, R″, R‴ = H)
Cycloheximide oxime (X = NOH, R′, R″, R‴ = H)
Cycloheximide semicarbazone ($X = N{-}NHC({=}O){-}NH_2$, R′, R″, R‴ = H)
ψ cycloheximide-I-acetate ($X = O{-}C({=}O){-}CH_3$, R′, R‴ = H)
α dihydrocycloheximide (X = OH—e, R′, R″, R‴ = H)
β dihydrocycloheximide (X = OH—a, R′, R″, R‴ = H)
Acetoxycycloheximide (X = O, $R' = O{-}C({=}O){-}CH_3$, R″, R‴=H)
Streptovitacin-A (X = O, R′ = OH, R″, R‴ = H)
Cycloheximide acetate (X = O, $R'' = {-}C({=}O){-}CH_3$, R′, R‴ = H)
N-methylcycloheximide (X = O, R′, R″ = H, $R''' = CH_3$)
N-methylcycloheximide acetate (X = O, R′ = H, $R'' = {-}C({=}O){-}CH_3$, $R''' = CH_3$)

Fig. 3. Structures of glutarimide derivatives. Cycloheximide, acetoxycycloheximide and streptovitacin A are naturally occurring antibiotics. The remaining compounds are derived from cycloheximide or are produced by organic synthesis. (Oxygen at R″ position is ketone in ψ cycloheximide-I acetate)

S. saki (SUZUKI, 1960). On the other hand, antitumor activity of the acetyl, propionyl, butyryl and benzoyl esters of acetoxycycloheximide is nearly as high as that of the parent antibiotic (RAO, 1962). It seems unlikely that any of these esters would be active, however, in the absence of esterases which release the parent antibiotic. For example, higher plants are sensitive to cycloheximide acetate, but they contain esterases which hydrolyze the esters (LEMIN and MAGEE, 1957; SISLER and SIEGEL, 1966), whereas cells of *S. pastorianus* which are highly sensitive to the parent antibiotic are deficient in such enzymes and apparently for this reason they are resistant to the ester (SISLER and SIEGEL, 1966). The oxime derivative of cycloheximide is only slightly toxic whereas the semicarbazone derivative is moderatly toxic to cells of *S. pastorianus* (Table 1). Toxicity in these cases again appears to depend upon release of the parent antibiotic. The release is known to be pH dependent in the case of the semicarbazone derivative. Toxicity of this derivative is about 2% of that of cycloheximide at pH 6.5, but it increases to about 60% as the pH is lowered to 3.5. The increase of free cycloheximide as the pH is lowered can be demonstrated chromatographically (SISLER and SIEGEL, 1966).

Methylation of the imide nitrogen of cycloheximide leads to complete loss of toxicity to *S. pastorianus* (Table 1), *S. saki* and *P. oryzae* (SUZUKI, 1960). Reduction of the carbonyl group of the cyclohexanone to produce α or β dihydrocycloheximide (Fig. 3) drastically reduces toxicity to *S. pastorianus* (Table 1) or to *S. saki* and *P. oryzae* (SUZUKI, 1960).

I. Structure-Activity Relationships

It is apparent, from the preceeding consideration of the structure of glutarimide derivatives, that the ketone-carbonyl, the hydroxyl, or the imide nitrogen groups cannot be removed or substituted without almost complete loss of activity. The least critical structural requirements appear to be in the moiety attached to the ketone-carbonyl group opposite the hydroxyethylglutarimide portion of the molecules. This is evident from a comparison of the structure of the biologically active compounds, cycloheximide and streptimidone.

In regard to the stereochemical isomers of cycloheximide involving the trisubstituted cyclohexanone ring (isocycloheximide, naramycin B and α-*epi*-isocycloheximide), it seems likely the ring configuration has more influence on activity than orientation of the methyl groups. The "normal" ring configuration in *l*-cycloheximide and *l*-α-*epi*-isocycloheximide is the mirror image of the "iso" configuration in *d*-isocycloheximide and *d*-naramycin B, but orientation of the hydroxyethylglutarimide side chain at position 6 is similar in all 4 isomers as is also the orientation of the hydroxyl group in the side chain. However, the conformational equilibrium position of the side chain is such that the carbonyl and hydroxyl groups are closer in the isomers with the "normal" ring configuration than in those with the "iso" configuration. Consequently, intramolecular hydrogen bonding is stronger in the former type isomer than in the latter (OKUDA, 1959; SUZUKI *et al.*, 1963). *l*-Cycloheximide and *l*-α-*epi*-isocycloheximide are both more active biologically than *d*-isocycloheximide or *d*-naramycin B. This may be due to the difference in distance between the carbonyl and hydroxyl group which could influence the affinity of the antibiotics for the biological site of action.

Dehydration of the cycloheximide molecule to from anhydrocycloheximide, a compound which lacks a hydroxyl group and is unsaturated between carbon 6 of the cyclohexanone ring and the α carbon of the ethylglutarimide side chain, leads to complete loss of toxicity to *S. pastorianus* (Table 1), *S. saki* and *P. oryzae* (SUZUKI, 1960). Reduction of the unsaturated linkage produces deoxycycloheximide, a compound also non-toxic to *S. saki* and *P. oryzae* (SUZUKI, 1960).

LEE and WILKIE (1965) report that anhydrocycloheximide is fully as toxic to *S. cerevisiae* as cycloheximide. This is at variance with the observation cited above. Possibly under the conditions of their experiments, rehydration of the molecule occurred.

III. Morphological and Cytological Effects

Although cycloheximide does not typically produce prominent morphological abnormalities in cells, such effects have been observed by GUNDERSEN (1961) in *Fomes annosus* and by GUNDERSEN and WADSTEIN (1962) in *S. pastorianus*. The antibiotic causes appreciable swelling of hyphal cells of *F. annosus* which is sometimes accompanied by cell lysis. At low concentrations it causes weakening of cell walls, giant cell formation, and cell rupture in growing cultures of *S. pastorianus*. These effects are possibly a consequence of inhibited protein synthesis, and may result from failure to synthesize wall protein.

Cycloheximide also causes aberrations in mitotic behavior in cells of pea and onion root tips (WILSON, 1950; HAWTHORNE and WILSON, 1952; HADDER and WILSON, 1958). The effect is distinct from that of colchicine and has been classified as prophase poisoning (WILSON, 1965). In a species of *Gymnosporangium* the antibiotic produces an effect on meiosis which suggests it may cause malfunctioning of the spindle (BERLINER and OLIVE, 1953).

It is not possible to say whether these aberrations result from a direct effect of the antibiotic in the mitotic or meiotic processes or from an indirect effect on some aspect of metabolism such as protein synthesis.

IV. Uptake of Cycloheximide by Yeast Cells

WESCOTT and SISLER (1964) studied uptake of cycloheximide by a sensitive yeast, *S. pastorianus*, and by a resistant yeast, *S. fragilis*, using a volume distribution technique. The sensitive yeast (sensitive to 1 μg/ml) concentrated cycloheximide more than 10 fold from solutions containing 0.1—1.0 μg/ml of the toxicant. A maximum accumulation of 7.9 μg/g of cells occurred when the external concentration was 10 μg/ml, although the efficiency of removal was less at this concentration than at 0.1—1.0 μg/ml. The antibiotic was apparently not concentrated by the resistant yeast (resistant to 1000 μg/ml), because the final concentration in the cellular volume was essentially the same as that in the extra-cellular solution. It was suggested, therefore, that cycloheximide penetrated the resistant yeast, but was not concentrated because of the lack of internal binding sites. These measurements were not sufficiently definitive, however, to eliminate the possibility that *S. fragilis* is impermeable to the antibiotic, because slight binding at the surface of the cells without penetration would give similar results. On the other hand, the conclusions of WESCOTT and SISLER are supported by the observation that the difference in sensitivity of the protein synthesizing systems in the 2 organisms to cycloheximide can readily explain the difference in sensitivity of the organisms to the antibiotic (see Section VI B).

Resistance of *S. fragilis* apparently does not result from an ability to detoxify the antibiotic, because there is no detectable loss of toxicant from solutions in which the organism is grown. GUNDERSEN and WADSTEIN (1962) were likewise unable to detect any detoxication of cycloheximide by a strain of *S. pastorianus* resistant to 5 μg/ml of the antibiotic.

V. Genetic Basis of Resistance to Cycloheximide

Yeasts grown in media containing cycloheximide usually develop resistance to the antibiotic. This was observed by WHIFFEN (1948) and by GUNDERSEN and WADSTEIN (1962) in *S. pastorianus*, and by MONREAL (1961) in *S. cerevisiae* var. *ellipsoideus*. Resistance to cycloheximide developed in the filamentous fungi, *F. annosus* (GUNDERSEN, 1962a), *Sclerotinia laxa*, and *Sclerotinia fructicola* (GROVER and MOORE, 1962). Resistance developed slowly as the organisms were transferred to media containing progressively higher concentrations of the antibiotic, but no highly resistant organisms were obtained in these particular studies.

The genetic basis of resistance to cycloheximide has been investigated in *S. cerevisiae* and *Neurospora crassa*. MIDDLEKAUF *et al.* (1957) analyzed genetic resistance to the antibiotic in a strain of *S. cerevisiae* and concluded that a single dominant gene conferred resistance. A much more extensive investigation of resistance in this organism was made by WILKIE and LEE (1965). Eight genes for resistance (to 0.5 μg/ml or greater) were shown to occur in various strains of the yeast. Four of these were semidominant, one was dominant, and three were recessive. Positive interaction between these genes in recombinant strains could be demonstrated. For instance, when crosses between strains possessing a different gene for resistance to 1 μg/ml of cycloheximide were made, the recombinants possessing both genes were resistant to 10 μg/ml of the antibiotic.

In addition to a variety of genes for resistance, recessive modifier genes were found which do not themselves confer resistance, but which modify activity of the resistance genes in a positive way. High levels of resistance were built up step-wise by ultraviolet induced mutations and selection on media containing successively higher concentrations of the antibiotic. The level of resistance seen in a first step mutant did not exceed 20 μg/ml of the antibiotic, but in 3 or 4 steps, strains resistant to 1000 μg/ml were obtained. Genetic analysis of a strain tolerant to 1000 μg/ml revealed the following genes controlling resistance. AC^r_7 conferring resistance to 1 μg/ml, ac^r_8 conferring resistance to 20 μg/ml, and an unlinked modifier, m_7, which increases resistance conferred by the interaction of AC^r_7 and ac^r_8 five fold. Genes AC^r_7 and ac^r_8 interact to produce a strain resistant to 200 μg/ml and in the presence of m_7, this resistance is increased to 1000 μg/ml.

The bases of cycloheximide resistance in *N. crassa* was studied by HSU (1963). Seven mutants resistant to the antibiotic were produced by ultraviolet irradiation. A 2:2 segregation for resistance and sensitivity in individual, unordered tetrads was obtained in each case when the mutants were crossed with the wild type. Resistance, therefore, was due to mutation of a single gene, but the mutant gene was located in linkage group I in some isolates whereas, in others it was located in linkage group V. The mutants, which were about 100 times as resistant as the wild type, were phenotypically indistinguishable. A cross between strains with resistance genes at different loci gave a 3:1 ratio of resistant to sensitive phenotypes in the progeny. Among the resistant segregants, one third were slow growers. These were subsequently shown to be highly resistant, double mutants. Apparently one wild type allele at either one of the 2 cycloheximide resistance loci in a single nucleus must be present for normal growth in the absence of the antibiotic. This was inferred from the observation that heterokaryons carrying mutant genes at both loci grew normally. The mutant alleles at both loci were dominant over their wild type alleles in heterokaryons.

Now that the inheritance of resistance to cycloheximide has been clarified in *S. cerevisiae* and *N. crassa* it may be possible to identify the factors of gene action which are involved. Positive interaction of genes might conceivably involve a lowered permeability combined with increased resistance at the site of action. It might be postulated that the several resistance genes in *S. cerevisiae* confer resistance to a corresponding number of separate sites of action of cycloheximide in the cells. But this seems unlikely, because 8 genes were shown which confer resistance to various levels of antibiotic in the range of 0.5—20 μg/ml. Therefore a mutant having a single gene conferring resistance to 20 μg/ml of the antibiotic should still contain sites which would be susceptible to concentrations of the toxicant less than 20 μg/ml.

VI. Reversal of Toxicity

Toxicity of cycloheximide to yeasts (KERRIDGE, 1958; COURSEN and SISLER, 1960) or to the fungus *Coccomyces hiemalis* (STARZYK, 1963) is easily reversed by washing the cells free of the antibiotic. Little loss of viability of *Coccomyces* spores occurs even after exposure for a day to 1—10 μg/ml of cycloheximide, but after 8 days, viability is reduced 88—92% relative to that of untreated spores. Inhibition of protein synthesis in mammalian L cells in suspension culture (ENNIS and LUBIN, 1964) or in rabbit reticulocytes (COLOMBO *et al.*, 1965) is likewise reversed when cells are washed free of the antibiotic.

On the other hand, attempts to reverse toxicity with metabolites has proved unsuccessful. Many metabolites added singly or in various combinations failed to reverse toxicity of cycloheximide to *S. pastorianus* (COURSEN, 1959). Vitamin A alcohol and acetate were slightly active, but the significance of this antagonim, if any, was not determined. In similar tests, COONEY and BRADLEY (1962) did not find any metabolites which counteracted the toxicity of the antibiotic to *Tetrahymena piriformis*. SMITH *et al.* (1960) were also unsuccessful in their attempts to reverse toxicity of streptovitacin A to KB human epidermoid carcinoma cells by a variety of metabolites. Uracil, xanthine, guanine, adenine and *p*-aminobenzoic acid slightly counteracted toxicity of cycloheximide to *F. annosus* (GUNDERSEN, 1962b). It is doubtful, however, whether these effects are of any significance, because purines, pyrimidines and nucleosides did not influence toxicity of glutarimide antibiotics to yeast (COURSEN, 1959), *Tetrahymena* (COONEY and BRADLEY, 1962), or mammalian cells (SMITH *et al.*, 1960).

Ferrous sulfate increases the effectiveness of cycloheximide in laboratory and field tests (FORD *et al.*, 1958). BLUMAUEROVÁ and STARKA (1959), on the other hand, demonstrated that heavy metal ions such as Fe, Mn and Zn counteract toxicity to some extent, and suggested that the antibiotic chelates these ions and is rendered less effective. Influence of these ions must not be very appreciable because several investigators (WHIFFEN, 1948; GUNDERSEN, 1962b; COONEY and BRADLEY, 1962) were unable to demonstrate an effect of heavy metal salts on toxicity of the antibiotic.

VII. Physiological and Biochemical Effects

A. Effect on Energy Metabolism and Amino Acid Synthesis

The effect of cycloheximide on respiratory metabolism has been studied in several species of yeast (SISLER and MARSHALL, 1957; KIELHÖFER and AUMANN, 1957; GRIEG *et al.*, 1958; KERRIDGE, 1958; BLUMAUEROVÁ and STARKA, 1959; TSUKADA *et al.*, 1962; WIDUCZYNSKI and STOPPANI, 1965) in filamentous fungi (WALKER and SMITH, 1952; MCCALLAN *et al.*, 1954; SISLER and MARSHALL, 1957), in the *T. pyriformis* (MEFFERD and LOEFER, 1954; COONEY and BRADLEY, 1962) and in mammalian tissue culture cells (ARNOW *et al.*, 1962). These studies showed that inhibition of respiration or glycolysis by concentrations of the antibiotic which prevented growth was usually slight and seldom exceeded 40%. However, a concentration (3.6 µg/ml) which completely inhibited germination of spores of *Myrothecium verrucaria* also inhibited respiration 85% (WALKER and SMITH, 1952).

In view of the fact that cycloheximide completely inhibits growth of a number of organisms without appreciable effects on respiration or glycolysis, it seems unlikely that its primary toxic effect is on these processes. The respiratory inhibition which does occur probably results from feedback effects of inhibition of some other process in the cells.

Other types of evidence also suggest that cycloheximide does not interfere primarily with energy metabolism or the synthesis of amino acids and Krebs cycle intermediates in sensitive cells. Incorporation of label from ^{14}C glucose into free amino acids and Krebs cycle acids in *S. pastorianus* was not markedly affected by the antibiotic, although distribution of label among these intermediates was somewhat altered (COURSEN and SISLER, 1960; SIEGEL and SISLER, 1964a). A marked inhibition of labelling of glutamine and of glutamic acid was the most prominent effect of cycloheximide. On the other hand, WIDUCZYNSKI and STOPPANI (1965) did not observe such an effect on the labelling of these amino acids in cells of *S. ellipsoideus* incubated with ^{14}C labelled glucose or acetate. Following a 90 minute incubation with these substrates, cycloheximide treated cells contained more label in the free amino acid and organic acid fractions than untreated cells. There was no apparent inhibition of labelling of any component within these fractions in the treated cells. The antibiotic (33 µg/ml) did not inhibit respiration or oxidative phosphorylation in rat liver mitochondria (LARDY *et al.*, 1958). These results are consistent with the observation that ^{32}P from inorganic orthophosphate is incorporated into ATP without difficulty by cells of *S. pastorianus* in the presence of cycloheximide (SIEGEL and SISLER, 1964a). Furthermore, the fact that 100 times as much cycloheximide is required to check motility of the alga, *Haematococcus lacustris*, as is required to stop cell division (ZEHNDER and HUGHES, 1958), also indicates that toxicity does not result from interference with energy production.

LATUASAN and BERENDS (1958) reported that cycloheximide is a potent inhibitor of alcohol and lactic dehydrogenases, but WESCOTT (1962) was unable to demonstrate any inhibitory effect of the antibiotic on the former enzyme. SEYDOUX and TURIAN (1962) detected marked accumulation of pyruvic and α ketoglutaric acids in cultures of *Neurospora sitophila* grown for 9 days in the presence of a 50% inhibitory dose (1 μg/ml) of cycloheximide. Very little accumulation of the acids occurred if thiamine was also added to the cultures; therefore, it was suggested the antibiotic may interfere with the synthesis or function of cocarboxylase.

Since cycloheximide inhibits protein synthesis (see Section VII B) it seems possible the accumulation of keto acids might occur as a secondary effect. The additional thiamine may aid in eliminating the acids by accelerating oxidative decarboxylation reactions.

B. Effect on Protein Synthesis

KERRIDGE (1958) demonstrated that cycloheximide is a potent inhibitor of protein synthesis in cells of *Saccharomyces carlsbergensis*. It has since been shown that the antibiotic also inhibits protein synthesis in other species of yeast (SIEGEL and SISLER, 1963, 1964a; FUKUHARA, 1965; WIDUCZYNSKI and STOPPANI, 1965; KJELLIN-STRABY and BOMAN, 1965), in *Aspergillus nidulans* (SHEPHERD, 1958), in mammalian cells (YOUNG *et al.*, 1963; ENNIS and LUBIN, 1964; BENNETT *et al.*, 1964; COLOMBO *et al.*, 1965) and in *T. piriformis* (COONEY and BRADLEY, 1962). The antibiotic inhibits adaptive synthesis of maltase (KERRIDGE, 1958; BRADLEY, 1962), and guanase (ROUSH and SHIEH, 1962) in yeast cells and adaptive synthesis of nitrate reductase in higher plants (HEWITT and AFRIDI, 1959). Antibody formation in mice (COONEY and BRADLEY, 1963) as well as protein synthesis and the estrogen response in the uterus of rats (GORSKI and AXMAN, 1964) are likewise inhibited by cycloheximide.

There can be little doubt that the toxic effects of the antibiotic are related to its effects on protein synthesis. Concentrations (0.5—1 μg/ml) which inhibit protein synthesis 80—90% in yeast (KERRIDGE, 1958; WIDUCZYNSKI and STOPPANI, 1965; KJELLIN-STRABY and BOMAN, 1965) and mammalian cells (ENNIS and LUBIN, 1964; BENNETT *et al.*, 1964), correspond closely to those concentrations (0.1—1 μg/ml) which strongly inhibit or completely prevent growth of highly sensitive organisms (WHIFFEN, 1948; KERRIDGE, 1958; COURSEN and SISLER, 1960; BRADLEY, 1962).

Acetoxycycloheximide is a highly effective inhibitor of protein synthesis in intact animals (YOUNG *et al.*, 1963). In tumor-bearing mice receiving 5 mg/kg of the antibiotic, incorporation of ^{14}C amino acids into protein of liver and ascites tumor cells was inhibited 95% and 96% respectively. Incorporation of amino acids into protein of rabbit liver cells was inhibited 88% when the animals were given a 0.5 mg/kg dose of antibiotic.

The mode of action of glutarimide antibiotics in the pathway to protein synthesis has been studied in several laboratories. SIEGEL and SISLER (1963, 1964b) showed that cycloheximide inhibited incorporation of amino acids into protein in a cell-free system from *S. pastorianus* and determined the site of inhibition in the system. The antibiotic did not inhibit amino acid activation or transfer of activated amino acids to s-RNA (soluble-RNA) but it prevented transfer of amino acids from amino acyl-s-RNA's into protein. Similar results were obtained by ENNIS and LUBIN (1964) using a cell-free system from rat liver. Cycloheximide and acetoxycycloheximide both inhibited polypeptide synthesis directed by either polyuridylic acid or by natural messenger RNA. High concentrations of the antibiotics did not inhibit synthesis of ^{14}C-phenylalanyl-s-RNA from ^{14}C-phenylalanine, but low concentrations prevented the transfer of ^{14}C-phenylalanine from s-RNA to polypeptide in the presence of polyuridylic acid. BENNETT *et al.* (1965) also concluded that inhibition of protein synthesis by cycloheximide in cell-free systems from cells of mouse Adenocarcinoma 755 occurred after formation of aminoacyl-s-RNA's. The glutarimide antibiotics, streptovitacin A, streptimidone and acetoxycycloheximide were also effective inhibitors in this system.

Very little is known of the precise mechanism by which glutarimide antibiotics inhibit the transfer of amino acids from aninoacyl-s-RNA's into polypeptide. WETTSTEIN *et al.* (1964) showed that cycloheximide inhibits the GTP dependent breakdown of ribosomal aggregates (polyribosomes) to monomers which normally accompanies protein synthesis *in vitro*. This effect is in contrast to that of puromycin which causes an accelerated release of monomers during amino acid incorporation *in vitro*. These data rule out the possibility that cycloheximide inhibits protein synthesis by damaging ribosomes in such a way as to cause their premature detachment from messenger RNA or by causing fragmentation of messenger RNA. Regarding the effect of cycloheximide on the breakdown of polyribosomes *in vitro*, the results of WILLIAMSON and SCHWEET (1965) obtained in cell-free systems with rabbit reticulocytes are consistent with those of WETTSTEIN *et al.* However, an actual decrease in monomeric ribosomes and an increase in polyribosomes was observed in the antibiotic treated preparations.

COLOMBO *et al.* (1965) studied the effect of cycloheximide on protein synthesis in intact rabbit reticulocytes where synthesis of DNA and RNA does not take place. The antibiotic inhibited protein synthesis in whole cells as well as in cell-free extracts. Studies were made to determine the effect of the toxicant on polyribosomes *in vivo*. Reticulocytes were incubated for 5 minutes with ^{14}C amino acids, cycloheximide was added, and the incubation continued for 5 additional minutes. Cells were then lysed and the polyribosomes analyzed by sucrose density gradient centrifugation. The ^{14}C and optical density profiles of polyribosomes isolated from treated cells were nearly identical with those of polyribosomes isolated from untreated cells. These experiments show that cycloheximide does not cause breakdown of polyribosomes while inhibiting protein synthesis, an observation which agrees with the results obtained in cell-free systems by WETTSTEIN *et al.* (1964) and by WILLIAMSON and SCHWEET (1965). In addition, the experiments also indicate that the antibiotic does not cause accelerated dissociation of growing peptide chains from polyribosomes, an observation previously made by ENNIS and LUBIN (1964) in cell-free systems. When the reticulocytes were incubated for an additional 30 seconds with 2.8×10^{-4} M puromycin, ^{14}C profiles of polyribosomes in the sucrose density gradients showed that almost complete removal of labelled peptide chains from polyribosomes of untreated cells had occurred, whereas only about 50% removal had occurred in polyribosomes from cycloheximide treated cells. Optical density profiles of the polyribosomes from treated and untreated cells, however, were almost identical. Complete removal of labelled peptides from polyribosomes of cycloheximide treated cells was accomplished after 5 minutes incubation with puromycin. These results suggest that cycloheximide slows down attachment of puromycin to the carboxyl end of the growing peptide chains, and thus slows down the release of the peptides from the polyribosomes.

On the other hand, WILLIAMSON and SCHWEET (1965) found that cycloheximide did not appreciably slow down the abortive release of peptide chains typically caused by puromycin, even though it strongly inhibited normal completion and release of the chains. Here it would appear that inhibition of the puromycin effect might have been detected had measurements been made at earlier intervals.

Polyribosomes of rabbit reticulocytes were dissociated into monoribosomes by treating the cells for 30 minutes with 10^{-2} M NaF (COLOMBO *et al.*, 1965). Reassembly of the polyribosomes took place when the cells were washed and reincubated with glucose and ^{14}C amino acids. The reassembly did not occur, however, in the presence of 10^{-4} M cycloheximide. The authors concluded, therefore, that cycloheximide inhibited a step in protein synthesis which was required for the initial binding of the messenger to ribosomes in a polyribosomal structure and for the advancement of the ribosomes along the messenger.

Results very similar to those of COLOMBO *et al.* were obtained by TRAKATELLIS *et al.* (1965) in systems from mouse liver cells. Polyribosomes from cells of cycloheximide treated animals performed as well in cell-free amino acid incorporating systems containing normal liver supernatants as those from treated animals. The breakdown of polyribosomes which occurred when mice were injected with actinomycin or ethionine was largely prevented by cycloheximide. Rapid reassembly of polyribosomes in cells of ethionine treated animals occurred after injection of methionine and ATP. However, reassembly was very slow in animals which were treated with cycloheximide.

The relationship between the inhibition of polyribosome assembly and inhibition of protein synthesis is not entirely clear. However, since the antibiotic interferes with protein synthesis by polyribosomes already assembled, it seems the inhibition of assembly is an effect rather than a cause of the inhibition of protein synthesis. Inhibition of the assembly process is probably caused by the slowing down of the movement of ribosomes relative to the messenger-RNA strand after they have become attached to it (TRAKATELLIS *et al.*, 1965). In other words, polyribosomes are assembled while ribosomes sequentially make their initial attachment to the same site on a messenger-RNA strand [at the point corresponding to the N-terminal amino acid of the peptide chain for which the messenger-RNA codes (WILLIAMSON and SCHWEET, 1965)] and then move along the strand as peptide synthesis proceeds. Cycloheximide would inhibit assembly if it prevented the first ribosomes attached, from moving away from the intitial attachment site.

Such an explanation is consistent with the observations of TRAKATELLIS *et al.* (1965) that some reassembly of light polyribosomes with few ribosomes per messenger-RNA strand takes place in the presence of cycloheximide, whereas reassembly of heavy polyribosomes with many ribosomes per strand is strongly inhibited. Since inhibition of any step in the synthesis of polypeptides from amino-acyl-s-RNA's would slow down movement of ribosomes along the messenger-RNA strand, these studies on polyribosome assembly do not identify the nature of interference of cycloheximide with protein synthesis. Interference might involve attachment of s-RNA to the decoding site or interference with the transfer of the growing peptide from the s-RNA to which it is attached, to the incoming amino-acyl-s-RNA. More refined studies of the amino acid incorporating system will be required to precisely fix the site of action of the antibiotic.

Table 1. *Relative effectiveness of glutarimide antibiotics and derivatives as inhibitors of growth of Saccharomyces pastorianus (in vivo) and as inhibitors of protein synthesis (in vitro*[1]*)*

Compounds	*In vitro* ED_{50} (µg/ml)	% Effec-tiveness[2]	*In vivo* ED_{50} (µg/ml)	% Effec-tiveness
l-Cycloheximide	0.36	100	0.028	100
dl-Cycloheximide	0.78	46	0.054	52
d-Naramycin-B[3]	1.05	34	0.11	26
d-Isocycloheximide	2.6	14	0.21	13
dl-α-*epi*-Isocycloheximide	—	—	0.12	24
dl-Neocycloheximide	>50	—	64	0.04
Inactone	7.5	5	0.36	8
Actiphenol	>50	—	>250	—
Streptimidone	1.4	26	0.084	33
Streptimidone acetate	>50	—	>250	—
Anhydrocycloheximide	—	—	>100	—
Cycloheximide oxime	>50	—	12.5	0.2
Cycloheximide semicarbazone	>50	—	1.4	2
Cycloheximide acetate	>50	—	>250	—
ψ-Cycloheximide-I-acetate	>50	—	>250	—
Streptovitacin-A	0.15	240	13.0	0.2
Acetoxycycloheximide	0.044	818	0.50	6
α-Dihydrocycloheximide	4.5	8	3.5	0.8
β-Dihydrocycloheximide	>50	—	52.0	0.05
N-methyl cycloheximide	—	—	>100	—
N-methyl cycloheximide acetate	>50	—	>250	—

[1] From SIEGEL *et al.* (1966).
[2] % effectiveness relative to that of *l*-cycloheximide.
[3] Contaminated with 25—33% *l*-cycloheximide.

Growth or protein synthesis *in vivo* are more sensitive to cycloheximide than protein synthesis *in vitro* (ENNIS and LUBIN, 1964; BENNETT *et al.*, 1964, 1965; SIEGEL and SISLER, 1965; SIEGEL *et al.*, 1966). The reason for this continues to be an interesting question, but it is unlikely that an explanation will alter present conclusions regarding the site of action of the antibiotic in cells or in the pathway to protein synthesis. Cycloheximide is nevertheless a very effective inhibitor of protein synthesis *in vitro*. The 50% inhibitory concentration in the *S. pastorianus* system ranges from 0.2—0.36 μg/ml, but inhibition is evident even at 0.05 μg/ml (SIEGEL and SISLER, 1963, 1965; SIEGEL *et al.*, 1966). Growth of *S. pastorianus* cells in liquid culture, on the other hand, is inhibited 50% by 0.028 μg/ml of the antibiotic.

Some glutarimide antibiotics are much more effective than cycloheximide in mammalian systems. Antitumor activity of acetoxycycloheximide and its acetyl propionyl, butyryl and benzoyl esters is 50—250 times higher than that of cycloheximide (RAO, 1962). Acetoxycycloheximide is also more potent than cycloheximide as an inhibitor of protein synthesis in intact animals (YOUNG *et al.*, 1963) and in mammalian cell-free systems (ENNIS and LUBIN, 1964; BENNETT *et al.*, 1965). The superiority of streptovitacin A over cycloheximide in mammalian systems is also quite evident. The concentration of the former antibiotic which produces 50% inhibition of growth of the KB strain of human epidermoid cells in tissue culture is 0.035 μg/ml whereas that of cycloheximide is 0.1 μg/ml (SMITH *et al.*, 1959). Streptovitacin A is more effective than cycloheximide as an antitumor agent in intact animals (EVANS *et al.*, 1960) and as an inhibitor of protein synthesis in mammalian cell-free systems (BENNETT *et al.*, 1965). It is also more than twice as toxic as cycloheximide to *T. vaginalis* (SOKOLSKI *et al.*, 1959).

On the other hand, cycloheximide is about 500 times as toxic to cells of *S. pastorianus* as streptovitacin A, but in a cell-free protein synthesizing system from the same organism, it is less than $^1/_2$ as effective as streptovitacin A (Table 1). In this regard, a striking contrast between cycloheximide and acetoxycycloheximide is also evident. The former antibiotic is more than 10 times as toxic to the cells as the latter, but it is only about $^1/_8$ as effective as the latter in the cell-free system. The relatively low toxicity of acetoxycycloheximide and streptovitacin A in comparison with that of cycloheximide has been observed in cells of *N. crassa* (SIEGEL *et al.*, 1966) and it has also been observed in *S. pastorianus* by SOKOLSKI *et al.* (1959) and by RAO and CULLEN (1960). Since acetoxycycloheximide and streptovitacin A are less toxic to whole cells than to the cell-free system, while the reverse is true for cycloheximide (Table 1), it appears that these 2 antibiotics may not penetrate the cells as readily as cycloheximide.

Other glutarimide antibiotics and derivatives (Table 1) generally follow the pattern of cycloheximide in being more effective *in vivo* than *in vitro*. The oxime and semicarbazone derivatives of cycloheximide are slightly toxic to cells of *S. pastorianus*, but not to the cell-free protein synthesizing system. Since activity of these derivatives is related to the amount of cycloheximide freed by a pH dependent hydrolysis (see Section II H) a difference in effectiveness in the two situations would be expected because growth measurements were made at pH 6.4, and cell-free protein synthesis was carried out at pH 7.5.

Most of the compounds listed in Table 1 were tested for toxicity to cells of the cycloheximide resistant yeast, *S. fragilis*, and as inhibitors in a cell-free amino acid incorporating system from this organism. However, none were toxic to the cells at 250 μg/ml or to the amino acid incorporating system at 50 μg/ml. These results suggest that difference in sensitivity of *S. pastorianus* and *S. fragilis* to glutarimide antibiotics is determined by some difference in their protein synthesizing systems. These results with the *S. fragilis* system are similar to those obtained by ENNIS and LUBIN (1964) in their studies of the cycloheximide resistant cells of *E. coli*. Protein synthesis in cell-free extracts of this organism was not inhibited by either cycloheximide or acetoxycycloheximide.

C. Effect on RNA and DNA Synthesis

1. *Acid Soluble Nucleotide and RNA Synthesis*

Concentrations of cycloheximide which drastically inhibit protein synthesis in yeast usually do not appreciably inhibit synthesis of acid soluble nucleotides or RNA in short term experiments. In fact, incorporation of labelled precursors into these fractions may actually be stimulated by cycloheximide under certain conditions. Incorporation of ^{14}C from glucose or ^{32}P from inorganic orthophosphate into acid soluble nucleotides and RNA of cells of *S. pastorianus* during a 40 minute incubation period was higher in cycloheximide treated than in untreated cells (SIEGEL and SISLER, 1964a). Stimulation of ^{14}C or ^{32}P incorporation into RNA was particularly evident because label was about $2^1/_2$ times higher in treated than in control cells. Results very similar to these were obtained by WIDUCZYNSKI and STOPPANI (1965) while following incorporation of ^{14}C-adenine by starved cells of *S. ellipsoideus*. Specific activity of adenine and guanine in RNA after 1 hour incubation was 7 times higher in treated cells than in untreated cells. Stimulation of labelling of adenine and guanine in the soluble nucleotides also occurred, but much less so than in RNA. In proliferating cells, on the other hand, a strong stimulation of incorporation of label into the soluble nucleotides was evident, but there was some inhibition of incorporation of label into nucleotides of RNA. Conversion of ^{14}C-adenine to ^{14}C-guanine in both starved and proliferating cells was accelerated by cycloheximide. In this connection, it might be noted that the stimulation of incorporation of ^{32}P from inorganic orthophosphate into acid soluble nucleotides by cycloheximide in *S. pastorianus* was most pronounced in the case of guanine nucleotides (SIEGEL and SISLER, 1964a).

Inhibition of RNA synthesis in yeast by cycloheximide, while absent or slight initially, becomes progressively greater with time. In *S. cerevisiae*, incorporation of ^{14}C-uracil into RNA was hardly affected by 25 µg/ml of the antibiotic during the first 20 minutes, but after 1 hour, inhibition was about 30%. On the other hand, inhibition of amino acids incorporation into protein was inhibited 95—100% throughout the experiment (FUKUHARA, 1965). Incorporation of ^{14}C-uracil into exponentially growing cells of a methionine mutant of *S. cerevisiae* was inhibited less than 20% by 5 µg/ml of cycloheximide after 30 minutes, but after 2 hours it was inhibited about 75%. However, incorporation of ^{14}C phenylalanine into protein was inhibited more than 95% at both time intervals (KJELLIN-STRABY and BOMAN, 1965). These results agree with those obtained earlier by KERRIDGE (1958) in *S. carlsbergensis*.

The effects of cycloheximide and acetoxycycloheximide on nucleotide and RNA synthesis in mammalian cells is very similar to those produced by cycloheximide in yeast cells. Both antibiotics markedly inhibited protein synthesis in tissue culture L cells, but even at concentrations 100 times greater than those producing maximum inhibition of protein synthesis, they did not affect incorporation of ^{14}C-uridine into RNA until after 90—120 minutes (ENNIS and LUBIN, 1964). Cycloheximide did not significantly inhibit incorporation of ^{14}C-orotic acid, ^{14}C-uridine or ^{14}C-adenine into RNA of mammalian cells under conditions where incorporation of these precursors into DNA was inhibited 70—90% (BENNETT *et al.*, 1964). As in the case of *S. ellipsoideus*, there was a striking increase in label in soluble adenine nucleotides in treated cells when ^{14}C-adenine was the precursor. Incorporation of ^{14}C-glycine or ^{14}C-formate into RNA was strongly inhibited which is in contrast to the observations for uridine, adenine, and orotic acid. However, a negative feedback effect of nucleotides accumulating because DNA synthesis is inhibited, probably explains the inhibition of glycine or formate incorporation into RNA (BENNETT *et al.*, 1964).

The effect of glutarimide antibiotics on RNA metabolism in intact animals has also been studied by several investigators. YOUNG *et al.* (1963) found incorporation of ^{32}P into acid soluble phosphorus compounds or into RNA of liver or kidney cells in intact rabbits was not inhibited in animals injected with a concentration of acetoxycycloheximide which strongly inhibited protein synthesis.

Cycloheximide did not inhibit normal incorporation of ^{3}H-cytidine into RNA of the uterus of immature rats, but it prevented the stimulation of ^{3}H-cytidine incorporation induced by injection of estradiol (GORSKI and AXMAN, 1964). Hormonal dependence of cycloheximide action in rats and mice was demonstrated by FIALA and FIALA (1965). Accumulation of RNA, particularly in the microsomal fraction, occurred in livers and adrenals of rats receiving a daily dose of 0.2 mg of cycloheximide for 7 days. The effect of cycloheximide on adrenal RNA was similar to that produced by ACTH. Administration of cycloheximide to hypophysectomized rats did not cause an increase in adrenal RNA, indicating the effect was ACTH-mediated. However, accumulation of RNA in the microsomal fraction of liver cells still occurred in the treated animals.

It is apparent from the results of experiments described thus far that cycloheximide has no major inhibitory effect on gross RNA synthesis in yeast and mammalian cells. These experiments, however, do not permit any conclusion regarding the effect of cycloheximide on the synthesis of different RNA species. This problem was studied by FUKUHARA (1965) and DE KLOET (1965). Using ^{14}C-uracil as a precursor, FUKUHARA showed that label in cells of *S. cerevisiae*, incubated in the presence of cycloheximide for 60 minutes, accumulated primarily in an RNA fraction which sedimented much more slowly than ribosomes in a sucrose density gradient. Furthermore, it was shown that none of this label was associated with newly synthesized protein. Label in untreated cells was found primarily in the ribosomal fraction, in association with newly synthesized protein. Analysis of total RNA extracted with phenol plus Duponol in a sucrose density gradient showed newly formed RNA in untreated cells to be ribosomal (24 S and 16 S) and transfer (4 S) types. The RNA from treated cells was of various types, the major portion of which corresponded to a size of about 16 S. The sedimentation profile of the RNA extracted from treated cells was very similar to that of high turnover RNA detected in untreated cells after short pulse (2—5 minutes) labelling with uracil. Normally, during extended incubation this RNA is converted into ribosomal and transfer RNA, but in cycloheximide treated cells it remained essentially unchanged after 1 hour.

Accumulation of RNA with abnormal sedimentation properties was observed by DE KLOET (1965) following incubation of protoplasts of *S. carlsbergensis* with cycloheximide. Following a 5 minute pulse with ^{14}C-uracil, label in both treated and untreated protoplasts was incorporated into rapidly sedimenting heterogeneous RNA. However, if the 5 minute incubation with labelled uracil was followed by a chase of unlabelled uracil for 60 minutes, the sedimentation pattern of the labelled RNA from treated protoplasts differed from that of labelled RNA from untreated protoplasts. Labelled RNA from treated protoplasts sedimented as a broad peak with its highest activity in front of the heaviest ribosomal RNA components. The pattern closely resembled that of pulse labelled (5 minutes) RNA from untreated protoplasts, with the exception of a peak of RNA of low molecular weight. In untreated protoplasts, label was found primarily in the ribosomal RNA fractions. Estimation of the base composition of the RNA from treated and untreated protoplasts indicated an accumulation of RNA in treated protoplasts with a more DNA-like composition than is normally found in yeast cells.

One apparent difference between the results of FUKUHARA (1965) and DE KLOET (1965) is the size of the RNA accumulating in the presence of cycloheximide, or produced normally during short pulse experiments. FUKUHARA found most of the label in RNA with sedimentation properties close to that of ribosomal RNA. If ribosomal RNA was present, then it seems the most obvious reason for the failure to incorporate it into ribosomes was the lack of ribosomal protein. DE KLOET, on the other hand, found label primarily in an RNA fraction heavier than ribosomal RNA components. Since the label in this fraction normally becomes transferred to the ribosomal components, it would seem that cycloheximide must interfere mainly with the conversion of this RNA to ribosomal RNA and/or with the synthesis of the ribosome rather than with the initial synthesis of RNA. Again it appears that failure to synthesize ribosomal protein was primarily responsible for the abnormal RNA pattern in cycloheximide treated protoplasts, especially since the effect became apparent only after an extended incubation period with the antibiotic.

FIALA and DAVIS (1965) studied the effect of cycloheximide on methylation of RNA in growing cells of *N. crassa*. The antibiotic inhibited incorporation of methyl groups from S-adenosylmethionine into ribosomal RNA and soluble RNA 94 and 68% respectively, whereas incorporation of uridine into these fractions was inhibited 58 and 15% respectively. However, the observed inhibition of RNA methylation may be only apparent because endogenous methionine probably accumulated in the treated cells where protein synthesis was blocked and competed with the externally supplied S-adenosylmethionine as a methyl donor.

KJELLIN-STRABY and BOMAN (1965) concluded that cycloheximide actually increases methylation of s-RNA in a methionine requiring mutant of *S. cereviseae*. The submethylated s-RNA normally synthesized in methionine depleted cells was largely converted to methylated s-RNA in the presence of cycloheximide. This conclusion was based on the observation that, *in vitro*, only about 10% as many methyl groups were incorporated per unit of s-RNA isolated from treated cells as was incorporated into s-RNA isolated from untreated cells. It was postulated that methionine released from breakdown of protein supplied the substrate for methylation in the treated cells.

2. *DNA Synthesis*

Cycloheximide markedly inhibits DNA synthesis in cells of *S. carlsbergensis* (KERRIDGE, 1958) and in cells of human epidermoid carcinoma (BENNETT *et al.*, 1964). In both cell types, the severity of inhibition of protein and DNA synthesis is similar. On the other hand, DNA synthesis in tissue culture L cells (ENNIS and LUBIN, 1964), and in cells of *S. pastorianus* (SIEGEL and SISLER, 1964a), is affected less by cycloheximide than protein synthesis. Inhibition of DNA synthesis begins immediately after addition of 2.5 μg/ml of cycloheximide to cells of *T. piriformis* in logarithemic growth, but inhibition of protein synthesis is not evident until several hours later (COONEY and BRADLEY, 1962). Such a delay in onset of inhibition of protein synthesis is in striking contrast to the rapid inhibition which occurs in other types of cells (KERRIDGE, 1958; SIEGEL and SISLER, 1964a; KJELLIN-STRABY and BOMAN, 1965; COLOMBO *et al.*, 1965).

BENNETT *et al.* (1964) made a detailed investigation of the effect of cycloheximide on DNA synthesis *in vitro* in systems prepared from mammalian cells. Although the antibiotic severely inhibited DNA synthesis in the whole cells, attempts to demonstrate inhibition *in vitro* were unsuccessful. Lack of any significant effect of cycloheximide on RNA synthesis in the cells suggested that inhibition on the pathway to DNA synthesis should be at some point beyond the formation of ribonucleotides. However, high levels of cycloheximide did not inhibit incorporation of deoxyribonucleoside monophosphates (dAMP, dGMP, dCMP and dTMP) into DNA in cell-free preparations. Acetoxycycloheximide and streptovitacin A were also ineffective in the system. Furthermore, supernatants prepared from cells exposed to cycloheximide overnight contained all the enzymes required to incorporate deoxythymidine monophosphate into DNA. Several types of experiments were carried out to provide evidence that cycloheximide binds to DNA *in vitro*, but all yielded negative results. The possibility that cycloheximide may interfere with DNA synthesis by preventing reduction of ribonucleotides to deoxyribonucleotides was not eliminated in these studies. A mixture of the 4 deoxynucleosides found in DNA did not reverse the inhibitory effects of cycloheximide, although it is not clear whether the attempts were made to reverse inhibition of growth or of DNA synthesis. Even though reduction of ribonucleotides to deoxyribonucleotides might be inhibited, attempts to reverse growth-inhibiting effects by adding a mixture of the 4 deoxyribonucleosides found in DNA, would, of necessity fail, because of the toxicity known to originate from the effects of the antibiotic on protein synthesis. BENNETT *et al.* concluded that inhibition of DNA synthesis must result from inhibition of a step not measured in the cell-free system employed or is a secondary effect of inhibited protein synthesis. With regard to the first possibility, it was suggested that cycloheximide might interfere with the process by which DNA is made ready, in the intact cell, to act as a template or primer for the polymerase reaction.

Whether inhibition of DNA synthesis results from an action independent of that on protein synthesis is not clear. The idea that inhibition of the protein synthesis is the primary basis for toxicity of glutarimide antibiotics is supported by the observation that cell-free protein synthesizing systems from resistant organisms are resistant to the antibiotics, whereas those from sensitive organisms are sensitive to the antibiotics (ENNIS and LUBIN, 1964; SIEGEL and SISLER, 1965; SIEGEL *et al.*, 1966).

References

ARNOW, P., S. H. BRINDLE, N. A. GIUFFRE, and D. PERLMAN: Effects of antibiotics, antitumor agents, and antimetabolites on the metabolism of mammalian cells in tissue culture. Antimicrobial Agents and Chemotherapy 1962, 731—739 (1963).

BENNETT, JR., L. L., D. SMITHERS, and C. T. WARD: Inhibition of DNA synthesis in mammalian cells by actidione. Biochim. et Biophys. Acta **87**, 60—69 (1964).

BENNETT, JR., L. L., V. L. WARD, and R. W. BROCKMAN: Inhibition of protein synthesis *in vitro* by cycloheximide and related glutarimide antibiotics. Biochim. et Biophys. Acta **103**, 478—485 (1965).

BERLINER, M. D., and L. S. OLIVE: Meiosis in *Gymnosporangium* and the cytological effects of certain antibiotic substances. Science **117**, 652—653 (1953).

BLUMAUEROVÁ, M., and J. STARKA: Reversal of antibiotic action of cycloheximide (actidione) by bivalent metal ions. Nature **183**, 261 (1959).

BRADLEY, S. G.: Relationship between sugar utilization and the action of cycloheximide on diverse fungi. Nature **194**, 315—316 (1962).

COLOMBO, B., L. FELICETTI, and C. BAGLIONI: Inhibition of protein synthesis by cycloheximide in rabbit reticulocytes. Biochem. Biophys. Research Commun **18**, 389—395 (1965).

COONEY, W. J., and S. G. BRADLEY: Action of cycloheximide on animal cells. Antimicrobial Agents and Chemotherapy-1961, 237—244 (1962).

COONEY, W. J., and S. G. BRADLEY: Effect of cycloheximide on the immune response. Antimicrobial Agents and Chemotherapy-1962, 1—9 (1963).

COURSEN, B. W.: Effect of the antibiotic, cycloheximide, on the growth and metabolism of *Saccharomyces pastorianus*. Ph.D. Thesis, University of Maryland 1959.

COURSEN, B. W., and H. D. SISLER: Effect of the antibiotic, cycloheximide, on the metabolism and growth of *Saccharomyces pastorianus*. Am. J. Botany **47**, 541—549 (1960).

DE KLOET, S. R.: Accumulation of RNA with DNA like base composition in *Saccharomyces carlsbergiensis* in the presence of cycloheximide. Biochem. Biophys. Research Commun **19**, 582—586 (1965).

EBLE, T. E., M. E. BERGY, C. M. LARGE, R. R. HERR, and W. G. JACKSON: Isolation, purification and properties of streptovitacins A and B. Antibiotics Ann. **1958/59**, 555—559 (1959).

ENNIS, H. L., and M. LUBIN: Cycloheximide: Aspects of inhibition of protein synthesis in mammalian cells. Science **146**, 1474—1476 (1964).

EVANS, J. S., J. CERU, and G. D. MENGEL: The *in vivo* antitumor activity of streptovitacins A, B, C_2 and D. Antibiotics Ann. **1959/60**, 962—965 (1960).

EVANS, J. S., G. D. MENGEL, J. CERU, and R. L. JOHNSTON: Biological studies on streptovitacin A, a new antitumor agent. Antibiotics Ann. **1958/59**, 565—571 (1959).

FIALA, E. S., and F. F. DAVIS: Preferential inhibition of synthesis and methylation of ribosomal RNA in *Neurospora crassa* by actidione. Biochem. Biophys. Research Commun **18**, 115—118 (1965).

FIALA, S., and E. FIALA: Hormonal dependence of actidione (cycloheximide) action. Biochim. et Biophys. Acta **103**, 699—701 (1965).

FORD, J. H., and W. KLOMPARENS: Cycloheximide (acti-dione) and its nonagricultural uses. Antibiotics & Chemotherapy **10**, 682—687 (1960).

FORD, J. H., W. KLOMPARENS, and C. L. HAMNER: Cycloheximide (actidione) and its agricultural uses. Plant Disease Reptr. **42**, 680—695 (1958).

FROHARDT, R. P., H. W. DION, Z. L. JAKUBOWSKI, A. RYDER, J. C. FRENCH, and Q. R. BARTZ: Chemistry of streptimidone, a new antibiotic. J. Am. Chem. Soc. **81**, 5500—5506 (1959).

FUKUHARA, H.: RNA synthesis of yeast in the presence of cycloheximide. Biochem. Biophys. Research Commun **18**, 297—301 (1965).

GORSKI, J., and M. C. AXMAN: Cycloheximide (actidione) inhibition of protein synthesis and the uterine response to estrogen. Arch. Biochem. Biophys. **105**, 517—520 (1964).

GREIG, M. E., R. A. WALK, and A. J. GIBBONS: Effect of actidione (cycloheximide) on yeast fermentation. J. Bacteriol. **75**, 489—491 (1958).

GROVER, R. K., and J. D. MOORE: Toximetric studies of fungicides against the brown rot organisms, *Sclerotinia fructicola* and *S. laxa*. Phytopathology **52**, 876—880 (1962).

GUNDERSEN, K.: Cycloheximide, the active substance in *Streptomyces griseus* antagonism against *Fomes annosus*. Acta Horti Gotoburgensis **24**, 1—24 (1961).

GUNDERSEN, K.: Induced resistance in *Fomes annosus* to the antibiotic cycloheximide. Acta Horti Gotoburgensis **25**, 1—32 (1962a).

GUNDERSEN, K.: The action mechanism of cycloheximide in *Fomes annosus*. Acta Horti Gotoburgensis **25**, 33—63 (1962b).

GUNDERSEN, K., and T. WADSTEIN: Morphological changes and resistance induced in *Saccharomyces pastorianus* by the antibiotic cycloheximide. J. Gen. Microbiol. **28**, 325—332 (1962).

HADDER, J. C., and G. B. WILSON: Cytological assay of c-mitotic and prophase poison actions. Chromosoma **9**, 91—104 (1958).

HAWTHORNE, M. E., and G. B. WILSON: The cytological effects of the antibiotic actidione. Cytologia (Tokyo) **17**, 71—85 (1952).

HERR, R. R.: Structure studies on streptovitacins A and B. Antibiotics Ann. **1958/59**, 560—564 (1959a).

HERR, R. R.: Structures of the streptovitacins. J. Am. Chem. Soc. **81**, 2595—2596 (1959b).

HEWITT, E. J., and M. M. R. K. AFRIDI: Adaptive synthesis of nitrate reductase in higher plants. Nature **183**, 57—58 (1959).

HIGHET, R. J., u. V. PRELOG: Stoffwechselprodukte von Actinomyceten. Helv. Chim. Acta **42**, 1523—1526 (1959).

HIRABAYASHI, A.: Studies on the antiamebic effect of protomycin, a new antibiotic isolated from the culture filtrate of a species of streptomycetes. J. Antibiotics (Japan), Ser. A **12**, 298—309 (1959).

HSU, K. S.: The genetic basis of actidione resistance in Neurospora. J. Gen. Microbiol. **32**, 341—347 (1963).

IGARASHI, S., and S. WADA: Fermicidin, an new antibiotic active against yeasts and trichomonas. [In Japanese] J. Antibiotics (Japan), Ser. B **7**, 221—225 (1954).

JOHNSON, F.: Glutarimide antibiotics. I. The synthesis of actiphenol. J. Org. Chem. **27**, 3658—3660 (1962).

JOHNSON, F., and A. A. CARLSON: Glutarimide antibiotics. Part VIII. A stereoselective synthesis of *dl-α-epi*-isocycloheximide. Tetrahedron Letters **14**, 885—889 (1965).

JOHNSON, F., W. D. GUROWITZ, and N. A. STARKOVSKY: Glutarimide antibiotics. Part II. The synthesis and stereochemistry of *dl*-neocycloheximide, a new isomer of cycloheximide. Tetrahedron Letters **25**, 1167—1171 (1962).

JOHNSON, F., N. A. STARKOVSKY, and W. D. GUROWITZ: Glutarimide antibiotics. VII. The synthesis of *dl*-neocycloheximide and the determination of the cyclohexanone ring stereochemistry of cycloheximide, its isomers, and inactone. J. Am. Chem. Soc. **87**, 3492—3500 (1965).

JOHNSON, F., N. A. STARKOVSKY, A. C. PATON, and A. A. CARLSON: Glutarimide antibiotics. IV. The total synthesis of *dl*- and *l*-cycloheximide. J. Am. Chem. Soc. **86**, 118—119 (1964).

KERRIDGE, D.: The effect of actidione and other antifungal agents on nucleic acid and protein synthesis in *Saccharomyces carlsbergensis*. J. Gen. Microbiol. **19**, 497—506 (1958).

KIELHÖFER, E., u. H. AUMANN: Untersuchungen über die Wirkung des Antibioticums Actidion auf Hefe im Vergleich mit anderen fungitoxischen Substanzen. Z. Lebensm.-Untersuch. u. Forsch. **105**, 283—296 (1957).

KJELLIN-STRABY, K., and H. G. BOMAN: Studies on microbial RNA. III. Formation of submethylated sRNA in *Saccharomyces cerevisiae*. Proc. Natl. Acad. Sci. U.S. **53**, 1346—1352 (1965).

KOHBERGER, D. L., M. W. FISHER, M. M. GALBRAITH, A. B. HILLEGAS, P. E. THOMPSON, and J. EHRLICH: Biological studies of streptimidone, a new antibiotic. Antibiotics & Chemotherapy **10**, 9—16 (1960).

KORNFELD, E. C., R. G. JONES, and T. V. PARKE: The structure and chemistry of actidione an antibiotic from *Streptomyces griseus*. J. Am. Chem. Soc. **71**, 150—159 (1949).

LARDY, H. A., D. JOHNSON, and W. C. MCMURRAY: Antibiotics as tools for metabolic studies. I. A survey of toxic antibiotics in respiratory, phosphorylating and glycolytic systems. Arch. Biochem. Biophys. **78**, 587—597 (1958).

LATUASAN, H. E., and W. BERENDS: The action mechanism of actidione. Rec. trav. chim. **77**, 416—422 (1958).

LEACH, B. E., J. H. FORD, and A. J. WHIFFEN: Actidione, an antibiotic of *Streptomyces griseus*. J. Am. Chem. Soc. **69**, 474 (1947).

LEE, B. K., and D. WILKIE: Sensitivity and resistance of yeast strains to actidione and actidione derivatives. Nature **206**, 90—92 (1965).

LEMIN, A. J., and J. H. FORD: Isocycloheximide. J. Org. Chem. **25**, 344—346 (1960).

LEMIN, A. J., and W. E. MAGEE: Degradation of cycloheximide derivatives in plants. Plant Disease Reptr. **41**, 447—448 (1957).

LINDNER, R. C., H. C. KIRKPATRICK, and T. E. WEEKS: Comparative inhibition of virus multiplication by certain types of chemicals. Phytopathology **49**, 802—807 (1959).

LOEFER, J. B., and T. S. MATNEY: Growth inhibition of free-living protozoa by actidione. Physiol. Zoöl. **25**, 272—276 (1952).

MCCALLAN, S. E. A., L. P. MILLER, and R. M. WEED: Comparative effect of fungicides on oxygen uptake and germination of spores. Contrib. Boyce Thompson Inst. **18**, 39—68 (1954).

MEFFERD, JR., R. B., and J. B. LOEFER: Inhibition of respiration in *Tetrahymena pyriformis S* by actidione. Physiol. Zoöl. **27**, 115—118 (1954).

MIDDLEKAUF, J. E., S. HINO, S. P. YANG, C. C. LINDEGREN, and G. LINDEGREN: Gene control of resistance vs. sensitivity to actidione in *Saccharomyces*. Genetics **42**, 66—71 (1957).

MONREAL, K.: Die Wirkung von Actidion auf *Saccharomyces cerevisiae* var *elipsoideus*. Angew. Botan. **35**, 24—60 (1961).

OKUDA, T.: Studies on streptomyces antibiotic, cycloheximide. VI. The absolute configuration of naramycin-A (cycloheximide) and its isomeric naramycin-B. Chem. Pharm. Bull. **7**, 671—679 (1959).

OKUDA, T., and M. SUZUKI: Absolute configuration of cycloheximide. Chem. Pharm. Bull. **9**, 1014—1016 (1961).

OKUDA, T., M. SUZUKI, Y. EGAWA, and K. ASHINO: Studies on streptomyces antibiotic, cycloheximide. II. Naramycin-B, an isomer of cycloheximide. Chem. Pharm. Bull. **7**, 27—30 (1959).

OKUDA, T., M. SUZUKI, T. FURUMAI, and H. TAKAHASHI: Studies on streptomyces antibiotic, cycloheximide. XVIII. Isomerization study of cycloheximides and thermal degradation of naramycin-B. Chemical support of the proposed absolute configuration of cycloheximides. Chem. Pharm. Bull. **11**, 730—736 (1963).

OSATO, T., Y. MORIKUBO, S. YAMAZAKI, T. HIKIJI, K. YANO, M. KANAO, T. OSONO, and H. UMEZAWA: Screening studies of antiviral substances produced by actinomycetes and new antiviral substances, niromycins. J. Antibiotics (Japan), Ser. A **13**, 97—109 (1960a).

OSATO, T., Y. MORIKUBO, and H. UMEZAWA: Production and extraction of niromycins, antiviral antibiotics. J. Antibiotics (Japan), Ser. A **13**, 110—113 (1960b).

PALMER, C., and T. E. MALONEY: Preliminary screening for potential algicides. Ohio J. Sci. **55**, 1—8 (1955).

PAUL, R., et S. TCHELITCHEFF: Constitution chimique de l'inactone. Synthèse partielle de trois isomères de l'actidione. Bull. soc. chim. France 1316 (1955).

RAO, K. V.: C-73: A metabolic product of *Streptomyces albulus*. J. Org. Chem. **25**, 661—662 (1960a).

RAO, K. V.: E-73: An antitumor substance. Part II. Structure. J. Am. Chem. Soc. **82**, 1129—1132 (1960b).
RAO, K. V.: E-73: An antitumor substance. Part III. Some derivatives. Antibiotics & Chemotherapy **12**, 123—127 (1962).
RAO, K. V., and W. P. CULLEN: E-73: An antitumor substance. Part I. Isolation and characterization. J. Am. Chem. Soc. **82**, 1127—1128 (1960).
ROUSH, A. H., and T. R. SHIEH: The inhibition of purine transport and the induced biosynthesis of enzymes in yeasts by actidione. Federation Proc. **21**, 147 (1962).
SEYDOUX, J., et G. TURIAN: Accumulation d'acide pyruvique et d'acide α-cetoglutarique et reversion partielle par l'aneurine chez neurospora traité à l'actidione. Path. Microbiol. **25**, 752—765 (1962).
SHEPHERD, C. J.: Inhibition of protein and nucleic acid synthesis in *Aspergillus nidulans*. J. Gen. Microbiol. **18**, IV (1958).
SIEGEL, M. R., and H. D. SISLER: Inhibition of protein synthesis *in vitro* by cycloheximide. Nature **200**, 675—676 (1963).
SIEGEL, M. R., and H. D. SISLER: Site of action of cycloheximide in cells of *Saccharomyces pastorianus*. I. Effect of the antibiotic on cellular metabolism. Biochim. et Biophys. Acta **87**, 70—82 (1964a).
SIEGEL, M. R., and H. D. SISLER: Site of action of cycloheximide in cells of *Saccharomyces pastorianus*. II. The nature of inhibition of protein synthesis in a cell-free system. Biochim. et Biophys. Acta **87**, 83—89 (1964b).
SIEGEL, M. R., and H. D. SISLER: Site of action of cycloheximide in cells of *Saccharomyces pastorianus*. III. Further studies on the mechanism of action and the mechanism of resistance in saccharomyces species. Biochim. et Biophys. Acta **103**, 558—567 (1965).
SIEGEL, M. R., H. D. SISLER, and F. JOHNSON: Relationship of structure to fungitoxicity of cycloheximide and related glutarimide derivatives. Biochem. Pharmacol. **15**, 1218—1223 (1966).
SISLER, H. D., and N. L. MARSHALL: Physiological effects of certain fungitoxic compounds on fungus cells. J. Wash. Acad. Sci. **47**, 321—329 (1957).
SISLER, H. D., and M. R. SIEGEL: Factors affecting toxicity of cycloheximide derivatives. Manuscript in preparation 1966.
SMITH, C. G.: Tissue culture. Bioassay methods for streptovitacin A. Proc. Soc. Exptl. Biol. Med. **100**, 757—759 (1959).
SMITH, C. G., W. L. LUMMIS, and J. E. GRADY: An improved tissue culture assay. I. Methodology and cytotoxicity of anti-tumor agents. Cancer Research **19**, 843—846 (1959).
SMITH, C. G., W. L. LUMMIS, and J. E. GRADY: Studies on the mode of action of streptovitacin A. Cancer Research **20**, 1394—1398 (1960).
SOKOLSKI, W. T., N. J. EILERS, and G. M. SAVAGE: Paper chromatography and microbiological assay of the streptovitacins. Antibiotics Ann. **1958/59**, 551—554 (1959).
STARZYK, M. J.: The effect of cycloheximide on the germination of conidia of *Coccomyces hiemalis*. Phytopathology **53**, 235 (1963).
SUGAWARA, R.: Protomycin, a new antibiotic of cycloheximide group. II. Production and properties. J. Antibiotics (Japan), Ser. A **16**, 115—120 (1963a).
SUGAWARA, R.: Protomycin, a new antibiotic of cycloheximide group. III. Degradation products. J. Antibiotics (Japan), Ser. A **16**, 167—171 (1963b).
SUZUKI, M.: Studies on streptomyces antibiotic, cycloheximide. X. Structure-antimicrobial activity relationship of cycloheximide and related compounds. [In Japanese.] Yakugaku Zasshi **80**, 1217—1222 (1960).
SUZUKI, M., Y. EGAWA, and T. OKUDA: Studies on streptomyces antibiotic, cycloheximide. XV. Hydroxycarbonylation of optically active 2,4-dimethylcyclohexanones with glutarimide-β-acetaldehyde. (Synthesis of isocycloheximide and its isomers.) Chem. Pharm. Bull. **11**, 582—588 (1963).
TRAKATELLIS, A. C., M. MONTJAR, and A. E. AXELROD: Effect of cycloheximide on polysomes and protein synthesis in the mouse liver. Biochemistry **4**, 2065—2071 (1965).

TSUKADA, Y., T. SUGIMORI, K. IMAI, and H. KATAGIRI: Action of cycloheximide on *Zygosaccharomyces soja*. J. Bacteriol. **83**, 70—75 (1962).

VAN TAMELEN, E. E., and V. HAARSTAD: Structure of the antibiotic streptimidone. J. Am. Chem. Soc. **82**, 2974—2975 (1960).

WALKER, A. T., and F. G. SMITH: Effect of actidione on growth and respiration of *Myrothecium verrucaria*. Proc. Soc. Exptl. Biol. Med. **81**, 556—559 (1952).

WELCH, J. J.: Rodent control. A review of chemical repellents for rodents. J. Agr. Food Chem. **2**, 142—149 (1954).

WESCOTT, E. W.: Uptake of cycloheximide by a sensitive and a resistant yeast and effect of the antibiotic on alcohol dehydrogenase. Ph.D. Thesis, University of Maryland 1962.

WESCOTT, E. W., and H. D. SISLER: Uptake of cycloheximide by a sensitive and a resistant yeast. Phytopathology **54**, 1261—1264 (1964).

WETTSTEIN, F. O., H. NOLL, and S. PENMAN: Effect of cycloheximide on ribosomal aggregates engaged in protein synthesis *in vitro*. Biochim. et Biophys. Acta **87**, 525—528 (1964).

WHIFFEN, A. J.: The production, assay, and antibiotic activity of actidione, an antibiotic from *Streptomyces griseus*. J. Bacteriol. **56**, 283—291 (1948).

WHIFFEN, A. J.: The activity *in vitro* of cycloheximide (actidione) against fungi pathogenic to plants. Mycologia **42**, 253—258 (1950).

WHIFFEN, A. J., N. BOHONOS, and R. L. EMERSON: The production of an antifungal antibiotic by *Streptomyces griseus*. J. Bacteriol. **52**, 610—611 (1946).

WIDUCZYNSKI, I., and A. O. M. STOPPANI: Action of cycloheximide on amino acid metabolism in *Saccharomyces ellipsoideus*. Biochim. et Biophys. Acta **104**, 413—426 (1965).

WILKIE, D., and B. K. LEE: Genetic analysis of actidione resistance in *Saccharomyces cerevisiae*. Genet. Res. Camb. **6**, 130—138 (1965).

WILLIAMSON, A. R., and R. SCHWEET: Role of the genetic message in polyribosome function. J. Mol. Biol. **11**, 358—372 (1965).

WILSON, G. B.: Cytological effects of some antibiotics. J. Heredity **41**, 227—231 (1950).

WILSON, G. B.: The assay of antimitotics. Chromosoma **16**, 133—143 (1965).

WOO, P. W. K., H. W. DION, and Q. R. BARTZ: The structure of streptimidone. J. Am. Chem. Soc. **83**, 3085—3087 (1961).

YOUNG, C. W., P. F. ROBINSON, and B. SACKTON: Inhibition of the synthesis of protein in intact animals by acetoxycycloheximide and a metabolic derangement concomitant with this blockage. Biochem. Pharmacol. **12**, 855—865 (1963).

ZEHNDER, A., and E. O. HUGHES: The antialgal activity of actidione. Can. J. Microbiol. **4**,399—408 (1958).

Chloramphenicol

F. E. Hahn

Chloramphenicol is of unique interest for a variety of reasons. It was the first broad-spectrum antibiotic introduced into medicinal use. It also was the first antibiotic to be completely synthesized by methods of organic chemistry and is still the only antibiotic which is industrially produced by chemical synthesis rather than by fermentation. The relative simplicity of the chemical molecule of chloramphenicol has rendered possible the synthesis of a large number of derivatives of the antibiotic, and the microbiological and biochemical study of many of these compounds has resulted in detailed theories of the relationships between structure and biological activity in the chloramphenicol series of compounds. Finally, the specific action of chloramphenicol upon microbial protein synthesis does not only present by itself an intriguing research problem in biochemistry and molecular biology but has rendered the antibiotic a versatile tool in experimental studies in which it is desired to block protein synthesis specifically in order to investigate other processes, notably the control and regulation of nucleic acid synthesis.

Advances in the knowledge of the mechanism of action of chloramphenicol have been reviewed by numerous authors, for example: BROCK (1961), DAVIS and FEINGOLD (1962), GALE (1963), HAHN (1964), NEWTON (1965), GOLDBERG (1965) and VAZQUEZ (1966a). The number of original experimental articles concerned with the action of chloramphenicol or having a bearing upon this problem is considerable; BROCK stated in 1961 that his bibliography on the subject of chloramphenicol contained more than 1000 items of a nonclinical nature. The present report is not meant to be bibliographically complete. Subjects have been selected for review and discussion that, in the opinion of the author, have significantly advanced the knowledge of the action of chloramphenicol and the formulation of hypotheses concerned with the underlying mechanisms.

Chloramphenicol is a fermentation product of *Streptomyces venezuelae* (EHRLICH *et al.*, 1947). EHRLICH and his associates (1952, 1953) have reported interesting studies on the ecology of the formation of chloramphenicol by this organism. Growth of *S. venezuelae* in natural *non-sterile* soil did not produce detectable amounts of chloramphenicol while identical growth of this organism in *sterilized* soil produced significant quantities of the antibiotic. These results may be interpreted as indications that chloramphenicol is not an "antibiotic" in the conventional sense of the word, i.e., a substance that is elaborated by one microorganism in response to its competition with other microorganisms for survival in a complex ecological environment.

The chemical structure of chloramphenicol (Fig. 1) was determined by REBSTOCK *et al.* (1949) and confirmed by synthesis (CONTROULIS *et al.*, 1949) and X-ray diffraction studies (DUNITZ, 1952). The close approximation (2.74 Å) of the two propane-diol oxygen atoms suggests the existence of a strong hydrogen bond between the two aliphatic hydroxyl groups in the crystallized antibiotic (DUNITZ, 1952); that this conformation of the molecule also exists in solution was concluded by JARDETZKY (1963) on the basis of proton resonance spectroscopic studies.

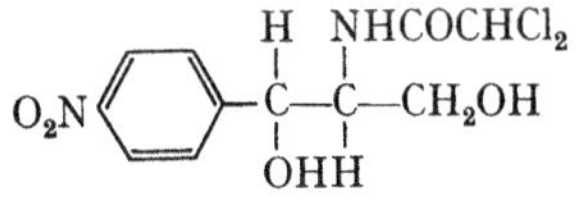

Chloramphenicol

Chloramphenicol possesses two asymmetric carbon atoms which give rise to four stereoisomers (Fig. 2) (REBSTOCK *et al.*, 1949). Only the natural antibiotic which is the D(—)*threo* stereoisomer has significant antimicrobial activity (MAXWELL and NICKEL, 1954).

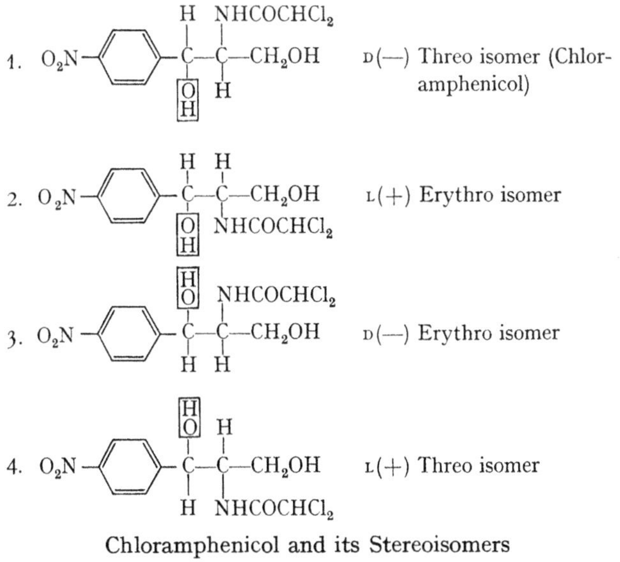

Chloramphenicol and its Stereoisomers

An unusual feature of the molecule of chloramphenicol is the aromatic nitro group. This author has reference to only two other nitro compounds of biological origin, β-nitropropionic acid (BUSH *et al.*, 1951) and 2-nitro-imidazole (NAKAMURA, 1955). While it was originally speculated that the nitro group in chloramphenicol was of unique importance to the action of the antibiotic (DANN *et al.*, 1950), subsequent studies (reviewed by HAHN *et al.*, 1956) have shown that a variety of electronegative groups can be substituted for the nitro group without drastic loss of antimicrobial activity.

Chloramphenicol is a broad-spectrum antibiotic (Table 1) which inhibits the growth of most bacteria, of rickettsiae, and of organisms of the psittacosis-lymphogranuloma group (MACLEAN *et al.*, 1949; SMADEL and JACKSON, 1947). Certain bacteria, notably members of the genera Clostridium and Pseudomonas are rather insensitive to the antibiotic, and euviruses, fungi, and yeasts are mostly resistant. A few exceptions to these generalizations are 1. a "curative" effect of chloramphenicol in bacteriophage-infected *Salmonella typhimurium* (TING, 1960), 2. an inhibition of the growth of the fungus *Scopulariopsis brevicaulis* by the antibiotic (BROADBENT and TERRY, 1958), and 3. a strong effect on the growth of *Candida albicans* by a close chemical relative of chloramphenicol (LONG and TROUTMAN, 1951).

Table 1. *Typical growth inhibitory concentrations of chloramphenicol for selected microorganisms* (After MCLEAN *et al.*, 1949)

Organism	Inhibiting concentration µg/ml
Bacillus anthracis	5
Bacillus subtilis	2.5
Clostridium perfringens	>500
Escherichia coli	2.5
Klebsiella pneumonia	0.5
Staphylococcus aureus	5
Proteus vulgaris	2.5
Pseudomonas aeruginosa	75
Salmonella typhosa	2.5
Shigella sonnei	2.5
Aspergillus niger	>1000
Histoplasma capsulatum	>1000
Saccharomyces cerevisiae	>1000
Endamoeba histolytica	1000 negative

Mammalian cells in culture are usually resistant to chloramphenicol (LEPINE *et al.*, 1950; FUSILLO *et al.*, 1952) but a few instances have been reported (DJORDJEVIC and SZYBALSKI, 1960; EAGLE and FOLEY, 1958; SMITH *et al.*, 1959) in which growth of certain human cells in culture was inhibited by the antibiotic at concentrations of the order of 10^{-4} M. The synthesis of antibody in cell cultures was also inhibited by chloramphenicol (AMBROSE and COONS, 1963).

The literature on the toxicity of chloramphenicol in animals has been reviewed recently (BROCK, 1964). The average LD_{50} of the antibiotic in adult mammals upon intravenous injection is approximately 160 mg/kg of body weight. Death from such large doses occurs within a few hours with symptoms of impaired respiration, decrease in blood pressure, and anoxia. This acute toxicity phenomenon appears to be unrelated to the mode of antimicrobial action of chloramphenicol although it has been observed that the antibiotic molecule and its microbiologically non-active enantiomer also display different toxicities in mammals. CHECCHI (1950) reported that the L-isomer of chloramphenicol had in mice only 30 to 50% of the toxicity of the D-isomer, chloramphenicol itself, while REUTNER *et al.* (1955) and NELSON and RADOMSKI (1954) reported, conversely that the L-isomer was more toxic than the natural D-isomer.

Chloramphenicol has a greater acute toxicity in newborn animals and infants than in mature mammals (KENT and WIDEMAN, 1959). The symptoms of death in newborn and mature animals are similar and the greater susceptibility at young ages has been attributed (KENT *et al.*, 1960) to an incompletely developed glucuronide conjugation system and, hence, to a less effective detoxification of chloramphenicol.

The literature on the toxicity of chloramphenicol in humans has been reviewed recently by YUNIS and BLOOMBERG (1964). The antibiotic produces blood dyscrasias of which several hundred cases have been reported. One can distinguish two types of bone marrow toxicity. One type has a rapid onset and occurs during treatment with chloramphenicol. It is dose-dependent, is characterized by a normocellular bone marrow and by certain cytological changes in peripheral blood that disappear when the administration of chloramphenicol is discontinued. The second type has a late onset from 2 weeks to 5 months, is not always related to the administered dosage of the antibiotic but produces aplastic bone marrow and has a fatal outcome. While chloramphenicol is the most frequent single cause of drug-induced aplastic anemia, the actual incidence is low (of the order of 1/200,000). There appears to be no clear-cut age dependency in developing aplastic anemia after chloramphenicol therapy but the incidence of this complication is significantly higher in females than in males (1.6:1).

The reversible hematopoietic depression caused by chloramphenicol can be regarded not so much as a "complication" but as a genuine pharmacological effect that may be related to the mode of action of the antibiotic. The biochemical or molecular basis of bone marrow aplasia from chloramphenicol however, remains unknown.

Chloramphenicol-treated bacteria do not differ in gross morphology from untreated control cells. HAHN *et al.* (1957) related the increase in *E. coli* nucleic acids during exposure to chloramphenicol to a marked increase in azure-A-thionyl chloride-positive structures that disappeared gradually when the organisms excreted excess RNA and recovered from the action of chloramphenicol. KELLENBERGER *et al.* (1958) studied the morphology of chloramphenicol-treated *E. coli* by electronmicroscopy of thin sections and described subtle changes in the nucleoid structure that were perhaps related to the observations of HAHN *et al.* (1957) under the light microscope.

Chloramphenicol as a Growth Inhibitor

Chloramphenicol can be regarded as a predominantly bacteriostatic agent. FASSIN *et al.* (1955) reported exceptions to this rule in that *Shigella flexneri* as well as an unidentified gram-positive sporeforming organism was rapidly killed by the antibiotic. The decrease in bacterial growth rate as a function of graded concentrations of chloramphenicol can be expressed in a typical dosage response correlation which can be converted into a straight line by a probit transformation (CIAK and HAHN, 1958); statistical handling of such data and calculation of the ED_{50} represent the most precise method by which the growth-inhibitory dose of chloramphenicol for a given organism can be determined.

ALLISON *et al.* (1962) have carried out a precise study of the changes in the total number as well as in the number of viable cells of *Escherichia coli* in liquid cultures in the presence of growth-inhibitory concentrations of chloramphenicol.

Total (automatic) cell count continued to increase for 14 generation times and approached an increment of 50%; viable count increased for only one to two generation times and then decreased to approximately 25% of the highest count that had been attained 1—2 generation times after the addition of chloramphenicol. Actual cell division of bacteria under the influence of chloramphenicol was observed under the microscope. These studies have shown that the view of chloramphenicol as a "bacteriostatic" agent in the literal sense of the term is an evident oversimplification of a more complex situation that does not become apparent in conventional turbidimetric inhibition analysis or routine plate counting with a fairly high standard deviation.

The growth of *Rickettsia tsutsugamushi* in mouse L cells in culture is immediately arrested by chloramphenicol, but it requires 3 weeks of continuous administration of the antibiotic to "cure" these cell cultures of their rickettsial infection (HOPPS *et al.*, 1959). Evidently, chloramphenicol acts as a rickettsiostatic agent rather than by killing *R. tsutsugamushi*.

In *Tetrahymena piriformis* chloramphenicol inhibits cell growth, i.e. increase in cell mass, especially in protein, but not cell division when these processes are experimentally dissociated by a temperature shift technique (LEE *et al.*, 1959). These results are somewhat remindful of the bacteriological findings of ALLISON *et al.* (1962).

Growth of the green alga, *Euglena gracilis* is not inhibited by chloramphenicol when the organism is grown heterotrophically, i.e. with carbon sources other than CO_2. The auxotrophic growth of *E. gracilis* with CO_2 as sole source of carbon is, however, inhibited by the antibiotic. This differential effect of chloramphenicol is the result of a specific inhibition of the synthesis of chloroplasts, i.e. of the photosynthesizing machinery of these cells (SMILLIE *et al.*, 1964). Similar studies with the green alga *Scenedesmus quadricauda* growing on carbonate in light have brought out the interesting observation that the enantiomer of chloramphenicol, the L(+) *threo* stereoisomer, was twice as active in reducing the growth rate of the test organism as was chloramphenicol itself (TAYLOR, 1965).

Finally, the formation of protein in mitochondria or mitochondrial preparations from a variety of chloramphenicol-resistant cells is sensitive to inhibition by the antibiotic (MAGER, 1960; KROON, 1963; WINTERSBERGER, 1965; HUANG *et al.*, 1966).

Effects of Chloramphenicol Upon Energy Metabolism

Chloramphenicol is without effect upon oxygen consumption of nongrowing bacterial suspensions (HAHN and WISSEMAN, 1951); respiration of bacteria in complete growth media is reduced by the antibiotic to the oxidation rates of non-growing cells (WISSEMAN *et al.*, 1954). Apparently this effect is a consequence of the inhibition of protein biosynthesis by chloramphenicol. Under these conditions, *Aerobacter aerogenes* accumulates a glycogen-like polymer as the result of a shunt mechanism of conserving a source of energy (SEGEL *et al.*, 1965).

The rate of glutamic acid oxidation in *Escherichia coli* is reduced by chloramphenicol (WISSEMAN *et al.*, 1950), but the oxidation of this amino acid goes to completion in the presence of the antibiotic while only 80% of the theoretical amount of oxygen is consumed by bacteria which oxidize glutamate in the absence of chloramphenicol (HAHN, unpublished data). These results reflect the action of the antibiotic upon protein synthesis and the failure to utilize glutamate for this process.

KOROTYAEV (1962) and KATAGIRI *et al.* (1960) have noted an influence of chloramphenicol upon the metabolism of pyruvate in *E. coli*. The antibiotic inhibited the aerobic dissimilation of pyruvate in intact cells but was less effective under anaerobic conditions or in cell-free extracts. KOROTYAEV (1961) attributes the effects of chloramphenicol in intact aerobic bacteria to the inhibition of a sequentially inducible formic acid dehydrogenase. HAHN (1952, unpublished data) has observed that the oxidation of pyruvate in *E. coli* proceeded at a linear rate until $^1/_2\,O_2$ per molecule of pyruvic acid had been consumed. This was followed by a lag in oxygen consumption and then by a secondary and exponential rise in oxygen consumption, suggesting a primary conversion of pyruvate to acetate by oxidative decarboxylation followed by induced enzyme synthesis. The secondary increase in oxygen consumption was inhibited by chloramphenicol but not the first linear uptake of oxygen. At high concentrations (1.1—6.1×10^{-3} M), chloramphenicol inhibited the respiration of human leukocytes (FOLLETTE *et al.*, 1956). Evidently, this reflects the toxicity of the antibiotic rather than a specific mode of action.

HAHN *et al.* (1955) have studied the action of chloramphenicol upon selected processes of bacterial energy metabolism and found essentially no effect on bioluminescence as an example of electron transfer, on phosphorylations involved in the dissimilation of glucose, and on motility as one example of energy utilization. Oxidative phosphorylation in a cell-free system of liver mitochondria also was insensitive to chloramphenicol (LOOMIS, 1950). It is concluded that the antibiotic at the growth-inhibitory concentration range between 10^{-5} and 10^{-4} M does not affect processes of energy generation and transduction directly and that the observations reviewed in this section are secondary events related to the inhibition of protein synthesis by chloramphenicol.

Effects of Chloramphenicol on Cell-Wall Biosynthesis

The incorporation of amino acids into bacterial cell wall polymers is not inhibited by chloramphenicol (HANCOCK and PARK, 1958; MANDELSTAM and ROGERS, 1958, 1959). An effect of the antibiotic on the incorporation of diaminopimelic acid into sporulating *Bacillus cereus* was noted by VINTER (1963) who considers this effect a consequence of an inhibition of induced enzyme synthesis by chloramphenicol.

Effects of Chloramphenicol on Aromatic Ring Biosynthesis

TRUHAUT *et al.* (1951) suggested that chloramphenicol interfered with some intermediate step in the biosynthesis of tryptophan and BERGMANN and SICHER (1952) postulated that the mode of action of chloramphenicol was an interference with the conversion of anthranilic acid to indole. The evidence for this idea was a limited reversal of the growth-inhibitory effects of chloramphenicol by addition of the respective essential metabolites to bacterial auxotrophs that required anthranilic acid, indole, or tryptophan for growth.

In wild-type *E. coli*, however, tryptophan fails to reverse the effect of the antibiotic on growth (HOPPS *et al.*, 1956); this renders it unlikely that the action of chloramphenicol, in general, is one of inducing tryptophan deficiency. GIBSON and his associates (GIBSON *et al.*, 1955, 1956; MCDOUGALL and GIBSON, 1958) have shown by chemical analysis that chloramphenicol but not its antibiotically non-active stereoisomers inhibits the biosynthesis of indole in a mutant of *E. coli* that accumulates indole as a result of a block in the conversion of indole to tryptophan. This effect was also observed when the antibiotic was added to non-growing suspensions of bacteria in which indole synthesis had been under way for hours and which evidently possessed a complete set of enzymes nesessary for indole synthesis. GIBSON and MCDOUGALL (1961) extended the study to include additional bacterial auxotrophs, accumulating indole-3-glycerol, anthranilic acid, or 5-dehydroshikimic acid, and concluded that chloramphenicol interfered in some reaction leading to the formation of 5-dehydroshikimic acid. Since tetracyclines produced effects identical to those of chloramphenicol, the inhibition of aromatic biosynthesis is not a specific mode of action of the latter antibiotic. The relationship between inhibitions of aromatic biosynthesis and an inhibition of protein synthesis warrants further study.

Inhibition of Protein Synthesis

Inhibition of protein biosynthesis is the mode of action of chloramphenicol. HAHN and WISSEMAN (1951) discovered that the antibiotic inhibits the induced synthesis of enzymes and concluded that this effect indicated an inhibition of protein synthesis as the general mode of action of the antibiotic. Sypherd and his associates (1962, 1963) found a preferential inhibition by chloramphenicol of the synthesis of inducible enzymes by comparison to that of constitutive enzymes. The same effect was, however, produced by a variety of other antibiotics and is plausibly the result of catabolite repression (PAIGEN, 1963; NAKADA and MAGASANIK, 1964) rather than of a specific action of chloramphenicol.

Direct proof of a general inhibition of bacterial protein synthesis by chloramphenicol was obtained through biochemical analysis by WISSEMAN *et al.* (1953, 1954) of *E. coli* and by GALE and FOLKES of *Staphylococcus aureus* (1953). Inhibition of protein synthesis in bacteria occurs at bacteriostatic concentrations of the antibiotic and is a highly specific effect since the formation of nucleic acids (WISSEMAN *et al.*, 1954; GALE and FOLKES, 1953), cell-walls (HANCOCK and PARK, 1958; MANDELSTAM and ROGERS, 1958, 1959), and polysaccharides (HOPPS *et al.*, 1954) continues in bacteria exposed to chloramphenicol. The specificity of the action of the antibiotic upon protein synthesis has led to widespread use of chloramphenicol as a biochemical tool.

The progressive resolution of the pathway and reaction mechanism of protein synthesis during the past decade has resulted in a delineation of the specific area of the reaction sequence in which chloramphenicol acts. The first step in protein synthesis, *viz.*, the activation of amino acids is not affected by chloramphenicol (DEMOSS and NOVELLI, 1955). The antibiotic also does not inhibit the synthesis of amino acyl transfer RNAs (LACKS and GROS, 1959); in the presence of chloramphenicol, amino acyl transfer RNAs accumulate in bacteria for the apparent reason that a more advanced step of the protein-synthesizing pathway is blocked.

The next phase in the reaction sequence is the formation of an assemblage of ribosomes, messenger RNA, and amino acyl transfer RNAs. The binding of these components to each other can be determined in cell-free experimental systems, and completely assembled systems are capable of polymerizing amino acids into polypeptides with the aid of enzymes, known as "transfer factors".

Polymerization of amino acids to polypeptides in such cell-free "incorporation systems" is inhibited by chloramphenicol (NIRENBERG and MATTHAEI, 1961; NATHANS and LIPMANN, 1961). This inhibition is a stereospecific effect of the molecule of the antibiotic since it is not observed with the three stereoisomers of chloramphenicol (RENDI and OCHOA, 1962). A detailed analysis of the reaction products of a ribosome-polyadenylic acid (poly A) system, synthesizing lysyl peptides in the absence or presence of chloramphenicol (JULIAN, 1965), has demonstrated that the antibiotic apparently inhibits the continuation of peptide chain formation rather than the initiation. The number of lysyl peptide chains formed was less reduced by chloramphenicol than was the average length of these chains: the predominant reaction products in chloramphenicol-inhibited systems were di- and tri-peptides while in the absence of the antibiotic, a second maximum of abundance of products with defined chain lengths was centered around the heptapeptide. JULIAN has interpreted his findings as an effect of chloramphenicol upon a peptide-forming step.

There exists, indeed, presumptive evidence that the antibiotic inhibits directly the type of peptide bond formation that occurs in protein synthesis. When puromycin, a structural and metabolic analogue of the amino acyl adenosine end group of amino acid-charged transfer RNA (YARMOLINSKY and DE LA HABA, 1959), is added to bacteria that are synthesizing protein (NATHANS, 1964), or to cell-free ribosome-poly U systems that synthesize polyphenylalanine (TRAUT and MONRO, 1964), the compound is incorporated into the growing peptide chains *in lieu* of the next incoming amino acid and peptidyl puromycin, i.e. incomplete peptide chains terminating with puromycin, is released from the ribosomal assemblage. Apparently, the growing peptide chain is transferred to puromycin in a manner analogous to that by which this chain is normally transferred to the amino groups of incoming amino acids in protein chain growth. Since peptide bond formation with puromycin does not require an interaction of a transfer RNA with the ribosome or the recognition of an anticodon in transfer RNA by a codon in messenger RNA, the puromycin reaction is a simplified model of peptide bond formation.

Chloramphenicol inhibits the formation of peptidyl puromycin in whole bacteria (NATHANS *et al.*, 1962; NATHANS, 1964) as well as in a cell-free ribosome-poly U system (TRAUT and MONRO, 1964), and the latter authors have inferred that the antibiotic acts as an inhibitor of a peptide bond forming enzyme. Such an enzyme has apparently been demonstrated in a cell-free system of mammalian origin (ARLINGHAUS *et al.*, 1964) but the identification of one of the "transfer factors" of bacterial origin (ALLENDE *et al.*, 1964) as a condensing enzyme has not as yet been accomplished. The conclusive testing of the hypothesis of TRAUT and MONRO (1964) awaits the resolution of the terminal enzymatic events of peptide bond synthesis in a chloramphenicol-sensitive microbial system.

Studies on the action of chloramphenicol in cell-free ribosomal systems that polymerize amino acids have led several authors to assume that the antibiotic acts on the ribosome (RENDI and OCHOA, 1962; KUCAN and LIPMANN, 1964). Especially the observation of SO and DAVIE (1963) that such an experimental system assembled from yeast ribosomes with *E. coli* enzymes was resistant to chloramphenicol while the corresponding homologous system with *E. coli* ribosomes was sensitive to the antibiotic, point to the ribosomes of sensitive cells as the site of action of chloramphenicol.

This idea has gained in probability through studies on the binding of ^{14}C-labelled chloramphenicol to ribosomes. VAZQUEZ reported that radioactive chloramphenicol binds to ribosomes of both *S. aureus* (1963) and *Bacillus megaterium* (1964a) and showed that the antibiotic combined preferentially with the 50s subunit of the ribosomal particle. The binding of chloramphenicol to ribosomes of susceptible bacteria is stereospecific (WOLFE and HAHN, 1964; VAZQUEZ, 1964b) and there exists a 1:1 equivalence between the number of ribosomes present and the number of chloramphenicol molecules bound (WOLFE and HAHN, 1965). At higher concentrations of the antibiotic, additional chloramphenicol appears to become bound to *E. coli* ribosomes (DAS *et al.*, 1966). Ribosomes from naturally chloramphenicol resistant cell types fail to bind the antibiotic and are of the "heavy", i.e. 80s category (VAZQUEZ, 1964b).

The stereospecificity of the ribosomal binding of chloramphenicol as well as the biological specificity of this binding to susceptible ribosomes support the hypothesis that the attachment of the antibiotic molecule to ribosomes is an essential prerequisite to the action of chloramphenicol upon protein synthesis.

This idea has important consequences for the interpretation of experimental studies and of proposed hypotheses concerning the influence of chloramphenicol upon the ribosomal binding of messenger RNA or upon the function of bound messenger RNA. RENDI and OCHOA (1962) had suggested that chloramphenicol interfered with the attachment of messenger RNA to ribosomes. This hypothesis was subsequently tested in OCHOA's laboratory for the attachment of poly A (SPEYER *et al.*, 1963), by JARDETZKY and JULIAN of polyuridylic acid (poly U) (1964), and by KUCAN and LIPMANN (1964) of poly UC; in no instance did chloramphenicol reduce significantly the quantities of polynucleotides bound to bacterial ribosomes. Since messenger RNA binds to the 30s ribosomal subunit (TAKANAMI and OKAMOTO, 1963) while chloramphenicol attaches to the 50s subunit (VAZQUEZ, 1964a), failure of chloramphenicol to reduce ribosomal binding of messenger RNA might plausibly be expected.

WEISBERGER *et al.* (1963, 1964) reported that a poly U-stimulated incorporation of phenylalanine in a cell-free system employing ribosomes from mammalian reticulocytes was inhibited by chloramphenicol; this inhibition could be gradually reversed by adding graded quantities of poly U simultaneously with, or *after*, chloramphenicol. The effect of 10^{-4} M chloramphenicol was overcome completely by the addition of 25µg/ml of polyuridylic acid. From these results, it was inferred that chloramphenicol and poly U were in competition for ribosomal binding sites. WEISBERGER and WOLFE (1964) showed that chloramphenicol did, indeed, interfere with the binding of poly U to reticulocyte ribosomes. The antibiotic also inhibited the binding of bacterial messenger RNA to the mammalian ribosomes, but the inhibition of amino acid incorporation in that particular system was not reversed by adding more messenger RNA. It should be noted that other workers (OCHOA and WEINSTEIN, 1964; KRUG as cited by KUCAN and LIPMANN, 1964) have been unable to demonstrate an effect of chloramphenicol on the poly U-stimulated polymerization of phenylalanine in mammalian ribosomal systems.

WOLFE and HAHN (1965) have tested the hypothesis of a competition between poly U and chloramphenicol for attachment to bacterial ribosomes. Neither was the inhibition of the polymerization of phenylalanine by chloramphenicol reversed by increasing the concentration of poly U in a bacterial ribosome system, nor did poly U reverse the binding of ^{14}C chloramphenicol to ribosomes. At the time of this writing, the apparent discrepancy between the results of WEISBERGER and his associates and those of the other authors, cited above, as concerns the effect of chloramphenicol on ribosomal binding of messenger RNA remain unresolved unless differences in the nature of bacterial and mammalian ribosomes are invoked as explanations of the different effects of chloramphenicol.

Cell-free amino acid incorporation systems containing synthetic polynucleotides as models of messenger RNA are generally less susceptible to chloramphenicol than is natural protein synthesis in intact cells. The nature of this difference in susceptibilities remains unknown. Chloramphenicol may alter the ribosome-messenger complex qualitatively in such a manner that polymerization of amino acids is inhibited. Two lines of evidence point in this direction. 1. Ribosomes to which natural messenger RNAs (viral RNAs) are added (OFENGAND and HASELKORN, 1962; KUCAN and LIPMANN, 1964) are more sensitive to chloramphenicol than those to which synthetic polynucleotides are supplied, and 2. the susceptibility of polynucleotide-containing ribosomal systems is strongly modified by the base composition of the synthetic polynucleotide employed (SPEYER *et al.*, 1963; KUCAN and LIPMANN, 1964). For example, the incorporation of a number of amino acids in ribosomal systems supplied with poly UCs of different quantitative base compositions was inhibited by chloramphenicol in direct proportion to the cytidylic acid content of these polymers (KUCAN and LIPMANN, 1964).

Furthermore, naturally messenger RNA-complexed ribosomal systems are less sensitive to chloramphenicol than those to which a messenger RNA is supplied *in vitro* (KUCAN and LIPMANN, 1964). It is difficult to interpret how the natural or synthetic nature of different messengers or their intrinsic or extrinsic nature modifies the response of amino acid polymerization systems to chloramphenicol. WOLFE and HAHN (1965) have proposed that ribosome-bound chloramphenicol is placed into a special stereometric position that enables the antibiotic to interfere specifically with the function of messenger RNA. An alternate explanation may be sought by considering the chloramphenicol effect to be in the nature of an allosteric mechanism in which binding of the antibiotic to the 50s subunit of the ribosomal particle influences events occurring on the 30s subunit although these events are a far distance away in terms of molecular dimensions. It has been suggested recently that natural messenger RNA contains termination codons which trigger the action of an esterase, hydrolyzing the ester bond between the carboxyl terminus of a completed protein molecule and the last transfer RNA molecule. This process "clears" the ribosome and yields the free protein; in contrast, synthetic polynucleotides used as messenger RNA models do not contain termination codons, and the peptides synthesized under the direction of these polynucleotides contain the last transfer RNA molecule still terminally esterified (Ganoza and Nakamoto, 1966). Since chloramphenicol is an inhibitor of bacterial esterases (Smith, *et al.*, 1949) a superior effect of the antibiotic might be expected upon protein synthesis with natural messenger RNA *in vivo* and *in vitro* if the drug were to interfere with the action of esterases that release completed protein chains.

Several authors have considered the possibility that chloramphenicol might interfere with protein synthesis by inhibiting the attachment of amino acyl transfer RNAs to the messenger-ribosome complex. The attachment of phenylalanyl transfer RNA to the poly U-ribosomes complex was not inhibited by chloramphenicol (Nakamoto *et al.*, 1963; Jardetzky and Julian, 1964; Suarez and Nathans, 1965) but Wolfe and Hahn reported (1965) a stereospecific inhibition by chloramphenicol (3×10^{-4} M) of the poly A-directed binding of lysyl transfer RNA to ribosomes. While the low magnitude of this effect (10—15%) appeared to rule it out as an explanation of the strong action of the antibiotic on the lysine incorporation system as recorded by Speyer *et al.* (1963), the subsequent finding of Julian (1965) that the antibiotic (2.1×10^{-4} M) actually inhibits peptide bond synthesis in this system by only 23% has rendered the observation of Wolfe and Hahn more significant. The possibility that chloramphenicol inhibits the binding of amino acyl transfer RNA to messenger-ribosome complexes has been discussed in detail by Goldberg (1965) and awaits the results of experimental testing.

Finally, the discrepancy between the sensitivities of protein biosynthesis *in vivo* and of amino acid polymerizations in ribosomal systems *in vitro* has led investigators (Das *et al.*, 1966; Dresden and Hoagland, 1966) to resume studies of the effect of the antibiotic in whole bacteria. These authors have concluded that chloramphenicol inhibits continued growth of nascent protein chains on the ribosomes and actually stabilizes polysomes under conditions under which they break down to individual ribosomes in the absence of the antibiotic. Further studies of the action of chloramphenicol in whole cells are likely to make contributions to the knowledge of its mechanism of action.

In summarizing the current state of knowledge concerning the mechanism of action of chloramphenicol upon protein synthesis, it can be stated that the antibiotic inhibits peptide chain extension rather than the initiation of the biosynthesis of protein molecules (Nathans, 1964; Traut and Monro, 1964; Julian, 1965; Das *et al.*, 1966). Any unitary hypothesis explaining the mechanism of action of chloramphenicol will have to take into account the following findings and conclusions.

1. Chloramphenicol binds to 70s ribosomes on their 50s subunits; this attachment is causally responsible for the inhibition of protein synthesis.

2. The relative potency of chloramphenicol is modified by the nature of the messenger RNA that is attached to the ribosomes. Complexes of 70s ribosomes with natural messenger RNA are more susceptible to the action of chloramphenicol

than are complexes with synthetic polynucleotides; the presence of cytidylic acid residues in such polynucleotides renders the ribosomal complexes more sensitive to inhibition of amino acid polymerization by the antibiotic.

3. In a simplified model system of peptide bond synthesis that does not require binding of a transfer RNA to ribosomes or recognition of a codeword by an anticodon, chloramphenicol inhibits the formation of peptidyl puromycin, i.e. it interferes with the formation of *one peptide bond.*

Chloramphenicol RNA

The continued biosynthesis of RNA in chloramphenicol-exposed bacteria in which protein synthesis is inhibited has stimulated investigations on the nature of this RNA and on the control and regulation of its biosynthesis. This work has been reviewed recently by VAZQUEZ (1966a). When chloramphenicol is removed from bacteria that have been synthesizing RNA for several generation times in the absence of protein synthesis, much of the newly synthesized RNA is broken down (HAHN *et al.*, 1957; NEIDHARDT and GROS, 1957) and eliminated from the bacterial cells in the form of purine and pyrimidine bases (HAHN and WOLFE, 1962). Even while being formed in chloramphenicol-exposed bacteria, RNA is subject to turnover but the rate of synthesis exceeds the rate of degradation and the result is a net increase in RNA as long as chloramphenicol is present (HOROWITZ *et al.*, 1958).

The degradation of RNA following the removal of chloramphenicol occurs in minimal medium and constitutes in physiological terms a recovery period (HAHN *et al.*, 1957; NEIDHARDT and GROS, 1957) which precedes a resumption of balanced growth and cell replication. When the recovery medium, however, is enriched with a complete complement of amino acids, no breakdown of RNA is observed (HORIUCHI *et al.*, 1958; ARONSON and SPIEGELMAN, 1961a) and the bacteria resume protein synthesis without delay, at first without concomitant RNA synthesis but soon accompanied by nucleic acid synthesis in the manner characteristic for balanced growth (ARONSON and SPIEGELMAN, 1961a); this situation is remindful of the kinetics of RNA and protein synthesis in bacteria that are "shifted down" to a poorer growth medium and temporarily possess a greater amount of RNA than is necessary to maintain balanced growth (NEIDHARDT, 1964).

Evidently all known categories of cellular RNA are synthesized in chloramphenicol-exposed bacteria. Formation of soluble RNA in such organisms (MIDGELEY, 1963) amounted to a considerable percentage (HAHN and CIAK, unpublished data) of the total increase in RNA.

RNA with compositional (HAHN and WOLFE, 1962; MIDGELEY, 1963) and functional properties of messenger RNA (WILLSON and GROS, 1964; OKAMOTO *et al.*, 1964) also accumulates in chloramphenicol-inhibited bacteria and is evidently subject to preferential breakdown after removal of the antibiotic (HAHN and WOLFE, 1962) in agrement with the well established lability of messenger RNA in bacteria. Several authors have actually suggested that chloramphenicol action protects messenger RNA from its usual decay by stabilizing the complex of the polymer with ribosomes (MIDGELEY and MCCARTHY, 1962; FAN *et al.*, 1964; WOESE *et al.*, 1963).

Ribosomal RNA is also synthesized by chloramphenicol-exposed bacteria and accumulates in the form of "chloramphenicol particles" (PARDEE *et al.*, 1957; NOMURA and WATSON, 1959; KURLAND *et al.*, 1962; SPIRIN, 1963; NOMURA and HOSOKOWA, 1965) of lesser protein content and lower sedimentation rates than normal 30s and 50s ribosomal subunits. When the RNA from chloramphenicol particles is isolated, its analytical properties differ slightly from those of normal 16s and 23s ribosomal RNAs possibly as the result of a lower content of methylated bases in chloramphenicol RNA by comparison to normal ribosomal RNA (DUBIN and ELKORT, 1964; GORDON *et al.*, 1964). It is possible that the ready resumption of protein synthesis in bacteria, in amino acid media after removal of chloramphenicol (HORIUCHI *et al.*, 1958; ARONSON and SPIEGELMAN, 1961a) serves to furnish ribosomal proteins that are necessary for the assemblage of complete ribosomes from the chloramphenicol particles (SPIRIN, 1963).

Finally, the ability of chloramphenicol to uncouple RNA synthesis from protein synthesis has led to the use of the antibiotic in studies on the regulation of RNA biosynthesis (reviewed by NEIDHARDT, 1964). Most bacteria require a complete complement of amino acids not merely for protein synthesis but also for RNA synthesis. This stringent requirement for amino acids can be partially (GROS and GROS, 1958) or completely (ARONSON and SPIEGELMAN, 1961b) overcome by supplying chloramphenicol to amino acid-requiring bacteria that are unable to synthesize RNA owing to the absence of an essential amino acid. Several authors have observed that addition of chloramphenicol to wild-type bacteria results in a distinctive stimulation of the rate of RNA synthesis (GALE and FOLKES, 1953; KURLAND and MAALØE, 1962; NEIDHARDT, 1964). A detailed discussion of the role of this chloramphenicol effect in hypotheses of the regulation of RNA synthesis in bacteria falls outside the scope of this review; the reader is referred to the article of NEIDHARDT (1964) for a detailed consideration of such hypotheses.

DNA Synthesis in Chloramphenicol-Exposed Bacteria

The role of protein synthesis in regulating DNA synthesis has been the subject of a considerable volume of study, recently reviewed by LARK (1963). While experiments with amino acid starvation of certain auxotrophs have suggested to some authors (for example, MAALØE, 1963) that initiation of each discrete round of cellular DNA replication requires the renewed synthesis of initiating proteins, experiments combining amino acid starvation and addition of chloramphenicol (KELLENBERGER *et al.*, 1962) have failed to show a limitation in the extent of DNA synthesis compatible with such a view. In a histidine-less mutant of *E. coli* starved with respect to this amino acid and exposed to chloramphenicol, chemical analysis showed that DNA nearly doubled in quantity, and density labelling followed by equilibrium centrifugation in a cesium chloride gradient proved that the DNA had undergone classical semi-conservative replication (NAKADA and RYAN, 1961). DNA which is synthesized in chloramphenicol-exposed bacteria exhibits type transforming activity identical to that of the DNA synthesized during normal growth (GOODGAL and MELECHEN, 1960) and, hence, can be considered to be biologically functional. Likewise, phage DNA synthesized in the presence of the antibiotic is utilized for the assemblage of viable phage after chloramphenicol is removed, and such DNA can also participate in genetic recombination (THOMAS, 1959).

Structure-Activity Relationships

Numerous chemical derivatives of chloramphenicol have been prepared and tested for antimicrobial activity. A tabulation of such compounds has been published by SHEMYAKIN (1961). Chloramphenicol analogues with different para-phenyl substituents have also been tested for their ability to inhibit amino acid polymerization in cell-free ribosomal systems (VAZQUEZ, 1966b). Rules determining structure-activity relationships in the chloramphenicol series of compounds have been derived independently by SHEMYAKIN *et al.* (1956) and by HAHN *et al.* (1956) and agree in their major conclusions.

These rules are summarized and discussed below in such a manner that the Roman numerals of the sections in the text correspond to those denoting the corresponding parts of the molecule of chloramphenicol in Fig. 3.

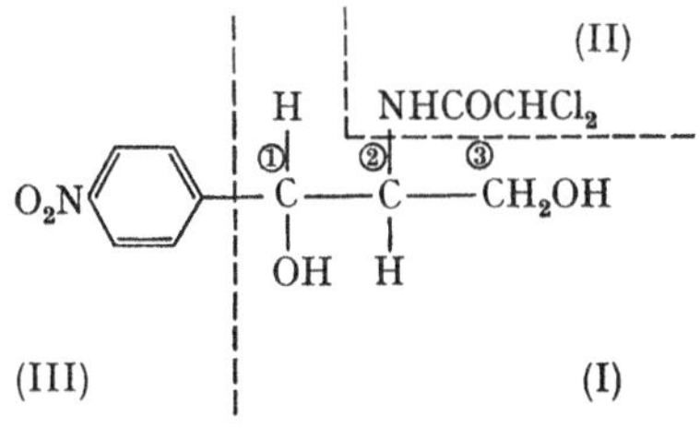

Chloramphenicol

I. The propanediol moiety of chloramphenicol and especially the stereochemical configuration of the substituents on the asymmetric carbon atoms 1 and 2 are absolutely essential for antimicrobial activity. Some diesters of chloramphenicol are active but actually may require restoration of the antibiotic molecule by hydrolysis of the ester bonds. In general, structural changes that affect the functional character of the hydroxyl groups or alter the length of the propane residue abolish the antibacterial activity. Since these groups are engaged in closing an alicyclic ring by hydrogen bonding in the antibiotic molecule (DUNITZ, 1952; JARDETZKY, 1963), such a result may be expected if this ring structure were essential for the action of chloramphenicol.

II. The dichloracetamido side chain can be varied only within rather narrow limits with moderate loss in antimicrobial activity provided that a strong electronegative character in the acyl residue is maintained and, more important, that the size of the acetyl group is not critically exceeded. If the dichloracetamide side chain is entirely deleted, the remaining "chloramphenicol base" has only about 2% of the activity of the intact antibiotic molecule.

III. The antibacterial potency is proportional to the relative electronegativity of the para-substituent of the phenyl group. Substitution of the nitro group by ionogenic groupings leads to complete loss of activity. The volume and geometry of the aromatic ring system are relatively unimportant. It is essential, however, that the substituted ring structure is resonating, perhaps in order to induce the hydroxyl group on the adjacent carbon atom 1 of the propanediol chain to engage in strong hydrogen bonding with the hydroxyl 3 of the chain. The lack of geometrical specificity of the aromatic ring systems in the chloramphenicol series suggests, that these systems are not engaged in specific interaction with the ribosomal binding site (or sites) of the antibiotic or its congeners. This lack also deemphasizes a formal similarity between chloramphenicol and uridylic acid that has been pointed out by JARDETZKY (1963) as the basis for a conjectured antimetabolic relationship between chloramphenicol and uridylic acid moieties in messenger RNA. HAHN (unpublished data) has synthesized dichloroacetyl serine, i.e. a chloramphenicol analogue in which the p-nitrophenyl residue is replaced by a carbonyl group. This substance did not show antibacterial activity. Other workers subsequently also synthesized the compound and found it to possess appreciable antitumor activity in mice (LEVI *et al.*, 1960).

There has been no lack of attemps to relate the structure of chloramphenicol to the structures of biologically important substances in order to deduce possible antimetabolite-metabolite relationships. WOOLLEY (1950) proposed that the antibiotic was an antagonist of phenylalanine. TRUHAUT *et al.* (1951) and BERGMANN and SICHER (1952) thought of chloramphenicol in relation to tryptophan. MENTZER *et al.* (1950) recognized a similarity to phenylserine, Molho and Molho-Lacroix compared chloramphenicol to a dipeptide, and Jardetzky, more recently regarded the antibiotic as an analogue of uridylic acid (1963). In no instance has experimental testing of these antimetabolite hypotheses produced more than marginal results to explain inhibition of growth and of protein synthesis by chloramphenicol in terms of antagonism of a metabolite. Clearly, the biochemical studies on the mechanism of action of chloramphenicol and the structure-activity studies in the chloramphenicol series of compounds remain unrelated and await the formulation of hypotheses that connect logically the two bodies of information.

Acquired Resistance to Chloramphenicol

Studies on the development of resistance to chloramphenicol have been recently reviewed by BROCK (1964). Chloramphenicol-resistant bacteria can be selectively bred by extensive series of cultural passages in the presence of increasing concentrations of the antibiotic (COFFEY *et al.*, 1950). Many studies (reviewed by BROCK, 1964) have shown that resistance to chloramphenicol is not infrequently accompanied by resistance to tetracyclines; this cross-resistance phenomenon is largely confined to enteric bacteria.

Genetic analysis has shown that the resistance to chloramphenicol is the result of a sequence of discrete gene mutations and is a cooperative polygenic phenomenon (CAVALLI and MACCACARO, 1950, 1952). Multistep resistant mutants are capable of transducing only to a degree of resistance corresponding to first-step resistance. This means that genes controlling single steps of resistance are not linked (BANIČ, 1959).

A non-chromosomal genetic basis of chloramphenicol resistance exists in the numerous instances in which resistance is conferred upon a bacterium by episomal transfer. The phenomenon is known as "infective heredity" and involves the intra- or inter-species transfer of hereditary factors, the episomes, that carry multiplicities of genetic properties, prominently multiple drug resistance including resistance to chloramphenicol (WATANABE, 1963).

One biochemical basis of chloramphenicol resistance has been shown to be an acquired impermeability to the antibiotic. This is the case when resistance is the result of multistep mutations but also when resistance results from episomal transfer (OKAMOTO and MIZUNO, 1964). In both instances, cell-free ribosomal systems of amino acid polymerization were susceptible to chloramphenicol regardless of whether such systems had been derived from sensitive or resistant bacteria.

Another biochemical basis of chloramphenicol resistance is the ability of resistant bacteria to degrade chloramphenicol (SADAO and OKETANI, 1962). Recently the presence of chloramphenicol-inactivating enzymes has been demonstrated in cell-free extracts of an episome-carrying strain of *E. coli* (OKAMOTO and SUZUKI, 1965). Enzymatic inactivation of the antibiotic required the addition of acetyl-coenzyme A, occurred in cell-free ribosomal systems for the polymerization of amino acids and, hence, could have given the fallacious impression of a true chloramphenicol-resistant protein synthesizing system.

Finally, several authors have reported the isolation of bacterial strains that were in part dependent upon chloramphenicol for growth (SZYBALSKI, 1953; GOCKE and FINLAND, 1950; SCHIØTT and STEDERUP, 1954). The genetic and biochemical basis of this dependency phenomenon would appear an interesting and important field for future investigation.

See addenda

References

ALLENDE, J. E., R. MONRO, and F. LIPMANN: Resolution of the *Escherichia coli* aminoacyl soluble ribonucleic acid transfer factor into two complementary fractions. Proc. Natl. Acad. Sci. U.S. **51**, 1211 (1964).

ALLISON, J. L., R. E. HARTMAN, R. S. HARTMAN, A. D. WOLFE, J. CIAK, and F. E. HAHN: Mode of action of chloramphenicol. VII. Growth and multiplication of *Escherichia coli* in the presence of chloramphenicol. J. Bact. **83**, 609 (1962).

AMBROSE, C. T., and A. H. COONS: Studies on antibody production. VIII. The inhibitory effect of chloramphenicol on the synthesis of antibody in tissue culture. J. Exptl. Med. **117**, 1075 (1963).

ARLINGHAUS, R., J. SHAEFFER, and R. SCHWEET: Mechanism of peptide bond formation in polypeptide synthesis. Proc. Natl. Acad. Sci. U.S. **51**, 1291 (1964).

ARONSON, A. I., and S. SPIEGELMAN: On the nature of the ribonucleic acid synthesized in the presence of chloramphenicol. Biochim. et Biophys. Acta **53**, 84 (1961a).

ARONSON, A. I., and S. SPIEGELMAN: Protein and ribonucleic acid synthesis in a chloramphenicol-inhibited system. Biochim. et Biophys. Acta **53**, 70 (1961b).

BANIČ, S.: Transduction to penicillin and chloramphenicol resistance in *Salmonella typhimurium*. Genetics **44**, 449 (1959).

BERGMANN, E. D., and S. SICHER: Mode of action of chloramphenicol. Nature **170**, 931 (1952).

BROADBENT, D., and D. A. TERRY: Effect of chloramphenicol on a fungus. Nature **182**, 1107 (1958).

BROCK, T. D.: Chloramphenicol. Bacteriol. Rev. **25**, 32 (1961).

BROCK, T. D.: Chloramphenicol. In: Experimental Chemotherapy, vol. III, p. 119. Academic Press 1964.

BUSH, M. T., O. TOUSTER, and J. E. BROCKMAN: The production of β-nitropropionic acid by a strain of *Aspergillus flavus*. J. Biol. Chem. **188**, 685 (1951).

CAVALLI, L. L., and G. A. MACCACARO: Chloromycetin resistance in *E. coli*, a case of quantitative inheritance in bacteria. Nature **166**, 991 (1950).

CAVALLI, L. L., and G. A. MACCACARO: Polygenic inheritance of drug-resistance in the bacterium, *Escherichia coli*. Heredity **6**, 311 (1952).

CHECCHI, S.: Sulla tossicita degli antipodi ottici e del composto racemico del cloramfenicolo sui topolini per somministrazione gastrica. Arch. ital. sc. farmacol. **3**, 3 (1950).

CIAK, J., and F. E. HAHN: Mechanisms of action of antibiotics. I. Additive action of chloramphenicol and tetracyclines on the growth of *Escherichia coli*. J. Bact. **75**, 125 (1958).

COFFEY, G. L., J. L. SCHWAB, and J. EHRLICH: In vitro studies of bacterial resistance to chloramphenicol (chloromycetin). J. Infectious Diseases **87**, 142 (1950).

CONTROULIS, J., M. C. REBSTOCK, and H. M. CROOKS: Chloramphenicol (Chloromycetin). V. Synthesis. J. Am. Chem. Soc. **71**, 2463 (1949).

DANN, O., H. ULRICH u. E. F. MÖLLER: Über die Bedeutung der Nitrogruppe im Chloromycetin. Z. Naturforsch. **5**, 446 (1950).

DAS, H., A. GOLDSTEIN, and L. KANNER: Inhibition by chloramphenicol of the growth of nascent protein chains in *Escherichia coli*. J. Mol. Pharm. **2**, 158 (1966).

DAVIS, B. D., and D. S. FEINGOLD: Antimicrobial agents: mechanism of action and use in metabolic studies. In: The Bacteria (ed. GUNSALUS), vol. 4, p. 343. 1962.

DEMOSS, J. A., and G. D. NOVELLI: An amino acid dependent exchange between inorganic pyrophosphate and ATP in microbial extracts. Biochim. et Biophys. Acta **18**, 592 (1955).

DJORDJEVIC, B., and W. SZYBALSKI: Genetics of human cell lines. III. Incorporation of 5-bromo- and 5-iododeoxyuridine into the DNA of human cells and its effect on radiation sensitivity. J. Exptl. Med. **112**, 509 (1960).

DRESDEN, M. H., and M. B. HOAGLAND: Effects of chloramphenicol on messenger-ribosome interactions in *E. coli*. Federation Proc. **25**, 582 (1966).

DUBIN, D. T., and A. T. ELKORT: Some abnormal properties of chloramphenicol RNA. J. Mol. Biol. **10**, 508 (1964).

DUNITZ, J. D.: The crystal structure of chloramphenicol and bromamphenicol. J. Am. Chem. Soc. **74**, 995 (1952).

EAGLE, H., and G. E. FOLEY: Cytotoxicity in human cell cultures as a primary screen for the detection of anti-tumor agents. Cancer Research **18**, 1017 (1958).

EHRLICH, J., Q. R. BARTZ, R. M. SMITH, D. A. JOSLYN, and P. R. BURKHOLDER: Chloromycetin, a new antibiotic from a soil actinomycete. Science **106**, 417 (1947).

EHRLICH, J., L. E. ANDERSON, H. L. COFFEY, and D. GOTTLIEB: *Streptomyces venezuelae*: soil studies. Antibiotics & Chemotherapy **2**, 595 (1952).

EHRLICH, J., L. E. ANDERSON, G. L. COFFEY, and D. GOTTLIEB: *Streptomyces venezuelae*: Further soil studies. Antibiotics & Chemotherap **3**, 1141 (1953).

FAN, D. P., A. HIGA, and C. LEVINTHAL: Messenger RNA decay and protection. J. Mol. Biol. **8**, 210 (1964).

FASSIN, W., R. HENGEL u. P. KLEIN: Bakteriostase und Bakterizidie als Alternativen des antibakteriellen Chloramphenicoleffektes. Z. Hyg. Infektionskrankh. **141**, 363 (1955).

FOLLETTE, J. H., P. M. SHUGARMAN, J. REYNOLDS, W. N. VALENTINE, and J. S. LAWRENCE: The effect of chloramphenicol and other antibiotics on Leukocyte respiration. Blood **11**, 234 (1956).

FUSILLO, M. H., J. F. METZGER, and D. M. KUHNS: Effect of chloromycetin and streptomycin on embryonic tissue growth in *in vitro* tissue culture. Proc. Soc. Exptl. Biol. Med. **79**, 376 (1952).

GALE, E. F.: Mechanism of antibiotic action. Pharmacol. Rev. **15**, 481 (1963).

GALE, E. F., and J. P. FOLKES: The assimilation of amino acids by bacteria. 15. Actions of antibiotics on nucleic acid and protein synthesis in *Staphylococcus aureus*. Biochem. J. **53**, 493 (1953).

GANOZA, M. C., and T. NAKAMOTO: Studies on the mechanism of polypeptide chain termination in cell-free extracts of *E. coli*. Proc. Natl. Acad. Sci. U.S. **55**, 162 (1966).

GIBSON, F., M. J. JONES, and H. TELTSCHER: Effect of antibiotics on indole synthesis by *Escherichia coli* 7—4. Nature **176**, 164 (1955).

GIBSON, F., and B. MCDOUGALL: The effect of chloramphenicol and oxytetracycline on the formation of intermediates in tryptophan biosynthesis. Australian J. Exptl. Biol. Med. Sci. **39**, 171 (1961).

GIBSON, F., B. MCDOUGALL, M. J. JONES, and H. TELTSCHER: The action of antibiotics on indole synthesis by cell suspensions of *Escherichia coli*. J. Gen. Microbiol. **15**, 446 (1956).

GOCKE, T. M., and M. FINLAND: Development of chloramphenicol-resistant and chloramphenicol-dependent variants of a strain of *Klebsiella pneumoniae*. Proc. Soc. Exptl. Biol. Med. **74**, 824 (1950).

GOLDBERG, I. H.: Mode of action of antibiotics. II. Drugs affecting nucleic acid and protein synthesis. Am. J. Med. **39**, 722 (1965).

GOODGAL, S. H., and N. E. MELECHEN: Synthesis of transforming DNA in the presence of chloramphenicol. Biochem. Biophys. Research Commun. **3**, 114 (1960).

GORDON, J., H. C. BOWMAN, and L. A. ISAKSSON: *In vivo* inhibition of RNA methylation in the presence of chloramphenicol. J. Mol. Biol. **9**, 831 (1964).

GROS, F., and F. GROS: Rôle des acides amines dans la synthese des acides nucléiques chez *Escherichia coli*. Exptl. Cell Res. **14**, 104 (1958).

HAHN, F. E.: Actions of antibiotics on protein synthesis. Proc. III. Intern. Congr. Chemotherapy 1964, p. 215.

HAHN, F. E., J. E. HAYES, C. L. WISSEMAN, H. E. HOPPS, and J. E. SMADEL: Mode of action of chloramphenicol. VI. Relation between structure and activity in the chloramphenicol series. Antibiotics & Chemotherapy **6**, 531 (1956).

HAHN, F. E., M. SCHAECHTER, W. S. CEGLOWSKI, H. E. HOPPS, and J. CIAK: Interrelations between nucleic acid and protein biosynthesis. I. Synthesis and fate of bacterial nucleic acids during exposure to, and recovery from the action of chloramphenicol. Biochim. et Biophys. Acta **26**, 469 (1957).

HAHN, F. E., and C. L. WISSEMAN: Inhibition of adaptive enzyme formation by antimicrobial agents. Proc. Soc. Exptl. Biol. Med. **76**, 533 (1951).

HAHN, F. E., C. L. WISSEMAN, and H. E. HOPPS: Mode of action of chloramphenicol. III. Action of chloramphenicol on bacterial energy metabolism. J. Bact. **69**, 215 (1955).

HAHN, F. E., and A. D. WOLFE: Mode of action of chloramphenicol. VIII. Resemblance between labile chloramphenicol-RNA and DNA of *Bacillus cereus*. Biochem. Biophys. Research Commun. **6**, 464 (1962).

HANCOCK, R., and J. T. PARK: Cell-wall synthesis by *Staphylococcus aureus* in the presence of chloramphenicol. Nature **181**, 1050 (1958).

HOPPS, H. E., E. B. JACKSON, J. X. DANAUSKAS, and J. E. SMADEL: Study on the growth of rickettsiae. IV. Effect of chloramphenicol and several metabolic inhibitors on the multiplication of *Rickettsia tsutsugamushi* in tissue culture cells. J. Immunol. **82**, 172 (1959).

HOPPS, H. E., C. L. WISSEMAN, and F. E. HAHN: Mode of action of chloramphenicol. V. Effect of chloramphenicol on polysaccharide synthesis by *Neisseria perflava*. Antibiotics & Chemotherapy **4**, 857 (1954).

HOPPS, H. E., C. L. WISSEMAN, F. E. HAHN, J. E. SMADEL, and R. HO: Mode of action of chloramphenicol. IV. Failure of selected natural metabolites to reverse antibiotic action. J. Bact. **72**, 561 (1956).

HORIUCHI, T., S. SUNAKAWA, and D. MIZUNO: Stability of nucleic acid synthesized in the presence of chloramphenicol in *E. coli* B under growing and resting conditions. J. Biochem. (Japan) **45**, 875 (1958).

HOROWITZ, J., A. LOMBARD, and E. CHARGAFF: Aspects of the stability of a bacterial ribonucleic acid. J. Biol. Chem. **233**, 1517 (1958).

HUANG, M., D. R. BIGGS, G. D. CLARK-WALTER, and A. W. LINNANE: Chloramphenicol inhibition of the formation of particulate mitochondrial enzymes of *Saccharomyces cerevisiae*. Biochim. et Biophys. Acta **114**, 434 (1966).

JARDETZKY, O.: Studies on the mechanism of action of chloramphenicol. I. The conformation of Chloramphenicol in solution. J. Biol. Chem. **238**, 2498 (1963).

JARDETZKY, O., and G. R. JULIAN: Chloramphenicol inhibition of polyuridylic acid binding to *E. coli* ribosomes. Nature **201**, 396 (1964).

JULIAN, G. R.: C^{14}-Lysine peptides synthesized in an *in vitro Escherichia coli* system in the presence of chloramphenicol. J. Mol. Biol. **12**, 9 (1965).

KATAGIRI, H., Y. SUZUKI, and T. TOCHIKURA: Studies on the action of antibiotics on bacterial metabolism V. On a site of the action of chloramphenicol. J. Antibiotics (Japan), Ser. A, **13**, 309 (1960).

KELLENBERGER, E., K. G. LARK, and A. BOLLE: Amino acid dependent control of DNA synthesis in bacteria and vegetative phage. Proc. Natl. Acad. Sci. U.S. **48**, 1860 (1962).

KELLENBERGER, E., A. RYTER, and J. SECHAUD: Electron microscope study of DNA-containing plasms. II. Vegetative and mature phage DNA as compared with normal bacterial nucleoids in different physiological states. J. Biophys. Biochem. Cytol. **4**, 671 (1958).

KENT, S. P., E. S. TUCKER, and A. TARANENKO: The toxicity of chloramphenicol in newborn versus adult mice. A. M. A. J. Diseases Children **100**, 400 (1960).

KENT, S. P., and G. L. WIDEMAN: Prophylactic antibiotic therapy in infants born after premature rupture of membranes. J. Am. Med. Ass. **171**, 1199 (1959).

KOROTYAEV, A. I.: Mechanism of action of levomycetin on pyruvate consumption by resting cells of *Escherichia coli* (Bacterium coli). Mikrobilogija **30**, 42 (1961).

KOROTYAEV, A. I.: The effect of levomycetin (L-chloramphenicol) on *Escherichia coli* enzyme systems, catalyzing the pyruvate metabolism. Biokhimiya **27**, 120 (1962),

KROON, A. M.: Protein synthesis in heart mitochondria. I. Amino acid incorporation into the protein of isolated beef-heart mitochondria and fractions derived from them by sonic oscillation. Biochim. et Biophys. Acta **72**, 391 (1963).

KUCAN, Z., and F. LIPMANN: Differences in chloramphenicol sensitivity of cell-free amino acid polymerization systems. J. Biol. Chem. **239**, 516 (1964).

KURLAND, C. G., and O. MAALØE: Regulation of ribosomal and transfer RNA synthesis. J. Mol. Biol. **4**, 193 (1962).

KURLAND, C. G., M. NOMURA, and J. D. WATSON: The physical properties of the chloromycetin particles. J. Mol. Biol. **4**, 388 (1962).

LACKS, S., and F. GROS: A metabolic study of the RNA-amino acid complexes in *Escherichia coli*. J. Mol. Biol. **1**, 301 (1959).

LARK, K. G.: Cellular control of DNA biosynthesis. In: Molecular Genetics (J. H TAYLOR, ed.). Academic Press 1963.

LEE, K. H., Y. O. YUZURIHA, and J. J. EILER: Studies on cell growth and cell division. II. Selective activity of chloramphenicol and azaserine on cell growth and cell division. J. Am. Pharm. Assoc., Sci. Ed. **48**, 470 (1959).

LEPINE, P., G. BARSKI, and J. MAURIN: Action of chloromycetin and of aureomycin on normal tissue cultures. Proc. Soc. Exptl. Biol. Med. **73**, 252 (1950).

LEVI, I., H. BLONDAL, and E. LOZINSKI: Serine derivative with antitumor activity. Science **131**, 666 (1960).

LONG, L. M., and H. D. TROUTMAN: Chloromycetin. Synthesis of alpha-dichloro-acetamido-beta-hydroxy-p-nitro-propiophenone. J. Am. Chem. Soc. **73**, 481 (1951).

LOOMIS, W. F.: On the mechanism of action of aureomycin. Science **111**, 474 (1950).

MAALØE, O.: Role of protein synthesis in the DNA replication cycle in bacteria. J. Cellular Comp. Physiol. **62**, Suppl. **1**, 31 (1963).

MAGER, J.: Chloramphenicol and chlortetracycline inhibition of amino acid incorporation into proteins in a cell-free system from *Tetrahymena pyriformis*. Biochim. et Biophys. Acta **38**, 150 (1960).

MANDELSTAM, J., and H. J. ROGERS: The incorporation of amino acids into the cell-wall mucopeptide of staphylococci and the effect of antibiotics on the process. Biochem. J. **72**, 654 (1959).
MANDELSTAM, J., and H. J. ROGERS: Chloramphenicol-resistant incorporation of amino-acids into staphylococci and cell-wall synthesis. Nature **181**, 956 (1958).
MAXWELL, R. E., and V. S. NICKEL: The antibacterial activity of the isomers of chloramphenicol. Antibiotics & Chemotherapy **4**, 289 (1954).
McDOUGALL, B., and F. GIBSON: The effect of the isomers of chloramphenicol on growth and indole synthesis by *Escherichia coli* 7—4. Australian J. Exptl. Biol. **36**, 245 (1958).
McLEAN, I. W., J. L. SCHWAB, A. B. HILLEGAS, and A. S. SCHLINGMAN: Susceptibility of micro-organisms to chloramphenicol (chloromycetin). J. Clin. Invest. **18**, 953 (1949).
MENTZER, C., P. MEUNIER et L. MOLHO-LACROIX: Faits de synergie et d'antagonisme entre la chloromycetine et divers amino-acides vis-a-vis de cultures d'*E. coli*. Compt. rend. soc. biol. **230**, 241 (1950).
MIDGLEY, J. E. M.: The kinetics of ribonucleic acid synthesis in *Escherichia coli*. Biochim. et Biophys. Acta **68**, 354 (1963).
MIDGLEY, J. E. M., and B. J. McCARTHY: The synthesis and kinetic behavior of deoxyribonucleic acid-like ribonucleic acid in bacteria. Biochim. et Biophys. Acta **61**, 696 (1962).
MOLHO, D., et L. MOLHO-LACROIX: Etude comparée de l'antagonisme entre quelques dérives de la phenylalanine et chloromycetine, la β-thienylalanine et la β-phenylserine. Bull. soc. chim. biol. **34**, 99 (1952).
NAKADA, D., and B. MAGASANIK: The roles of inducer and catabolite repressor in the synthesis of β-galactosidase by *Escherichia coli*. J. Mol. Biol. **8**, 105 (1964).
NAKADA, D., and F. J. RYAN: Replication of deoxyribonucleic acid in non-dividing bacteria. Nature **189**, 398 (1961).
NAKAMOTO, T., T. W. CONWAY, J. E. ALLENDE, G. J. SPYRIDES, and F. LIPMANN: Formation of peptide bonds-I peptide formation from aminoacyl-s-RNA. Cold Spring Harbor Symposia Quant. Biol. **28**, 227 (1963).
NAKAMURA, S.: Structure of azomycin, a new antibiotic. Pharm. Bull. (Tokyo) **3**, 379 (1955).
NATHANS, D.: Puromycin inhibition of protein synthesis: incorporation of puromycin into peptide chains. Proc. Natl. Acad. Sci. U.S. **51**, 585 (1964).
NATHANS, D., and F. LIPMANN: Amino acid transfer from aminoacylribonucleic acids to protein on ribosomes of *Escherichia coli*. Proc. Natl. Acad. Sci. U.S. **47**, 497 (1961).
NATHANS, D., G. VON EHRENSTEIN, R. MONRO, and F. LIPMANN: Protein synthesis from aminacyl-soluble ribonucleic acid. Federation Proc. **21**, 127 (1962).
NEIDHARDT, F. C.: The regulation of RNA synthesis in bacteria. In: Progress in Nucleic Acid Research and Molecular Biology, vol. 3, p. 145. Academic Press 1964
NEIDHARDT, F. C., and F. GROS: Metabolic instability of the ribonucleic acid synthesized by *Escherichia coli* in the presence of chloromycetin. Biochim. et Biophys. Actas, **25**, 513 (1957).
NELSON, A. A., and J. L. RADOMSKI: Comparative pathological study in dogs of feeding of six broad-spectrum antibiotics. Antibiotics & Chemotherapy **4**, 1174 (1954).
NEWTON, B. A.: Mechanisms of antibiotic action. Ann. Rev. Microbiol. **19**, 209 (1965).
NIRENBERG, M. W., and J. H. MATTHAEI: Dependence of cell-free protein synthesis in *E. coli* upon naturally occurring or synthetic polyribonucleotides. Proc. Natl. Acad. Sci. U.S. **47**, 1588 (1961).
NOMURA, M., and K. HOSOKOWA: Biosynthesis of ribosomes. Fate of chloramphenicol particles and of pulse-labelled RNA in *Escherichia coli*. J. Mol. Biol. **12**, 242 (1965).
NOMURA, M., and J. D. WATSON: Ribonucleoprotein particles within chloromycetin-inhibited *Escherichia coli*. J. Mol. Biol. **1**, 204 (1959).
OCHOA JR., M., and I. B. WEINSTEIN: Polypeptide synthesis in a subcellular system derived from the L1210 mouse ascites leukemia. J. Biol. Chem. **239**, 3834 (1964).

OFENGAND, J., and R. HASELKORN: Viral RNA-dependent incorporation of amino acids into protein by cell-free extracts of *E. coli*. Biochem. Biophys. Research **6**, 469 (1962).

OKAMOTO, K., Y. SUGINO, and M. NOMURA: Synthesis and turnover of phage messenger RNA in *E. coli* infected with bacteriophage T4 in the presence of chloromycetin. J. Mol. Biol. **5**, 527 (1962).

OKAMOTO, S., and D. MIZUNO: Mechanism of chloramphenicol and tetracycline resistance in *Escherichia coli*. J. Gen. Microbiol. **35**, 125 (1964).

OKAMOTO, S., and Y. SUZUKI: Chloramphenicol-dihydrostreptomycin-, and kanamycin-inactivating enzymes from multiple drug-resistant *Escherichia coli* carrying episome 'R'. Nature **208**, 1301 (1965).

PAIGEN, K.: Changes in the inducibility of galactokinase and β-galactosidase during inhibition of growth in *Escherichia coli*. Biochim. et Biophys. Acta **77**, 318 (1963).

PARDEE, A. B., K. PAIGEN, and L. S. PRESTIDGE: A study of the ribonucleic acid of normal and chloromycetin-inhibited bacteria by zone electrophoresis. Biochim. et Biophys. Acts. **23**, 162 (1957).

REBSTOCK, M. C., H. M. CROOKS, J. CONTROULIS, and Q. BARTZ: Chloramphenicol (Chloromycetin). IV. Chemical studies. J. Am. Chem. Soc. **71**, 2458 (1949).

RENDI, R., and S. OCHOA: Effect of chloramphenicol on protein synthesis in cell-free preparations of *Escherichia coli*. J. Biol. Chem. **237**, 3711 (1962).

REUTNER, T. F., R. E. MAXWELL, K. E. WESTON, and J. K. WESTON: Chloramphenicol toxicity studies in experimental animals. Part 1. The effects of chloramphenicol and various other antibiotics on malnutrition in dogs with particular reference to the hematopoietic system. Antibiotics & Chemotherapy **5**, 679 (1955).

SADAO, M., and S. OKETANI: Studies on chloramphenicol inactivation by microorganisms. II. Relation between chloramphenicol inactivation and chloramphenicol resistance in various microorganisms. Nippon Saikingaku Zassh. **17**, 294 (1962).

SCHIØTT, C. R., and A. STENDERUP: Terramycin-, aureomycin-, and chloromycetin-dependent bacteria isolated from patients. Acta Pathol. Microbiol. Scand. **34**, 410 (1954).

SEGEL, I. H., J. CATTANEO, and N. SIGAL: The regulation of glycogen synthesis in *Aerobacter aerogenes*. Colloq. intern. centre natl. recherche. sci. (Paris) **124**, 337 (1965).

SHEMYAKIN, M. M.: Khimia antibiotikov, vol. I. Moscow: Academy of Sciences, U.S.S.R. 1961.

SHEMYAKIN, M. M., M. N. KOLOSOV, M. M. LEVITOV, K. I. GERMANOVA, M. G. KARAPETIAN, IU. B. SHVETSOV, and E. M. BAMDAS: Studies on the chemistry of chloromycetin (Levomycetin). VIII. Dependence of antimicrobial activity of chloromycetin on its structure and mechanism of action of chloromycetin. Zhur. Obshchei Khim. **26**, 773 (1956).

SMADEL, J. E., and E. B. JACKSON: Chloromycetin, an antibiotic with chemotherapeutic activity in experimental rickettsial and viral infections. Science **106**, 418 (1947).

SMILLIE, R. M., W. R. EVANS, and H. LYMAN: Metabolic events during the formation of a photosynthetic from a nonphotosynthetic cell. Brookhaven Symposia Biol. **16**, 89 (1963).

SMITH, C. G., W. L. LUMMIS, and J. E. GRADY: An improvised tissue culture assay. II. Cytotoxicity studies with antibiotics, chemicals, and solvents. Cancer Research **19**, 847 (1959).

SMITH, G. N., C. S. WORREL, and A. I. SWANSON: Inhibition of bacterial esterases by chloramphenicol (chloromycetin). J. Bact. **58**, 803 (1949).

So, A. G., and E. W. DAVIE: The incorporation of amino acids into protein in a cell-free system from yeast. Biochemistry **2**, 132 (1963).

SPEYER, J. F., P. LENGYEL, C. BASILIO, A. J. WAHBA, R. S. GARDNER, and S. OCHOA: Synthetic polynucleotides and the amino acid code. Cold Spring Harbor Symposia Quant. Biol. **28**, 559 (1963).

SPIRIN, A. S.: In vitro formation of ribosome-like particles from Cm-particles and protein. Cold Spring Harbor Symposia Quant. Biol. **28**, 267 (1963).

SUAREZ, G., and D. NATHANS: Inhibition of aminoacyl-sRNA binding to ribosomes by tetracycline. Biochem. Biophys. Research Commun. **18**, 743 (1965).

SYPHERD, P. S., N. STRAUSS, and H. P. TREFFERS: The preferential inhibition by chloramphenicol of induced enzyme synthesis. Biochem. Biophys. Research Commun. **7**, 477 (1962).

SYPHERD, P. S., and N. STRAUSS: Chloramphenicol-promoted repression of β-galactosidase synthesis in *Escherichia coli*. Proc. Natl. Acad. Sci. U.S. **49**, 400 (1963).

SZYBALSKI, W.: Genetic studies on microbial cross-resistance to toxic agents. II. Gross resistance of *Micrococcus pyogenes* var. *aureus* to thirty-four antimicrobial drugs. Antibiotics & Chemotherapy **3**, 1095 (1963).

TAKANAMI, M., and T. OKAMOTO: Interaction of ribosomes and synthetic polyribonucleotides. J. Mol. Biol. **7**, 323 (1963).

TAYLOR, F. J.: The effect of chloramphenicol on the growth of *Scenedesmus quadricauda*. J. Gen. Microbiol. **39**, 275 (1965).

THOMAS, R.: Effects of chloramphenicol on genetic replication in bacteriophage. Virology **9**, 275 (1959).

TING, R. C.-Y.: A curing effect of chloramphenicol on bacteria infected with bacteriophage. Virology **12**, 68 (1960).

TRAUT, R. R., and R. E. MONRO: The puromycin reaction and its relation to protein synthesis. J. Mol. Biol. **10**, 63 (1964).

TRUHAUT, R., S. LAMBIN et M. BOYER: Contribution a l'etude du mecanisme d'action de la chloromycetine vis-a-vis-d'*Eberthella typhi*. Role du tryptophane. Bull. soc. chim. biol. **33**, 387 (1951).

VAZQUEZ, D.: Antibiotics which affect protein synthesis: the uptake of C^{14}-chloramphenicol by bacteria. Biochem. Biophys. Research. Commun. **12**, 409 (1963).

VAZQUEZ, D.: The binding of chloramphenicol by ribosomes from *Bacillus megaterium*. Biochem. Biophys. Research Commun. **15**, 464 (1964a).

VAZQUEZ, D.: Uptake and binding of chloramphenicol by sensitive and resistant organisms. Nature **203**, 257 (1964b).

VAZQUEZ, D.: Mode of action of chloramphenicol and related antibiotics. 16th Symp. Soc. Gen. Microbiol. 169, 1966a.

VAZQUEZ, D.: Antibiotics affecting chloramphenicol uptake by bacteria. Their effect on amino acid incorporation in a cell-free system. Biochim. et Biophys. Acta **114**, 289 (1966b).

VINTER, V.: Spores of microorganisms. Chloramphenicol-sensitive and penicillin-resistant incorporation of C^{14}-diaminopimelic acid into sporulating cells of *Bacillus cereus*. Experientia **19**, 307 (1963).

WATANABE, T.: Infective heredity of multiple drug resistance in bacteria. Bacteriol. Rev. **27**, 87 (1963).

WEISBERGER, A. S., S. ARMENTROUT, and S. WOLFE: Protein synthesis by reticulocyte ribosomes. I. Inhibition of polyuridylic acid-induced ribosomal protein synthesis by chloramphenicol. Proc. Natl. Acad. Sci. U.S. **50**, 86 (1963).

WEISBERGER, A. S., and S. WOLFE: Effect of chloramphenicol on protein synthesis. Federation Proc. **23**, 976 (1964).

WEISBERGER, A. S., S. WOLFE, and S. ARMENTROUT: Inhibition of protein synthesis in mammalian cell-free systems by chloramphenicol. J. Exptl.Med. **120**, 161 (1964).

WILLSON, C., and F. GROS: Protein synthesis with an *Escherichia coli* system in vitro. Biochim. et Biophys. Acta **80**, 478 (1964).

WINTERSBERGER, E.: Proteinsynthese in isolierten Hefe-Mitochondrien. Biochem. Z. **341**, 409 (1965).

WISSEMAN, C. L., F. E. HAHN, H. HOPPS, and J. E. SMADEL: Chloramphenicol inhibition of protein synthesis. Federation Proc. **12**, 466 (1953).

WISSEMAN, C. L., H. L. LEY, and F. HAHN: Action of chloramphenicol on microorganisms. Bacteriol. Proc. **1950**, 94.

WISSEMAN, C. L., J. E. SMADEL, F. E. HAHN, and H. E. HOPPS: Mode of action of chloramphenicol. I. Action of chloramphenicol on assimilation of ammonia and on synthesis of proteins and nucleic acids in *Escherichia coli*. J. Bact. **67**, 662 (1954).

WOESE, C., S. NAOMO, R. SOFFER, and F. GROS: Studies on the breakdown of mRNA. Biochem. Biophys. Research Commun. **11**, 435 (1963).

WOLFE, A. D., and F. E. HAHN: Studies on chloramphenicol, ribosomes, and an amino acid incorporation system of *E. coli* origin. Federation Proc. **23**, 269 (1964).

WOLFE, A. D., and F. E. HAHN: Mode of action of chloramphenicol. IX. Effects of chloramphenicol upon a ribosomal amino acid polymerization system and its binding to bacterial ribosome. Biochim. et Biophys. Acta **95**, 146 (1965).

WOOLLEY, D. W.: A study of non-competitive antagonism with chloromycetin and related analogues of phenylalanine. J. Biol. Chem. **185**, 293 (1950).

YARMOLINSKY, M. B., and G. DE LA HABA: Inhibition by puromycin of amino acid incorporation into protein. Proc. Natl. Acad. Sci. U.S. **44**, 885 (1959).

YUNIS, A. A., and G. R. BLOOMBERG: Chloramphenicol toxicity: Clinical features and pathogenesis. Progr. Hematol. **4**, 138 (1964).

Tetracyclines

Allen I. Laskin

The tetracyclines are the prototypes of the broad spectrum antibiotics, so-called because they inhibit the growth of a wide range of microorganisms, including many gram-positive and gram-negative bacteria, species of rickettsia and mycoplasma (PPLO), certain protozoa and large viruses. In Table 1 are listed some representative data on the minimum inhibitory concentration (M.I.C.) of the tetracyclines, in μg/ml, against a variety of microorganisms. The M.I.C. ranges presented encompass most of the data reported in the literature (e.g.

Table 1. *Some microorganisms inhibited by tetracyclines*

	Organisms	M.I.C. (μg/ml)
Bacteria, gram-positive	*Bacillus anthracis*	0.05—0.4
	Bacillus cereus	0.05—0.4
	Staphylococcus aureus	0.05—0.4
	Streptococcus faecalis	0.2—0.5
	Streptococcus pyogenes	0.05—0.2
	Diplococcus pneumoniae	0.1—0.2
Bacteria, gram-negative	*Escherichia coli*	0.2—3.0
	Salmonella schottmuelleri	0.2—3.0
	Proteus vulgaris	10—100
	Pseudomonas aeruginosa	1—100
	Neisseria gonorrhoeae	0.1—2.0
	Borrelia recurrentis	1.0—25
	Haemophilus aegyptius	0.4—6.25
Protozoa	*Trichomonas foetus*	25—100
	Trichomonas vaginalis	100—250
	Entamoeba histolytica	2—200
Mycoplasma (PPLO)	chronic respiratory disease of poultry	[1]
	PPLO in tissue culture	2.5—20[3]
Rickettsia	scrub typhus	[1]
	Rocky Mountain spotted fever	[1]
	epidemic louse-borne typhus	[1]
Viruses and *Bedsoniae*	Rous sarcoma	[2]
	lymphogranuloma venereum	[1]
	feline pneumonitis	[1]
	psittacosis	[1]

[1] Tetracyclines effective against experimental or human infections.
[2] Inactivated by exposure to antibiotic.
[3] Hooser *et al.* (1964).

DEL LOVE *et al.*, 1954; WELCH *et al.*, 1954; REEDY *et al.*, 1955; BOHONOS *et al.*, 1953; SPECTOR, 1957) and are also representative of results obtained at The Squibb Institute for Medical Research (BASCH, unpublished data). It should be noted that although the tetracyclines have in general very similar antimicrobial spectra (DEL LOVE *et al.*, 1954; BOHONOS *et al.*, 1953), there have been reported some significant quantitative differences. Thus, the chlorinated compounds, chlortetracycline and demethylchlortetracycline, were found to be considerably more active than oxytetracycline and tetracycline against a variety of staphylococci, streptococci and pneumococci (WELCH *et al.*, 1954; REEDY *et al.*, 1955; McCORMICK *et al.*, 1957 and 1960; GARROD and WATERWORTH, 1960) and coliforms (KIRBY *et al.*, 1961).

The several names of the antibiotics, their chemical formulae, producing organisms and the abbreviations used in this article are presented in Table 2, and the structures are diagrammed in Fig. 1.

Table 2

Abbreviation Producing Organism	Generic (and other names)	Chemical name and molecular formula
CTC — *Streptomyces aureofaciens*	chlortetracycline (7-chlorotetracycline)	7-chloro-4-(dimethylamino)-1,4,4a,5,5a,6,11,12a-octahydro-3,6,10,12,12a-pentahydroxy-6-methyl-1,11-dioxo-2-naphthacenecarboxamide $C_{22}H_{23}ClN_2O_8$
OTC — *Streptomyces rimosus*	oxytetracycline (hydroxytetracycline, 5-hydroxytetracycline)	4-(dimethylamino)-1,4,4a,5,5a,6,11,12a-octahydro-3,5,6,10,12,12a-hexahydroxy-6-methyl-1,11-dioxo-2-naphthacene-carboxamide $C_{22}H_{24}N_2O_9$
TC — *Streptomyces viridifaciens*	tetracycline	4-(dimethylamino)-1,4,4a,5,5a,6,11,12a-octahydro-3,6,10,12,12a-pentahydroxy-6-methyl-1,11-dioxo-2-naphthacene-carboxamide $C_{22}H_{24}N_2O_8$
DMTC — variant of *Streptomyces aureofaciens*	demethylchlortetracycline (6-demethyl-chlortetracycline; 7-chloro-6-demethyl-tetracycline)	7-chloro-4-(dimethylamino)-1,4,4a,5,5a,6,11,12a-octahydro-3,6,10,12,12a-pentahydroxy-1,11-dioxo-2-naphthacenecarboxamide $C_{22}H_{21}N_2O_8$

A number of reviews concerning the mode of action of tetracyclines have appeared since the introduction of these antibiotics. The contribution by HOBBY (1953) to a symposium on mode of action of antibiotics discussed some of the early data on CTC and OTC, and UMBREIT (1953) mentioned some aspects of the mechanism of action of these compounds. Shortly thereafter, EAGLE and SAZ (1955) cited the relevant literature on the subject as part of a comprehensive general review on antibiotics. An interesting review by HAHN (1959) on modes of action of antibiotics seriously considered the problems of the multiple reactions of the tetracyclines, and presented his own studies on the relationships and similarities between the modes of action of the tetracyclines and of chloramphenicol. These studies were again discussed in a subsequent review by HAHN (1961) concerning the inhibition of protein synthesis by antibiotics. In their book on the actinomyces, WAKSMAN and LECHEVALIER (1962) included a brief review of modes of action, including information on the tetracyclines. GALE'S review on mechanisms of antibiotic action (1963) included a brief discussion of the tetracyclines, listing them among those antibiotics "whose primary effect is inhibition of protein synthesis".

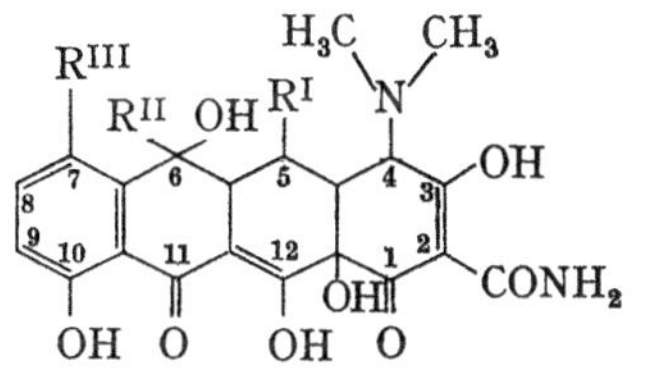

R^I	R^{II}	R^{III}	
H	CH_3	H	Tetracycline
OH	CH_3	H	Oxytetracyline
H	CH_3	Cl	Chlortetracycline
H	H	Cl	Demethylchlortetracycline

Fig. 1. Structures of tetracycline antibiotics

A particularly thoughtful and well-presented paper by SNELL and CHENG (1961) included a discussion of much of the significant information on the subject, and JACKSON (1964) covered the topic comprehensively in a later review. GOLDBERG (1965) emphasized the more recent work on the inhibition of protein synthesis by the tetracyclines, especially in cell-free systems.

Since the appearance of the original reports on the tetracyclines, a large number of derivatives, degradation products and similar compounds, having a wide range of antibiotic activity, have been described. The present discussion will concern itself largely with the four antibiotics which are used extensively in the clinic: chlortetracycline (CTC), oxytetracycline (OTC), tetracycline (TC) and demethylchlortetracycline (DMCT). Of these, CTC, OTC and TC have been the subject of most of the studies concerning modes of action. The close chemical similarity among these antibiotics (Fig. 1), their similar antibiotic spectra (DEL LOVE *et al.*, 1954; BOHONOS *et al.*, 1953), and the mutual cross-resistance which often develops to them (HERRELL *et al.*, 1950; PANSY *et al.*, 1950; FUSILLO and ROMANSKY, 1951; WRIGHT and FINLAND, 1954) have led to the general assumption that the mechanisms by which the tetracyclines inhibit the growth of microbial cells are similar, if not identical. Although a number of differences have been reported in some of the effects of the various tetracyclines (SNELL *et al.*, 1958), the preponderance of evidence would appear to support the assumption. It must be realized, however, that any attempt to define *the* mode of action of an antibiotic may be futile, and this is perhaps especially true of the tetracyclines. HAHN (1959) and SNELL and CHENG (1961) have presented excellent discussions on the problem of assigning a single mode of action to a molecule containing as many reactive groups as do the tetracycline antibiotics. The latter authors consider that the question "what is *the* mode of action of . . . tetracycline?" is both unanswerable and meaningless, and directed their efforts toward "looking into specific biological systems for clues as to the *order* and *conditions* under which one, several, or all of [the reported] mechanisms might apply . . ." Although they grant that for any given biological system there is probably one reaction which is most sensitive to the antibiotic (Snell *et al.*, 1958; Hahn, 1959), they point out that this is not necessarily the key reaction in every biological system. In an attempt to eliminate unimportant or secondary effects, Hahn (1959) adopted a general set of criteria which a physiological process must fulfill in order to be considered the key process whose inhibition leads to the overall result of growth inhibition: 1. The inhibited reaction must be of vital necessity for the economy of the microbial cell. 2. The inhibition must be produced specifically in organisms whose growth is susceptible to the action of the drug. 3. The inhibition must be produced by an antibiotic concentration that is of the same order as the growth inhibitory concentration range. 4. The degree of inhibition must approach an all-or-none effect. 5. The inhibition must depend upon the specific chemical structure of the antibiotic molecule in precisely the same manner as does the growth-inhibitory effect. Similar criteria have been used, either conciously or not, by most investigators studying modes of action of antibiotics, and they are the basis of some of the considerations which follow.

A number of the effects of the tetracyclines which have been reported in the literature are listed in Tables 3—8. These listings are in no sense meant to be complete, but are presented as representative of the range and variety of effects which have been observed. The classifications of the reactions are somewhat arbitrary, *e.g.* it was not always possible to ascertain whether an observed inhibition of a particular enzyme activity was due to inhibition of enzyme formation, inhibition of the enzymatic reaction, or some other secondary effect. Wherever possible, an indication of the amount of antibiotic used in the experiments is given (in μg/ml).

Table 3. *Inhibition by tetracyclines of bacterial oxidation and respiration*

Reference	Organism	Antibiotic	Activity inhibited
Wagner (1950)	*Mycobacterium smegmatis*	CTC (1—100)[1]	oxidation of benzoate and catechol
Ajl (1953)	*Escherichia coli*	CTC, OTC ("minute amounts")	oxidation of acetic, pyruvic, di- and tricarboxylic acids and other substrates
Bernheim and de Turk (1952)	*Pseudomonas aeruginosa*	CTC, OTC (5)	oxidation of phenylalanine, tyrosine and phenylserine
Karp and Snyder (1952)	Murine and epidemic typhus rickettsia	CTC (100—300) OTC (200—300)	oxidation of glutamate; respiration
McCullough and Beal (1952)	*Brucella* spp.	CTC (100—250)	oxidation of glucose, pyruvate, D-fructose, D-xylose and D-trehalose

[1] Amount of antibiotic used (in μg/ml) is indicated by the figures in parentheses.

Table 3. (Continued)

Reference	Organism	Antibiotic	Activity inhibited
OSTEAUX *et al.* (1952)	*E. coli*, *Ps. aeruginosa* and *Proteus vulgaris*	CTC (240)	oxidation of tricarboxylic acid cycle intermediates; respiration
PORRO and SONCIN (1953a)	*E. coli*	CTC (3.0) OTC (30)	oxidation of acetoacetate
WONG *et al.* (1953)	*E. coli*	CTC, OTC	terminal respiration
BERNHEIM (1954a) (also see BERNHEIM and DE TURK, 1953b)	*Ps. aeruginosa*	CTC, OTC (0.12—0.5)	oxidation of benzoic acid
PORRO and SONCIN (1954)	*E. coli*	CTC, OTC (30)	O_2 uptake in the presence of glutamic acid
ARORA and KRISHNA MURTI (1955b)	*Vibrio comma*	CTC, OTC, TC (500)	oxidation of tricarboxylic acid cycle intermediates
JOHNSON and COLMER (1957)	*Azotobacter vinelandii*	CTC (10) TC (90)	respiration
SRIKANTAN *et al.* (1957)	*Pasturella pestis*	CTC, OTC, TC (1000)	oxidation of glucose and serine
KRASKIN and STERN (1957)	*E. coli*	OTC (100—200)	oxidation of gluconate
SHAHANI (1957)	*Streptococcus lactis*	OTC (100)	pyruvate utilization and aerobic carbohydrate metabolism
SNELL and CHENG (1958) (see also SNELL and CHENG 1961)	*Staph. aureus* and *E. coli*	OTC (1.25)	respiration
YEE *et al.* (1958)	*Shigella flexneri*	OTC (20—100)	oxidation of glutamate
GUILLAUME and OSTEUX (1959)	*Proteus mirabilis*	CTC (25—75)	utilization of glucose and acetate (25) and oxalacetate (75)
FEDOROV and SEGI (1961)	*Azotobacter vinelandii*	CTC, OTC, TC (100)	respiration
KATAGIRI *et al.* (1959, 1961)	*E. coli*	CTC, OTC, TC (*ca.* 150—450)	oxidation of glucose, pyruvate, acetate, succinate, fumarate, lactate, etc.

Table 4. *Inhibition by tetracyclines of microbial enzyme systems*

Reference	Organism	Antibiotic	Activity inhibited
OSTEAUX and LATURAZE (1952)	*Clostridium welchii*	CTC (0.2) OTC (0.1)	"pyruvic hydrogenlyase"
SAZ and SLEI (1953a and b, 1954a) also SAZ and MARMUR (1953)	*E. coli*	CTC (10—100)	nitro-reductase

Table 4. (Continued)

Reference	Organism	Antibiotic	Activity inhibited
SLOANE (1953)	*Mycobacterium smegmatis*	CTC, OTC (approx. 0.5—2)	hydroxylase (aniline *p*-aminophenol)
ARORA and KRISHNA MURTI (1955a)	*E. coli*	CTC, OTC (200—1000)	tryptophanase
MICHEL and FRANÇOIS (1956)	intestinal flora of pig	CTC (10)	amino acid decarboxylase
LIEBFREID (1957)	*E. coli* and *Shigella* spp.	CTC	catalase and certain dehydrogenases
ROKOS *et al.* (1959a)	*Aspergillus oryzae*	CTC (40—80)	α-amylase
GOLDMAN (1960)	*Mycobacterium tuberculosis*	OTC (80—100)	alanine dehydrogenase
FUWA (1963)	*Mycrococcus lysodeikticus*	CTC, OTC, TC	polynucleotide phosphorylase
MOROZ and SHIBAEVA (1964)	*S. aureus*	CTC (3.9)	dehydrogenase

Table 5. *Inhibition by tetracyclines of enzyme formation in bacteria*

Reference	Organism	Antibiotic	Activity inhibited
HAHN and WISSEMAN (1951)	*E. coli*	CTC, OTC (20)	adaptive enzymes
CHANDLER *et al.* (1951, 1952)	*S. albus* and *S. aureus*	CTC (0.05—1.56)	penicillinase
BERNHEIM (1954a)	*Ps. aeruginosa*	CTC, OTC (0.12—0.5)	benzoic acid oxidase
GRUNBERGER *et al.* (1954)	*E. coli* and *Streptococcus fecalis*	CTC, OTC (0.075—0.15)	glutamic acid decarboxylase and tyrosine decarboxylase
CREASER (1955)	*S. aureus*	CTC (0.1) OTC (0.03) TC (0.03)	β-galactosidase
MELNYKOVYCH and SNELL (1958)	*E. coli*	OTC 0.1)	arginine decarboxylase
SRIKANTAN *et al.* (1958)	*Pasteurella pestis*	CTC, OTC, TC (250)	aldolase (OTC and TC inhibited, CTC stimulated)
MELNYKOVYCH and JOHANSSON (1959)	*E. coli*	CTC, OTC (0.04)	lysine decarboxylase
NAKAYA and TREFFERS (1959)	*E. coli*	OTC (0.018—0.23)	β-galactosidase D-serine deaminase
ALEXANDER (1960)	*E. coli*	CTC (0.3—1.0)	glutamic acid decarboxylase
KATAGIRI *et al.* (1961)	*Aerobacter aerogenes*	CTC, OTC (100)	citrate oxidizing enzymes

Table 6. *Inhibition by tetracyclines of various mammalian systems*

Reference	Organism	Antibiotic	Activity inhibited
LOOMIS (1950)	rat liver or rabbit kidney mitochondria	CTC (200)	uncoupling of oxidative phosphorylation
BRODY and BAIN (1951)	rat liver and brain particulate preparations	CTC (90)	uncoupling of oxidative phosphorylation
VAN METER and OLESON (1951)	rat liver homogenates	CTC (50)	inhibition of respiration
VAN METER *et al.* (1952)	rat liver mitochondria	CTC (50)	uncoupling of oxidative phosphorylation and inhibition of respiration
GHATEK and KRISHNA MURTI (1953)	rat kidney extract	OTC	inhibition of alkaline phosphatase
MULLI *et al.* (1953)	beef liver	CTC (0.05)	inhibition of citrate breakdown
PORRO and SONCIN (1953b)	rat kidney, rabbit heart	CTC, OTC (30)	inhibition of respiration and acetoacetate oxidation
ZIMMERMAN and HUMOLLER (1953)	rat liver homogenates	CTC	inhibition of choline oxidase, stimulation of citrate dehydrogenase
ARORA and KRISHNA MURTI (1954)	pig heart homogenates (also pigeon breast)	OTC	inhibition of succinic oxidase, cytochrome oxidase and succinic dehydrogenase
BRODY *et al.* (1954)	rat liver and brain mitochondria	CTC, OTC, TC (100—200)	uncoupling of oxidative phosphorylation and inhibition of octanoate oxidation
HUMOLLER and ZIMMERMAN (1954)	rat liver	CTC	inhibition of betaine aldehyde oxidase
GREEN *et al.* (1956)	rat liver	CTC	inhibition of nitroreductase
VONK *et al.* (1957)	hog intestinal mucosa	CTC (100)	inhibition protease
ROKOS *et al.* (1958), MALEK *et al.* (1959) and ROKOS *et al.* (1959a and b)	dog pancreas	CTC (50)	inhibition of lipase, α-amylase
YAGI *et al.* (1959) (see also YAGI *et al.*, 1956)	hog kidney	CTC (100)	inhibition of D-amino acid oxidase
VYSHEPAN and ZUEVA (1959)	rat heart	CTC (24)	inhibition of ATP-ase of rat cardiac myosin

Table 6. (Continued)

Reference	Organism	Antibiotic	Activity inhibited
ARORA and KRISHNA MURTI (1960)	goat liver	CTC (3.33—6.67) OTC (0.113—6.67)	inhibition of purified catalase
PORFIRIEVA (1961)	rat liver tissue slices	CTC (125)	inhibition of urea formation
BELDING and KERN (1963)	cat gastric mucosa	OTC (2000)	inhibition of urease

Table 7. *Miscellaneous reactions of the tetracyclines*

Reference	Organism	Antibiotic	Activity
FAGUET and EDLINGER (1951)	*S. aureus* — bacteriophage system	CTC (0.5—2.5)	inhibition of phage-induced lysis
AGARWALA *et al.* (1952)	purified plant enzyme	CTC (100—4000)	inhibition of urease
BERNHEIM and DE TURK (1952)	*Ps. aeruginosa*	CTC, OTC (100)	inhibition of deamination of phenylalanine, tyrosine and phenylserine
MIURA (1952)	*S. aureus*	OTC	inhibition of specific activity of acid-soluble organic phosphorus fraction, inhibition of phosphorylation
NETIEN *et al.* (1952)	lentils, peas and rapeseed	CTC, OTC (5)	inhibition of biosynthesis of chlorophyll
WEIL (1952)	*Serratia marcesens*	CTC (10—40) OTC (5—20)	inhibition of prodigiosin formation
ALTENBERN (1953)	*E. coli* — (T 3) bacteriophage	CTC (2.5)	lowering of adsorption of phage and suppression of phage growth
BERNHEIM and DE TURK (1953a)	*Mycobacterium tuberculosis* BCG	CTC, OTC (100—400)	inhibition of deamination and desulfuration of cysteine
MIURA *et al.* (1953)	*S. aureus*	CTC, OTC (1.0)	inhibition of incorporation of P^{32} into organic phosphates
OLITZKI (1954)	*Salmonella typhi*	CTC (1000)	inhibition of hydrogen sulfide production
REGE and SREENIVASAN (1954)	*Lactobacillus casei*	CTC (0.003)	inhibition of RNA and DNA synthesis
DELAMATER *et al.* (1955)	*Bacillus megaterium*	CTC, OTC (2.0)	nuclear abberations

Table 7. (Continued)

Reference	Organism	Antibiotic	Activity
GIBSON *et al.* (1956) (see also GIBSON and MCDOUGALL, 1961)	*E. coli*	CTC, OTC, TC (0.1)	inhibition of indole synthesis
BACHRACH *et al.* (1958)	*Proteus vulgaris*	CTC (30) TC (100)	depression of formation of isoamyl and isobutyl amines
SNELL and CHENG (1958) (see also SNELL and CHENG, 1959; SNELL and CHENG, 1961; CHENG and SNELL, 1962)	*E. coli*	OTC (2.5)	accumulation of glutamic acid, inhibition of D-glutamic acid incorporation into cell walls
SAZ and MARTINEZ (1958)	*E. coli*	CTC (0.5—5.0)	inhibition of electron transport
YEE *et al.* (1958)	*Shigella flexneri*	CTC (20—100)	inhibition of membrane transport of glutamate
MANDELSTAM and ROGERS (1959)	*S. aureus*	CTC (100)	inhibition of cell wall mucopeptide synthesis
MARSH and KELLEY (1959)	nematode	OTC, TC (<1.0)	inhibition of inorganic pyrophosphatase
MELNYKOVYCH and JOHANSSON (1959)	*E. coli*	CTC (0.83)	retardation of inactivation of arginine decarboxylase
ALEXANDER (1960)	*E. coli*	CTC (0.3—1.0)	reduction of vitamin B_6 uptake
TANNER (1960)	*Salmonella typhi*	TC (100)	modification of antigenic structure
KATAGIRI *et al.* (1961)	*E. coli*	CTC (20)	inhibition of aerobic phosphorylation
BROCK (1962)	*Bacillus cereus*	TC (10)	inhibition of sporulation
DOUGHTY and HAYASHI (1962)	*Strep. pyogenes*-Cl phage	CTC (100)	enhancement of phage-induced lysis
KOROTYAEV (1962)	*E. coli*	CTC, OTC	inhibition of anaerobic pyruvate consumption
VINTER (1962)	*B. cereus* and *B. megaterium*	CTC, OTC, TC (5)	inhibition of Ca^{++} incorporation, dipicolinic acid synthesis, and sporulation
BELDING and KERN (1963)	jackbean meal	OTC (300)	inhibition of urease
FREEMAN and CIRCO (1963)	various fungi	CTC, OTC, TC	alterations (especially decreases) in amino acid pools
HAYANO (1952)	*Strep. hemolyticus*	CTC (0.08) OTC (0.24)	streptolysin production

Table 8. *Inhibition by tetracyclines of specific protein synthesis in bacteria*

Reference	Organism	Antibiotic	Activity inhibited
KINDLER *et al.* (1956)	*Clostridium parabotulinum*	CTC, OTC (100)	toxin production
YOUNATHAN and BARKULIS (1957)	*Strep. pyogenes*	CTC, OTC, TC (0.02)	streptolysin S′
HINTON and ORR (1960)	*S. aureus*	OTC, TC (0.05)	α-hemolysin production
SAKAGUCHI *et al.* (1960)	*Cl. botulinum*	OTC (0.05—0.2)	toxin production
BROCK (1963)	*Strep. pyogenes*	CTC, TC (1.0)	M protein synthesis

Respiration and Oxidation

The effects of the tetracyclines on a wide variety of reactions involving respiration and various oxidation processes in microbial (Table 3) and mammalian (Table 6) systems have been reported. As can be seen from the data in the tables, the concentrations of antibiotics required (or reported) to be inhibitory was in many instances much greater than those required for growth inhibition. In addition, many of these effects appear to be secondary to other reactions. For example, KARP and SNYDER (1952) postulated that the inhibition by OTC and CTC of respiration in two rickettsial species was due to an interference with energy transfer mechanisms. The inhibition of gluconate oxidation in *E. coli* by OTC observed by KRASKIN and STERN (1957) was attributed to a competitive inhibition of DPN in the electron transport system mediating the oxidation. The inhibition of oxidation of benzoic acid in *Pseudomonas aeruginosa* by low levels (0.12—0.5) of CTC and OTC (BERNHEIM and DE TURK, 1953b; BERNHEIM, 1954a) was later attributed (BERNHEIM, 1954b) to inhibition of the synthesis of a specific component of the enzyme system. YEE *et al.* (1958) determined that the depression of oxidation of glutamate in tetracycline-treated *Shigella flexneri* cells was not a result of inhibition of any of the enzymatic steps (glutamate oxidation by broken cell suspensions or by cell-free extracts was not inhibited by tetracyclines). They suggested that the antibiotics interfered with the mechanisms involved in membrane transport of glutamate. They reported further that the inhibition was reversed by Mg^{++}, Fe^{++} and Fe^{+++}. The ability of the tetracyclines to bind metallic ions, a phenomenon which will be discussed later in more detail, was also invoked to explain the inhibition by tetracyclines of respiration and oxidative phosphorylation in mammalian systems (LOOMIS, 1950; BRODY and BAIN, 1951; VAN METER and OLESON, 1951; VAN METER *et al.*, 1952; BRODY *et al.*, 1954).

SNELL and CHENG (1958 and 1961) observed inhibition of respiration by OTC in both *S. aureus* and *E. coli*, but suggested that the "inhibition of O_2 uptake is a rather general phenomenon resulting from more intricate (enzymatic) disturbances in the metabolism of the cell".

In no instance among these effects on oxidation and respiration is there compelling evidence to suggest that a primary site of inhibition is involved.

Specific Enzyme Systems

The reports on inhibitions by the tetracyclines of specific enzyme systems (Tables 4 and 6) are also confounded by indications of other contributory factors. Again, metal binding phenomena appear to be involved in many of these systems. The inhibition of nitroreductase in *E. coli* (SAZ and SLEI, 1953a and b, 1954a; SAZ and MARMUR, 1953), of α-amylases (ROKOS *et al.*, 1958, 1959a and b; MALEK *et al.*, 1959), of *Mycobacterium tuberculosis* alanine dehydrogenase (GOLDMAN, 1960) and of *Micrococcus lysodeikticus* polynucleotide phosphorylase (FUWA, 1963) will be discussed further in relation to metal binding. It is doubtful, however, that any of these enzyme reactions can be considered to be the major site of tetracycline inhibition.

Glutamate Accumulation and Cell-wall Synthesis

SNELL and his coworkers applied a systematic technique for studying mode of action, comparing the metabolism of radioisotopically labelled indicator compounds (e. g. acetate-2-^{14}C) in antibiotic-inhibited and in control cells (SNELL *et al.*, 1958). It was noted that OTC-inhibited cells accumulated glutamic acid (SNELL and CHENG, 1958), and all of the glutamic acid which accumulated was of the D-configuration (SNELL and CHENG, 1959). As D-glutamic acid was known to be a component of the bacterial cell wall, and considering the A ring of OTC as an analog of glutamic acid, it was postulated (SNELL and CHENG, 1961) that OTC could act by competitive inhibition with D-glutamic acid during the process of cell wall synthesis. It was further demonstrated (SNELL and CHENG, 1961; CHENG and SNELL, 1962) that OTC inhibited the incorporation of D-glutamic acid into cell wall and membrane material. These authors also felt that the data of GALE and FOLKES (1953a) on inhibition by CTC of the formation of "combined glutamate" could have been interpreted as inhibition of cell wall synthesis as well as protein synthesis. PARK (1958) observed that under conditions favoring incorporation of various amino acids into the mucopolysaccharide-peptide component of *S. aureus* cell walls, and under which incorporation into protein is greatly reduced, 50 μg/ml of CTC resulted in an 85% inhibition of lysine incorporation into cell wall material. At lower concentrations, however, CTC inhibited protein synthesis with no effect on cell wall synthesis. MANDELSTAM and ROGERS (1959) reported that no cell-wall mucopeptide synthesis was detectable in *S. aureus* cells treated with 100 μg/ml of CTC.

HASH (1963) and HASH *et al.* (1964), on the other hand, found that lower levels of TC and CTC (5 μg/ml) not only inhibited the incorporation of alanine into protein of *S. aureus* but actually accelerated its incorporation into the cell wall. Earlier, HASH and DAVIES (1962) had observed by electron microscopy that tetracycline-treated *S. aureus* cells had greatly thickened cell walls, and they had postulated an acceleration, rather than an inhibition of cell wall synthesis. It would appear, therefore, that inhibition of cell wall synthesis is not a primary mechanism of tetracycline inhibition.

Chelation of Metal Ions

The ability of tetracyclines to bind metallic ions has long been a major consideration in studies on mode of action. VAN METER and OLESON (1951) and

VAN METER *et al.* (1952) found that the inhibitory effects of CTC on respiration and oxidative phosphorylation in rat liver mitochondria could be reversed by Mg^{++}. Alkaline phosphatase from rat kidney tissue was protected from OTC inactivation by Mg^{++} (GHATAK and KRISHNA MURTI, 1953). BRODY *et al.* (1954) attributed the *in vitro* inhibition by the tetracyclines of oxidative phosphorylation in rat liver, kidney and brain mitochondria (BRODY and BAIN, 1951) to the ability of the antibiotics to bind Mg^{++}. SONCIN (1953) reported that Mg^{++} reversed the inhibition by tetracyclines of respiration, glucolysis and multiplication of *E. coli*. The inhibition by CTC and OTC of formation of a benzoic acid oxidase system in *Pseudomonas aeruginosa* (BERNHEIM, 1954a) was found to be reversed by the addition of Fe^{++} or Mn^{++} (BERNHEIM, 1954b).

In an interesting series of studies, SAZ and his coworkers reported the effects of CTC and OTC on a cell-free system from *E. coli* which reduces the nitro groups of chloramphenicol to the corresponding arylamines (SAZ and SLEI, 1953a and b, 1954a and b; SAZ and MARMUR, 1953). CTC (10—100 μg/ml) inhibited the reaction, whereas OTC had little effect. The inhibition by CTC could be reversed by manganese, and it was concluded that the inhibition resulted from a binding by CTC of manganese, presumably by the formation of a chelate. The enzyme, after purification, was found to be a pyridine nucleotide-linked, loosely dissociable flavin mononucleotide-containing flavoprotein with a requirement for Mn^{++}. When the cell-free enzyme system from a CTC-resistant mutant of *E. coli* was examined, it was found to be much more resistant to CTC inhibition than was the enzyme from the sensitive strain (SAZ *et al.*, 1956). The difference was attributed to a much firmer binding of flavin and Mn^{++} by the resistant enzyme system (SAZ and MARTINEZ, 1956).

An extensive series of studies was carried out by WEINBERG (1954a and b; 1955a and b; 1957) on the influence of organic salts and chelating agents on the ability of the tetracyclines to inhibit microbial growth, and he has summarized these and other reports in the literature in a review (WEINBERG, 1957). Fe^{++} reversed tetracycline inhibition in all eleven genera tested, and Mg^{++} was effective in reversing inhibition in *Pseudomonas, Escherichia, Proteus, Bacillus* and *Staphylococcus*. Other ions were active in only an occasional genus. JOHNSON and COLMER (1957) reported that Mg^{++} reversed CTC and TC inhibition of respiration in *Azotobacter vinelandii*. YEE *et al.* (1958) found that the inhibition of glutamate oxidation in *Shigella flexneri* cells treated with CTC, OTC or TC was reversed by Mg^{++}, Fe^{++}, and Fe^{+++}. The inhibition of the polynucleotide phosphorylase of *Micrococcus lysodeikticus* was attributed by FUWA (1963) to the binding of Mg^{++}.

PRICE *et al.* (1957a) attributed the antagonistic activity of milk against CTC and OTC to the high concentrations of inorganic ions, especially Ca^{++} and Mg^{++} present in milk. Casein was also found to play a role in the antagonism. They proposed (PRICE *et al.*, 1957b) that the mechanism of inactivation could be through the formation of an antibiotic-metal ion complex.

According to another group of reports, chelation of metal ions would appear to be necessary for inhibitory activity of tetracyclines. LITTLE *et al.* (1953) found that Mn^{++} enhanced the inhibition of the protozoan *Colpeda cucullus* by CTC. WEINBERG (1954a, 1954b) observed moderate enhancement of growth inhibition of *Ps. aeruginosa* with low concentrations of Mn^{++} or with high concentrations of Fe^{++}. ROKOS *et al.* (1958, 1959b) reported that bivalent cations were necessary for the inhibition of hydrolases by CTC. The inhibition by CTC of ATP-ase from rat heart myosin (VYSHEPAN and ZUEVA, 1959) depended upon the concentration of Mg^{++}. GOLDMAN (1960) suggested that in his studies, the metal chelate of OTC was the actual inhibitor of the alanine dehydrogenase of *Mycobacterium tuberculosis*. KOHN (1961) demonstrated a divalent metal ion-mediated binding of TC to DNA and to serum albumin and suggested that tetracyclines may exert some of their biological effects by complexing with macromolecules through metal ions.

The specific nature of the binding of inorganic ions by tetracyclines has been the subject of a number of investigations. The marked tendency of OTC to form complexes with certain inorganic salts was noted by REGNA *et al.* (1951). ALBERT (1953) and ALBERT and REES (1956) studied in some detail the affinity of CTC, OTC and TC for metallic ions. ALBERT (1958) concluded that "... chelation is likely to play a part in [the mode of action of tetracyclines] because substances with [affinity] constants of this magnitude could not fail to compete for metals in the tissues". Further studies on the details of tetracycline binding have been carried out by CONOVER (1956), DOLUISIO and MARTIN (1963) and others, and will be mentioned in the discussion to follow.

An examination of the antibiotic activities of the large number of tetracycline analogs which have been prepared to date leads to some generalizations as to which parts of the molecule are necessary for biological activity. When the 11, 12 chromophore is disrupted (e.g. the isotetracyclines), biological activity is lost. The 2-carboxamido substituent is also necessary for activity, but the "upper periphery" (carbons 4—7) can be subjected to many changes without loss of activity (STEPHENS *et al.*, 1958). If the 4-dimethylamino group, however, is completely removed, the resulting dedimethylamino derivatives retain only about 10% of the antibiotic activity of the parent compounds. Moreover, the 4-dimethylamino group must retain its configuration; the 4-epi-derivatives are of a very low order of activity. These same parts of the molecule have also been implicated in the metal-binding properties of the tetracyclines. CONOVER (1956) found that the primary site of metal complexing was the β-diketone system between the 11 and 12 positions. When the 11—12 system is absent, as in the isotetracyclines, Ca^{++} is no longer bound, but DOLUISIO and MARTIN (1963) showed that Cu^{++}, Ni^{++} and Zn^{++} can be bound by the isotetracyclines. They concluded that chelation with these ions occurs by coordination with the 4-dimethylamino group and either the 12a-or 3-hydroxyl group. DOLUISIO and MARTIN (1963) attempted to correlate the metal binding properties and the antibacterial activity of various tetracycline analogs. The potent antibacterial agents (CTC, OTC, TC and DMCTC) and anhydro CTC formed 2:1 complexes with Cu^{++}, Ni^{++} and Zn^{++}, whereas the 4-epitetracyclines, which are approximately 5% as active, and iso-CTC, with essentially no bioactivity, formed 1:1 complexes with these ions. COLAIZZI, *et al.* (1965) used a model enzyme system to investigate the possibility that tetracyclines inhibit bacterial growth by inhibiting metalloflavoenzymes responsible for oxidative phosphorylation by chelation of enzyme bound metal ions (SAZ and MARTINEZ, 1956 and 1958; MIURA *et al.*, 1952). They studied the effects of a series of biologically active and inactive tetracycline analogs on a purified metalloflavoenzyme, NADH-cytochrome *c* oxidoreductase. Many of the known structure-activity relationships of the tetracyclines correlated with their activity in this system. Epimerization of the 4-dimethylamino group and modification of the 2-carboxamide group, which lead to biologically inactive compounds, also resulted in compounds inactive against the model system. Other biologically inactive derivatives, however (isotetracycline, tetracycline methiodide and dedimethylaminotetracycline), inhibited the enzyme at least as well as the parent tetracyclines. The authors suggested that the biological inactivity of these derivatives might be explained by inability to enter bacterial cells.

The correlation between metal-binding properties of the tetracycline derivatives and their antibiotic potency appears to be far from complete. Although there seems to be little doubt that the metal-binding properties of tetracyclines are involved in a wide variety of the reactions attributed to these antibiotics, there is no convincing evidence that these are the key reactions involved in growth inhibition, especially inhibition by low concentrations of the antibiotics.

Reversal by Metabolites

Attempts have been made to elucidate the mode of action of the tetracyclines by seeking metabolites which reverse their inhibitory effect. FOSTER and PITTILLO (1953a) found that complex organic supplements added to the media were able to reverse CTC inhibition of *E. coli*. They subsequently (FOSTER and PITTILLO 1953b) proposed that riboflavin was one of the significant reversing agents, and that CTC competitively inhibited both the synthesis and utilization of riboflavin in the cells. YAGI *et al.* (1956, 1959) reported that CTC inhibited D-amino acid oxidase by binding to the riboflavin moiety of flavin adenine dinucleotide (FAD). HUGUCHI and BOLTON (1959) demonstrated the binding of OTC to riboflavin as well as to desoxyribonucleic acid and adenylic acid. It is possible that riboflavin (and other molecules) can inactivate the tetracyclines simply by physically removing the antibiotic from the medium in the form of a complex.

STANECKI *et al.* (1958) were able to reverse the inhibitory action of CTC against *S. aureus* with filtrates from CTC-resistant strains of *Pseudomonas* and *Proteus*, and they suggested that the filtrates could either be supplying a necessary metabolite missing in the antibiotic-inhibited culture or could be exerting a blocking effect upon the antibiotic.

Synthesis of Specific Enzymes and Other Proteins

In Tables 5 and 8 are listed a variety of enzymes and other proteins, the production of which has been reported to be inhibited by tetracyclines. These inhibitions are characterized in general by the very small quantities of antibiotic required for the inhibition. Taken together, these phenomena might be suggestive that protein synthesis represents a particularly sensitive site of tetracycline action. The following section considers in some detail the inhibition of protein synthesis by tetracyclines.

Protein Synthesis

One of the earliest reports in the literature relating to the mode of action of the tetracyclines was the abstract of a paper by GALE and PAINE (1950) claiming that CTC completely inhibited protein synthesis in *Staphylococcus aureus*. Since that time, the hypothesis that inhibition of protein synthesis is the major mechanism by which the tetracyclines exert their antibacterial activity has been widely accepted and is the basis for most of the recent research in this area. At about the same time, WAGNER (1950) reported that adaptive enzyme formation in *Mycobacteria* was inhibited by CTC, and shortly thereafter, HAHN and WISSEMAN (1951) reported similar results for *E. coli*, in which OTC and CTC inhibited adaptive enzyme formation. They attributed this to a general inhibition of cellular protein synthesis. Subsequently, during the course of a comprehensive series of studies on amino acid assimilation by bacteria, GALE and his coworkers investigated in some detail the effects of tetracyclines on protein synthesis and on other cell functions. GALE and PAINE (1951) demonstrated that CTC added to washed cells of *Staphylococcus aureus* markedly inhibited the intracellular formation of "combined glutamate", and at higher concentrations inhibited free glutamate accumulation. In these studies, 100% inhibition of the former was observed with 0.07 mM CTC, and 50% inhibition with 0.014 mM CTC. Glutamate accumulation was inhibited by 0.2 mM CTC. GALE and FOLKES (1953a) next reported that the treatment of washed cells of *S. aureus* with bactericidal levels of CTC and OTC resulted in inhibition of total protein synthesis and stimulation of RNA synthesis. Fifty percent inhibition of protein synthesis required only 0.2 μg/ml of CTC or 0.4 μg/ml of OTC, but inhibition of the other reactions studied (glucose fermentation, nucleic acid synthesis, and free glutamic acid accumulation) required 100 to 1000 times the minimum growth inhibitory levels of these antibiotics. When protein synthesis was measured as a function of glutamic-C^{14} acid incorporation by washed cell suspensions, CTC was again found to be inhibitory (GALE and FOLKES, 1953b). The incorporation of phenylalanine-C^{14} was even more sensitive to the action of CTC and OTC than was the incorporation of glutamate (GALE and FOLKES, 1953c). In a disrupted cell system, both CTC and OTC (10^{-3}—10^{-5} M) inhibited the incorporation of glycine into protein (GALE and FOLKES, 1957). PARK (1958) also reported that protein synthesis in *S. aureus* was inhibited by CTC. The concentrations required for inhibition of protein synthesis were lower than those required for inhibition of synthesis of the mucopolysaccharide-peptide component of cell walls. MANDELSTAM and ROGERS (1959), in similar studies, reported that the synthesis of proteins, nucleic acids and cell wall mucopeptide were all inhibited by rather high (100 μg/ml) levels of CTC.

JONES and MORRISON (1962, 1963) studied the effects of tetracycline and oxytetracycline on growth inhibition of *Aerobacter aerogenes* under various conditions, and proposed two modes of action for these antibiotics. Mode I, found in unaerated cultures, is concerned with an interference with hydrogen transfer processes. Mode II inhibition, under aeration conditions, is considered a derangement of protein synthesis. Subsequently, BENBOUGH and MORRISON (1965) proposed a third mode of action for the chlorinated derivatives related to the metabolism of D-glutamate (see also SNELL and CHENG, 1961).

CIAK and HAHN (1958) (also see HAHN, 1959 and 1961) demonstrated that the effects of mixtures of chloramphenicol and either OTC or CTC on the growth rate of *E. coli* were additive. They interpreted these results as a concurrent blocking of different metabolic pathways which contribute to protein synthesis.

BROCK (1963) found that TC and CTC fell into the group of antibiotics which inhibited M protein synthesis in *Streptococcus pyogenes* at the same concentration at which they inhibited growth (1 μg/ml) and inferred that growth inhibition was a result of inhibition of protein synthesis. YEE and GEZON (1963) reported that CTC inhibited protein synthesis in *Shigella flexneri*. As little as 0.1 μg/ml resulted in significant inhibition, and almost complete inhibition (94%) was observed in the presence of 0.5 ml/ml. A marked stimulation of RNA production was observed in CTC treated cells and it was determined that it was the soluble RNA synthesis which was stimulated; the production of ribosomal RNA was reduced.

In growing cultures of *E. coli* and *B. cereus* studied by ČERNÝ and HABERMANN (1964) protein synthesis was blocked immediately upon the addition of 20—50 μg/ml of TC, whereas nucleic acid synthesis continued. Abnormally large amounts of RNA accumulated in the cells. The authors speculated that the cessation of protein synthesis caused by TC made available amino acids which are required for the normal nucleic acid biosynthesis, allowing unrestricted nucleic acid production for a period of about an hour. Accumulation of RNA in cells treated with CTC was also observed in the earlier GALE and FOLKES (1953a) experiments with *S. aureus*, and the RNA accumulation caused by CTC in *E. coli* was the subject of a more detailed recent study by HOLMES and WILD (1965).

The effects of tetracyclines on the incorporation of alanine-C^{14} into cell wall and protein of *S. aureus* were studied by HASH (1963) and HASH *et al.* (1964), who found that TC and CTC at 5 μg/ml inhibited the incorporation of alanine into protein, but accelerated incorporation into the cell wall. Even at 0.1 μg/ml, TC inhibited incorporation into protein by about 70%, and at 0.5 μg/ml inhibition was greater than 90%. The inhibition by TC was complete within 5 minutes of adding the antibiotic. The incorporation of glutamate-C^{14} and lysine-C^{14} was also inhibited by tetracycline; the inhibition of glutamate was the most pronounced of the three. The rapidity and extent of inhibition and the fact that only very low levels were required led them to the conclusion that inhibition of protein synthesis was the primary site of antibiotic action.

Several studies on the effect of the tetracyclines on protein synthesis in mammalian systems have been reported. NIKOLOV and ILKOV (1961) found that in chlortetracycline-fed rabbits (20 mg/kg/day for 10 days) the incorporation of methionine-S^{35} into liver, gastric mucosa, kidney and spleen proteins was markedly inhibited. FRANKLIN (1963b), however, was unable to observe any effect on either induction of tryptophan pyrollase or on the incorporation of leucine-C^{14} into liver protein of rats after a single injection of CTC (20 mg/100 g) or after prolonged oral dosage (20 mg/100 g for 10 days). Since FRANKLIN (1962, 1963a) had previously observed inhibition of leucine-C^{14} incorporation into ribosomal protein in cell-free rat liver preparations, he postulated that the absence of a CTC effect in intact animals might be explained by an inability of the drug to reach the site of protein biosynthesis in the liver *in vivo*. Subsequently, WEISBERGER *et al.* (1964) reported that although TC had no effect on "endogenous" protein synthesis (i.e. in the absence of added template RNA) in a cell-free system prepared from rabbit reticulocytes, there was appreciable inhibition (75%) of the incorporation of amino acids stimulated by added template RNA in the presence of relatively low levels of TC (0.01 μmoles/ml). In general, it would appear that protein synthesis in mammalian cells can also be inhibited by the tetracyclines, but much higher concentrations are required. SHILS (1962), in a paper on the metabolic aspects of tetracycline therapy in humans, suggested that the increased urinary loss of nitrogen occasionally noted in some patients may be interpreted as a manifestation of a general inhibition of protein synthesis. According to his interpretation, the decreased utilization of amino acids for protein synthesis could lead to an increased load of the products of amino acid metabolism being presented for excretion by the kidney.

It was not long after the first major steps were taken toward a more precise understanding of the details of protein biosynthesis that information on the activity of antibiotics upon the various specific reactions involved began to appear. These reactions may be outlined as follows:

1. Amino acid activation and attachment to sRNA.

2. Formation of the ribosome-messenger-aminoacyl-sRNA complex. This has often been considered as consisting of two steps: a) the attachment of messenger RNA to the ribosomes and b) the binding of aminoacyl-sRNA to the ribosome-messenger RNA complex (the "binding reaction").

3. Transfer of amino acids from sRNA to the growing peptide chain (formation of peptide bonds).

Reactions 2 and 3 have been referred to as the "transfer reaction", *i.e.* the transfer of amino acid from aminoacyl-sRNA to protein, and all three taken together can be considered as the "overall amino acid incorporation reaction". RENDI and OCHOA (1961) made brief mention of their observation that both chloramphenicol and OTC inhibited the transfer of leucine-C^{14} from aminoacyl-sRNA to protein in *E. coli* preparations, but neither antibiotic had any effect on the transfer reaction with rat liver ribosomes. In a more detailed study on the effect of chloramphenicol on protein synthesis in *E. coli* cell-free systems, they (RENDI and OCHOA, 1962) again mentioned that OTC had an inhibitory effect, similar to that of chloramphenicol, on the transfer reaction.

Contrary results were reported by FRANKLIN (1962) who found that CTC inhibited the overall incorporation of leucine-C^{14} into protein in cell-free rat liver preparations, and demonstrated that the sensitive step was the transfer reaction. FRANKLIN (1963a) suggested that the difference in these reports may have been due to the relative insensitivity of the rat liver system to CTC and that the concentration used by RENDI and OCHOA (1961) may have been too low to demonstrate the inhibition. Incorporation of leucine-C^{14} into protein in *E. coli* cell-free systems was found to be much more sensitive to CTC than was the incorporation into rat liver systems over the entire range of concentrations tested (FRANKLIN, 1963a). Again, no effect of CTC was found on the attachment of amino acid to sRNA; the subsequent transfer to protein appeared to be the sensitive step in both the *E. coli* and rat liver preparations. OTC and TC were found to be as effective as CTC in the *E. coli* system, and somewhat less effective than CTC in the rat liver system. The amino acid, which in the presence of CTC is not transferred to ribosomes, was shown to be largely retained on the sRNA. In another publication, FRANKLIN (1964) reported that CTC had no marked effect on the "energy-dependent" binding of sRNA labelled with uracil-C^{14} and cytosine-C^{14} to rat liver ribosomes, but he felt that such an inhibition might have been obscured by the high level of "energy-free" binding in his experiments.

LASKIN and CHAN (1964) studied the effects of various tetracyclines on polyuridylic acid (poly U)-directed phenylalanine incorporation in *E. coli* cell-free systems. The synthesis of polyphenylalanine in such systems, with poly U acting as the "messenger RNA", has been used as a model of protein synthesis for a wide variety of studies on the detailed steps in the protein biosynthetic pathway. A *general* similarity was noted in the degree of inhibition caused by TC, OTC, CTC and DMCTC, but the chlorinated derivatives were consistently more inhibitory than were either TC or OTC. These results were reminiscent of many reports in the literature (*e.g.* WELCH *et al.*, 1954; REEDY *et al.*, 1955; MCCORMICK *et al.*, 1957 and 1960; GARROD and WATERWORTH, 1960; KIRBY *et al.*, 1961) that the chlorinated tetracyclines are 2—3 times as potent against several species of bacteria as are TC or OTC. Moreover, the activity of dedimethylamino-OTC (DDA-OTC) which was about 10% as active as TC in inhibiting growth of *E. coli*, was also reflected in the cell-free system, in which 10 μg/ml of DDA-OTC was required to inhibit to the same extent as 1 μg/ml of TC (LASKIN and CHAN, 1964). The close parallel between the relative potencies of these antibiotics against whole cells and in the cell-free systems lends further support to the hypothesis that the primary mode of action of the tetracyclines is their effect on protein synthesis. LASKIN and CHAN (1964) also demonstrated that tetracycline, at levels of 10 to 100 μg/ml, had no effect on the steps involving activation of phenylalanine-C^{14} and transfer to sRNA, but the subsequent transfer of radioactivity from ^{14}C-phenylalanyl-sRNA to the ribosomes was the sensitive step. Shortly thereafter, TRAUT and MONRO (1964) also noted that CTC inhibited the poly U-directed transfer of phenylalanine from sRNA to polypeptide in an *E. coli* system and similar results have since been reported from several laboratories (e.g. SUAREZ and NATHANS, 1965; HIEROWSKI, 1965; CLARK and CHANG, 1965).

In addition, HIEROWSKI (1965) found that CTC inhibited amino acid incorporation directed by other synthetic nucleotides and copolymers (lysine by poly A, proline by poly C, phenylalanine by poly UA and poly UC), and by various other RNA templates (from f2 bacteriophage, turnip yellow mosaic virus and tobacco mosaic virus). CLARK and CHANG (1965) reported that TC inhibited both polyphenylalanine and hemoglobin synthesis in a cell-free rabbit reticulocyte system.

With the introduction of a simple, rapid and sensitive method for determining specific messenger-directed binding of aminoacyl-sRNA to ribosomes (NIRENBERG and LEDER, 1964) a number of workers investigated the effects of tetracyclines upon this reaction. The technique depends upon the fact that ribosomes bind to Millipore membrane filters, and if a reaction mixture containing ribosomes, polynucleotide and ^{14}C-aminoacyl-sRNA is passed through the filter, any aminoacyl-sRNA which binds to the ribosome-polynucleotide complex (due to the presence of the appropriate codon) can be subsequently detected on the filter.

WOLFE and HAHN (1965a) reported only slight inhibition by OTC of the binding of phenylalanyl-sRNA to poly U-charged *E. coli* ribosomes. SUAREZ and NATHANS (1965), however, first by a method utilizing the sedimentation of ribosome-messenger-aminoacyl-sRNA complex by centrifugation at 105,000 g for 2 hours, and then using the NIRENBERG and LEDER technique, demonstrated inhibition of the binding reaction by TC. They used ^{14}C-N-acetyl-phenylalanyl-sRNA for their experiments in order to exclude the possibility that acid-soluble peptides were formed on the ribosomes under the conditions used. The maximum inhibition of binding which was observed was about 50%, even though concentrations of tetracycline as high as 2×10^{-4} M were tested. Tetracycline had no effect on the binding of the polynucleotide template to the ribosomes. The fact that tetracycline inhibited the binding to the extent of only 50%, although it inhibits the overall incorporation reaction almost completely, led these authors to speculate that the antibiotic interferes with only one of the two postulated sRNA binding sites on the ribosome (WARNER and RICH, 1964; ARLINGHAUS *et al.*, 1964). Similar results were reported at about the same time by HIEROWSKI (1965), who, using sucrose gradient centrifugation, found that CTC inhibited the binding of ^{14}C-phenylalanyl-sRNA to *E. coli* ribosomes by *ca.* 60%, but had no effect on the binding of ^{14}C-poly U.

CLARK and CHANG (1965) using rabbit reticulocyte ribosomes and purified binding enzyme, found that TC inhibited the binding reaction by about 40%, as measured by the membrane filter technique. Furthermore, as in the *E. coli* experiments reported by HIEROWSKI (1965), preincubation of ribosomes with tetracycline did not result in an inhibition of binding of ^{14}C-poly U. The inhibition of polyphenylalanine synthesis by TC was not altered by variations of poly U concentration, again indicating that TC does not appear to compete with messenger RNA for sites on the ribosome. TC did not affect the formation of puromycin peptides, a reaction which does not appear to require additional binding of aminoacyl-sRNA, but it did inhibit the completion of partial chains, which does require additional aminoacyl-sRNA binding. CLARK and CHANG concluded that TC inhibits the binding of aminoacyl-sRNA to messenger RNA-containig ribosomes.

LAST (1965) studied the binding reaction using the membrane filter technique in an attempt to find a correlation between the antibiotic potency of several tetracyclines and their ability to inhibit binding. Among the antibiotics tested, the order of effectiveness in inhibiting growth, amino acid incorporation, and aminoacyl-sRNA binding to ribosomes was the same, with only one exception. A possible permeability factor was suggested to explain the fact that 5,6-anhydro-TC was relatively more effective in inhibiting growth than in inhibiting the cell-free systems. In these experiments, the extent of inhibition reached as high as 75%, and LAST questioned the suggestion previously made by SUAREZ and NATHANS (1965) that interference of one of the two sRNA binding sites on the ribosomes was the mechanism of inhibition. LASKIN and CHAN (1966), also using the membrane filter technique, found that under a variety of conditions of Mg^{++} concentration, ribosome concentration, polynucleotide concentration, antibiotic concentration and preincubation, tetracycline inhibition of aminoacyl-sRNA binding rarely exceeded 30%. The reasons for the variations among the results reported are not known, but it would seem that care must be exercised in interpreting the results of the membrane filter experiments.

VAZQUEZ (1963) reported that neither OTC nor CTC inhibited the binding of chloramphenicol to *S. aureus* or *B. megaterium* ribosomes, suggesting that binding of the tetracyclines (if it occurs), might be at a different site on the ribosomes. He later reported that the chloramphenicol binding site was on the 50 S subunit (VAZQUEZ, 1964). WOLFE and HAHN (1965b) confirmed this observation using

E. coli ribosomes. CONNAMACHER and MANDEL (1965) determined that TC binds to the 30 S subunit of both *E. coli* and *B. cereus* ribosomes, both *in vivo* and *in vitro*. Since TC also was observed to bind to the 70 S ribosomes, they concluded that TC did not obstruct the site of association of the 30 S and 50 S subunits. Mg^{++} was deemed not to be essential for the binding, since 10^{-4} M EDTA added to preparations prior to antibiotic addition reduced the binding by only 20%. TC added to ribosomes prior to the addition of C^{14}-poly U resulted in only a 20% decrease of poly U binding, indicating that TC does not act by prevention of the attachment of messenger RNA to the ribosome. LAST *et al.* (1965), were not able to demonstrate binding of TC to *E. coli* ribosomes by the method of WOLFE and HAHN (1965 b) or by sucrose density gradient ultracentrifugation.

Studies with Resistant *E. coli* Strains

One approach to the study of mode of action has been to compare the properties of antibiotic-resistant and sensitive strains. A few recent studies of this nature will be mentioned in connection with inhibition by tetracyclines of protein synthesis. YOKOTA and AKIBA (1962a) concluded that the resistance of *E. coli* strains carrying a multiple drug resistance factor (WATANABE and FUKASAWA, 1961) was due to a decrease in the TC-permeability of the cells, since amino acid incorporation into ribosomes from resistant cells was sensitive to TC. The resistance of a strain obtained by repeated subculturing in the presence of increasing concentrations of TC ("artificial TC-resistant strain"), however, was thought to be due to a change in "internal metabolic pathways". In a subsequent study, YOKOTA and AKIBA (1962b), investigated the ultracentrifugal pattern of ribosomes isolated from sensitive and resistant strains grown in the presence of TC, or ribosomes isolated and then incubated with TC. They concluded that TC acted by destruction of sensitive ribosomes, perhaps by chelation of Mg^{++} necessary for maintaining their integrity. Ribosomes from the resistant strain carrying the TC-resistance factor were also destroyed by TC, but ribosomes from the "artificial TC-resistant strain" appeared to differ, consisting exclusively of 20 S particles which were not affected by TC. A second mechanism of TC-resistance was suggested, whereby the ribosomes of resistant cells developed resistance to TC action.

LASKIN and CHAN (1964) studied the effects of tetracyclines on cell-free systems derived from a clinical isolate of *E. coli* resistant to more than 100 μg/ml of tetracycline. (In the same test the sensitive strain, *E. coli* B, was inhibited by 0.2 μg/ml.) Poly U-directed phenylalanine incorporation in these preparations was about as sensitive to the tetracyclines as were the preparations from the sensitive strain. OKAMOTO and MIZUNO (1964) also reported that cell-free systems from two resistant strains were not resistant to TC. One strain was developed by *in vitro* passage in chloramphenicol-containing medium and exhibited considerable cross-resistance to TC; the second was resistant by virtue of carrying the multiple drug resistance factor. Similar results were subsequently reported by FRANKLIN (1965) with a resistant strain selected by serial passage in CTC-containing medium. LAST (1965), found that extracts from resistant and sensitive cells were equally sensitive to CTC both as to the overall amino acid incorporation and the binding reaction.

Although the work of YOKODA and AKIBA (1962a and b) suggests two mechanisms of resistance to the tetracyclines, the other studies reported all point to some mechanism whereby the resistant cell can keep the antibiotic from reaching the sensitive site. ARIMA and IZAKI (1963) described the accumulation of a large amount of OTC, dependent upon an energy yielding system, in OTC-sensitive *E. coli* cells. The cells of the multiple drug resistant strain of *E. coli*, however, accumulated significantly less OTC, and cells of a more highly resistant strain accumulated no significant amount of antibiotic (IZAKI and ARIMA, 1963). These results were confirmed by FRANKLIN and GODFREY (1965), who found that resistant *E. coli* cells (developed by the serial passage method) accumulated much less CTC and TC than did the sensitive cells. There was no evidence to suggest that this could be a result of a specific TC-excretion system in resistant cells. Most of the evidence, therefore, favors the proposal that tetracycline resistance is due to an alteration in permeability, perhaps due to a change in a specific active transport system.

It would appear that the most convincing evidence points to protein biosynthesis as the most significant target of the tetracyclines. The inhibition occurs at the ribosome, and is manifested by an interference with the formation of the necessary complex between ribosome, messenger-RNA and aminoacyl-sRNA, perhaps by inhibition of the binding of the latter to the ribosome-messenger RNA complex.

See addendum

References

AGARWALA, S. C., C. R. KRISHNA MURTI, and D. L. SHRIVASTAVA: Studies on enzyme inhibition in relation to drug action. I. Effect of certain antibiotics on urease. J. Sci. Ind. Research (India) **11** B, 1965 (152).

AJL, S.: As cited in: Symposium on the mode of action of antibiotics. Bacteriol. Rev. **17**, 17 (1953).

ALBERT, A.: Avidity of Terramycin and Aureomycin for metallic cations. Nature **172**, 201 (1953).

ALBERT, A.: Metal binding in chemotherapy: The activation of metals by chelation. In: The strategy of chemotherapy. Eighth Symposium of the Society for General Microbiology, Cambridge, England, 1958, p. 112.

ALBERT, A., and C. W. REES: Avidity of the tetracyclines for the cations of metals. Nature **177**, 433 (1956).

ALEXANDER, B.: Effect of chlortetracycline on vitamin B_6 and amino acid decarboxylase in bacteria from the alimentary tract of the chick. Appl. Microbiol. **8**, 69 (1960).

ALTENBERN, R. A.: The action of Aureomycin on the *Escherichia coli* bacteriophage T_3 system. J. Bacteriol. **65**, 288 (1953).

ARIMA, K., and K. IZAKI: Accumulation of oxytetracycline relevant to its bacteriocidal action in the cells of *Escherichia coli*. Nature **200**, 192 (1963).

ARLINGHAUS, R., J. SHAEFFER, and R. SCHWEET: Mechanism of peptide bond formation in polypeptide synthesis. Proc. Natl. Acad. Sci. U.S. **51**, 1291 (1964).

ARORA, K. L., and C. R. KRISHNA MURTI: Enzyme inhibition studies in relation to drug action. VI. Action of certain antibacterial agents on the succinic oxidase system J. Sci. Ind. Research (India) **13** B, 482 (1954).

ARORA, K. L., and C. R. KRISHNA MURTI: Enzyme inhibition in relation to drug action. VII. Action of certain antibacterial agents on tryptophanase. J. Sci. Ind. Research (India) **14** C, 6 (1955a).

ARORA, K. L., and C. R. KRISHNA MURTI: Enzyme inhibition studies in relation to drug action. VIII. Action of certain antibacterial agents on the tricarboxylic acid cycle of *Vibrio comma*. J. Sci. Ind. Research (India) **14**C, 66 (1955b).

ARORA, K. L., and C. R. KRISHNA MURTI: Enzyme inhibition studies in relation to drug action. IX. Action of certain antibacterial agents on catalase. J. Sci. Research (India) **19**C, 103 (1960).

BACHRACH, U., M. SEGAL, and R. ROZANSKY: Effect of tetracyclines on formation of amines by bacteria. Proc. Soc. Exptl. Biol. Med. **97**, 874 (1958).

BELDING, M., and F. KERN, JR.: Inhibition of urease by oxytetracycline. J. Lab. Clin. Med. **61**, 560 (1963).

BENBOUGH, J., and G. A. MORRISON: Bacteriostatic actions of some tetracyclines. J. Pharm. and Pharmacol. **17**, 409 (1965).

BERNHEIM, F.: The effect of certain antibiotics on the formation of an adaptive enzyme in a strain of *Pseudomonas aeruginosa*. J. Pharmacol. Exptl. Therap. **110**, 115 (1954a).

BERNHEIM, F.: The effect of certain metal ions and chelating agents on the formation of an adaptive enzyme in *Pseudomonas aeruginosa*. Enzymologia **16**, 351 (1954b).

BERNHEIM, F., and W. E. DE TURK: The effect of chloramphenicol and certain other drugs on the oxidation of aromatic amino acids by a strain of *Pseudomonas aeruginosa*. J. Pharmacol. Exptl. Therap. **105**, 246 (1952).

BERNHEIM, F., and W. E. DE TURK: An aerobic cysteine desulfurase in a mycobacterium. Enzymologia **16**, 69 (1953a).

BERNHEIM, F., and W. E. DE TURK: Factors which affect the oxidation of benzoic acid by a strain of *Pseudomonas aeruginosa*. J. Bacteriol. **65**, 65 (1953b).

BOHONOS, N., A. C. DORNBUSH, L. I. FELDMAN, J. H. MARTIN, E. PELCAK, and J. H. WILLIAMS: *In vitro* studies with chlortetracycline, oxytetracycline and tetracycline. Antibiotics Ann. **1953/54**, 49 (1953).

BROCK, T. D.: Inhibition of endotrophic sporulation by antibiotics. Nature **195**, 309 (1962).

BROCK, T. D.: Effect of antibiotics and inhibitors on M protein synthesis. J. Bacteriol. **85**, 527 (1963).

BRODY, T. M., and J. A. BAIN: The effect of Aureomycin and Terramycin on oxidative phosphorylation. J. Pharmacol. Exptl. Therap. **103**, 388 (1951).

BRODY, T. M., R. HURWITZ, and J. A. BAIN: Magnesium and the effect of the tetracycline antibiotics on oxidative processes in mitochondria. Antibiotics & Chemotherapy **4**, 864 (1954).

ČERNÝ, R., and V. HABERMANN: On the effects of tetracycline on the biosynthesis of proteins and nucleic acids with *Escherichia coli* and *Bacillus cereus*. Collection Czech Chem. Commun. **29**, 1326 (1964).

CHANDLER, C. A., V. Z. DAVIDSON, P. H. LONG, and J. J. MONNIER: Studies on resistance of staphylococci to penicillin: The production of penicillinase and its inhibition by the action of aureomycin. Bull. Johns Hopkins Hosp. **89**, 81 (1951).

CHANDLER, C. A., and E. VON DER GALTZ: Studies of the effect of aureomycin on the production of penicillinase by staphylococci. Bull. Johns Hopkins Hosp. **91**, 475 (1952).

CHENG, L., and J. F. SNELL: Studies in metabolic spectra. IV. Effects of tetracyclines, some of their derivatives, and chloramphenicol on accumulation of glutamic acid in *Escherichia coli*. J. Bacteriol. **83**, 711 (1962).

CIAK, J., and F. E. HAHN: Mechanisms of action of antibiotics. I. Additive action of chloramphenicol and tetracyclines on the growth of *Escherichia coli*. J. Bacteriol. **75**, 125 (1958).

CLARK, JR., J. M., and A. Y. CHANG: Inhibitors of the transfer of amino acids from aminoacyl soluble ribonucleic acid to proteins. J. Biol. Chem. **240**, 4734 (1965).

COLAIZZI, J. L., A. M. KNEVEL, and A. N. MARTIN: Biophysical study of the mode of action of the tetracycline antibiotics. J. Pharm. Sci. **54**, 1425 (1965).

CONNAMACHER, R. H., and H. G. MANDEL: Binding of tetracycline to the 30S ribosomes and to polyuridylic acid. Biochem. Biophys. Research Commun. **20**, 98 (1965).

CONOVER, L. H.: In: Symposium on Antibiotics and Mould Metabolites. Chem. Soc. Special Publication No. 5, p. 48. London, England 1956.

Creaser, E. H.: The induced (adaptive) biosynthesis of β-galactosidase in *Staphylococcus aureus*. J. Gen. Microbiol. **12**, 288 (1955).

De Lamater, E. D., M. E. Hunter, W. Szybalski, and V. Bryson: Chemically induced aberrations of mitosis in bacteria. J. Gen. Microbiol. **12**, 203 (1955).

DelLove, Jr., B., S. S. Wright, E. M. Purcell, T. W. Mou, and M. Finland: Antibacterial action of tetracycline: Comparisons with oxytetracycline and chlortetracycline. Proc. Soc. Exptl. Biol. Med. **85**, 25 (1954).

Doluisio, J. T., and A. N. Martin: Metal complexation of the tetracycline hydrochlorides. J. Med. Chem. **6**, 16 (1963).

Doughty, C. C., and J. A. Hayashi: Enzymatic properties of a phage-induced lysin affecting group A streptococci. J. Bacteriol. **83**, 1058 (1962).

Eagle, H., and A. K. Saz: Antibiotics. Ann. Rev. Microbiol. **9**, 173 (1955).

Faguet, M., et E. Edlinger: Antibiotiques et lyse bactériophagique. VII. L'action de l'aureomycin sur la lyse bactériophagique étudiée au microbiophotométre. Ann. inst. Pasteur **80**, 281 (1951).

Fedorov, M. V., and I. Segi: Effect of certain antibiotics on the physiological activity of *Azotobacter chroococcum*. Mikrobiologiya **30**, 275 (1961).

Foster, J. W., and R. F. Pittillo: Reversal by complex natural materials of growth inhibition caused by antibiotics. J. Bacteriol. **65**, 361 (1953a).

Foster, J. W., and R. F. Pittillo: Metabolite reversal of antibiotic inhibition, especially reversal of Aureomycin inhibition by riboflavin. J. Bacteriol. **66**, 478 (1953b).

Franklin, T. J.: The inhibition of protein synthesis by chlortetracycline in cell-free systems. Biochem. J. **84**, 110P (1962).

Franklin, T. J.: The inhibition of incorporation of leucine into protein of cell-free systems from rat liver and *Escherichia coli* by chlortetracycline. Biochem. J. **87**, 449 (1963a).

Franklin, T. J.: Absence of effect of chlortetracycline administration on amino acid incorporation and enzyme synthesis in the liver of the intact rat. Biochim. et Biophys. Acta **76**, 138 (1963b).

Franklin, T. J.: The effect of chlortetracycline on the transfer of leucine and "transfer" ribonucleic acid to rat-liver ribosomes *in vitro*. Biochem. J. **90**, 624 (1964).

Franklin, T. J., and A. Godfrey: Resistance of *Escherichia coli* to tetracycline. Biochem. J. **94**, 54 (1965).

Freeman, B. A., and R. Circo: Effect of tetracyclines on the intracellular amino acids of molds. J. Bacteriol. **86**, 38 (1963).

Fusillo, M. H., and M. J. Romansky: The simultaneous increase in resistance of bacteria to Aureomycin and Terramycin upon exposure to either antibiotic. Antibiotics & Chemotherapy **1**, 107 (1951).

Fuwa, I.: Inhibition of polynucleotide phosphorylase by tetracycline and its derivatives. J. Antibiotics (Japan), Ser. B **16**, 171 (1963).

Gale, E. F.: Mechanisms of antibiotic action. Pharmacol. Rev. **15**, 481 (1963).

Gale, E. F., and J. P. Folkes: The assimilation of amino-acids by bacteria. 15. Actions of antibiotics on nucleic acid and protein synthesis in *Staphylococcus aureus*. Biochem. J. **53**, 493 (1953a).

Gale, E. F., and J. P. Folkes: The assimilation of amino-acids by bacteria. 18. The incorporation of glutamic acid into the protein fraction of *Staphylococcus aureus*. Biochem. J. **55**, 721 (1953b).

Gale, E. F., and J. P. Folkes: The assimilation of amino acids by bacteria. 19. The inhibition of phenylalanine incorporation in *Staphylococcus aureus* by chloramphenicol and p-chlorophenylalanine. Biochem. J. **55**, 730 (1953c).

Gale, E. F., and J. P. Folkes: The assimilation of amino acids by bacteria. 24. Inhibitors of incorporation of glycine in disrupted staphylococcal cells. Biochem. J. **67**, 507 (1957).

Gale, E. F., and T. F. Paine: Effect of inhibitors and antibiotics on glutamic acid accumulation and on protein synthesis in Staphylococcus aureus. Biochem. J. **47**, XXVI (1950).

GALE, E. F., and T. F. PAINE: The action of inhibitors and antibiotics on the accumulation of free glutamic acid and the formation of combined glutamate in *Staphylococcus aureus*. Biochem. J. **48**, 298 (1951).

GARROD, L. P., and P. M. WATERWORTH: The relative merits of the four tetracyclines. Antibiotics Ann. **1959/60**, 440 (1960).

GHATAK, S., and C. R. KRISHNA MURTI: Enzyme inhibition studies in relation to drug action. IV. Action of certain antibiotics on alkaline phosphatase. J. Sci. Ind. Research (India) **12**B, 160 (1953).

GIBSON, F., and B. MCDOUGALL: The effect of chloramphenicol and oxytetracycline on the formation of intermediates in tryptophan biosynthesis. Australian J. Exptl. Biol. Med. Sci. **39**, 171 (1961).

GIBSON, F., B. MCDOUGALL, M. J. JONES, and H. TELTSCHER: The action of antibiotics on indole synthesis by cell suspensions of *Escherichia coli*. J. Gen. Microbiol. **15**, 446 (1956).

GOLDBERG, I. H.: Mode of action of antibiotics. II. Drugs affecting nucleic acid and protein synthesis. Am. J. Med. **39**, 722 (1965).

GOLDMAN, D. S.: The inhibition of alanine dehydrogenase by metal chelates of tetracyclines. J. Biol. Chem. **235**, 616 (1960).

GREEN, M. N., J. B. JOSIMOVICH, K. C. TSOU, and A. M. SELIGMAN: Nitroreductase activity of animal tissues and of normal and neoplastic human tissues. Cancer **9**, 176 (1956).

GRÜNBERGER, D., J. ŠKODA, and F. ŠORM: Mechanism of antibiotic action. V. Effect of chloramphenicol, chlortetracycline, and oxytetracycline on the synthesis of glutamic acid decarboxylase in *Escherichia coli*, and of tyrosine decarboxylase in *Streptococcus faecalis*. Chem. listy **48**, 1711 (1954).

GUILLAUME, J., et R. OSTEUX: Mode d'action de l'aureomycine. Inhibition du métabolisme du glucose et des acides du cycle citrique chez *Proteus mirabilis*. Compt. rend. **249**, 2643 (1959).

HAHN, F. E.: Modes of action of antibiotics. Proc. Fourth Intern. Congr. Biochem., Vienna 1958, **5**, 104 (1959).

HAHN, F. E.: Inhibition of protein synthesis by antibiotics. Antimicrobial Agents Ann. 1960, 310 (1961).

HAHN, F. E., and C. L. WISSEMAN, JR.: Inhibition of adaptive enzyme formation by antimicrobial agents. Proc. Soc. Exptl. Biol. Med. **76**, 533 (1951).

HASH, J. H.: Effects of tetracyclines on the incorporation of C^{14}-alanine into *Staphylococcus aureus*. Federation Proc. **22**, 301 (1963).

HASH, J. H., and M. C. DAVIES: Electron microscopy of *Staphylococcus aureus* treated with tetracycline. Science **138**, 828 (1962).

HASH, J. H., M. WISHNICK, and P. A. MILLER: On the mode of action of the tetracycline antibiotics in *Staphylococcus aureus*. J. Biol. Chem. **239**, 2070 (1964).

HAYANO, M.: Action of antibiotics and other substances on the formation of streptolysin S by *Streptococcus hemolyticus*. Japan, J. Bacteriol. **7**, 319 (1952).

HERRELL, W. E., F. R. HEILMAN, and W. E. WELLMAN: Some bacteriologic, pharmacologic, and clinical observations on Terramycin. Ann. N.Y. Acad. Sci. **53**, 448 (1950).

HIEROWSKI, M.: Inhibition of protein synthesis by chlortetracycline in the *E. coli in vitro* system. Proc. Natl. Acad. Sci. U.S. **53**, 594 (1965).

HINTON, N. A., and J. H. ORR: The effect of antibiotics on the toxin production of *Staphylococcus aureus*. Antibiotics & Chemotherapy **10**, 758 (1960).

HOBBY, G. L.: The mode of action of Terramycin and Aureomycin. Bacteriol. Rev. **17**, 29 (1953).

HOLMES, I. A., and D. G. WILD: The synthesis of ribonucleic acid during inhibition of *Escherichia coli* by chlortetracycline. Biochem. J. **97**, 277 (1965).

HOOSER, L. E., E. V. DAVIS, M. L. MOORE, and R. A. SIEM: Elimination of pleuropneumonia-like organisms from embryonic human lung tissue culture with tetracycline. J. Bacteriol. **87**, 237 (1964).

HUGUCHI, T., and S. BOLTON: The solubility and complexing properties of oxytetracycline and tetracycline. III. Interactions in aqueous solution with model compounds, biochemicals, metals, chelates, and hexametaphosphate. J. Am. Pharm. Assoc. Sci. **48**, 557 (1959).

HUMOLLER, F. L., and H. J. ZIMMERMAN: Factors influencing betaine aldehyde oxidase activity of rat livers. Am. J. Physiol. **177**, 279 (1954).

IZAKI, K., and K. ARIMA: Disappearance of oxytetracycline accumulation in the cells of multiple drug-resistant *Escherichia coli*. Nature **200**, 384 (1963).

JACKSON, F. L.: Mode of action of tetracyclines. In: Experimental Chemotherapy (ed. R. J. SCHNITZER and F. HAWKING), vol. III. New York and London: Academic Press 1964.

JOHNSON, E. J., and A. R. COLMER: The relation of magnesium ion to the inhibition of the respiration of *Azotobacter vinelandii* by chlortetracycline, tetracycline, and 2,4-dichlorrophenoxyacetic acid. Antibiotics & Chemotherapy **7**, 521 (1957).

JONES, J. G., and G. A. MORRISON: The bacteriostatic actions of tetracycline and oxytetracycline. J. Pharm. Pharmacol. **14**, 808 (1962).

JONES, J. G., and G. A. MORRISON: Inhibitions by tetracycline and oxytetracycline of the consumption of pyruvate by *Aerobacter aerogenes*. J. Pharm. Pharmacol. **15**, 34 (1963).

KARP, A., and J. C. SNYDER: *In vitro* effect of Aureomycin, Terramycin and chloramphenicol on typhus rickettsiae. Proc. Soc. Exptl. Biol. Med. **79**, 216 (1952).

KATAGIRI, H., T. TOCHIKURA, and Y. SUZUKI: Microbiological studies of *coli-aerogenes* bacteria. VI. The action of antibiotics on bacterial respiration and α-ketoglutaric acid fermentation. Bull. Agr. Chem. Soc. Japan **23**, 322 (1959).

KATAGIRI, H., Y. SUZUKI, and T. TOCHIKURA: Studies on the action of antibiotics on bacterial metabolism. II. Effect of dihydrostreptomycin, chloramphenicol and oxytetracycline upon the aerobic carbohydrate metabolism by *Escherichia coli*. J. Antibiotics (Japan), Ser. A **13**, 155 (1960).

KATAGIRI, H., Y. SUZUKI, and T. TOCHIKURA: Studies on the action of antibiotics on bacterial metabolism. VII. Tetracyclines and bacterial respiration. Antibiotics (Japan), Ser. A **14**, 134 (1961).

KINDLER, S. H., J. MAGER, and N. GROSSOWICZ: Toxin production by *Clostridium parabotulinum* type A. J. Gen. Microbiol. **15**, 394 (1956).

KIRBY, W. M. M., C. E. ROBERTS, and R. E. BURDICK: Comparison of two new tetracyclines with tetracycline and demethylchlortetracycline. Antimicrobial Agents and Chemotherapy 1961, 286 (1961).

KOHN, K. W.: Mediation of trivalent metal ions in the binding of tetracycline to macromolecules. Nature **191**, 1156 (1961).

KOROTYAEV, A. I.: Effect of antibiotics on pyruvate consumption by resting cells of *Escherichia coli*. Mikrobiologiya **31**, 24 (1962).

KRASKIN, K. S., and A. M. STERN: Terramycin inhibition of gluconate oxidation by *Escherichia coli*. J. Bacteriol. **73**, 608 (1957).

LASKIN, A. I., and W. M. CHAN: Inhibition by tetracyclines of polyuridylic acid directed phenylalanine incorporation in *Escherichia coli* cell-free systems. Biochem. Biophys. Research Commun. **14**, 137 (1964).

LASKIN, A. I., and W. M. CHAN: The effects of vernamycins on aminoacyl-transfer RNA binding to *Escherichia coli* ribosomes. Antimicrobial Agents and Chemotherapy 1965, 321 (1966).

LAST, J. A.: Personal communication 1965.

LAST, J. A., K. IZAKI, and J. F. SNELL: The failure of tetracycline to bind *Escherichia coli* ribosomes. Biochim. et Biophys. Acta **103**, 534 (1965).

LEIBFRIED, E. L.: The effect of streptomycin and chlortetracycline on catalase and certain dehydrogenases of *Escherichia coli* and *Shigella*. Antibiotiki **2**, 21 (1957).

LITTLE, P. A., J. J. OLESON, and J. H. WILLIAMS: Factors influencing the sensitivity of protozoa to antibiotics. Antibiotics & Chemotherapy **3**, 29 (1953).

LOOMIS, W. F.: On the mechanism of action of Aureomycin. Science **111**, 474 (1950).

MALEK, P., J. ROKOS, M. BURGER, J. KOLC, and P. PROCHAZKA: The effect of antibiotics of the teteracycline group on enzymes and the practical clinical significance thereof. In: Antibiotics Ann. **1958/59**, 221 (1959).

MANDLESTAM, J., and H. J. ROGERS: The incorporation of amino acids into the cell-wall mucopeptide of staphylococci and the effect of antibiotics on the process. Biochem. J. **72**, 654 (1959).

MARSH, C. L., and G. W. KELLEY: Studies in helminth enzymology. II. Properties of an inorganic pyrophosphatase from *Ascaridia galli*, a nematode parasite of chickens. Exptl. Parasitol. **8**, 274 (1959).

MCCORMICK, J. R. D., N. O. SJOLANDER, U. HIRSCH, E. R. JENSEN, and A. P. DOERSCHUK: A new family of antibiotics: the demethyltetracyclines. J. Am. Chem. Soc. **79**, 4561 (1957).

MCCORMICK, J. R. D., E. R. JENSEN, P. A. MILLER, and A. P. DOERSCHUK: The 6-deoxytetracyclines: Further studies on the relationship between structure and antibacterial activity in the tetracycline series. J. Am. Chem. Soc. **82**, 3381 (1960).

MCCULLOUGH, N. B., and G. A. BEAL: Antimetabolic action of sulfadiazine and certain antibiotics for brucella. J. Infectious Diseases **90**, 196 (1952).

MELNYKOVYCH, G., and K. R. JOHANSSON: Effects of chlortetracycline on the stability of arginine decarboxylase in *Escherichia coli*. J. Bacteriol. **77**, 638 (1959).

MELNYKOVYCH, G., and E. E. SNELL: Nutritional requirements for the formation of arginine decarboxylase in *Escherichia coli*. J. Bacteriol. **76**, 518 (1958).

MICHEL, M., and A. C. FRANÇOIS: Influence de la chlortétracycline sur les decarboxylase de la flore intestinale du porc. Comp. rend. **242**, 1770 (1956).

MIURA, Y., Y. NAKAMURA, H. MATSUDAIRA, and T. KOMEIJI: The mode of action of Terramycin. Antibiotics & Chemotherapy **2**, 152 (1952).

MIURA, Y., Y. NAKAMURA, Y. YOSHIZAWA, and H. MATSUDAIRA: Comparative studies on the phosphorus metabolism of staphylococci in the presence of chlortetracycline and oxytetracycline. Antibiotics & Chemotherapy **3**, 822 (1953).

MOROZ, A. F., and I. V. SHIBAEVA: The effect of levomycetin and chlortetracycline on the dehydrogenase activity of staphylococci sensitive and resistant to these antibiotics. Antibiotiki **9**, 232 (1964).

MULLI, K., K. UHLENBROOCK u. L. LUDWIG: Zum wirkungsmechanismus des Aureomycin. Arzneimittel-Forsch. **3**, 559 (1953).

NAKAYA, R., and H. P. TREFFERS: The growth rates and adaptive enzyme activities of chloramphenicol- and oxytetracycline-resistant *Escherichia coli*. Antibiotics Ann. **1958/59**, 865 (1959).

NETIEN, G., P. HUTINEL, and O. SOTTY: Action de l'auréomycine et de la terramycine sur la biogénèse de la chlorophylle au cours de la germination. Compt. rend. soc. biol. **146**, 1337 (1952).

NIKOLOV, T. K., and A. T. ILKOV: Effect of chlortetracycline on methionine-^{35}S incorporation into macroorganism proteins. Abstracts of Communications, V. Internat. Congr. Biochem. (Moscow) 1961, p. 44.

NIRENBERG, M., and P. LEDER: RNA codewords and protein synthesis. The effect of trinucleotides upon the binding of sRNA to ribosomes. Science **145**, 1399 (1964).

OKAMATO, S., and D. MIZUNO: Mechanism of chloramphenicol and tetracycline resistance in *Escherichia coli*. J. Gen. Microbiol. **35**, 125 (1964).

OLITZKI, A. L.: Hydrogen sulfide production by non-multiplying organisms and its inhibition by antibiotics. J. Gen. Microbiol. **11**, 160 (1954).

OSTEUX, R., et J. LATURAZE: Mode d'action des antibiotiques: Antagonisme entre le groupe auréomycin-chloromycétine-terramycine et la biotine chez *Clostridium welchii*. Compt. rend. **234**, 677 (1952).

OSTEUX, R., J. LATURAZE et J. BÜRCK: Action inhibitrice de l'auréomycine sur la respiration bactérienne et l'oxydation des acides du cycle citrique. Compt. rend. **235**, 554 (1952).

PANSY, F. E., P. KAHN, J. F. PAGANO, and R. DONOVICK: The relationship between Aureomycin, chloramphenicol and Terramycin. Proc. Soc. Exptl. Biol. Med. **75**, 618 (1950).

PARK, J. T.: Inhibition of cell-wall synthesis in *Staphylococcus aureus* by chemicals which cause accumulation of wall precursors. Biochem. J. **70**, 2P (1958).

PORFIRIEVA, R. P.: The influence of chlortetracycline on urea formation in the liver. Antibiotiki **6**, 127 (1961).

PORRO, A., e SONCIN: Antibiotici e ossidazione dell'acido acetacetico prodotta dall' *E. coli*. Arch. intern. pharmacodynamie **95**, 64 (1953a).

PORRO, A., e E. SONCIN: Antibiotici e ossidazione dell'acido acetoacetico prodotta dai tessuti. Arch. intern. pharmacodynamie **95**, 497 (1953b).

PORRO, A., e E. SONCIN: Azione di alcuni antibiotici sul metabolismo dell'acido glutammico nell'*E. coli*. Arch. intern. pharmacodynamie **99**, 481 (1954).

PRICE, K. E., Z. ZOLLI, JR., J. C. ATKINSON, and H. G. LUTHER: Antibiotic antagonists. I. The effect of certain milk constituents. Antibiotics & Chemotherapy **7**, 672 (1957a).

PRICE, K. E., Z. ZOLLI, JR., J. C. ATKINSON, and H. G. LUTHER: Antibiotic antagonists. II. Mode of inhibitory action of divalent cations for oxytetracycline. Antibiotics & Chemotherapy **7**, 689 (1957b).

REEDY, R. J., W. A. RANDALL, and H. WELCH: Variations in the antimicrobial activity of the tetracyclines. II. Antibiotics & Chemotherapy **5**, 115 (1955).

REGE, D. V., and A. SREENIVASAN: Influence of folic acid and vitamin B_{12} on the impairment of nucleic acid synthesis in *Lactobacillus casei* by Aureomycin. Nature **173**, 728 (1954).

REGNA, P. P., I. A. SOLOMONS, K. MURAI, A. E. TIMRECK, K. J. BRUNINGS, and W. A. LAZIER: The isolation and general properties of Terramycin and Terramycin salts. J. Am. Chem. Soc. **73**, 4211 (1951).

RENDI, R., and S. OCHOA: Enzyme specificity in activation and transfer of amino acids to ribonucleoprotein particles. Science **133**, 1367 (1961).

RENDI, R., and S. OCHOA: Effect of chloramphenicol on protein synthesis in cell-free preparations of *Escherichia coli*. J. Biol. Chem. **237**, 3711 (1962).

ROKOS, J., M. BURGER, and P. PROCHÁZKA: Effect of calcium ions on the inhibition of hydrolases by chlortetracycline. Nature **181**, 1201 (1958).

ROKOS, J., M. BURGER, and P. PROCHÁZKA: Effect of chlortetracycline on the activity of α-amylases. Antibiotiki **4**, 3 (1959a).

ROKOS, J., P. MÁLEK, M. BURGER, P. PROCHÁZKA, and J. KOLC: The effect of divalent metals on the inhibition of pancreatic lipase by chlortetracycline. Antibiotics & Chemotherapy **9**, 600 (1959b).

SAKAGUCHI, G., S. SAKAGUCHI, T. KAWABATA, Y. NAKAMURA, T. AKANO, and K. SHIROMIZU: Influence of oxytetracycline upon the toxin production of type *E Clostridium botulinum*. Japan J. Med. Sci. & Biol. **13**, 13 (1960).

SAZ, A. K., and J. MARMUR: The inhibition of organic nitro-reductase by Aureomycin in cell-free extracts. Proc. Soc. Exptl. Biol. Med. **82**, 783 (1953).

SAZ, A. K., and L. M. MARTINEZ: Enzymatic basis of resistance to Aureomycin. I. Differences between flavoprotein nitro reductase of sensitive and resistant *Escherichia coli*. J. Biol. Chem. **223**, 285 (1956).

SAZ, A. K., and L. M. MARTINEZ: Enzymatic basis of resistance to Aureomycin. II. Inhibition of electron transport in *Escherichia coli* by Aureomycin. J. Biol. Chem. **233**, 1020 (1958).

SAZ, A. K., and R. B. SLIE: Inhibition of organic nitro reductase by chlortetracycline in bacterial cell-free extracts. Antibiotics Ann. **1953/54**, 303 (1953a).

SAZ, A. K., and R. B. SLIE: Manganese reversal of Aureomycin inhibition of bacterial cell-free nitro-reductase. J. Am. Chem. Soc. **75**, 4626 (1953b).

SAZ, A. K., and R. B. SLIE: The inhibition of organic nitro-reductase by Aureomycin in cell-free extracts. II. Cofactor requirements for the nitro-reductase enzyme complex. Arch. Biochem. Biophys. **51**, 5 (1954a).

SAZ, A. K., and R. B. SLIE: Reversal of Aureomycin inhibition of bacterial cell-free nitro reductase by manganese. J. Biol. Chem. **210**, 407 (1954b).

SAZ, A. K., L. W. BROWNELL, and R. B. SLIE: Aureomycin-resistant cell-free nitroreductase from aureomycin-resistant *Escherichia coli*. J. Bacteriol. **71**, 421 (1956).

SHAHANI, K. M.: Carbohydrate and pyruvate metabolism of oxytetracycline-sensitive and oxytetracycline-resistant organisms. Antibiotics Ann. **1956/57**, 523 (1957).
SHILS, M. E.: Some metabolic aspects of tetracyclines. Clin. Pharmacol. Therap. **3**, 321 (1962).
SLOANE, N. H.: Biological activity of a metabolite of *p*-aminobenzoic acid (PABA) in a hydroxylating system. J. Am. Chem. Soc. **75**, 6352 (1953).
SNELL, J. F., and L. CHENG: Studies in metabolic spectra. II. Application of metabolic spectra to the investigation of the mode of action of oxytetracycline. Antibiotics Ann. **1957/58**, 538 (1958).
SNELL, J. F., and L. CHENG: Studies in metabolic spectra. III. The accumulation of D-glutamic acid in oxytetracycline-treated *Escherichia coli*. Antibiotics & Chemotherapy **9**, 159 (1959).
SNELL, J. F., and L. CHENG: Studies on modes of action of tetracycline. (II). Develop. Ind. Microbiol. **2**, 107 (1961).
SNELL, J. F., F. Z. THANASSI, and D. A. SYPOWICZ: Studies in metabolic spectra. I. Mode of action of tetracycline antibiotics. Antibiotics & Chemotherapy **8**, 57 (1958).
SONCIN, E.: Fenomeni di interferenza tra elettroliti e antibiotici. III. Ione magnesio e aureomycina, terramicina, chloramfenicolo. Arch. intern. pharmacodynamie **94**, 346 (1953).
SPECTOR, W. S. (ed.): Handbook of toxicology. Philadelphia: W. B. Saunders Co. 1957.
SRIKANTAN, T. N., S. C. AGARWALA, and D. L. SHRIVASTAVA: Studies in the enzyme make-up of *Pasteurella pestis*. III. Oxidative metabolism of virulent and avirulent strains. Indian J. Med. Research **45**, 151 (1957).
SRIKANTAN, T. N., C. R. KRISHNA MURTI, and D. L. SHRIVASTAVA: Studies on the enzyme make-up of *Pasteurella pestis*. VI. Aldolase activity of virulent and avirulent strains. Indian J. Med. Research **46**, 1 (1958).
STANECKI, J., J. FAST, and T. KRZYWY: Inactivation of the bacteriostatic action of chlortetracycline by substances produced by bacterial metabolism. Antibiotics & Chemotherapy **8**, 167 (1958).
STEPHENS, C. R., K. MURAI, K. J. BRUNINGS, and R. B. WOODWARD: Acidity constants of the tetracycline antibiotics. J. Am. Chem. Soc. **78**, 4155 (1956).
SUAREZ, G., and D. NATHANS: Inhibition of aminoacyl-sRNA binding to ribosomes by tetracycline. Biochem. Biophys. Research Commun. **18**, 750 (1965).
TANNER, J.: Contribution a l'étude de l'action des antibiotiques sur l'immunité. Action de la tetracycline sur les antigènes de *Salmonella* typhi. Ann. inst. Pasteur **98**, 772 (1960).
TRAUT, R. R., and R. E. MONRO: The puromycin reaction and its relation to protein synthesis. J. Mol. Biol. **10** 63 (1964).
UMBREIT, W. W.: Mechanisms of antibacterial action. Pharmacol. Revs **5**, 275 (1953).
VAN METER, J. C., and J. J. OLESON: Effect of Aureomycin on the respiration of normal rat liver homogenates. Science **113**, 273 (1951).
VAN METER, J. C., A. SPECTOR, J. J. OLESON, and J. H. WILLIAMS: *In vitro* action of Aureomycin on oxidative phosphorylation in animal tissues. Proc. Soc. Exptl. Biol. Med. **81**, 215 (1952).
VAZQUEZ, D.: Antibiotics which effect protein synthesis: The up-take of ^{14}C-chloramphenicol by bacteria. Biochem. Biophys. Research Commun. **12**, 409 (1963).
VAZQUEZ, D.: The binding of chloramphenicol by ribosomes from *Bacillus megaterium*. Biochem. Biophys. Research Commun. **15**, 464 (1964).
VINTER, V.: Spores of microorganisms. X. Interference of tetracycline antibiotics with sporogenesis of bacilli. Folia Microbiol. **7**, 275 (1962).
VONK, M. A., L. W. MCELROY, and R. T. BERG: The effect of ingested chlortetracycline on some hydrolases and organs associated with the digestive process in growing pigs. I. Assay methods for protease, amylase, and cellulase activity. Can. J. Biochem. and Physiol. **35**, 181 (1957).
VYSHEPAN, E. D., and V. S. ZUEVA: The effect of chlortetracycline on the enzymatic hydrolysis of adenosinetriphosphoric acid. Biokhimiya **24**, 833 (1959).

WAGNER, W. H.: Über den hemmenden Einfluß von Aureomycin auf den oxydativen Abbau aromatischer Substanzen durch saprophytare Mycobakterien. Naturwissenschaften **22**, 525 (1950).
WAKSMAN, S. A., and H. LECHEVALIER: Modes of action of antibiotics. In: *The actinomycetes*, vol. 3. Baltimore: Williams & Wilkins Co. 1962.
WARNER, J. R., and A. RICH: The number of soluble RNA molecules on reticulocyte ribosomes. Proc. Nat. Acad. Sci. U.S. **51**, 1134 (1964).
WATANABE, T., and T. FUKASAWA: Episome-mediated transfer of drug resistance in *Enterobacteriaceae*. I. Transfer of resistance factors by conjugation. J. Bacteriol. **81**, 669 (1961).
WEIL, A. J.: Inhibition of pigment formation of *Serratia marcescens* by chloramphenicol, Aureomycin and Terramycin. Proc. Soc. Exptl. Biol. Med. **79**, 539 (1952).
WEINBERG, E. D.: The reversal of the toxicity of oxytetracycline (Terramycin) by multivalent cations. J. Infectious Diseases **95**, 291 (1954a).
WEINBERG, E. D.: The influence of inorganic salts on the activity *in vitro* of oxytetracycline. Antibiotics & Chemotherapy **4**, 35 (1954b).
WEINBERG, E. D.: The effect of Mn^{++} and antimicrobial drugs on sporulation of *Bacillus subtilis* in nutrient broth. J. Bacteriol. **70**, 289 (1955a).
WEINBERG, E. D.: Futher studies on metallic ion reversal of oxytetracycline; reactivation of drug-inactivated cells by Mg^{++}. Antibiotics Ann. **1954/55**, 169 (1955b).
WEINBERG, E. D.: The mutual effects of antimicrobial compounds and metallic cations. Bacteriol. Rev. **21**, 46 (1957).
WEISBERGER, A. S., S. WOLFE, and S. ARMENTROUT: Inhibition of protein synthesis in mammalian cell-free systems by chloramphenicol. J. Exptl. Med. **120**, 161 (1964).
WELCH, H., W. A. RANDALL, R. J. REEDY, and E. J. OSWALD: Variations in antimicrobial activity of the tetracyclines. Antibiotics & Chemotherapy **4**, 741 (1954).
WOLFE, A. D., and F. E. HAHN: Influence of inhibitors of protein synthesis on the messenger-directed binding of amino acyl-s-RNA to ribosomes. Federation Proc. **24**, 217 (1965a).
WOLFE, A. D., and F. E. HAHN: Mode of action of chloramphenicol. IX. Effects of chloramphenicol upon a ribosomal amino acid polymerization system and its binding to bacterial ribosomes. Biochim. et Biophys. Acta **95**, 146 (1965b).
WONG, D. T. O., S. BARBAN, and S. J. AJL: Inhibition of respiration by Aureomycin and Terramycin. Antibiotics & Chemotherapy **3**, 607 (1953).
WRIGHT, S. S., and M. FINLAND: Cross-resistance among three tetracyclines. Proc. Soc. Exptl. Biol. Med. **85**, 40 (1954).
YAGI, K., J. OKUDA, T. OZAWA, and K. OKADA: Inhibitory mechanism of chlortetracycline on D-amino acid oxidase. Science **124**, 273 (1956).
YAGI, K., J. OKUDA, T. OZAWA, and K. OKADA: Mechanism of inhibition of D-amino acid oxidase. I. Inhibitory action of chlortetracycline. Biochim. et Biophys. Acta **34**, 372 (1959).
YEE, R. B., and H. M. GEZON: Ribonucleic acid of chloramphenicol-treated *Shigella flexneri*. J. Gen. Microbiol. **32**, 299 (1963).
YEE, R. B., S. F. PAN, and H. M. GEZON: Studies on the metabolism of *Shigella*. III. The inhibition of the oxidation of glutamate by Aureomycin. J. Bacteriol. **75**, 56 (1958).
YOKOTA, T., and T. AKIBA: Studies on the mechanism of transfer of drug resistance in bacteria. 22. Influence of chloramphenicol and tetracycline on the ^{14}C-amino acid incorporation by ribosomes isolated from the drug sensitive and multiple resistant strain of *E. coli*. Med. and Biol. (Japan) **64**, 9 (1962a).
YOKATA, T., and T. AKIBA: Studies on the mechanism of transfer of drug resistance in bacteria. 23. Mechanisms of the antibacterial action of tetracycline and the tetracycline resistance in the artificial, TC-resistant strain of *E. coli*. Med. and Biol. (Japan) **64**, 39 (1962b).
YOUNATHAN, E. S., and S. S. BARKULIS: Effect of some antimetabolites on the production of streptolysin S'. J. Bacteriol. **74**, 151 (1957).
ZIMMERMAN, H. J., and F. L. HUMOLLER: Effect of Aureomycin on choline oxidase and other enzyme systems of rat liver. Am. J. Physiol. **175**, 468 (1953).

Tenuazonic Acid

Harold T. Shigeura

While investigating the metabolic products of *Alternaria tenuis* Auct, ROSETT *et al.* (1957) observed that a fraction from the culture filtrate gave a strong orange-red ferric chloride color. The material which was very soluble in organic solvent was ketonic and acidic in nature. Its rotation $[\alpha]_{5461}^{19^\circ}$ in methanol was —124°. Analysis of the compound indicated the molecular formula $C_{10}H_{15}O_2N$. On long standing, the rotation of the product slowly became less negative, and the substance eventually crystallized. The purified crystalline substance also corresponded to the formula $C_{10}H_{15}O_2N$ and had very similar chemical properties to the original material. However, it was found to be dextrorotatory, $[\alpha]_{5461}^{22^\circ} +23°$. The name of tenuazonic acid was proposed for the metabolic product and iso-tenuazonic acid for the isomer. Tenuazonic acid titrated sharply as a monobasic acid, contained no methoxyl group and formed a semicarbazone, m.p. 187—189° and was found to be converted into the iso-acid by boiling with aqueous alkali.

Subsequently, STICKINGS (1959) made a detailed study of the structure of tenuazonic acid and concluded that the substance was 3-acetyl-5-*sec*-butyl-tetramic acid (I) with the configuration about the two asymmetric centers corresponding to that in L-isoleucine. Tenuazonic acid is believed to be the first substituted tetramic acid isolated from natural sources.

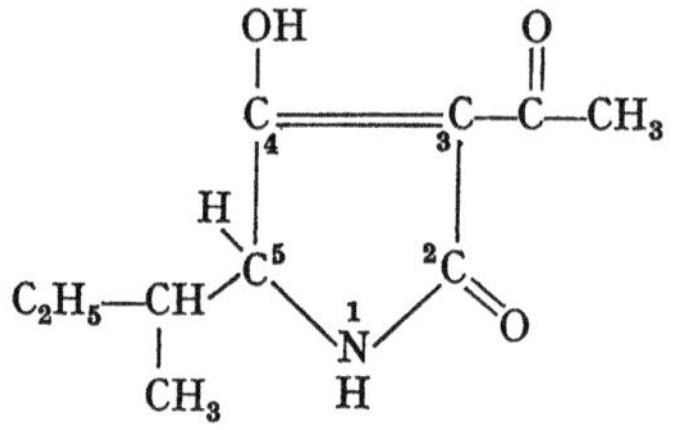

(I)

The structure of tenuazonic acid has recently been verified by total synthesis from L-isoleucine and diketene (HARRIS *et al.*, 1965).

In 1964, GITTERMAN *et al.* reported that the fermentation broth of *Alternaria tenuis* Auct inhibited the growth of human adenocarcinoma (H. Ad. #1) growing in the embryonated egg. With the aid of this assay system, the isolation of the active substance from the broth was reported by KACZKA *et al.* (1964). The filtered fermentation broth was acidified to pH 1—2 and extracted with ethyl acetate. The ethyl acetate solution was extracted with 5% sodium bicarbonate. After acidification to pH 2, the sodium bicarbonate solution was extracted with petroleum ether (30—60°).

The solvent residue was dissolved in Skellysolve B and N,N′-dibenzylethylenediamine (DBED) was added until there was no further precipitation. The oily precipitate was dissolved in acetone and crystallized by the addition of benzene. Titration of the acid with aqueous $NaHCO_3$ and lyophilization of the solution gave a monosodium salt. The material was identified as tenuazonic acid by microanalytical tests, and ultraviolet and infrared absorption measurements and was indistinguishable from authentic tenuazonic acid supplied by Dr. C. E. STICKINGS.

Tenuazonic acid has also been found to be synthesized by *Aspergillus tamarii* and a member of the Sphaeropsidales.

Metabolic Activities of Tenuazonic Acid

GITTERMAN *et al.* (1964) reported that tenuazonic acid at a dosage of 0.25 mg/egg inhibited the growth of human adenocarcinoma growing in the embryonated egg. In this system, it was found that tenuazonic acid was 20 times as active as hadacidin or 6-mercaptopurine, 2 times as active as azaserine and 1/20 as active as triethylene melamine. The substance, however, was only slightly active against human tumor A-42 growing in the embryonated egg and KB cells in culture. It had no effect on Sarcoma 180 in the mouse.

Tenuazonic acid was active against the following animal tumors *in vivo* (mg/kg/day): Ridgeway osteogenic sarcoma (100—200), carcinoma 1025 (100 to 200), Ehrlich ascites carcinoma (50—100) and Friend virus leukemia (50—100) (Personal Communication from K. Sugiura, quoted in paper of GITTERMAN *et al.*, 1964).

The first indication on the mode of action of tenuazonic acid was obtained in experiments using radioactive amino acids (SHIGEURA and GORDON, 1963). Fasted male Sprague-Dawley rats weighing 100—110 g were injected intraperitoneally with tenuazonic acid at a dosage of 500 mg/kg and a labeled amino acid. After 60 minutes, the total proteins were obtained from liver, spleen, thymus and intestinal mucosa and purified. Under these conditions, it was found that the incorporation of glycine-U-^{14}C into the proteins of these organs was inhibited by 93, 89, 90 and 92%, respectively. When L-lysine-^{14}C was used as the labeled precursor, the per cent inhibition of protein synthesis in the corresponding organs was 67, 52, 64 and 65%, respectively.

When experiments were done with suspensions of Ehrlich ascites cells, it was observed that at 2.4 mM tenuazonic acid, the incorporation of ^{14}C-labeled glycine, formate, L-leucine, L-phenylalanine, L-lysine and L-valine into total proteins was inhibited by 50—80%. These results suggested that the antibiotic acted as an inhibitor of a reaction in the protein synthetic process common to all the precursors rather than as an antagonist of a single amino acid. With cell-free systems of ascites cells, tenuazonic acid at 0.8 mM inhibited the incorporation of both L-leucine and L-valine into proteins by about 60%.

Since tenuazonic acid was found to inhibit the over-all proteosynthetic process in Ehrlich ascites and rat liver cells, a detailed study was undertaken to determine the specific locus of action of the antibiotic. When the pH 5 precipitates of the 12,000 × g supernatant fluids of Ehrlich ascites and rat liver cells were incubated with labeled amino acids, a source of energy, and varying concentrations of tenuazonic acid, it was observed that the antibiotic at concentrations that were previously found to inhibit amino acid incorporation into microsomes did not suppress the formation of aminoacyl-soluble RNA. On the contrary, addition of tenuazonic acid resulted in slight but noticeable increases in the specific activities of aminoacyl-soluble RNA. It was also concluded from these results that the generation of high energy phosphate bonds and subsequent activation of amino acids with ATP to form aminoacyl-AMP were not affected by the antibiotic. The results, therefore, implicated the site of action of tenuazonic acid to be at a stage subsequent to the formation of aminoacyl-soluble RNA.

The effect of tenuazonic acid on amino acid transfer from ^{14}C-leucine-labeled pH 5 precipitate to microsomes was next studied. When the pH 5 precipitate containing labeled aminoacyl-soluble RNA was incubated with microsomes and varying concentrations of the antibiotic, it was observed that the transfer of lebeled amino acid to microsomes was partially inhibited. However, the per cent inhibition was reduced only to approximately one-half of that obtained with whole cells and crude cell-free extracts.

Because of these results, further studies on the effect of tenuazonate on this reaction were made by using purified ribonucleoprotein particles or ribosomes instead of microsomes. It was found that the markedly inhibitory effect of tenuazonate on amino acid incorporation into microsomes observed earlier with crude systems appeared to decrease upon further purification of the system. The results suggested that the pathway involving the incorporation of amino acids into ribosomal proteins was not the major site of action of tenuazonic acid.

The effect of tenuazonic acid on the release *in vitro* of labeled proteins of Ehrlich ascites microsome into the supernatant fluid was next examined. In the presence of the antibiotic, the energy-dependent release of proteins from the microsomes into the supernatant fluid was inhibited. Puromycin has been reported to stimulate the release of newly formed proteins and peptides from prelabeled ribosomes obtained from various sources (MORRIS and SCHWEET, 1961; LAMBERG, 1962; ALLEN and ZAMECNIK, 1962). The comparative effects of tenuazonic acid and puromycin on the microsomal protein releasing activity in ascites cells was studied. As shown in Fig. 1, in the presence of puromycin, the specific activity of microsomes dropped precipitously after a few minutes of incubation. Tenuazonic acid, on the other hand, inhibited the release of proteins. Thus, the principal site of action of the antibiotic appeared to be related to the release of newly formed proteins from the microsomes into the cell sap. It is conceivable that microsomes prevented from releasing newly synthesized proteins would be unable to accept amino acids from transfer RNA. Such a situation may explain the inhibition of amino acid incorporation into microsomal proteins observed with crude cell extracts and the increase in specific activity of soluble RNA with increasing concentration of tenuazonic acid.

A striking difference in the activities of tenuazonic acid and puromycin was subsequently observed with whole cells (GITTERMAN *et al.*, 1964). As indicated before, tenuazonic acid inhibited the growth of human adenocarcinoma #1 with an ED_{60} value of 225 μg/egg. Under these conditions, tenuazonic acid appeared to be without toxic effects on the embryo. On the other hand, puromycin did not affect the tumor even at concentrations that resulted in high embryo mortality. Similar studies with other normal and tumor cells have not yet been done.

Tenuazonic acid at a concentration of 0.3 mM inhibited the incorporation of leucine-^{14}C into ferritin and haemoglobin by 70 to 80% (MATIOLI and EYLAR, 1964). From these experiments, the authors concluded that ferritin was synthesized by erythropoietic cells.

MILLER *et al.* (1963) reported that tenuazonic acid at comparatively high concentrations showed antiviral activity. The substance was active against enteroviruses (poliovirus MEF-1, ECHO-9, Coxsackie B_1), respiratory virus (parainfluenza-3, Salisbury HGP), vaccinia, herpes simplex HF and „B" virus. It was inactive in tissue culture against polyoma virus and in the mouse against Asian influenza, rabies and Friend leukemia virus. It is interesting to note that tenuazonic acid was inactive against 31 strains of bacteria, 48 strains of yeast and *Trichomonas vaginalis in vitro.* It was, however, active against *Entamoeba histolytica in vitro.*

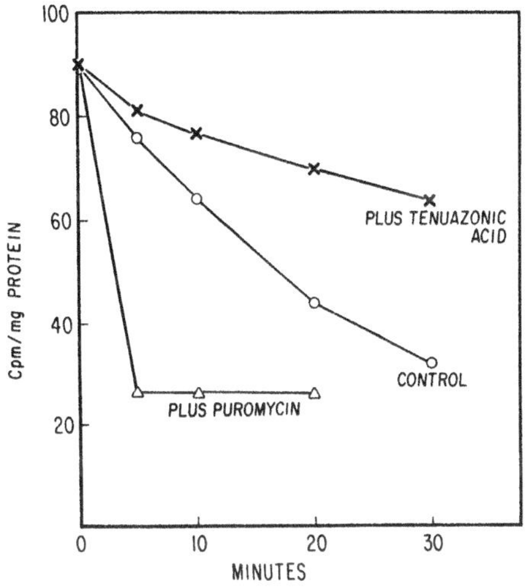

Fig. 1. Microsomes prelabeled with L-leucine-^{14}C and suspended in unlabeled 105,000×g supernatant fluid was incubated with 75 μmoles of PGA, 8 μmoles of ATP and 13 μmoles of tenuazonic acid or 1.5 μmoles of puromycin in a total volume of 7.6 ml. Aliquots were removed at specified intervals and microsomes were separated and measured for radioactivity.

Congeners of Tenuazonic Acid

A large number of tetramic acids (Table 1) with various substituents at the 1, 3 and 5 positions have been synthesized and reported by HARRIS *et al.* (1965). At a concentration of 2 mM, none of the synthetic compounds was as active as tenuazonic acid in inhibiting the incorporation of L-leucine-U-^{14}C into proteins in whole ascites cells (SHIGEURA and GORDON, unpublished observations).

GITTERMAN (1965) examined the antitumor activity of these congeners of tenuazonic acid against human adenocarcinoma growing in the embryonated egg. Compounds substituted at the C-5 position had less than 5% of the antitumor activity of tenuazonic acid while N-methyl substituted 3-acetyl-5-*sec*-butyl-tetramate was 15% as active. Other substitutions at N-1 and C-3 positions resulted in compounds that were not active against H.Ad. #1. The cytotoxic activities of the C-5 substituted tetramates against KB cells correlated with antitumor activities in the egg system. None of the compounds was as active as tenuazonic acid (ED_{60} = 126 μg/egg) in either H.Ad. #1 or KB systems.

GITTERMAN (1965), however, found that several of the N-substituted tetramates were considerably more active than tenuazonic acid against *Bacillus megaterium.* The results suggested that in this system, the N-substituted tetramates may be acting on processes other than protein synthesis. The inactivity of tenuazonic acid against several strains of bacteria and yeast offers an opportunity to study the possible differences in the over-all proteosynthetic process of mammalian and microbial cells. Since microbial cells are essentially devoid of endoplasmic reticulum, the likelihood that the action of tenuazonic acid on protein synthesis is related to the function of membranes is suggested by the results. Furthermore, the observation that the congeners of tenuazonic acid were inactive indicated the highly specific structural requirement for inhibition of release of newly-synthesized microsomal proteins.

Table 1. *Effect of congeneric tetramic acids on the incorporation of L-leucine-^{14}C into proteins in whole Ehrlich ascites cells*

Congeneric tetramic acids	% Inh.[1]
3-Acetyl tetramic acid	12
3-Acetyl-5-methyl tetramic acid	11
3-Acetyl-5-ethyl tetramic acid	16
3-Acetyl-5,5-dimethyl tetramic acid	0
3-Acetyl-5-isopropyl tetramic acid	0
3-Acetyl-5-N-butyl tetramic acid	0
D-allo tenuazonic acid	9
3-Acetyl-5-tertbutyl tetramic acid	0
3-Acetyl-5-isobutyl tetramic acid	9
3-Acetyl-5-N-pentyl tetramic acid	0
3-Acetyl-5-phenyl tetramic acid	7
3-Acetyl-5-spirotetramethylene tetramic acid	0
3-Acetyl-1,5-trimethylene tetramic acid	0
3-Acetyl-N-methyl tenuazonic acid	0
3-Acetyl-N-benzyl tenuazonic acid	0
3-Acetyl-5-(1-ethylpropyl)-N-benzyl tetramic acid	0

[1] Per cent inhibition of L-leucine-U-^{14}C incorporation into total proteins in intact Ehrlich ascites cells. Under these conditions, the per cent inhibition by 1 mM tenuazonic acid was 70%.

Concentration of substituted tetramic acid was 2 mM.

Summary

Tenuazonic acid (3-acetyl-5-*sec*-butyltetramic acid), isolated from the culture filtrate of *Alternaria tenuis* Auct., inhibited the growth of a number of human and rodent tumors. The principal site of action of this antibiotic in mammalian cells appeared to be related to the suppression of protein synthesis; more precisely, the inhibition of release of nascent proteins from the microsomes into the cell sap. The compound, was inactive against several species of bacteria and yeast. Tenuazonic acid appeared to have no direct effect on nucleic acid synthesis.

References

ALLEN, D. W., and P. C. ZAMECNIK: The effect of puromycin on rabbit reticulocyte ribosomes. Biochim. et Biophys. Acta **55**, 865 (1962).

GITTERMAN, C. O.: Antitumor, cytotoxic and antibacterial activities of tenuazonic acid and congeneric tetramic acids. J. Med. Chem. **8**, 483 (1965).

GITTERMAN, C. O.. E. L. DULANEY, E. A. KACZKA, G. W. CAMPBELL, D. HENDLIN, and H. B. WOODRUFF: The human tumor-egg host system. III. Tumor-inhibitory properties of tenuazonic acid. Cancer Research **24**, 440 (1964).

HARRIS, S. A., L. V. FISHER, and K. FOLKERS: The synthesis of tenuazonic acid and congeneric tetramic acids. J. Med. Chem. **8**, 478 (1965).
KACZKA, E. A., C. O. GITTERMAN, E. L. DULANEY, M. C. SMITH, D. HENDLIN, H. B. WOODRUFF, and K. FOLKERS: Discovery of inhibitory activity of tenuazonic acid for growth of human adenocarcinoma-1. Biochem. Biophys. Research. Commun. **14**, 54 (1964).
LAMBERG, M. R.: The *in vitro* release of protein from *Escherichia coli* ribosomes. Biochim. et Biophys. Acta **55**, 719 (1962).
MATIOLI, G. T., and E. H. EYLAR: The biosynthesis of apoferritin by reticulocytes. Proc. Natl. Acad. Sci. U.S. **52**, 508 (1964).
MILLER, F. A., W. A. RIGHTSEL, B. J. SLOAN, J. EHRLICH, J. C. FRENCH, and Q. R. BARTZ: Antiviral activity of tenuazonic acid. Nature **200**, 1338 (1963).
MORRIS, A. J., and R. S. SCHWEET: Release of soluble protein from reticulocyte ribosomes. Biochim. et Biophys. Acta **47**, 415 (1961).
ROSETT, T., R. H. SANKHALA, C. E. STICKINGS, M. E. U. TAYLOR, and R. THOMAS: Studies in the biochemistry of micro-organisms. 103. Metabolites of *Alternaria tenuis* Auct.: Culture filtrate products. Biochem. J. **67**, 390 (1957).
SHIGEURA, H. T., and C. N. GORDON: The biological activity of tenuazonic acid. Biochemistry **2**, 1132 (1963).
STICKINGS, C. E.: Studies in the Biochemistry of Micro-organisms. 106. Metabolites of *Alternaria tenuis* Auct.: The structure of tenuazonic acid. Biochem. J. **72**, 332 (1959).

Macrolide antibiotics — Spiramycin, Carbomycin, Angolamycin, Methymycin and Lancamycin

D. Vazquez

Introduction

The term macrolide has been applied to members of a group of structurally related antibiotics produced by species of streptomyces. All macrolide antibiotics (Woodward, 1957) contain a large lactone ring (aglycone of 12 to 22 atoms) which contain few double bonds and no nitrogen atoms; they have one or more sugars which can be amino sugars, non-nitrogenous sugars or both. In the widest sense however, the term macrolide has been ascribed to all the antibiotics containing a large lactone ring; in this sense the polyene antibiotic and antibiotics of streptogramin A and streptogramin B groups can be also termed macrolides. This article will be restricted to the "classical" macrolides of Woodward (1957) and related compounds discovered after 1957.

In 1950 Brockmann and Henkel described the isolation of picromycin the first known macrolide antibiotic. Since then, more than thirty antibiotics, classified as macrolides or suspected macrolides have discovered. Many of the streptomyces species which produce macrolide antibiotics produce two ore more of these compounds which are usually distinguished for purposes of nomenclature by the addition of letters or figures to the name of the original complex antibiotic, e.g. erythromycin A, B and C. In many cases the chemical structures are not yet known and only in the case of oleandomycin is the complete configuration known (Celmer, 1965a). The best known macrolides are shown in Table 1. Where the sugar configuration has not been determined, the configuration given in Table 1 is that predicted by Celmer (1965b, c) on the basis of his model for the macrolides.

The macrolide antibiotics have been considered as a homogeneous group of compounds. Their chemical compositions are related and their antibacterial spectra are similar. All macrolides are preferentially active against Gram-positive bacteria and cross resistance between different macrolides has been reported. However some of them differ in certain chemical and physical properties; thus most of the macrolide antibiotics are basic substances but some are neutral compounds; some are fairly soluble in water whereas others are very insoluble in water but soluble in ethanol. These differences between the macrolides are reflected in their modes of action which will be discussed later in this chapter.

Three of the macrolide antibiotics (erythromycin, spiramycin and oleandomycin) have been used clinically and also as supplements in animal feeding. Tylosin is used in preservation of food and also as supplement in animal feeding.

Table 1. *The macrolide group of antibiotics*

Antibiotic	Formula	Lactone ring atoms	Sugars components: Amino sugars	Sugars components: Non-nitrogenous sugars	References
Angolamycin	$C_{50}H_{89}O_{18}N$	Unknown	Unknown	Unknown	CORBAZ *et al.* (1955)
Carbomycin A	$C_{42}H_{67}O_{16}N$	17	β-D-Mycaminose	α-L-Mycarose	WOODWARD (1957)
Carbomycin B	$C_{42}H_{67}O_{15}N$	17	β-D-Mycaminose[1]	α-L-Mycarose[1]	WOODWARD (1957)
Chalcomycin	$C_{35}H_{56}O_{14}$	16	None	β-D-Mycinose and β-D-Chalcose	see JORDAN, chapter
Erythromycin A	$C_{37}H_{67}O_{13}N$	14	β-D-Desosamine	α-L-Cladinose	see HAHN, chapter
Erythromycin B	$C_{37}H_{67}O_{12}N$	14	β-D-Desosamine	α-L-Cladinose	see HAHN, chapter
Erythromycin C	$C_{36}H_{65}O_{13}N$	14	β-D-Desosamine[1]	α-L-Cladinose[1]	see HAHN, chapter
Lancamycin	$C_{42}H_{72}O_{16}$	14	None	β-D-Chalcose and 4-O-Acetyl-L-arcanose	GÄUMANN *et al.* (1960)
Leucomycin A_1	$C_{46}H_{81}O_{17}N$	22	β-D-Mycaminose[1]	α-L-Mycarose[1]	WATANABE *et al.* (1960); WATANABE (1961)
Macrocin	$C_{46}H_{79}O_{17}N$	18	β-D-Mycaminose[1]	α-L-Mycarose[1] and another one	HAMILL and STARK (1964)
Methymycin	$C_{25}H_{43}O_{7}N$	12	β-D-Desosamine[1]	None	DJERASSI and ZDERIC (1956)
Narbomycin	$C_{28}H_{47}O_{7}N$	14	β-D-Desosamine	None	PRELOG *et al.* (1962)
Neomethymycin	$C_{25}H_{43}O_{7}N$	12	β-D-Desosamine[1]	None	DJERASSI and HALPERN (1958)
Niddamycin	$C_{40}H_{65}O_{14}N$	17	β-D-Mycaminose[1]	α-L-Mycarose[1]	UMEZAWA (1964)
Oleandomycin	$C_{35}H_{61}O_{12}N$	14	β-D-Desosamine	α-L-Oleandrose	see HAHN, chapter
Picromycin	$C_{25}H_{43}O_{7}N$	12	β-D-Desosamine[1]	None	ANLIKER and GUBLER (1957); BROCKMANN and OSTER (1957)
Relomycin	$C_{45}H_{79}O_{17}N$	18	β-D-Mycaminose[1]	α-L-Mycarose[1] and another one	UMEZAWA (1964)
Spiramycin I	$C_{45}H_{76}O_{15}N_2$	19	β-D-Mycaminose[1] and isomycamine	α-L-Mycarose[1]	PAUL and TCHELITCHEFF (1965)
Spiramycin II	$C_{47}H_{78}O_{16}N_2$	19	β-D-Mycaminose and isomycamine	α-L-Mycarose	PAUL and TCHELITCHEFF (1965)
Spiramycin III	$C_{48}H_{80}O_{16}N_2$	19	β-D-Mycaminose and isomycamine	α-L-Mycarose	PAUL and TCHELITCHEFF (1965)
Tylosin	$C_{45}H_{77}O_{17}N$	18	β-D-Mycaminose[1]	α-L-Mycarose[1] and β-D-Mycinose	MORIN and GORMAN (1964)

[1] Configuration predicted on the basis of the model of CELMER (1965b, 1965c) for the macrolide antibiotics.

Dr. F. E. HAHN describes the mode of action of erythromycin and oleandomycin. Dr. D. C. JORDAN writes independently on the mode of action of chalchomycin. Spiramycin, carbomycin, methymycin, angolamycin and lancamycin[1] will be considered in this chapter.

Spiramycin

The antibiotic complex spiramycin is produced by a species of streptomyces now classified as *Streptomyces ambofaciens* (PINNERT-SINDICO *et al.*, 1954/55). Synonyms for spiramycin are: rovamycin, sequamycin, selectomycin, 5337 R.P., and provamycin. Spiramycin is basic, slightly soluble in water, and soluble in most organic solvents. Three difference components can be separated from the complex by countercurrent distribution: spiramycin I, spiramycin II and spiramycin III (Fig. 1). These components are basic but form salts which are very soluble

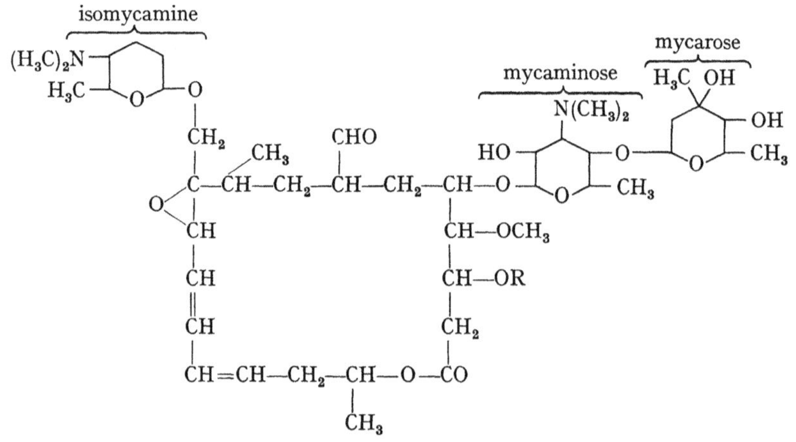

R= —H Spiramycin I
R= —CO—CH_3 Spiramycin II
R= —CO—CH_2—CH_3 Spiramycin III

Fig. 1. The structures of spiramycins I, II and III

in water. The mycarose can be removed chemically from the spiramycin I, II and III to form three new antibiotics known respectively as neospiramycins I, II and III. From the neospiramycins I, II and III the antibiotics forocidins I, II and III are formed by removing the isomycamine residue (PAUL and TSCHELITCHEFF, 1965). Only the spiramycin complex has been used clinically. Biological studies using the spiramycin complex but not the individual antibiotics have been reported; as these compounds are closely related it is probable that they have a similar mode of action.

Spiramycin is active *in vitro* mainly against Gram-positive bacteria and in general has a much reduced activity against Gram-negative organisms (Table 2); *Haemophilus pertussis* is an exception in that, although Gram-negative, it is very sensitive to spiramycin (GASTAL, 1958). *In vivo* the antibiotic is very effective in

[1] The anglicized version lancamycin has been adopted as it conforms to the nomenclature of all other macrolides.

Table 2. *In vitro inhibitory concentrations of spiramycin, carbomycin, angolamycin, methymycin and lancamycin*

Organism	*In vitro* inhibitory concentration µg/ml				
	Spira-mycin	Carbo-mycin	Angola-mycin	Methy-mycin	Lanca-mycin
Gram-positive bacteria:					
Bacillus megaterium	—	—	0.1—1	—	100
Bacillus subtilis	3	0.36	—	730	—
Staphylococcus aureus	1	0.22	10	40	100
Streptococcus pyogenes	0.6	0.08	10	10.5	100
Streptococcus faecalis	1	1.3	>100	1875	>100
Diplococcus pneumoniae	0.2	0.07	—	6.0—50	—
Corynebacterium diphteriae	3	—	100	20	100
Mycobacterium sp. 607	23	—	—	—	—
Mycobacterium tuberculosis	—	<50	>100	1875	—
Gram-negative bacteria:					
Escherichia coli	31	100	>100	1875	>100
Aerobacter aerogenes	31	100	—	1875	—
Neisseria catarrhalis	10	—	—	—	—
Klebsiella pneumoniae	33	3	>100	3.2	100
Pseudomonas aeruginosa	>1500	60	>100	1875	>100
Proteus vulgaris	>1500	100	—	1875	—
Yeasts:					
Candida albicans	—	100	100	—	>100
Protozoa:					
Endamoeba histolytica		>100	10—100	—	125

Data taken from CORBAZ *et al*,. 1955; GÄUMANN *et al.*, 1960; DONIN *et al.*, 1954; ENGLISH *et al.*, 1952; PAGANO, WEINSTEIN and MCKEE, 1953; PINNER-SINDICO *et al.*, 1954/55).

protecting mice against lethal infections of *Staphylococcus aureus*, *Diplococcus pneumoniae* and *Streptococcus pyogenes;* although *in vitro* experiments have shown that spiramycin is less active than other macrolides, *in vivo* spiramycin has a higher activity than erythromycin or carbomycin. The toxicity of spiramycin in mice is low, LD_{50} 1.5—2 g/kg (PINNERT-SINDICO *et al.*, 1954/55; GASTAL, 1958; MANIAR and EIDUS, 1961).

Cross resistance of a laboratory strain of *Staphylococcus aureus* has been found between erythromycin and spiramycin (JONES *et al.*, 1956; GARROD and WATERWORTH, 1956). Nevertheless CHABBERT *et al.* (1956) found that when a number of strains of *S. aureus* resistant to erythromycin were studied, some were sensitive to spiramycin. HUDSON *et al.* (1956) also found that most of their clinical isolates of erythromycin-resistant *S. aureus* were sensitive to spiramycin.

In vitro spiramycin is bacteriostatic and its minimum growth inhibitory concentration does not depend significantly on the inoculum size (GARROD and WATERWORTH, 1956). However, at concentrations 4—10 times its minimum growth inhibitory concentration spiramycin is bactericidal. This behaviour of spiramycin contrasts with that of other bacteriostatic antibiotics, like chloramphenicol, which even at 100 times their minimum growth inhibitory concentration remain bacteriostatic (LUTZ *et al.*, 1957). Spiramycin antagonises and interferes with the inhibitory action of penicillin and streptomycin on bacteria (MATHIEU and FAGUET, 1958).

In vitro erythromycin and chalcomycin inhibit bacterial growth by blocking protein synthesis (BROCK and BROCK, 1959; TAUBMAN, YOUNG and CORCORAN, 1963; JORDAN, 1963). Similar findings have been observed with spiramycin by D. VAZQUEZ (unpublished). VIDEAU (1958) found that spiramycin is taken up by *Staphylococcus aureus* when incubated in a suitable medium at 37°; on the other hand there is no uptake at 4° or by killed bacteria. Spiramycin prevents the uptake of ^{14}C-chloramphenicol by bacteria, and in cell-free systems prevents the binding of ^{14}C-chloramphenicol to ribosomes (VAZQUEZ, 1966a), suggesting that spira-

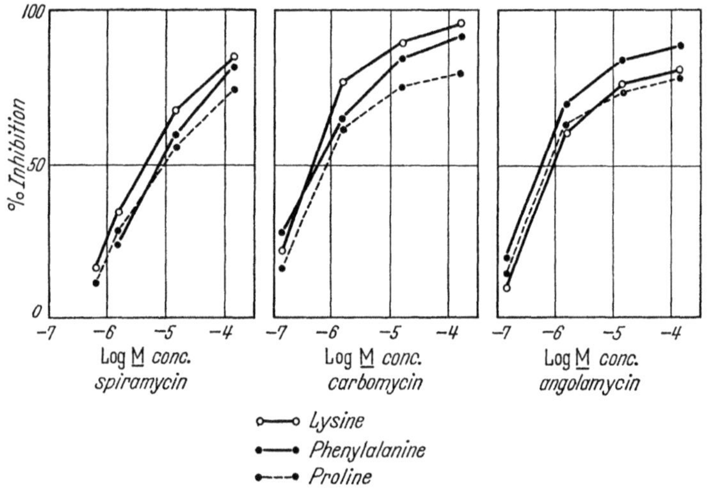

Fig. 2. Effects of spiramycin, carbomycin and angolamycin on polynucleotide directed incorporation of amino acids. Amino acid incorporation from lysine, prolyl-s-RNA and phenylalanyl-s-RNA was directed by poly A, poly C and poly U respectively (VASZQUEZ, 1966b)

mycin, like chloramphenicol, can act on the ribosomes. Chloramphenicol is bound reversibly to ribosomes but spiramycin is strongly bound and ribosomes treated with spiramycin are unable to bind ^{14}C-chloramphenicol even after being repeatedly washed with buffer (VAZQUEZ, 1966a).

By binding to ribosomes, spiramycin might inhibit protein synthesis at the ribosome level. Indeed it has been found that amino acid incorporation is inhibited by spiramycin in bacterial cell-free systems in which synthetic polynucleotides are used as m-RNA. The formation of aminoacyl-s-RNA is unaffected but the reaction(s) following the formation of aminoacyl-s-RNA and occurring before the completion of synthesis of the peptide on the ribosomes are blocked (Fig. 2) (VAZQUEZ, 1966b).

Carbomycin and Angolamycin

Carbomycin (synonym: magnamycin, M-4209) was first obtained from culture filtrates of *Streptomyces halstedii* (TANNER *et al.*, 1952). Other workers independently obtained the same antibiotic from *S. hygroscopicus* (PAGANO *et al.*, 1953) and from *S. albireticuli* (MIYAKE *et al.*, 1959). The carbomycin produced by *S. halstedii* is a complex mixture containing carbomycin A with a smaller proportion of carbomycin B (HOCHSTEIN and MURAI, 1954). The structures of carbomycin A and carbomycin B are shown in Fig. 3 (WOODWARD, 1957). Both antibiotics are closely related basic substances and are sparingly soluble in water but soluble in ethanol; they form soluble salts with hydrochloric acid. Carimbose which also has an antibacterial action, is formed by chemical removal of mycarose isovalerate from carbomycin A.

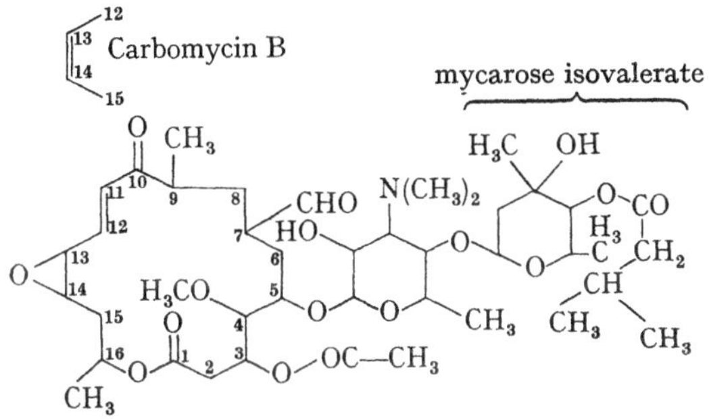

Fig. 3. The structures of carbomycins A and B

Like the other macrolide antibiotics, carbomycin is mainly active against Gram-positive bacteria (Table 2). Anti-rickettsial and antiviral activities of carbomycin have been reported (PAGANO *et al.*, 1953; WONG *et al.*, 1953) and at high concentrations the antibiotic is active against protozoa (SENECA and IDES, 1953). The antibiotic is bacteriostatic at the minimum growth inhibitory concentration but bactericidal when its concentration is increased by 4—10 fold (LUTZ *et al.*, 1957). Like chloramphenicol, carbomycin antagonises the bactericidal effect of penicillin (COLEMAN *et al.*, 1953). Complete cross resistance of bacteria between erythromycin and carbomycin has been reported (FINLAND *et al.*, 1952; FUSILLO *et al.*, 1953; JONES *et al.*, 1956) but a small percentage of erythromycin-resistant mutants are sensitive to carbomycin and *vice versa* (HSIE *et al.*, 1955/56). *In vivo*, carbomycin protects mice against the lethal effect of *Streptococcus pyogenes*, *Diplococcus pneumoniae* and *Staphylococcus aureus* (ENGLISH *et al.*, 1953). This protective effect of carbomycin is much less than that of spiramycin (MANIAR and EIDUS, 1961). The toxicity of carbomycin to mice and rats is small, LD_{50} 3 g/kg.

Angolamycin is a basic antibiotic, sparingly soluble in water but soluble in ethanol, and produced by a newly isolated species of streptomyces classified as *Streptomyces eurythermus*. The antibiotic has two sugar components which are released by acid hydrolysis but its chemical structure has not yet been elucidated. Like other macrolides angolamycin is active mainly against Gram-positive bacteria (Table 2). It is also active *in vivo* and protects mice against lethal infections of *Streptococcus pyogenes*. The toxicity of angolamycin for mice is 1 g/kg (CORBAZ *et al.*, 1955).

Carbomycin and angolamycin inhibit uptake of ^{14}C-chloramphenicol by *Bacillus megaterium* and also the binding of ^{14}C-chloramphenicol to bacterial ribosomes (VAZQUEZ, 1966a). Thus, carbomycin, angolamycin and chloramphenicol may act at related sites on the ribosomes. Indeed, carbomycin and angolomycin inhibit amino acid incorporation directed by synthetic polynucleotides in bacterial cell-free system (Fig. 2). The patterns of inhibition of the different amino acids are not the same for carbomycin or angolamycin and chloramphenicol which suggests that the sites of action on the ribosome are not identical. Carbomycin and angolamycin do not inhibit the formation of aminoacyl-s-RNA but prevent formation of the peptide on the ribosome (VAZQUEZ, 1966b).

Methymycin and Lancamycin

Methymycin was first isolated from a strain of *Streptomyces venezuelae*. The antibiotic is a base, insoluble in water but soluble in ethanol. It forms salts soluble in water (DONIN *et al.*, 1953/54). This antibiotic has an amino sugar attached to the macrolactone ring but contains no non-nitrogenous sugar (Table 1). Methymycin was the first macrolide to be chemically characterised (Fig. 4) (DJERASSI and ZDERIC, 1956).

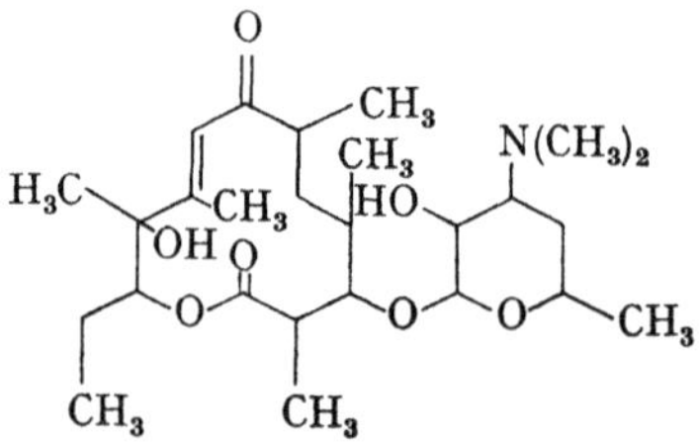

Fig. 4. The structure of methymycin

Methymycin has an antibacterial spectrum similar to but less active, weight for weight, than other macrolide antibiotics (Table 2) (DONIN *et al.*, 1953/54).

Lancamycin was first obtained from culture filtrates of a strain of *Streptomyces violaceoniger*. Lancamycin is sparingly soluble in water and soluble in ethanol; it is a neutral compound and on acids hydrolysis yields two non-nitrogenous sugars but no amino sugars (Table 1) (Fig. 5). *In vitro* lancamycin is only slightly active against Gram-positive organisms and practically inactive

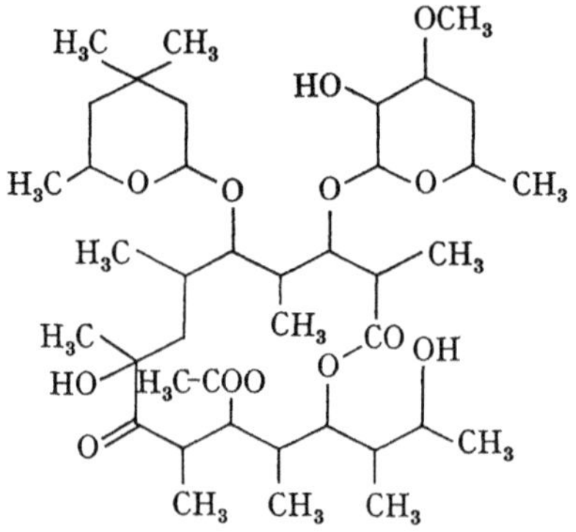

Fig. 5. The structure of lancamycin

against Gram-negative bacteria (Table 2). *In vivo* it is tolerated by mice and is not toxic when administered subcutaneously at 2 g/kg but is efective even at 1 g/kg in protecting mice against lethal infections of *Streptococcus pyogenes* or *Staphylococcus aureus* (GAUMANN *et al.*, 1960).

Methymycin and lancamycin reduce the uptake of ^{14}C-chloramphenicol by bacteria and the binding of this antibiotic to ribosomes. These effects of methymycin and lancamycin are readily reversible and smaller than for most of the other macrolides tested (VAZQUEZ, 1966a). These antibiotics inhibit proline and lysine incorporation, directed respectively by poly C and poly A, in bacteria cell-free systems but do not significantly affect the incorporation of phenylalanine directed by poly U (Fig. 6) (FAZQUEZ, 1966b).

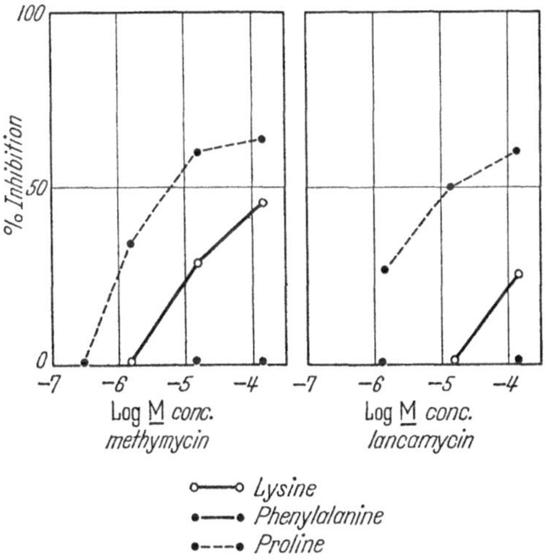

Fig. 6. Effects of methymycin and lancamycin on polynucleotide directed incorporation of amino acids. Amino acid incorporation from lysine, prolyl-s-RNA and phenylalanyl-s-RNA was directed by poly A, poly C and poly U respectively (VAZQUEZ, 1966b)

Discussion

All the macrolides studied have a number of features in common but they also show some interesting differences. These antibiotics are mainly active against Gram-positive bacteria but there are considerable differences between the inhibitory concentrations *in vitro* and methymycin and lancamycin have a very little activity. Of the five antibiotics considered above, only spiramycin has marked antibacterial action *in vivo*, which may be even higher than the *in vivo* activity of other macrolide antibiotics that are more active than spiramycin *in vitro*. As a general rule it appears that bacteria exhibit cross resistance to the macrolide antibiotics although erythromycin-resistant bacteria are frequently sensitive to spiramycin and occasionally sensitive to carbomycin.

It was previously thought that the basicity of the macrolides, which is due to their amino sugars residues, was related in some way to their mode of action, but this idea must be modified in view of the discovery of neutral macrolide antibiotics (chalcomycin and lancamycin). Chemical removal of the sugars from the macrolide antibiotics results in a decrease in their antibacterial activity.

Chloramphenicol binds to the 50 S subunit of the 70 S ribosomes (VAZQUEZ, 1964) and by doing so inhibits protein synthesis. All the macrolide antibiotics tested (spiramycin, carbomycin, angolamycin, methymycin, lancamycin, erythromycin and oleandomycin) inhibit the binding of ^{14}C-chloramphenicol to ribosomes, suggesting that these antibiotics also act on the 50 S ribosome subunit. There are quantitative differences between macrolides and whereas the attachment of lancamycin and methymycin to the ribosomes is feeble, spiramycin is firmly bound. This firm binding of spiramycin may be the cause of the reported bactericidal effect of this antibiotic at concentrations higher than the minimum inhibitory concentrations.

The macrolide antibiotics inhibit protein synthesis in bacteria by binding to ribosomes. This inhibition lies in the complex reaction(s) following formation of aminoacyl-s-RNA and prior to completion of the complete peptide on the ribosomes. The extent of the inhibition by spiramycin, carbomycin and angolomycin of amino acid incorporation in cell-free systems does not depend on the amino acid incorporated or the synthetic polynucleotide acting as m-RNA. Erythromycin and oleandomycin inhibit amino acid incorporation directed by poly C and poly A to a greater extent than that directed by poly U. Lancamycin and methymycin inhibit incorporation of some amino acids but do not inhibit phenylalanine incorporation directed by poly U. The different macrolides do not present the same pattern of inhibition of amino acid incorporation in cell-free systems and it may be that they do not all act at precisely the same site on the ribosomes.

The inhibition of protein synthesis by the macrolide antibiotics might occur at one of a number of steps including:

1. Formation of the m-RNA-ribosomes-aminoacyl-s-RNA complex;
2. Growth of the peptide;
3. Release of the peptide.

There is no evidence as yet on the nature of the step inhibited by the macrolide antibiotics considered in this article. It is unlikely that they inhibit protein synthesis at step (3) above since they also inhibit protein synthesis in cell-free systems in which there is no detachment of peptides from the ribosomes. It has been shown that the macrolide antibiotics which are able to inhibit polyphenylalanine synthesis in a cell-free system (erythromycin, spiramycin, carbomycin, angolamycin and oleandomycin) cause a slight reduction in the binding of phenylalanyl-s-RNA to ribosomes directed by poly U (D. VAZQUEZ, unpublished result). However, this inhibition is less than the corresponding inhibition of phenylalanine incorporation by the same antibiotics. It has recently been found that phenylalanyl-RNA binds also to the individual 30 S ribosome subunits in the presence of poly U (SUZUKA *et al.*, 1965); this binding is not affected by the macrolide antibiotics (D. VAZQUEZ, unpublished result).

Detailed studies on the effect of the macrolides considered above on metabolic processes other than protein synthesis have not been reported. Consequently inhibition of protein synthesis may not be the only mechanism by which these antibiotics can inhibit bacterial growth.

Thanks are due to my colleagues of the Sub-Department of Chemical Microbiology for their help and stimulating discussions. Particularly valuable were the criticisms of Dr. D. KERRIDGE and Prof. E. F. GALE, F. R. S. Thanks are also given to the Imperial Chemical Industries for a Fellowship.

See addendum

References

ANLIKER, R., u. K. GUBLER: Stoffwechselprodukte von Actinomyceten. Die Konstitution des Kromycins ein Abbauprodukt des Pikromycins. Helv. Chim. Acta **40**, 1768 (1957).

BROCK, T. D., and M. L. BROCK: Similarity in mode of action of chloramphenicol and erythromycin. Biochim. et Biophys. Acta **33**, 274 (1959).

BROCKMANN, H., u. W. HENKEL: Pikromycin ein neues Antibiotikum aus Actinomyceten. Naturwissenschaften **37**, 138 (1950).

BROCKMANN, H., u. R. OSTER: Antibiotica aus Actinomyceten. XXXVIII. Zur Konstitution des Pikromycins und Kromycins (Pikromycin, VI). Chem. Ber. **90**, 605 (1957).

CELMER, W. D.: Macrolide stereochemistry. I. The total absolute configuration of oleandomycin. J. Am. Chem. Soc. **87**, 1797 (1965a).

CELMER, W. D.: Macrolide stereochemistry. II. Configurational assignments at certain centers in various macrolide antibiotics. J. Am. Chem. Soc. **87**, 1799 (1965b).

CELMER, W. D.: A configurational model for macrolide antibiotics. J. Am. Chem. Soc. **87**, 1801 (1965c).

CELMER, W. D.: Basic stereochemical research topics in the macrolide antibiotics. In: Biogenesis of antibiotic substances, ed by Z. VANĚK and Z. HOŠŤÁLEK. New-York and London: Academic Press 1965c.

CHABBERT, Y.: Antagonisme *in vitro* entre l'erythromycine et la spiramycine. Ann. Inst. Pasteur **90**, 787 (1956).

CORBAZ, R., L. ETTLINGER, E. GÄUMANN, W. KELLER-SCHIERLEIN, L. NEIPP, V. PRELOG, P. REUSSER u. H. ZÄHNER: Stoffwechselprodukte von Actinomyceten. Angolamycin. Helv. Chim. Acta **38**, 1202 (1955).

COLEMAN, V. R., J. B. GUNNISON, and E. JAWETZ: Participation of erythromycin and carbomycin in combined antibiotic action *in vitro*. Proc. Soc. Exptl. Biol. Med. **83**, 668 (1953).

DJERASSI, C., and O. HALPERN: Macrolide antibiotics. VII. The structure of neomethymycin. Tetrahedron **3**, 255 (1958).

DJERASSI, C., and J. A. ZDERIC: The structure of the antibiotic methymycin. J. Am. Chem. Soc. **78**, 6390 (1956).

DONIN, M. N., J. PAGANO, J. D. DUTCHER, and C. M. MCKEE: Methymycin, a new crystalline antibiotic. Antibiotics Ann. **1953/54**, 179.

ENGLISH, A. R., M. F. FIELD, S. R. SZENDY, N. J. TAGLIANI, and R. A. FITTS: Magnamycin. I. *In vitro* studies. Antibiotics & Chemotherapy **2**, 678 (1952).

FINLAND, M., C. WILCOX, and E. M. PURCELL: Cross resistance to antibiotics: Effect of exposures of bacteria to carbomycin or erythromycin *in vivo*. Proc. Soc. Exptl. Biol. Med. **81**, 725 (1952).

FUSILLO, M. H., H. E. NOYES, E. J. PULASKI, and J. Y. S. TOM: Antimicrobial spectrum and cross resistance studies of erythromycin and carbomycin. Antibiotics & Chemotherapy **3**, 581 (1953).

GARDOCKI, J. F., S. Y. P'AN, A. L. RAPUZZI, G. M. FANELLI, and E. K. TIMMENS: Magnamycin: toxicity in experimental animals. Antibiotics & Chemotherapy **3**, 55 (1953).

GARROD, L. P., and P. M. WATERWORTH: Behaviour *in vitro* of some new antistaphylococcal antibiotics. Brit. Med. J. **1956, II** 61.

GASTAL, R.: Action de la spiramycine sur l'infection expérimentale de la souris par *H. pertussis*. Ann. Inst. Pasteur **94**, 636 (1958).

GÄUMANN, E., R. HÜTTER, W. KELLER-SCHIERLEIN, L. NEIPP, V. PRELOG u. H. ZÄHNER: Stoffwechselprodukte von Actinomyceten. Helv. Chim. Acta **43**, 601 (1960).

HOCHSTEIN, F. A., and K. MURAI: Magnamycin B, a second antibiotic from *Streptomyces halstedii*. J. Am. Chem. Soc. **76**, 5080 (1954).

HSIE, J.-Y., R. KOTZ, and W. NUSSER: Analysis of cross resistance to erythromycin and carbomycin in *Micrococcus pyogenes* var. *aureus*. Antibiotics Ann. **1955/56**, 773.

HUDSON, D. G., G. M. YOSHIHARA, and W. M. M. KIRBY: Spiramycin. Clinical and laboratory studies. A.M.A. Arch. Internal Med. **97**, 57 (1956).

JONES, W. F., R. L. NICHOLS, and M. FINLAND: Development of resistance and cross-resistance *in vitro* to erythromycin, carbomycin, spiramycin, oleandomycin and streptogramin. Proc. Soc. Exptl. Biol. Med. **93**, 388 (1956).

JORDAN, D. C.: Effect of chalcomycin on protein synthesis by *Staphylococcus aureus*. Can. J. Microbiol. **9**, 129 (1929).

LUTZ, A., O. GROOTEN et J. HOFFERER: Evolution et modifications de la résistance des staphylocoques pathogènes à six antibiotiques usuels de 1950 à 1956. L'action comparée *in vitro* de l'érythromycine, de la magnamycine, de la spiramycine, de la novobiocine (albamycine) et de l'oléandomycine. Ann. Inst. Pasteur **92**, 778 (1957).

MANIAR, A. C., et L. EIDUS: Un des facteurs influençant l'action des antibiotiques. Ann. Inst. Pasteur **101**, 887 (1961).

MATHIEU, N., et M. FAGUET: Activité *in vitro* de la spiramycine en association avcc la tétracycline, l'érythromycine, la pénicilline, la streptomycine sur la multiplication de *Staphylococcus aureus* étudiée au microbiophotomètre. Ann. Inst. Pasteur **94**, 69 (1958).

MIYAKE, A., H. IWASAKI, T. TAKEWATA, M. SHIBATA, and K. NAKAZAWA: Production of tertiomycin A by *Streptomyces albireticuli*. J. Antibiotics (Japan), Ser. A **12**, 59 (1959).

MORIN, R. B., and M. GORMAN: The partial structure of tylosin, a macrolide antibiotic. Tetrahedron Letters, p. 2339 (1964).

PAGANO, J. F., M. J. WEINSTEIN, and C. M. MCKEE: An anti-rickettsial antibiotic from a streptomycete, M-4209. I. Biological caracterizations. Antibiotics & Chemotherapy **3**, 899 (1953).

PAUL, R., et S. TCHELITCHEFF: Structure de la spiramycine. VI. Etablissement de la formule développée. Bull. soc. chim. France, p. 650 (1965).

PINNERT-SINDICO, S., L. NINET, J. PREUD'HOMME, and C. COSAR: A new antibiotic, spiramycin. Antibiotics Ann. **1954/55**, 724.

PRELOG, V., A. M. GOLD, G. TALBOT u. A. ZAMOJSKI: Stoffwechselprodukte von Actinomyceten. Über die Konstitution der Narbomycins. Helv. Chim. Acta **45**, 4 (1962).

SENECA, H., and D. IDES: The effect of magnamycin on protozoa and spermatozoa. Antibiotics & Chemotherapy **3**, 117 (1953).

SUZUKA, I., H. KAJI, and A. KAJI: Binding of specific RNA to 30 S subunits. Comparison with the binding to 70 s ribosomes. Biochem. Biophys. Research Commun. **21**, 187 (1965).

TANNER, F. W., A. R. ENGLISH, T. M. LEES, and J. B. ROUTIEN: Some properties of magnamycin, a new antibiotic. Antibiotics & Chemotherapy **2**, 441 (1952).

TAUBMAN, S. B., F. E. YOUNG, and J. W. CORCORAN: Antibiotic glycosides. IV. Studies on the mechanism of erythromycin resistance in *Bacillus subtilis*. Proc. Natl. Acad. Sci. U.S. **50**, 955 (1963).

UMEZAWA, H.: Recent advances in chemistry and biochemistry of antibiotics. Tokyo 1964. Microbial Chemistry Research Foundation.

VAZQUEZ, D.: The binding of chloramphenicol by ribosomes from *Bacillus megaterium*. Biochem. Biophys. Research Commun. **15**, 464 (1964).

VAZQUEZ, D.: Binding of chloramphenicol to ribosomes. The effect of a number of antibiotics. Biochim. et Biophys. Acta **144**, 277 (1966a).
VAZQUEZ, D.: Antibiotics affecting chloramphenicol uptake by bacteria. Their effect on amino acid incorporation in a cell-free system. Biochim. et Biophys. Acta **114**, 289 (1966b).
VIDEAU, D.: Sur le mode d'action des antibiotiques. Cas particulier de la spiramycine. Ann. Inst. Pasteur **94**, 709 (1958).
WATANABE, T.: Studies on leucomycin. IV. Isolation of mycaminose from the acid hydrolysate. Bull. Chem. Soc. Japan **34**, 15 (1961).
WATANABE, T., H. NISHIDA, J. ABE, and K. SATAKE: Studies on leucomycin. Bull. Chem. Soc. Japan **33**, 1104 (1960).
WONG, S. C., C. C. JAMES, and A. FINLAY: The action of carbomycin (magnamycin) on some viral and rickettsial infectial infections. Antibiotics & Chemotherapy **3**, 741 (1953).
WOODWARD, R. B.: Struktur und Biogenese der Makrolide. Eine neue Klasse von Naturstoffen. Angew. Chem. **69**, 50 (1957).

Erythromycin and Oleandomycin

F. E. Hahn

Erythromycin

Erythromycin (Fig. 1) is the most important member of a group of antibiotics known as macrolides. Structural characteristics of this group are 1. large lactone rings, 2. keto groups, and 3. amino sugars in glycosidic linkages. The mode of action of erythromycin has been subject to only relatively few studies which have, however, shown that the antibiotic is a specific inhibitor of protein synthesis. Reviews on erythromycin have been published by FORFAR and MACCABE (1957) and by GRUNDY (1964).

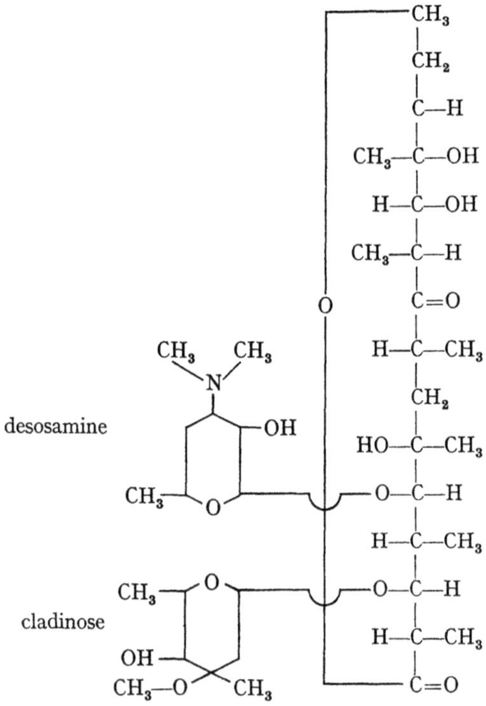

Fig. 1. Erythromycin

The antibiotic is a fermentation product of *Streptomyces erythreus* (MCGUIRE *et al.*, 1952). Its chemistry has been reviewed briefly by CHAIN (1957) and quite extensively by SHEMYAKIN (1961). The structure of erythromycin has been elucidated in a series of brilliant studies in the laboratory of E. H. FLYNN, and the structural formula depicted in Fig. 1 has been assigned to the antibiotic (WILEY *et al.*, 1957). Erythromycin is a weak basic, crystalline substance which is only slightly soluble in water and looses its biological activity at pH values below 5. Since the molecule of the antibiotic does not lend itself readily to organic synthetic studies, detailed theories of structure-activity relationships have not been developed for erythromycin. The free hydroxyl group of the desosamine moiety can be esterified with propionic acid yielding propionyl erythromycin which is an active antibiotic (GRIFFITH *et al.*, 1958).

Erythromycin is a medium-spectrum antibiotic which is active against many gram-positive bacteria but only against few gram-negative bacteria (POWELL *et al.*, 1953). Table 1 lists examples of sensitivities of microorganisms to the antibiotic.

Table 1. *Sensitivities of selected microorganisms to erythromycin*
(Data form SHEMYAKIN, 1961 and WALTER and HEILMEYER 1965)

Organism	Inhibitory concentration μg/ml
Streptococci	0.01—0.3
Neisseria gonorrhoeae	0.1—0.8
Corynebacterium diphtheriae	0.01—1
Clostridia	0.2—0.6
Staphylococcus aureus	0.3—0.7
Bacillus anthracis	0.3—1.0
Bacillus subtilis	0.5
Klebsiella pneumoniae	5
Mycobacterium tuberculosis	40
Aerobacter aerogenes	50
Nocardia asteroides	50—100
Escherichia coli	50—100
Serratia marcescens	100
Proteus vulgaris	>100

Natural resistance of *Proteus mirabilis* is apparently the result of an impermeability of the organism to erythromycin. The minimal growth inhibitory concentration of the antibiotic for the intact bacterium was of the order of 1000 μg/ml while the stable L-forms of *P. mirabilis* were inhibited by 1 μg/ml (TAUBENECK, 1962). Erythromycin has a significant effect against *Rickettsia prowazecki* as well as against the "large viruses" of meningopneumonitis and lymphogranuloma venereum; "small viruses" are not affected (POWELL *et al.*, 1953). *Entamoeba histolytica* is inhibited by 125—500 μg/ml of the antibiotic (MCCOWEN *et al.*, 1953) but yeasts and filamentous fungi are quite resistant to erythromycin (POWELL *et al.*, 1953). Leptospira loose their motility when exposed to >1 μg/ml of the antibiotic (GOLDBERG and LOGUE, 1956). The literature on the antimicrobial spectrum of erythromycin has been reviewed by MUSSGNUG (1956).

The antibiotic is predominantly bacteriostatic (OTTO *et al.*, 1961) although bactericidal effects have been demonstrated against a few bacteria (*Corynebac-*

terium diphtheriae, Bordetella pertussis, and streptococci) (HEILMAN *et al.*, 1952). HAIGHT and FINLAND (1962a) have reported that the bactericidal effect of erythromycin upon *Staphylococcus aureus* was only observed when the antibiotic was added to actively multiplying bacteria while no cell death from erythromycin occurred in the stationary phase of growth or at 4 C.

Erythromycin has been shown to cause bleaching of *Euglena gracilis* when added to this alga during active growth in light (EBRINGER, 1962). The depigmented cells can be grown heterotrophically (EBRINGER, 1963) for at least 16 months in the absence of the antibiotic and in light without greening.

The toxicity of erythromycin and other macrolides has recently been reviewed (GRUNDY, 1964). Among the major antibiotics, erythromycin appears to be the least toxic. The LD_{50} in laboratory mammals of erythromycin hydrochloride when injected intravenously is of the order of 200 to 400 mg/kg (ANDERSON *et al.*, 1952, 1955). Such toxic doses produce clonic convulsions, prostration, and respiratory depression. Death either occurs within one hour or the animals recover completely. In man, erythromycin also is relatively non-toxic. Mild gastrointestinal symptoms and very occasional urticaria or other mild allergies are the only reported toxic manifestations (WELCH *et al.*, 1957).

NAKAGAWA (1960) found an inhibition of the oxygen uptake of "resting" *B. subtilis* oxidizing glucose, glucose-6-phosphate, succinate, pyruvate, citrate, malate, and α-ketoglutarate in the presence of 1 μg/ml of erythromycin. D-amino acid oxidase and cytochrome oxidase were not inhibited, and the antibiotic had no effect on oxygen consumption of *Escherichia coli*.

An inhibition of protein synthesis is the most plausible biochemical explanation of the antimicrobial action of erythromycin. BENIGNO *et al.* (1954) were the first to carry out a comparative study of the effects of erythromycin and oxytetracycline in *S. aureus*. The two drugs caused an accumulation of bacterial nucleic acids, a strong inhibition of increase in total bacterial mass, and a slight decline in the number of viable cells. The authors interpreted their observations as indications of a specific inhibition of protein synthesis. NAKAGAWA carried out a similar study (1960) and found that induced synthesis of β-galactosidase as well as protein synthesis in general was inhibited by erythromycin in *E. coli* while the biosyntheses of DNA and RNA were not affected. The mode of action of erythromycin was also investigated independently by BROCK and BROCK (1959) in *E. coli*, using a high concentration of the antibiotic (1.4×10^{-3} M) and confirming that protein synthesis was inhibited while DNA and RNA synthesis continued; the authors also called attention to a similarity between the modes of action of erythromycin and chloramphenicol and stated that the effects of these two antibiotics upon bacterial growth were additive.

Erythromycin inhibits the polymerization of phenylalanine in polyuridylic acid-directed systems of ribosomes and enzymes of *Bacillus subtilis* (TAUBMAN *et al.*, 1963a), *E. coli* (WOLFE and HAHN, 1964), and mammalian reticulocytes (WEISBERGER *et al.*, 1964). TAUBMAN *et al.* (1963a) also showed that the synthesis of amino acyl transfer RNAs by enzymes from *B. subtilis* was not sensitive to erythromycin.

Evidently, the antibiotic binds to bacterial ribosomes. TANAKA and TERAOKA (1966) showed that pre-treatment of *E. coli* ribosomes with the antibiotic rendered these ribosomes incapable of functioning subsequently in the polyadenylic acid-directed synthesis of oligolysins when they were washed, dialyzed, and tested in polymerization experiments. When erythromycin was added directly to such experiments, the size distribution of the synthesized oligolysins was shifted to smaller lengths, primarily tripeptides and dipeptides. The identical observation has been reported by JULIAN (1965) for chloramphenicol, adding to the evidence for an apparent similarity between the modes of action of these structurally unrelated antibiotics. Additional evidence in favor of this idea is provided by the observations of VAZQUEZ (1963, 1966) and of WOLFE and HAHN (1965) that erythromycin inhibits the specific binding of ^{14}C-chloramphenicol to bacterial ribosomes. Whether chloramphenicol inhibits, conversely, the ribosomal binding of erythromycin awaits testing.

The mechanistic details of the action of erythromycin upon protein synthesis remain to be elucidated. WOLFE and HAHN (1964) have observed that erythromycin precipitated RNA and certain synthetic polyribonucleotides and have noticed more recently (unpublished observations) that the antibiotic interfered with the polyuridylic acid-directed binding to ribosomes of phenylalanyl transfer RNA.

Resistance to erythromycin emerges in bacteria during serial cultural passages in the presence of increasing concentrations of the antibiotic (HAIGHT and FINLAND, 1962b; HEILMAN *et al.*, 1952). This resistance is retained upon continued cultural passage in the absence of erythromycin. Sensitive bacteria can be transformed to erythromycin resistance by DNA from resistant bacteria; at least five different regions of a single transforming DNA molecule were involved in the transformation of pneumococcus (IYER and RAVIN, 1962) indicating that resistance is probably a polygenic phenomenon. Resistance to erythromycin in staphylococci can also be transduced by bacteriophages (NIWA, 1963).

TAUBMAN *et al.* (1963b) have studied the biochemical basis of the resistance of *B. subtilis* to erythromycin. The resistant strain had been selectively bred on erythromycin-containing culture plates and its DNA was capable of transforming the sensitive parent strain to erythromycin resistance. The resistant organism did not degrade erythromycin nor was it markedly impermeable to the antibiotic. Cell-free ribosomal systems from these bacteria, polymerizing lysine, valine, or leucine were *sensitive* when they were derived from the *sensitive* parent strain of *B. subtilis* but were *resistant* to erythromycin when derived from the *resistant* mutant cells. Since no combinations between ribosomes from resistant bacteria with enzymes from the sensitive organism or *vice versa* were tested and no attempt was reported to hybridize the ribosomal subunits from resistant and sensitive *B. subtilis*, the experiments auf TAUBMAN *et al.* (1963b) only suggest that resistance or sensitivity resided in one or several of the reactants of the cell-free amino acid polymerization systems. In view of the studies of TANAKA and TERAOKA (1966) on ribosomal binding of erythromycin, it is worthy of consideration that resistance or sensitivity to erythromycin is a genetically controlled property of ribosomes.

Cross-resistance between erythromycin and other macrolides has been reviewed by GRUNDY (1964). SZYBALSKI noted (1954) a tendency of bacteria to become cross-resistant to erythromycin and tetracyclines. If the keto-enol systems in both classes of antibiotics were involved in binding to the same biological sites of action, cross-resistance might plausibly be based upon structural changes in such common binding sites.

Oleandomycin is another of the macrolide antibiotics. Widespread interest in oleandomycin was aroused by the publicizing of claims (WELCH, 1957) that combinations of this antibiotic, especially with tetracycline (ENGLISH *et al.*, 1956) were synergistic and could be used rationally as a method of attacking the problem of resistant organisms. It is surprising that the ensuing controversy did not lead to critical testing for potentiation, additivity, or mutual interference as exemplified by studies on tetracycline-chloramphenicol combinations (CIAK and HAHN, 1958) nor to extensive studies on the mode of action of oleandomycin. Only most recently have certain observations pointed to an inhibition of protein synthesis as a possible mode of action of the antibiotic.

The antibiotic is a fermentation product of *Streptomyces antibioticus* (SOBIN *et al.*, 1955). The structure of oleandomycin has been determined by HOCHSTEIN *et al.* (1960), and the chemistry of the antibiotic has been reviewed in detail by SHEMYAKIN (1961). Fig. 2 shows the structural formula assigned to the drug; the 14-membered lactone ring differs in minor detail from a similar ring system in erythromycin. The neutral sugar moiety, oleandrose, is unique for the antibiotic while the amino sugar, desosamine, is the same as in the molecule of erythromycin.

Table 2. *Sensitivities of selected bacteria to oleandomycin*

Organism	Inhibitory concentration μg/ml
Staphylococcus aureus	0.2—1.6
Bacillus subtilis	0.4
Staphylococcus albus	0.8
Bacillus anthracis	0.8
Neisseria meningitides	1.6
Streptococcus faecalis	1.6
Hemophilus influenzae	3.12
Corynebacterium diphtheriae	6.25
Clostridium tetani	6.25
Neisseria gonorrhoeae	25
Aerobacter aerogenes	>100
Proteus vulgaris	>100
Pseudomonas aeroginosa	>100
Salmonella typhosa	>100

Oleandomycin is a medium-spectrum antibiotic with an antibacterial spectrum resembling that of erythromycin and other macrolides. Table 2 lists examples of sensitivities of microorganisms to oleandomycin (SOBIN *et al.*, 1955; ENGLISH and MCBRIDE, 1958).

The antibiotic is active against *Leptospira icterohaemorrhagiae in vitro* (COOK and THOMPSON, 1957) but the test data are irregular and do not afford a transformation into a dosage response correlation.

The optimum for the antibacterial action of oleandomycin is at pH 8.5; decreasing the hydrogen ion concentration to pH 5.5 decreases the activity 1000-fold (WATERWORTH, 1959). The antibiotic is predominantly bacteriostatic although a delayed bactericidal effect upon gram-positive cocci has been observed (HOBBY and LENERT, 1958).

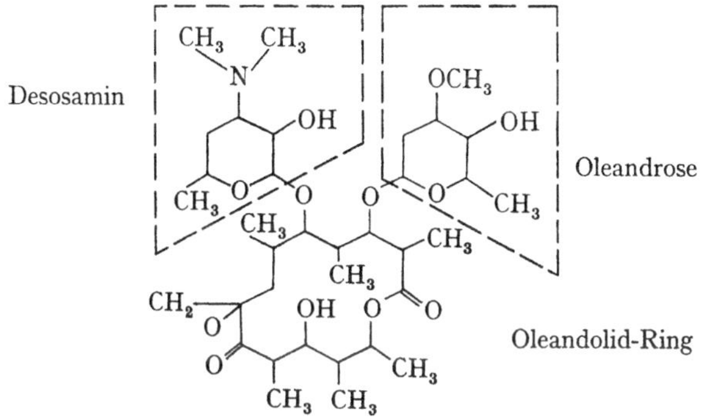

Fig. 2. Structure of oleandomycin

Oleandomycin exhibits low toxicity resembling that of erythromycin. Upon intravenous injection, the LD_{50} for rats was of the order of 500 mg/kg (SORENSEN *et al.*, 1957). Such lethal does cause signs of ataxia and increased excitability leading to tonic and clonic convulsions and death within 5 minutes. Surviving animals recover completely within 15 minutes. Extended oral administration produced no evidence of any organ-specific toxicity. In man, oleandomycin also is relatively non-toxic. In a very small percentage of patients (0.3%) mild gastro-intestinal symptoms were seen. There have been a few observations on hepatic dysfunction associated with triacetyl oleandomycin therapy (ROBINSON, 1962; MONTES *et al.*, 1964) which disappear, however, upon withdrawal of the drug.

Oleandomycin, like erythromycin and other macrolides (spiramycin, carbomycin), inhibits the binding of radioactive chloramphenicol to bacterial ribosomes *in vitro* (VAZQUEZ, 1966a). The polyuridylic acid-directed polymerization of phenylalanine was inhibited by 14%, the polyadenylic acid-directed polymerization of lysine by 45%, and the polycytidylic acid-directed polymerization of proline by 84% in an *Escherichia coli* ribosomes system in which oleandomycin was present at a concentration of 1.5×10^{-4} M (VAZQUEZ, 1966b). The results suggest that oleandomycin is an inhibitor of protein biosynthesis but this idea requires testing in whole sensitive bacteria.

JONES *et al.* (1956) have demonstrated the emergence of high resistance to oleandomycin upon 5 to 6 serial transfers of *S. aureus* in media containing increasing concentrations of the antibiotic. These bacteria also developed cross-resistance to other macrolide antibiotics.

ENGLISH *et al.* (1956) claimed that a 2:1 mixture of tetracycline and oleandomycin exerted a synergistic effect upon staphylococci; GARROD (1957) found no indication that such was the case. The use of only one combination of the two antibiotics as well as the determination of "minimal inhibitory concentrations" as an indicator of activity makes it difficult to evaluate if results on "synergism" indicate merely a possible *additive effect* or, more unlikely, an actual *potentiation* of the partial activities of the two drugs. A critical study of growth rates and handling of the data for a variety of drug pairs according to the isobologram method of Loewe as exemplified by the work of Ciak and Hahn (1958) would probably provide a conclusive answer.

See addendum

References

Anderson, R. C., P. N. Harris, and K. K. Chen: The toxicity and distribution of "Ilotycin". J. Am. Pharm. Assoc. Sci. Ed. **41**, 555 (1952).

Anderson, R. C., P. N. Harris, and K. K. Chen: Further toxicological studies with Ilotycin. J. Am. Pharm. Assoc., Sci. Ed. **44**, 199 (1955).

Benigno, P., A. Porro e L. Cima: Azione dell'ossitetraciclina e dell'eritromicina sul metabolismo fosforato dell "Staphilicoccus aureus". Atti accad. nazl. Lincei **16**, 773 (1954).

Brock, T. D., and M. L. Brock: Similarity in mode of action of chloramphenicol and erythromycin. Biochim. et Biophys. Acta **33**, 274 (1959).

Chain, E. B.: Chimica e biochimica du nuovi antibiotici. Giorn. ital. chemioterap. **4**, 213 (1957).

Ciak, J., and F. E. Hahn: Mechanism of action of antibiotics. I. Additive action of chloramphenicol and tetracyclines on the growth of Escherichia coli. J. Bacteriol. **75**, 125 (1958).

Cook, A. R., and P. E. Thompson: The effects of oleandomycin, carbomycin, and penicillin G on *Leptospira icterohaemorrhagiae* in vitro and in experimental animals. Antibiotics & Chemotherapy **7**, 425 (1957).

English, A. R., and T. J. McBride: Triacetyloleandomycin: biological studies. Antibiotics & Chemotherapy **8** 424 (1958).

English, A. R., T. J. McBride, G. van Halsema, and M. Carlozzi: Biologic studies on PA 775, a combination of tetracycline and oleandomycin with synergistic activity. Antibiotics & Chemotherapy **6**, 511 (1956).

Erbringer, L.: Erythromycin-induced bleaching of *Euglena grazilis*. J. Protozool. **9**, 373 (1962).

Erbringer, L.: Apochloroza buniek *Euglena grazilis* indukovana erythromycinom. Biologia (Bratislava) **18**, 371 (1963).

Forfar, J. O., and A. F. MacCabe: Erythromycin, a review. Antibiot. et Chemother. (Basel) **4**, 115 (1957).

Garrod, L. P.: The erythromycin group of antibiotics. Brit. med. J. **1957 II**, 57.

Goldberg, H. S., and J. T. Logue: Antibiotic sensitivity of leptospira as indicated by loss of motility. Antibiotics & Chemotherapy **6**, 19 (1956).

Griffith, R. S., V. C. Stephens, R. N. Wolfe, W. S. Boniece, and C.-C. Lee: Preliminary studies on propionyl erythromycin. Antibiotic Med. & Clin. Therapy **5**, 609 (1958).

Grundy, W. E.: The macrolides (erythromycin group). Exptl. Chemoth. Acad. Press **3**, 171 (1964).

Haight, T. H., and M. Finland: Observations on mode of action of erythromycin. Proc. Soc. Exptl. Biol. Med. **81**, 188 (1952a).

Haight, T. H., and M. Finland: Resistance of bacteria to erythromycin. Proc. Soc. Exptl. Biol. Med. **81**, 183 (1952b).

Heilman, F. R., W. E. Herrell, W. E. Wellman, and J. E. Geraci: Some laboratory and clinical observations on a new antibiotic, erythromycin (Lotycin). Proc. Staff Meetings Mayo Clinic **27**, 285 (1952).

Hobby, G. L., and T. F. Lenert: Observations on the mode of action of oleandomycin. Antibiotics & Chemotherapy **8**, 219 (1958).

Hochstein, F. A., H. Els, W. D. Celmer, B. L. Shapiro, and R. B. Woodward: The structure of oleandomycin. J. Am. Chem. Soc. **82**, 3225 (1960).

IYER, V. N., and A. W. RAVIN: Factors influencing recombination and the expression of recombinants during transformation to erythromycin resistance. VIIIth Internat. Congr. for Microbiology, Abstracts, Montreal, Quebec, Canada 1962, Abstract No. A 5.5, p. 27.

JONES, W. F., R. L. NICHOLS, and M. FINLAND: Development of resistance and cross-resistance *in vitro* to erythromycin, carbomycin, spiramycin, oleandomycin, and streptogramin. Proc. Soc. Exptl. Biol. Med. **93**, 388 (1956).

JULIAN, G. R.: C^{14}-lysine peptides synthesized in an *in vitro Escherichia coli* system in the presence of chloramphenicol. J. Mol. Biol. **12**, 9 (1965).

McCOWEN, M. C., M. E. CALLENDER, J. F. LAWLIS, and M. C. BRANDT: The effects of erythromycin (Ilotycin, Lilly) against certain parasitic organisms. Am. J. Trop. Med. Hyg. **2**, 212 (1953).

McGUIRE, J. M., R. L. BUNCH, R. C. ANDERSON, H. E. BOAZ, E. H. FLYNN, H. M. POWELL, and J. W. SMITH: "Ilotycin" a new antibiotic. Antibiotics & Chemotherapy **2**, 281 (1952).

MONTES, L. F., J. W. MIDDLETON, and A. FISHER: Hepatic dysfunction and fixed-drug eruption due to triacetyloleandomycin. Lancet **1964** No. 7334, 662.

MUSSGNUG, G.: Erythromycin. Arzneimittel-Forsch. **6**, 468 (1956).

NAKAGAWA, H.: Mode of action of erythromycin. Chem. Abstr. **54**, 11154a (1960).

NIWA, C.: Transduction of erythromycin-resistance in staphylococcus. Nippon Saigingaku Zasshi **18**, 21 (1963).

OTTO, R. H., E. F. ALFORD, W. E. GRUNDY, and J. C. SYLVESTER: Antibiotic bactericidal studies. Bactericidal and bacteriostatic tests with various antibiotics. Antimicrobial Agents Ann. **1960**, 104 (1960).

POWELL, H. M., W. S. BONIECE, R. C. PITTENGER, R. L. STONE, and C. G. GULBERTSON: Laboratory studies on 'Ilotycin'. Antibiotics & Chemotherapy **3**, 165 (1953).

ROBINSON, M. M.: Hepatic dysfunction associated with triacetyloleandomycin and propionyl erythromycin ester lauryl sulfate. Am. J. Med. Sci. **243**, 502 (1962).

SHEMYAKIN, M. M.: Khimia Antibiotikov, Vol. I, Acad. Sci. U.S.S.R., Moscow, 601, 641 (1961).

SO, A. G., J. W. BODLEY, and E. W. DAVIE: Influence of environment on the specificity of polynucleotide-dependent amino acid incorporation into polypeptide. Biochemistry **3**, 1977 (1964).

SOBIN, B. A., A. R. ENGLISH, and W. D. CELMER: P.A. 105, A new antibiotic. Antibiotics Annual **1954/55**, 827 (1955).

SORENSEN, O. J., R. A. FISKEN, T. F. REUTNER, K. WESTON, and J. K. WESTON: Experimental toxicological studies on oleandomycin. Antibiotics & Chemotherapy **7**, 419 (1957).

SZYBALSKI, W.: Genetic studies on microbial cross-resistance to toxic agents. Appl. Microbiol. **2**, 57 (1954).

TANAKA, K., and H. TERAOKA: Binding of erythromycin to *Escherichia coli* ribosomes. Biochim. et Biophys. Acta **114**, 204 (1966).

TAUBENECK, U.: Susceptibility of *Proteus mirabilis* and its stable L-forms to erythromycin and other macrolides. Nature **196**, 195 (1962).

TAUBMAN, S. B., A. G. SO, F. E. YOUNG, E. W. DAVIE, and J. W. CORCORAN: Effect of erythromycin on protein biosynthesis in *Bacillus subtilis*. Antimicrobial Agents and Chemotherapy 1963, 395 (1963a).

TAUBMAN, S. B., F. E. YOUNG, and J. W. CORCORAN: Antibiotic glycosides. IV. Studies on the mechanism of erythromycin resistance in *Bacillus subtilis*. Proc. Natl. Acad. Sci. U.S. **50**, 955 (1963b).

VAZQUEZ, D.: Antibiotics which affect protein synthesis: the uptake of ^{14}C-chloramphenicol by bacteria. Biochem. Biophys. Research Commun **12**, 409 (1963).

VAZQUEZ, D.: Binding of chloramphenicol to ribosomes. The effect of a number of antibiotics. Biochim. et Biophys. Acta **114**, 277 (1966a).

VAZQUEZ, D.: Antibiotics affecting chloramphenicol uptake by bacteria. Their effect on amino acid incorporation in a cell-free system. Biochim. et Biophys. Acta **114**, 289 (1966b).

WALTER, A. M., and L. HEILMEYER: Antibiotika-Fibel. Stuttgart: Georg Thieme 1965.
WATERWORTH, P. M.: The antibacterial properties of leucomycin. Antibiotics & Chemoth. **10**, 101 (1960).
WEISBERGER, A. S., S. WOLFE, and S. ARMENTROUT: Inhibition of protein synthesis in mammalian cell-free systems by cloramphenicol. J. Exptl. Med. **120**, 161 (1964).
WELCH, H.: Opening remarks. Antibiotics Ann. **1956/57**, 1 (1957).
WELCH, H., C. N. LEWIS, H. I. WEINSTEIN, and B. B. BOECKMAN: Severe reactions to antibiotics. A nationwide survey. Antibiotic Med. & Clin. Therapy **4**, 800 (1957).
WILEY, P. F., K. GERZON, E. H. FLYNN, M. V. SIGAL, O. WEAVER, U. C. QUARCK, R. R. CHAUVETTE, and R. MONAHAN: Erythromycin. X. Structure of erythromycin. J. Am. Chem. Ass. **79**, 6062 (1957).
WOLFE, A. D., and F. E. HAHN: Erythromycin: mode of action. Science **143**, 1445 (1964).
WOLFE, A. D., and F. E. HAHN: Mode of action of chloramphenicol. IX. Effects of chloramphenicol upon a ribosomal amino acid polymerizing system and its binding to bacterial ribosome. Biochim. et Biophys. Acta **95**, 146 (1965).

The Streptogramin Family of Antibiotics*

D. Vazquez

The classification of antibiotics in the streptogramin family has been reviewed briefly by LESTER SMITH (1963). All the antibiotics of this family are closely related in composition, mode of action and antibacterial spectra. Streptogramin itself was first obtained from culture filtrates of a species of streptomyces, now classified as *Streptomyces graminofaciens* (CHARNEY *et al.*, 1953) and since then other closely related antibiotics have been described, for example, staphylomycin, ostreogrycin, synergistin, mikamycin, pristinamycin and vernamycin. These antibiotics are mixtures of two or more different active compounds and there are numerous reports of the isolation and properties of the individual components. All streptogramins can be placed in two major groups A and B (Table 1). The antibiotics in group A show a marked synergism with those in group B in their activity against Gram-positive bacteria and consequently all the complex antibiotics of this family have a markedly higher activity than the individual components. Viridogrisein, unlike all the other members of the family, is not a complex antibiotic but is included in group B because its chemical structure and properties are related to others in the group. Of the single components of the streptogramin family, viridogrisein is, in general, the most active.

The antibiotics of the streptogramin family are sparingly soluble in water and petroleum ether, slightly soluble in methanol, ethanol, acetone and benzene and very soluble in chloroform. Viridogrisein has a higher solubility in water (1 mg/ml) than other members of the family.

Some complex antibiotics of the streptogramin family (mikamycin, staphylomycin and pristinamycin) have been used clinically.

Antibiotics of group A

These antibiotics are obtained from the complex antibiotics of the streptogramin family after removal by crystallization of the group B substances. All the antibiotics in group A are similar to each other. The most probable structure of ostreogrycin A is shown in Fig. 1 (DELPIERRE *et al.*, 1966). None of the structures of other compounds in group A has yet been completely elucidated, but from chemical and physical data it is thought that ostreogrycin A, streptogramin A, staphylomycin M_I and synergistin A-1 are closely related and may be identical.

The antibiotics in group A are preferentially active against Gram-positive cocci (Table 2); their action is bacteriostatic in the cases of *Bacterium agri* and *Staphylococcus aureus* (YAMAGUCHI, 1961; VAZQUEZ, 1966c;, CHABBERT and ACAR,

* This paper was written while the author was in residence at the University of Cambridge, Department of Biochemistry, Sub-department of Chemical Microbiology.

Table 1. *The streptogramin family of antibiotics*

Antibiotic complex (synonyms)	Individual components				Source, isolation and chemistry	
	Group A		Group B			
	Antibiotic	Synonym	Antibiotic	Synonym	Streptomyces strain producer	References
Ostreogrycin (E 129)	Ostreogrycin A	Streptogramin A[1] Staphylomycin M_I[1] Synergistin A-1[1]	Ostreogrycin B	Streptogramin B[1] Synergistin B-1 Mikamycin B Pristinamycin I_A Vernamycin B_α	*Streptomyces ostreogriseus*	Ball *et al.*, 1958 Gream, 1961 Sarin, 1962 Eastwood, Snell and Todd, 1960 Delpierre *et al.*, 1966
	Ostreogrycin G					
	Ostreogrycin C		Ostreogrycin B_1	Vernamycin B_γ		
	Ostreogrycin D		Ostreogrycin B_2	Vernamycin B_β Pristinamycin I_B		
	Ostreogrycin Q		Ostreogrycin B_3			
Streptogramin	Streptogramin A		Streptogramin B		*Streptomyces graminofaciens*	Charney *et al.*, 1953 Vazquez, 1964b, 1966c
Staphylomycin (Virgimycin)	Staphylomycin M_I Staphylomycin M_{II}		Staphylomycin S		*Streptomyces virginiae*	De Somer and van Dijck, 1955 Vanderhaeghe *et al.*, 1957 Vanderhaeghe and Parmentier, 1960

[1] Identification not completed but based on comparison of physical and chemical properties of these compounds.

Table 1. (Continued)

Antibiotic complex (synonyms)	Individual components				Source, isolation and chemistry	
	Group A		Group B		Streptomyces strain producer	References
	Antibiotic	Synonym	Antibiotic	Synonym		
Synergistin (PA 114)	Synergistin A-1		Synergistin B-1 Synergistin B-3		*Streptomyces olivaceus*	CELMER and SOBIN, 1956 HOBBS and CELMER, 1960
Mikamycin	Mikamycin A		Mikamycin B		*Streptomyces mitakaensis*	ARAI *et al.*, 1956 WATANABE, 1960 WATANABE, 1961
Pristinamycin (Pyostacin) (7293 RP)	Pristinamycin II_A Pristinamycin II_B		Pristinamycin I_A Pristinamycin I_B		*Streptomyces pristinae spiralis*	BENAZET *et al.*, 1962 PREUD'HOMME *et al.*, 1965
Vernamycin	Vernamycin A		Vernamycin B_α Vernamycin B_β Vernamycin B_γ Vernamycin B_δ Doricin		*Streptomyces loidensis*	BODANSZKY and ONDETTI, 1963 BODANSZKY and SHEEHAN, 1964
			Viridogrisein	Etamycin	*Streptomyces sp.* *Streptomyces griseus* *Streptomyces lavendulae*	BARTZ *et al.*, 1955 HEINEMANN *et al.*, 1955 ARNOLD, JOHNSON and MAUGER, 1958 SHEEHAN, ZACHAU and LAWSON, 1958

1965; VIDEAU, 1965). However, mixtures of these compounds with antibiotics of either group B or the tetracycline family are bactericidal against *S. aureus* (VAZQUEZ, 1966c). On the other hand antibiotics of group A protect bacteria against the bactericidal action of streptomycin.

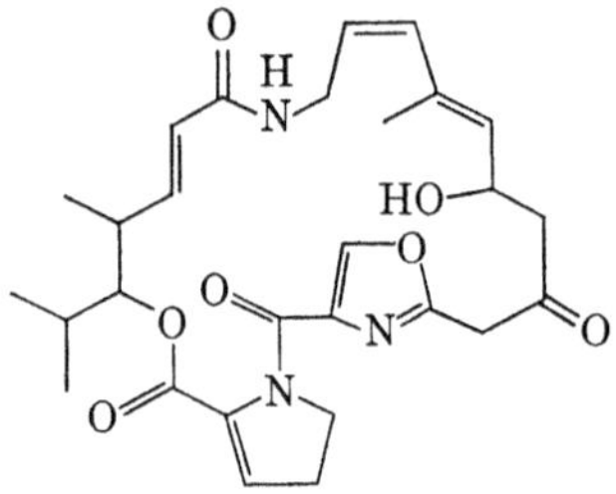

Fig. 1. The structure of ostreogrycin A

In vivo studies have shown that these antibiotics have little activity in protecting mice against experimental infections with a virulent strain of *S. aureus*. They are not toxic to mice when injected intraperitoneally at doses of 350 mg/kg daily (BESSELL *et al.*, 1958; TANAKA *et al.*, 1959, 1961).

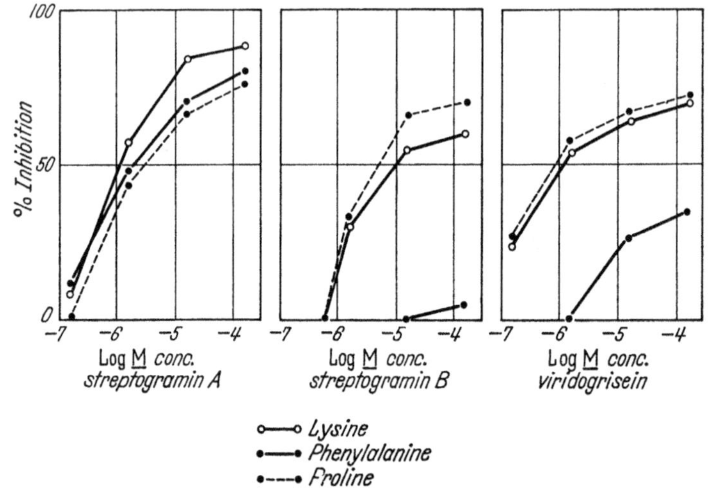

Fig. 2. Effects of viridogrisein and the streptogramin antibiotics on polynucleotide directed incorporation of amino acids. Amino acid incorporation from lysine, prolyl-s-RNA and phenylalanyl-s-RNA was directed by poly A, poly C and poly U respectively (VAZQUEZ, 1966b)

CHENG, VAN STRATEN and SNELL (1960) found a considerable increase in the rate of glucose oxidation by *Escherichia coli* (1.44 × 18^8 bacteria/ml) in the presence of 0.5 μg of synergistin A-1/ml; no effect by synergistin A-1 was found if the concentration of bacteria or the antibiotic were changed. These results have not been confirmed by other workers. VAZQUEZ (1966c) found no effect of these antibiotics on endogenous respiration oxidation of ethanol or glucose or anaerobic fermentation of glucose by *S. aureus*.

At growth inhibitory concentrations, antibiotics in group A inhibit protein synthesis without inhibiting either nucleic acid or cell wall synthesis or accumulation of low molecular weight constituents in the "pool" (Table 3); the inhibitory effect on protein synthesis can be detected within 30 sec of addition of the antibiotic (YAMAGUCHI, 1961; VAZQUEZ, 1966c; ENNIS, 1965a).

The overall effects of chloramphenicol and the antibiotics in group A are very similar. ^{14}C-chloramphenicol is taken up by bacteria and bound to their ribosomes; both uptake by bacteria and binding to ribosomes of ^{14}C-chloramphenicol are inhibited by antibiotics in group A. Binding of ^{14}C-chloramphenicol to ribosomes is readily reversible whereas ribosomes treated with antibiotics A are unable to bind ^{14}C-chloramphenicol even after repeated washings. Since it is known that the site of action of chloramphenicol is the 50 S subunit of the 70 S ribosome these results suggest that antibiotics A also act on the 50 S subunit of the ribosome (VAZQUEZ, 1963, 1964a, 1966a, 1964c and 1966c). This suggestion is supported by other experimental evidence. The inhibitory effect of antibiotics of group A on protein synthesis has been confirmed by studies of amino acid incorporation in cell-free systems (YAMAGUCHI and TANAKA, 1964; LASKIN and MAY CHAN, 1964; VAZQUEZ, 1966c; ENNIS, 1965b). LASKIN and MAY CHAN (1964) have also reported that, in the absence of synthetic polynucleotides, amino acid incorporation directed by natural m-RNA attached to the ribosomes is not inhibited by vernamycin A. On the other hand YAMAGUCHI and TANAKA (1964) have reported inhibition of leucine incorporation by mikamycin A under similar condi-

Table 2. *In vitro inhibitory concentrations of the antibiotics in groups A and B*

Organism	Inhibitory concentrations in μg/ml								
	Viridogrisein	Streptogramin		Synergistin		Staphylomycin		Mikamycin	
		A	B	A-1	B-1	M_I	S	A	B
Bacteria, Gram-positive:									
Bacillus megaterium	—	40.00	3.00	—	—	—	—	800.00	20.00
Bacillus subtilis	2.50	—	—	100.00	3.12	50.00	13.00	800.00	10.00
Staphylococcus aureus	0.31	6.00	10.00	0.78	6.25	5.00	125.00	20.00	100.00
Sarcina lutea	—	—	—	—	—	2.50	14.00	—	—
Streptococcus pyogenes	0.63	—	—	0.19	50.00	—	—	40.00	40.00
Bacteria, Gram-negative:									
Escherichia coli	>200.00	40.00	100.00	—	—	—	—	>800.00	>800.00
Hemophilus pertussis	5.00	—	—	—	—	—	—	4.00	100.00

(Data taken from: HEINEMANN *et al.*, 1955; EHRLICH *et al.*, 1955; VAZQUEZ, 1964b; VAN DIJCK, VANDERHAEGHE and DE SOMER, 1957; TANAKA *et al.*, 1961; ENGLISH *et al.*, 1956.)

tions. Antibiotics of group A, unlike chloramphenicol, do not show differential inhibition of proline, lysine or phenylalanine incorporation directed respectively by poly C, poly A and poly U (Fig. 2) (VAZQUEZ, 1966b). They do not inhibit the activation of amino acids or formation of aminoacyl-s-RNA (LASKIN and MAY CHAN, 1964; VAZQUEZ, 1966b). These results suggest that antibiotics of group A inhibit protein synthesis at the level of peptide growth on the ribosome. This might possibly be a consequence of their binding to the 50 S subunit of the ribosomes. It has recently been found that in the presence of poly U phenylalanyl-sRNA binds not only to the 70 S ribosomes but also to preparations of 30 S ribosomes subunits (SUZUKA, KAJI and KAJI, 1965; D. VAZQUEZ, unpublished result). Antibiotics of group A reduce binding of phenylalanyl-sRNA to the 70 S ribosomes but not to the 30 S ribosome subunit (D. VAZQUEZ, unpublished result).

Table 3. *The effect of viridogrisein and the streptogramin antibiotics on the incorporation of radioactive compounds into cellular fractions*

^{14}C-labelled compound	Antibiotic	% control incorporation				
		μg/ml	Pool	NA*	Protein	Wall
(U-^{14}C) Glycine	Streptogramin A	6.0	100	100	26	100
	Streptogramin A	20.0	100	100	12	100
L-(U-^{14}C) Glutamic acid	Streptogramin A	6.0	120	100	27	100
	Streptogramin A	20.0	128	100	11	100
(8-^{14}C) Adenine	Streptogramin A	6.0	126	204	—	—
	Streptogramin A	20.0	121	189	—	—
(U-^{14}C) Glycine	Streptogramin B	10.0	77	59	54	57
	Streptogramin B	30.0	73	49	43	46
L-(U-^{14}C) Glutamic acid	Streptogramin B	10.00	83	57	52	58
	Streptogramin B	30.00	76	46	40	48
(8-^{14}C) Adenine	Streptogramin B	10.00	74	61	—	—
	Streptogramin B	30.00	69	58	—	—
(U-^{14}C) Glycine	Streptogramin	0.6	100	100	34	100
	Streptogramin	2.0	100	100	11	100
L-(U-^{14}C) Glutamic acid	Streptogramin	0.6	118	100	35	100
	Streptogramin	2.0	127	100	10	100
(8-^{14}C) Adenine	Streptogramin	0.6	130	206	—	—
	Streptogramin	2.0	120	176	—	—
(U-^{14}C) Glycine	Viridogrisein	5.0	100	72	14	89
L(U-^{14}C) Glutamic acid	Viridogrisein	5.0	100	59	12	78
(8-^{14}C) Adenine	Viridogrisein	5.0	50	50	—	—

NA* total nucleic acid.

The effect of the streptogramin antibiotics was studied in *Staphylococcus aureus*. Samples were taken after 15 minutes of incubation.

The effect of viridogrisein was studied in *Bacillus megaterium*. Samples were taken after 30 minutes of incubation.

(Data taken from GARCIA MENDOZA, 1965; VAZQUEZ, 1966c.)

Antibiotics of group B

Antibiotics of group B are obtained as crystalline compounds from methanolic solutions of the complex antibiotics. The chemical structures of some of the group B compounds have been determined (Fig. 3). The basic structures consist

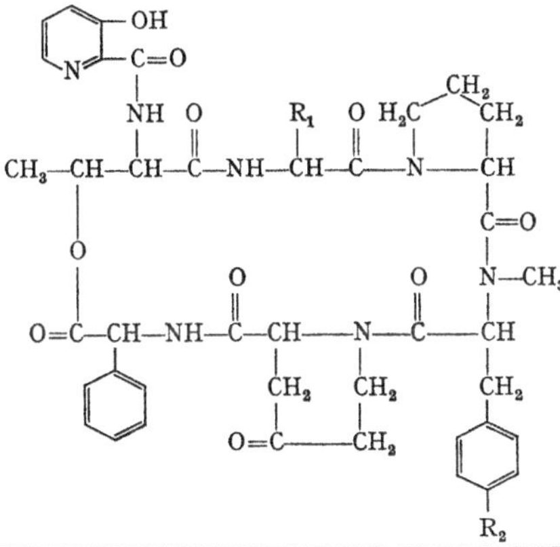

	Staphylomycin S	Vernamycin B_δ	Ostreogrycin B	Ostreogrycin B_1	Ostreogrycin B_2
R_1	$-CH_2-CH_3$	$-CH_3$	$-CH_2-CH_3$	$-CH_3$	$-CH_2-CH_3$
R_2	$-H$	$-NH-CH_3$	$-N(CH_3)_2$	$-N(CH_3)_2$	$-NH-CH_3$

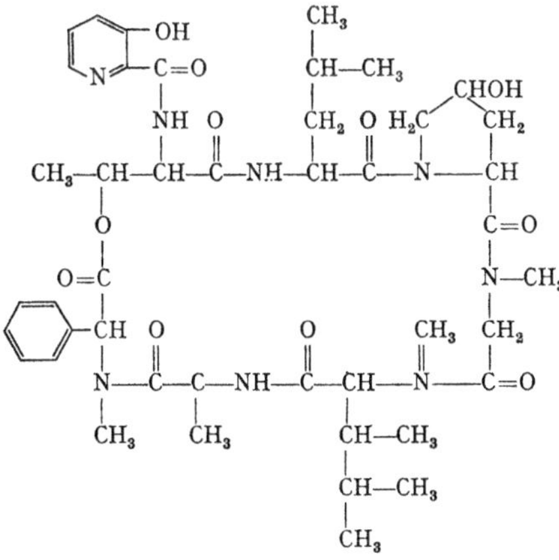

Viridogrisein

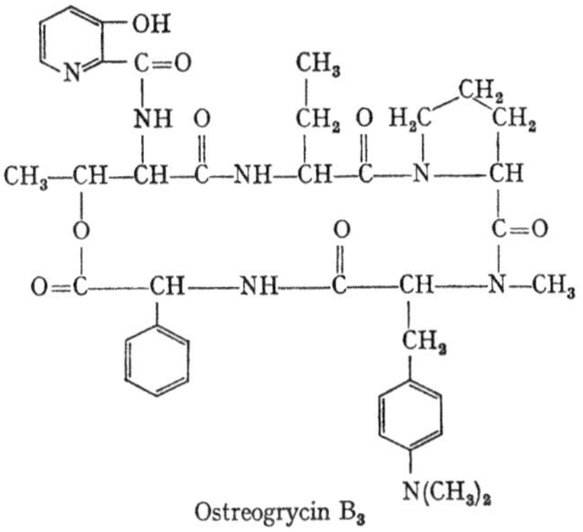

Ostreogrycin B_3

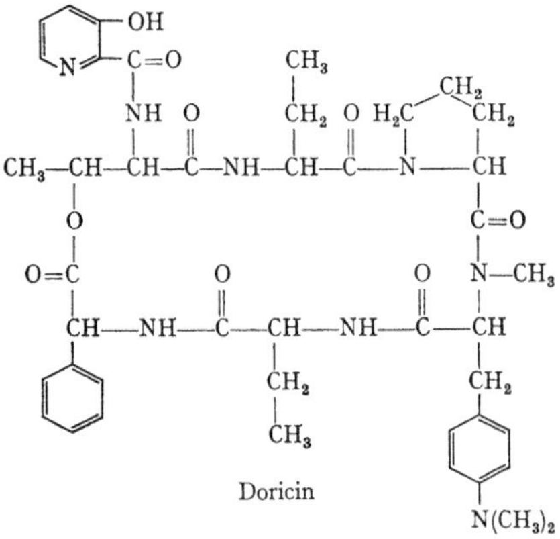

Doricin

Fig. 3. The structures of certain antibiotics of the streptogramin B group of a polypeptide containing unusual amino acids linked through the hydroxyl of threonine to form a macrocyclic lactone ring. In addition all antibiotics in group B contain 3-hydroxypicolinic acid linked to the cyclic peptide and may act as chelating agents as a result. It is possible that when the detailed chemical structure of all the individual antibiotics of group B are known, some of the minor compounds isolated by different workers will prove to be identical.

These antibiotics are mainly active against Gram-positive bacilli (Table 2) and are bacteriostatic to *S. aureus* and *Bacterium agri* (YAMAGUCHI, 1961; VAZQUEZ, 1966c; CHABBERT and ACAR, 1965; GARCIA-MENDOZA, 1965; VIDEAU, 1965; DUBOST and PASCAL, 1965). It has been reported that ostreogrycin B is highly bactericidal against *S. aureus* (GARROD and WATERWORTH, 1956), but this result was probably due to impurities of ostreogrycin A or ostreogrycin G in the preparation and has not been confirmed by other workers. The antibiotics in group B are not active against Gram-negative bacteria, yeasts, fungi and protozoa. At low concentration viridogrisein does not affect growth of seedlings of wheat but causes complete bleaching; the apochlorotic effect of viridogrisein is reduced by copper ions (CERCOS, 1964).

Cross resistance between antibiotics in group B and the macrolide antibiotics has been reported (GARROD and WATERWORTH, 1956; TANAKA *et al.*, 1959, 1961; CHABBERT and ACAR, 1965; ACTOR, BASCH and JAMBOR, 1963).

In vivo studies have shown that most of the antibiotics in group B have little activity in protecting mice against *S. aureus* and *Diplococcus pneumoniae* infections. Viridogrisein is an exception and when administered orally or parenterally prevents death of mice which have been experimentally infected with *Haemophilus pertussis* or *Diplococcus pneumoniae.* Antibiotics in group B are toxic to mice only in high doses (2—3 g/kg) BESSELL *et al.*, 1958; TANAKA *et al.*, 1959; EHRLICH *et al.*, 1955; HEINEMANN *et al.*, 1955).

CHENG, VAN STRATEN and SNELL (1960) found a three-fold increase in the rate of glucose oxidation by *E. coli* (1.44×10^8 bacteria/ml) in the presence of 0.5 μg of synergistin B-1/ml, but no effect by synergistin B-1 was observed if the concentrations of the antibiotic or the bacteria were changed. However, no effect of the antibiotics in group B has been found by other workers on endogenous respiration, oxidation of ethanol or glucose, or anaerobic fermentation of glucose by *S. aureus*. These antibiotics do not cause leakage of UV absorbing material from the cell (GARCIA-MENDOZA, 1965; VAZQUEZ, 1966c).

Antibiotics in group B, at growth inhibitory concentrations, inhibit protein synthesis and reduce not only nucleic acid and cell wall synthesis but also affect the accumulation of low molecular weight constituents in the pool (Table 3). However, protein synthesis is somewhat more sensitive than the other processes and its inhibition can be detected within 30 sec of adding the antibiotics whereas the effect on the other processes is not established until after 1—2 minutes. The syntheses of both RNA and DNA are affected by these antibiotics (GARCIA-MENDOZA, 1965; VAZQUEZ, 1966c). This inhibition is not due to a direct effect on DNA-dependent DNA or RNA polymerases as cell free preparations of these enzymes are not affected by the antibiotics (ELLIOTT, 1964; WARING, 1965). YAMAGUCHI (1961) found a slight inhibition of protein synthesis in the presence of high concentration of mikamycin B, but not significant effect on nucleic acid synthesis. He suggested that this inhibitory effect on protein synthesis by mikamycin B was probably due to traces of mikamycin A contaminating the mikamycin B and considered that mikamycin B was not an inhibitor of protein synthesis. In further work YAMAGUCHI (1963a, 1963b) reported that protein synthesis was not significantly inhibited by mikamycin B in *S. aureus*, was partially inhibited in *Micrococcus lysodeikticus* and completely blocked in *Bacillus subtilis*. No inhibitory effect of mikamycin B in protein synthesis was found in cell-free systems of *E. coli* by YAMAGUCHI and TANAKA (1964); they concluded that the antibiotic probably has different modes of action in different organisms.

Antibiotics in group B reduce the uptake of ^{14}C-chloramphenicol by bacteria but do not prevent the binding of this antibiotic to ribosomes. The reported finding that ostreogrycin B inhibits binding of ^{14}C-chloramphenicol to ribosomes has been found, in later work, to be due to impurities of ostreogrycin A in the preparation (VAZQUEZ, 1963, 1964a, 1966a).

In cell-free systems, antibiotics in group B do not significantly affect activation of amino acids or formation of aminoacyl-s-RNA (LASKIN and MAY CHAN, 1964; GARCIA-MENDOZA, 1965; VAZQUEZ, 1966b) but inhibit incorporation of proline and lysine directed by poly C and poly A respectively. Viridogrisein is the only one of the group which inhibits phenylalanine incorporation directed by poly U and this inhibition is always smaller than that obtained for the other amino acids (Fig. 2). The inhibition of protein synthesis by these antibiotics occurs after the formation of aminoacyl-s-RNA and before the formation of the complete peptide on the ribosome (VAZQUEZ, 1966b). In preliminary studies LASKIN and MAY CHAN (1965) found that vernamycin B_α partially inhibits the binding of aminoacyl-s-RNA to ribosomes. However this result could not be confirmed by D. VAZQUEZ (unpublished result) who showed that antibiotics in group B do not reduce either the rate or the total binding of phenylalanyl-s-RNA to ribosomes or to preparations of 30s ribosome subunits in the cell-free system of NIRENBERG and LEDER (1964), but cause an enhancement in these bindings.

Complex antibiotics of the streptogramin family

The antibiotic complexes of the streptogramin family are closely related but do not have a defined composition. For the same antibiotic complex the ratio of components of group A to components of group B is variable and depends not only on the growth conditions of the streptomyces producing the antibiotics but also on the methods used to obtain the complex and to estimate the individual components.

The reported ratio of group A components to group B components is 5—9/1 for mikamycin (TANAKA *et al.*, 1961; YAMAGUCHI, 1961), 16/1 for staphylomycin (THOMSEN, 1963), 2—5/1 for streptogramin (VAZQUEZ, 1964b) and 2—3/1 for pristinamycin (PREUD'HOMME *et al.*, 1965). However the antibacterial activity and spectra of these antibiotic complexes do not change significantly with wide range of the ratio so that results obtained with different complex mixtures can be compared. For convenience the various antibiotic mixtures will be referred to below as "streptogramins".

It would seem obvious that the mixture of two or more compounds will affect metabolic processes which are inhibited by the individual antibiotics. However in the case of the synergistic complex of "streptogramins" the effects of the separate components are negligible when tested at the concentration in which they occur in the complex at its minimal growth inhibitory concentration.

The inhibitory spectra of various of the complex antibiotics are shown in Table 4; the antibiotics have no significant inhibitory action on fungi, yeasts, protozoa and Gram-negative bacteria. *Haemophilus pertussis* and *Neisseria gonorrhoeae* are exceptions in being as sensitive to the complex antibiotics as most Gram-positive bacteria.

Although YAMAGUCHI (1961) and ENNIS (1965a) found that the "streptogramins" have a bacteriostatic effect on *Bacterium agri* and *S. aureus*, a number of workers have reported that these antibiotics are bactericidal on growing *S. aureus* (CHARNEY *et al.*, 1953; BENAZET *et al.*, 1962; MURAT and PELLERAT, 1965; VAZQUEZ, 1966c). It is unlikely that different "streptogramins" have different effects on bacterial viability and it is possible that the reported differences are due to variations in the test organisms or experimental conditions.

"Streptogramins" prevent the bactericidal effect of penicillin, probably by inhibiting bacterial growth. Also, their bactericidal effect is completely prevented by chloramphenicol or erythromycin and partially prevented by penicillin; puromycin has no effect while aureomycin and terramycin increase the "streptogramin" action. When growth of *S. aureus* is prevented by using a medium from which glutamic acid has been omitted, the bactericidal effect of the "streptogramins" is not significantly reduced (VAZQUEZ, 1966c; CHABBERT and ACAR, 1965). These findings suggest that the complex streptogramin antibiotics can exert their bactericidal effect on *S. aureus* under conditions where growth is reduced and that the action of chloramphenicol and erythromycin in preventing the killing effect cannot be explained simply on the basis that they inhibit bacterial growth.

Contradictory reports have appeared on the occurrence of cross-resistance between the "streptogramins" and the macrolide antibiotics. JONES, NICHOLS and FINLAND (1956) found that *S. aureus* strains made resistant *in vitro* to macrolide antibiotics were not resistant to streptogramin, but strains of *S. aureus* made resistant to streptogramin were also resistant to the macrolide antibiotics. ENGLISH *et al.* (1956) found cross-resistance between synergistin and the macrolides in a laboratory strain of *S. aureus* but not in a number of erythromycin-resistant clinical isolates of *S. aureus*. Partial cross-resistance between pristinamycin, lincomycin and the macrolide antibiotics has been found by BARBER and WATERWORTH (1965). TANAKA *et al.* (1961) found partial cross-resistance between mikamycin and the macrolide antibiotics whereas cross-resistance between staphylomycin or ostreogrycin and erythromycin has not been found by other workers (GARROD and WATERWORTH, 1956; DE SOMER and VAN DIJCK, 1955).

The "streptogramins" are active when administered orally, subcutaneously or intraperitoneally in protecting mice against infections by *S. aureus*, *Streptococcus pyogenes* and *Diplococcus pneumoniae*. The toxicity of the antibiotics to mice is small when administered orally (2—2.5 g/kg) but higher when administered intraperitoneally (450 mg/kg) (VERWEY, WEST and MILLER, 1958; TANAKA *et al.*, 1961, 1962; ENGLISH *et al.*, 1956; BALL *et al.*, 1958; DE SOMER and VAN DIJCK, 1955; BENAZET *et al.*, 1962; BENAZET and COSAR, 1965).

The "streptogramins" have no effect on endogenous respiration, oxidation of ethanol or glucose, or anaerobic fermentation of glucose (VAZQUEZ, 1962). These antibiotics inhibit bacterial growth by blocking protein synthesis (Table 3); unlike chloramphenicol the inhibitory effect on protein synthesis is not readily reversible, and removal of the streptogramin is followed by only a slight increase in the rate of protein synthesis. The antibiotics do not significantly affect accumulation in the "pool" of low molecular weight constituents or the synthesis of nucleic acid and cell-wall material. The inhibitory effect of the antibiotics on protein synthesis can be detected within 2 minutes of addition. In the presence of the complex antibiotics there is an increase in nucleic acid content which is due to RNA. The synthesis of DNA is unaffected by minimum growth inhibitory concentrations of the "streptogramins" but is reduced in the presence of high concentrations (VAZQUEZ, 1962, 1966c; ENNIS, 1965a). In cell-free systems, these antibiotics have no effect on either DNA-dependent DNA polymerase or DNA-dependent RNA polymerase (ELLIOTT, 1963; WARING, 1965).

In bacterial cell-free systems the "streptogramins" inhibit amino acid incorporation, and have an additive effect, but no synergism could be demonstrated between the antibiotics in group A and B in these systems by YAMAGUCHI and TANAKA (1964), LASKIN and MAY CHAN (1964) and VAZQUEZ (1966c). However ENNIS (1965b) claims to have found synergism between antibiotics in groups A and B when they are present at certain critical concentrations. This finding has to be confirmed by other workers and, it seems rather unlikely that it is related to the synergism in intact bacteria as ENNIS (1965b) himself found that in some experiments, antibiotics of group A were more active than the complex mixtures in cell-free systems.

Mechanism of the Synergistic Effect of the Mixtures of Antibiotics in Groups A and B

The overall effects of streptogramin on *S. aureus* are similar to those of streptogramin A with three main differences: *1.* The minimum growth inhibitory concentration of streptogramin for *S. aureus* is 10% of that of streptogramin A alone. This is due to the synergistic effect of the streptogramin components A and B as an identical result can be obtained with a mixture of these antibiotics in proportions equivalent to those of the streptogramin complex. *2.* Whereas streptogramins A and B are separately bacteriostatic on *S. aureus*, the synergistic mixture is bactericidal. It is not known why the action of the synergistic mixture should be bactericidal, but it seems improbable that there is any direct connection between the bactericidal action and synergism as such since: a) Mixtures of group A antibiotics and tetracyclines are also bactericidal (VAZQUEZ, 1966c) but are not synergistic (ENGLISH *et al.*, 1956); b) mixtures of antibiotics in groups A and B have a synergistic inhibitory effect on *Bacterium agri* and certain strains of *S. aureus* and are bacteriostatic on these organisms (YAMAGUCHI, 1961; ENNIS, 1965a); and c) chloramphenicol protects bacteria against the bactericidal effect of a mixture of streptogramins A and B but does not affect the enhanced inhibitory effect of this mixture on protein synthesis (VAZQUEZ, 1966c). *3.* A lag period of 1—2 minutes is found before the synergistic mixture is effective whereas the action of growth inhibitory concentrations of either streptogramin A or B when tested separately on bacterial protein synthesis can be detected within 30 sec of incubation. This suggests that the delay in onset of the synergistic action is not explicable on the basis that the antibiotics require time to cross the permeability barrier of the bacteria (Vazquez, 1966c).

Otherwise, studies on the site of action of the streptogramin antibiotics have been useful in suggesting a possible mechanism of the synergistic action. Direct studies on binding of streptogramin A or streptogramin B to bacterial organelles have not been reported. However, streptogramin A and, to a lesser extent, streptogramin B reduce the uptake of ^{14}C-chloramphenicol by bacteria. Also, streptogramin B enhances the inhibitory effect of streptogramin A on the uptake of ^{14}C-chloramphenicol by Gram-positive organisms. Consequently it is thought that the reduction in ^{14}C-chloramphenicol uptake may be taken as a measure of uptake of the streptogramin antibiotics (Vazquez, 1966c).

Streptogramin A, but not streptogramin B, prevents binding of ^{14}C-chloramphenicol to bacterial ribosomes in cell-free systems. Streptogramin B enhances the effect of streptogramin A; a dialyzable, low molecular weight, heat stable constituent of the bacterial soluble fraction is required for this enhancement (Vazquez, 1966c). In Gram-positive bacteria the synergistic effect of streptogramin A and streptogramin B is more marked when bacteria are preincubated with the antibiotics prior to breakage of the cells and the addition of ^{14}C-chloramphenicol to the cell-sap. The binding of chloramphenicol to ribosomes is reduced by pretreatment of the cells with streptogramin A even at 4^0, but the enhancement of the inhibitory effect by streptogramin B will occur only if conditions are such that growth would normally take place in the absence of the antibiotics. On the other hand, streptogramin A and streptogramin B show no synergistic inhibitory effect on the growth of *E. coli* and in this organism pretreatment of intact cells with the mixture of the streptogramins does not enhance the effect of streptogramin A in preventing subsequent binding of ^{14}C-chloramphenicol to ribosomes (Vazquez, 1966c).

As streptogramin B enhances the binding of streptogramin A on the ribosomes and the inhibitory effect of the streptogramin complex appears to occur at the ribosome level, it seems probable that the synergism of the streptogramin antibiotics in Gram-positive bacteria is due to an enhancement by streptogramin B of the binding of streptogramin A to the ribosomes.

Discussion

The antibacterial activities of the different antibiotics within the same group of the streptogramin family are of the same order; viridogrisein is an exception in that it is more active than related antibiotics. Mikamycins are apparently less active than the other antibiotics of the family (Tables 2 and 4); this could be due to the fact that solid media were used to assay mikamycin activity whereas liquid media were used for all other antibiotics.

A partial cross resistance in bacteria has been reported between the complex antibiotics of the streptogramin family and the macrolide antibiotics. In general this cross resistance would appear to be related to the group B components of the

Table 4. *In vitro inhibitory concentrations of the complex antibiotics of the streptogramin family*

Organism	Inhibitory concentrations in µg/ml				
	Strepto-gramin	Syner-gistin	Staphylo-mycin	Mika-mycin	Pristina-mycin
Bacteria Gram-positive:					
Bacillus megaterium	2.00	—	—	64.00	—
Bacillus subtilis	—	0.78	1.00	32.00	0.70
Staphylococcus aureus	0.60	0.19	0.20	4.00	0.20
Sarcina lutea	—	—	0.10	1.00	—
Streptococcus pyogenes	0.05	0.08	0.07	—	0.10
Streptococcus faecalis	1.49	0.39	0.50	—	0.20
Diplococcus pneumoniae	0.25	3.12	0.07	6.00	0.15
Corynebacterium diphteriae	0.04	0.39	—	1.00	0.02
Mycobacterium sp. 607	11.00	6.25	—	280.00	—
Mycobacterium tuberculosis	5.00	—	20.00	200.00	—
Bacteria Gram-negative:					
Salmonella typhosa	11.80	100.00	—	1600.00	—
Escherichia coli	40.00	100.00	—	1600.00	50.00
Aerobacter aerogenes	—	100.00	100.00	—	250.00
Hemophilus pertussis	0.04	3.12	—	—	—
Neisseria gonorrheae	—	3.12	—	—	0.20
Pseudomonas aeruginosa	50.00	100.00	—	1600.00	250.00
Yeasts:					
Saccharomyces cerevisiae	85.00	—	—	1600.00	—
Candida albicans	—	100.00	100.00	1600.00	—
Fungi:					
Aspergillus niger	85.00	—	—	—	—
Aspergillus oryzae	—	—	—	1600.00	—
Protozoa:					
Trichomonas vaginalis	490.00	—	—	—	—
Trichophyton sulfureum	—	100.00	—	—	—

(CHARNEY *et al.*, 1953; VERWEY, WEST and MILLER, 1958; ENGLISH *et al.*, 1956; DE SOMER and VAN DIJCK, 1955; TANAKA *et al.*, 1958; BENAZET *et al.*, 1962).

"streptogramins". In early work on the mode of action of antibiotics, importance was placed on cross resistance between antibiotics as it was considered that cross resistance between two antibiotics meant a similarity in their site(s) or mode of action. However, it is now known that some bacterial strains carry a drug resistant episome which confers resistance to a number of drugs with completely unconnected sites or modes of action (WATANABE, 1963) and consequently it no longer follows that antibiotics showing cross resistance are necessarily related in their site(s) or modes of action.

Antibiotics in group A are inhibitors of protein synthesis. The accumulation of RNA in the presence of the antibiotics is not a direct effect of the antibiotics. An increase in the rate of RNA accumulation has also been observed in bacteria treated with chloramphenicol and it is thought to be a secondary effect following inhibition of protein synthesis. The RNA which accumulates in bacteria treated with chloramphenicol is mainly ribosomal RNA (accumulated due to an alteration of the control mechanism) and messenger-RNA (protected from decay when protein synthesis is blocked) (see reviews by HAHN in this book and VAZQUEZ, 1966d). It is likely that a similar situation occurs when protein synthesis is inhibited by streptogramin.

Antibiotics in group A inhibit the binding of chloramphenicol to the 50S subunit of the ribosomes, probably by binding to the same ribosomal subunit; consequently their site of action could be on the 50S ribosome subunit. By binding to ribosomes, antibiotics in group A may inhibit protein synthesis at one of a number of steps including: 1. Formation of the m-RNA-ribosome-aminoacyl-s-RNA complex; 2. growth of the peptide; 3. detachment of the peptide.

It has been found in cell-free systems that antibiotics in group A reduce the binding of phenylalanyl-s-RNA to ribosomes (D. VAZQUEZ, unpublished result); however this inhibition is smaller than the inhibition of phenylalanine incorporation by the same antibiotics. In cell-free systems, these antibiotics inhibit amino acid incorporation under experimental conditions in which there is no release of the peptides formed on the ribosome; it is therefore unlikely that their main action is to prevent the release of the complete peptide. They may inhibit the binding of m-RNA to ribosomes or the formation of a functional m-RNA-ribosomes-aminoacyl-s-RNA complex. They may inhibit peptide growth on the ribosome by such action as: a) inhibition of either of the two enzymes involved in the last steps of protein synthesis (ALLENDE *et al.*, 1964; ARLINGHAUS, SHAEFFER and SCHWEET, 1964) or b) alteration of the ribosomal structure as has been postulated for streptomycin (DAVIES *et al.*, 1964) and chloramphenicol (VAZQUEZ, 1966d). Antibiotics in group A may not attach to ribosomes at precisely the same site as chloramphenicol but their effect on the 70 S ribosomes is very similar to that of chloramphenicol.

Antibiotics in group B are also inhibitors of protein synthesis. *In vitro* studies have shown that these antibiotics have also some inhibitory effect on nucleic acid and cell wall synthesis. The inhibitory effect on nucleic acid synthesis occurs in intact cells and the antibiotics have no demonstrable effect on cell-free DNA-dependent DNA or RNA-polymerases. The inhibitory effect of these antibiotics on protein synthesis is located in the reactions which follow the formation of aminoacyl-s-RNA and precede the formation of the complete polypeptides on the ribosome.

A number of antibiotics believed to act on the 50S ribosome subunit (chloramphenicol, macrolides, lincomycin, antibiotics of group A) reduce the binding to ribosomes of either phenylalanyl-s-RNA or chloramphenicol. As antibiotics of group B do not inhibit the binding to ribosomes of either chloramphenicol or aminoacyl-s-RNA it is probable that they do not act on the 50S ribosome subunit. Antibiotics of group B may well act on the enzymic reactions leading to protein synthesis or on the 30S ribosome subunit. Indeed it has been found that antibiotics of group B enhance the binding of phenylalanyl-s-RNA to 30S ribosome subunits directed by poly U (D. VAZQUEZ, unpublished result).

The overall effects of the "streptogramin" mixtures are very similar to those of antibiotics in group A. The results reported above suggest that the synergism of A and B antibiotics can be explained by an enhancement by component B of the binding of component A to ribosomes.

Thanks are due to Dr. D. KERRIDGE and Prof. E. F. GALE, F.R.S., for advice during the preparation of this manuscript. Thanks are also given to the Imperial Chemical Industries for a Fellowship.

See addendum

References

ACTOR, P., H. BASCH, and W. P. JAMBOR: Synergistic activity of vernamycins *in vitro* and *in vivo*. Bacteriol. Proc. **1963**, 94.

ALLENDE, J. E., R. MONRO, and F. LIPMANN: Resolution of the *Escherichia coli* aminoacyl-s-RNA transfer factor into two complementary fractions. Proc. Natl. Acad. Sci. U.S. **51**, 1211 (1964).

ARAI, M., S. NAKAMURA, Y. SAKAGAMI, K. FUKUHARA, and H. YONEHARA: A new antibiotic, mikamycin. J. Antibiotics (Japan), Ser. A **9**, 193 (1956).

ARLINGHAUS, R., J. SHAEFFER, and R. SCHWEET: Mechanism of peptide bond formation in polypeptide synthesis. Proc. Natl. Acad. Sci. U.S. **51**, 1291 (1964).

ARNOLD, R. B., A. W. JOHNSON, and A. B. MAUGER: The structure of viridogrisein (etamycin). J. Chem. Soc. **1958**, 4466.

BALL, S., B. BOOTHROYD, K. A. LEES, A. H. RAPER, and E. LESTER SMITH: Preparation and properties of an antibiotic complex E 219. Biochem. J. **68**, 24P (1958).

BARBER, M., and P. M. WATERWORTH: Antibacterial activity of lincomycin and pristinamycin: A comparison with erythromycin. Brit. Med. J. **1964II**, 603.

BARTZ, Q. R., J. STANDIFORD, J. D. MOLD, D. W. JOHANNESSEN, A. RYDER, A. MARETZKI, and T. H. HASKELL: Griseoviridin and viridogrisein: isolation and characterization. Antibiotics Ann. **1954/55**, 777.

BENAZET, F., et C. COSAR: Etude chez l'animal des constituants de la pristinamycine (7293 R.P.). Ann. Inst. Pasteur **109**, 281 (1965).

BENAZET, F., C. COSAR, M. DUBOST, L. JULOU et D. MANCY: Un nouvel antibiotique, la pristinamycine (7293 R.P.). Semaine hôp. **38**, 13 (1962).

BESSELL, J., K. H. FANTES, W. HEWITT, P. W. MUGGLETON, and J. P. R. TOOTILL: The analysis and evaluation of the synergistic components of antibiotic E 129. Biochem. J. **68**, 24P (1958).

BODANSKY, M., and M. A. ONDETTI: Structure of the vernamycin B group of antibiotics. Antimicrobial Agents and Chemotherapy, p. 360 (1963).

BODANSZKY, M., and J. T. SHEEHAN: Structure of doricin, a peptide related to the vernamycin B group. Antimicrobial Agents and Chemotherapy, p. 38 (1963).

CELMER, W. D., and B. A. SOBIN: The isolation of two synergistic antibiotics from a single fermentation source. Antibiotics Ann. **1955/56**, 437.

CERCOS, A. P.: Effects of etamycin upon seedling growth and chlorophyll production. Phytopathology **54**, 741 (1964).

CHABBERT, Y. A., et J. F. ACAR: Interactions bacteriostatiques et bactericides chez les antibiotiques du groupe de la streptogramine. Ann. Inst. Pasteur **107**, 777 (1965).

CHARNEY, J., W. P. FISHER, CH. CURRAN, R. A. MACHLOWITZ, and A. A. TYTELI: Streptogramin, a new antibiotic. Antibiotics & Chemotherapy **3**, 1283 (1953).

CHENG, L., S. VAN STRATEN, and J. F. SNELL: Metabolic spectra. VI. An evaluation of the synergistic action between PA 114 A and B *in vitro*. Antibiotics & Chemotherapy **10**, 671 (1960).

DAVIES, J., W. GILBERT, and L. GORINI: Streptomycin, supression, and the code. Proc. Natl. Acad. Sci. U.S. **51**, 883 (1964).

DELPIERRE, G. R., F. W. EASTWOOD, G. E. GREAM, D. G. I. KINGSTON, P. S. SARIN, LORD TODD, and D. H. WILLIAMS: The structure of ostreogrycin A. Tetrahedron Letters **4**, 369 (1966).

DE SOMER, P., and P. VAN DIJCK: A preliminary report on antibiotic number 899, a streptogramin-like substance. Antibiotics & Chemotherapy **5**, 632 (1955).

DUBOST, M., et C. PASCAL: Méthodes de dosage des constituants de la pristinamycine dans les liquides biologiques. Ann. Inst. Pasteur **109**, 290 (1965).

EASTWOOD, F. W., R. K. SNELL, and L. TODD: Antibiotics of the E 129 (ostreogrycin) complex. Part I. The structure of E 129B. J. Chem. Soc. **1960**, 2286.

ELLIOTT, W. H.: The effects of antimicrobial agents on deoxyribonucleic acid polymers. Biochem. J. **86**, 562 (1963).

ENGLISH, A. R., T. J. MCBRIDGE, and G. VAN HALSEMA: Biologic studies on the PA 114 group of antibiotics. Antibiotics Ann. **1955/56**, 422.

ENNIS, H. L.: Inhibition of protein synthesis by polypeptide antibiotics. I. Inhibition in intact bacteria. J. Bacteriol. **90**, 1102 (1965a).

ENNIS, H. L.: Inhibition of protein synthesis by polypeptide antibiotics. II. *In vitro* protein synthesis. J. Bacteriol. **90**, 1109 (1965b).

GARCIA-MENDOZA, C.: Studies on the mode of action of etamycin (viridogrisein). Biochim. et Biophys. Acta **97**, 394 (1965).

GARROD, L. P., and P. M. WATERWORTH: Behaviour *in vitro* of some new antistaphylococcal antibiotics. Brit. Med. J. **1956II**, 61.

GREAM, G. E.: Structural studies on ostreogrycin A. Ph. D. Thesis, Cambridge University, England 1961.

HEINEMAN, B., A. GOUREVITCH, J. LEIN, D. L. JOHNSON, M. A. KAPLAN, D. VANAS, and I. R. HOOPER: Etamycin, a new antibiotic. Antibiotics Ann. **1954/55**, 728.

HOBBS, D. C., and W. D. CELMER: Structure of the antibiotics PA 114 B-1 and PA 114 B-3. Nature **187**, 598 (1960).

JONES, W. F., R. L. NICHOLS, and M. FINLAND: Development of resistance and cross-resistance *in vitro* to erythromycin, carbomycin, spiramycin, oleandomycin and streptogramin. Proc. Soc. Exptl. Biol. Med. **93**, 388 (1956).

KNUDSEN, M. P., R. W. SARBER, A. S. SCHLINGMAN, R. M. SMITH, and J. K. WESTON: Griseoviridin and viridogrisein: Biologic studies. Antibiotics Ann. **1954/55**, 790.

LASKIN, A. I., and W. MAY CHAN: Inhibition by vernamycin A of amino acid incorporation in *Escherichia coli* cell-free systems. Antimicrobial Agents and Chemotherapy, p. 485 (1964).

LASKIN, A. I., and W. MAY CHAN: Effects of vernamycins on aminoacyl-transfer RNA binding to *Escherichia coli* ribosomes. Antimicrobial Agents and Chemotherapy **1965**, 321.

LESTER SMITH, E.: The ostreogrycins. A family of synergistic antibiotics. J. Gen. Microbiol. **33**, 111 (1963).

MURAT, M., et J. PELLERAT: Etude comparative des pouvoirs bactériostatiques et bactéricide de la pristinamycine, de la méthicilline et de la pénicilline sur un certain nombre de souches de staphylocoques et de streptocoques hemolytiques. Ann. Inst. Pasteur **109**, 317 (1965).

NIRENBERG, M., and P. LEDER: RNA codewords and protein synthesis. The effect of trinucleotides upon the binding of sRNA to ribosomes. Science **145**, 1399 (1964).

PREUD'HOMME, J., A. BELLOC, Y. CHARPENTIÉ et P. TARRIDEC: Un antibiotique formé de deux de composants à synergie d'action: la pristinamycine. Compt. rend. **260**, 1309 (1965).

SARIN, P. S.: Structural studies on the antibiotics ostreogrycin A and G. Ph. D. Thesis, Cambridge University, England 1962.

SHEEHAN, J. C., H. G. ZACHAU, and W. B. LAWSON: The structure of etamycin. J. Am. Chem. Soc. **80**, 3349 (1958).

SUZUKA, I., H. KAJI, and A. KAJI: Binding of specific sRNA to 30s subunits. Comparison with the binding to 70s ribosomes. Biochem. Biophys. Research Commun. **21**, 187 (1965).

TANAKA, N., N. MIYAIRI, K. WATANABE, N. SHINJO, T. NISHIMURA, and H. UMEZAWA: Biological studies on mikamycin. II. Laboratory investigations of mikamycin A and mikamycin B. J. Antibiotics (Japan), Ser. A **12**, 290 (1959).

TANAKA, N., N. MIYAIRI, T. NISHIMURA, and H. UMEZAWA: Activity of mikamycins, angustmycins and emimycin against antibiotic-resistant staphylococci. J. Antibiotics (Japan), Ser. A **14**, 18 (1961).

TANAKA, N., N. SHINJO, N. MIYAIRI, and H. UMEZAWA: Biological studies on mikamycin. J. Antibiotics (Japan), Ser. A **11**, 127 (1958).

TANAKA, N., H. YAMAKI, H. YAMAGUCHI, and H. UMEZAWA: Biologic studies on mikamycin. III. Influence of blood on the activity against experimental infections. J. Antibiotics (Japan), Ser. A **15**, 28 (1962).
THOMSEN, V. F.: The *in vitro* activity of staphylomycin. Acta Path. Microbiol. Scand. **57**, 120 (1963).
VANDERHAEGHE, H., P. VAN DIJCK, G. PARMENTIER, and P. DE SOMER: Isolation and properties of the components of staphylomycin. Antibiotics & Chemotherapy **7**, 606 (1957).
VANDERHAEGHE, H., and G. PARMENTIER: The structure of factor S of staphylomycin. J. Am. Chem. Soc. **82**, 4414 (1960).
VAN DIJCK, P., H. VANDERHAEGHE, and P. DE SOMER: Microbiologic study of the components of staphylomycin. Antibiotics & Chemotherapy **7**, 625 (1957).
VAZQUEZ, D.: Antibiotics which affect protein synthesis: The uptake of ^{14}C-chloramphenicol by bacteria. Biochem. Biochys. Research Commun. **12**, 409 (1963).
VAZQUEZ, D.: Uptake and binding of chloramphenicol by sensitive and resistant organisms. Nature **203**, 257 (1964a).
VAZQUEZ, D.: The mode of action of streptogramin. Ph. D. Thesis, Cambridge University, Cambridge, England 1964b.
VAZQUEZ, D.: The binding of chloramphenicol by ribosomes from *Bacillus megaterium*. Biochem. Biophys. Research. Commun. **15**, 464 (1964c).
VAZQUEZ, D.: Binding of chloramphenicol to ribosomes. The effect of a number of antibiotics. Biochim. et Biophys. Acta **144**, 277 (1966a).
VAZQUEZ, D.: Antibiotics affecting chloramphenicol uptake by bacteria. Their effect on amino acid incorporation in a cell-free system. Biochim. et Biophys. Acta **114**, 289 (1966b).
VAZQUEZ, D.: Studies on the mode of action of the streptogramin antibiotics. J. Gen. Microbiol. **42**, 93 (1966c).
VAZQUEZ, D.: Mode of action of chloramphenicol and related antibiotics. Symposium Soc. Gen. Microbiol. **16**, 169 (1966d).
VERWEY, W. F., M. K. WEST, and A. K. MILLER: Laboratory studies of streptogramin. Antibiotics & Chemotherapy **8**, 500 (1958).
VIDEAU, D.: La pristinamycine et le phénomène de bactériopause. Ann. Inst. Psteur **108**, 602 (1965).
WARING, K. J.: The effect of antimicrobial agents on ribonucleic acid polymerase. Mol. Pharmacol. **1**, 1 (1965).
WATANABE, K.: Studies on mikamycin. V. *In vitro* synergistic action and differential assay of mikamycin components. J. Antibiotics (Japan), Ser. A **13**, 62 (1960).
WATANABE, K.: Studies on mikamycin. VII. Structure of mikamycin B. J. Antibiotics (Japan), Ser. A **14**, 14 (1961).
WATANABE, T.: Infective heredity of multiple drug resistance in bacteria. Bacteriol. Rev. **27**, 87 (1963).
YAMAGUCHI, H.: Action mechanism of mikamycins. I. Effect of mikamycins on protein and nucleic acid metabolisms. J. Antibiotics (Japan), Ser. A **14**, 313 (1961).
YAMAGUCHI, H.: Action mechanism of mikamycins. II. Effect of mikamycins on incorporation of ^{14}C-L-leucine into ribonucleic acid and protein in various microorganisms. J. Antibiotics (Japan), Ser. A **16**, 92 (1963a).
YAMAGUCHI, H.: Action mechanism of mikamycins. III. Further studies on the site of action of mikamycins. J. Antibiotics (Japan), Ser. A **16**, 97 (1963b).
YAMAGUCHI, H., and N. TANAKA: Selective toxicity of mikamycins inhibitors of protein synthesis. Nature **201**, 499 (1964).

Fucidin

C. L. Harvey, C. J. Sih, and S. G. Knight

This volume attests to the fact that we are now entering a period in which our knowledge about the mode of action of antibiotics is increasing at a rapid rate. This increase is largely the result of an increased understanding of cellular physiology and better techniques for its study. However, there have been but few studies on the mechanism of action of the steroid antibiotics, probably because only a few are known. In brief, there are two antifungal steroid antibiotics: viridan produced by *Trichoderma iride*, and eburicoic acid produced by a basidiomycete; and three antibacterial steroid antibiotics: helvolic acid produced by *Aspergillus fumigatus*, cephalosporin P_1 produced by *Cephalosporium salmosynnematum*, and fusidic acid produced by *Fusidium coccineum*. At this time, fusidic acid seems to be the steroid antibiotic with greatest therapeutic potential. It was isolated by GODTFREDSEN *et al.* (1962), and tentatively characterized by GODTFREDSEN and VANGEDAL (1962); recently the chemical structure has been modified to that shown in Fig. 1 (GODTFREDSEN, personal communication). Fig. 1 shows that the three antibacterial steroid antibiotics, helvolic acid, fusidic acid, and cephalosporin P_1, are chemically related. They each contain a tetracyclic ring with an identical side chain which has an *alpha, beta* unsaturated carboxylic acid and a *beta* oriented acetoxyl group on carbon 16.

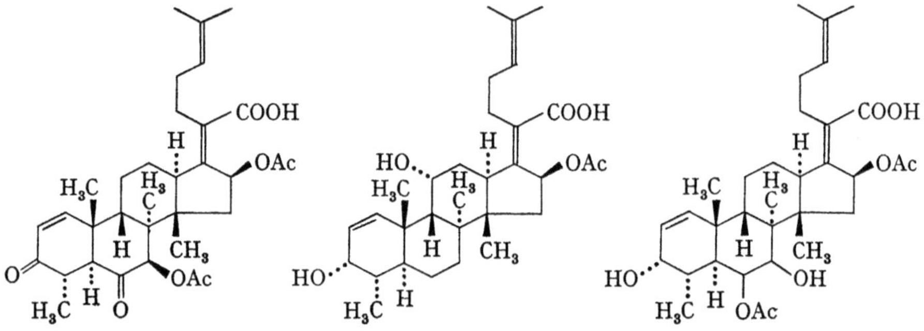

(I) (II) (III)

Fig. 1. Structures of the steroidal antibiotics. *I*. Helvolic acid; *II*. Fusidic acid; *III*. Cephalosporin P_1

Fusidic acid was shown by GODTFREDSEN *et al.* (1962) to be active against gram positive bacteria but not against gram negative bacteria and fungi, and cross resistance with cephalosporin P_1 was found.

Although the three antibiotics in Fig. 1 have a similar structure and antibacterial spectrum, there is a quantitative difference in activity. RITCHIE *et al.* (1951) showed that cephalsporin P_1 was 16 times more active against *Staphylococcus aureus* than helvolic acid and BARBER and WATERWORTH (1962) found that fusidic acid was more active against a number of gram positive bacteria than was cephalosporin P_1. Fusidic acid is very insoluble in water while the sodium and potassium salts are soluble. For this reason, fusidic acid is used clinically as the sodium salt which has been designated fucidin by the manufacturer (Leo Pharmaceutical Products, Copenhagen, Denmark).

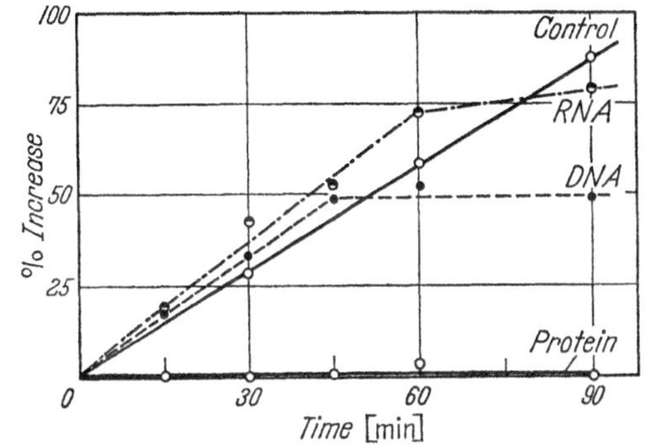

Fig. 2. The effect of fucidin on the synthesis of DNA, RNA, and protein in growing cells of *Staphylococcus aureus*. The cells were grown (generation time of 1.6 hours) in tryptose-phosphate broth (Difco). At mid-log phase (0 time), 10 µg/ml of fucidin was added and samples were taken every 15 minutes. o —— o DNA, RNA and protein of control; • —— • DNA after addition of fucidin; ◒ —— ◒ RNA after addition of fucidin; o —— o Protein after addition of fucidin

Preliminary work by HARVEY *et al.* (1965) showed that fucidin inhibited protein synthesis in whole cells of *S. aureus* and in cell-free extracts of *Escherichia coli*; a recent paper by YAMAKI (1965) has confirmed this. YAMAKI showed that fucidin and helvolinic acid (a hydrolysis product of helvolic acid) inhibited protein synthesis directed by both polyuridylic acid or endogenous messenger in cell-free extracts of *E. coli* and *Mycobacterium* 607. He proposed that the primary effect of these antibiotics was in blocking protein synthesis.

The following is a summary of extensive research on the mode of action of fucidin. The details of the methods used in this research have been published by HARVEY (1966) and by HARVEY *et al.* (1966).

The addition of 10 µg/ml of fucidin to slowly growing (generation time of 1.6 hr) cells of *S. aureus* stopped growth only after the optical density had increased 100—150%. The addition of this concentration of the antibiotic never caused lysis of the cells. However, Fig. 2 shows that after the addition of fucidin, RNA increased 75% and stopped, DNA increased 40—50% and stopped, and measurable protein synthesis was stopped at once. The synthesis of cell wall mucopeptide was not stopped by 10 µg/ml of fucidin since L-lysine-^{14}C was still incorporated into the mucopeptide in the absence of incorporation into cytoplasmic protein. This continued synthesis of cell wall mucopeptide most likely accounts for the 100—150% increase in optical density after the addition of fucidin. Similar results were obtained by HANCOCK and PARK (1958) upon the addition of chloramphenicol to growing cells of *S. aureus*.

The antibacterial spectrum of fucidin closely follows the separation of bacteria by the gram reaction; gram positive cells are sensitive and gram negative are not. *E. coli* C was insensitive to 100 μg fucidin/ml under the assay conditions used for *S. aureus* and L-phenylalanine-^{14}C was incorporated into the protein fraction. However, incorporation of the L-phenylalanine into spheroplasts of *E. coli* C was inhibited by 10 μg/ml of fucidin and in the absence of fucidin the amino acid was incorporated. Hence, resistance to fucidin by this strain of *E. coli*, and perhaps other resistant bacteria, would seem to be the result of the lack of cell wall permeability and not enzymatic degradation of the antibiotic or a basic difference in the reaction which is inhibited. To test this hypothesis, the effect of fucidin on three different cell-free protein synthesizing systems was determined. The three systems were those of NIRENBERG (1963) in *E. coli*, FRIEDMAN and WEINSTEIN (1964) in *Bacillus stearothermophilus*, and BRETTHAUER *et al.* (1963) in a diploid yeast, *Saccharomyces fragilis* × *S. dobzhanskii*. The cell free incorporation of phenylalanine-^{14}C into polyphenylalanine-^{14}C when directed by polyuridylic acid was inhibited 77—85% by fucidin in the three systems. In the *E. coli* system, ^{14}C-polyphenylalanine synthesis was inhibited nearly 100% by 4×10^{-3} M fucidin and not at all by 2×10^{-5} M. Fucidin at all concentrations was approximately twice as inhibitory as equal amounts of chloramphenicol. The rest of the work on inhibition of protein synthesis in cell free systems was done with *E. coli* preparations, since they have been studied very extensively and much of our current knowledge about protein synthesis has been obtained by studying this organism.

Fucidin at 4×10^{-4} M inhibited the incorporation of phenylalanine-^{14}C, alanine, tyrosine, and lysine 54 to 59% by ribosomes plus endogenous messenger RNA. Similar results were obtained in cell free systems directed by polyuridylic acid. Fucidin was inhibitory to polyphenylalanine synthesis when added either before or after the polyuridylic acid messenger. Studies then were made to determine the specific step in protein synthesis that was inhibited by fucidin. The first step in protein synthesis consists of the activation of amino acids by specific enzymes and ATP to form aminoacyl-adenylates, followed by the transfer of the amino acid to its specific soluble RNA (HOAGLAND, *et al.*, 1957). Experiments showed that 1 mM fucidin had no effect on the activation and transfer of phenylalanine to phenylalanyl-soluble RNA; whereas, this concentration of the antibiotic caused 70—80% inhibition of polyphenylalanine synthesis. Further experiments showed that fucidin did not prevent the attachment of polyuridylic acid-C^{14} to the ribosomes in the formation of polyribosomes; hence the formation of this functional unit of protein synthesis (GILBERT, 1963) was not blocked.

The next step in protein synthesis is a specific binding of aminoacyl soluble RNA to the ribosomes in the presence of complementary template (SPYRIDES, 1964). This binding takes place before the polymerization of the amino acids and is considered to be the final step before the formation of the peptide chain. The procedure of NIRENBERG and LEDER (1964) was used to determine the effect of fucidin on the binding of aminoacyl soluble RNA to *E. coli* C ribosomes. Fucidin concentrations of 0.2 mM and 2.0 mM had no effect on the binding of phenylalanyl-^{14}C soluble RNA to the polyuridylic acid complex.

In an attempt to reverse or at least decrease the inhibitory effect of fucidin, different components that are known to be necessary for protein synthesis were added in varying amounts to the complete mixture. Varying the concentration of ribosomes 200 fold and the concentration of the supernatant fraction 8 fold had no effect on the inhibition caused by 0.1 mM fucidin. The optimum amount of magnesium ions necessary for protein synthesis was not displaced by 0.1 mM fucidin, indicating that the antibiotic did not act as a chelating agent. Likewise, inhibition of synthesis was not changed by concentrations of phenylalanyl-^{14}C soluble RNA from 31 μg to 250 μg, a 20 fold increase in polyuridylic acid, an 11 fold increase in guanosine triphosphate. Spermidine at a concentration of 60 μg and 600 μg did not inhibit the synthesis. In further attempts to locate the region of inhibition by fucidin, it was found that total inhibition of protein synthesis by fucidin plus chloramphenicol or streptomycin was additive. Thus, polyphenylalanine formation was inhibited 37% by 0.1 mM fucidin and 17% by 0.2 mM chloramphenicol; the same concentrations of fucidin and chloramphenicol when added together inhibited protein synthesis 52%. Streptomycin at a concentration of 0.02 mM inhibited protein synthesis 54%, but streptomycin plus 0.1 mM fucidin inhibited 94%. Thus, it seems apparent that fucidin inhibits protein synthesis at a different site than does either chloramphenicol or streptomycin.

Finally, a series of experiments were done to determine if fucidin was irreversibly bound to or inactivated by some component of the supernatant or the ribosome fraction. Ribosomes that were incubated with fucidin for 10 minutes and removed by centrifugation at 107,000 × g for 2 hours were as efficient in forming polyphenylalanine as ribosomes that had not been exposed to fucidin. Furthermore, ribosomes and supernatant fraction to which fucidin had been added, and then removed by dialysis, were as active as the controls. Fucidin, therefore, does not inhibit protein synthesis by inactivating or irreversibly binding with and inactivating ribosomes or supernatant fraction.

One of the difficulties in assigning a mode or site of action to an antibiotic is separating the primary reaction from the secondary ones. This often can only be done by careful studies of the kinetics of intermediary and cellular reactions. Where this has been done, the drug has been assigned a single mode of action; other effects have been secondary. One of the most useful techniques, and one used here, has been to lengthen the generation time and thereby make possible the separation of the numerous reactions envolved. This was done by growing the cells slowly at suboptimal temperatures. In the study of the mode of action of fucidin, the immediate and most apparent effect of the drug was inhibition of cytoplasmic protein synthesis in slowly growing cells. Inhibition of DNA and RNA synthesis occurred later and has been considered secondary. Likewise, the 100—150% increase in optical density and the increase of cell-wall mucopeptide after the addition of fucidin indicates that inhibition of cell wall mucopeptide synthesis was secondary. Hash, *et al.* (1964) found a similar situation in studying the action of tetracycline on growing cells of *S. aureus*. In regard to the delay in the inhibition of DNA synthesis, Kurland and Maaløe (1962) believe that synthesis stops only after the completion of a division cycle because new protein is needed to start the next cycle- this may be the situation in the delayed inhibition of DNA synthesis by fucidin.

Although the main objective of this work was to find the mode of action of fucidin, a useful and interesting secondary finding was that a lack of permeability of *E. coli* to the antibiotic was responsible for resistance. Fucidin was inactive against whole cells of *E. coli* at concentrations up to 100 μg/ml, whereas protein synthesis in spheroplasts of *E. coli* was inhibited by 10 μg/ml, the same amount needed to inhibit whole cells of *S. aureus*. The spheroplasts did not lyse. Furthermore, fucidin, which like other steroid antibiotics is an anionic surface active compound, did not cause "leakage" from *S. aureus* of compounds absorbing at 260 mμ, a general test for membrane damage.

All of the data gathered from the work on inhibition of protein synthesis in cell free systems from *E. coli* C indicate that fucidin does not irreversibly bind to any known constituent that is needed for *in vitro* protein synthesis. Any binding, if indeed binding occurs, must be extremely reversible, and at the same time damaging to the system. Although binding of fucidin to any of the components needed for protein synthesis and the actual point of inhibition could not be shown, the possible mechanisms of action were narrowed.

Fucidin did not effect the specific activation or transfer of phenylalanine to soluble RNA and the formation of the polysomes, and the binding of phenylalanyl soluble RNA to this complex was not inhibited. At this stage in protein synthesis, the ternary complex has been formed and the actual synthesis of the peptide chain is about to start, if no inhibitor is present. Fucidin, therefore, must effect the *final* polymerization of the amino acids after the formation of the ternary complex. This stage may be arbitrarily divided into three steps, 1. initiation of the peptide chain by polymerization of amino acids, 2. the movement of the ribosome to the successive codons, and 3. the release of the completed peptide chain from the ribosome. The exact mechanisms by which these steps take place are not known. Further research on the mode of action of fucidin and on the terminal steps of protein synthesis will be mutually helpful in solving these intriguing basic problems. Indeed, studies on the mode of action of a number of different antibiotics might greatly clarify, and contribute to, our knowledge of basic metabolic reactions.

This work was supported by a predoctoral fellowship, 1-Fl-GM-22, 761-01 from the National Institutes of Health to C. L. HARVEY, and by grant AI-01201-09 from the National Institutes of Health to S. G. KNIGHT.

References

BARBER, M., and P. W. WATERWORTH: Antibacterial activity *in vitro* of fucidin. Lancet **1962**, 931.

BRETTHAUER, R. K., L. MARCUS, J. CHALOUPKA, H. O. HALVORSON, and R. M. BOCK: Amino acid incorporation into protein by cell-free extracts of yeast. Biochemistry **2**, 1079 (1963).

FRIEDMAN, S. M., and I. B. WEINSTEIN: Lack of fidelity in the translation of synthetic polynucleotides. Prod. Natl. Acad. Sci. U.S. **52**, 988 (1964).

GILBERT, W.: Polypeptide synthesis in *Escherichia coli*. 1. Ribosomes and the active complex. J. Mol. Biol. **6**, 374 (1963).

GODTFREDSEN, W. O., S. JAHNSEN, H. LORCK, K. ROHOLT, and L. TYBRING: Fusidic acid, a new antibiotic. Nature **193**, 987 (1962).

GODTFREDSEN, W. K., and S. VANGEDAL: The structure of fusidic acid. Tetrahedron **18**, 1029 (1962).

HANCOCK, R., and J. T. PARK: Cell-wall synthesis of *Staphylococcus aureus* in the presence of chloramphenicol. Nature **181**, 1050 (1958).
HARVEY, C. L.: The mode of action of fucidin. Ph. D. Thesis, University Wisconsin, Madison 1966.
HARVEY, C. L., C. J. SIH, and S. G. KNIGHT: The mode of action of fusidic acid. Bacteriol. Proc. 3 (1965).
HARVEY, C. L., C. J. SIH, and S. G. KNIGHT: On the mode of action of fusidic acid. Biochemistry **5**, 3320 (1966).
HASH, J. H., M. WISHNICK, and P. A. MILLER: On the mode action of the tetracycline antibiotics in *Staphylococcus aureus*. J. Biol. Chem. **239**, 2070 (1964).
HOAGLAND, M. B., P. C. ZAMECNICK, and M. L. STEPHENSON: Intermediate reactions in protein synthesis. Biochim. et Biophys. Acta **24**, 215 (1957).
KURLAND, C. G., and O. MAALØE: Regulation of ribosomal and transfer RNA synthesis. J. Mol. Biol. **4**, 193 (1962).
NIRENBERG, M. W.: Cell-free protein synthesis directed by messenger RNA. In: S. P. COLWICK, and N. O. KAPLAN (eds.), Methods of enzymology, vol. 6. p. 17. New York: Academic Press, Inc. 1963.
NIRENBERG, M., and P. LEDER: RNA codewords and protein synthesis; the effect of trinucleotides upon the binding of sRNA to ribosomes. Science **145**, 1399 (1964).
RITCHIE, A. C., N. SMITH, and H. W. FLOREY: Some biological properties of cephalosporin P_1. Brit. J. Pharmacol. **6**, 430 (1951).
SPYRIDES, G. J.: The effect of univalent cations on the binding of sRNA to the template-ribosome complex. Proc. Natl. Acad. Sci. U.S. **51**, 1220 (1964).
YAMAKI, H.: Inhibition of protein synthesis by fusidic and helvolinic acids, steroidal antibiotics. J. Antibiotics (Japan), Ser. A, **18**, 228 (1965).

Sparsomycin

Libor Slechta

Sparsomycin is one of the antibiotics produced by *Streptomyces sparsogenes* var. *sparsogenes* (OWEN, DIETZ and CAMIENER, 1962). It has been isolated as crystalline material from the culture filtrates and has the molecular formula $C_{31}H_{21}N_3O_6S_2$ (ARGOUDELIS and HERR, 1962) but its structure is not yet known.

Biological Properties

Sparsomycin inhibits the growth of both Gram-positive and Gram-negative bacteria (Table 1) and has also a weak antifungal activity. It has a marked cytotoxic effect on KB cells in tissue culture and has been, therefore, evaluated *in vivo* as an antitumor agent (Table 2). The antitumor effect of sparsomycin was only found at toxic or very nearly toxic levels. Recently PITTILLO *et al.* (1965), have reported that sparsomycin modified the effect of ionizing irradiation on *Escherichia coli*. Depending on concentration, the antibiotic either afforded a slight protection or markedly potentiated the radiation damage to the cells.

Table 1. *Antibacterial spectrum of sparsomycin* (OWEN, DIETZ and CAMIENER, 1962)

Microorganism	Growth Medium[1]	MIC[2] (μg/ml)		
		16 hours	24 hours	40 hours
Bacillus subtilis	BH 1	10	10	10
Lactobacillus casei	BH 1	10	12.5	12.5
Streptococcus faecalis	BH 1	25	25—50	50
Klebsiella pneumoniae	BH 1	25	25	25
Proteus vulgaris	BH 1	10	12.5—25	25
Escherichia coli	BH 1	25	25	25
Salmonella galinarum	BH 1	5—10	5—10	6.3—12.5

[1] BH 1: Brain heart infusion broth (Difco).
[2] MIC- Minimal inhibitory concentration.

Mechanism of Action

The mode of action of sparsomycin in bacteria has been examined by SLECHTA (1965) and in reticulocytes by COLOMBO, FELICETTI and BAGLIONI (1965). In the study with growing *E. coli* as the model system, the antibiotic had primarily a bacteriostatic effect which was followed by a slow bactericidal effect. The inhibition of bacterial growth by this antibiotic led to a release of several free L-amino acids from the cells into the growth medium. As shown in Table 3, the amounts of released amino acids were dependent on the extent of growth inhibition.

Measurements of DNA, RNA and protein synthesis in cells with partially inhibited growth indicated that protein synthesis was the primary site of action of sparsomycin and demonstrated the dissociation of protein and RNA synthesis. In these experiments, the growth and DNA synthesis were inhibited to the same degree, RNA synthesis was inhibited less and protein synthesis more than growth. The differential inhibitory effect of sparsomycin on RNA and protein synthesis in bacteria was also demonstrated by measuring the incorporation of appropriate radioactive precursors. Results of such experiments (Fig. 1) show not only marked inhibition of protein synthesis as compared with RNA synthesis (15 minutes'

Table 2. *In vivo antitumor activity of sparsomycin*[1] (OWEN, DIETZ, and CAMIENER, 1962)

Tumor[2]	mg/kg Dose	Per cent Inhibition[3]	Deaths
Sarcoma 180 (solid)	0.5	31	0/5
	1.0	32	2/5
Sarcoma 180 (ascitic)	0.5	98—99	1—2/5
Ridgeway osteogenic sarcoma	0.5	28—37	0/5
	0.25	39	0/5
Bashford carcinoma 63	0.5	30—40	0/5
Carcinoma 1025	0.25	46	0/5
	0.5	43	2/5
Ehrlich carcinoma (ascitic)	0.5	90—98	1—2/5
Glioma 26	0.5	25—33	0—1/5
Walker carcinoma 256	0.5	50—72	2/5
Flexner Jobling carcinoma	0.5	53	0/5
Iglesias sarcoma	0.25	35	1/5
Babcock rat-kidney tumor	0.5	32—46	0—1/5

[1] Tumor data presented in this table furnished by K. SUGIURA at the Sloan-Kettering Institute for Cancer Research, Rye, N.Y.

[2] Tumors exhibiting less than a 25% inhibition at 0.5 mg/kg were mammary adenocarcinoma E 0771, Mecca lymphosarcoma, Miyono adenocarcinoma, Wagner osteogenic sarcoma, Ehrlich carcinoma (solid), Lewis lung carcinoma, Harding Bassey melanoma, Murphy-Sturm lymphosarcoma, and Crabb hamster sarcoma.

[3] The per cent inhibition values shown above for solid tumors were calculated using tumor-diameter measurements; 25% inhibition was considered significant. The values for ascitic tumors were calculated from tumor weight; 58% inhibition was considered significant.

Table 3. *Amino acids released by E. coli in the presence of sparsomycin during 4 hours incubation* (SLECHTA, 1965)

Conc. of sparsomycin in medium	Inhibition of growth	µMoles of amino acid in 100 ml of medium							
		Aspartic acid	Serine	Glutamic acid	Glycine	Alanine	Valine	Isoleucine	Leucine
0	0%	0.207	0.000	0.315	0.000	1.650	0.550	0.000	0.000
6 µg/ml	45%	0.330	0.115	1.205	0.200	2.675	3.537	0.100	0.365
9 µg/ml	74%	0.317	0.195	3.025	0.975	4.850	3.030	0.192	0.727
12 µg/ml	89%	0.370	0.287	7.625	1.062	5.700	1.812	0.205	0.747
15 µg/ml	96%	0.345	0.950	9.825	1.065	4.700	1.172	0.240	0.682

incubation), but also the continuation of RNA synthesis after the protein synthesis came to a stop.

It was of interest, therefore, to examine the RNA synthesized under these conditions. The cells, incubated for 15 minutes with sparsomycin to stop the protein synthesis, were exposed for various lengths of time to radioactive precursors of RNA. Extracts were prepared by grinding the cells with alumina and were analyzed by the sucrose density gradient centrifugation. The results of a 1 minute pulse experiment with tritiated uridine (Fig. 2) showed the precursor incorporated

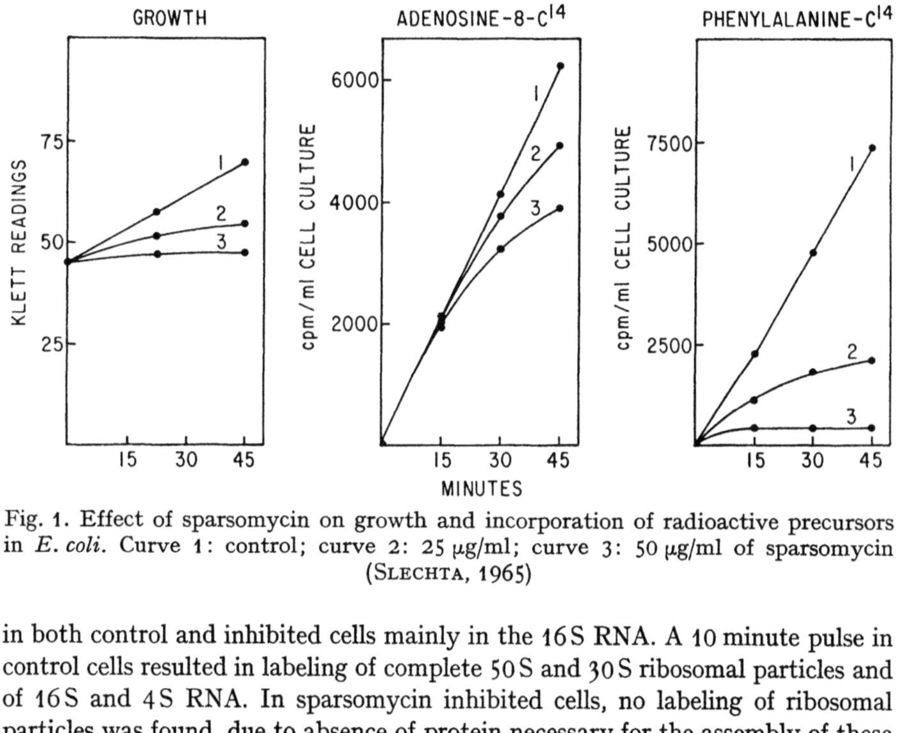

Fig. 1. Effect of sparsomycin on growth and incorporation of radioactive precursors in *E. coli*. Curve 1: control; curve 2: 25 μg/ml; curve 3: 50 μg/ml of sparsomycin (SLECHTA, 1965)

in both control and inhibited cells mainly in the 16S RNA. A 10 minute pulse in control cells resulted in labeling of complete 50S and 30S ribosomal particles and of 16S and 4S RNA. In sparsomycin inhibited cells, no labeling of ribosomal particles was found, due to absence of protein necessary for the assembly of these units. Radioactive uridine was found only in 16S RNA and 4S RNA (Fig. 3). A longer exposure of inhibited cells to RNA precursors led to a very strong labeling of 4S RNA. After a 60 minute pulse with ^{32}P, more than 90% of the incorporated radioactivity was found in the 4S RNA peak. Direct analysis of the inhibited cells proved that the labeling of 4S RNA was the result of actual accumulation and not due to turnover.

The function of 4S RNA ("transfer" RNA) molecules in the cellular metabolism is to accept specific amino acids and to transfer these into the protein synthesizing units (polysomes). Accumulation of 4S RNA in the cells inhibited by sparsomycin suggested experiments to show whether it can be charged with amino acids *in vivo*. Cells were incubated with sparsomycin to stop protein synthesis completely and then pulsed for several hours with various radioactive amino acids. With one exception, no radioactivity was found associated with the 4S RNA isolated from those cells, which indicated the absence of the charging reaction. The exception was methionine labeled in the methyl group with ^{14}C.

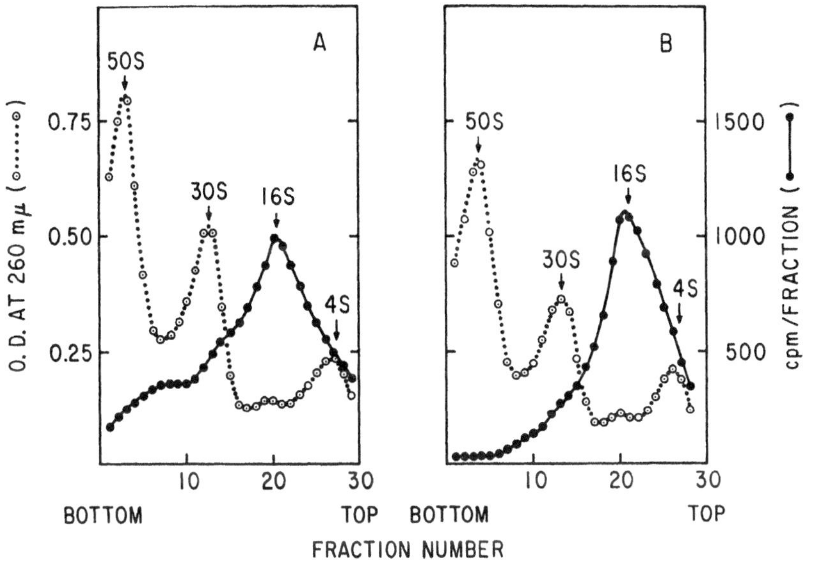

Fig. 2. Sedimentation analysis of extracts from control (A) and sparsomycin inhibited cells (B) given 1 minute exposure to tritiated uridine (SLECHTA, 1965)

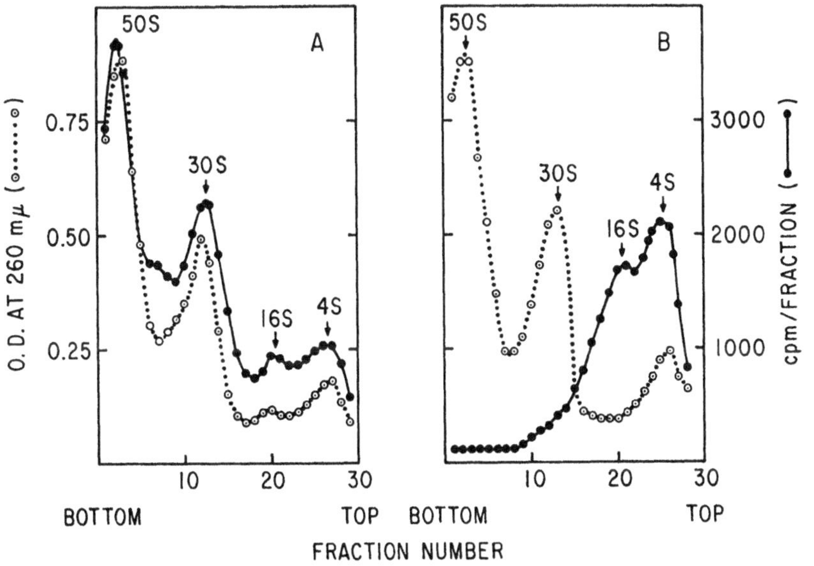

Fig. 3. Sedimentation analysis of extracts from control (A) and sparsomycin inhibited cells (B) given 10 minute exposure to tritiated uridine (SLECHTA, 1965)

Incubation with methyl labeled methionine, but not methionine-2-^{14}C, led to labeling of 4 S RNA in sparsomycin inhibited cells. In view of the well documented methylation of transfer RNA by methyl groups from methionine (BISWAS, EDMONDS and ABRAMS, 1961), this observation was taken as support for the notion of transfer RNA accumulating in the inhibited cells. From these results it was concluded that sparsomycin inhibited the growth of the bacteria by interfering with the early stages of the protein synthesis.

COLOMBO, FELICETTI and BAGLIONI (1965) studied the effect of sparsomycin on protein synthesis in rabbit reticulocytes *in vitro*. Using whole cells, the authors found no inhibitory effect on the hemoglobin synthesis, even with very high concentrations of the antibiotic. However, in the cell-free system, sparsomycin completely inhibited the protein synthesis at the level of 3 μg/ml and it was postulated that the antibiotic did not penetrate inside the intact reticulocytes. The inhibition of protein synthesis by sparsomycin in the cell-free system also prevented the breakdown of polysomes.

See addendum

References

ARGOUDELIS, A. D., and R. R. HERR: Sparsomycin, a new antitumor antibiotic. II. Isolation and characterization. Antimicrobial Agents and Chemotherapy, p. 780 (1962).

BISWAS, B. B., M. EDMONDS, and R. ABRAMS: Methylation of the purines of soluble RNA with methyl labeled methionine. Biochem. Biophys. Research Commun. **6**, 146 (1961).

COLOMBO, B., L. FELICETTI, and C. BAGLIONO: Inhibition of protein synthesis by antibiotics in reticulocytes. Biochim. et Biophys. Acta (in press) (1965).

OWEN, S. P., A. DIETZ, and G. W. CAMIENER: Sparsomycin, a new antitumor antibiotic. I. Discovery and biological properties. Antimicrobial Agents and Chemotherapy, p. 772 (1962).

PITTILLO, R. F., M. LUCAS, C. WOOLLEY, R. T. BLACKWELL, and C. MONCRIEF: Sparsomycin modification of the lethal action of ionizing irradiation on *Escherichia coli*. Nature **205**, 773 (1965).

SLECHTA, L.: Mode of action of sparsomycin in *E. coli B*. Antimicrobial Agents and Chemotherapy 326 (1965).

Rifamycins

Laura Frontali and Giorgio Tecce

Rifamycins[1] are a group of closely related antibiotics produced by a *Streptomyces* strain first isolated in "Lepetit Research Laboratories" (Milan, Italy) from a soil sample collected near St. Raphael (France). The strain was cultured in shakeflasks and the fermentations broths showed high activity against gram-positive bacteria and *Mycobacterium tuberculosis* (SENSI *et al.*, 1959). A limited activity against gram-negative bacteria was also present. A detailed description of this strain was reported by MARGALITH and BERETTA (1960); its cultural and biochemical characteritics led these Authors to conclude that this strain constitutes a new species which was named *Streptomyces mediterranei.*

A chromatographic study of the fermentation broths showed that at least five antibiotic substances were produced by *S. mediterranei*. Only one of these, rifamycin B, an acid, could be easily separated and crystallized. Its neutral salts were very stable and soluble. On the contrary, the other antibiotics were very difficult to separate and purify; their crude mixture, which was very unstable and variable in composition, was indicated as "rifamycin complex" (SENSI *et al.*, 1960a).

Rifamycin B proved to be the most interesting natural rifamycin and was obtained in the almost pure state under special fermentation conditions (MARGALITH, 1961).

In aerated aqueous solutions rifamycin B undergoes an "activation" due to the formation of a derivative, called rifamycin S, which is much more active than rifamycin B. During the activation process, rifamycin B is oxidized into rifamycin O, which is in turn hydrolyzed to rifamycin S; rifamycin S can easily be reduced to rifamycin SV (SENSI *et al.*, 1960b; SENSI *et al.*, 1960c; SENSI *et al.*, 1961). The correlations between these rifamycins are summarized in Fig. 1.

The structural formulae of these four rifamycins are reported in Fig. 2 (PRELOG, 1963a; PRELOG, 1963b; PRELOG, 1963c; OPPOLZER *et al.*, 1964; BRUFANI *et al.*, 1964) This type of structure is unusual, and rifamycins are a family of antibiotics structurally completely different from all other known antibiotics. An extensive review on the chemical and pharmacological properties of rifamycins has been published by SENSI (1964).

Several derivatives of natural rifamycins were prepared in the attempt to obtain a higher antibacterial activity. Since the splitting off of the glycolic acid moiety from the molecule of rifamycin B resulted in an increase of the antimicrobial activity (rifamycins S and SV), it was hypothesized that the free

[1] In early literature the name "rifomycin" was adopted. This name was afterwards changed to avoid confusion with the commercial names of other antibiotics.

carboxyl group could play the role of hindering or internally binding the groups principally responsible for the antibiotic activity. Therefore esthers and amides of rifamycin B were prepared, which had very high antimicrobial activity (SENSI *et al.*, 1962). The diethylamide of rifamycin B or rifamide (earlier referred to also as rifamycin M_{14}) showed, in some cases, higher activity than rifamycin SV itself (PALLANZA *et al.*, 1965).

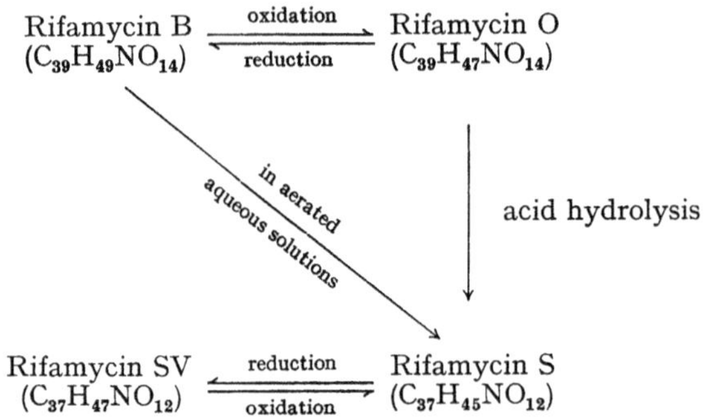

Fig. 1. Correlations between rifamycins B, O, S and SV

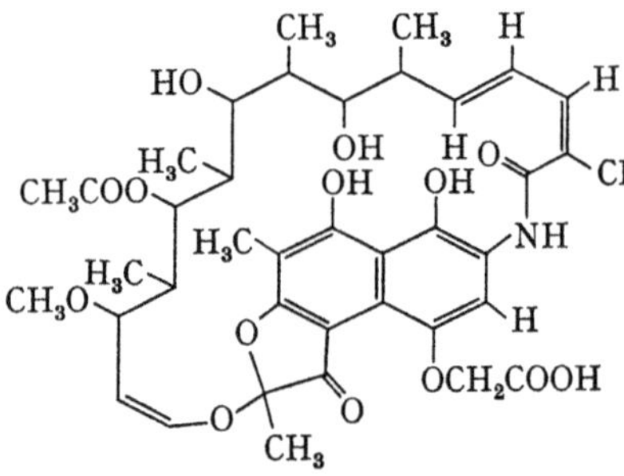

Rifamycin B $C_{39}H_{49}NO_{14}$

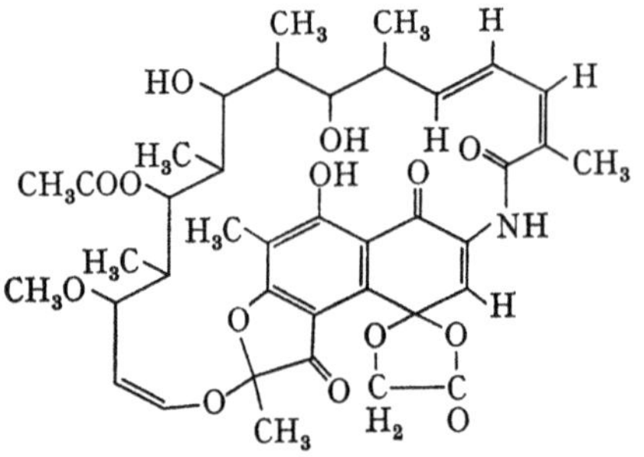

Rifamycin O $C_{39}H_{47}NO_{14}$

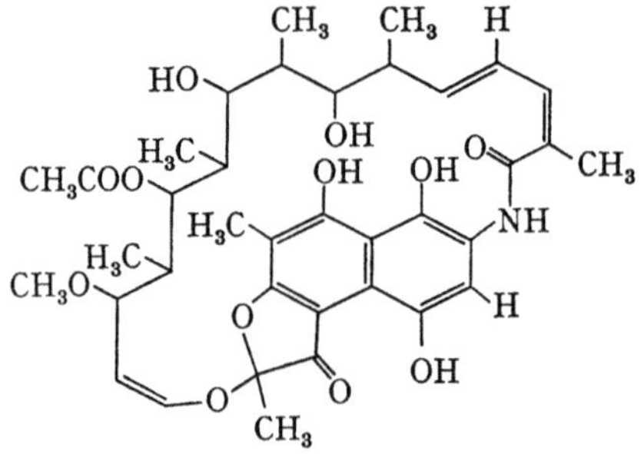

Rifamycin SV $C_{37}H_{47}NO_{12}$

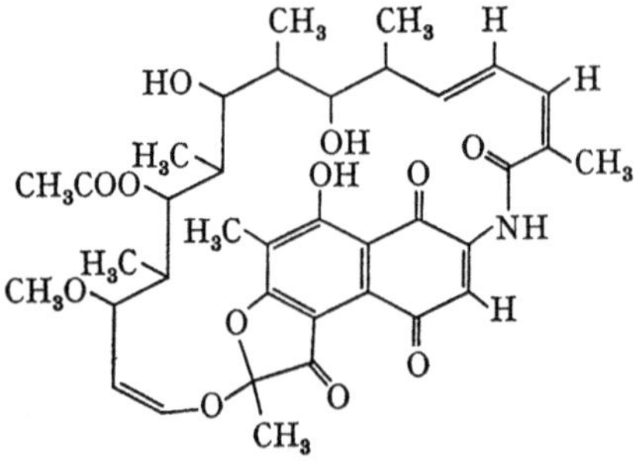

Rifamycin S $C_{37}H_{45}NO_{12}$

Fig. 2. Structural formulae of rifamycins B, O, S and SV

The antibiotic that is used therapeutically is rifamycin SV; an extensive review on its antimicrobial activity, pharmacological and therapeutical properties has been published by BERGAMINI and FOWST (1965). Most of the work on the mechanism of action of rifamycins was performed with rifamycin SV and with the diethylamide of rifamycin B.

Chemical and Chemico-Physical Properties

Rifamycin B crystallizes from ethyl acetate as brilliant yellow prismatic needles. It has no definite melting point; decomposes in the range 160—164°C and does not melt until 300°C; is scarcely soluble in most usual solvents; and it forms neutral and monobasic salts with organic and inorganic bases (SENSI *et al.*, 1960a).

Rifamycin SV occurs as small orange yellow crystals without a well defined melting point (decomposes at 140°C and does not melt up to 300°C). Rifamycin SV is sparingly soluble in water, but soluble in bicarbonate solution; it is very soluble in methanol, ethanol, acetone, and ethyl acetate; soluble in ethyl ether; and scarcely soluble in petroleum ether. In aqueous solutions, rifamycin SV is in equilibrium with rifamycin S unless a reducing substance such as ascorbic acid is present. The preparation and properties of rifamide have been described by MAGGI *et al.* (1965).

Antimicrobial Activity

The *in vitro* activity of rifamycin B when assayed by the serial dilution technique, is due, at least in part, to the active transformation product. When the effect of rifamycin B was studied on a continuous culture in a turbidostatic system, the effect of the antibiotic could be measured in a very short time by continuously determining the generation time; under these conditions, "activation" effect was negligible and no significant influence of rifamycin B on the growth rate of several microorganisms was observed (ORLANDO, SCHIESSER and TECCE, unpublished results). The same conclusion was drawn by FÜRESZ and TIMBAL (1963) from different experiments. The minimal inhibitory concentration of rifamycins S and SV and rifamide against some gram-positive and gram-negative bacteria is reported in Table 1.

The *in vivo* activity of rifamycin SV on experimental infections has been reviewed by BERGAMINI and FOWST (1965).

In Table 2 the *in vitro* sensitivity of spirocheta, mycetes and protozoa to rifamycin SV is reported.

Bacteriostatic concentrations of rifamycin SV do not exert any activity on rabbit monocyte cultures (BASILICO, 1962). The data on the emergence of strains resistent to rifamycin SV have been reviewed by BERGAMINI and FOWST (1965).

Acute and Chronic Toxicity to Animals

Acute toxicity of rifamycin SV was tested on three animal species by different routes of administration (MAFFII *et al.*, 1961; SENSI *et al.*, 1960b); the LD_{50} values are given in Table 3.

Subacute and chronic toxicity tests were carried out in rats. No alterations or significant changes in body weight were observed in rats treated orally for

Table 1. *Minimal inhibitory concentrations of rifamycins SV, S, and rifamide*[1]

Microorganism	Rifamycin SV M.I.C. (μg/ml)	Rifamycin S M.I.C. (μg/ml)	Rifamide M.I.C. (μg/ml)
Staphylococcus pyogenes aureus ATCC 6538	0.005	0.005	0.01
Streptococcus faecalis ATCC 10541	0.05	0.09	0.1
Streptococcus haemolyticus C 203	0.0025	0.0025	
Neisseria gonorrhoeae ATCC 9826	0.1		0.05
Sarcina lutea ATCC 9341	0.01		0.05
Bacillus subtilis ATCC 6633	0.075	0.075	0.05
Klebsiella pneumoniae ATCC 10031	25	25	20
Escherichia coli McLEOD ATCC 10536	50	12	10
Aerobacter aerogenes ATCC 8724	200		20
Pseudomonas aeruginosa ATCC 10145	50	25	50
Proteus vulgaris X 19 H ATCC 881	25	25	20
Salmonella typhi M 507	150		20
Brucella melitensis ATCC 4309	2.5		2
Pasteurella pestis ATCC 87 NIH	10		
Mycobacterium tuberculosis var. *hominis* H 37 RV ATCC 9360	0.05	0.05	0.2

[1] From SENSI (1964) and from PALLANZA *et al.* (1965).

Table 2. *In vitro sensitivity of microorganisms to rifamycin SV*[1]

Microorganism	Minimum inhibiting concentration (mcg/ml)
Treponema pallidum NICHOLS	Between 100 and 1000
Candida albicans	Between 100 and 1000
Trichosporum cutaneum	Between 100 and 1000
Nocardia asteroides	Between 10 and 100
Leishmania tropica	Between 10 and 100
Entamoeba histolytica	< 10
Trichomonas vaginalis	> 1000

[1] From BERGAMINI and FOWST (1965)

Table 3. *Acute toxicity of rifamycin SV in three species of animals*[1]

Animal species	Administration route	LD_{50} (mg/kg)	Confidence limits
Mouse	Oral	2,120	1,876—2,395
	Subcutaneous	1,080	982—1,188
	Intraperitoneal	625	579—675
	Intravenous	550	482—627
	Intracerebral	5.8	
Rat	Oral	2,680	2,680—3,350
	Subcutaneous	1,120	1,018—1,232
	Intraperitoneal	480	465—496
Dog	Intravenous	350	

[1] From BERGAMINI and FOWST (1965)

168 days, intraperitoneally for 30 days, or subcutaneously for 1—6 months at daily dosages from 50 to 200 mg/kg (MAFFII *et al.*, 1961).

The acute toxicity of rifamycin S is higher (SENSI *et al.*, 1960b) and the local tolerance to its subcutaneous or intramuscular administration is very poor.

Rifamycins are mainly eliminated through the bile and to a lesser extent through the urine (FÜRESZ and SCOTTI, 1960 and 1961; MAFFII *et al.*, 1961).

Effects of Rifamycins on Cells

The effect of sub-inhibiting concentrations (0.05 μg/ml) of rifamycin SV on the morphology of *Mycobacterium tuberculosis* was observed under the electron microscope (NITTI *et al.*, 1961). After 96 hours incubation, the appearance of a

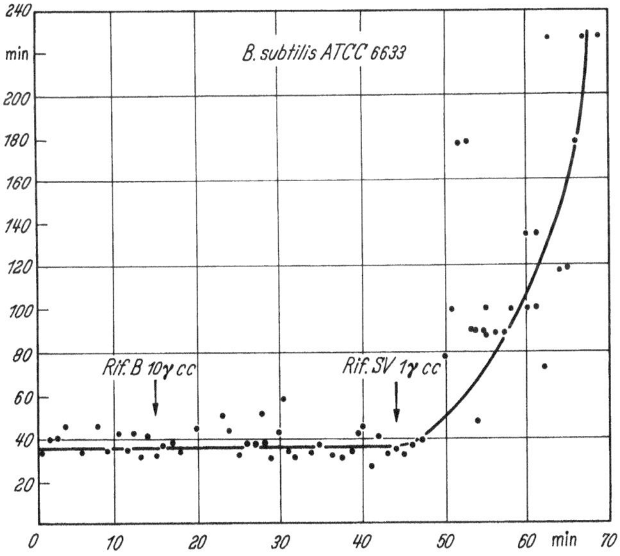

Fig. 3. Generation time of *Bacillus subtilis* strain ATCC 6633 before and after the addition of rifamycins B and SV

circumscribed, variously located swelling was observed, together with a marked increase of the electronic density. In cultures containing inhibiting concentrations, lysis of the bacterial body started within 96 hours; irregular images of multiple effraction of the cellular walls and afterwards some cellular shadows could be observed.

The appearance of swellings and of filamentous forms was also observed in cultures of *Bacillus subtilis* (FRONTALI and LEONI, unpublished results).

As previously mentioned, the effect of rifamycins B ans SV on the growth rate of several microorganisms was tested by determining the generation time in the turbidostatic apparatus described by GRAZIOSI (1956). The short time required by this type of determination permits to avoid errors due to the chemical transformation of the antibiotic, alterations in the chemical composition of the medium or selection of mutants.

The effects of rifamycins B and SV on the generation time of *Bacillus subtilis* is reported in Fig. 3. Similar results have been obtained with *Bacillus cereus* and

Staphylococcus pyogenes aureus (ORLANDO, SCHIESSER and TECCE, unpublished results).

The action of rifamycin SV on the oxidation of various substrates by resting cells of *Bacillus subtilis* and of *Staphylococcus pyogenes aureus* was studied by the usual manometric technique of Warburg. Results showed that rifamycin SV is an effective inhibitor of O_2 uptake in the presence of pyruvate, glucose, succinate, fumarate and acetate. Anaerobic fermentation of glucose was also inhibited. On the contrary, endogenous respiration was not affected by the antibiotic; see Fig. 4 (LEONI and TECCE; FÜRESZ and TIMBAL, unpublished results). The effect of rifamycin B on respiration was less than that of rifamycin SV.

High concentrations (10^{-3} M) of rifamycin SV exert an inhibitory effect on the respiration of rat liver mitochondria as measured in a Warburg apparatus. Investigators who have studied the influence of rifamycin SV on *in vitro* tissue respiration processes hypothesize that the antibiotic, owing to the presence of the hydroquinone group, might act on the respiratory chain at a level between the pyridine nucleotides and cytochrome oxidase (GINOULHIAC and BONOMI, 1964).

The possibility of an effect of rifamycins on the cell permeability of bacteria has not been directly investigated, but several experimental findings could be very well explained by alterations of cell permeability caused by the antibiotic; among these are the inhibition by rifamycin SV of the oxidation of exogenous, but not of endogenous substrates and the inhibition by the diethylamide of rifamycin B of the incorporation of ^{14}C uracil into TCA insoluble material by *B. subtilis* cells.

Effects on Cell Free Extracts

The action of rifamycin SV and of rifamide (diethylamide of rifamycin B) on protein synthesis was investigated by testing their effect on the incorporation of ^{14}C amino acids into proteins by cell-free extracts of *Bacillus subtilis* strain ATCC 6633. Extracts were prepared at first following the method described by TISSIÈRES *et al.* (1960) and afterwards following the method reported by MATTHAEI and NIRENBERG (1961); the results reported in Table 4 indicate that rifamycins are effective inhibitors of the incorporation of amino acids into proteins at molar concentrations lower than those which produce the same inhibition by chloramphenicol or by other antibiotics active on protein synthesis (FRONTALI *et al.*, 1964). Separate experiments showed that rifamycins do not affect the activation of amino acids or the energy supplying system (FRONTALI *et al.*, 1964).

However when crude extracts prepared following the method reported by TISSIÈRES were used with a ten fold increased ATP concentration, the inhibiting action of rifamycin disappeared. In order to exert this protection, ATP had to be added to the reaction mixture at the same time as rifamycin; incubation of rifamycin with the extract before the addition of ATP allowed the inhibition to take place (LEONI and TECCE, 1963). These results, which suggest a competition between rifamycin SV and ATP at the level of the ribosomes or of the enzymes involved in the last stages of protein synthesis, were not obtained when the effect of rifamycins was studied in the presence of tenfold increased ATP concentrations,

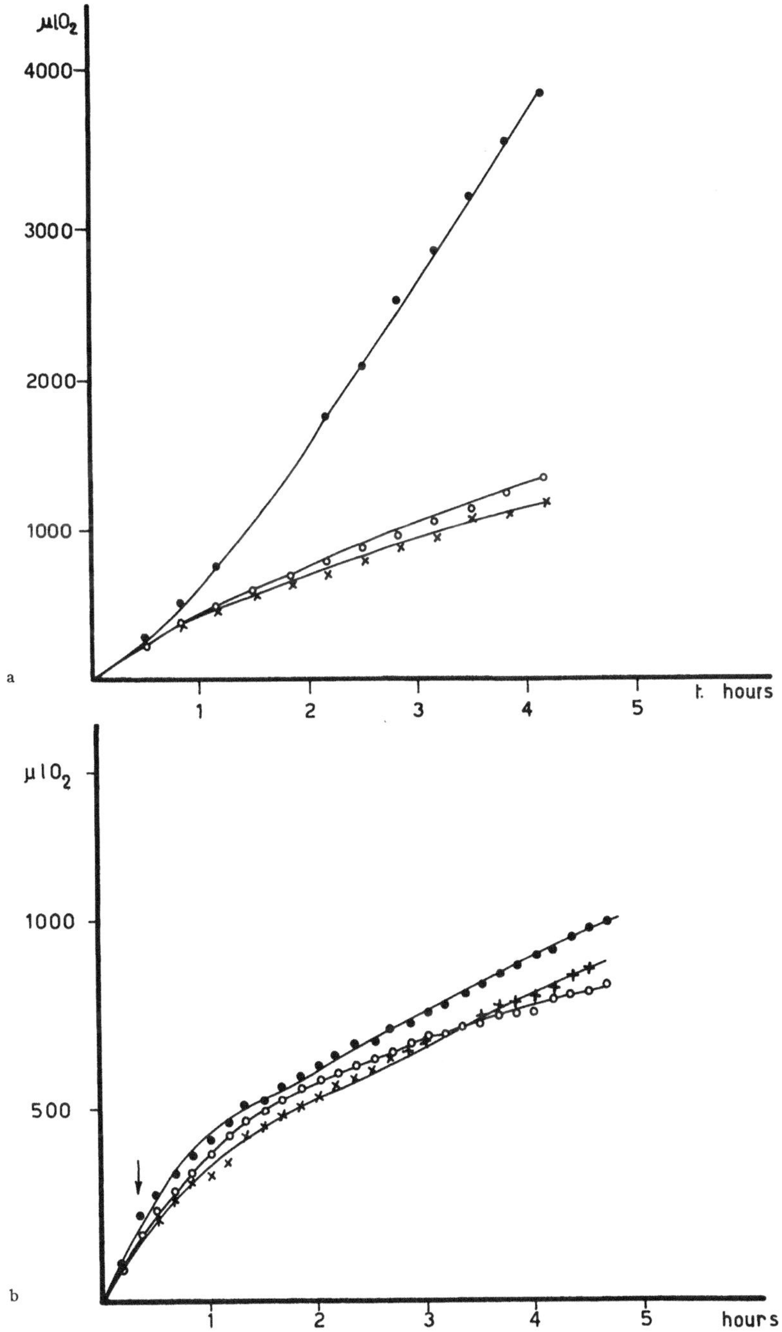

Fig. 4. Effect of rifamycin SV on the oxidation of glucose (a) and on the endogenous respiration (b) of resting *B. subtilis* cells. Experimental conditions: phosphate buffer M/15 pH 7, glucose 10 μmoles in (a), 0.2 or 2 μg/ml rifamycin SV, 3 mg in (a) and 10 mg in (b) wet weight *B. subtilis* cells per flask, 20% KOH 0.2 ml in center well; total volume 2.2 ml. Temperature 37 C; gas phase air. No antibiotic •—•—•; rifamycin SV 0.2 μg/ml ○—○—○; rifamycin SV2 μg/ml ×—×—×

Table 4. *^{14}C-L-isoleucine incorporation into protein by cell-free B. subtilis preparations*

Exp. No.		Additions	C.p.m./mg protein	Percentage inhibition
1	Complete mixture		880	
	Complete mixture	+0.03 μmole/ml rifamycin SV	467	59
	Complete mixture	+0.15 μmole/ml rifamycin SV	347	76
	Complete mixture	+0.03 μmole/ml rifamide	423	65
	Complete mixture	deproteinized at zero time	178	
2	Complete mixture		1,500	
	Complete mixture	+0.03 μmole/ml rifamycin SV	1,020	40
	Complete mixture	+0.03 μmole/ml rifamide	636	72
	Complete mixture	deproteinized at zero time	300	

The reaction mixture contained the following in μmole/ml. In exp. 1: 10 tris-HCl pH 7.4; 10 magnesium acetate; 40 KCl; 0.34 ^{14}C-L-isoleucine (specific activity 2.68×10^6 c.p.m./μmole); 0.2 GTP; 1 ATP; 10 phosphoenolpyruvate; 84 μg/ml pyruvate kinase; 120 μg/ml DNA prepared by the method of MARMUR (1961); 2 mg/ml homogenate protein prepared by the method of TISSIÈRES *et al.* (1960). In exp. 2: 100 tris-HCl pH 7.4; 12 magnesium acetate; 50 KCl; 6 mercaptoethanol; 0.05 each of 20 L-amino-acids minus isoleucine; 0.17 ^{14}C-L-isoleucine (specific activity 2.68×10^6 c.p.m./μmole); 0.03 GTP; 1 ATP; 5 phosphoenolpyruvate; 20 μg/ml pyruvate kinase; 120 μg/ml DNA; 1.2 and 0.6 mg S-105 and ribosomal protein prepared following the method of MATTHAEI and NIRENBERG (1961). In both cases the reaction was stopped with perchloric acid by the method of OFENGAND *et al.* (1962). Radioactivity was determined by a windowless gas-flow-counter. From FRONTALI *et al.* (1964).

on systems prepared according to MATTHAEI and NIRENBERG. The cause of this behaviour remains to be elucidated.

Since the incorporation of amino acids into proteins by *B. subtilis* extracts is dependent on the addition of DNA to the reaction mixture, the results of the experiments reported in Table 4 do not allow one to decide whether the inhibition of amino acid incorporation into proteins is connected with an effect of the antibiotic on the synthesis of messenger RNA or with an inhibition of protein synthesis at the ribosomal level. The observation that rifamide causes a strong inhibition of ^{14}C-uracil incorporation into TCA insoluble material by *B. subtilis* cells (CALVORI *et al.*, 1965), cannot be considered as a conclusive evidence in favour of the first hypothesis, since the observed results might be consequence of an alteration of cell permeability. Alternatively, the decrease of RNA synthesis might be a secondary effect of the inhibition of protein synthesis.

On the other hand, when natural or synthetic messengers are added to the incubation mixture the results reported in Tables 5 and 6 are obtained.

The inhibition of either RNA or polyuridylic acid (poly U) dependent amino acid incorporation into proteins fully supports the hypothesis that the site of rifamycin action is at the level of ribosomes. The fact that the inhibitory action of rifamycin strongly decreases when ribosomes are preincubated with poly U suggests the possibility that rifamycin might affect the interaction between ribosomes and messenger RNA.

When ribosomes extracted from cells of *B. subtilis* which have been in contact with rifamide for 60 minutes, are examined in the analytical ultracentrifuge a

Table 5. *Effect of rifamide on ^{14}C-L-phenylalanine incorporation into proteins in the presence of DNA and RNA*

	Additions	C.p.m./mg protein	Percentage inhibition
Complete mixture		210	
Complete mixture	+0.03 μmoles/ml rifamide	210	
Complete mixture	+100 μg/ml DNA	2,500	
Complete mixture	+100 μg/ml DNA +0.03 μmoles/ml rifamide	670	80
Complete mixture	+2 mg/ml RNA	1,350	
Complete mixture	+2 mg/ml RNA +0.03 μmoles/ml rifamide	420	81

The reaction mixture contained the following, in μmoles/ml: 100 tris-HCl, pH 7.4; 12 magnesium acetate; 50 ammonium acetate; 6 mercaptoethanol; 1 ATP; 5 phosphoenolpyruvate; 20 μg/ml pyruvate kinase; 0.05 each of 20 L-amino-acids minus L-isoleucine; 0.03 GTP; 0.07 ^{14}C-L-Isoleucine (specific activity 6.5×10^6 c.p.m./μmole); 2 mg/ml S-30 protein. Total volume 250 μl. Samples were incubated at 37 C for 45 minutes, and the reaction was stopped with perchloric acid by the method of OFENGAND (1962). Radioactivity was determined by a windowless gas-flow counter. From CALVORI *et al.* (1965).

Table 6. *Effect of rifamycin on ^{14}C-L-phenylalanine incorporation into proteins in the presence of polyuridylic acid*

	Additions	C.p.m./mg protein	Percentage inhibition
Complete mixture		450	
Complete mixture	+0.03 μmoles/ml rifamide	370	
Complete mixture	+80 μg/ml poly U	4,150	
Complete mixture[1]	+0.03 μmoles/ml rifamide +80 μg/ml poly U	1,050	84
Complete mixture[2]	+80 μg/ml poly U +0.03 μmoles/ml rifamide	2,670	40

The reaction mixture contained the following, in μmoles/ml: 100 tris-HCl, pH 7.4; 12 magnesium acetate; 50 ammonium acetate; 6 mercaptoethanol; 1 ATP; 5 phosphoenolpyruvate; 20 μg/ml pyruvate kinase; 0.05 each of 20 L-amino-acids minus L-phenylalanine; 0.03 GTP; 0.03 ^{14}C-L-penylalanine (specific activity 74×10^6 c.p.m./μmole); 2 mg/ml S-30 protein. Total volume was 250 μl. Samples were incubated at 37 C for 45 minutes, and the reaction was stopped with perchloric acid by the method of OFENGAND *et al.* (1962). Radioactivity was determined by a windowless gas-flow conter.

[1] Rifamycin was incubated for 5 minutes at room temperature in the complete assay mixture before addition of poly U.

[2] Poly U was incubated for 5 minutes at room temperature in the complete assay mixture before addition of rifamycin. From CALVORI *et al.* (1965).

sharp modification of normal sedimentation pattern can be observed. The Schlieren diagram of the sedimentation velocities (Fig. 5) shows the absence of the 70 and 100 S components in the extracts from *B. subtilis* cells treated with diethylamide of rifamycin B.. (CALVORI *et al* 1966). This effect was not observed *in vitro* when rifamide was added to the extracts of untreated cells, in the presence of absence of the complete Matthaei and Nirenberg system. The ,,*in vitro*" dissociation and association of ribosomal subunits at various. Mg^{++} concentrations is not affected by rifamycin.

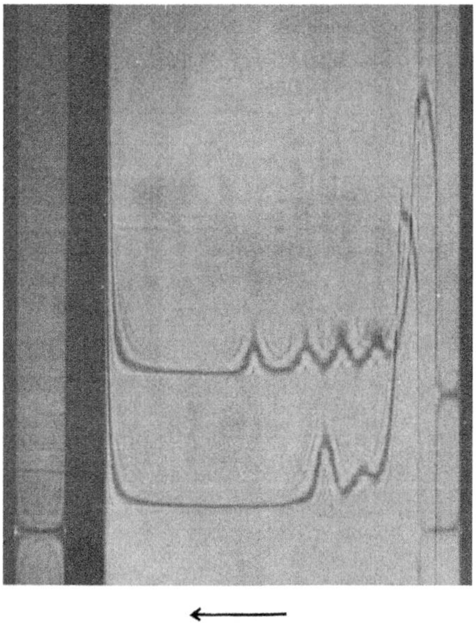

Fig. 5. Schlieren diagram of a sedimentation velocity analysis of ribosomes extracted from rifamycin treated (lower curve) and untreated (upper curve) *B. subtilis* cells. *B. subtilis* cells were collected during the logarithmic growth phase, washed and incubated at 37 C in a medium containing 20 μg/ml rifamide. In the control (upper curve) growth was stopped by the addition of penicillin. After 60 minutes incubation cells were collected, disrupted by grinding with alumina. The extract suspended in 0.01 M Tris HCl buffer containing 0.01 M Mg^{++} was centrifuged for 1 hour at 30,000 xg and examined in a Spinco Model E analytical ultracentrifuge at 31,410 rev/minutes. Photograph taken after 20'. (From CALVORI *et al.*, 1966)

The effects of different rifamycins are very similar and it seems reasonable to assume that their mechanism of action is the same. The inhibition of respiration exhibits some peculiar features which suggest the possibility that this effect is secondary to a modification of cell permeability. In fact, fermentation and respiration are both affected, but the inhibition cannot be located only at the level of the Embden Meyerhof scheme, since O_2 uptake in the presence of pyruvate or acetate is also strongly reduced. Moreover, endogenous respiration is not modified by rifamycins.

The inhibition of protein synthesis in *in vitro* systems seems to be the most important specific effect of rifamycins; at least it is difficult to consider it as a consequence of other effects. Since the activation of amino acids is not affected by rifamycins and the inhibition of protein synthesis also takes place in the presence of added natural or synthetic messengers, the site of rifamycin action should be at the level of the formation of polypeptide chains on ribosomes. The influence of the preincubation of ribosomes with poly U suggests the possibility that rifamycins might interfere with the attachment of messengers to ribosomes.

As to the effect on ribosomes, it does not take place *in vitro*, therefore the inhibition of protein synthesis in cell-free extracts cannot be a consequence of a "splitting" of the ribosomes. The reverse is possible; namely that the inhibition of protein synthesis leads to the *in vivo* formation of ribosomal subunits in which some protein is lacking. Therefore the subunits fail to associate to form 70 S units. If this is the case, the effect of rifamycins, on ribosomes would be a consequence of the preferential inhibition of the synthesis of a ribosomal protein. Sometimes the presence of subunits with lowered sedimentation coefficients was observed.

This work was partially supported by a grant from C. N. R.

References

BASILICO, E., e C. GRASSI: Attività antitubercolare della rifamicina SV nella monocitocultura. Giorn. ital. tuberc. **16**, 66 (1962).

BERGAMINI, N., and G. FOWST: Rifamycin SV: a review. Arzneimittel-Forsch. **15**, 1951 (1965).

BRUFANI, M., W. FEDELI, G. GIACOMELLO, and A. VACIAGO: X ray determination of the structure of rifamycin. Accad. naz. Lincei, R.C. Classe Sci. fis. mat. nat. **36**, 113 (1964).

CALVORI, C., L. FRONTALI, L. LEONI, and G. TECCE: Effect of rifamycin on protein synthesis. Nature **207**, 417 (1965).

CALVORI, C., L. FRONTALI, L. LEONI, and G. TECCE: In preparation (1966).

FRONTALI, L., L. LEONI, and G. TECCE: Action of rifamycin on incorporation of aminoacids into proteins in cell-free systems from *B. subtilis*. Nature **203**, 84 (1964).

FÜRESZ, S., and R. SCOTTI: Rifomycin. IV. Some laboratory and clinical experiences with rifomycin B. Antibiotics Ann. **1959/60**, 285 (1960).

FÜRESZ, S., and R. SCOTTI: Rifomycin. XX. Further studies on rifomycin SV: *in vitro* activity, absorption and elimination in man. Farmaco, Ed. sci. **16**, 262 (1961).

FÜRESZ, S., and M. T. TIMBAL: Antibacterial activity of rifamycins. Internat. Symposium on Rifamycins, Milan 1963, Chemotherapia **7**, 200 (1963).

GINOULHIAC, E., and U. BONOMI: VI Int. Congr. Biochem., New York City 1964.

GRAZIOSI, F.: Metodo per la coltura continua di batteri in turbidostato. Giorn. microbiol. **1**, 491 (1956).

LEONI, L., e G. TECCE: Azione della rifamicina SV sulle reazioni della sintesi proteica. Internat. Symposium on Rifamycins, Milan 1963. Chemoterapia **7**, 194.

MAFFII, G., P. SCHIATTI, G. BIANCHI, and M. G. SERRALUNGA: Rifomycin. XVIII. Pharmacological studies with rifomycin SV. Changes in respiratory activity of mitochondria induced by rifomycins. Farmaco, Ed. sci. **16**, 235 (1961).

MAGGI, N., G. G. GALLO e P. SENSI: Proprietà chimiche e chimico fisiche della dietilammide della rifamicina B. Farmaco **20**, 147 (1965).

MARGALITH, P., and G. BERETTA: Rifomycin. XI. Taxonomic study on *Streptomyces mediterranei* nova species. Mycopathol. et Mycol. Appl. **13**, 321 (1960).

MARGALITH, P., and H. PAGANI: Rifomycin. XIV. Production of rifomycin B. Appl. Microbiol. **9**, 325 (1961).

MARMUR, J.: A procedure for the isolation of DNA from microorganisms. J. Mol. Biol. **3**, 208 (1961).

MATTHAEI, H. J., and M. W. NIRENBERG: Characteristics and stabilization of DNAase sensitive protein synthesis in *E. coli* extracts. Proc. Nat. Acad. Sci. U.S. **47**, 1580 (1961).

NITTI, V., R. VIRGILIO, e A. MINNI: Attività della rifomicina SV sui micobatteri in vitro. Arch. tisiol. mal. app. respirat. (Naples) **16**, 1023 (1961).

OFENGAND, J., and R. HASELKORN: Viral RNA dependent incorporation of amino acids into protein by cell-free extracts of *E. coli*. Biochem. Biophys. Research Comm. **6**, 469 (1962).

OPPOLZER, W., V. PRELOG u. P. SENSI: Konstitution des Rifamycins B und verwandter Rifamycine. Experientia **20**, 336 (1964).

PALLANZA, R., S. FÜRESZ, M. T. TIMBAL, and G. CARNITI: *In vitro* bacteriological studies on rifamycin B diethylamide (rifamide). (In the press 1965.)

PRELOG, V.: Über die Konstitution der Rifamycine. Internat. Symposium on Rifamycins. Milan, June 5—6. Chemotherapia **7**, 133 (1963a).

PRELOG, V.: Constitution of rifamycins. Symposium on Chemistry and Biochemistry of Fungi and Yeast, Dublin, July 18—20, p. 551. London: Butterworths 1963 (1963c).

PRELOG, V.: Constitution of rifamycins. Pure Appl. Chem. **7**, 551 (1963b).
SENSI, P.: A family of new antibiotics, rifamycins. Res. Progr. Org. Biol. Med. Chem. **1**, 337 (1964).
SENSI, P., R. BALLOTTA, and A. M. GRECO: Rifomycin. V. Rifomycin O, a new antibiotic of the rifomycin family. Farmaco, Ed. sci. **15**, 228 (1960c).
SENSI, P., R. BALLOTTA, and G. G. GALLO: Rifomycin. XV. Activation of rifomycin B and rifomycin O. Production and properties of rifomycin S and rifomycin SV. Farmaco, Ed. sci. **16**, 165 (1961).
SENSI, P., A. M. GRECO, and R. BALLOTTA: Rifomycins. I. Isolation and properties of rifomycin B and rifomycin complex. Antibiotics Ann. **1959/60**, 262 (1960a).
SENSI, P., N. MAGGI, R. BALLOTTA, S. FÜRESZ, R. PALLANZA, and V. ARIOLI: Rifamycins. XXXV. Amides and hydrazides of rifamycin B. J. Medicinal Chem. **7**, 596 (1962).
SENSI, P., P. MARGALITH, and M. T. TIMBAL: Rifomycin, a new antibiotic. Preliminary report. Farmaco, Ed. sci. **14**, 146 (1959).
SENSI, P., M. T. TIMBAL, and G. MAFFII: Rifomycin. IX. Two new antibiotics of rifomycin family: Rifomycin S and rifomycin SV. Preliminary report. Experientia **16**, 412 (1960b).
TISSIÈRES, A., D. SCHLESSINGER, and F. GROS: Amino acid incorporation into proteins by *E. coli* ribosomes. Proc. Natl. Acad. Sci. U.S. **46**, 1450 (1960).

Nucleocidin

J. R. Florini

Attention was first attracted to nucleocidin by its very great activity against trypanosomes. Subsequent investigations revealed that the toxicity of this antibiotic was too great to allow its extensive therapeutic use; consequently relatively little work has been done on its mode of action. However, its structural similarity to puromycin led to the suggestion that it might inhibit protein synthesis. Investigations of this possibility have revealed that nucleocidin is an extremely potent inhibitor of protein synthesis *in vivo*. In cell-free systems, however, its potency is not remarkably greater than that of other antibiotics. Although the mechanism by which nucleocidin inhibits protein synthesis has not been fully explained, some apparently unique properties of the process have been discovered.

Streptomyces calvus, Lederle strain T 3018, is a new species of *Streptomyces* (Backus *et al.*, 1957) isolated from a soil sample obtained in Dinepur, India. Fermentation liquors from this organism were highly active in the mouse antitrypanosome test (Hewitt *et al.*, 1953); this observation prompted intensive fermentation studies. The pure crystalline antibiotic was ultimately isolated using its activity against *Streptococcus pyogenes* var. *haemolyticus* as an assay (Thomas *et al.*, 1956—1957). The empirical formula was $C_{11}H_{16}N_6O_8S$. Examination of the hydrolysis products, pKa, and various specific group reactions led Waller *et al.* (1957) to suggest a preliminary structure for nucleocidin which differs only slightly from the structure given below (J. B. Patrick and W. E. Meyer, 1965). This compound is the first instance of a sulfamate in ester linkage in a naturally-occurring compound.

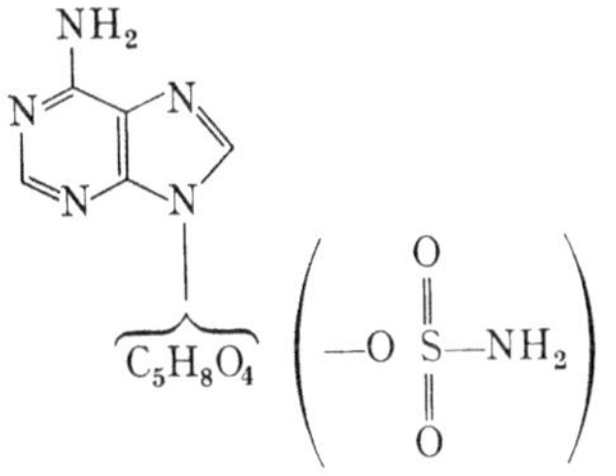

Antibiotic Activity

The effect of nucleocidin which attracted the most interest was its remarkable activity against trypanosomes. Table 1 contains data from Hewitt *et al.* (1956—1957) comparing the effects of nucleocidin and puromycin in protecting mice against *Trypanosoma equiperdum*. Nucleocidin was approximately 4000 times as active as puromycin. The same authors demonstrated that nucleocidin was 40 times as active as antrycide or suramin sodium. They reported "nucleocidin is

Table 1. *Effectiveness of nucleocidin and puromycin against Trypanosoma equiperdum in mice*[1]

Compound	Dose mg/kg intraperitoneal[2]	ST_{50}[3]	S_{30}[4]	Activity
Puromycin	200	>30	70	Curative
	100	10	10	Suppressive
	50	9	10	Suppressive
	25	7	10	Suppressive
Nucleocidin	0.2	>30	60	Curative
	0.1	>30	100	Curative
	0.05	>30	60	Curative
	0.02	8	0	Suppressive
	0.01	7	10	Suppressive
Control	—	4	0	—

[1] Data from HEWITT *et al.* (1956—1957).
[2] Injected 3 to 5 hours after inoculation with trypanosomes.
[3] Median Survival Time — number of days following inoculation at which 50% of the mice remained.
[4] Per Cent Survival for 30 days — per cent of mice which survived for 30 days after inoculation; relapse after this time is rare.

by far the most effective substance against experimental infections with *T. equiperdum* in mice that has been tested in these laboratories".

HEWITT *et al.* (1956—1957) also reported that an appreciable residue of nucleocidin remained after intramuscular injection of the antibiotic, as "70% of the mice inoculated with trypanosomes on the day following treatment were protected for at least two weeks". However, when inoculation was done one or two weeks after treatment with the antibiotic, no protection was observed.

TOBIE (1957) demonstrated that nucleocidin was active (at doses of 0.15 mg/kg) in curing infections of *T. congolense*, *T. equinum*, and *T. gambiense* in rats and mice. This was the first antibiotic shown to be highly active against *T. congolense*. STEPHEN and GRAY (1960) observed that nucleocidin had considerable activity against *T. vivax* in West African zebu cattle; however, the infection was not cured and relapses occurred 18—33 days after treatment.

Nucleocidin was active against both Gram-positive and Gram-negative bacteria, as shown in Table 2. This table demonstrates the high activity against *S. pyogenes* var. *hemolyticus* which provided a means of assay during the isolation of nucleocidin.

Toxicity to Animals

Detailed studies on the toxicity of nucleocidin have not been published, but the available data make it clear that this is an extremely toxic antibiotic. HEWITT *et al.* (1956—1957) found the LD_{50} in mice to be 0.2 mg/kg by intraperitoneal injection and 2.0 mg/kg by oral administration. Subcutaneous doses of 2.5 and 5.0 mg/kg were lethal to rabbits. In very limited experiments with rats, FLORINI *et al.* (1966) found that intraperitoneal injection of nucleocidin at 0.8 mg/kg was consistently lethal, whereas 0.4 mg/kg caused no deaths. The most striking toxicity of nucleocidin was exhibited in young bovines, in which "0.05 mg/kg

Table 2. *Antibacterial activity of nucleocidin**

Organism	μg/ml giving complete inhibition of growth
Gram-positive	
Bacillus cereus	4—8
Bacillus subtilis	2—4
Corynebacterium flaccumfaciens	1—2
Corynebacterium xerose	8—16
Micrococcus pyogenes var. *albus*	2—8
Micrococcus pyogenes var. *aureus*	2—16
Sarcina lutea	4—8
Streptococcus faecalis	1—2
Streptococcus mitia	2—8
Streptococcus pyogenes var. *haemolyticus*	0.05—0.1
Gram-negative	
Agrobacterium tumefaciens	0.25
Alcaligenes faecalis	128
Erwinia amylovora	0.5—1
Erwinia carotovora	4—16
Escherichia coli	8—16
Klebsiella pneumoniae	64
Proteus vulgaris	4—8
Pseudomonas aeruginosa	64—128
Pseudomonas glycinea	16
Pseudomonas solanacearum	4—16
Pseudomonas tabaci	0.5—1
Pseudomonas torelliana	4—16
Salmonella gallinearum	8—16
Salmonella pullorum	4—8
Salmonella typhosa	16
Serratia marcescens	4

* From Table 1 of Thomas *et al.* (1956—1957). Growth was measured after 16 hour incubation in trypticase soy broth at pH 7.2.

produced death, marked toxicity reactions, and changes in the blood picture. Mild toxic symptoms were produced at 0.025 mg/kg, and a 0.01 mg/kg dose was essentially asymptomatic" (Hewitt *et al.*, 1956—1957). The nature of the toxic symptoms occurring after administration of nucleocidin, the time before death occurred, and any probable causes of death have not been described in most cases. Florini *et al.* (1966) noted that rats receiving intraperitoneal injection of 0.8 mg/kg of nucleocidin died within two to four hours.

Biochemical Effects

Lardy *et al.* (1958) reported that nucleocidin had no effect on respiration or phosphorylation by isolated liver mitochondria using glutamate as substrate. Iyer and Szybalski (1958) observed that nucleocidin had no significant mutagenic activity on *E. coli*. Florini *et al.* (1966) found no inhibition by nucleocidin of RNA synthesis in a cell-free preparation from rat liver nuclei.

The effects of nucleocidin on amino acid incorporation into protein have not been studied widely because only small quantities of the material have been available and because its toxicity has precluded extensive therapeutic use[1]. Its structural similarity to puromycin and its greater antibiotic potency (Table 1) led us to hope that nucleocidin might be a very potent inhibitor of protein synthesis. However, comparative studies on effects of these two antibiotics on amino acid incorporation into protein (using a relatively purified system consisting of liver polyribosomes, pH 5 fraction, and partially purified transfer enzymes) demonstrated (Fig. 1) that nucleocidin was no more potent than puromycin in inhibiting the process. This experiment also revealed that there was no effect of nucleocidin until 5—10 minutes after incubation was begun. Thus inhibition by nucleocidin apparently required prior occurence of a process which occurred no more rapidly than peptide bond formation.

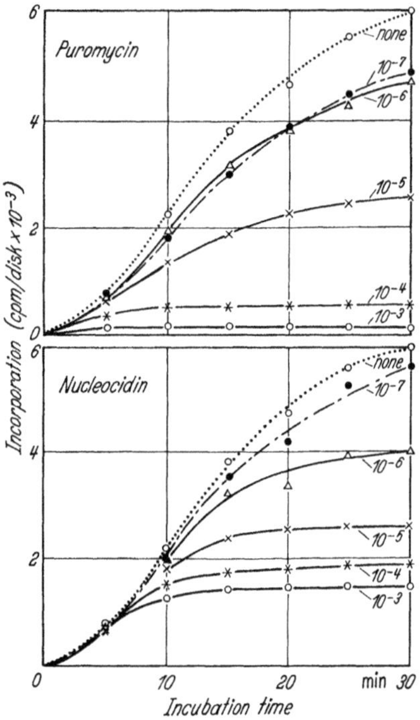

Fig. 1

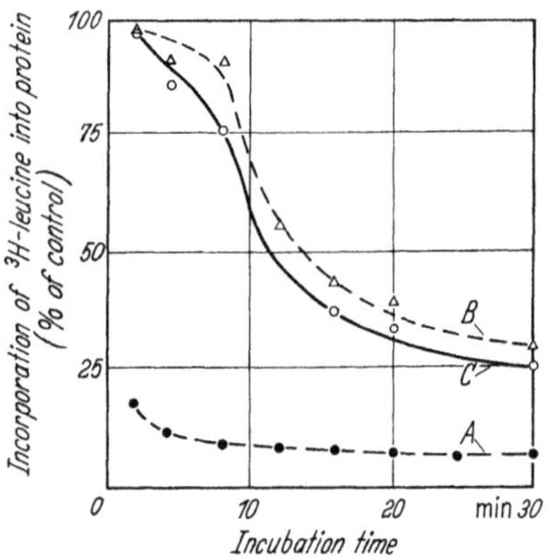

Fig. 2

Fig. 1. Effects of nucleocidin and puromycin on the time course of ^{3}H-leucine incorporation into protein by cell-free preparations from rat liver. Inhibitors (to give the molar concentrations indicated in the figure) and reactants were mixed with tissue components at zero time; incubations and analyses were conducted as described by FLORINI *et al.* (1966)

Fig. 2. Effect of preincubation with 10^{-4} M nucleocidin on ^{3}H-leucine incorporation into protein by liver preparations. Curve *A*, complete system preincubated with nucleocidin; curve *B*, complete system preincubated without nucleocidin; Curve *C*, ribosomes omitted from complete system during preincubation and added back at zero time (FLORINI *et al.*, 1966)

As these results suggest, preincubation of the complete system with nucleocidin before addition of the radioactive amino acid caused elimination of the lag period and a striking increase in inhibition of amino acid incorporation (Fig. 2, Curves A

[1] All data on the effects of nucleocidin on protein synthesis presented in this chapter are from the studies of FLORINI, BIRD, and BELL (1965, 1966).

and B). If any component of the incorporating system was omitted during the preincubation, the results were the same as if no preincubation had occurred (Fig. 2, Curve C). The requirement for ribosomes indicated that nucleocidin was not simply converted to an "active form" during the preliminary incubation. Ribosomes reisolated by centrifugation through 1.0 M sucrose after preincubation with nucleocidin were less active than similarly reisolated control ribosomes; activity was assayed either by measuring incorporation of free leucine-^{3}H or transfer of label from leucyl-^{3}H-sRNA into protein. This last observation is important, because addition of nucleocidin to a "transfer reaction" assay system (containing polyribosomes, leucyl-^{3}H-sRNA, and partially purified transfer enzymes) had no effect on the labeling of protein. Rather surprisingly, addition of a heat-labile component of the soluble fraction (or the pH 5 precipitate) was necessary to achieve inhibition of the transfer reaction by nucleocidin. Thus the lowered activity of reisolated ribosomes measured by the transfer reaction could not be attributed to non-specific contamination of the ribosomes with nucleocidin. When incubation of these reisolated ribosomes was done in the presence of pH 5 fraction (and absence of nucleocidin), the inhibition was quickly reversed and incorporation soon proceeded as rapidly as in controls.

Additional attempts to elucidate the mechanism of action of nucleocidin gave negative results. Thus, nucleocidin had no effect on the binding of sRNA-^{32}P to ribosomes. Preliminary experiments on the binding of leucyl-^{3}H-sRNA to ribosomes (FLORINI *et al.*, 1965) had been interpreted to indicate that nucleocidin inhibited this binding; however, parallel studies with other antibiotics and direct measurement of the binding of sRNA-^{32}P led to the conclusion (FLORINI *et al.*, 1966) that the techniques used for the earlier measurements did not give valid results.

When leucine incorporation was stimulated by addition of poly UG (3:1), the relationship of nucleocidin to per cent inhibition was the same as in the unstimulated system. Thus nucleocidin apparently did not specifically affect binding to ribosomes of synthetic messenger RNA. Incubation with nucleocidin had no effect on the sucrose gradient profiles of reisolated ribosomes; apparently nucleocidin did not affect the progression of ribosomes along the messenger RNA strand (NOLL *et al.*, 1963).

Analysis by centrifugation of ribosomes through sucrose gradients revealed that nucleocidin inhibited incorporation of labeled amino acids into peptides associated with polyribosomes, but neither inhibited nor caused premature release of prelabeled peptides. Prior incubation with nucleocidin did not inhibit the puromycin-induced release of peptides from ribosomes. This observation suggests that the adenine of nucleocidin and the dimethyl adenine of puromycin do not interact with the same site on the ribosome.

Consideration of all of our results with nucleocidin led to the conclusion that nucleocidin forms a complex with ribosomes which is inactive in peptide bond formation. Formation of this complex requires the some conditions that are required for peptide bond formation; in addition, a heat-labile soluble component (which was precipitated at pH 5) is also essential. The complex apparently dissociates under the conditions of its formation. Binding of either sRNA or messenger RNA to this complex is apparently not inhibited, nor is progression of ribosomes down the messenger RNA molecule. The specific aspect of peptide bond formation which is inhibited in nucleocidin-ribosomes has not been determined.

Studies (Table 3) on the effects of nucleocidin on amino acid incorporation into protein *in vivo* indicate that its effects *in vitro* are not simply artifacts of the assay procedure. Indeed, nucleocidin is the most potent inhibitor of protein synthesis *in vivo* reported to date. Young *et al.* (1963) reported that cycloheximide at 50 mg/kg, acetoxycycloheximide at 5 mg/kg, or puromycin at 5 hourly doses of 75 mg/kg caused approximately 90% inhibition of amino acid incorporation into liver proteins. Inhibition of protein labeling *in vivo* by nucleocidin cannot be attributed to an effect on amino acid accumulation by liver; radioactivity accumulation in the TCA-soluble portion of liver was not inhibited (Table 3).

Table 3. *Effect of nucleocidin on ^{3}H-leucine incorporation into liver protein in vivo*[1]

Experiment	Nucleocidin injected (mg/kg)	Radioactivity in liver fractions		
		TCA-soluble (dpm/mg liver)	Protein	
			dpm/mg protein ($\times 10^{-5}$)	% inhibition
1	None	1420 ± 56[2]	30.8 ± 0.6[2]	—
	0.05	1370 ± 32	28.0 ± 2.4	9.1
	0.25	1720 ± 105	9.2 ± 0.4	70.3
2	None	2380 ± 41	82.0 ± 1.9	—
	0.20	3100 ± 41	12.4 ± 0.6	84.8
	0.40	3785 ± 47	13.3 ± 47	83.7

[1] Data from Florini *et al.* (1966). Nucleocidin was injected 2 hours before ^{3}H-leucine. The rats were decapitated one (Exp. 1) or two (Exp. 2) hours after administration of the radioactive amino acid.

[2] Mean ± standard error (3 rats/group).

Nucleocidin appears to offer some advantages as an inhibitor of protein synthesis *in vivo*. The low dosage required, lack of violent reaction of animals receiving doses sufficient to inhibit protein synthesis (by contrast, see Young *et al.*, 1963), and failure of nucleocidin to affect the other biochemical systems in which it has been tried, indicate that it would be useful in studies on effects of hormones, etc., in which puromycin is very extensively employed. Unfortunately, very little nucleocidin is now available, and its lack of commercial utility and the low yield from cultures of *Streptomyces calvus* (Backus *et al.*, 1957) offer little reason to hope that more will be available in the future.

References

Backus, E. J., H. D. Tresner, and T. H. Campbell: Antibiotics & Chemotherapy **7**, 532 (1957).

Florini, J. R., H. H. Bird, and Paul H. Bell: Federation Proc. **24**, 1975 (1965).

Florini, J. R., H. H. Bird, and Paul H. Bell: J. Biol. Chem. **241**, 1091 (1966).

Hewitt, R. I., W. S. Wallace, A. R. Gumble, E. R. Gill, and J. H. Williams: Am. J. Trop. Med. Hyg. **2**, 254 (1953).

HEWITT, R. I., A. R. GUMBLE, L. H. TAYLOR, and W. S. WALLACE: Antibiotics Ann. **1956/57**, 722.
IYER, V. N., and W. SZYBALSKI: Appl. Microbiol. **6**, 23 (1958).
LARDY, H. A., D. JOHNSON, and W. C. McMURRAY: Arch. Biochem. Biophys. **78**, 587 (1958).
NOLL, H., T. STAEHELIN, and F. O. WETTSTEIN: Nature **198**, 632 (1963).
PATRICK, J. B., and W. E. MEYER: Personal communication 1965.
STEPHEN, L. E., and A. R. GRAY: J. Parasitol. **46**, 509 (1960).
THOMAS, S. O., V. L. SINGLETON, J. A. LOWERY, R. W. SHARPE, L. M. PRUESS, J. N. PORTER, J. H. MOWAT, and N. BOHONOS: Antibiotics Ann. **1956/57**, 716.
TOBIE, E. J.: J. Parasitol. **43**, 291 (1957).
WALLER, C. W., J. B. PATRICK, W. FULMOR, and W. E. MEYER: J. Am. Chem. Soc. **79**, 1011 (1957).
YOUNG, C. W., P. F. ROBINSON, and B. SACKTOR: Biochem. Pharmacol. **12**, 855 (1963)

Blasticidin S

Tomomasa Misato

Blasticidin S is one of a group of antibiotics that are produced by *Streptomyces griseochromogenes* (TAKEUCHI, HIRAYAMA *et al.*, 1958); other members are blasticidin a, b, and c (FUKUNAGA, MISATO *et al.*, 1955). Blasticidin S inhibits various species among the bacteria and fungi at concentrations between 5 and 100 µg per ml. These sensitive species include both some Gram-positive and Gram-negative bacteria, even members of the genus *Pseudomonas*. Most fungi are not inhibited at low antibiotic concentrations but some, such as *Piricularia oryzae*, are inhibited at 10 µg or less. The inhibition of this pathogenic fungus lead to its use as a protective and therapeutic agent in the control of the blast disease of rice. The effect of the antibiotic is greater on the mycelial than on the spore phase of the fungus (Table 1) and the fungicide is therefore applied to the rice blades after infection has occurred (MISATO, ISHII *et al.*, 1959).

Table 1. *Effect of blasticidin S on spore germination and mycelial growth of Piricularia oryzae*

Blasticidin S concentration (mcg/ml)	Spore		Mycelium	
	Inhibition rate on germination	Inhibition rate on O_2 uptake	Inhibition rate on growth	Inhibition rate on O_2 uptake
0.01	20.3	0.0	22.3	0.0
0.1	27.5	5.7	80.1	55.4
1.0	90.1	45.5	96.2	59.7
10.0	100.0	40.9	100.0	58.4

The toxicity of blasticidin S is rather high with a peroral LD_{50} in rats of 39.5 mg per kg body weight. It causes a severe irritation of the eyes in people. The antibiotic is not toxic to fish and thus it can be used in rice paddys and also near fish ponds which are vital to the food resources of Japan.

Chemical Structure

Blasticidin S free base has a molecular formula of $C_{17}H_{26}O_5N_8$. The chemical structure was established by H. YONEHARA *et al.* as shown in Fig. 1 (OTAKA, TAKEUCHI *et al.*, 1965). It consists of a new nucleoside designated as cytosinine ($C_{10}H_{12}O_4N_4$) and a new amino acid blastidic acid ($C_7H_{16}O_2N_4$). The antibiotic can be prepared by the simple procedure, involving absorption on cation exchange resin and elution with hydrochloric acid. After concentration under vacuum, the crude hydrochloride is obtained from which a crystalline free base or commercially used benzylaminobenzene sulfonate can be prepared.

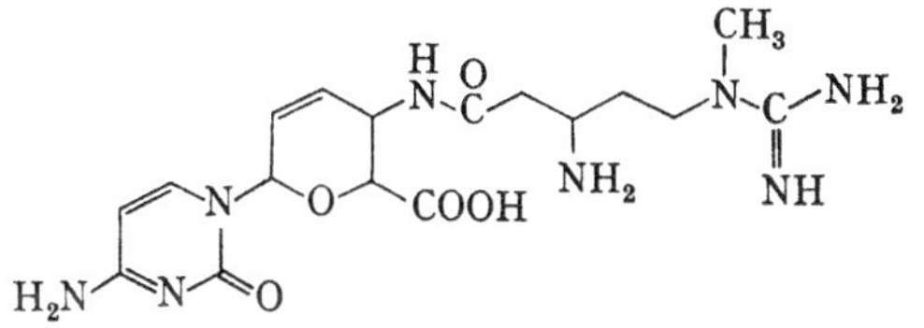

Fig. 1. Chemical structure of blasticidin S

Effect on Protein Synthesis of *Piricularia oryzae*

The antibiotic inhibits oxygen consumption by *Piric. oryzae*. Oxygen uptake was inhibited to a greater extent in mycelium than in spores when either glucose, pyruvate, succinate or glutamate were used as substrates (Table 1) (MISATO, ISHII *et al.*, 1961a). The extent of inhibition was almost constant through concentrations of 0.1 to 100 μg per ml. There was no inhibitory effect on the succinic acid oxidation by mitochondria of *Piric. oryzae* even at 500 μg per ml. Blasticidin S had no effect on glycolysis, succinic acid dehydrogenation, oxidative phosphorylation, or on the incorporation of ^{32}P into nucleic acids (Table 2). The effects on oxygen consumption were therefore considered as secondary.

Table 2. *Effect of blasticidin S on the metabolism of Piricularia oryzae*

Growth — (Agar dilution streak method) — minimum inhibitory conc., 5 ppm.
(Shaking liquid culture) — minimum inhibitory conc., 0.1 ppm.
Respiration (Spore, Mycellium) — partially inhibition at 1—100 ppm.
Electron transport system — no inhibition at 100 ppm.
Succinic dehydrogenase — no inhibition at 100 ppm.
Oxidative phosphorylation — no inhibition at 100 ppm.
Incorporation of ^{32}P into the nucleic acid — no inhibition at 2 ppm.
Incorporation of ^{14}C-amino acid into the protein fraction — 100% inhibition at 1 ppm.

MISATO, OKIMOTO *et al.* (1961b) noticed that blasticidin S caused a marked decrease in the incorporation of glutamic acid-^{14}C into the protein fraction of mycelium. The inhibition occurred at levels of antibiotic about the same as the minimum inhibitory growth concentrations (1 μg per ml). This suggested that the

Table 3. *Effect of blasticidin S on ^{32}P-ATP exchange, s-RNA-^{14}C-amino acid formation and over all incorporation of Piricularia oryzae*

Conc. of blasticidin S (ppm)	^{32}P-ATP exchange[1]	s-RNA-^{14}C-amino acid formation[1]	Over all incorporation[2]
0	850[1]	412[1]	920[2]
1	450	363	80
10	0	279	—

[1] cpm/10 mg protein-N/10 minute incubation.
[2] cpm/10 mg protein-N/15 minute incubation.

primary effect was on protein synthesis. Studies by HUANG, MISATO *et al.* (1964a) with cell-free extracts of *Piric. oryzae* showed that the incorporation of amino acids-^{14}C was almost completely prevented by the antibiotic at 1 µg per ml. Amino

$$\text{amino acid} \xrightarrow{\text{ATP}} \text{AMP-amino acid} \xrightarrow{\text{sRNA}} \text{sRNA-amino acid} \xrightarrow[\uparrow \atop \text{blasticidin S}]{\text{ribosome}} \text{protein}$$

Fig. 2. The action site of blasticidin S on protein synthesis

acid activation and the transfer of activated amino acid to soluble RNA was inhibited to a lesser degree at this concentration (Table 3). The data indicated that the probable site of action of blasticidin S is the final step in protein synthesis which occurs on the ribosomal fraction (Fig. 2). Its action is thus similar to puromycin and chloramphenicol on *Escherichia coli.* Further studies, however, revealed differences in the action of these three antibiotics on fungi (HUANG, MISATO *et al.*, in press 1965a). Blasticidin S completely inhibited amino acid incorporation into *Piric. oryzae* but had little effect on the incorporation into *Pellicularia sasakii* (Table 4). Chloramphenicol partially inhibited the incorporation into *Piric. oryzae* and completely in *Pellic. sasakii*. Puromycin had no effect on *Piric. oryzae* even at 100 µg per ml but partially inhibited the process in *Pellic. sasakii* at the lower concentrations and caused complete inhibition at 100 µg.

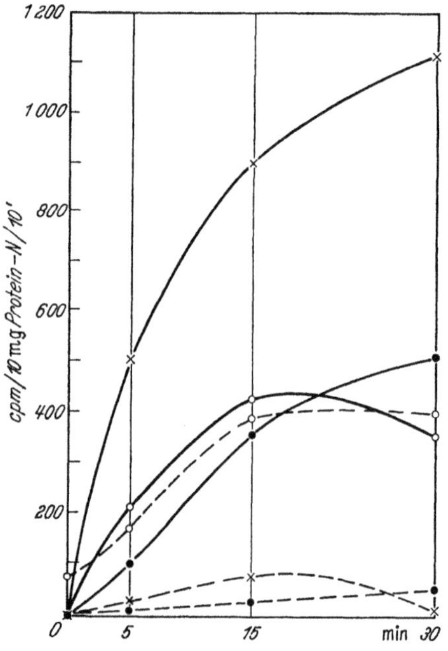

Fig. 3. Effect of blasticidin S on ^{14}C-amino acid incorporation into microsomal protein of blasticidin S tolerant and sensitive colones of Piric. oryzae, and Pellic. sasakii in cell free systems. ×—× Sensitive clone of Piric. oryzae. × --- × Sensitive clone of Piric. oryzae + blasticidin S. •——• Tolerant clone of Piric. oryzae. • --- • Tolerant clone of Piric. oryzae + blasticidin S. ○——○ Pellic. sasakii. ○ --- ○ Pellic. sasakii + blasticidin S

Investigations of NAKAMURA and SAKURAI (1962) revealed that *Piric. oryzae* became resistant to blasticidin S when it was grown in media with successively higher concentrations of the antibiotic. The acquired resistance to the antibiotic was associated with a loss in pathogenicity to the rice plant. The tolerance of the derived clone of fungus to blasticidin S seems to be based on a difference in permeability from that of the normal sensitive parent (HUANG, MISATO and ASUYAMA, 1964b). Amino acid incorporation into ribosomal protein by intact cells of the tolerant clone was not inhibited even at a concentration of antibiotic of 1000 µg/ml (Fig. 3) whereas protein synthesis in cell-free extracts of this clone was inhibited at 1 µg. Inhibition of protein synthesis in the normal sensitive strain of *Piric. oryzae* was the same in the whole cell as in the cell-free extract. The insensitivity of *Pellic. sasakii* to blasticidin S is not caused by the impermeability of the cell membrane but is probably due to a somewhat different metabolic pathway of protein synthesis.

Table 4. *Effect of blasticidin S, chloramphenicol and puromycin on* ^{14}*C-amino acid incorporation into microsomal protein of Piric. oryzae and Pellic. sasakii in cell free system*

Antibiotics	Concentration (mcg/ml)	Piricularia oryzae	Pellicularia sasakii
Blasticidin S	1	complete inhibition	no effect
	10	complete inhibition	no effect
	100	complete inhibition	partial inhibition
Chloramphenicol	1	no effect	partial inhibition
	10	partial inhibition	complete inhibition
	100	partial inhibition	complete inhibition
Puromycin	1	no effect	partial inhibition
	10	no effect	partial inhibition
	100	no effect	complete inhibition

Action on Plants

Blasticidin S is toxic to plants at high concentrations. When rice plants are sprayed with solutions having concentrations exceeding 40 µg/ml, yellowish (chlorotic) spots are produced on the leaves within several days. The chlorotic spots change into brown necrotic spots in extreme cases. Phytotoxicity also occurs on soybean, apple, pear, peach, Chinese cabbage, cucumber, tomato, and other plants, when the plants are sprayed with solutions containing 10 µg/ml or more of blasticidin S. The monobenzylaminobenzensulfonate derivative was found by ASAKAWA *et al.* (1963) to be least phytotoxic to rice plant. This salt is now being used as the active ingredient of commercial blasticidin S preparations. Moreover, HASHIMOTO *et al.* (1963) suggested that the relative contents of non-protein N, which consists mainly of amino acids and RNA, were increased in trated plants. The increase in tryptophane was especially marked. The chlorophyll content of rice plants treated with low concentration of blasticidin S was also increased, whereas the chlorophyll in the leaf blades having phytotoxic spots was markedly decreased.

HUANG *et al.* (1965b) found that the multiplication of chlorella was inhibited by blasticidin S at 2—4 ppm, although the cells usually continued to grow to 3—4 times the size of the untreated cells, even after 40 hours treatment with blasticidin S. The growth of the cells was inhibited by 100 ppm and the large cells sometimes contained 4 nuclei. The large cells began to grow when blasticidin S was removed from the culture. These results indicated that the inhibition by blasticidin S on chlorella was similar to 8-azaguanine. Azaguanine belonged to type III of Tamiya's classification on the effect of chemical agents on chlorella (TAMIYA *et al.*, 1962).

Effect on RNA Metabolism

The RNA content was increased in the blasticidin S treated cells of green plants and in *Piric. oryzae*, while their protein synthesis was completely inhibited. From further experiments on RNA metabolism in *Saccharomyces sake*, HASHIMOTO *et al.* (1965) suggested that in the organism the RNA content was also increased by concentrations of blasticidin S which inhibited protein synthesis. The accumulated RNA was stable and could also be utilized for normal metabolism, when the cell began to grow. These phenomena were similar to the effects of puromycin on *Pseudomonas fluorescens*. However, when a ^{32}P-labelled microsome fraction that had been synthesized in the presence of blasticidin S was run in an electrophoretic apparatus, it contained a significant amount of a radioactive substance which migrated more rapidly to the anode than did the nontreated microsome fraction. This fast running substance was considered to be ribonucleoprotein particles having abnormal properties.

Effect on Plant Virus

In a preliminary report, KITANI *et al.* (1963) stated that the rate of infection of rice plants with stripe virus, which is transmissible by a leafhopper, *Delphacodes striatella* FALLEN, was reduced by blasticidin S. HIRAI and SHIMOMURA (1965) observed that blasticidin S at a low concentration had a high inhibitory effect on the synthesis of tobacco mosaic virus (TMV). The antibiotic inhibited TMV multiplication in tobacco leaf discs about 50% at 0.05 ppm but caused no chemical injury to leaves. The same concentration of the antibiotic almost completely inhibited local lesions caused by TMV either on *Nicotiana glutinosa* or Pinto bean. They further investigated the inhibitory mechanism of blasticidin S against TMV multiplication. RNA content in noninfected tobacco leaf discs treated with the antibiotic was increased compared with that in untreated discs. Blasticidin S also increased the incorporation rates of uracil-^{14}C into nucleic acids of noninfected and infected leaf discs, although the amount of TMV-RNA was reduced by the treatment. The incorporation rates of amino acids-^{14}C into proteins of noninfected and infected leaf discs were not reduced but were even increased at these concentrations of the antibiotic; the total amounts of normal and TMV proteins were reduced by the treatment. They suggested that the synthesis of enzymes associated with the polymerization of TMV-RNA might be inhibited by blasticidin S.

References

ASAKAWA, M., T. MISATO, and K. FUKUNAGA: Studies on the prevention of the phytotoxicity of blasticidin S. Pesticide and Technique (Tokyo) **8**, 24—30 (1963).

FUKUNAGA, K., T. MISATO, I. ISHII, and M. ASAKAWA: Blasticidin. A new anti-phytopathogenic fungal substance. Bull. Agr. Chem. Soc. Japan **19**, 181—188 (1955).

HASHIMOTO, K., M. KATAGIRI, and T. MISATO: Studies on the phytotoxic action of an antiblastic antibiotic, blasticidin S. I. The effect of blasticidin S on the content of free amino acids, proteins and nucleic acids in rice leaf and yeast. J. Agr. Chem. Soc. Japan **37**, 245—250 (1963).

HASHIMOTO, K., and M. MISATO: Studies on the microsomes of yeast cells treated with blasticidin S. J. Antibiotics (Japan), Ser. A **18**, 77—81 (1965).

HIRAI, T., and T. SHIMOMURA: Blasticidin S, an effective antibiotic against plant virus multiplication. Phytopathology **55**, 291—295 (1965).

HUANG, K. T., T. MISATO, and H. ASUYAMA: Effect of blasticidin S on protein synthesis of Piricularia oryzae. J. Antibiotics (Japan), Ser. A **17**, 65—70 (1964a).
HUANG, K. T., T. MISATO, and H. ASUYAMA: Effects of protein synthesis inhibitors, blasticidin S, puromycin and chloramphenicol on Piricularia oryzae and Pellicularia sasakii. J. Antibiotics (Japan), Ser. A (in press) (1965a).
HUANG, K. T., T. MISATO, and H. ASUYAMA: Selective toxicity of blasticidin S to Piricularia oryzae and Pellicularia sasakii. J. Antibiotics (Japan), Ser. A **17**, 71—74 (1964b).
HUANG, K. T., T. MISATO, and H. ASUYAMA: Effect of blasticidin S on the growth and protein synthesis of Chlorella ellipsoidea. J. Antibiotics (Japan), Ser. A (in press) (1965b).
KITANI, S., and A. KISO: Studies on the chemical prevention against rice stripe virus disease. Ann. Phytopath. Soc. Japan **28**, 293 (1963) (Abstr.).
MISATO, T., I. ISHII, M. ASAKAWA, Y. OKIMOTO, and K. FUKUNAGA: Antibiotics as protectant fungicides against rice blast. II. The therapeutic action of blasticidin S. Ann. Phytopath. Soc. Japan **24**, 302—306 (1959).
MISATO, T., I. ISHII, M. ASAKAWA, Y. OKIMOTO, and K. FUKUNAGA: Antibiotics as protectant fungicides against rice blast. III. Effect of blasticidin S on respiration of Piricularia oryzae. Ann. Phytopath. Soc. Japan **26**, 19—24 (1961a).
MISATO, T., Y. OKIMOTO, I. ISHII, M. ASAKAWA, and K. FUKUNAGA: Antibiotics as protectant fungicides against rice blast. IV. Effect of blasticidin S on the metabolism of Piricularia oryzae. Ann. Phytopath. Soc. Japan **26**, 25—30 (1961b).
NAKAMURA, H., and L. SAKURAI: Tolerance of Piricularia oryzae on blasticidin S. Ann. Phytopath. Soc. Japan **27**, 84 (1962) (Abstr.).
OTAKE, N., S. TAKEUCHI, T. ENDO, and H. YONEHARA: The structure of blasticidin S. Tetrahedron Letters No 19, 1411—1419 (1965).
TAKEUCHI, S., K. HIRAYAMA, K. UEDA, H. SAKAI, and H. YONEHARA: Blasticidin S, a new antibiotic. J. Antibiotics (Japan), Ser. A **11**, 1—5 (1958).
TAMIYA, H., Y. MORIMURA, and M. YOKOTA: Effects of various antimetabolites upon the life cycle of Chlorella. Arch. Mikrobiol. **42**, 4—16 (1962).

Lincomycin*

F. N. Chang and B. Weisblum

Lincomycin, an antibiotic produced by *Streptomyces lincolnensis var. lincolnensis,* has the following structure (HOEKSEMA *et al.*, 1964).

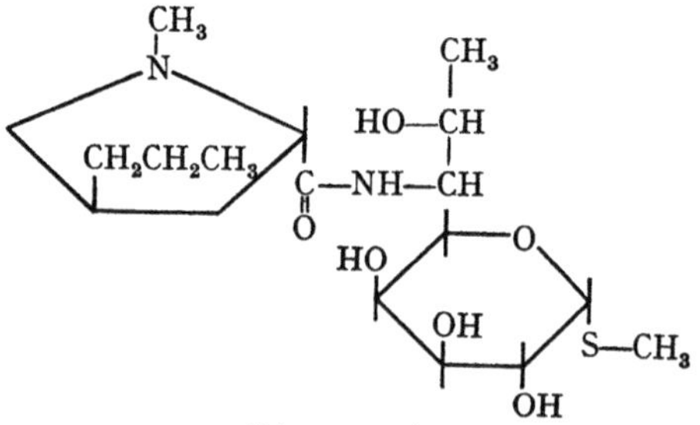

Lincomycin

The activity spectrum of lincomycin tested *in vitro* against some representative strains of bacteria is presented in Table 1. Gram-positive bacteria are more sensitive than gram-negative bacteria both *in vivo* and *in vitro* (LEWIS, CLAPP, and GRADY, 1962). Intact yeast cells *in vitro* (*Saccharomyces* and *Candida* species) and KB

Table 1. *In vitro spectrum of lincomycin tested by tube dilution*
(Based on LEWIS, CLAPP, and GRADY 1962)

	Organism	No. of strains	Minimum inhibitory concentration of lincomycin (μg/ml) after 18 hr. incubation	
			Range	Average
Gram-positive	*Staphylococcus aureus*	41	0.36—2.8	1.25
	Diplococcus pneumoniae	5	0.08—0.72	0.34
	β-Streptococcus	8	0.04—0.72	0.21
	α-Streptococcus	3	0.17—0.92	0.31
	Streptococcus faecalis	2	1.4—46.0	23.7
	Clostridium	2	0.36—1.4	0.88
Gram-negative	*Coli-Aerogenes*	5	>92	—
	Proteus	6	>92	—
	Pseudomonas	3	>92	—
	Salmonella	9	>92	—

* This work was supported by Research Grant GB 3080 from the National Science Foundation.

cells grown in tissue culture are insensitive at 100 μg/ml (J. E. GRADY, personal communication). The minimum inhibitory concentrations for *Mycoplasma* species were: less than 0.04 μg/ml for *M. hominis*, less than 0.62 μg/ml for *M. arthritidis*, and less than 1.2 μg/ml for *M. gallisepticum* (L. J. HANKA, personal communication). The initial rate of protein synthesis in a cell-free system from rabbit reticulocytes was unaffected by 10^{-4} lincomycin (BAGLIONI, 1966).

The antibacterial properties of various chemically modified forms of lincomycin have been studied by MASON and LEWIS (1964). Antibacterial activity tested by the *S. lutea* tube dilution assay is strongly dependent on the substituents attached to the sulfur- and ring nitrogen atoms. N-ethyl lincomycin is as active as the parent compound, while N-demethyl-lincomycin is only 10% as active. S-ethyl lincomycin is 130% as active as lincomycin while dethiomethyl lincomycin is inactive.

GRAY *et al.* (1964) reported that the LD_{50} for intraperitoneal administration in mice is greater than 1000 mg/kg and greater than 4000 mg/kg for oral administration in rats. At 50 mg/kg no teratogenic effects in dogs were noted.

At a concentration of 50 μg/ml, JOSTEN and ALLEN (1964) found an immediate cessation of lysine incorporation into protein by intact cells of *S. aureus in vitro*, whereas RNA synthesis stopped only after a 15 minute lag. Most of the lysine incorporated in the lincomycin-inhibited cultures was found in cell wall glycopeptide. The incorporation of lysine into the bacterial cell wall occurs by a different mechanism from that utilized by the cell for lysine incorporation into protein (ITO and STROMINGER, 1964). On the other hand, glycine incorporation into cell wall glycopeptide has a few features in common with protein synthesis. Cell-free extracts of *S. aureus* which synthesize glycopeptide require an sRNA-like molecule to which glycine is charged prior to peptide bond formation (MATSUHASHI, DIETRICH, and STROMINGER, 1965). A similar reaction is also utilized in the incorporation of threonine by cellfree extracts of *Micrococcus roseus* (ROBERTS and STROMINGER, 1966). These reactions are not inhibited by lincomycin at levels of 100 μg/ml and 1000 μg/ml respectively (M. MATSUHASHI, W. ROBERTS and J. L. STROMINGER, personal communications).

Additional details concerning the mechanism of lincomycin action in cell-free extracts of *B. stearothermophilus* have been reported by CHANG, SIH and WEISBLUM (1966). *B. stearothermophilus* was used as the test organism because cell-free extracts were found to be more active in protein synthesis than those prepared from *S. aureus* or *B. subtilis*.

It was observed that:

1. Protein synthesis, as measured by poly U-directed polyphenylalanine synthesis, is sensitive to lincomycin in extracts of *B. stearothermophilus*, but not in *E. coli* (Fig. 1).

2. The site of lincomycin action is on the ribosome (Table 2), more specifically, on the 50S subunit (Fig. 2).

3. The binding of phenylalanine-sRNA to the ribosome-messenger complex is inhibited by lincomycin (Fig. 3).

The possibility that gram-negative bacteria may inactivate lincomycin has not been ruled out. This consideration is of special interest because of the recent description of a cell-free antibiotic inactivating system obtained from certain antibiotic-resistant strains of *E. coli*, OKAMOTO and SUZUKI (1965).

Table 2. *Inhibition of protein synthesis by lincomycin in systems reconstituted from homologous and heterologous ribosomes and supernatants*

Ribosomes	Supernatant	^{14}C phenylalanine incorporation (cpm)			% Inhibition
		—poly U	+poly U —Lincomycin	+poly U +Lincomycin $10^{-4}M$	
E. coli	*P. coli*	130	3660	5220	0
B. stearo	*B. stearo*	210	3280	*490*	85
E. coli	*B. stearo*	160	5120	4730	9
B. stearo	*E. coli*	110	1100	*256*	77
E. coli	none		50		
none	*E. coli*		92		
B. stearo	none		104		
none	*B. stearo*		70		

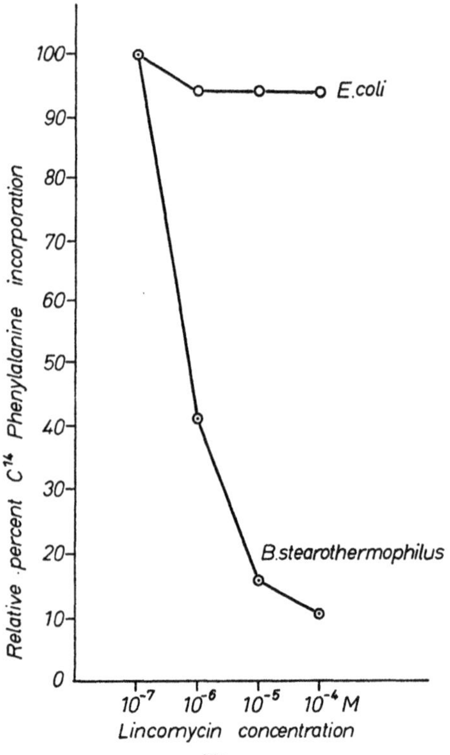

Fig. 1

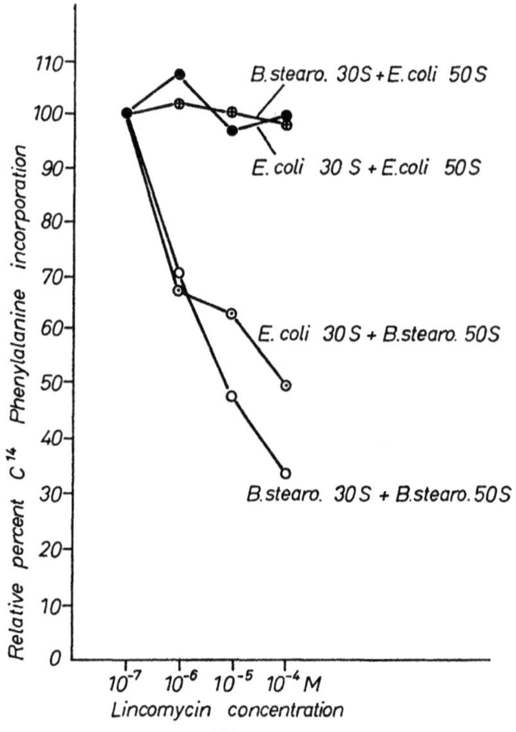

Fig. 2

Fig. 1. Inhibition of poly U-directed polyphenylalanine synthesis in bacterial cell-free extracts as a function of lincomycin concentration

Fig. 2. Lincomycin sensitivity of polyphenylalanine synthesis in system reconstructed from hybrid ribosomes which contain heterologous 30 S and 50 S subunits. *E. coli* and *B. stearothermophilus* were used as source of resistant and sensitive subunits, respectively. The data suggest that the 50 S subunit of *B. stearothermophilus* is the site of lincomycin action because polyphenylalanine synthesis is inhibited only when 50 S subunits from *B. stearothermophilus* were used

A number of different antibiotics which inhibit protein synthesis at the ribosome can compete with each other with respect to ribosomal binding or antagonize each other with respect to inhibition of protein synthesis. For example, VASQUEZ (1966), has shown that the binding of chloramphenicol to the 50 S ribosomal subunit is inhibited by lincomycin. Tetracycline which acts on the 30 S subunit

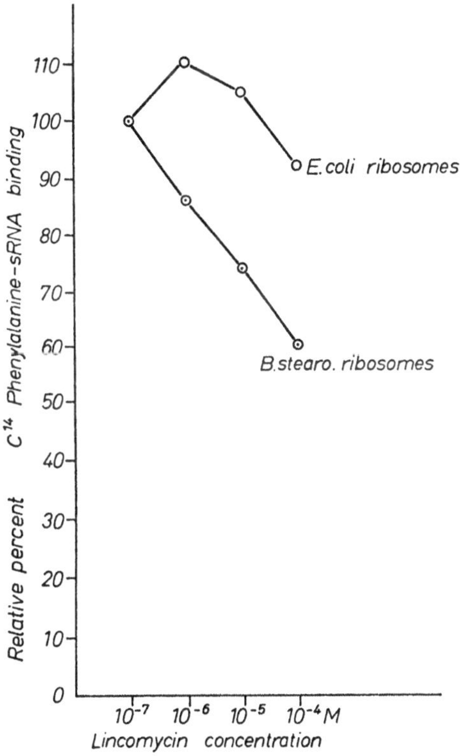

Fig. 3

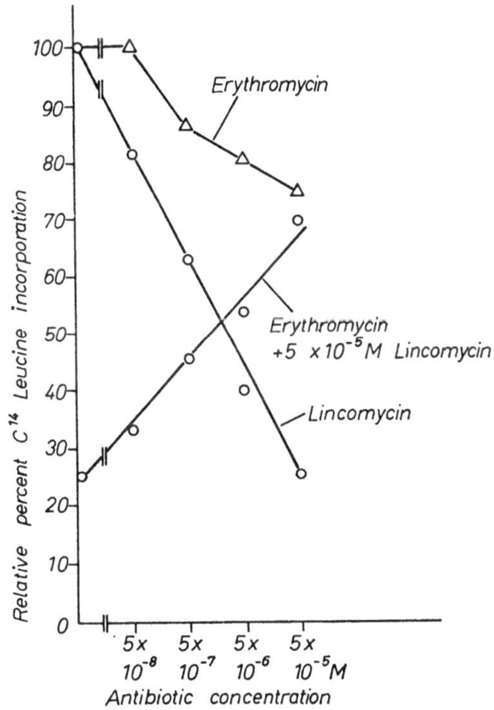

Fig. 4

Fig. 3. Inhibition of ^{14}C-phe-sRNA binding to ribosomes from *E. coli* and *B. stearothermophilus* as a function of lincomycin concentration. Ribosomes from *B. stearothermophilus* are inhibited at one hundreth the dose required to inhibit *E. coli* ribosomes

Fig. 4. Inhibition by lincomycin of poly UC-directed ^{14}C leucine incorporation in a cell-free extract of *B. stearothermophilus;* antagonistic action of erythromycin. Leucine incorporation is inhibited by increasing concentrations of lincomycin as well as erythromycin up to 5×10^{-5} *M*. At this inhibitory concentration of lincomycin, the addition of increasing amounts of erythromycin partly restores the level of leucine incorporation

was not found to inhibit chloramphenicol-binding. Streptomycin, as well as kanamycin and neomycin which probably also act on the 30 S subunit because of their pharmacological similarity to streptomycin, likewise did not prevent chloramphenicol-binding by ribosomes.

Antagonism between lincomycin and erythromycin *in vitro* has been reported by BARBER and WATERWORTH (1964) and by GRIFFITH *et al.* (1965). The latter observed a decreased zone of inhibition near the lincomycin disc of lincomycin and erythromycin sensitivity discs were placed in proximity on a plate seeded with erythromycin-resistant *S. aureus*. In the presence of erythromycin (0.6 μg/ml) the minimum inhibitory concentration of lincomycin was increased at least 10-fold (from less than 0.3 μg/ml in the absence of erythromycin to greater than 3 μg/ml in the presence of erythromycin). Transformation products of lincomycin and erythromycin were not detectable in the broth recovered from cultures of *S. aureus* which had been incubated with these antibiotics. Lincomycin-erythromycin antagonism can also be observed in relation to protein synthesis in cell-free extracts (F. N. CHANG and B. WEISBLUM, (1967). In particular, leucine incorporation by *B. stearothermophilus* extracts, inhibited to 25% of the original level by $5 \times 10^{-5} M$ lincomycin, can be restored by the addition of erythromycin (Fig. 4). The inhibition by lincomycin of poly U-directed ^{14}C phenylalanine-sRNA-binding to *B. stearothermophilus* ribosome was also found to be reversible by erythromycin (Fig. 5).

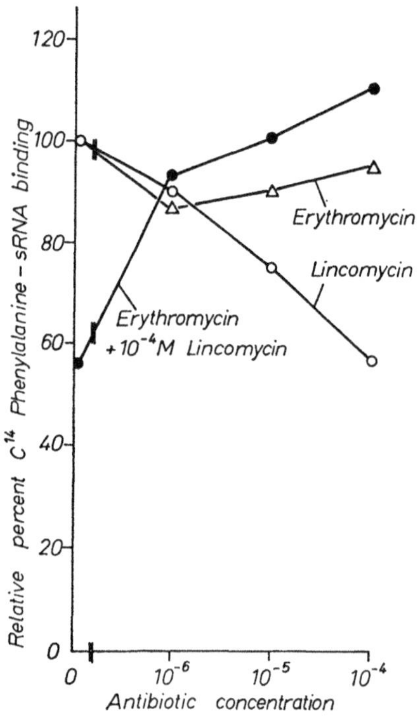

Fig. 5. Inhibition by lincomycin of poly U-directed ^{14}C phenylalanine-sRNA binding to *B. stearothermophilus* ribosomes; antagonistic action of erythromycin. ^{14}C phenylalanine-sRNA binding is inhibited about 45% at $10^{-4} M$ lincomycin. At this inhibitory concentration of lincomycin, the addition of increasing amounts of erythromycin up to $10^{-4} M$ restores the level of ^{14}C phenylalanine-sRNA binding to 110% o its control value.

These results indicate that the antagonism between lincomycin and erythromycin occurs at the ribosome and not, e.g., at the site involved in transport across the bacterial cell membrane. The chemical nature of these antibiotic antagonisms will have to be characterized more extensively. It would be of interest to knowwhether antagonistic pairs compete for the same binding site on the ribosome or whether one antibiotic induces configurational changes in the ribosome which preclude binding of antibioticsat different sites.

The binding of lincomycin-^{14}C to ribosomes of *B. stearothermophilus* was studied with respect to ribosomal subunit specificity and the stability of the lincomycin-ribosome complex. Ammonium or potassium but not calcium or magnesium ions are required for optimal binding. Lincomycin binds to the 50 S subunit of *B. stearothermophilus* but not to the 30 S subunit nor to the 70 S ribosome of *E. coli*. By dilution of the complex, it is possible to show that the binding of lincomycin-^{14}C to ribosomes is revesible (25 C). Lincomycin-^{14}C can be displaced from the ribosome by lincomycin-^{12}C or erythromycin but not by chlortetracycline.

Chlortetracycline which also inhibits the sRNA binding reaction has been found to act at the 30 S subunit (SUZUKA, KAJI, and KAJI, 1965). The combined inhibitory effects of lincomycin and chlortetracycline on the binding reaction are additive (F. N. CHANG and B. WEISBLUM, unpublished data).

A knowledge of the specificity of lincomycin action and its interaction with other antibiotics is directly applicable to clinical situations. The specific effects of lincomycin on the 50 S ribosomal subunit provide us with another tool to study 50 S subunit function and its role in the translation of genetic information.

References

BAGLIONI, C.: Inhibition of protein synthesis in reticulocytes by antibiotics. III. Mechanism of action of sparsomycin. Biochim. et Biophys. Acta **129**, 642 (1966).

BARBER, M., and P. M. WATERWORTH: Antibacterial activity of lincomycin and pristinamycin: A comparison with erythromycin. Brit. Med. J. **1964II**, 603.

CHANG, F. N., D. J. SIH, and B. WEISBLUM: Lincomycin, an inhibitor of aminoacyl sRNA binding to ribosomes. Proc. Natl. Acad. Sci. U.S. **55**, 431 (1966).

CHANG, F. N., and B. WEISBLUM: The specificity of lincomycin binding to ribosomes. Biochemistry (1967, in press).

GRAY, J. E., A. PURMALIS, and E. S. FEENSTRA: Animal toxicity studies of a new antibiotic, lincomycin. Toxicol. and Appl. Pharmacol. **6**, 476 (1964).

GRIFFITH, L. J., W. E. OSTRANDER, C. G. MULLINS, and D. E. BESWICK: Drug antagonism between lincomycin and erythromycin. Science **147**, 746 (1965).

HOEKSEMA, H., B. BANNISTER, R. D. BIRKENMEYER, F. KAGAN, B. J. MAGERLEIN, F. A. MACKELLEAR, W. SCHROEDER, G. SLOMP, and R. R. HERR: Chemical studies on lincomycin. I. The structure of lincomycin. J. Am. Chem. Soc. **86**, 4223 (1964).

IITO, E., and J. L. STROMINGER: Enzymatic synthesis of the peptide in bacterial uridine nucleotides. III. Purification and properties of L-lysine adding enzyme. J. Biol. Chem. **239**, 210 (1964).

JOSTEN, J. J., and P. M. ALLEN: The mode of action of lincomycin. Biochem. Biophys. Research Commun. **14**, 241 (1964).

LEWIS, C. H. W. CLAPP, and J. E. GRADY: *In vitro* and *in vivo* evaluation of lincomycin a new antibiotic. In: Antimicrobial agents and chemotherapy (M. FINLAND and G. SAVAGE, eds.), p. 570—582. Michigan: Braun-Brumfield Inc. 1962.

MASON, D. J., and C. LEWIS: Biological activity of the lincomycin-related antibiotics. In: Antimicrobial agents and chemotherapy (M. FINLAND and G. SAVAGE, eds.), p. 7—12. Michigan: Braun-Brumfield Inc. 1964.

MATSUHASHI, M., C. P. DIETRICH, and J. L. STROMINGER: Incorporation of glycine into the cell wall glycopeptide in *Staphylococcus aureus:* Role of sRNA and lipid intermediates. Proc. Natl. Acad. Sci. U.S. **54**, 587 (1965).

OKAMOTO, S., and Y. SUZUKI: Chloramphenicol-, dihydrostreptomycin, and kanamycin-inactivating enzymes from multiple drug-resistant *Escherichia coli* carrying episome "R". Nature **208**, 1301 (1965).

ROBERTS, W. S. L., and J. L. STROMINGER: Requirement of sRNA for L-threonine incorporation into the cell wall glycopeptide in *Micrococcus roseus*. Federation Proc. **25**, 403 (1966).

SUZUKA, I., H. KAJI, and A. KAJI: Binding of specific sRNA to 30 S ribosomal subunitseffect of 50 S ribosomal subunits. Biochem. Biophys. Research Commun. **21**, 187 (1965).

VASQUEZ, D.: Binding of chloramphenicol to ribosomes; The effect of a number of antibiotics. Biochim. et Biophys. Acta **114**, 277 (1966).

Chalcomycin

D. C. Jordan

Chalcomycin, is a fermentation product of a culture of *Streptomyces* now regarded as a new strain of *Streptomyces bikiniensis*. This organism differs from the description of *S. bikiniensis* given by JOHNSTONE and WAKSMAN (1948) in that it produces chalcomycin; has oblong spores; produces no soluble pigment in Czapek's agar and produces a dark grey pigment, instead of a dark brown pigment, in nutrient agar (COFFEY *et al.*, 1965). Two different isolates of this strain are maintained by Parke, Davis and Company (05020 and 05071) and by the Northern Utilization Research and Development Division, U.S. Department of Agriculture, Peoria, Illinois (NRRL 2737 and NRRL 2738).

This essentially neutral antibiotic contains only carbon, hydrogen and oxygen, has a molecular weight of about 600—700, and is soluble in organic solvents (FROHARDT *et al.*, 1962). It is slightly soluble in water (to approximately 7 mg/ml) but more concentrated solutions can be prepared by dissolving the antibiotic in methanol or ethanol and diluting with water to 5—10% alcohol (EHRLICH, *personal communication*). Neutral solutions are stable at room temperature for about 6 weeks. A microbial assay procedure has been described by COFFEY *et al.* (1965).

With the help of data accumulated from previous studies (including those of WOO, DION and BARTZ, 1961; DION, WOO and BARTZ, 1962; and WOO, DION and JOHNSON, 1962) WOO, DION and BARTZ (1964a, b, c) have established the structural formula of chalcomycin. The molecule (Fig. 1) contains two carbohydrate residues, chalcose and mycinose. Since the antistaphylococcal potency of chalcomycin can be decreased by prior exposure of this compound to ethylene oxide it may be that groups essential for its antibacterial properties are susceptible to alkylation (HOEPRICH, 1962). The antibiotic is not rendered ineffective by bacterial penicillinases.

Chalcomycin is active against certain gram-positive bacteria, principally *Staphylococcus aureus* and *Streptococcus pyogenes* (COFFEY *et al.*, 1965) which are inhibited by 0.4 μg/ml or less. The antistreptococcal activity of chalcomycin is unusual in that it is limited to Lancefield groups A, C and G, strains of streptococci in groups B, D, E and F being relatively resistant. The reason for this phenomenon is unknown, but it may be related to permeability differences among the streptococci. *Corynebacterium diphtheriae* and *Diplococcus pneumoniae* require 50 μg chalcomycin/ml for inhibition, whereas strains of *Aerobacter, Brucella, Escherichia, Klebsiella, Paracolobactrum, Pasteurella, Proteus, Pseudomonas, Salmonella* and *Shigella* are insensitive to 100 μg/ml. The antibiotic is inactive at less than 200 μg/ml against a variety of pathogenic molds, protozoa and viruses.

The potent effect of chalcomycin on staphylococci was stressed by HOEPRICH (1962), who found that 192 of 193 tellurite-positive, human-associated staphylococci were inhibited by 0.10 μmoles (60 μg)/ml, whereas several species of *Mycobacterium* and *Enterococcus*, in addition to many gram-negative bacteria, were resistant to 0.250 μmoles (150 μg)/ml. HOEPRICH concluded that at a concentration of 0.01 μmoles/ml the antistaphylococcal potency of chalcomycin was similar to that of phenoxymethylpenicillin, benzylpenicillin and neomycin and superior to that of aminocarboxybutylpenicillin, dihydrostreptomycin and kanamycin.

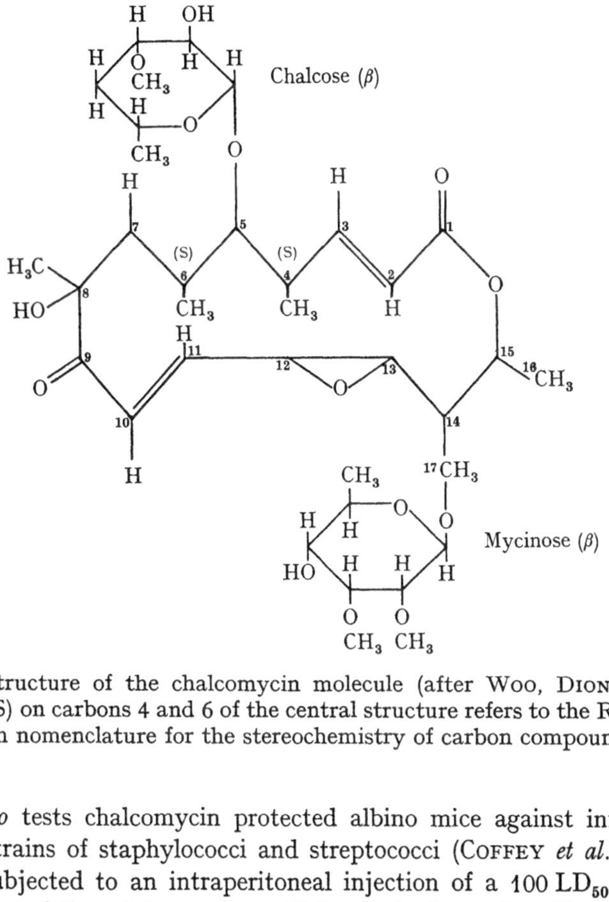

Fig. 1. The structure of the chalcomycin molecule (after WOO, DION and BARTZ, 1964c). The (S) on carbons 4 and 6 of the central structure refers to the R-S configuration nomenclature for the stereochemistry of carbon compounds

In *in vivo* tests chalcomycin protected albino mice against infection by a number of strains of staphylococci and streptococci (COFFEY *et al.*, 1965). The mice were subjected to an intraperitoneal injection of a 100 LD_{50} dose of the infective agent, followed by an immediate single dose of antibiotic. The 50% effective dose (ED_{50}) ranged from 13 to 53 mg chalcomycin/kg body weight orally and from 8 to 47 mg/kg subcutaneously, against 8 different strains of *S. aureus*. The ED_{50} for protection against a strain of *S. pyogenes* was about 88 mg/kg orally and 55 mg/kg subcutaneously, for a single dose.

Chalcomycin is well tolerated by rats, mice, dogs and monkeys (COFFEY *et al.*, 1965). The 50% lethal dose (LD_{50}) for white mice has been reported as more than 2500 mg/kg for acute oral administration and 498 ± 1.9 mg/kg for intravenous administration. Chronic oral toxicity tests in rats, dogs and monkeys showed that the antibiotic could be tolerated, with no detectable irreversible abnormalities, at daily doses, respectively, of 1805, 200 and 400 mg/kg for 4 to 6 weeks.

Chalcomycin is presently under clinical investigation but the results have not yet been published (EHRLICH, *personal communication*).

Information on the mode of action of chalcomycin is meagre. HOEPRICH (1962) found no pattern of bacterial cross-resistance or susceptibility among chalcomycin, phenoxymethylpenicillin and neomycin, suggesting that chalcomycin had a different inhibitory mechanism than either of the other two antibiotics. In addition, since chalcomycin failed to produce protoplasts from staphylococci, it was inferred that this antibiotic was not an inhibitor of cell-wall synthesis.

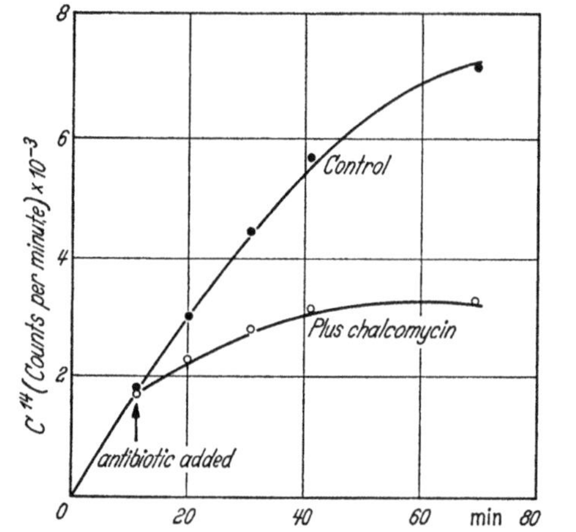

Fig. 2. Effect of chalcomycin on the uptake of glycine-2-^{14}C into the trypsin-sensitive protein of *Staphylococcus aureus* (JORDAN, 1963)

JORDAN (1963), using the technique of PARK and HANCOCK (1960), studied the influence of chalcomycin at a concentration of 22.4 μg/mg cell dry weight on the uptake of glycine-2-^{14}C into the intracellular pool, ethanol-soluble "protein" and lipid, trypsin-solubilized protein, and cell wall mucopeptide of a pathogenic strain of *S. aureus* sensitive to the antibiotic at a level of 0.5—1.0 μg/ml. In addition, any possible effect on the uptake of ^{32}P-labelled orthophosphate into the cellular deoxyribonucleic acid (DNA) and ribonucleic acid (RNA) was investigated by a slight modification of the method of HANAWALT (1959). At the concentration of chalcomycin employed, the action was bactericidal. Although chalcomycin is primarily bacteriostatic with staphylococci at a concentration of 0.6 μg/ml, there is a marked increase in the bactericidal effect as the concentration increases to 6 μg/ml (HOEPRICH, 1962). For at least 1 hr after the addition of the antibiotic to logarithmic-phase cells there was no demonstrable effect on the passage of glycine into the intracellular pool, upon the incorporation of this acid into the ethanol-soluble "protein" or lipid, or upon the incorporation of ^{32}P into either DNA or RNA. However, within 10 minutes of adding chalcomycin there was a marked inhibition in the synthesis of trypsin-sensitive protein (Fig. 2), which became absolute within a 40 minutes contact period. Although there was a slight decrease in the uptake of glycine into the wall mucopeptide after the addition of the antibiotic this was assumed to be associated with the decreased synthesis of a trypsin resistant "protein" commonly associated with the mucopeptide (PARK and HANCOCK, 1960) and which may represent some portion of the plasma membrane.

Continued studies indicated that chalcomycin exerted little or no effect on the amino acid activating capacity of cellular extracts of staphylococci (Table 1) but that the antibiotic caused a striking depression in the passage of radioactivity from glycine-2-^{14}C to both cellular s-RNA and ribosomes (Table 2).

Table 1. *Effect of chalcomycin on ^{32}P-ATP exchange*

	ATP[1] synthesis		
	No added amino acids no chalcomycin	Added amino acids no chalcomycin	Added amino acids plus chalcomycin
Run A[2]	132×10^3	423×10^3	423×10^3
Run B[2]	185×10^3	508×10^3	510×10^3
Percent inhibition			None

[1] Counts per minute/μmole.
[2] Run A 100 μg chalcomycin/mg cell dry weight. Run B 500 μg chalcomycin/mg cell dry weight. The amount of radioactivity initially added was higher in run B than in run A.
See JORDAN (1963) for experimental details.

From these results it was concluded that chalcomycin inhibited protein synthesis via an interference in the transfer of activated amino acids to the cellular s-RNA. The problem of whether or not the interference is directed against the actual transfer or against the s-RNA remains to be elucidated.

Table 2. *Effect of chalcomycin on the transfer of glycine-2-^{14}C to the s-RNA and ribosomes of Staphylococcus aureus 71435*

	Specific activity			
	s-RNA[1]		Ribosomes[1]	
	Control	plus chalcomycin	Control	plus chalcomycin
	1916	774	356	208
Percent inhibition	59.7		41.6	

[1] Counts per minute/mg dry weight.

References

COFFEY, G. L., L. E. ANDERSON, J. D. DOUROS, A. L. ERLANDSON, JR., M. W. FISHER, R. J. HANS, R. F. PITTILLO, D. K. VOGLER, K. S. WESTON, and J. EHRLICH. Chalcomycin, a new antibiotic: biological studies. Can. J. Microbiol. **9**, 665 (1965).

DION, H. W., P. W. K. WOO, and Q. R. BARTZ: Chemistry of mycinose: 6-deoxy-2,3-di-O-methyl-D-allose. J. Am. Chem. Soc. **84**, 880 (1962).

FROHARDT, R. P., R. F. PITTILLO, and J. EHRLICH: Chalcomycin and its fermentation production. U.S. Patent 3,065,137, Nov. 20 (1962).

HANAWALT, P.: Use of phosphorus-32 in microassay for nucleic acid synthesis in *Escherichia coli*. Science **130**, 386 (1959).

HOEPRICH, P. D.: In vitro antibacterial potency of chalcomycin. Antimicrobial agents and chemotherapy-1961. Am. Soc. Microbiol., Ann Arbor, Michigan, p. 481—490 (1962).

JOHNSTONE, D. B., and S. A. WAKSMAN: The production of streptomycin by *Streptomyces bikiniensis*. J. Bacteriol. **55**, 317 (1948).

JORDAN, D. C.: Effect of chalcomycin on protein synthesis by *Staphylococcus aureus*. Can. J. Microbiol. **9**, 129 (1963).

PARK, J. T., and R. HANCOCK: A fractionation procedure for studies on the synthesis of cell wall mucopeptide and other polymers in cells of *Staphylococcus aureus*. J. Gen. Microbiol. **22**, 249 (1960).

WOO, P. W. K., H. W. DION, and Q. R. BARTZ: Chemistry of chalcose, a 3-methoxy-4,6 dideoxyhexose. J. Am. Chem. Soc. **83**, 3352 (1961).

WOO, P. W. K., H. W. DION, and Q. R. BARTZ: Partial structure of chalcomycin. I. A C_{18} chalcoxyloxy moiety. J. Am. Chem. Soc. **86**, 2724 (1964a).

WOO, P. W. K., H. W. DION, and Q. R. BARTZ: Partial structure of chalcomycin. II. A C_{17} mycinosyloxy moiety. J. Am. Chem. Soc. **86**, 2724 (1964b).

WOO, P. W. K., H. W. DION, and Q. R. BARTZ: The structure of chalcomycin. J. Am. Chem. Soc. **86**, 2726 (1964c).

WOO, P. W. K., H. W. DION, and L. F. JOHNSON: The stereochemistry of chalcose, a degradation product of chalcomycin. J. Am. Chem. Soc. **84**, 1066 (1962).

Hadacidin

Harold T. Shigeura

In addition to certain normal cellular metabolites that exert control over the biosynthesis of nucleic acids, a large number of substances synthesized chemically or obtained from natural sources have now been demonstrated to interfere with the ultimate formation of these macro-molecules. These inhibitors, which are structurally related to purines, pyrimidines and amino acids, have been found to antagonize the metabolism of a corresponding normal substrate. Furthermore, the modes of action of some of these antimetabolites have been elucidated. This review pertains to hadacidin, a structural analogue of L-aspartic acid, isolated from the fermentation fluid of *Penicillium frequentans* and subsequently found to inhibit the biosynthesis *de novo* of adenylic acid.

Discovery, Isolation and Characterization of Hadacidin

Gitterman *et al.* (1962) reported that the fermentation broth of *Penicillium frequentans* Westling suppressed the growth of human adenocarcinoma (H.Ad. # 1) growing in the embryonated egg. For the isolation of the active component (Kaczka *et al.*, 1962), three liters of the filtered fermentation medium were lyophilized. The dried material was triturated with methanol and the methanol extract was evaporated to dryness. The residue was then dissolved in water and precipitated with ethanol. Repeated recrystallization from water with ethanol yielded a pure salt corresponding to $C_3H_4NO_4Na$. The substance gave a positive test with ferric chloride and an atypical ninhydrin product. It was optically inactive and its ultraviolet absorption spectrum showed only end-absorption. Two acid groups with pK of 3.5 and 9.1 were determined by potentiometric titration. The substance in the acid form was found to decompose into formic acid and hydroxyaminoacetic acid. The antitumor agent was thus characterized as N-formyl hydroxyaminoacetic acid (I).

$$\mathrm{H{-}\overset{\overset{\displaystyle O}{\|}}{C}{-}\overset{\overset{\displaystyle OH}{|}}{N}{-}CH_2\,COOH}$$

(I)

Hydroxyaminoacetic acid in a mixture of formic acid acetic anhydride was converted to a compound indistinguishable from N-formyl hydroxyaminoacetic acid obtained from the broth of *Penicillium frequentans*. Because of its activity against H.Ad. #1, the trivial name of hadacidin was assigned to this new compound.

Hadacidin was also reported to be produced by the following species of *Penicillium: P. aurantio-violaceum, P. caseicolum, P. crustosum, P. implicatum, P. janthinellum, P. lividum, P. purpurescens, P. spinulosum, P. trzebinskii,* and *P. turbatum* (Dulaney and Gray, 1962).

Metabolic Effects of Hadacidin

An extensive study on the effect of hadacidin on the growth of human adenocarcinoma in the embryonated egg has been made by GITTERMAN *et al.* (1962). Fifty per cent inhibition (ID_{50}) was obtained at a dosage level of 3.3 mg per egg. In this system, hadacidin was found to be as active as azaserine and 6-mercaptopurine but about 100—200 times less active than an alkylating agent, triethylene melamine. The inhibitory effect of hadacidin on the growth of H.Ad. #1 was confirmed by MERKER *et al.* (1963) with tumors growing in cortisone-treated Swiss mice. Inhibition was obtained at a total daily intraperitoneal dosage of 6 g per kg/day administered for 7 days. The growth of Skiff's bronchogenic carcinoma, A-42 (GITTERMAN *et al.*, 1962) and sarcoma HS-1 (HARRIS *et al.*, 1962) were also found to be suppressed by hadacidin.

Carcinoma 1025, Ehrlich carcinoma, Harding-Passey melanoma, Jensen sarcoma and Walker carcinosarcoma 256 were only slightly inhibited, while sarcoma 180, mammary adenocarcinoma E-0771, Mecca lymphoma, Ridgeway osteogenic sarcoma, Lewis lung carcinoma, Friend virus leukemia, Crabb hamster sarcoma and Fortner pancereas adenocarcinoma were not inhibited by hadacidin (Personal Communication from K. Sugiura, quoted in ELLISON, 1963).

ELLISON (1963) performed preliminary clinical trials of hadacidin on 17 patients with various types of cancer. The material administered in single oral doses of 100 to 500 mg/kg daily caused leukocyte depression in 11 patients and platelet depression without leukocyte fall in one patient. Gastrointestinal tract abnormalities were observed in 6 cases. Though decreases in leukocyte count occurred regularly in chronic granulocytic leukemia, the trials were not sufficient to determine whether or not clinical benefit will result from the use of hadacidin. The effects of fractional doses given orally at 6-hour intervals on drug levels in serum and urine were studied recently (ELLISON, 1965).

An interesting reaction was observed by DIXON *et al.* (1965) when hadacidin was used in combination with ionizing irradiation. They noted that the lethal effects of irradiation on Ca 755, KB and HeLa cells were potentiated by hadacidin and the degree of potentiation was found to be related to the dose of both X-ray and hadacidin. Under similar conditions, however, no potentiation of the lethal effect of X-ray was seen with Sa-180 cells.

The first indication of the manner of action of hadacidin was obtained in studies *in vivo* with rats injected with ^{14}C-labeled precursors of nucleic acids (SHIGEURA and GORDON, 1962a). When hadacidin was administered intraperitoneally to a rat at a dosage of 2 g/kg rat, the incorporation after 4 hours of glycine-2-^{14}C into ribonucleic acid and deoxyribonucleic acid of spleen, thymus and intestinal mucosa was inhibited. An extensive study of this observation was carried out in experiments *in vitro* with Ehrlich ascites tumor cells. When hypoxanthine-8-^{14}C was incubated with whole ascites cells for 30 minutes at 37° in the presence of 1 mM hadacidin, the incorporation of the labeled substance into ribonucleic acid was suppressed by about 80%. Subsequent studies demonstrated that the uptake of ^{14}C-labeled glycine, formate and hypoxanthine into adenylic acid obtained from the perchloric acid-insoluble fraction was markedly inhibited whereas the incorporation of the same precursors into guanylic acid was not affected. These results indicated that the site of inhibition was between inosinic acid and perchloric acid-insoluble RNA. Studies with cell-free extracts of ascites cells showed that the conversion of hypoxanthine-8-^{14}C into adenylic acid was inhibited by hadacidin and this effect was partially reversed by the simultaneous addition of L-aspartic acid. The latter observation indicated that, in Ehrlich ascites cells, hadacidin antagonized the function of aspartic acid in the conversion of inosinate to adenylosuccinate catalyzed by adenylosuccinate synthetase (inosine-5'-phosphate: L-aspartate ligase). Evidence to support this view was obtained with the enzyme obtained from *Escherichia coli* B and these results are discussed below.

Another substance which is known to adversely affect the biosynthesis of adenine nucleotides in rats is ethionine (SHULL, 1962; VILLA-TREVINO, SHULL and FARBER, 1963). These workers showed that the inhibitory effect of ethionine was overcome by methionine, adenine, adenosine, adenosine nucleotides and inosine. SHULL and VILLA-TREVINO (1964) have now demonstrated that the reversing effect of inosine was nullified when hadacidin was simultaneously administered to the rat, also indicating that hadacidin prevented the conversion of inosine into adenosine nucleotides.

Hadacidin at 4 to 6 mM inhibited the growth of cultured KB cells by 50% (ID_{50}) and the effect was reversed by L-aspartate and adenine (NEUMAN and TYTELL, 1963). Pyruvate, α-ketobutyrate and oxalacetate were also found to antagonize the inhibitory effect of hadacidin. The reason for the latter effect, however, is not understood.

Hadacidin at a concentration of 0.7 mg/ml inhibited the growth of *Escherichia coli* B by about 50% and the inhibition was completely reversed by adenine or adenosine (SHIGEURA, 1963). In agreement with the data obtained in studies with mammalian cells, these results indicated that hadacidin interfered with the formation of adenine or adenine derivatives in this micro-organism.

As mentioned earlier, the locus of action of hadacidin in Ehrlich ascites cells appeared to be in the conversion of inosinic acid to adenylosuccinic acid in the pathway *de novo* of adenylic acid formation. In order to define further the site of inhibition by hadacidin, the enzyme adenylosuccinate synthetase (inosine-5'-phosphate: L-aspartate ligase) was prepared from logarithmically growing *E. coli* B. In the presence of equimolar amounts of hadacidin and L-aspartate, the conversion of inosinate to adenylosuccinate by adenylosuccinate synthetase was completely blocked (SHIGEURA and GORDON, 1962b). Furthermore, in the presence of a constant amount of hadacidin, the per cent inhibition was found to decrease with increasing amounts of L-aspartate. A quantitative appraisal of the competitive nature of inhibition by hadacidin was obtained by determining the reaction velocity as a function of varying L-aspartate concentration. The data when plotted according to the method of LINEWEAVER and BURK (1936), demonstrated that the inhibition of adenylosuccinate synthetase by hadacidin was competitively reversed by L-aspartate. From these graphs, the apparent K_m value at pH 8.0 for L-aspartate and K_i for hadacidin were found to be 1.5×10^{-4} M and 4.2×10^{-6} M, respectively. The ratio (K_m to K_i) of the constants, calculated to be 35, indicated that hadacidin was a relatively potent competitor of L-aspartate in this enzyme system.

The subsequent reaction, the conversion of adenylosuccinate to adenylic acid, catalyzed by adenylosuccinase was not affected by hadacidin.

The specificity of the biological action of hadacidin was shown by the fact that a similar type of reaction in purine biosynthesis in which L-aspartate also participated; namely, the amidation of 5-amino-4-imidazolecarboxylic acid ribonucleotide to 5-amino-4-imidazole-N-succinocarboxamide ribonucleotide was not inhibited by hadacidin. Furthermore, the activity of L-aspartate in pyrimidine biosynthesis was only weakly inhibited by hadacidin. Hadacidin showed no direct effect on the synthesis of proteins (SHIGEURA and GORDON, 1962c).

The effects of several compounds structurally similar to hadacidin (Table 1) were examined for possible inhibitory effects on adenylosuccinate synthetase from *E. coli* B (SHIGEURA, 1963b). Only N-formyl-α-hydroxyaminopropionate significantly inhibited the activity of the enzyme when the ratio of concentration of inhibitor to L-aspartate was 1:5. The results obtained when equimolar concentrations of L-aspartate and various test compounds were used are shown in Table 1. The percentage inhibition exerted by N-acetylhydroxyaminopropionate, N-acetylhydroxyaminoacetate, hydroxyaminoacetate, N-formylaminoacetate and N-formylhydroxyaminoacetamide was 90, 30, 23, 8 and 4%, respectively. The remaining compounds were inert. The inhibition by N-formyl-α-hydroxyaminopropionate was also competitively reversed by L-aspartate. The apparent K_i of N-formyl-α-hydroxyaminopropionate was found to be 8.7×10^{-6} M, indicating that hadacidin was about twice as potent as N-formyl-α-hydroxyaminopropionate in inhibiting the activity of adenylosuccinate synthetase.

Table 1. *Effects of analogues of hadacidin on the activity of adenylosuccinate synthetase*

Compound	% Inhibition
N-Formylhydroxyaminoacetamide	4
Sodium hydroxyaminoacetate	23
Sodium N-formylaminoacetate	8
Sodium N-acetylhydroxyaminoacetate	30
Sodium N-formyl-α-hydroxyaminopropionate	90
Sodium N-formyl-α-hydroxyaminobutyrate	0
Sodium N-formyl-α-hydroxyaminocaproate	0
Sodium N-formyl-l-hydroxyaminocyclopentane-l-carboxylate	0
Sodium N-formyl-α-hydroxyamino-β-phenylpropionate	0
Sodium N-formyl-β-hydroxyamino-β-phenylpropionate	0
Sodium-N-formyl-β-hydroxyamino-β-(o-chlorophenyl)-propionate	0
Sodium N-formyl-β-hydroxyamino-β-(p-nitrophenyl)-propionate	0
Sodium hadacidin	100

The effects of hadacidin when used in combination with various antitumor agents on the growth of *E. coli* B were also investigated (SHIGEURA and GORDON, 1962c). 2,6-Diaminopurine, azaserine, 5-fluorouracil, puromycin, psicofuranine, aminopterin and amethopterin potentiated the inhibitory activity of hadacidin. On the other hand, hadacidin antagonized the action of 6-mercaptopurine and 6-azauracil. The unusual effect on the micro-organism caused by the joint action of hadacidin and 6-azauracil was examined further (SHIGEURA, 1963a). The antagonistic effect of hadacidin on the inhibitory activity of 6-azauracil was partially reversed by adenine, adenosine, deoxyadenosine, inosine and L-aspartate. A number of other purines and pyrimidines were without effect. These results suggested that the mechanism of the process was in some manner related to the inhibition by hadacidin of purine biosynthesis *de novo*. This concept was supported by the observation that the inhibition caused by 6-azauracil alone was enhanced by exogenously added adenine. Furthermore, hadacidin did not antagonize the inhibitory effect of 6-azauridine on a 6-azauracil-resistant strain of *E. coli* B. It may be concluded that the inhibition due to hadacidin alone; namely, the suppression of formation of AMP or other adenine derivatives in some manner accounted for the reversal of 6-azauracil inhibition by hadacidin.

The antagonistic effect of hadacidin against 6-mercaptopurine is not understood. It is interesting to note that 6-mercaptopurine is converted to the 5'-monophosphate via GMP pyrophosphorylase; whereas, 2,6-diaminopurine (a compound potentiated by hadacidin) is phosphorylated via AMP pyrophosphorylase. Whether this observation is of significance remains to be investigated.

The unexpected potentiating and antagonistic effects of hadacidin on the metabolism of certain antitumor agents have raised some intriguing questions as to the interrelationship of these compounds with normal metabolites. Future studies along these lines may contribute to a better understanding of drug metabolism and thereby provide a more rational approach to chemotherapy.

PITTILLO *et al.* (1965) demonstrated that hadacidin potentiated the lethal effects of ionizing irradiation on proliferating cells of *E. coli* ATCC 9637, *E. coli* B (ORNYL), *Salmonella typhimurium* SR-11 and *Serratia marcescens* ATCC 274. It was also observed that two alkylating agent-resistant strains of *E. coli* were both sensitive to the radio-potentiating action of hadacidin.

GRAY *et al.* (1964) observed that hadacidin exerted a dwarfing effect on pea and bean plants. A foliage spray of the substance inhibited the growth of both stems and roots and delayed flowering of the plants. Chloroplast formation in nondividing, dark-grown Euglena cells was markedly inhibited by 2.5—15 mM hadacidin (MEGO, 1964). The extent of inhibition was proportional to the concentration of hadacidin in the medium and the inhibition was reversed by adenine and L-aspartate.

Summary

Hadacidin (N-formyl hydroxyaminoacetic acid) has been found to be synthesized by several species of penicillium and experiments *in vivo* and *in vitro* have shown that this relatively simple compound suppressed the growth of animal, bacterial and plant cells. Although direct evidence for its role as an antagonist of L-aspartic acid in the conversion of inosinic acid to adenylosuccinic acid has been obtained only with *E. coli* B cells, the primary site of action of hadacidin appears to be similar in animal and plant cells studied so far, that is, the inhibition by hadacidin of adenylic acid synthesis.

Certain other reactions in which aspartic acid also participated were either only weakly or not at all affected. The synthesis of carbamyl aspartate was apparently only mildly suppressed; whereas, the formation of 5-amino-4-imidazole-N-succinocarboxamide ribonucleotide was not affected. The utilization of aspartic acid in protein synthesis was not antagonized by hadacidin, possibly due to the inability of hadacidin to be activated by L-aspartate activating enzyme. The L-aspartate-α-ketoglutarate transamination reaction was also inert to the influence of the antibiotic.

References

DIXON, G. J., M. M. BLACKWELL, and F. M. SCHABEL: Hadacidin potentiation of lethal action of ionizing irradiation. I. Effect of mammalian tumor cells in culture. Proc. Soc. Exptl. Biol. Med. **118**, 521 (1965).

DULANEY, E. L., and R. A. GRAY: Penicillia that make N-formylhydroxyaminoacetic acid, a new fungal product. Mycologia **54**, 476 (1962).

ELLISON, R. R.: Preliminary clinical trials of hadacidin, a new tumor-inhibitory substance. Clinical Pharm. & Therap. **4**, 326 (1963).

ELLISON, R. R.: Clinical pharmacologic study of hadacidin (NSC-521778). Cancer Chemotherapy Reports **46**, 37 (1965).

GITTERMAN, C. O., E. L. DULANEY, E. A. KACZKA, D. HENDLIN, and H. B. WOODRUFF: The human tumor-egg host system. II. Discovery and properties of a new antitumor agent, hadacidin. Proc. Soc. Exptl. Biol. Med. **109**, 852 (1962).

GRAY, R. A., G. W. GAUGER, E. L. DULANEY, E. A. KACZKA, and H. B. WOODRUFF: Hadacidin, a new plant-growth inhibitor produced by fermentation. Plant Physiol. **39**, 204 (1964).

HARRIS, J. J., M. N. TELLER, E. YAP-GUEVARA, and G. W. WOOLLEY: Effects of hadacidin on human tumors grown in eggs and rats. Proc. Soc. Exptl. Biol. Med. **110**, 1 (1962).

KACZKA, E. A., C. O. GITTERMAN, E. L. DULANEY, and K. FOLKERS: Hadacidin, a new growth-inhibitory substance in human tumor systems. Biochem. **1**, 340 (1962).

LINEWEAVER, H., and D. BURK: The determination of enzyme dissociation constants. J. Am. Chem. Soc. **56**, 658 (1934).

MEGO, J. L.: The effect of hadacidin on chloroplast development in non-dividing euglena cells. Biochim. et Biophys. Acta **79**, 221 (1964).

MERKER, P. C., J. S. SARINO, R. ANIDO, M. BOWIE, and G. W. WOOLLEY: Effect of hadacidin on a transplantable human epidermoid carcinoma. In: J. E. SYLVESTER (ed.), Antimicrobial Agents and Chemotherapy, p. 749. Ann Arbor (Michigan): Braun-Brumfield, Inc. 1963.

NEUMAN, R. E., and A. A. TYTELL: Inhibitory effects of hadacidin on KB cell cultures. Proc. Soc. Exptl. Biol. Med. **112**, 57 (1963).

PITTILLO, R. F., and F. C. MONCRIEF: Hadacidin potentiation of lethal action of ionization irradiation. II. Effect of proliferating Gram-negative bacteria. Proc. Soc. Exptl. Biol. Med. **118**, 525 (1965).

SHIGEURA, H. T.: 6-Azauracil inhibition of *Escherichia coli* B and its reversal by hadacidin. Arch. Biochem. Biophys. **100**, 472 (1963a).

SHIGEURA, H. T.: Structural modifications of hadacidin and their effects on the activity of adenylosuccinate synthetase. J. Biol. Chem. **238**, 3999 (1963b).

SHIGEURA, H. T., and C. N. GORDON: Hadacidin, a new inhibitor of purine biosynthesis. J. Biol. Chem. **237**, 1932 (1962a).

SHIGEURA, H. T., and C. N. GORDON: The mechanism of action of hadacidin. J. Biol. Chem. **237**, 1937 (1962b).

SHIGEURA, H. T., and C. N. GORDON: Further studies on the activity of hadacidin. Cancer Research **22**, 1356 (1962c).

SHULL, K. H.: Hepatic phosphorylase and adenosine triphosphate levels in ethionine-treated rats, J. Biol. Chem. **237**, PC 1735 (1962).

SHULL, K. H., and S. VILLA-TREVINO: The effects of hadacidin and inosine on hepatic protein synthesis and adenosine triphosphate levels in ethionine-treated rats. Biochem. Biophys. Research. Commun. **16**, 101 (1964).

VILLA-TREVINO, S., K. H. SHULL, and E. FARBER: The role of adenosine triphosphate deficiency in ethionine-induced inhibition of protein synthesis. J. Biol. Chem. **238**, 1757 (1963).

Psicofuranine

Ladislav J. Hanka

Psicofuranine (Fig. 1) is an antibiotic which was first described by SCHROEDER and HOEKSEMA (1959) and EBLE *et al.* (1959). The compound closely resembles angustmycin C described by YÜNTSEN (1958). It is produced in fermentation by *Streptomyces hygroscopicus* var. *decoyicus*. The taxonomy and the fermentation conditions were reported by VAVRA *et al.* (1959); *in vivo* antibacterial activity was studied by LEWIS *et al.* (1959). It protected mice from experimental infections with *Streptococcus haemolyticus*, *Staphylococcus aureus*, and *Escherichia coli* when administered orally or subcutaneously. However, psicofuranine showed essentially no

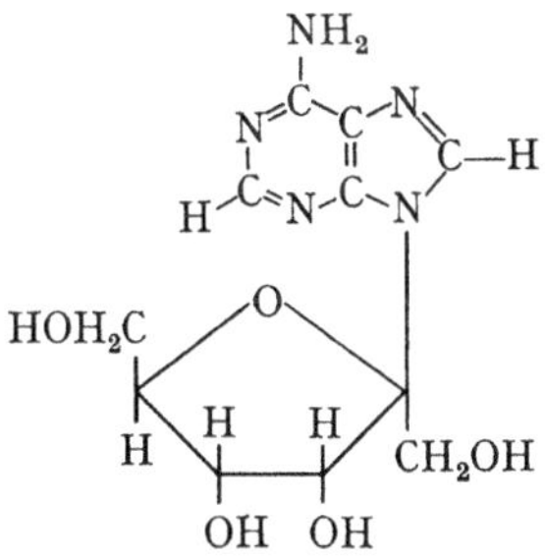

Fig. 1. Structure of psicofuranine (6-amino-9-D-psicofuranosylpurine)

in vitro activity against the same microorganism when tested on conventional media. *In vitro* activity was demonstrated using special media and assay techniques described by HANKA *et al.* (1959, 1960). A method for chemical determination of psicofuranine in blood plasma and serum was reported by FORIST *et al.* (1959). Psicofuranine was not inhibitory to the KB cells in tissue culture. Pharmacologic studies including the absorption and excretion of psicofuranine in the dog were done by WALLACH and THOMAS (1959), who reported that psicofuranine was absorbed following oral and intramuscular administration. Most of the drug was excreted through the kidney; biliary excretion was negligible. Free psicofuranine was absorbed in animals but not in man. In the form of psicofuranine tetraacetate it was absorbed in man, however.

EVANS and GRAY (1959) reported that orally administered psicofuranine allowed an increase in the number of survivors and caused tumor regressions in rats bearing Walker adenocarcinoma, Murphy-Sturm lymphosarcoma, Jensen sarcoma, or Guerin tumor. Psicofuranine was, however, inactive in tumor-bearing mice. Those authors reported a low order toxicity of psicofuranine both in mice and rats. The toxicity of psicofuranine was, however, of considerable importance in man. A significant number of cancer patients treated with psicofuranine or psicofuranine tetraacetate developed pericarditis in the studies done by Costa *et al.* (1961), Yates and Olson (1961), and Talley and Carlson (1963). It is interesting that Talley and Carlson (1963) did not find any such toxic manifestations in rat, dog, monkey (*Cebus apella*), or chicken. This certainly makes psicofuranine a rather unique drug and might well be directly related to its peculiar mode of action.

Magee and Eberts (1961) reported that psicofuranine caused a marked regression of Walker 256 adenocarcinoma in rats and caused a distinct drop in utilization of phosphate-P^{32} uptake by the tumors.

The mechanism of action of psicofuranine was first studied by Hanka (1960) using the technique of quantitative reversal of antimicrobial action against *Staphylococcus aureus*. In a semi-synthetic medium (Hanka and Burch, 1960), he was able to reverse the antimicrobial activity of psicofuranine by several compounds containing purine bases. The most effective reversing agents were guanine and guanosine and the reversal was noncompetitive (Table 1). Once the concentration of guanine in the medium reached 5 µg/ml, even a psicofuranine concentration of 1000 µg/ml did not cause inhibition in agar or liquid media.

Table 1. *Zones of inhibition (mm) of S. aureus by psicofuranine in the presence of guanine or guanosine in the growth media* (Hanka, 1960)

Compound Tested	Conc. (µg/ml)	Concentration of psicofuranine (µg/ml)				
		10	20	40	80	160
Control	—	15.5	18	21	24	27
Guanine	2.5	0	0	trace	21	24.5
	5.0	0	0	0	0	0
Guanosine	2.5	trace	16	18	21	24.5
	5.0	0	0	0	0	19

Hanka also found that the inhibition of *S. aureus* by psicofuranine can be partially overcome by addition of adenosine or inosine in the growth media. Both those compounds were considerably less effective than guanine, however. This obviously indicates that psicofuranine is not directly involved in the biosynthesis of any one of these two compounds. Xanthosine has shown little effect and the addition of pyrimidine-base nucleosides did not help the microorganism to overcome the effect of psicofuranine.

Hanka interpreted this evidence in the light of current concepts of purine synthesis as presented in Schema 1 (Magasanik *et al.*, 1957; Mager and Magasanik, 1958; Carter and Cohen, 1956; Lagerkvist, 1958; Moyed and Magasanik, 1957) and concluded that the main effect of psicofuranine in *S. aureus* was interference with biosynthesis of guanosine-5′-phosphate from xanthosine-5′-phosphate. This interpretation was later verified by the investigations of Slechta (1960a, 1960b), and Udaka and Moyed (1963).

Slechta (1960a, 1960b) studied the mechanism of psicofuranine action with *Escherichia coli* B. In his first investigation, Slechta (1960a) demonstrated that the effect of psicofuranine was bacteriostatic and the cells would grow even at high concentrations of the drug after an extended lag phase. He studied the capacity of the common purine and pyrimidine compounds to reverse the inhibition of *E. coli* by psicofuranine. The results of this study are summarized in Table 2. It can be seen that guanine-containing compounds were by far the most effective reversing agents. This is in agreement with the results found by HANKA (1960) with *S. aureus*. In the same investigation SLECHTA found that, in the presence of psicofuranine and growing cells of *E. coli*, xanthosine accumulated in the growth medium. He also reported that the incorporation of C^{14}-labeled glycine into purine bases was markedly changed in the presence of psicofuranine. These findings led SLECHTA to conclude that the principal effect of psicofuranine in *E. coli* is the interference with the bioconversion of xanthosine-5′-phosphate to guanosine-5′-phosphate.

Schema 1 (HANKA, 1960)

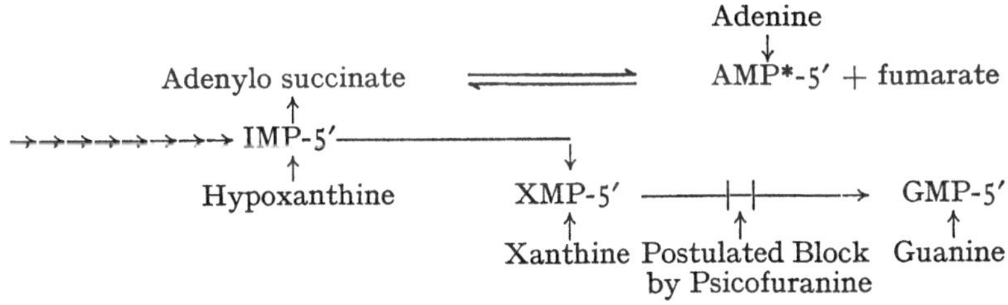

* The abbreviations used throughout this chapter are: AMP, adenosine monophosphate; GMP, guanosine monophosphate; IMP, inosine monophosphate; XMP, xanthosine monophosphate; and PP, pyrophosphate.

In his second investigation (1960b) he worked with cell-free extracts of *E. coli* and demonstrated that xanthosine-5′-phosphate aminase activity was inhibited by psicofuranine (Fig. 2). These findings were supported by the fact that in the intact *E. coli* the conversion of C^{14}-labeled xanthosine-5′-phosphate to guanosine-5′-phosphate was inhibited by psicofuranine.

Table 2. *Prevention of the inhibitory action of psicofuranine (100 μg/ml) on the growth of E. coli B by purines and pyrimidines present in the medium* (SLECHTA, 1960a) (The growth was measured after 8 hours)

Reversing compound (10 μg/ml)	Growth in % of the Control	Reversing compound (10 μg/ml)	Growth in % of the Control
Adenine	14.5	Adenosine-5′-phosphate	6
Guanine	102	Guanosine-5′-phosphate	102
Hypoxanthine	2	Cytidine-5′-phosphate	2
Xanthine	4	Uridine-5′-phosphate	2
Cytosine	4	Deoxyadenosine	4
Uracil	2	Deoxyguanosine	75
Thymine	4	Deoxycytidine	4
Adenosine	4	Thymidine	2
Guanosine	100	Deoxyadenosine-5′-phosphate	4
Inosine	4	Deoxyguanosine-5′-phosphate	62.5
Xanthosine	4	Deoxycytidine-5′-phosphate	4
Cytidine	1	Thymidine-5′-phosphate	2
Uridine	1	No additions	2

MOYED (1961) studied the effect of psicofuranine against *E. coli* on the enzymatic level. He offered a plausible explanation for the bacteriostatic effect of psicofuranine. He showed that the production of both IMP dehydrogenase and XMP aminase are controlled by the levels of GMP through a feedback control mechanism. He postulated that the inhibition of XMP aminase by psicofuranine causes a reduction of growth rate by reducing the supply of GMP. However, with the increasing depletion of GMP, the formation of XMP aminase will start to increase quickly due to the derepression and the growth of the organism will be resumed regardless of the presence of psicofuranine.

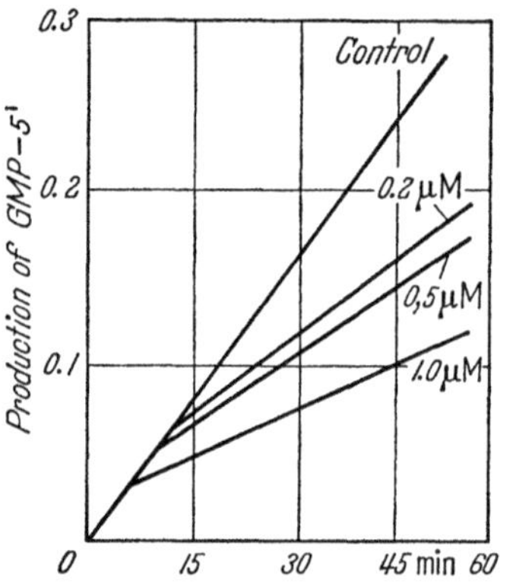

Fig. 2. Inhibition of xanthosine-5'-phosphate aminase by psicofuranine (SLECHTA, 1960b) (amounts of the drug [in μM] are given in the Figure)

UDAKA and MOYED (1963) conducted an extensive study on the inhibition of XMP aminase by psicofuranine in the wild type of *E. coli* B and in psicofuranine resistant mutants of this organism. They found that the level of XMP aminase in some resistant strains (type B-24) was about six times higher than in the parent organism when both strains were grown without an exogenous supply of guanine (Table 3). However, they also found resistant mutants (type B-35) with greatly reduced XMP aminase activity. Yet those mutants did not manifest guanine deficiency. The formation of both IMP dehydrogenase and XMP aminase in both types of mutants was susceptible to repression by guanosine. The authors further established that the XMP aminases of sensitive and resistant strains of *E. coli* are substantially more inhibited by psicofuranine in the presence of pyrophosphate, which is one of the products of the XMP amination. The authors concluded that the inhibition by psicofuranine is at least a two step process consisting of: 1. a reversible, pyrophosphate-dependent reaction between the drug and the aminase; and 2. an irreversible reaction, requiring xanthosine-5'-phosphate. In the psicofuranine-

Table 3. *Enzymes of GMP synthesis in extracts of psicofuranine-sensitive and -resistant organisms* (UDAKA and MOYED, 1963)

Experiment	Strain	Addition to growth medium	Specific Activity $\times 10^{-6}$	
			IMP Dehydrogenase	XMP Aminase
1	B		3.6	4.3
	B	Guanosine, 100 mcg/ml	1.2	2.2
	B-24		1.0	26.1
	B-24	Guanosine, 100 mcg/ml	0.2	3.6
2	B		2.7	5.3
	B	Guanosine, 50 mcg/ml	1.9	3.2
	B-35		3.1	0.6
	B-35	Guanosine, 50 mcg/ml	1.9	

resistant mutant the aminase is apparently unable to undergo the second, irreversible reaction. The study of the kinetic constants of the enzymatic reaction indicated that psicofuranine acts as a noncompetitive inhibitor.

FUKUYAMA and MOYED (1964) reported that the binding of psicofuranine by the xanthosine-5'-phosphate aminase was strongly stimulated by a substrate, xanthosine-5'-phosphate, and by one of the products of the reaction, inorganic pyrophosphate.

$$XMP + ATP + NH_3 \xrightarrow{Mg^{++}} GMP + AMP + PPi$$

The inhibited reaction mixture contained equimolar amounts of xanthosine-5'-phosphate, pyrophosphate and psicofuranine. Increasing the concentrations of ATP and NH_3 in the reaction mixture reduced the inhibitory effect of psicofuranine without affecting its binding to the enzyme. The authors showed again that the primary interaction between psicofuranine and the enzyme is a noncompetitive process. From the lack of competition for binding sites on the enzyme between psicofuranine and xanthosine-5'-phosphate, they concluded that the enzyme apparently had a specific site for the binding of psicofuranine. The existence of such a specific site raised the possibility of desensitizing the enzyme to psicofuranine without changing its other functions. KURAMITSU and MOYED (1964) studied the effect of three protein-modifying agents on xanthosine-5'-phosphate aminase obtained either from a parent strain of *Escherichia coli* or from its mutant partially resistant to psicofuranine. They found that urea, mercaptoethanol and ethylene glycol were able to desensitize the enzyme. The enzyme from the parent strain was less readily desensitized than that from the mutant. This desensitization was usually accompanied by a partial loss of its enzymatic activity. Both the desensitization and the enzyme inactivation were reversible. The authors suggest that the psicofuranine binding site on the enzyme is distinct from the substrate binding site but the distinction between the psicofuranine site and the substrate sites on the enzyme was not quite complete.

In their most recent study KURAMITSU and MOYED (1966) investigated the possibility of altering the enzyme selectively in such a way that its catalytic properties and its sensitivity to inhibition by psicofuranine would be affected differently. If such a selective alteration of the enzyme could be demonstrated, it would constitute an additional evidence for the existence of a distinct psicofuranine binding site on the enzyme. Using three distinctly different agents in their study (urea, 2-mercaptoethanol and methylene blue), the authors found that such a selective alteration of xanthosine-5'-phosphate aminase was indeed possible. They concluded that psicofuranine increased the availability of sulfhydryl groups of the enzyme for reaction with sulfhydryl reagents. The authors suggested that the psicofuranine binding site is not an essential part of the active center of the aminase. Nevertheless, they felt that the drug may be influencing the active center of the enzyme by distorting its tertiary structure.

Summary

Psicofuranine is an antibiotic whose principal effect in bacteria is the inhibition of xanthosine-5'-phosphate aminase. The inhibition of bacteria by psicofuranine can be most effectively prevented by several guanine-containing compounds.

The primary interaction between the xanthosine-5′-phosphate aminase and psicofuranine is noncompetitive and readily reversible. The binding of psicofuranine by the enzyme was strongly stimulated by xanthosine-5′-phosphate and by pyrophosphate. The enzyme can be selectively desensitized to psicofuranine without altering its catalytic properties. It appears that the enzyme has a specific site for binding of psicofuranine.

Acknowledgments. The author wishes to acknowledge the kind cooperation of the following publishers in granting us the permission to reprint materials from previous publications:

1. American Society for Microbiology as the editor of the Journal of Bacteriology (printed by Williams and Wilkins Co., Baltimore 2, Maryland). Table 1 and Schema 1. Reference: HANKA (1960).
2. Pergamon Press, Inc., Long Island City, New York as the editor of Biochemical Pharmacology. Table 2. Reference: SLECHTA (1960a).
3. Academic Press, Inc., New York, New York as the editor of Biochemical and Biophysical Research Communications. Fig. 2. Reference: SLECHTA (1960b).
4. The American Society of Biological Chemists, Inc. as the publisher of The Journal of Biological Chemistry. Table 3. Reference: UDAKA and MOYED (1963).

References

CARTER, C. E., and L. J. COHEN: The preparation and properties of adenylosuccinase and adenylosuccinic acid. J. Biol. Chem. **222**, 17—30 (1956).

COSTA, G., J. F. HOLLAND, and J. W. PICKREN: Acute pericarditis produced by psicofuranine, a nucleoside analogue. New Engl. J. Med. **265**, 1143—1146 (1961).

EBLE, T. E., H. HOEKSEMA, G. A. BOYACK, and G. M. SAVAGE: Psicofuranine. I. Discovery, isolation, and properties. Antibiotics & Chemotherapy **9**, 419—420 (1959).

EVANS, J. A., and J. E. GRAY: Psicofuranine. VI. Antitumor and toxicopathological studies. Antibiotics & Chemotherapy **9**, 675—684 (1959).

FORIST, A. A., S. THEAL, and H. HOEKSEMA: Psicofuranine. VII. Chemical determination in plasma and serum. Antibiotics & Chemotherapy **9**, 685—689 (1959).

FUKUYAMA, T. T., and H. S. MOYED: A separate antibiotic-binding site in xanthosine-5′-phosphate aminase: Inhibitor- and substrate-binding studies. Biochemistry **3**, 1488—1492 (1964).

HANKA, L. J.: Mechanism of action of psicofuranine. J. Bacteriol. **80**, 30—36 (1960).

HANKA, L. J., and M. R. BURCH: Improved assay for psicofuranine. Antibiotics & Chemotherapy **10**, 484—487 (1960).

HANKA, L. D., M. R. BURCH, and W. T. SOKOLSKI: Psicofuranine. IV. Microbiological assay. Antibiotics & Chemotherapy **9**, 432—435 (1959).

KURAMITSU, H., and H. S. MOYED: Desensitization of guanosine-5′-phosphate synthetase to inhibition by an antibiotic. Biochem. et Biophys. Acta **85**, 504—506 (1964).

KURAMITSU, H., and H. S. MOYED: To be published in J. Biol. Chem. Personal communication by H. S. MOYED. 1966.

LAGERKVIST, U.: Biosynthesis of guanosine-5′-phosphate. I. Xanthosine-5′-phosphate as an intermediate. J. Biol. Chem. **233**, 138—142 (1958a).

LAGERKVIST, U.: Biosynthesis of guanosine-5′-phosphate. II. Amination of xanthosine-5′-phosphate by purified enzyme from pigeon liver. J. Biol. Chem. **233**, 143—149 (1958b).

LEWIS, C. N., H. R. REAMES, and L. E. RHULAND: Psicofuranine. II. Studies in experimental animal infections. Antibiotics & Chemotherapy **9**, 421—426 (1959).

MAGASANIK, B., H. S. MOYED, and L. B. GEHRING: Enzymes essential for the biosynthesis of nucleic acid guanine; inosine-5′-phosphate dehydrogenase of *Aerobacter aerogenes*. J. Biol. Chem. **226**, 339—350 (1957).

MAGEE, W. F., and F. S. EBERTS: Studies with psicofuranine in the tumor-bearing rat. Cancer Research **21**, 611—619 (1961).

MAGER, J., and B. MAGASANIK: Conversion of guanosine-5'-phosphate (G 5' P) to inosine-5'-phosphate (I 5' P) as part of the biosynthetic cycle. Federation Proc. **17**, 267 (1958).

MOYED, H. S.: Interference with feedback control of enzyme activity. Cold Spring Harbor Symposia Quant. Biol. **26**, 323—329 (1961).

MOYED, H. S., and B. MAGASANIK: Enzymes essential for the biosynthesis of nucleic acid guanosine; xanthosine-5'-phosphate aminase of *Aerobacter aerogenes*. J. Biol. Chem. **226**, 351—363 (1957).

SCHROEDER, W., and H. HOEKSEMA: A new antibiotic, 6-amino-9-d-psicofuranosylpurine. J. Am. Chem. Soc. **81**, 1767 (1959).

SLECHTA, L.: Studies on the mode of action of psicofuranine. Biochem. Pharmacol. **5**, 96—107 (1960a).

SLECHTA, L.: Inhibition of xanthosine-5'-phosphate aminase by psicofuranine. Biochem. Biophys. Research Commun. **3**, 596—598 (1960b).

TALLEY, R. W., and R. G. CARLSON: Polyserositis induced by psicofuranine in man and comparative toxicity in the rat, mouse, dog, chicken, and monkey. Toxicol. Appl. Pharmacol. **5**, 235—246 (1963).

UDAKA, S., and H. S. MOYED: Inhibition of parental and mutant xanthosine-5'-phosphate aminases by psicofuranine. J. Biol. Chem. **238**, 2797—2803 (1963).

VAVRA, J. J., A. DIETZ, B. W. CHURCHILL, P. SIMINOFF, and H. J. KOEPSELL: Psicofuranine. III. Production and biological studies. Antibiotic & Chemotherapy **9**, 427—431 (1959).

WALLACH, D. P., and R. C. THOMAS: Psicofuranine. VIII. Some pharmacological observations. Antibiotics & Chemotherapy **9**, 722—729 (1959).

YATES, R. C., and K. B. OLSON: Drug induced pericarditis. New Eng. J. Med. **265**, 274—277 (1961).

YÜNTSEN, H.: Studies in Angustmycins. VIII. The structure of Angustmycin C. J. Antibiotics (Japan), Ser. A **11**, 244—249 (1958).

Angustmycin A

Armand J. Guarino

Angustmycin A[1] is a nucleoside produced by *Streptomyces hygroscopius*, and its isolation from this organism has usually been found to be associated with angustmycin C (psicofuranine). Angustmycin A was originally identified as 6-amino-9-(L-1,2-fucopyranoseenyl)-purine by YÜNTSEN *et al.* (1958).

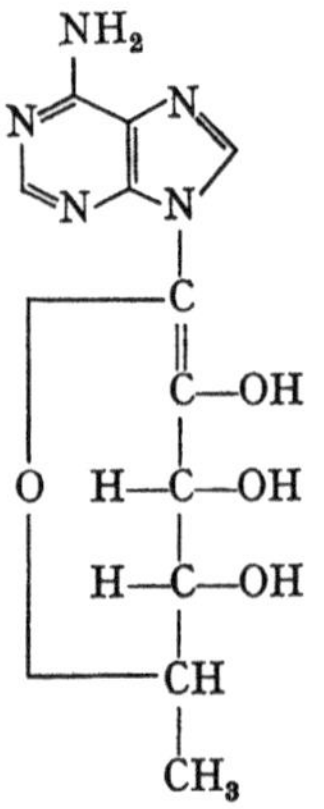

Angustmycin A according to YÜNTSEN *et al.*

More recently HOCKSEMA *et al.* (1964) in studies involving the structure of decoyinine isolated from *Streptomyces*, established that angustmycin A and decoyinine were the same compound. From nuclear magnetic resonance stud, ies on this compound and its derivatives, periodate oxidations, hydrolysis- and fermentation data, they concluded that the structure for angustmycin A and decoyinine is that indicated below.

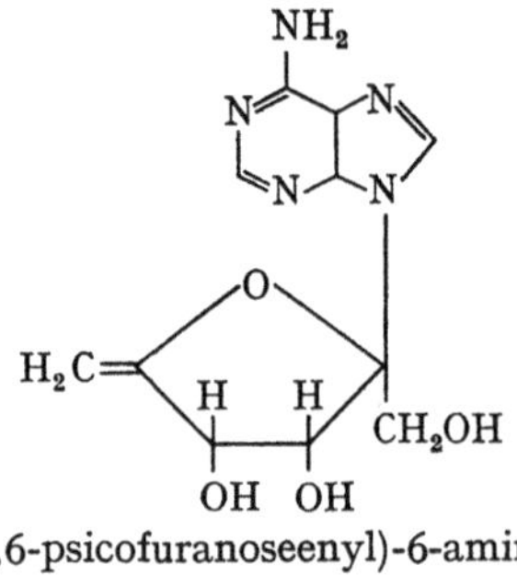

9-B-D-(5,6-psicofuranoseenyl)-6-amino purine

[1] Decoyinine is a synonym for angustmycin A.

It should be noted that this is a nucleoside of adenine containing an unsaturated hexose substituted for deoxyribose or ribose which are the more common sugars associated with nucleosides. The striking similarity between its structure and that of psicofuranine should also be noted. In fact, the addition of a water molecule across the double bond of decoyinine may yield psicofuranine. Whether this compound originates from psicofuranine in this organism by a dehydrase type of reaction or whether psicofuranine originates by hydration of decoyinine is not known at the present time. The details of biosynthesis of psicofuranine are described in Volume II.

For purposes of discussion in this section, the structure proposed by HOCKSEMA *et al.* (1964) is accepted as the correct one. Angustmycin A and decoyinine are undoubtedly the same coumpound, and will be used interchangeably throughout this section.

The first reports of the antibiotic properties of angustmycin A were reported by YÜNTSEN (1954), and as mentioned earlier, this nucleoside along with angustmycin C was obtained from broth filtrates of *S. hygroscopicus* var. angustmyceticus. In these studies, angustmycin A was reported to have antimicrobial activity exclusively against mycobacteria (YÜNTSEN *et al.*, 1956). Although it exerted antibiotic activity in synthetic media, its activity decreased in organic media. This has the implication that certain antagonists to this compound are present in the organic media. TANAKA *et al.* (1959) investigated the effects of various vitamins and nucleic acid derivatives with regard to their ability to overcome inhibition caused by angustmycins. The gram positive organisms examined were sensitive to angustmycin A in concentrations of 10—200 mcg/ml, but gram-negative organisms were more resistant. When assayed for their ability to overcome angustmycin A inhibited *Bacillus subtilis* and Mycobacterium 607 growth, only guanine or its nucleoside had the ability to reverse the inhibition by the method employed. Other compounds tested in this study were thiamine, nicotinamide, pyridoxine, pantothenic acid, biotin, folic acid, adenine, uracil, and thymine. The nucleosides of guanine and adenine were also able to reverse the inhibiting action of angustmycin A, but guanine as its nucleoside was much more potent in its ability to reverse inhibition than adenosine.

TANAKA *et al.* (1961 a) continued studies in which the activity of this compound, along with a variety of other antibiotics, was tested for its potency on antibiotic resistant, coagulase-positive staphylococci. Both laboratory as well as clinical resistant strains were used. Of some 20 resistant strains tested, variously resistant to penicillin, streptomycin, tetracycline, chloramphenical, and erythromycin, angustmycin A showed some activity against these organisms, but was not as effective as angustmycin C (psicofuranine). TANAKA *et al.* (1961 b) published a procedure for a differential assay for angustmycin A and C.

In addition to the bacterial studies carried out decribed above, TANAKA *et al.* (1961 c) studied the activity of angustmycin against experimental infections and tumors in animals. Both angustmycin C and A exhibited considerable effects against staphylococcal and streptococcal infections in mice, although angustmycin C was more effective than A. Both compounds exhibited considerable activity against Walker adenocarcinoma 256 in rats, and much less activity against adenocarcinoma 755, Ehrlich carcinoma, and sarcoma 180 of solid forms in mice. In the technique used, no inhibition of tumor growth *in vivo* was observed with ascitic tumors including Yoshida sarcoma, Ehrlich carcinoma and sarcoma 180.

TANAKA (1963) published evidence, in keeping with his earlier observations, that the angustmycins may inhibit the process of biosynthesis of guanosine monophosphate from xanthosine monophosphate. This metabolic transformation is certainly involved in explaining the mode of action of angustmycin C (psicofuranine) which is reviewed in another section. Similar to what had been found for angustmycin C, angustmycin A inhibited cultures of *B. subtilis* were found to contain xanthosine. So in this respect the mode of action of this compound appears to be quite similar to that of psicofuranine, namely it inhibits the amination of xanthosine-5'-phosphate (XMP) to form guanosine-5'-phosphate (GMP). As was pointed out above, because of the close similarity of structure of these two compounds, it is conceivable that only one of the compounds is the metabolically active one and that the inhibiting action of one of these in a given organism could in large measure be due to its conversion to the other.

HOCKSEMA *et al.* (1964) presented preliminary evidence indicating that decoyinine may be converted to psicofuranine, while SUHADOLNIK (unpublished, personal communication) has data to indicate that psicofuranine may be converted to decoyinine, but in each study it was not indicated which compound is more metabolically active.

BLOCH and NICHOL (1964a) found that decoyinine decreased the growth of *S. faecalis* by 50% at 5×10^{-6} M in a purine and pyrimidine-free medium. Of a number of compounds tested, guanine and guanosine were most effective in reversing this inhibition and did so competitively. Adenosine and adenine, although they had some ability to reverse the inhibiting effect of decoyinine were much less effective, while xanthine, xanthosine, and hypoxanthine were without effect. This competitive action of guanine and its nucleosides suggest again the selective impairment of guanine metabolism by this analog and is in agreement with the earlier work cited above by TANAKA *et al.* (1959) for angustmycin A.

As an extension of this work, BLOCH and NICHOL (1964b) studied the effect of decoyinine on ribose phosphate pyrophosphokinase activity. In cell-free extracts of *S. faecalis* no phosphorolysis of decoyinine occurred. Decoyinine was found to inhibit the conversion of XMP to GMP in cell-free extracts of this organism in a manner analogous to that described for psicofuranine. When they incubated a cell-free extract of this organism with ribose-5-phosphate, ATP, and radioactive guanine, then GMP, GDP, and GTP were formed and demonstrated chromatographically. When decoyinine was added to such a mixture, guanine nucleotide formation was inhibited. If 5-phosphoribosyl pyrophosphate (PRPP) was added to a cell-free preparation instead of ATP and ribose-5-phosphate in the presence of guanine, GMP alone was formed. When decoyinine was added to this preparation, the formation of GMP was not inhibited. Nucleoside kinase activity was not detectable in these preparations, nor was there any evidence that decoyinine was converted to its nucleotides. This makes it rather unlikely that the conversion of the guanine to the nucleotides occurred by either a nucleoside phosphorylase or kinase pathway. These studies imply that decoyinine exerts its inhibiting effect on this enzyme system in the synthesis of PRPP from ATP and ribose-5-phosphate.

It has also been pointed out that decoyinine exerts an inhibiting effect on the conversion of XMP to GMP, a conversion which also requires ATP. The authors suggest that decoyinine may act by occupying the ATP-site in reactions involving pyrophosphate cleavage from ATP. In fact, they postulate the same mechanism for an explanation of psicofuranine inhibition.

In contrast to the work described for cordycepin it seems that decoyinine functions as an antagonist without prior conversion to its nucleotide. The similarity of its structure to psicofuranine, and preliminary evidence for the possible interconversion of these compounds do not allow us to state at the present time whether one species is more active than the other, or whether they are both active without being interconverted. In any event they appear to have a striking similarity in their possible modes of action.

References

BLOCH, A., and C. A. NICHOL: Studies on decoyinine. A nucleoside analog. Federation Proc. **23**, 324 (1964a).

BLOCH, A., and C. A. NICHOL: Inhibition of ribosephosphate pyrophosphokinase activity by decoyinine, an adenine nucleoside. Biochim. Biophys. Research Commun. **16**, 400 (1964b).

HOCKSEMA, H., G. SLOMP, and E. E. VAN TAMELEN: Angustmycin A and decoyinine. Tetrahedron Letters **1964** (27—28), 1787.

TANAKA, N.: Mechanism of action of angustmycins, nucleoside antibiotics. J. Antibiotics (Japan), Ser. A **16**, 163 (1963).

TANAKA, N., N. MIYAIRI, and H. UMEZAWA: Studies on antagonists to angustmycins. J. Antibiotics (Japan), Ser. A. **13**, 265 (1959).

TANAKA, N., N. MIYAIRI, T. NISHIMURA, and H. UMEZAWA: Activity of mikamycins, angustmycins and emimycin against antibiotic-resistant Staphylococci. J. Antibiotics (Japan), Ser. A **14**, 18 (1961a).

TANAKA, N., N. MIYAIRI, and H. UMEZAWA: Differential bioassay of angustmycins A and C. J. Antibiotics (Japan), Ser. A **14**, 23 (1961b).

TANAKA, N., T. NISHIMURA, H. YAMAGUCHI, and H. UMEZAWA: Activity of angustmycins against experimental infections and transplantable tumors. J. Antibiotics (Japan), Ser. A **14**, 98 (1961c).

YÜNTSEN, H., K. OHKUMA, Y. ISHII, and H. YONEHARA: Studies on angustmycin. III. J. Antibiotics (Japan), Ser. A **9**, 195 (1956).

YÜNTSEN, H.: Studies on angustmycins. VII. The structure of angustmycin A. J. Antibiotics (Japan), Ser. A **11**, 233 (1958).

YÜNTSEN, H., H. YONEHARA, and H. UI: Studies on a new antibiotic, angustmycin. I. J. Antibiotics (Japan), Ser. A **7**, 113 (1954).

Cordycepin

Armand J. Guarino

The early work of CUNNINGHAM *et al.* (1951) described the isolation of cordycepin from the culture broth of *Cordyceps militaris* (Linn) LINK. and for approximately ten years this organism provided the chief source of cordycepin for the studies to be reported below. More recently FREDERIKSEN *et al.* (1965) reported on its isolation from another strain of the same organism [*Cordyceps militaris* (L. Ex. Fr.) LINK.] and KACZKA *et al.* (1964a) reported on the isolation and identification of this compound from cultures of *Aspergillus nidulans* (EIDAM) WINT. To date, these appear to be the only organisms from which the nucleoside has been identified. Several routes for the chemical synthesis of this compound have been reported by TODD and ULBRICHT (1960), LEE *et al.* (1961) and WALTON *et al.* (1964).

It should be mentioned at the outset of this discussion the structure originally proposed by BENTLEY *et al.* (1951) was that of a nucleoside containing adenine and a branched chain 3-deoxypentose. This structure (I) is indicated below. Many of the studies to be discussed regarding the mechanism of action of cordycepin have been reported, assuming the structure proposed by BENTLEY *et al.* (1951). More recently KACZKA *et al.* (1964b) showed by IR and NMR spectroscopy that the active metabolite derived from *A. nidulans*, synthetic 3'-deoxyadenosine, and two samples of cordycepin obtained from different sources, were identical.

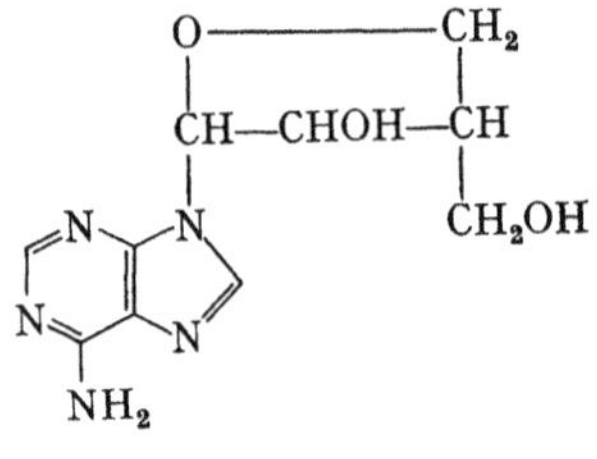

(I)

(I) Structure of cordycepin as proposed by BENTLEY *et al.*

FREDERIKSEN *et al.* (1965) have also obtained spectral and enzymatic evidence that the compound isolated from *Cordyceps militaris* (L. Ex. Fr.) LINK. is also 3'-deoxyadenosine. Indirect evidence for the identity of cordycepin and 3'-deoxyadenosine has come from the work of SUHADOLNIK and CORY (1964) who reported on the isolation of formaldehyde following periodate oxidation of the phenylhydrazide of cordyceponolactone. Periodate oxidation of this compound should not give formaldehyde if cordycepin had the structure originally proposed by

BENTLEY *et al.* (1951). Unpublished work of GUARINO and PRAJSNAR (1964) has demonstrated the formation of malonaldehyde as an intermediate in the complete oxidation of the sugar derived from cordycepin and the ultimate consumption of five mols of periodate per mol of sugar oxidized. Not only are these results in contrast to those expected for the originally proposed structure, but indeed support the conclusion that cordycepin is identical to 3'-deoxyadenosine. It is important to recognize that all studies to date regarding the antitumor or antibiotic activity of cordycepin and 3'-deoxyadenosine are indeed with the same compound. The structure we shall accept for the rest of the chapter is that of 3'-deoxyadenosine [II].

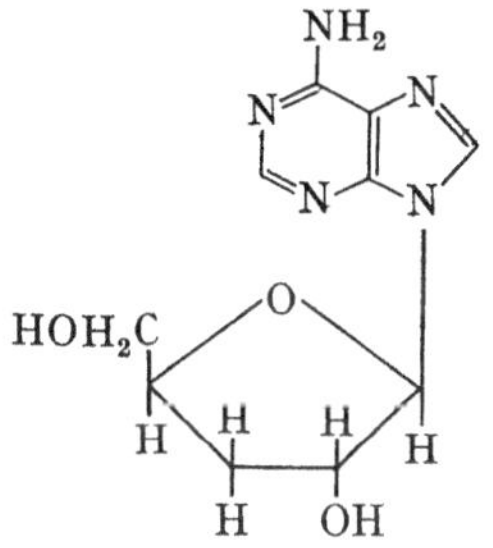

(II)

(II) 3'-deoxyadenosine (Cordycepin)

That *Cordyceps militaris* might produce an antibiotic was deduced from the observation that the residue of host tissue on which this organism grew in its normal habitat was resistant to decay. In the report of CUNNINGHAM *et al.* (1951) cordycepin in aqueous solutions at concentrations of 10 μg/ml to 100 μg/ml was found to inhibit the growth of *Bacillus subtilis*, strain 6752 N.C.T.C. in bouillion broth. Of 45 strains of this organism tested, 43 were inhibited in bouillion broth to varying degrees by cordycepin at a concentration of 1.0 mg/ml. They also reported that it inhibited the growth of the avian-tubercle bacillus at a concentration of 0.1 mg/ml in Youman's medium while with Dubos-Tween-albumin medium it inhibits a bovine-type tubercle bacillus at a dilution of 1:60,000. In this study it was reported that cordycepin did not inhibit the development of *Staphylococcus aureus Oxf.* H., *Sarcina lutea, Escherichia coli, B. welchii, Streptococcus haemolyticus, Strep. faecalis, Shigella flexneri,* or *Pasteurella septica.*

With the exception of the detailed work to be reported below on the possible mechanism of action of this compound on the growth of *B. subtilis*, little else has been done in intact bacterial systems. However, considerable work has been carried out with mammalian systems including the Ehrlich mouse ascites tumor cell, KB cells in tissue culture, H. Ep. No. 1 human tumor cells in tissue culture, chick fibroblasts in tissue culture, as well as studies in cell-free systems derived from these cells or bacterial cells.

First, some generalizations might be made regarding the mechanism of action of this compound before citing specific work that tends to support these generalizations. One may well ask the question regarding the mechanism of action of such a compound whether the compound itself is the active "culprit" as administered, or does the organism convert it to a more active form. For cordycepin, it would appear to be the latter. As indicated in its structure, cordycepin is a nucleoside but in the work reviewed to date there seems to be little indication that in this form it is capable of exerting its growth inhibiting effect. Rather, it would appear that a phosphorylated form of the compound may be a more potent inhibitor than the free nucleoside itself. Whether this is as the mono-, di-, or triphosphate derivative is by no means clear. For example in one cell-free bacterial system it has been shown that 3'-deoxy AMP[1] inhibits an enzyme catalyzing an early step in purine biosynthesis, while in another bacterial system, 3'-deoxy ATP has been shown to have an inhibiting effect on the polymerization of nucleotides to nucleic acids. As to the "level" of phosphorylation, there seems to be no certainty.

In trying to understand the mechanism of action of any compound like this it becomes apparent there may be multiple sites of action, not necessarily relating to species differences alone but possible multiple sites within a given organism. Perhaps we are too preoccupied with trying to define "the" site, and should be content with the fact that many sites may exist. That site which is affected at the lowest concentration of inhibitor may not be "the" site of action.

Bacterial Systems

In addition to the studies reported above by CUNNINGHAM *et al.*(1951) the only other work with this antibiotic carried out with intact microorganisms is the work of ROTTMAN and GUARINO (1964a). They showed that cordycepin inhibited the growth of *B. subtilis* (ATCC 10783) at concentrations ranging from 10 μg/ml to 500 μg/ml when growth was measured turbidimetrically. At lower concentrations (10 μg/ml) the organism was able to overcome the inhibition, and eventually achieved growth commensurate with uninhibited cultures. Because of the structural similarity of cordycepin to 2'-deoxyadenosine a logical guess as to its mode of action would relate to an involvement in nucleic acid synthesis. A series of studies were carried out to see what types of compounds had the ability to overcome the growth inhibiting effects. When the concentration of adenosine or guanosine was 10 μg/ml and cordycepin 100 μg/ml, they were able to restore

[1] Abbreviations used in this section are:

3'-deoxy AMP	3'-deoxyadenosine-5'-phosphate
3'-deoxy ADP	3'-deoxyadenosine-5'-diphosphate
3'-deoxy ATP	3'-deoxyadenosine-5'-triphosphate
2'-deoxy AMP	2'deoxyadenosine-5'-monophosphate
2'-deoxy ADP	2'-deoxyadenosine-5'-diphosphate
2'deoxy ATP	2'deoxyadenosine-5'-triphosphate
AMP	adenosine-5'-phosphate
ADP	adenosine-5'-diphosphate
ATP	adenosine-5'-triphosphate
2'-deoxy CTP	deoxycytidine-5'-triphosphate
CTP	cytidine-5'-triphosphate
RNA	ribonucleic acid
DNA	deoxyribonucleic acid
DON	6-diazo-5-oxonorleucine
PRPP	5-phosphoribosyl pyrophosphate
GAR	glycinamide ribonucleotide
FGAR	formylglycinamide ribonucleotide

growth to approximately 70% of uninhibited cultures. The free purines, adenine and guanine, as well as their deoxyribonucleoside derivatives were also effective, although less so than their ribonucleosides. Two major sites of inhibition could be implicated as a result of these studies. One would involve pathways by which purines are synthesized *de novo* while the other might involve pathways by which *de novo* synthesized purines are interconverted. 5-Amino-4-imidazole carboxamide (see below) was able to overcome the growth inhibiting properties of cordycepin

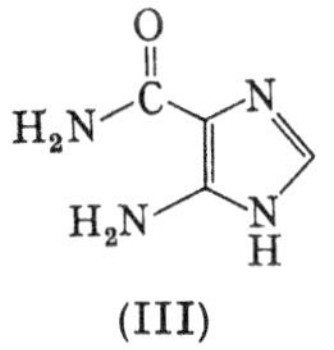

(III)

(III) 5-amino-4-imidazole carboxamide

although a higher concentration was needed. This implied that the metabolic block involved a step before completion of the purine ring, and consequently did not involve purine interconversion. Another line of evidence indicating that the metabolic block did not involve purine interconversions came from the failure to demonstrate either in the cells or in the media of inhibited cells any ultra-violet absorbing material which might have been expected. A similar study by SLECHTA (1960) on psicofuranine inhibition of growth lead to the conclusion that there was an accumulation of xanthosine in the media of inhibited cultures.

Utilizing intact cells, ROTTMAN and GUARINO (1964a) were able to show that the reversal of cordycepin inhibition by adenosine was competitive. The inhibited growth rate was proportional to the ratio of the cordycepin to adenosine and not to the absolute amount of cordycepin present. The amino group on the six position of cordycepin appeared to be necessary for optimal inhibition. When 3'-deoxy-inosine was tested as a growth inhibiting substance, it was found to be only one-tenth as effective as cordycepin.

At lower concentrations of the inhibitor, *B. subtilis* was able to overcome the growth inhibiting effect. In this study this was attributed to two possible sites: first, that *B. subtilis* has the ability to cleave the nucleoside to adenine and cordycepose, and second, that it has the ability to deaminate the nucleoside to the less effective inhibitor, 3'-deoxyinosine. Proof for these possibilities came from an experiment in which cordycepin 8-^{14}C was incubated with *B. subtilis* cells and hypoxanthine-^{14}C and adenine-^{14}C was identified in the media of the inhibited cultures. Whether the deamination occurred at the nucleoside or free base level was not investigated, although it was presumed to be the former.

Utilizing intact cells, ROTTMAN and GUARINO (1964b) studied the uptake of purine precursors such as formate-^{14}C or glycine-^{14}C into the nucleic acid purines of *B. subtilis* in the presence and absence of cordycepin. The incorporation of formate-^{14}C into the purines of ribonucleic acid and deoxyribonucleic acid was greatly diminished in the presence of cordycepin. This decrease was more than that which could be attributed to isotope dilution by the adenine which would result by cleavage of the N-glycosidic bond of cordycepin. The incorporation of 5-amino-4-imidazole-(2-^{14}C)-carboxamide into the nucleic acids of *B. subtilis* was studied and the specific activities of the purines isolated in the presence of cordycepin were found to be lower than those of the control cells. The difference was attributed in this case to an isotope dilution effect in which the adenine arising from cordycepin was diluting the isotope.

The lower specific activities noted in the nucleic acid purines when formate was used as a precursor again supports the concept that the metabolic block in this organism was occurring at a stage prior to completion of the purine ring. In this study an attempt was made to detect the accumulation of intermediates involved in *de novo* purine synthesis by studying the acid-soluble fractions of this organism by radioautography after the administration of either glycine-^{14}C or formate-^{14}C. Although there was a general lowering of radioactivity in all areas of the chromatogram in the inhibited cultures, there were no areas where specific compounds were found to accumulate. This would imply that the metabolic block must be very early in the stage of purine biosynthesis, at some stage prior to the incorporation of glycine. Further evidence for this concept came from an experiment in which the accumulation of radioactivity from glycine-^{14}C into formylglycinamide ribonucleotide (FGAR) was studied in cells inhibited with 6-diazo-5-oxonorleucine in the presence and absence of cordycepin (6-diazo-5-oxonorleucine inhibits reaction 5 thereby causing the accumulation of FGAR). In the cordycepin inhibited cultures the FGAR isolated was only one-tenth as radioactive as the uninhibited culture, again indicating a block early in the stage of purine synthesis. The reactions being discussed are outlined below:

It was postulated that these results are consistent with an inhibition of reactions 2 or 3 above. The inhibition of reaction 1 would also explain the results observed in these studies. Reaction 1 has subsequently been shown to be inhibited by cordycepin triphosphate in extracts of Ehrlich ascites tumor cells (OVERGAARD-HANSEN, 1964).

As a continuation of the results utilizing intact cell preparations of bacteria, ROTTMAN and GUARINO (1964c) proceeded to study an enzyme purified from both pigeon liver and *B. subtilis* that catalyzes reaction 2 (phosphoribosyl pyrophosphate amidotransferase). Since the inhibition of an early step was implied from these studies, and because WYNGAARDEN and ASHTON (1959) reported on the inhibition of phosphoribosyl pyrophosphate amidotransferase by AMP, it seemed likely that a possible site of action of cordycepin would be as its monophosphate derivative and on this reaction. The enzymes purified from *B. subtilis* and pigeon liver were found to be inhibited by cordycepin monophosphate and the inhibition was competitive with PRPP. *B. subtilis* had the ability to convert cordycepin to its monophosphate derivative. The free nucleoside exerted no inhibiting effect on the purified enzyme. On this basis, ROTTMAN and GUARINO concluded that the growth inhibiting effects observed in their *B. subtilis* experiments could be explained by the inhibition of reaction 2 which is catalyzed by phosphoribosyl pyrophosphate amidotransferase.

Other studies have been done with purified enzymes obtained from bacterial sources. SUHADOLNIK and CORY (1965) reported that with a polymerase purified from *E. coli* 3′-deoxy ATP effects DNA synthesis by inhibiting the incorporation of either tritium labelled 2′-deoxy ATP or tritium labelled deoxy CTP into an acid-insoluble product. The authors presented evidence that 3′-deoxy ATP may

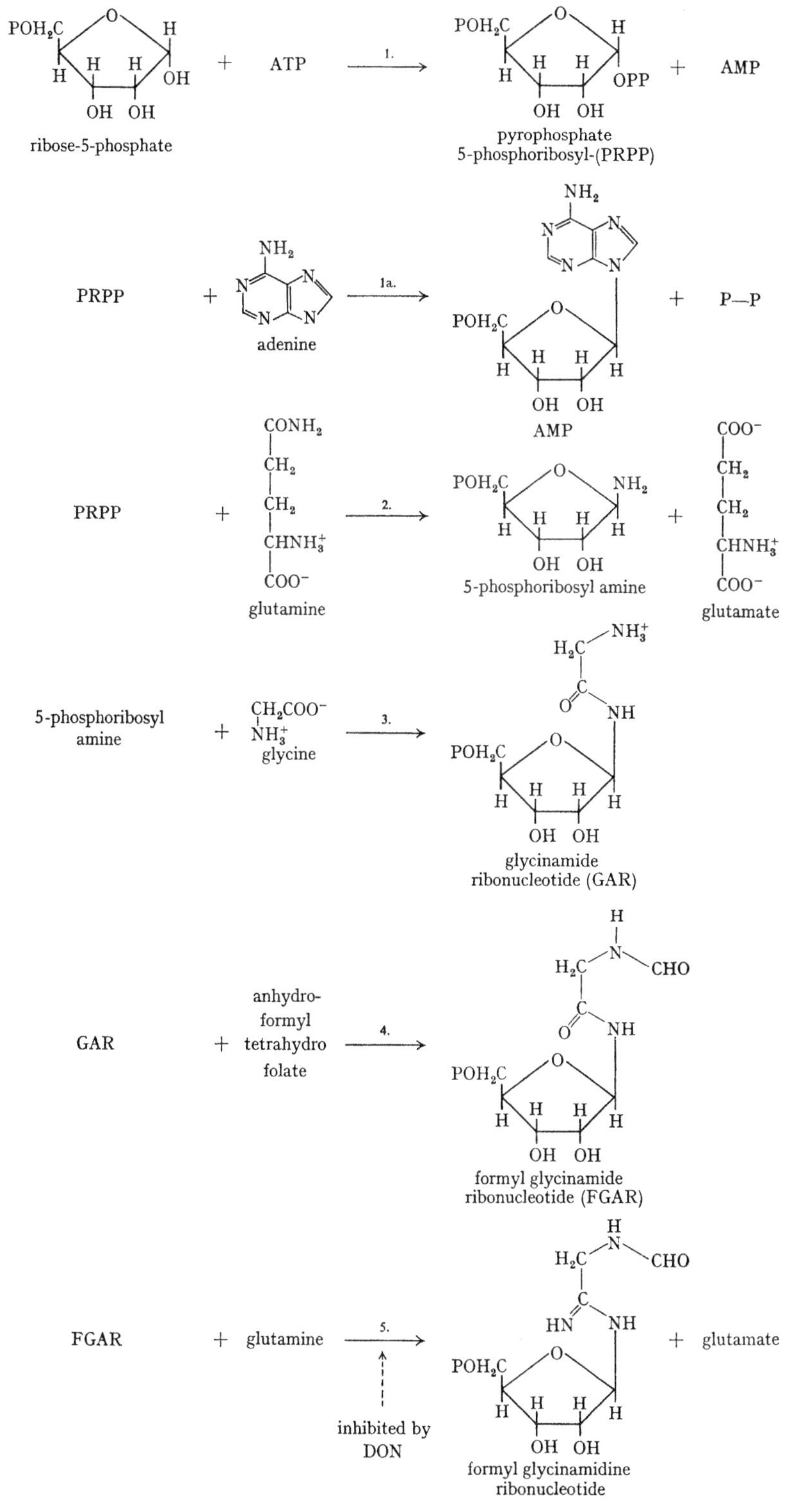
ribose-5-phosphate
ATP
1.
AMP
pyrophosphate
5-phosphoribosyl-(PRPP)
PRPP
adenine
1a.
P—P
AMP
PRPP
glutamine
2.
5-phosphoribosyl amine
glutamate
5-phosphoribosyl amine
glycine
3.
glycinamide ribonucleotide (GAR)
GAR
anhydro-formyl tetrahydro folate
4.
formyl glycinamide ribonucleotide (FGAR)
FGAR
glutamine
5.
inhibited by DON
glutamate
formyl glycinamidine ribonucleotide

be incorporated by the *E. coli* DNA polymerase into a polymeric form. It should be pointed out, however, that the growth of *E. coli* is not inhibited by this antibiotic. Even if cordycepin becomes incorporated into the DNA of this organism the mechanism by which the "fraudulent" DNA exerted its growth inhibiting effects is not yet understood. If the possibility exists that cordycepin can be incorporated into the DNA molecule, as these indirect results seem to indicate, it implies that such a polymer, at least where internally bound 3'-deoxyribose is concerned, must have some 2'-5'-phosphodiester bonds rather than the conventional 3'-5'-phosphodiester bonds known to occur in RNA and DNA.

Another bacterial site which has been considered comes from the work of SHIGEURA and BOXER (1964) who studied the incorporation of 3'-deoxy ATP into RNA by a purified RNA polymerase obtained from *Micrococcus lysodeikticus*. The incorporation of 3'-deoxy ATP ^{14}C was limited. When the RNA so synthesized was subjected to alkaline hydrolysis and fractionation, all of the radioactivity was found in the nucleoside fraction and practically none in the nucleotide fraction. These results are in keeping with the hypothesis that the incorporated 3'-deoxyadenosine was in a terminal position of the growing nucleotide chain, and prevented further elongation of the polymer. As an extension of this work SHIGEURA and GORDON (1965) investigated the effects of 3'-deoxyadenosine as its mono-, di-, and triphosphate derivatives on the RNA polymerase purified from *M. lysodeikticus*. They found that the mono-, and diphosphate derivatives of 3'-deoxyadenosine were without effect on the DNA directed RNA and polyadenylate formation, while the triphosphate derivative inhibited these reactions. The authors point out that the results indicated the 3'-deoxy ATP competed with ATP in various polymerization reactions.

Mammalian Systems

A large number of the growth inhibitory studies carried out with cordycepin have been done in mammalian systems, particularly the Ehrlich Mouse Ascites Tumor both *in vivo* and *in vitro* and also various other cell lines in tissue culture. One of the first observations involving the Ehrlich Ascites Tumor was reported by JAGGER *et al.* (1961) in which they demonstrated an increased survival time of mice bearing the tumor when given cordycepin. Two basic types of experiments were carried out in this study. The first involved experiments in which the tumor and drug (or saline) administrations were started on the same day and drug or saline injections were continued daily for 7 days and stopped. The second involved experiments in which the tumor was allowed to develop for periods of time before drug or saline injections were started. After various intervals, the drug or saline injections were repeated daily until seven had been administered. In both types of experiments, survival time was used as one of the parameters to determine growth inhibition or antitumor activity. In the first series of experiments it was noted that significant increase in survival times over those of controls was achieved when the level of cordycepin administered was 15 to 200 mg/kg body weight. In the second series of experiments it was demonstrated that at a fixed dose level of 150 mg/kg of body weight, the survival time of animals receiving cordycepin was increased significantly over those of control animals when the interval between tumor inoculation and drug inoculation was as much as five days. With regard to the toxicity of this compound in mice in this study, a single dose of 900 mg/kg of body weight was tolerated and seemed to have no outward harmful effects. When the drug was administered daily over a seven day period at a dosage up to 300 mg/kg of body weight it was found to be uniformly tolerated. When both tumor and drug were simultaneously administered this tolerance was lowered to 150 mg/kg body weight. This study pointed out the striking similarity of this compound to 2′-deoxyadenosine and postulated that it was serving as an antimetabolite.

KLENOW (1963a) utilizing suspensions of Ehrlich acites tumor cells was able to show that when the cells were incubated in the presence of cordycepin, he was able to isolate in the acid-soluble fraction obtained from these cells three compounds which he identified as the mono-, di-, and triphosphate derivatives of cordycepin. This was the first demonstration of a living system capable of phosphorylating this nucleoside. The author also pointed out that the compound identified as cordycepin diphosphate was capable of reacting in the pyruvate kinase reaction and could accept phosphate from phosphoenolpyruvate. This served to demonstrate that the phosphorylated derivative of this compound can participate in reactions similar to those reported for other nucleotides. KLENOW (1963b) also found that when tumor cells were incubated with lower concentrations of cordycepin (0.5—1.0 μmole/ml), the triphosphate derivative accumulates in the cells and the incorporation of orthophosphate-^{32}P into DNA is not inhibited. At higher concentrations of cordycepin (1.6—2.0 μmoles/ml), in addition to the accumulation of cordycepin triphosphate, there also begins to occur an accumulation of the mono- and diphosphate derivatives. In addition, two other notable events occur. First, there is a decrease in the acid-soluble pool of ribonucleotides extractable from the cells, and second there is a pronounced inhibition of incorporation of ^{32}P into the nucleic acids. It should be pointed out that these cells possess a potent deaminase which deaminates cordycepin as efficiently as adenosine and deoxyadenosine; but in spite of this, significant quantities of the non-deaminated compound can be isolated as the phosphorylated derivatives. The author concludes that cordycepin triphosphate does not inhibit the biosynthesis of DNA. This is based on the fact that the incorporation of ^{32}P into DNA is not inhibited in experiments when cordycepin triphosphate accumulates in the cells. This would seem to indicate that cordycepin monophosphate and cordycepin diphosphate concentrations increase as the cordycepin concentration is increased in the suspending medium and has the added implication that it is one of these compounds rather than the triphosphate derivative which is the more immediate inhibiting substance. The decreased incorporation of ^{32}P into nucleic acids, and the diminished ribonucleotide pool would also support this conclusion. The data reported in this study could be explained by the proposal of ROTTMAN and GUARINO (1964b) assuming the monophosphate derivative was the "active" form of the inhibitor.

A suggestion that cordycepin diphosphate is the "active" form of the inhibitor comes from the work of FREDERIKSEN (1963) who studied the inhibition of RNA and DNA synthesis in suspensions of Ehrlich ascites tumor cells by cordycepin-N′-oxide. This oxide is slowly reduced to cordycepin. In agreement with the work of KLENOW, FREDERIKSEN found that the accumulated triphosphate derivative of cordycepin at levels as high as 2.5—3.0 μmoles/gm of cells had no effect on DNA synthesis. However, the diphosphate derivative at 1 μmole/g of cells is postulated by FREDERIKSEN to be the inhibitor. He further postulated that the diphosphate inhibits the rephosphorylating system and as a consequence causes a slow decrease in the adenine nucleotide pool which is observed in these experiments.

Again using suspensions of Ehrlich ascites tumor cells KLENOW and OVERGAARD-HANSEN (1964) showed that under conditions in which cordycepin triphosphate was allowed to accumulate and under conditions that did not significantly inhibit the incorporation ^{32}P into the DNA of the cells, the incorporation of adenine-^{14}C into the DNA was markedly inhibited. They showed that this difference could not be ascribed to an inhibition of passage of adenine through the cell membrane. They concluded these results could be explained by the sequence of reactions known to be responsible for the incorporation of adenine into the acid soluble pool, reactions 1 and 1a. In a recent paper by OVERGAARD-HANSEN (1964) in which extracts of the cells were made it was demonstrated that cordycepin triphosphate produced a pronounced inhibition on the incorporation of adenine into adenine phosphates. The author localized which of the two reactions is involved. At no concentration of cordycepin triphosphate was any inhibiting effect observed on the formation of AMP from adenine and PRPP, and consequently he postulated that it was the synthesis of PRPP from ribose-5-phosphate and ATP that was involved. Since *de novo* synthesized purines as well as intact purines require PRPP in their over all incorporation into nucleic acids it is difficult to explain how adenine incorporation is inhibited while the incorporation of *de novo* precursors is not, if the sole site of inhibition involves the synthesis of PRPP. In any event this work of OVERGAARD-HANSEN also seems to support the concept that cordycepin as a phosphate derivative exerts an inhibiting effect early in the stage of purine synthesis if one will consider the synthesis of PRPP as one of the early reactions.

Further work by KLENOW and FREDERIKSEN (1964) utilizing the Ehrlich ascites tumor cells studied the effect of cordycepin triphosphate on the enzyme catalyzing the DNA-dependent synthesis of RNA. The enzyme responsible for this reaction, purified from these cell nuclei, was assayed by studying the incorporation of AMP-^{32}P into an acid insoluble product (RNA). The enzyme which they obtained was dependent on the presence of all four nucleoside triphosphates. For instance the omission of CTP or GTP from the reaction mixture strongly inhibited the incorporation. The presence of 3′-deoxy ATP almost completely prevented the incorporation of AMP-^{32}P into the acid-precipitable fraction (RNA). This effect was still observed when the molar ratio of ATP-^{32}P/3′deoxy-ATP was 25. Of a number of possibilities which could account for these results, the incorporation of 3′-deoxy AMP either in an internucleotide linkage or into free 3′-OH end groups of polyribonucleotides seems to be excluded on the basis of an experiment in which 3′-deoxy ATP-^{32}P was used in a complete system minus ATP-^{32}P. No detectable incorporation of ^{32}P into an acid-precipitable form (RNA) was noted. As will be seen below this may not be the case in other systems.

FREDERIKSEN and KLENOW (1964) have extended these studies on the enzyme catalyzing the DNA dependent synthesis of RNA by examining the possible effect of 3'-deoxy ATP on the RNA synthesis in whole cells. Under conditions in which 3'-deoxy ATP accumulated to the extent of 1.4 μmoles/g of cells, the incorporation of ^{32}P into RNA was partially inhibited. The maximum inhibition observed was about 50% after an induction period of about 60 minutes. Further fractionation of the RNA was carried out and three major fractions were obtained, cytoplasmic RNA and two fractions representing nuclear RNA. In these studies it was shown that not only was there inhibition of incorporation of ^{32}P into total RNA but specifically into cytoplasmic RNA and one of the nuclear RNA fractions. The other nuclear fraction of RNA showed no inhibition of incorporation.

Recent work by SHIGEURA and GORDON (1965) also demonstrated that 3'deoxyadenosine inhibited the incorporation of formate, glycine, hypoxanthine, adenine, and guanine, into the RNA of intact Ehrlich ascites cells. The ribonucleic acid was hydrolyzed in alkali and the incorporation of these labeled precursors into the ribonucleic acid purine nucleotides was determined. Whether the precursor being studied was a *de novo* purine precursor or an intact purine, 3'-deoxyadenosine definitely inhibited the incorporation of all precursors alike. This to some degree negates the objections cited below as to whether intact purines or *de novo* precursors serve as valid indices of nucleic acid synthesis in an intact system.

Tissue Culture Studies

The work cited so far has related either to bacterial systems or the Ehrlich mouse ascites tumor cell. Two groups have studied cordycepin inhibition utilizing cells maintained in tissue culture. RICH *et al.* (1965) found that cordycepin inhibits the growth of human tumor cells (H. Ep. No. 1) grown in culture. Their data indicated that the inhibition is cytostatic rather than cytocidal. Exposure of these cells to inhibiting concentrations of cordycepin did not markedly effect the protein, RNA or DNA content of these cells. However, a two to four-fold depression of the incorporation of adenosine-8-^{14}C into RNA and DNA was observed, and the authors note that this data is not in accord with the suggestion that the sensitive site for growth inhibition is early in the pathway of purine biosynthesis. One might take exception to this conclusion by asking the question: What precursor can validly be used as an index of DNA or RNA synthesis in a cell? Normally, potential precursors for nucleic acid synthesis such as adenine or adenosine are considered to be on "salvage pathways" by which *de novo* synthesized heterocyclic rings may be reutilized for nucleic acid synthesis. When such a precursor is used as an index of nucleic acid synthesis, and an inhibition is noted, it may be due to a true inhibition of nucleic acid synthesis or an inhibition of a specific enzyme or enzyme system that can take this precursor into the "main line" of nucleic acid synthesis. The fact that protein, RNA, and DNA synthesis in this study do not seem to be markedly altered, suggests the possibility that an enzyme or enzyme systems responsible for utilizing preformed purines may account for the results obtained with adenosine-8-^{14}C and that the nucleic acid synthesis in the cells may not be appreciably altered.

As an extension of this investigation CORY *et al.* (1965) studied the incorporation of cordycepin into the DNA and RNA of growing H. Ep. No. 1 cells in tissue culture. When these cells were incubated with tritiated cordycepin, the RNA and

DNA were found to be radioactive. The nucleic acids were subjected to fractionation, and then subjected to hydrolysis. Radioactive cordycepin was then isolated from both the terminal and internal positions of the RNA. In the case of DNA the location of the cordycepin is not known, but cordycepin was incorporated into this polymer. As had been mentioned earlier, the presence of cordycepin in phosphodiester linkage in the RNA of these cells creates a unique situation in that such a linkage must be 2'-5' because cordycepin does not possess a free hydroxyl group at position 3. In these studies the isolation of cordycepin as a mononucleotide from the RNA is a bit surprising because the RNA fraction was hydrolyzed in alkali according to standard procedures. The alkali lability of RNA under these conditions, in contrast to the stability of DNA under the same conditions, resides in the ability of cyclic ester formation to the available free hydroxyl group in RNA. Such hydroxyl groups are not available in the case of DNA. It is this transient formation of the cyclic ester then that accounts for the lability of RNA and stability of DNA. A 2'-5'-phosphosdiester bond must be involved if cordycepin is internally bound in RNA. Because there is no available free hydroxyl group with which it can form the cyclic intermediate, it is strange that it is degraded to a mononucleotide under these conditions. In light of present knowledge, one might rather predict that it would come out as a dinucleotide or oligonucleotide. Of course 3'-deoxynucleotides may behave quite different than the 2'-deoxynucleotides in regard to their alkali lability.

In any event it would appear that if cordycepin is actually capable of being incorporated into DNA and RNA, then one might predict that the "fraudulent" nucleic acid so formed at some later stage in metabolism might have a cytostatic (or in the case of DNA, a cytocidal) effect.

Other cells in tissue culture that have been used to study the growth inhibiting property of cordycepin are KB cells and chick embryo fibroblast cells. GITTERMAN *et al.* (1965) studied the effects of cordycepin on the incorporation of uridine-^{3}H into the acid-insoluble fractions of these two types of cells. In essence the authors showed that cordycepin exerted its cytotoxic effect within 1—2 days and indeed was an effective inhibitor of uridine-^{3}H incorporation in both cell systems. These results certainly seem to indicate interference with RNA synthesis similar to that reported in the Ehrlich ascites tumor cell.

It seems to become apparent in going over the available literature that cordycepin, like many other growth inhibiting substances may have multiple sites of action, and as was pointed out earlier in this chapter, perhaps we are too preoccupied with finding "The" site. One point studies seem to indicate is that the nucleoside per se is not active, and in all probability the phosphorylated compound is the active "culprit". Whether this is the mono-, di-, or triphosphate derivative seems to vary depending upon the system being studied. To date all studies have focused on pathways of nucleic acid synthesis as being the most logical site for the inhibition.

In one study cited above it seems that 3'-deoxy ATP is a potent inhibitor of RNA synthesis, probably by being incorporated in competition with ATP, and thus terminates further growth of the polynucleotide chain. Another study seems to indicate that this nucleotide may actually be incorporated into an internucleotide link. Who is right? Both investigations used different systems, and each one may be correct for his system. There obviously is a good deal more work to be done with this compound. Its ability, if true, to participate actually as a component in polynucleotide structure may have more basic importance to the field of biology than understanding the exact mechanism by which it inhibits growth.

See Addendum

References

BENTLEY, H. R., K. G. CUNNINGHAM, and F. S. SPRING: CORDYCEPIN: A metabolic product from cultures of *Cordyceps militaris* (LINN.) Link. Part II. The structure of cordycepin. J. Chem. Soc. **1951**, 2301.

CORY, J. G., R. J. SUHADOLNIK, B. RESNICK, and M. RICH: Incorporation of cordycepin (3'-deoxyadenosine) into ribonucleic acid and deoxyribonucleic acid of human tumor cells. Biochim. et Biophys. Acta **103**, 646 (1965).

CUNNINGHAM, K. G., S. A. HUTCHINSON, W. MANSON, and F. S. SPRING: Cordycepin, a metabolic product from cultures of *Cordyceps militaris* (LINN.) Link. Part I. Isolation and characterisation. J. Chem. Soc. **1951**, 2299.

FREDERIKSEN, S.: Inhibition of ribonucleic acid and deoxyribonucleic acid synthesis in Ehrlich ascites cells by cordycepin-N^1-oxide. Biochim. et Biophys. Acta **76**, 366 (1963).

FREDERIKSEN, S., and H. KLENOW: Differential inhibition by 3'-deATP of nuclear and cytoplasmic RNA fractions of Ehrlich ascites tumor cells *in vitro*. Biochem. Biophys. Research. Commun. **17**, 165 (1964).

FREDERIKSEN, S., H. MALLING, and H. KLENOW: Isolation of 3'-deoxyadenosine (cordycepin) from the liquid medium of *Cordyceps militaris* (L. Ex Fr.) Link. Biochim. et Biophys. Acta **95**, 189 (1965).

GITTERMAN, C. O., R. W. BURG, G. E. BOXER, D. MELTZ, and J. HITT: Relation of structure to activity of purine 3'-deoxynucleosides in KB cell and chick embryo fibroblast cell cultures. J. Med. Chem. **8**, 664 (1965).

JAGGER, D. V., N. M. KREDICH, and A. J. GUARINO: Inhibition of Ehrlich mouse ascites tumor growth by cordycepin. Cancer Research, **21**, 216 (1961).

KACZKA, E. A., E. L. DULANEY, C. O. GITTERMAN, H. B. WOODRUFF, and K. FOLKERS: Isolation and inhibitory effects on KB cell cultures of 3'-deoxyadenosine from *Aspergillus nidulans* (EIDAM) Wint. Biochem. Biophys. Research Commun. **14**, 452 (1964a).

KACZKA, E. A., N. R. TRENNER, B. ARISON, R. W. WALKER, and K. FOLKERS: Identification of cordycepin, a metabolite of *Cordyceps militaris*, as 3'-deoxyadenosine. Biochem. Biophys. Research Commun. **14**, 456 (1964b).

KLENOW, H.: Formation of the mono-, di- and triphosphate of cordycepin in Ehrlich ascites-tumor cells *in vitro*. Biochim. et Biophys. Acta **76**, 347 (1963a).

KLENOW, H.: Inhibition by cordycepin and 2-deoxyglucose of the incorporation of [^{32}P] orthophosphate into the nuclei acids of Ehrlich ascites-tumor cells *in vitro*. Biochim. et Biophys. Acta **76**, 354 (1963b).

KLENOW, H., and S. FREDERIKSEN: Effect of 3'-deoxyATP (cordycepin triphosphate) and 2'-deoxyATP on the DNA-dependent RNA nucleotidyltransferase from Ehrlich ascites tumor cells. Biochim. et Biophys. Acta **87**, 495 (1964).

KLENOW, H., and K. OVERGAARD-HANSEN: Effect of cordycepin triphosphate on the incorporation of [8-^{14}C] adenine and [^{32}P] orthophosphate into the acid-soluble ribotides of Ehrlich ascites tumor cells *in vitro*. Biochim. et Biophys. Acta **80**, 500 (1964).

LEE, W. W., A. BENITEZ, C. D. ANDERSON, L. GOODMAN, and B. R. BAKER: Potential anticancer agents. LV. Synthesis of 3'-amino-2',3'-dideoxyadenosine and related analogs. J. Am. Chem. Soc. **83**, 1906 (1961).

OVERGAARD-HANSEN, K.: The inhibition of 5-phosphoribosyl-1-pyrophosphate formation by cordycepin triphosphate in extracts of Ehrlich ascites tumor cells. Biochim. et Biophys. Acta **80**, 504 (1964).

RICH, M. A., P. MEYERS, G. WEINBAUM, J. G. CORY, and R. J. SUHADOLNIK. Inhibition of human tumor cells by cordycepin. Biochim. et Biophys. Acta **95**, 194 (1965).

ROTTMAN, F., and A. J. GUARINO: Studies on the inhibition of *Bacillus subtilis* growth by cordycepin. Biochim. et Biophys. Acta **80**, 632 (1964a).

ROTTMAN, F., and A. J. GUARINO: The inhibition of purine biosynthesis *de novo* in *Bacillus subtilis* by cordycepin. Biochim. et Biophys. Acta **80**, 640 (1964b).

ROTTMAN, F., and A. J. GUARINO: The inhibition of phosphoribosyl-pyrophosphate amidotransferase activity by cordycepin monophosphate. Biochim. et Biophys. Acta **89**, 465 (1964c).

SHIGEURA, H. T., and G. E. BOXER: Incorporation of 3′-deoxyadenosine-5′-triphosphate into RNA by RNA polymerase from *Micrococcus lysodeikticus*. Biochem. Biophys. Research Commun. **17**, 758 (1964).

SHIGEURA, H. T., and C. N. GORDON: The effects of 3′-deoxyadenosine on the synthesis of ribonucleic acid. J. Biol. Chem. **240**, 806 (1965).

SLECHTA, L.: Studies on the mode of action of psicofuranine. Biochem. Pharmacol. **5**, 96 (1960).

SUHADOLNIK, R. J., and J. G. CORY: Further evidence for the biosynthesis of cordycepin and proof of the structure of 3-deoxyribose. Biochim. et Biophys. Acta **91**, 661 (1964).

SUHADOLNIK, R. J., and J. G. CORY: Effect of cordycepin triphosphate (3′-deoxyadenosine-5′-triphosphate) on the *E. coli* DNA polymerase system. Abs. 150th Meeting Am. Chem. Soc. 86C (1965).

TODD, A., and T. L. V. ULBRICHT: Deoxynucleosides and related compounds. IX. Synthesis of 3′-deoxy-adenosine. J. Chem. Soc. 3275 (1960).

WALTON, E., R. F. NUTT, S. R. JENKINS, and F. W. HOLLY: 3′-Deoxynucleosides. I. A synthesis of 3′-deoxyadenosine. J. Am. Chem. Soc. **86**, 2952 (1964).

WYNGAARDEN, J. B., and D. M. ASHTON: The regulation of activity of phosphoribosylpyrophosphate amidotransferase by purine ribonucleotides: A potential feedback control of purine biosynthesis. J. Biol. Chem. **234**, 1492 (1959).

Azaserine and 6-Diazo-5-Oxo-L-Norleucine (DON)

R. F. Pittillo and D. E. Hunt

Introduction

The discovery of azaserine in culture filtrates of *Streptomyces fragilis* (Anderson *et al.*, 1956) was announced by Ehrlich *et al.* (1954); and its inhibitory activity against Crocker Mouse Sarcoma 180 was described (Stock *et al.*, 1954). 6-Diazo-5-oxo-L-norleucine(DON), produced by an unidentified *Streptomyces*, was discovered shortly thereafter (Ehrlich *et al.*, 1956; Clark, Reilly and Stock, 1956). Azaserine occupies a unique position in the historical development of antibiotics: it is the first antibiotic whose discovery was the direct result of a systematic search for tumor-inhibiting antibiotics. Although equivocal clinical utility has been demonstrated against various malignancies, both of these antibiotics have proved to be valuable research tools and significant biochemical advances have resulted from their discovery.

Structurally, azaserine and DON are quite similar: azaserine has been identified as O-diazoacetyl-L-serine (Fusari *et al.*, 1954a and b); and DON as 6-diazo-5-oxo-L-norleucine (Dion *et al.*, 1956). They bear an obvious structural similarity to glutamine.

Azaserine *DON* *Glutamine*

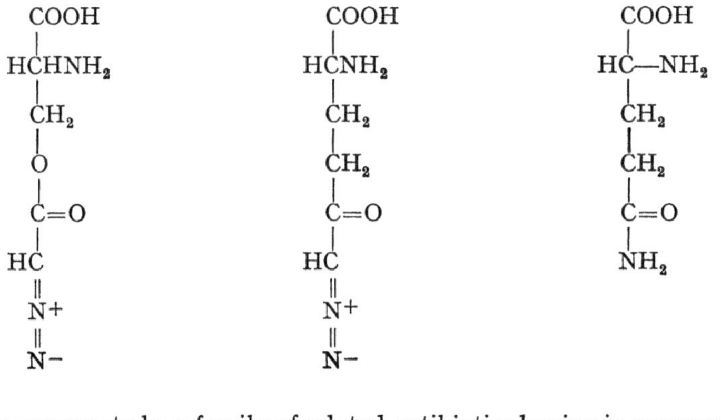

There appears to be a family of related antibiotics having in common the diazo moiety since alazopeptin, produced by *Streptomyces griseoplanus* (deVoe *et al.*, 1957; Barg *et al.*, 1957), has been characterized as L-alanyl-(6-diazo-5-oxo)-L-norleucyl-(6-diazo-5-oxo)-L-norleucine (Patterson *et al.*, 1965) and duazomycin A (Rao *et al.*, 1960) has been identified as N-acetyl DON (Rao, 1962).

Biological Activities of Azaserine and DON

The *in vitro* antimicrobial activities of both azaserine and DON have been reported (EHRLICH *et al.*, 1956; COFFEY *et al.*, 1954). Representative data reported by these workers are summarized in Table 1. Interesting differences in the antimicrobial activity of azaserine and DON were found. In the complex culture media used, *Acetobacter aceti, Bacillus subtilis, Clostridium perfringens, Clostridium septicum, Corynebacterium diphtheriae* and *Diplococcus pneumoniae* were most sensitive to DON. Five strains of *Clostridium* and the H_{37} Rv strain of *Mycobacterium tuberculosis* var. *hominis* were found to be quite sensitive to azaserine. Modest antifungal activity *in vitro* was observed with both azaserine and DON. Both antibiotics showed little or no activity *in vitro* against African and South American trypanosomes or *Trichomonas foetus*, or in mice with experimentally induced shistosomiasis. However, azaserine is effective *in vivo* against other protozoal infections, notably *Plasmodium lophurae* (MCCARTHY, BAYLES and THOMPSON, 1957) and *Trypanosoma equiperdum* (JAFFRE, 1963; NAKAMURA,

Table 1. *Activity of azaserine and DON against selected microorganisms*

Species	Azaserine concentration (µg/ml medium) causing		DON concentration (µg/ml medium) causing	
	Complete inhibition of growth	50% inhibition	Complete inhibition of growth	50% inhibition
A. Bacteria				
Gram-positive				
Bacillus cereus	25	—	>100	—
Bacillus megaterium	10	—	50	—
Bacillus subtilis	>100	—	1.56	—
Clostridium feseri	0.5	—	25	—
Micrococcus pyogenes var. *aureus*	>100	>100	>100	>50
Gram-negative				
Acetobacter aceti	25	—	0.39	—
Aerobacter aerogenes	>100	54	>100	>50
Agrobacterium tumefaciens	10	3.6	>100	>50
Brucella suis	>100	—	>100	—
Escherichia coli	50	—	>100	—
Neisseria catarrhalis	25	—	25	—
Proteus vulgaris	>100	9.1	>100	>50
Pseudomonas aeruginosa	>100	—	>100	—
Salmonella typhosa	50	76	>100	11.8
Shigella sonnei	—	12.8	—	20
Acid-fast				
Corynebacterium diphtheriae	>100	—	12.5	—
Mycobacterium tuberculosis var. *hominis*	3.13 to >100	—	>100	—

1956). DON did not alter the cytopathogenic effects of a variety of human viruses in monkey kidney cultures. Inhibition of some algae by both azaserine and DON has been reported (BARKER *et al.*, 1956; TOMISEK *et al.*, 1957; VAN DER MEULEN and BASSHAM, 1959; AARONSON, 1959) as well as the inhibition of growth of various plant cells (NORMAN, 1955, 1959; TRUHANT and DEYSSON, 1957; AMMANN and SAFFERMAN, 1958; BENBADIS, 1965). Both azaserine and DON adversely affect fecundity in various insects (CRYSTAL, 1963; GROSCH, 1963) and have been observed to exert a variety of teratogenic effects in chick embryos, rat litters, rabbits and dogs (DAGG and KARNOFSKY, 1955; FRIEDMAN, 1957; KARNOFSKY and LACON, 1962; MURPHY and KARNOFSKY, 1962; PREISLER, 1960; THIERSCH, 1957a and b).

Azaserine and DON have been exhaustively evaluated in a variety of experimental tumor systems. Representative data are given in Table 2. CLARKE, REILLY and STOCK (1956) found that both DON and azaserine are potent inhibitors of Sarcoma 180 but that inhibition with either agent persists only as long as the

Table 1. (Continued)

Species	Azaserine concentration (μg/ml) causing inhibition of growth			DON concentration (μg/ml) causing inhibition of growth		
	Complete	Partial	None	Complete	Partial	None
B. Fungi						
Alternaria sp.		1000	500	—	—	200
Aspergillus fumigatus	31.3	3.9—15.6	2.0	—	—	200
Blastomyces dermatitidis			250	>100	12.5	6.25
Candida krusei	250	31.3—125	15.6	200	50	25
Candida monosa	62.5	15.6—31.3	7.8	>200	6.25	3.12
Candida mycoderma (*Mycoderma vini*)	250	31.3—125	15.6	>200	50	25
Cercospora beticola	250	125	62.5	>200	50	25
Debaryomyces matruchoti		1000	500	—	—	200
Endomycopsis fibuliger	62.5	31.2	15.6	>200	50	25
Fomes geotropus	1000	500	250	>200	6.25	3.12
Fusarium oxysporum		1000	500	—	—	200
Hansenula anomala		500—1000	250	>200	100	50
Microsporum gypseum			250	—	—	200
Mucor racemosus		500—1000	250	—	—	200
Nocardia asteroides			250	>200	200	100
Pichia chodati	1000	62.5—500	31.3	—	—	200
Poria luteofibrata	125	—	62.5	—	—	
Rhizopus nigricans	500	250	125	200	25	12.5
Saccharomyces cerevisiae var. *ellipsoideus*	62.5	15.6—31.3	7.8	>200	25	12.5
Streptomyces griseus			1000	—	—	200
Syncephalastrum sp.	1000	125—500	62.5	—	—	200
Torulopsis rotundata			1000	>200	12.5	6.25
Trichophyton mentagrophytes var. *gypseum*			250	—	—	200

Table 2. *Comparative antitumor activity of azaserine and DON in representative tumor systems*

Tumor system	% Reduction in tumor size at optimum dosage[1]		References
	Azaserine	DON	
Walker Carcino-sarcoma 256	70 (approx.)	70 (approx.)	LOUSTALOT, DESAULLES, and MEIER (1958)
Rous Sarcoma	69	90	JOHNSON, BAKER and WRIGHT (1958)
Flexner-Jobling Carcinoma	70 (approx.)	70 (approx.)	JOHNSON, BAKER and WRIGHT (1958)
Sarcoma 180	42	38	CLARKE, REILLY and STOCK (1957)
	% Increase in life span[1]		
CH_3 70429 (Mouse plasma cell tumor)	70	>70	POTTER and LAW (1957)
Leukemia L1210	38	40	LASTER and GRISWOLD (personal communication)

[1] Compared to controls at comparable time intervals.

host mice remained under therapy. Of the two, azaserine was far less effective. In general, the greater activity of DON toward a variety of tumors has been reported by numerous workers. These compounds have been evaluated against a vast spectrum of tumors including human tumors in embryonated eggs, human epidermoid carcinoma (H.Ep.-3) in Swiss mice, various transplantable human tumors in the rat and hamster, Rous Sarcoma in the chicken, a variety of mammary tumors, and leukemias in rodents. Complete information and details of the antitumor activity or inhibition of experimental tumors by these agents may be found in the following references: GRISWOLD *et al.*, 1963; HARRIS, 1962; HUTCHISON *et al.*, 1962; LE PAGE and HOWARD, 1963; MERKER *et al.*, 1962; SUGIURA, 1962; TARNOWSKI and STOCK, 1957; TELLER, 1962; WOOLLEY, 1962.

With the recognition of the involvement of both azaserine and DON in purine metabolism (see below) numerous attempts have been made to obtain therapeutic potentiation with azaserine or DON in combination with various purine analogs both in experimental systems and in humans. Thus TARNOWSKI and STOCK (1957) investigated the effect of combinations of azaserine and DON with purine analogues and other metabolites on the growth of mouse mammary carcinomas. 6-Chloropurine and azaserine (SARTORELLI and BOOTH, 1961, 1963) 6-thioguanine and azaserine (SARTORELLI and LE PAGE, 1958), and various combinations of 6-mercaptopurine, 6-thioguanine, 4-APP (4-aminopyrazolo [3,4-*d*] pyrimidine) and azaserine (HENDERSON and FUNGA, 1960, 1961) have all been tested in diverse systems. Consistent therapeutic potentiation with the combination of azaserine plus 6-mercaptopurine has been reported both in experimental systems and in children with acute leukemia (BURCHENAL, MURPHY and TAN, 1956; BURCHENAL *et al.*, 1955). WHEELER, SCHABEL and SKIPPER (1956) found that some B_6 antagonists enhanced the inhibition of *Escherichia coli*, Sarcoma 180, and Adenocarcinoma 755 by azaserine (SKIPPER and SCHABEL, unpublished observations,

1954). The utility of both azaserine and DON in the management of various human neoplasms must await more definitive *in vivo* evaluations (SKIPPER *et al.*, 1964). A summary of the biological and clinical data accumulated on both azaserine and DON has been prepared by DUVAL (1960a and b).

REILLY (1954a, 1958) found that azaserine was enzymatically destroyed by mouse and rat tissues, particularly liver, kidney and spleen. The degradation of azaserine was evidenced by loss of activity, ultraviolet adsorption, and the liberation of a keto-acid and 1 mole of ammonia for each mole of azaserine destroyed. The enzyme is specific. Azaserine, but not DON or 19 other amino acids, was destroyed. The keto-acid formed has been identified as pyruvic acid (JACQUEZ and SHERMAN, 1962).

The incorporation of radiolabeled formate or glycine into nucleic acids of normal and neoplastic cells *in vivo* was found to be inhibited by azaserine; however, it did not inhibit similar incorporation of preformed purines (BENNETT, SCHABEL, and SKIPPER, 1956). HARTMAN, LEVENBERG and BUCHANAN (1955) demonstrated that both azaserine and DON inhibited inosinic acid biosynthesis from its elemental precursors in extracts of pigeon liver. Inhibition of this system by azaserine resulted in the enhanced accumulation of an intermediate of purine biosynthesis, 2-formamido-N-ribosylacetamide-5'-phosphate (formylglycinamide ribotide). Subsequent isotope studies with mouse tissues confirmed that azaserine inhibited incorporation of glycine into purines and showed that adenine utilization was increased (FERNANDES, LE PAGE and LINDNER, 1956; BENNETT, SCHABEL and SKIPPER, 1956). Azaserine inhibition of *de novo* purine biosynthesis with concomitant accumulation of formylglycinamide ribonucleotide and ribonucleoside was also demonstrated in *Escherichia coli* (TOMISEK, KELLY and SKIPPER, 1956). Similar effects were demonstrated in tumor cells *in vivo* (GREENLEES and LE PAGE, 1956); however, glutamine partially reversed the inhibition (LEVENBERG, MELNICK and BUCHANAN, 1957). Subsequently, both azaserine and DON were found to compete with glutamine for an enzyme site, and both inhibitors combined irreversibly with the enzyme (BUCHANAN, 1958). LEVENBERG, MELNICK and BUCHANAN (1957) studied the effects of azaserine and DON on the enzymatic reactions involved in the *de novo* biosynthesis of inosinic acid in pigeon liver extract and concluded that the synthesis of formylglycinamidine from glutamine and formylglycinamide was the most sensitive reaction. GOLDTHWAIT (1956) using pigeon liver extract demonstrated that the reaction of glutamine with ATP to form phosphoribosylamine was sensitive to azaserine attack. The sensitivity of this site was confirmed by LEVENBERG, MELNICK and BUCHANAN (1957) but was found to be less marked than the inhibition of the amination of formylglycinamide ribonucleotide. These findings were extended by ANDERSON, LEVENBERG, and LAW (1957) to the mouse plasma cell neoplasm 70429: the incorporation of glycine-C^{14} into acid-soluble purines was inhibited as were the conversions of formylglycinamide ribonucleotide and aminoimidazole carboxamide ribonucleotide (ANDERSON and LAW, 1960).

DON has been demonstrated to have similar effects on purine metabolism. Incorporation of formate and glycine into nucleic acids is inhibited by DON in *Escherichia coli* (MAXWELL and NICKEL, 1957) and in various mammalian cells, both *in vitro* (BARCLAY, GARFINKEL and PHILLIPPS, 1962) and *in vivo* (MOORE and HURLBERT, 1961). Extensive data have been presented which show DON to be a more potent inhibitor of *de novo* purine biosynthesis than azaserine (BARG *et al.*, 1957; BROCKMAN and ANDERSON, 1962; HARTMAN, 1962). Fig. 1 illustrates the sites in *de novo* purine biosynthesis which are inhibited by these antibiotics.

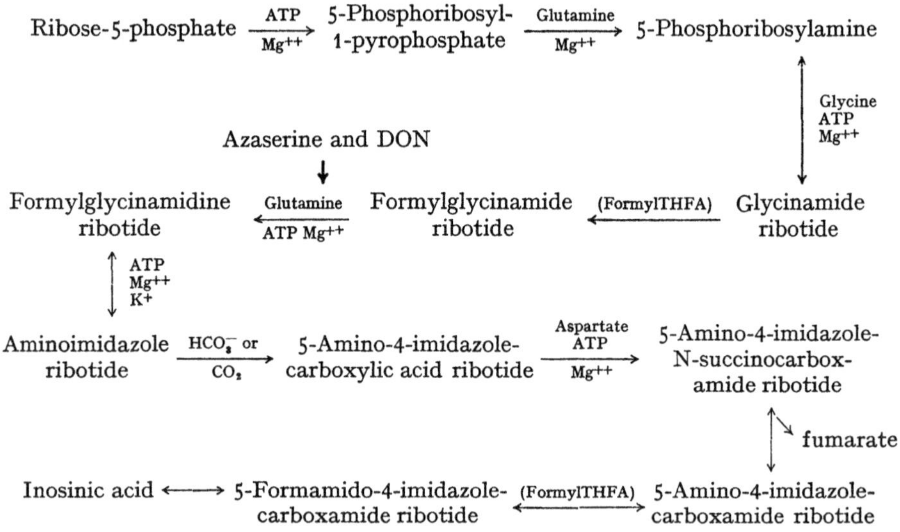

Fig. 1. Azaserine and DON sensitive sites in *de novo* purine biosynthesis

A significant step forward in elucidating the mechanism of action of azaserine has been taken by BUCHANAN'S group. They have reported that azaserine combines irreversibly with a sulfhydryl grouping on the enzyme that catalyzes the conversion of formylglycinamide ribotide (in the presence of glutamine) to formylglycinamidine ribotide (DAWID, FRENCH and BUCHANAN, 1963; FRENCH, DAWID and BUCHANAN, 1963; FRENCH *et al.*, 1963). DON was not included in the study.

The sensitivity of other glutamine requiring reactions to azaserine and DON has been investigated. Azaserine competitively inhibits the amination of xanthylic acid to guanylic acid in an enzyme preparation from calf thymus (ABRAMS and BENTLEY, 1959). The amination of the nicotinic acid moiety of adenine dinucleotide in DPN was shown to require glutamine or ammonium salts in a yeast enzyme preparation (PREISS and HANDLER, 1958). LANGAN, KAPLAN and SHUSTER (1959) observed that azaserine administered *in vivo* produced a decrease in liver DPN levels.

Elucidation of the mechanism of action of azaserine in bacteria has been complicated by the observed reversing activity of amino acids, especially the aromatic amino acids. REILLY (1954b) reported that the inhibitory effect of azaserine on the growth of *Escherichia coli* could be blocked by any one of the three aromatic amino acids, L-tryptophan, L-tyrosine or L-phenylalanine, but that the inhibitory effect of azaserine on the growth of the yeast *Kloeckera brevis* was best antagonized by the basic amino acids (KOHBERGER *et al.*, 1955; REILLY, 1956). The reversing action of aromatic amino acids on azaserine inhibition of *Escherichia coli* was also noted by MAXWELL and NICKEL (1954) and KAPLAN and STOCK (1954). The data of KAPLAN, REILLY, and STOCK (1959) suggested that azaserine interfered with the metabolism of shikimic acid. In both *Escherichia coli* and *Aerobacter aerogenes*, glutamine is required for the amination of shikimic acid to anthranilic acid (RIVERA and SRINIVASAN, 1962) and both azaserine and DON have been reported to inhibit this reaction (SRINIVASAN, 1959). Consequently, the biosynthesis of *p*-aminobenzoic acid from shikimic acid has been found to be inhibited by both of these antibiotics (SRINIVASAN and WEISS, 1961). In another strain of *Escherichia coli* inhibition by azaserine was antagonized by histidine as well as by urocanic acid and formamidinoglutaric acid (HEDEGAARD, THOAI, and ROCHE, 1959; HEDEGAARD *et al.*, 1959a and b). MAXWELL and NICKEL (1957) reported that inhibition of *Escherichia coli* growth by DON, unlike inhibition by azaserine, was not reversed by aromatic amino acids but was reversed by the free purine bases and their corresponding nucleosides. It was also noted that slight reversal of DON inhibition of *Escherichia coli* was afforded by L-histidine, L-ornithine, L-lysine, L-arginine, and L-glutamine and of azaserine inhibition of *Escherichia coli* by methionine. KAPLAN, REILLY and STOCK (1959) found that the combination of any one of the aromatic amino acids with either L-arginine or DL-histidine exerted greater blocking of inhibition by azaserine than the aromatic amino acids alone. This work was extended by other workers who suggested that the activity of histidine in reversing inhibition by azaserine could be a consequence of this antibiotic's inhibiting the synthesis of histidine from purine precursors (PITTILLO, 1961; PITTILLO and QUINNELLY, 1962). Azaserine inhibition of cell division of *Tetrahymena piriformis*, which requires preformed purines for growth, could be reversed by phenylalanine but not by glutamine (LEE, YUZURIHA, and EILER, 1959; LEE and YUZURIHA, 1964). Similarly, in *Escherichia coli* B 96, a mutant strain requiring preformed purines for growth, it was noted that only aromatic amino acids reversed inhibition of growth by azaserine. However, in a phenylalanine requiring strain, *Escherichia coli* M 83-5, the aromatic amino acids, as well as histidine and purines all individually reversed inhibition by azaserine (PITTILLO and QUINNELLY, 1962).

In tumor cells both azaserine and DON are actively transported by an amino acid transport system; and glycine, glutamine and tryptophan competed with azaserine for this transport system (JACQUEZ, 1957, 1958). Phenylalanine or DON were not included in this study. BROCK and BROCK (1961) postulated that in *Escherichia coli* the aromatic amino acids blocked entry of azaserine into the cell. That such blockage by phenylalanine is the sole explanation for its reversing activity appears unlikely in view of the work of TOMISEK, REID and SKIPPER (1959) which shows that phenylalanine prevented azaserine inhibition of aminoimidazolecarboxamide synthesis in a cell-free system. Similarly, GOTS and GOLLUB (1956) demonstrated that phenylalanine was an active reversing agent even when added after preincubation with azaserine.

The most probable explanation of the activity of aromatic amino acids in reversing azaserine inhibition in bacteria is that this antibiotic competes with these amino acids for a site on a transport system and, in all likelihood, competes with these amino acids in critical but as yet undefined areas within the cell. It has been demonstrated that nondividing *Escherichia coli* cells are rapidly killed by azaserine but are refractory to DON. Inhibition of such cells by azaserine can be reversed by the aromatic amino acids but not by glutamine (Narkates and Pittillo, 1964). Furthermore, such cells of *Escherichia coli* readily take up radiolabeled phenylalanine from the environment but do not transport radiolabeled glutamine across the cell membrane (Pittillo and Narkates, unpublished observations, 1965). These observations suggest that azaserine and DON enter the cell by different transport mechanisms.

In spite of the vast amount of work that has been done on the mechanisms of action of azaserine and DON it is impossible at this time to completely delineate the role of these antibiotics in cell metabolism. In many respects, they seem to behave in an identical manner, such as in the inhibition of *de novo* purine biosynthesis in a variety of cells; but in other respects there are sharp differences in biological response to these antibiotics. Notable in the latter category are the differences relative to resistance, cross-resistance and collateral sensitivity (see Reviews by Hutchison, 1963; Brockman, 1963) and the radiomimetic and mutagenic properites of azaserine which are lacking in DON (Iyer and Szybalski, 1958, 1959; Pittillo, Narkates and Burns, 1965). Perhaps further work and reflection will resolve these problems.

Acknowledgments. This work was supported in part by the Cancer Chemotherapy National Service Center, National Cancer Institute, National Institutes of Health Contract No. PH 43-65-594. The capable assistance of Miss Mary Virginia Wright and Mrs. Mary Tucker Weir is appreciatively acknowledged.

References

Aaronson, S.: Mode of action of azaserine on *Gaffkya homari*. J. Bacteriol. **77**, 548 (1959).

Abrams, R., and M. Bentley: Biosynthesis of nucleic acid purines. III. Guanosine 5'-phosphate formation from xanthosine 5'-phosphate and L-glutamine. Arch. Biochem. Biophys. **79**, 91 (1959).

Ammann, C. A., and R. S. Safferman: The onion test as a possible screening method for antitumor agents. Antibiotics & Chemotherapy **8**, 1 (1958).

Anderson, L. E., J. Ehrlich, S. H. Sun, and P. R. Burkholder: Strains of *Streptomyces*, the sources of azaserine, elaiomycin, griseoviridin, and viridogrisein. Antibiotics & Chemotherapy **6**, 100 (1956).

Anderson, E. P., and L. W. Law: Biochemistry of cancer. Ann. Rev. Biochem. **29**, 577 (1960).

Anderson, E. P., B. Levenberg, and L. W. Law: Purine biosynthesis in azaserine-sensitive and -resistant lines of the mouse plasma cell neoplasm 70429. Federation Proc. **16**, 145 (1957).

Barclay, R. K., E. Garfinkel, and M. Phillipps: Effects of 6-diazo-5-oxo-L-norleucine on the incorporation of precursors into nucleic acids. Cancer Res. **22**, 809 (1962).

Barg, W., E. Boggiano, N. Sloane, and E. C. de Renzo: Inhibitors of *de novo* formyl glycinamide ribotide synthesis in pigeon liver extracts. Federation Proc. **16**, 150 (1957).

Barker, S. A., J. A. Bassham, M. Calvin, and U. A. Quark: Sites of azaserine inhibition during photosynthesis by *Scenedesmus*. J. Am. Chem. Soc. **78**, 4632 (1956).

Benbadis, M. C.: Modality of the resumption of mitotic activity in the radicular meristem of *Allium sativum* after moderate treatment with azaserine; comparison with the action of triethylene melamine. Compt. Rend. Soc. Biol. **260**, 268 (1965).

Bennett, Jr., L. L., F. M. Schabel, Jr., and H. E. Skipper: Studies on the mode of action of azaserine. Arch. Biochem. Biophys. **64**, 423 (1956).

BROCK, T. D., and M. L. BROCK: Reversal of azaserine by phenylalanine. J. Bacteriol. **81**, 212 (1961).

BROCKMAN, R. W.: Mechanisms of resistance to anticancer agents. In: A. HADDOW and S. WEINHOUSE (eds.), Advances in cancer research, vol. 7, p. 129. New York: Academic Press, Inc. 1963.

BROCKMAN, R. W., and E. P. ANDERSON: Biochemical effects of duazomycin A in the plasma cell neoplasm 70429. Proc. Am. Assoc. Cancer Research **3**, 307 (1962) (Abstract 32).

BUCHANAN, J. M.: The interference of azaserine in purine biosynthesis. In: G. E. W. WOLSTENHOLME and C. M. O'CONNOR (eds.), p. 75—88. Ciba foundation symposium on amino acids and peptides with antimetabolic activity. London: J. & A. Churchill, Ltd. 1958.

BURCHENAL, J. H., M. L. MURPHY, and C. T. C. TAN: Treatment of acute leukemia. Pediatrics **18**, 643 (1956).

BURCHENAL, J. H., M. L. MURPHY, C. T. C. TAN, M. YUCEOGLU, and D. A. KARNOFSKY: Combination therapy of acute leukemia with azaserine and mercaptopurine. Am. J. Diseases Children **90**, 644 (1955).

CLARKE, D. A., H. C. REILLY, and C. C. STOCK: A comparative study of 6-diazo-5-oxo-L-norleucine and O-diazoacetyl-L-serine on Sarcoma 180. Antibiotics & Chemotherapy **7**, 653 (1957).

COFFEY, G. L., A. B. HILLEGAS, M. P. KNUDSEN, H. J. KOEPSELL, J. E. OYAAS, and J. EHRLICH: Azaserine: microbiological studies. Antibiotics & Chemotherapy **4**, 775 (1954).

CRYSTAL, M. M.: The induction of sexual sterility in the screwworm fly by antimetabolites and alkylating agents. J. Econ. Entomol. **56** 468 (1963).

DAGG, C. P., and D. A. KARNOFSKY: Teratogenic effects of azaserine on the chick embryo. J. Exptl. Zool. **130**, 555 (1955).

DAWID, I. B., T. C. FRENCH, and J. M. BUCHANAN: Azaserine-reactive sulfhydryl group of 2-formamido-*N*-ribosylacetamide-5'-phosphate: L-glutamine amido-ligase (adenosine diphosphate). II. Degradation of azaserine-C^{14}-labeled enzyme. J. Biol. Chem. **238**, 2178 (1963).

DE VOE, S. E., N. E. RIGLER, A. J. SHAY, J. H. MARTIN, T. C. BOYD, E. J. BACKUS, J. H. MOWAT, and N. BOHONOS: Alazopeptin: production, isolation, and chemical characteristics. In: H. WELCH and F. MARTI-IBAÑEZ (eds.), Antibiotics annual, p. 730—735. New York: Medical Encyclopedia 1957.

DION, H. W., S. A. FUSARI, Z. L. JAKUBOWSKI, J. G. ZORA, and Q. R. BARTZ: 6-Diazo-5-oxo-L-norleucine, a new tumor-inhibitory substance. II. Isolation and characterization. J. Am. Chem. Soc. **78**, 3075 (1956).

DUVAL, L. R.: New agent data summaries: azaserine. Cancer Chemoth. Rept. **7**, 65 (1960a).

DUVAL, L. R.: New agent data summaries: 6-diazo-5-oxo-L-norleucine. Cancer Chemoth. Rept. **7**, 86 (1960b).

EHRLICH, J., L. E. ANDERSON, G. L. COFFEY, A. B. HILLEGAS, M. P. KNUDSEN, H. J. KOEPSELL, D. L. KOHBERGER, and J. E. OYAAS: Antibiotic studies of azaserine. Nature **173**, 72 (1954).

EHRLICH, J., G. L. COFFEY, M. W. FISHER, A. B. HILLEGAS, D. L. KOHBERGER, H. E. MACHAMER, W. A. RIGHTSEL, and F. R. ROEGNER: 6-Diazo-5-oxo-L-norleucine, a new tumor inhibitory substance. Antibiotics & Chemotherapy **6**, 487 (1956).

FERNANDES, J. F., G. A. LE PAGE, and A. LINDNER: The influence of azaserine and 6-mercaptopurine on the *in vivo* metabolism of ascites tumor cells. Cancer Research **16**, 154 (1956).

FRENCH, T. C., I. B. DAWID, and J. M. BUCHANAN: Azaserine reactive sulfhydryl group of 2-formamido-*N*-ribosylacetamide 5'-phosphate: L-glutamine amido-ligase (adenosine diphosphate). III. Comparison of degradation products with synthetic compounds. J. Biol. Chem. **238**, 2186 (1963).

FRENCH, T. C., I. B. DAWID, R. A. DAY, and J. M. BUCHANAN: Azaserine-reactive sulfhydryl group of 2-formamido-*N*-ribosylacetamide 5'-phosphate: L-glutamine amido-ligase (adenosine diphosphate). I. Purification and properties of the enzyme from *Salmonella typhimurium* and the synthesis of L-azaserine-C^{14}. J. Biol. Chem. **238**, 2171 (1963).
FRIEDMAN, M. H.: The effect of O-diazoacetyl-L-serine (azaserine) on the pregnancy of the dog; a preliminary report. J. Am. Vet. Med. Assoc. **130**, 159 (1957).
FUSARI, S. A., R. P. FROHARDT, A. RYDER, T. H. HASKELL, D. W. JOHANNESSEN, C. C. ELDER, and Q. R. BARTZ: Azaserine, a new tumor-inhibitory substance. Isolation and characterization. J. Am. Chem. Soc. **76**, 2878 (1954a).
FUSARI, S. A., T. H. HASKELL, R. B. FROHARDT, and Q. R. BARTZ: Azaserine, a new tumor-inhibitory substance. Structural studies. J. Am. Chem. Soc. **76**, 2881 (1954b).
GOLDTHWAIT, D. A.: 5-Phosphoribosylamine, a precursor of glycinamide ribotide. J. Biol. Chem. **222**, 1051 (1956).
GOTS, J. S., and E. G. GOLLUB: Purine metabolism in bacteria. IV. L-azaserine as an inhibitor. J. Bacteriol. **72**, 858 (1956).
GREENLEES, J., and G. A. LE PAGE: Purine biosynthesis and inhibitors in ascites cell tumors. Cancer Research **16**, 808 (1956).
GRISWOLD, D. P., W. R. LASTER, JR., M. Y. SNOW, F. M. SCHABEL, JR., and H. E. SKIPPER: Experimental evaluation of potential anticancer agents. XII. Quantitative drug response of SA 180, Ca 755, and leukemia L 1210 systems to a standard list of active and inactive agents. Cancer Research, Suppl. (part. 2), **23**(4), 271 (1963).
GROSCH, D. S.: Insect fecundity and fertility: chemically induced decrease. Science **141**, 732 (1963).
HARRIS, J. J.: The effect of NSC survey compounds on human tumors in embryonated eggs. Cancer Research, Suppl. (part 2), **22**(1), 1 (1962).
HARTMAN, S. C.: Glutamine-phosphoribosyl pyrophosphate amidotransferase (GPA). Federation Proc. **21**, 244 (1962).
HARTMAN, S. C., B. LEVENBERG, and J. M. BUCHANAN: Involvement of ATP, 5-phosphoribosylpyrophosphate and L-azaserine in the enzymatic formation of glycinamide ribotide intermediates in inosinic acid biosynthesis. J. Am. Chem. Soc. **77**, 501 (1955).
HEDEGAARD, J., S. MASPERO-SEGRE, N. V. THOAI, and J. ROCHE: Influence of histidine and its metabolites on biosynthesis of purines by *Escherichia coli* B. IV. Action on cultures inhibited by azaserine. Compt. Rend. Soc. Biol. **153**, 767 (1959a).
HEDEGAARD, J., S. MASPERO-SEGRE, N. V. THOAI, and J. ROCHE: Influences of histidine and its metabolites on biosynthesis of purines by *Escherichia coli* B. V. Mode of action in cultures inhibited by azaserine. Compt. Rend. Soc. Biol. **153**, 954 (1959b).
HEDEGAARD, J., N. V. THOAI, and J. ROCHE: The influence of histidine on the biosynthesis of purines in *Escherichia coli*. Arch. Biochem. Biophys. **83**, 183 (1959).
HENDERSON, J. R., and I. G. FUNGA: Inhibition of ascites tumor growth by 4-aminopyrazolo[3,4-*d*]pyrimidine in combination with azaserine, 6-mercaptopurine, and thioguanine. Cancer Research **20**, 1618 (1960).
HENDERSON, J. R., and I. G. FUNGA: Treatment of ascites tumors with 4-aminopyrazolo[3,4-*d*]pyrimidine alone and in combination with azaserine, thioguanine, and 6-mercaptopurine. Cancer Research (part 2), **21**(3), 7 (1961).
HUTCHISON, D. J.: Cross resistance and collateral sensitivity studies in cancer chemotherapy. In: A. HADDOW and S. WEINHOUSE (eds.), Advances in cancer research, vol. 7, p. 235. New York: Academic Press, Inc. 1963.
HUTCHISON, D. J., D. L. ROBINSON, D. MARTIN, O. L. ITTENSOHN, and J. DILLENBERG: Effects of selected cancer chemotherapeutic drugs on the survival times of mice with L 1210 leukemia: relative responses of antimetabolite-resistant strains. Cancer Research, Suppl., (part 2), **22**(1), 57 (1962).

IYER, V. N., and W. SZYBALSKI: Mechanism of chemical mutagenesis. I. Kinetic studies on the action of triethylene melamine (TEM) and azaserine. Proc. Natl. Acad. Sci. U.S. **44**, 446 (1958).

IYER, V. N., and W. SZYBALSKI: Mutagenic effect of azaserine in relation to azaserine resistance in *E. coli*. Science **129**, 839 (1959).

JACQUEZ, J. A.: Active transport of O-diazoacetyl-L-serine and 6-diazo-5-oxo-L-norleucine in Ehrlich ascites carcinoma. Cancer Research **17**, 890 (1957).

JACQUEZ, J. A.: Concentrative uptake of 6-diazo-5-oxo-L-norleucine by sarcoma 180, liver and muscle *in vivo*. Proc. Soc. Exptl. Biol. Med. **99**, 611 (1958).

JACQUEZ, J. A., and J. H. SHERMAN: Enzymatic degradation of azaserine. Cancer Research **22**(1), 56 (1962).

JAFFRE, J. J.: *In vivo* activity of L-azaserine against *Trypanosoma equiperdum*. J. Protozool. **10**, 340 (1963).

JOHNSON, I. S., L. A. BAKER, and H. F. WRIGHT: Possible utility of the Rous Sarcoma for antitumor screening. Ann. N.Y. Acad. Sci. **76**, 861 (1958).

KAPLAN, L., H. C. REILLY, and C. C. STOCK: Action of azaserine on *Escherichia coli*. J. Bacteriol. **78**, 511 (1959).

KAPLAN, L., and C. C. STOCK: Azaserine, an inhibitor of amino acid synthesis in *Escherichia coli*. Federation Proc. **13**, 239 (1954).

KARNOFSKY, D. A., and C. R. LACON: Survey of cancer chemotherapy service center compounds for teratogenic effect in the chick embryo. Cancer Research, Suppl. (part 2), **22**(1), 84 (1962).

KOHBERGER, D. L., H. C. REILLY, G. L. COFFEY, A. B. HILLEGAS, and J. EHRLICH: Azaserine assay with *Kloeckera brevis*. Antibiotics & Chemotherapy **5**(2), 59 (1955).

LANGAN, T. A., N. O. KAPLAN, and L. SHUSTER: Formation of the nicotinic acid analogue of diphosphopyridine nucleotide after nicotinamide administration. J. Biol. Chem. **234**, 2161 (1959).

LEE, K. H., and Y. YUZURIHA: Studies on cell growth and cell division III. Action of azaserine on cell division. J. Pharm. Sci. **53**, 290 (1964).

LEE, K. H., Y. O. YUZURIHA, and J. J. EILER: Studies on cell growth and cell division. II. Selective activity of chloramphenicol and azaserine on cell growth and cell division. J. Am. Pharm. Assoc. **48**, 470 (1959).

LE PAGE, G. A., and N. HOWARD: Chemotherapy studies of mammary tumors of C_3H mice. Cancer Research **23**, 622 (1963).

LEVENBERG, B., I. MELNICK, and J. M. BUCHANAN: Biosynthesis of the purines. XV. The effect of aza-L-serine and 6-diazo-5-oxo-L-norleucine on inosinic acid biosynthesis *de novo*. J. Biol. Chem. **225**, 163 (1957).

LOUSTALOT, P., P. A. DESAULLES, and R. MEIER: Characterization of the specificity of action of tumor-inhibiting compounds. Ann. N.Y. Acad. Sci. **76**, 838 (1958).

MAXWELL, R. E., and V. S. NICKEL: Filament formation in *Escherichia coli* induced by azaserine and other antineoplastic agents. Science **120**, 270 (1954).

MAXWELL, R. E., and V. S. NICKEL: 6-Diazo-5-oxo-L-norleucine, a new tumor inhibitory substance. V. Microbiologic studies of mode of action. Antibiotics & Chemotherapy **7**, 81 (1957).

MCCARTHY, D. A., A. BAYLES, and P. E. THOMPSON: The effect of azaserine against *Plasmodium lophurae* in chicks and attempts to antagonize this effect with metabolites. J. Parasitol. **43**, 283 (1957).

MERCKER, P. C., P. ANIDO, J. SARINO, and G. W. WOOLLEY: A study of human epidermoid carcinoma (H.Ep. No. 3) growing in conditioned Swiss mice. III. Chemotherapy with selected chemicals and observations on diet, food intake, and drug toxicities. Cancer Research, Suppl. (part 2) **22**(1), 9 (1962).

VAN DER MEULEN, P. Y. F., and J. A. BASSHAM: Study of inhibition of azaserine and diazoöxonorleucine (DON) on the algae *Scenedesmus* and *Chlorella*. J. Am. Chem. Soc. **81**, 2233 (1959).

MOORE, E. C., and R. B. HURLBERT: Biosynthesis of ribonucleic acid (RNA), cytosine, and RNA purines: differential inhibition by diazoöxonorleucine. Cancer Research **21**, 257 (1961).

MURPHY, M. L., and D. A. KARNOFSKY: Effect of azaserine and other growth-inhibiting agents on fetal development of the rat. Cancer **9**, 955 (1962).
NAKAMURA, M.: Amoebicidal action of azaserine. Nature **178**, 1119 (1956).
NARKATES, A. J., and R. F. PITTILLO: Inhibition of nonproliferating *Escherichia coli* by azaserine. In: J. C. SYLVESTER (ed.), p. 439—446, Antimicrobial agents and chemotherapy, 1963. Ann Arbor: Braum-Brumfield, Inc. American Society for Microbiology 1964.
NORMAN, A. G.: Inhibition of root growth by azaserine. Science **121**, 213 (1955).
NORMAN, A. G.: Inhibition of root growth and cation uptake by antibiotics. Soil Sci. Soc. Am. Proc. **23**, 368 (1959).
PATTERSON, E. L., B. L. JOHNSON, S. E. DEVOE, and N. BOHONOS: Structure of the antitumor antibiotic alazopeptin (Abstract 38), p. 18. In: Abstracts of papers presented at the fifth interscience conference on antimicrobial agents and chemotherapy 1965.
PITTILLO, R. F.: Studies on the antimicrobial nature of action of azaserine. In: P. GRAY, B. TABENKIN and S. G. BRADLEY (eds.), Antimicrobial agents annual, p. 276—287, 1960. New York: Plenum Press 1961.
PITTILLO, R. F., A. J. NARKATES, and J. BURNS: Microbiological evaluation of 1,3-bis (2-chloroethyl)-1-nitrosourea. Cancer Res. **24**, 1222 (1964).
PITTILLO, R. F., and B. G. QUINNELLY: Further studies on the antimicrobial nature of action of azaserine. In: M. FINLAND and G. M. SAVAGE (eds.), Antimicrobial agents and chemotherapy, p. 245—253, 1961. Detroit: American Society for Microbiology 1962.
POTTER, M., and L. W. LAW: Studies of a plasma cell neoplasm of the mouse. I. Characterization of neoplasm 70429, including its sensitivity to various antimetabolites with the rapid development of resistance to azaserine, DON, and N-methyl formamide. J. Natl. Cancer Inst. **18**, 413 (1957).
PREISLER, O.: Effect of cytostatic agents on the genital development of rabbits. Arch. Gynäkol. **192**, 501 (1960).
PREISS, J., and P. HANDLER: Biosynthesis of disphosphopyridine nucleotide. II. Enzymatic aspects. J. Biol. Chem. **233**, 493 (1958).
RAO, K. V.: Chemistry of the duazomycins. I. Duazomycins A. In: M. FINLAND and G. M. SAVAGE (eds.), Antimicrobial agents and chemotherapy, 1961, p. 178—183. Detroit: American Society for Microbiology 1962.
RAO, K. V., S. C. BROOKS, JR., M. KUGELMAN, and A. A. ROMANO: Duazomycins A, B, and C, three antitumor substances. I. Isolation and characterization. In: H. WELCH and F. MARTI-IBAÑEZ (eds.), Antibiotics annual, p. 943—948. New York: Medical Encyclopedia 1960.
REILLY, H. C.: Inactivation of azaserine by a liver enzyme. Federation Proc. **13**, 279 (1954a).
REILLY, H. C.: The effect of amino acids upon the antimicrobial activity of azaserine. Proc. Am. Assoc. Cancer Res. **1**, 40 (1954b).
REILLY, H. C.: Effect of test medium upon the demonstration of antimicrobial activities of certain antibiotics. Bacteriol. Proc. **9**, 72 (1956).
REILLY, H. C.: Some aspects of azaserine, 6-diazo-5-oxo-L-norleucine and β-2-Thienylalanine. In: G. E. W. WOLSTENHOLME and C. M. O'CONNOR (eds.), Ciba foundation symposium on amino acids and peptides with antimetabolic activity, p. 62—74. London: J. and. A. Churchill, Ltd. 1958.
RIVERA, A., and P. R. SRINIVASAN: 3-Enolpyruvylshikimate 5-phosphate, an intermediate in the biosynthesis of anthranilate. Proc. Natl. Acad. Sci. U.S. **48**, 864 (1962).
SARTORELLI, A. C., and B. A. BOOTH: Comparative studies on the *in vivo* action of 6-chloropurine,6-chloropurine ribonucleoside, and 6-chloro-9-ethylpurine on sarcoma 180 ascites cells. J. Parmacol. Exptl. Ther. **134**, 123 (1961).
SARTORELLI, A. C., and B. A. BOOTH: Some factors affecting the tumor-inhibitory properties of combinations of azaserine and 6-chloropurine. Biochem. Pharmacol. **12**, 847 (1963).

SARTORELLI, A. C., and G. A. LE PAGE: Inhibition of ascites cell growth by combinations of 6-thioguanine and azaserine. Cancer Res. **18**, 938 (1958).

SKIPPER, H. E.: Perspectives in cancer chemotherapy: therapeutic design. Cancer Res. **24**, (8), 1295 (1964).

SRINIVASAN, P. R.: Enzymatic synthesis of anthranilic acid from shikimic acid-5-phosphate and L-glutamine. J. Am. Chem. Soc. **81**, 1772 (1959).

SRINIVASAN, P. R., and B. WEISS: The biosynthesis of *p*-amino-benzoic acid: studies on the origin of the amino group. Biochem. Biophys. Acta **51**, 597 (1961).

STOCK, C. C., H. C. REILLY, S. M. BUCKLEY, D. A. CLARKE, and C. P. RHOADS: Azaserine, a new tumor inhibitory substance: studies with Crocker mouse sarcoma 180. Nature **173**, 71 (1954).

SUGIURA, K.: Studies in a spectrum of mouse, rat, and hamster tumors. Cancer Res., Suppl. (part 2) **22**(1), 93 (1962).

TARNOWSKI, G. S., and C. C. STOCK: Effects of combinations of azaserine and 6-diazo-5-oxo-L-norleucine with purine analogs and other antimetabolites on the growth of two mouse mammary carcinomas. Cancer Res. **17**, 1033 (1957).

TELLER, M. N.: Chemotherapy of transplantable human tumors in the rat. Cancer Res., Suppl. (part 2) **22**(1), 25 (1962).

THIERSCH, J. B.: Effect of O-diazo acetyl-L-serine on rat litter. Proc. Soc. Exptl. Biol. Med. **94**, 27 (1957a).

THIERSCH, J. B.: Effect of 6-diazo-5-oxo-L-norleucine (DON) on the rat litter *in utero*. Proc. Soc. Exptl. Biol. Med. **94**, 33 (1957b).

TOMISEK, A. J., H. J. KELLY, and H. E. SKIPPER: Chromatographic studies of purine metabolism. I. The effect of azaserine on purine biosynthesis in *E. coli* using various C^{14}-labeled precursors. Arch. Biochem. Biophys. **64**(2), 437 (1956).

TOMISEK, A., M. R. REID, W. A. SHORT, and H. E. SKIPPER: Studies on the photosynthetic reaction. III. The effects of various inhibitors upon growth and carbonate-fixation in *Chlorella pyrenoidosa*. Plant Physiol. **32**, 7 (1957).

TOMISEK, A. J., M. R. REID, and H. E. SKIPPER: Chromatographic studies of purine metabolism. IV. Reversal of azaserine-induced inhibition by phenylalanine and tryptophan. Cancer Res. **19**, 489 (1959).

TRUHANT, R., and G. DEYSSON: Use of the plant cell as test object for the control of cancer by application of radiomimetics. Bull. assoc. franç. étude cancer. **44**, 221 (1957).

WHEELER, G. P., F. M. SCHABEL, JR., and H. E. SKIPPER: Potentiated inhibition of *Escherichia coli* by certain combinations of agents. Proc. Soc. Exptl. Biol. Med. **92**, 396 (1956).

WOOLLEY, G. W.: Chemotherapy of transplantable human tumors in the hamster. Cancer Res., Suppl. (part 2), **22**(1), 34 (1962).

Tubercidin and Related Pyrrolopyrimidine Antibiotics

George Acs and Edward Reich

The pyrrolopyrimidine ribosides constitute a newly characterized class of cytotoxic nucleoside antibiotics. Because their discovery and the elucidation of their structure have occurred so recently, relatively little information concerning the biological properties of these interesting compounds has accumulated. This

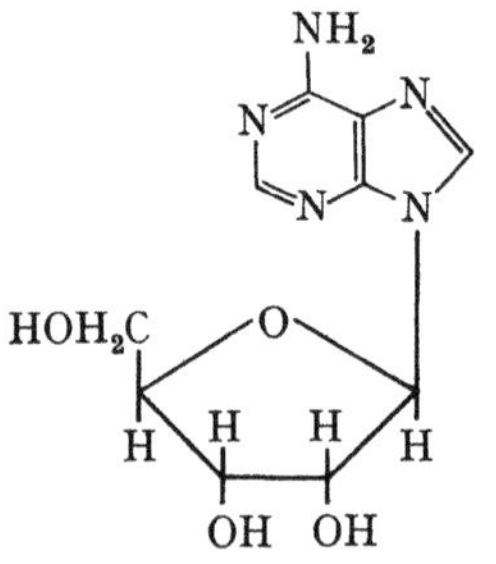

Adenosine

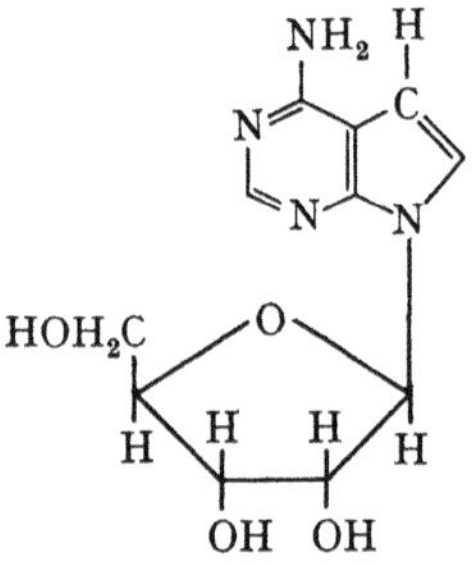

Tubercidin

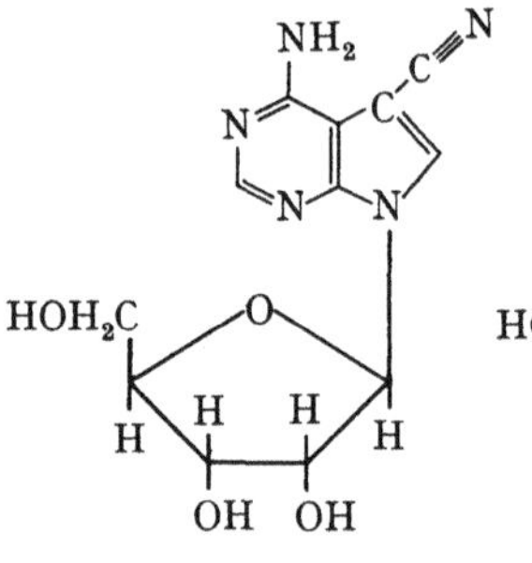

Toyocamycin

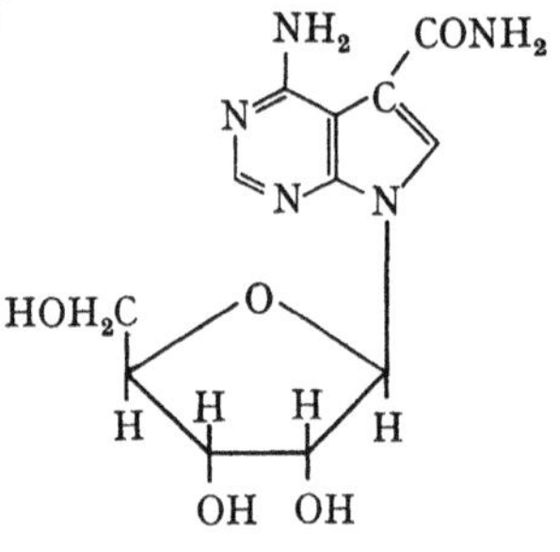

Sangivamycin

article summarizes briefly some exploratory experiments on the metabolism and mode of action of the pyrrolopyrimidine antibiotics. Tubercidin was discovered in Japan by ANZAI *et al.* (1957) and its structure was established by SUZUKI and MARUMO (1961a and b). It is produced by *Streptomyces tubercidicus*. The discovery and characterization of toyocamycin and sangivamycin are described by NISHIMURA *et al.* (1956) and by RAO (1963). Tubercidin inhibits the growth of several microorganisms including *Mycobacterium tuberculosis*, is toxic to many vertebrate species, and is powerfully cytotoxic to vertebrate cell lines in culture (ANZAI *et al.*, 1957; ACS *et al.*, 1964; OWEN *et al.*, 1964).

All three antibiotics are analogues of adenosine and are excellent substrates for adenosine kinase. The remarkable stability of the glycosidic bond in the pyrrolopyrimidine ribosides (MIZUNO *et al.*, 1961), and the complete lack of toxicity of the tubercidin aglycone (ACS *et al.*, 1964; DAVOLL, 1960), make it almost certain that these antibiotics enter cellular metabolism by being converted to the corresponding nucleoside monophosphate through phosphorylation at the 5′-position by adenosine kinase. This assumption could be proved if mutant cells resistant to the antibiotics could be isolated and shown to lack adenosine kinase or to have an enzyme of altered specificity. No such mutants have been reported to date. It may be significant in this respect that *Escherichia coli*, extracts of which have little or no detectable adenosine kinase, is resistant to high levels of tubercidin, (SLECHTA personal communication).

Several lines of evidence show that phosphorylated derivatives of the pyrrolopyrimidines are present in susceptible cells:

1. The acid-soluble fraction of washed mouse fibroblasts previously exposed to radioactive tubercidin for a few hours contains most of the radioactivity extracted from the medium. Virtually all the intracellular radioactivity is accounted for by tubercidin 5′-mono, -di-, and triphosphates, only traces of the free nucleoside being found in the acid soluble fraction (ACS *et al.*, 1964).

2. Mammalian erythrocytes exposed to radioactive tubercidin *in vivo* or *in vitro* accumulate tubercidin nucleotides (SMITH *et al.*, 1966).

3. Tubercidin is incorporated into the nucleic acids of a susceptible bacterium, *Streptococcus faecalis* (BLOCH *et al.*, 1966).

4. Cultures of growing mouse fibroblasts incubated with radioactive tubercidin incorporate small but definite amounts of tubercidin into cellular RNA and DNA. Likewise, tubercidin is incorporated into the virus-directed RNA synthesized in fibroblasts infected with Mengovirus (ACS *et al.*, 1964).

Finally, fibroblasts growing in the presence of 2′-deoxytubercidin incorporate some of this analogue into DNA (ACS *et al.*, 1964). Since all known nucleic acid polymerases require nucleoside-5-triphosphates for nucleic acid synthesis, these findings show that the 5′-triphosphates of tubercidin and 2′-deoxytubercidin are formed within the cell and are accessible both to nuclear and cytoplasmic poly-

	Tu	Toyo	Sang.
Hexokinase (yeast)	+	+	+
Myokinase (rabbit muscle)	+	+	O
Phosphoenolpyruvate kinase (rabbit muscle)	+	+	O
RNA polymerase (E. coli)	+	+	+
Polynucleotide phosphorylase (E. coli)	+	—	—
DNA polymerase (E. coli) (Mn^{++} reaction)	+	—	+
Aminoacyl s-RNA synthetases (rabbit liver)	—	O	*
Aminoacyl s-RNA synthetases (E. coli)	—	O	O
Myosin ATP-ase (rabbit muscle)	+	O	O
Terminal C-C-A-sRNA pyrophosphorylase (rabbit liver)	+	+	+
Adenosine kinase (rabbit liver) — as nucleoside	+	+	+
— as triphosphate	+	O	O

+ = functions as substrate; — = not a substrate; * = a competitive inhibitor of the over-all reaction; O = not tested.

merizing systems. Preliminary experiments (Reich *et al.*, unpublished results) indicate that toyocamycin is also incorporated into cellular RNA (but not DNA), and that sangivamycin is incorporated into both nucleic acids by purified enzymes.

The close resemblance between tubercidin and adenosine suggests that tubercidin nucleotides should substitute for adenine nucleotides in a variety of reactions. The enzymes listed below have been tested for their ability to use pyrrolopyrimidine nucleotides as substrates (Acs *et al.*, 1964). Affinity constants (Km) have not been determined for any of these; however, the conditions selected, and the reaction velocities observed make it unlikely that these differ by as much as an order of magnitude from the values for the corresponding adenine nucleotides.

In addition to participating in the reactions listed above, the following properties of pyrrolopyrimidine nucleotides should be noted:

1. Tubercidin-5′-monophosphate has been observed to give rise to the corresponding analogue of diphosphopyridine nucleotide when incubated with cell-free extracts of bacterial cells (Bloch *et al.*, 1966).

2. Tubercidin supresses the biosynthesis of purine nucleotides in cultures of mouse fibroblasts (Reich *et al.*, unpublished results), and in ascites cells (Henderson *et al.*, 1965). It has not been established whether this inhibition is due to false feed-back inhibition or to interference with the synthesis of specific precursors, such as glutamine and phosphoribosylpyrophosphate, required for purine formation.

3. A homopolymer of tubercidin monophosphate and copolymers of tubercidin monophosphate, and uridylic acid have been synthesized. The coding properties of these polymers for polypeptide synthesis in cell-free systems are indistinguishable from the corresponding adenine-containing polymers (Reich *et al.*, unpublished results).

4. When tubercidin is incorporated into the end-groups of s-RNA in place of adenosine, the resulting s-RNA functions normally with respect to aminoacylation by activating enzymes, association with ribosome-synthetic polynucleotide complexes, and transfer of amino acids into polypeptide. Comparable substitution of adenosine by toyocamycin or sangivamycin decreases the amino acid acceptor activity of s-RNA (Reich *et al.*, unpublished results).

The data available to date permit no definite conclusions concerning the primary biological action of tubercidin. Since tubercidin-nucleotides can replace adenine nucleotides in so many reactions, it appears possible that the cytotoxicity, and/or antibacterial action might be the cumulative result of quantitative effects involving numerous cellular processes. An additional possibility is that one or more cellular functions are inhibited (competitively, by false repression or false feed-back inhibition) by some tubercidin nucleotide. Moreover, the primary biological action of tubercidin and its relatives may well vary among different cell-types. For example, the observation that *Streptococcus faecalis* can be protected against the toxic action of tubercidin by a mixture of amino acids, nucleosides, ribose-5-phosphate and pyruvate has prompted the suggestion that the primary action of the antibiotic is due to interference with pyridine-nucleotide dependent reactions (Bloch *et al.*, 1966). No such protective effect is seen in mammalian cell systems.

Several observations suggest that the toxicity of these antibiotics to mammalian cells derives, at least in part, from their incorporation into nucleic acids. When mouse fibroblasts are exposed to tubercidin, morphological changes which closely resemble a typical viral cytopathogenic effect develop within a few hours (REICH *et al.*, unpublished results). These changes are prevented by actinomycin which blocks the incorporation of tubercidin into RNA, but does not inhibit either the cellular uptake of the antibiotic, nor its phosphorylation or incorporation into DNA. A second related finding concerns the effect of tubercidin on Mengovirus growth in mouse fibroblasts. When Mengovirus infection proceeds in the presence of appropriate concentrations of tubercidin viral RNA is synthesised, a typical viral cytopathogenic effect is observed, and tubercidin is incorporated into the viral RNA. However, the production of infective progeny virus is profoundly inhibited.

These results should not be interpreted as suggesting that all cellular effects of tubercidin in mammalian cells can be explained by its incorporation into RNA. For example, the antibiotic strongly inhibits DNA synthesis and especially protein synthesis; and these effects follow antibiotic administration too promptly to be accounted for by the production of faulty RNA.

The pyrrolopyrimidine antibiotics deserve to be studied in greater detail for several reasons:

1. The study of these analogues will yield additional information about pathways of nucleotide metabolism in normal cells.

2. Changes in structure of the pyrrolopyrimidine nucleus markedly affect the metabolism of the antibiotic. Thus, whereas tubercidin strongly inhibits all cellular macromolecule synthesis and is incorporated into both DNA and RNA, toyocamycin selectively inhibits only cellular RNA synthesis, and is not incorporated into DNA in intact cells or enzyme preparations.

3. Both toyocamycin and sangivamycin are readily converted by mammalian cells and enzymes to the corresponding nucleoside polyphosphates. This demonstrates that the introduction of even large and complex functional groups at the corresponding position of the nucleus does not deter the entry of the altered nucleosides into cellular nucleotide metabolism. Moreover, the functional groups of these two antibiotics provide exceptionally favorable starting material for the production of a wide variety of chemical modifications and derivatives.

All the above considerations suggest that the study of this family of antibiotics may provide some insights which could ultimately facilitate the rational design of specific chemotherapeutic and antiviral agents. In addition, pyrrolopyrimidine nucleotides will be useful reagents for exploring the substrate specificity of nucleotide metabolizing enzymes.

References

ACS, G., E. REICH, and M. MORI: Biological and biochemical properties of the analogue antibiotic tubercidin. Proc. Natl. Acad. Sci. U.S. **52**, 493 (1964).

ANZAI, K., and S. MARUMO: A new antibiotic, tubercidin. J. Antibiotics (Japan), Ser. A, **10**, 201 (1957).

ANZAI, K., G. NAKAMURA, and S. SUZUKI: A new antibiotic, tubercidin. J. Antibiotics (Japan), Ser. A **10**, 201 (1957).

Bhuyan, B. K., H. E. Renis, and C. G. Smith: A collagen plate assay for cytotoxic agents. II. Biological studies. Cancer Research **22**, 1131—1136 (1962).
Bloch, A., R. Y. Leonard, and C. A. Nichol: On the mode of action of the nucleoside antibiotic tubercidin. Federation Proc. **25**, 454 (1966).
Brindle, S. A., N. A. Gjuffre, B. J. Amrein, R. C. Millonig, and D. Perlman: Antibiotic sensitivity of Ehrlich ascites cells grown in tissue culture. Antimicrobial Agents and Chemotherapy 159—161 (1961).
Davoll, J.: Pyrrolo[2,3-d]pyrimidines. J. Chem. Soc. **1960**, 131.
Henderson, J. F., and M. K. Y. Khoo: On the mechanism of feedback inhibition of purine biosynthesis *de novo* in Ehrlich ascites tumor cells *in vitro*. J. Biol. Chem. **240**, 3104 (1965).
Ikehara, M., and Eiko Ohtsuka: Stimulation of the binding of aminoacyl-sRNA to ribosomes by tubercidin (7-deazaadenosine) and N^6-dimethyladenosine containing trinucleoside diphosphate analogs. Biochem. Biophys. Research. Commun. **21**, No. 3, 257—264 (1965).
Nakamura, G.: Studies on antibiotic actinomycetes. II. J. Antibiotics (Japan) Ser. A **14**, 90 (1961).
Nishimura, H., K. Katagiri, K. Sato, M. Mayama, and N. Shimaoka: Toyocamycin, a new anti-candida antibiotics. J. Antibiotics (Japan), Ser. A **9**, 60 (1956).
Ohkuma, K.: Chemical structure of toyocamycin. J. Antibiotics (Japan), Ser. A **13**, 361 (1960).
Ohkuma, K.: Chemical structure of toyocamycin. J. Antibiotics (Japan), Ser. A **14**, 345 (1961).
Owen, S. P., and C. G. Smith: Cytotoxicity and antitumor properties of the abnormal nucleoside tubercidin. Cancer Chemoth. Rep. **36**, 19 (1964).
Rao, K. V.: Antimicrobial Agents and Chemotherapy 77 (1963).
Reich, E., and G. Acs: Unpublished results.
Renis, H. E., H. G. Johnson, and B. K. Bhuyan: A collagen plate assay for vytotoxic agents. I. Methods. Cancer Research **22**, 1126—1130 (1962).
Slechta, L.: Personal communication.
Smith, C. G., W. L. Lummis, and J. E. Grady: An improved tissue culture assay. II. Cytotoxicity studies with antibiotics, chemicals, and solvents. Cancer Research **19**, 847—852 (1959).
Smith, C. G., L. M. Reineke, and H. Harpootlian: Uptake of tubercidin and seven-deazainosine by human blood cells. Abstract: Proc. Am. Soc. Cancer Research **7**, 66 (1966).
Suzuki, S., and S. Marumo: Chemical structure of tubercidin. J. Antibiotics (Japan), Ser. A **13**, 360 (1960).
Suzuki, S., and S. Marumo: Chemical structure of tubercidin. J. Antibiotics (Japan), Ser. A **14**, 34 (1961a).
Suzuki, S., and S. Marumo: Chemical structure of tubercidin. J. Antibiotics (Japan), Ser A **14**, 34 (1961b).

Sideromycins

J. Nüesch and F. Knüsel

In recent years, substances containing iron and showing a broad absorption band, with an absorption maximum between 420 and 440 mμ, have been isolated from cultures of various microorganisms (BICKEL *et al.*, 1960a; PRELOG, 1963; KELLER-SCHIERLEIN *et al.*, 1964). Within this group of naturally occurring substances can be found some which display antibiotic properties, whereas others antagonise this antibiotic activity and actually promote the growth of certain micro-organisms. Chemical studies have revealed that all these substances are iron (III)-trihydroxamate complexes. For this reason, BICKEL *et al.* (1960a) designated them collectively as "siderochromes". Subsequently, ZÄHNER *et al.* (1962) subdivided them on the basis of their biological properties into the following categories:

a) Sideromycins; i.e. siderochromes displaying antibiotic activity.

b) Sideramines; i.e. siderochromes which competitively antagonise the antibiotic effect of the sideromycins and which also exert a growth-promoting action on certain micro-organisms.

c) Siderochromes whose biological properties are as yet unknown.

The sideromycins were first to be discovered. Grisein was described by REYNOLDS *et al.* in 1947. In 1951 GAUSE and BRAZHNIKOVA published a paper on albomycin, a new sideromycin which is closely related to, or possibly identical with, grisein. Both these antibiotics have a relatively broad spectrum of antibacterial activity. BICKEL *et al.* (1960a) described ferrimycin and other sideromycins with a narrow spectrum of action that was confined to Gram-positive bacteria. Other antibiotics of this type were later discovered (HASKELL *et al.*, 1963; TSUKIURA *et al.*, 1964). Thus, sideromycins have been obtained only from a few species of actinomycetes. The sideramines, by contrast, have a wide distribution and can be isolated from micro-organisms belonging to various systematic groups (ZÄHNER *et al.*, 1962). There are three main features which distinguish the sideromycins from other antibiotics; they display cross-resistance to one another; their action can be competitively antagonised by structurally related, microbial metabolites (sideramines); and sideromycin-sensitive bacterial populations show a very marked tendency to develop resistance to them.

BICKEL *et al.* (1960a) divided the sideromycins into three groups on the basis of their spectrum of activity and their paperchromatographic behaviour:

Group 1: Sideromycins active against Gram-positive and Gram-negative bacteria.

Groups 2 and 3: Sideromycins active against Gram-positive bacteria only. Groups 2 and 3 differ in their paperchromatographic behaviour (BICKEL *et al.*, 1960a).

Table 1. *The producers of sideromycins (from* KELLER-SCHIERLEIN *et al.*, 1964*)*

Group of sidero-mycins	Species	Strain No.	Sideromycin	Literature
1	*S. griseus* WAKSMAN and HENRICI	G-25	Grisein	REYNOLDS *et al.* (1947)
				REYNOLDS and WAKSMAN (1948)
	S. griseus	6 strains	Grisein	OKAMI (1950)
				UMEZAWA *et al.* (1949)
	A. subtropicus KUDRINA et KOCHETKOVA	39,738	Albomycin	GAUSE and BRAZHNIKOVA (1951)
	Species similar to *S. griseus*	I A-1787	Similar to grisein	THRUM (1957)
2	*S. aureofaciens* Duggar	ETH 22083	Antibiotic A 22765	ZÄHNER *et al.* (1960)
	S. aureofaciens	ETH 22765	Antibiotic A 22765	ZÄHNER *et al.* (1960)
	S. aureofaciens	ETH 22931	Antibiotic A 22765	BICKEL *et al.* (1960a)
	S. olivochromogenes (WAKSMAN) WAKSMAN and HENRICI		Succinimycin	HASKELL *et al.* (1963)
	S. albaduncus TSUKIURA *et al.*	13246	Danomycin	TSUKIURA *et al.* (1964)
3	*S. griseoflavus* (KRAINSKY) WAKSMAN and HENRICI	ETH 9578	Ferrimycin	BICKEL *et al.* (1960b)
	S. griseoflavus	ETH 15311	Ferrimycin	ZÄHNER *et al.* (1960)
	S. lavendulae (WAKSMAN and CURTIS) WAKSMAN and HENRICI	ETH 14677	Ferrimycin	ZÄHNER *et al.* (1960)
	S. lavendulae	ETH 21510	Ferrimycin	ZÄHNER *et al.* (1960)
				BICKEL *et al.* (1960b)
	S. galilaeus ETTLINGER *et al.*	ETH 18822	Ferrimycin	ZÄHNER *et al.* (1960)
				BICKEL *et al.* (1960b)
2 or 3	*S. sp.*	LA 5352	Antibiotic LA 5352	SENSI and TIMBAL (1958)
	S. sp.	LA 5937	Antibiotic LA 5937	SENSI and TIMBAL (1958)

Producers of sideromycins have so far been found only among the actinomycetes. Table 1 lists the various antibiotics and the micro-organisms which produce them.

HÜTTER (1963) assigned the albomycin-producing *Streptomyces subtropicus* KUDRINA and KOCHETKOVA to the species *Streptomyces griseus* WAKSMAN and HENRICI. Thus, all the Streptomyces strains producing the sideromycins in group 1 belong to the species *Streptomyces griseus*. The sideromycins in groups 2 and 3, on the other hand, have been obtained from strains of various species belonging to the genus *Streptomyces* WAKSMAN and HENRICI.

The method by which producer-strains are cultured for the fermentation of sideromycins does not differ to any marked extent from that employed in the production of other antibiotics. The processes are based on submerged, aerobic cultivation in fermenters, using various complex nutrient media. The carbohydrate sources and iron content of the media appear to play an important role. Like the sideramines, the sideromycins are presumably released into the culture solution in their iron-free form. Generally the yield is extremely small, averaging between 1 and 100 mcg./ml. Frequently a sideramine is produced in addition to the sideromycin (REYNOLDS *et al.*, 1947; REYNOLDS and WAKSMAN, 1948; BRINBERG and GRINYUK, 1959; BICKEL *et al.*, 1960b).

Chemistry

The sideromycins are readily soluble in strongly polar solvents such as water, dimethylformamide, glycol, and methylcellosolve. Some of them are also soluble in methanol; however, all the sideromycins are completely insoluble in less polar solvents. All of them are highly soluble in phenol as well as in mixtures of phenol and lipoid solvents (e.g. chloroform). The sideromycins can be extracted with the aid of such mixtures. By diluting the extracts with ether it is possible to expel the antibiotics from the organic phase and to extract them with water (KELLER-SCHIERLEIN *et al.*, 1964). Adsorption on charcoal and the use of ion-exchangers are also suitable for isolating sideromycins. Often combinations of various methods are employed (REYNOLDS and WAKSMAN, 1948; BICKEL *et al.*, 1960b; HASKELL *et al.*, 1963; TSUKIURA *et al.*, 1964).

It is usually very difficult to purify the sideromycins contained in crude extracts. The great difficulty in preparing these antibiotics in pure form is chiefly due to the low yields in culture media. The crude extracts contain large quantities of inactive components from the nutrient solution, as well as fermentation products displaying similar physico-chemical properties, and these impurities prove troublesome. Furthermore some of the sideromycins are quite unstable over a wide range of pH levels.

The sideromycins can be roughly classified into groups by reference to their basicity, their behaviour with respect to adsorbents and precipitants, and their partition coefficients in suitable solvents. Accurate characterisation is possible with the aid of paper-chromatography and electrophoresis (BICKEL *et al.*, 1960b). The classic methods of characterisation (melting point, infra-red spectrum, etc.) are only of limited value in the case sideromycins. The general properties of the sideromycins, as outlined above, make it difficult to identify them by physico-chemical means. Hence, for this group of antibiotics, biological identification by reference to the competitive antagonism between sideromycins and sideramines is of major importance.

According to Keller-Schierlein *et al.* (1964), only ferrimycin A_1 and δ_2-albomycin and a few of its transformation products have been subjected to close chemical study. Relatively little is known at present about the chemical constitution of the other sideromycins.

In all the siderochromes, the trivalent iron is bound into a complex by three hydroxamic-acid groups. These iron complexes are stable over a broad pH range (pH 2—10). This pH-stability of the iron complex, however, is not matched by a similar stability of the antibiotic activity over the whole pH range. As a rule, the mildest method of removing the iron from sideromycins or siderochromes is by the use of 8-hydroxyquinoline or cupferron (Bickel *et al.*, 1960b; Haskell *et al.*, 1963). The iron-free siderochromes selectively bind ferric-ions, and display a very high complex-stability constant and selectivity. Other metallic ions, however, give low stability constants (Zähner *et al.*, 1962). The biological activity of the iron-free sideromycins is discussed later. Investigations designed to determine the chemical constitution of ferrimycin A_1 and δ_2-albomycin showed that structurally the sideromycins are closely related to their antagonists, the sideramines (Keller-Schierlein *et al.*, 1964; Bickel *et al.*, 1965). This structural affinity probably has an important bearing on the mode of action of the sideromycins.

All sideramines contain iron as an iron (III)-trihydroxamate complex. The iron-free parent substances of the sideramines obtained from Streptomyces differ fundamentally from those which originate from fungi. Those from Streptomyces possess three aminohydroxylamino-alkane and three carboxylic acid residues, succinic acid and acetic acid. Ferrioxamine D_1, N-acetylated ferrioxamine B, is an exception. The constitution of the main representative from the group of Streptomyces sideramines is shown in Fig. 1. The basic and the acid elements in its structure are interlinked by peptide and hydroxamic-acid bonds in such a way that there is a free amino group at one end and an acetyl residue at the other end. The hydroxamic-acid groups are divided by chains, which are sufficiently long to ensure that a stable, octahedral iron (III)-complex can be formed. The sideramines produced by fungi, on the other hand, are cyclic hexapeptides. The iron-free parent substance consists of 6 amino-acids, i.e. three molecules of L-δ-N-hydroxyornithine and three molecules of glycine (or serine and glycine in a molecular ratio of 2:1 or 1:2), and three carboxylic acids. The 9 basic and 9 acid groups of structural elements are interlinked by peptide and hydroxamic-acid bonds. The three hydroxamate groups responsible for binding the iron are formed from the binding of the carboxylic acids with the δ-N-hydroxyornithine residues; they contain, in the δ-position, the nitrogen atom which is present as a hydroxylamino group (Fig. 2, Keller-Schierlein *et al.*, 1964).

The sideromycins with a broad antibacterial spectrum include the antibiotics albomycin and grisein. Grisein, which was first described by Reynolds *et al.* (1947), was partially purified by Kühl *et al.* (1951). After painstaking processing, the authors obtained a highly active, crude, amorphous powder which was readily soluble in water and phenol, but completely insoluble in all other commonly employed organic solvents. It showed absorption maxima at 265 mμ $\left(E_{1\,cm}^{1\%} = 108\right)$ and 420 mμ $\left(E_{1\,cm}^{1\%} = 28.9\right)$. Potentiometric titration revealed that it was a weak acid. Elemental analyses best fit the empirical formula $C_{40}H_{61}O_{20}N_{10}SFe$ (mol. weight: 1090). The iron, bound in trivalent form, was successfully removed from the acid stable complex by treating it with 8-hydroxyquinoline. The iron-

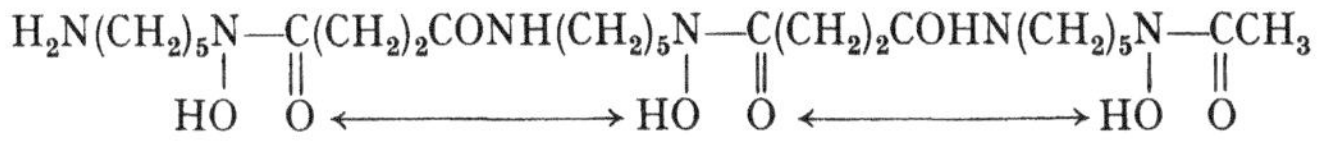

Desferrioxamine B

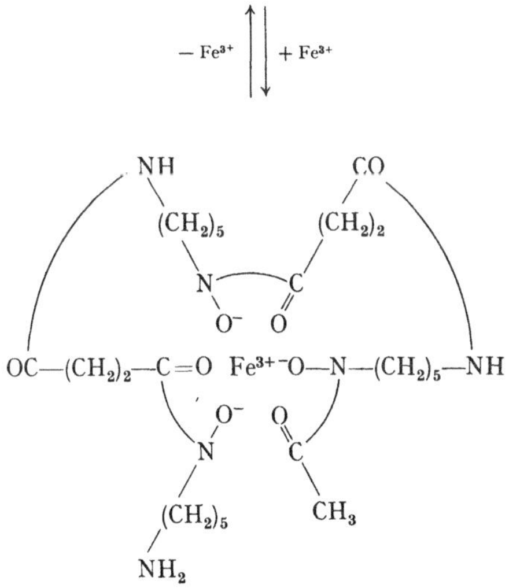

Ferrioxamine B

Fig. 1. Ferrioxamine B, a typical sideramine from a Streptomycete

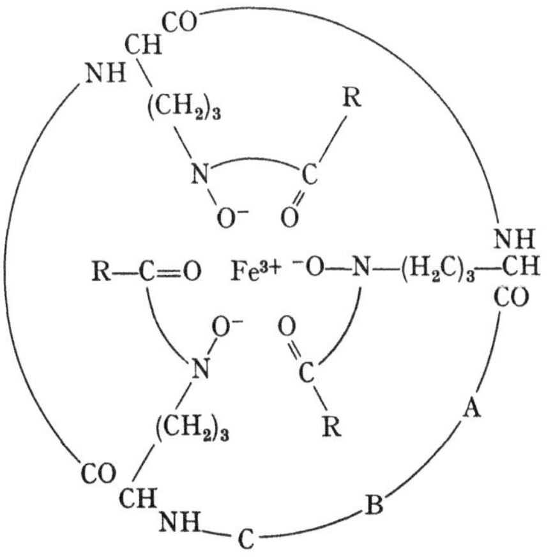

Fig. 2. Structures of sideramines from fungi

free grisein was colourless, but showed a lower specific activity than the iron-containing form. It could be converted to the iron-containing form by adding a stoichiometric quantity of $FeCl_3$. An excess of iron (III) ions resulted in a grisein-Fe complex which was sparingly soluble in water; it contained 7.6% iron and displayed reduced activity.

The albomycin described by GAUSE and BRAZHNIKOVA (1951) showed essentially the same features as grisein. According to STAPLEY and ORMOND (1957), the grisein and albomycin preparations contain four components endowed with antibiotic activity. The ratios between the four components varied considerably from one preparation to another. TURKOVÀ *et al.* (1962) demonstrated that, of the components of the albomycin mixture, only the comparatively unstable δ_2-component is of biogenetic origin, whereas the other components are transformation products. These findings suggest that the ratio of the components in the mixture may depend to a large extent on the methods of purification and enrichment employed, and that albomycin and grisein are in all probability identical.

BICKEL *et al.* (1960a) found that grisein, albomycin, and the antibiotic 1787 reported by THRUM (1957), which is similar to grisein, resembled one another by paper-chromatography. All the antibiotics in group 1 show a relatively high stability over a pH range of 4—10.5 (ŠEVČIK, 1963).

It was not until δ_2-albomycin had been produced in pure form that it became possible to undertake detailed studies of its chemical constitution (KELLER-SCHIERLEIN *et al.*, 1964). The results of degradation reactions and analyses indicate that the empirical formula is probably $C_{39}H_{62}N_{12}O_{20}SFe$ (KRYSIN and PODDUBNAYA, 1963).

Hydrolysis of the iron-free parent of δ_2-albomycin resulted in the appearance of some structural elements which were the same as those found in various sideramines of fungal origin.

According to KELLER-SCHIERLEIN *et al.* (1964), δ_2-albomycin is a substituted ferrichrome. The residues so far identified are a pyrimidine base (3-methylcytosine), which is responsible for the UV absorption at 265 mμ and is linked to the cyclohexapeptide by an SO_4 group, as well as serine and a methyl group (cf. Fig. 2, KELLER-SCHIERLEIN *et al.*, 1965). δ_2-albomycin thus shows a very close structural affinity to the sideramines of fungal origin.

As a general rule, the sideramines can be clearly subdivided by reference to the micro-organisms which produce them and to their chemical constitutions. Cyclopolypeptide sideramines have been obtained only from fungi, and aminohydroxylamino-alkane types only from actinomycetes. In the case of the sideromycins, however, this biogenetic specificity is not consistently observed, as witnessed by the example of albomycin, which, though obtained from *Streptomyces*, is chemically related to the fungal sideramines.

The sideromycins of group 2 show marked differences from those of group 1 in regard to their spectrum of antibiotic activity and their paper-chromatographic behaviour (BICKEL *et al.*, 1960a). Typical representatives are the antibiotic A 22,765 (BICKEL *et al.*, 1960a; GÄUMANN *et al.*, 1961), succinimycin (HASKELL *et al.*, 1963), and danomycin (TSUKIURA *et al.*, 1964). These antibiotics cannot be distinguished from one another by paper-chromatography (Personal communication: F. BENZ and H. BICKEL, CIBA Ltd.). The pH-stability of the antibiotics in this group (cf. Fig. 3) contrasts with that of the ferrimycins (sideromycins of group 3). These antibiotics show a pronounced maximum of stability at pH levels of 5—7, whereas it is precisely within this pH range that the ferrimycins display a minimum of stability (Fig. 4). The two groups also differ in their paper-chromatographic behaviour.

Little is yet known about the chemical constitution of the sideromycins in this group. Like all siderochromes, they show a typical absorption maximum at 425—435 mμ. HASKELL *et al.* (1963) and TSUKIURA *et al.* (1964) have discussed their general chemico-physical properties and described a few products of hydrolysis.

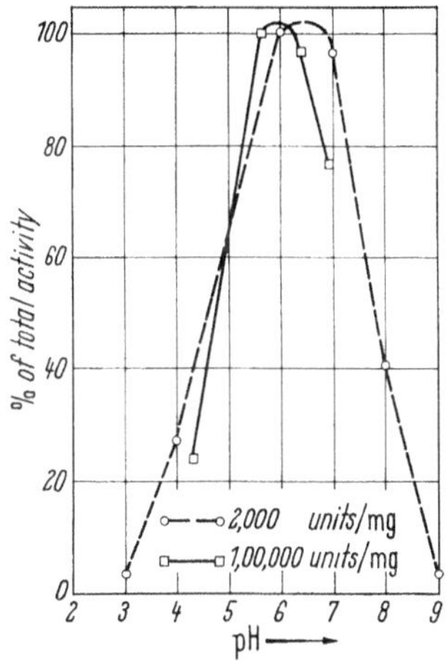

Fig, 3

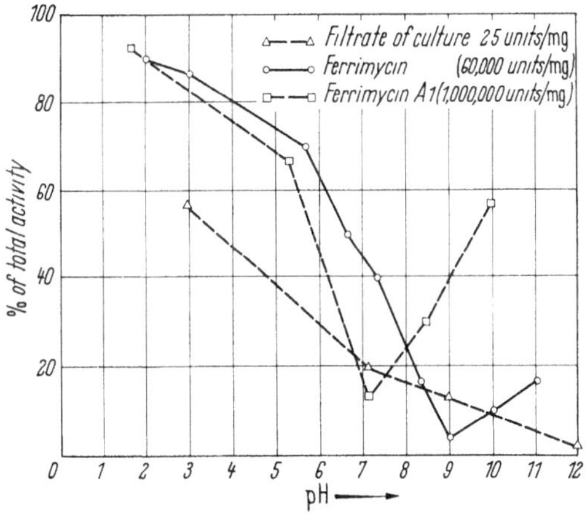

Fig. 4

Fig. 3. Succinimycin activity in aqueous buffer solutions after 24 hours at various pH values (25°) (From HASKELL *et al.*, 1963)

Fig. 4. Antibiotic activity of ferrimycin after 24 hours at 25°C in various aqueous buffer solutions

Typical sideromycins of group 3 are the ferrimycins, which belong to the category of sideromycins with a narrow spectrum of activity confined to Gram-positive bacteria. The ferrimycins are unstable over a wide pH-range, and show minimum stability at pH 7 (Fig. 4). When inactivated, the ferrimycins are transformed into compounds which possess the same properties as sideramines (BICKEL *et al.*, 1960b).

In contrast to succinimycin, the ferrimycins display not only the typical UV-absorption maximum at 430 mμ, but also maxima at 230 and 319 mμ (HASKELL *et al.*, 1963). The ferrimycins are formed as mixtures of various components. BICKEL *et al.* (1965) have succeeded in elucidating the constitution of ferrimycin A_1 which has the empirical formula $C_{41}H_{65}N_{10}O_{14}Fe$. On the basis of chemical and spectroscopic studies of products of hydrolysis from the iron-free parent substance of ferrimycin A_1, it has also been possible to elucidate the structure of this antibiotic. BICKEL *et al.* (1965) have demonstrated that ferrimycin A_1 is a form of 5-amino-3-hydroxylbenzoyl-ferrioxamine B with a substitution at the aromatic nitrogen atom (Fig. 5). In contrast to δ_2-albomycin, which is structurally related to the fungal sideramines, ferrimycin A_1 has a close affinity with the sideramines

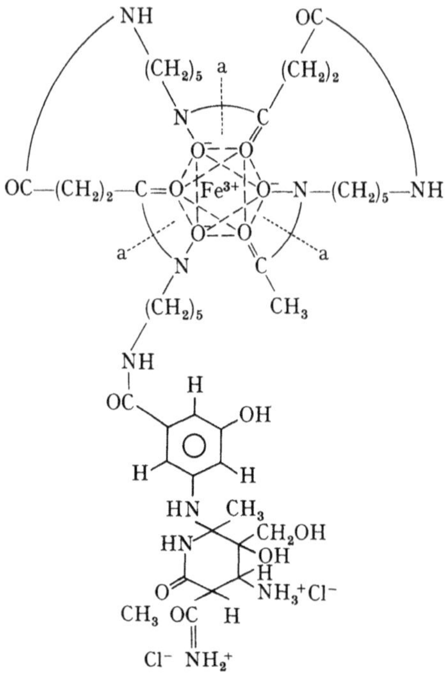

$C_{41}H_{67}O_{14}N_{10}Cl_2Fe$

Ferrimycin A_1

Fig. 5. Structure of ferrimycin A1 (From BICKEL *et al.*, 1965)

produced by actinomycetes. Its chemical configuration also accounts for the fact that this antibiotic can easily be transformed into a sideramine.

Biological Activity

Biological methods are virtually the only ones suitable for quantitative assays and for general qualitative analyses of the sideromycins. In theory it should also be possible to assay the sideromycins by reference to the typical absorption which they show at 420—440 mμ. In practice, however, this method of chemical determination is of no value, because all siderochromes display this absorption and because the sideromycins are usually available in only very small quantities.

An assay for the sideromycins is based on the competitive antagonism between the sideromycins and the sideramines (ZÄHNER *et al.*, 1960). Generally speaking, all sideromycin-sensitive bacteria are suitable for use as test organisms. Two strips — one soaked in a sideromycin solution and the other in a sideramine solution — are placed crosswise on a Petri dish which has been inoculated in the usual manner. After incubation, the competitive antagonism is revealed as illustrated in Fig. 6. Characteristic of a competitive antagonism is the fact that the ratio between the concentration of metabolite and antimetabolite (in this instance, between sideramine and sideromycin) which leads to complete de-antagonism, remains constant over a broad range of concentrations. The action exerted by the sideramines in this test results in a wedge-shaped zone of bacterial growth within the halo of inhibition produced by the sideromycin. The line bounding the area of bacterial growth represents the geometric location of those points at which there is a constant sideramine/sideromycin concentration ratio producing complete de-antagonism.

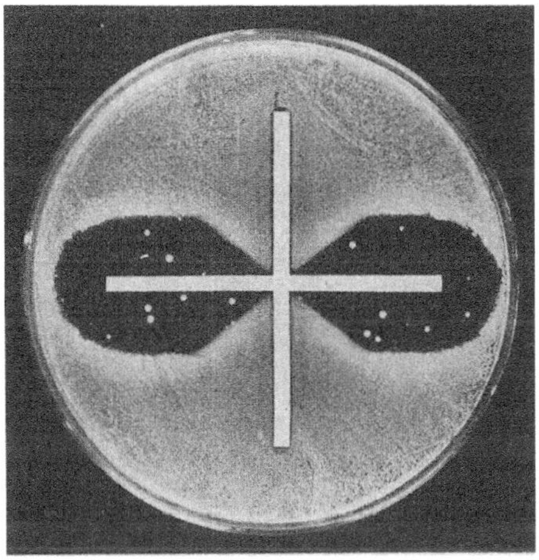

Fig. 6. The antagonism test (Bonifas). Test organism: *Staphylococcus aureus* SG 511. Horizontal strip: A 22,765 1 mg/ml; Vertical strip: Ferrioxamine 1 mg/ml

This test can be employed to identify an antibiotic suspected of being a sideromycin, and also — by using known sideromycins — to identify a sideramine. When carrying out the test it is important to note that the action of broad-spectrum sideromycins (group 1) on Gram-negative bacteria can be antagonised only by sideramines of the ferrichrome type (ZÄHNER *et al.*, 1960).

Agar-diffusion tests using filter discs or cups are most suitable for quantitative determinations of sideromycins. Here again, all sideromycin-sensitive bacteria can be employed as test organisms, e.g. *Staphylococcus aureus*, *Bacillus subtilis*, etc. Quantitative evaluation of the diffusion tests can be effected either by means of the 4-point method or by plotting standard curves. Fig. 7 shows standard curves for ferrimycin and antibiotic A 22,765. A mathematical comparison between the regression coefficients of both dose-effect curves reveals no significant difference, so that the curves may therefore be regarded as parallel. Within concentrations of 5—625 mcg/ml the curves are invariably linear.

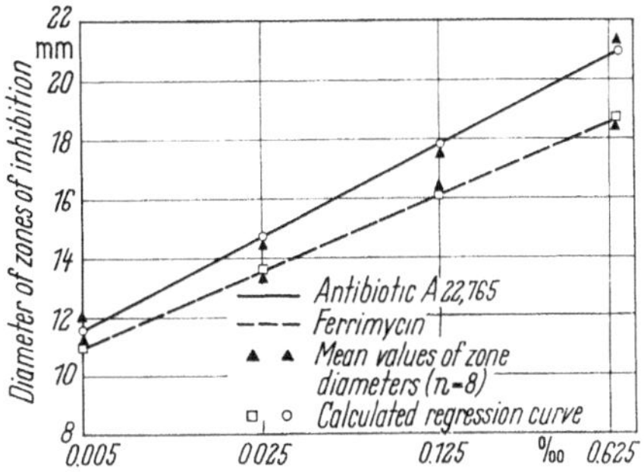

Fig. 7. Dose-effect curves for agar diffusion tests with ferirmycin and antibiotic A 22,765. ○—○ Antibiotic A 22,765; ▲—▲ Ferrimycin; □--□ Calculated regression curve; ▲--▲ Mean values of zone diameters (n=8)

The classic type of serial dilution test is not suitable for determining the minimal growth-inhibiting concentration of sideromycins, because bacterial resistance to these antibiotics develops very rapidly indeed, with the result that one cannot evaluate their activity by reference to the degree of turbidity (REYNOLDS and WAKSMAN, 1948). TSUKIURA *et al.* (1964) have employed an agar dilution test. In our experience, however, it is with the gradient-plate streak assay that the best results are obtained (Fig. 8). With the aid of this test it is possible to assay various micro-organisms on a single plate and to observe the type of action of each antibiotic. The use of a biophotometer has also proved of great value for continuous observation of the influence exerted by the antibiotics on the growing cell population (COULTAS and HUTCHINSON, 1962).

GAUSE (1955) and REYNOLDS and WAKSMAN (1948) reported that albomycin and grisein display marked bacteriostatic activity. In our laboratories, similar experiments were undertaken with ferrimycin, antibiotic A 22,765, and albomycin. When the growth of a sensitive bacterial population was studied biophotometrically under the influence of a sideromycin, pronounced static inhibition lasting 6 hours was observed. The growth curve obtained with albomycin differed from the control curve only inasmuch as the lag-phase was more prolonged (Fig. 9). This also illustrates why it is impossible to determine the effect of sideromycins in serial dilution tests using fluid media. SACKMANNN *et al.* (1962) noted a decrease in the number of microorganisms capable of multiplication when they added ferrimycin to a *Staph. aureus* broth culture in a concentration of 1 mcg/ml Within 5 hours the growth rate was reduced to one-tenth (Fig. 10). This effect is not attributable to agglomeration of the bacteria. Studies of bacterial respiration in the Warburg apparatus clearly revealed that only static inhibition of growth occurs, and that the microorganisms are not actually destroyed; although the number of staphylococci

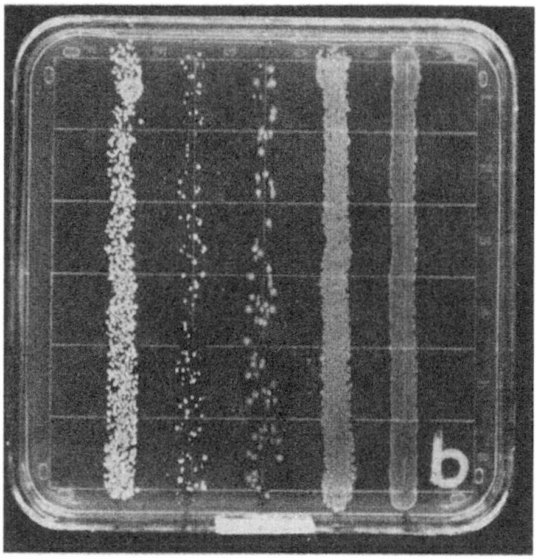

Fig. 8. Gradient plate streak assay. Brain-heart infusion agar with antibiotic A 22,765 in a concentration range from 0—1 mcg/ml. Test organisms (from left to rigth): *Staph. aureus* SG 511, *Staph. aureus* Z 2070, B. subtilis Z 2016, B. megatherium, Strept. faecalis

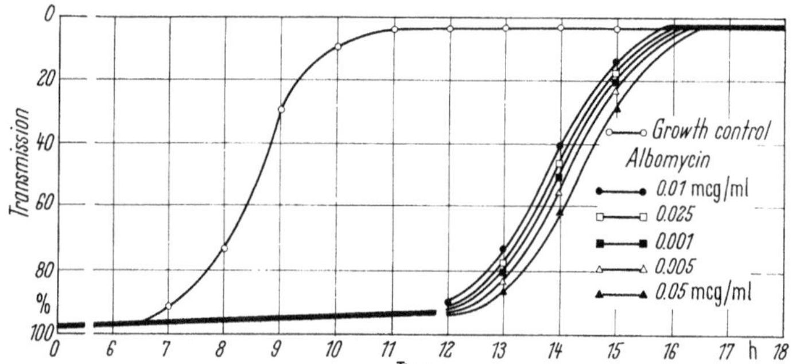

Fig. 9. Inhibition of growth of *E. coli* by various concentrations of albomycin (aerobic culture in BHIB pH 7.2)

capable of multiplication diminishes throughout the whole period, residual respiration remains constant (Fig. 11). Similar conclusions may be drawn from evidence showing that the antibiotic can easily be washed out, whereupon the bacteria are able to grow again. In short, the sideromycins may be described as antibiotics with a bacteriostatic effect which is confined to proliferating cells.

According to GAUSE and BRAZHNIKOVA (1951) and GAUSE (1955), the following bacteria are sensitive to albomycin:

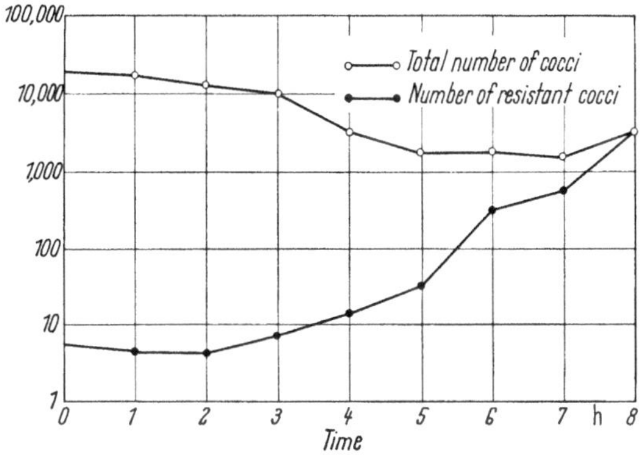

Fig. 10. Influence of ferrimycin on a broth culture of *Staph. aureus* (From SACKMANN *et al.*, 1962).

Staphylococci, *Bacillus subtilis*, *Sarcina subflava*, some — but not all — strains of *Streptococcus pyogenes*, *Aerobacter aerogenes*, *Escherichia coli*, pneumococci, *Klebsiella* and *Shigella* bacteria. Meningococci and *Haemophilus pertussis* are less sensitive. On the other hand, albomycin has a very marked inhibitory effect *in vitro* on *Spirochaeta sogdiana*. *Listeria*, tubercle bacilli, and *Bacillus mycoides* are said to be insensitive. Albomycin has generally proved effective against bacteria resistant to the commoner antibiotics such as penicillin, streptomycin, the tetracyclines, and erythromycin.

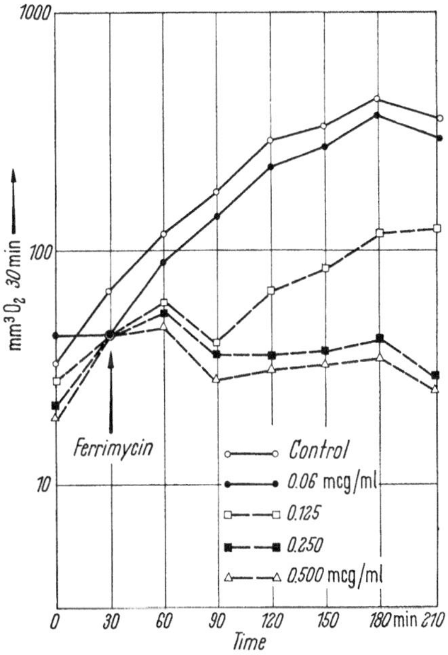

Fig. 11. Oxygen uptake of a proliferating culture of *Staph. aureus* under the influence of ferrimycin

The minimum inhibitory concentration in the case of staphylococci was approx. 0.002 mcg./ml. STAPLEY and ORMOND (1957) made a microbiological comparison between albomycin and grisein. In the light of the results outlined in Table 2, these authors concluded that the antibacterial activity of these two antibiotics is identical. Similar experiments carried out by REYNOLDS and WAKSMAN (1948) with culture filtrates of a grisein-producing Streptomyces yielded the same spectrum of activity. Thus the sideromycins of group 1 have a relatively broad spectrum of antibacterial activity and their specific activity (minimum inhibitory concentration) is very high. These sideromycins show no cross-resistance with the main antibiotics used in clinical practice.

Table 2. *Spectra of activity of albomycin and grisein*

Test organism	Zone of inhibition in mm	
	Albomycin 91,000 U/mg 5 mcg/ml	Grisein 41,000 U/mg 5 mcg/ml
Staphylococcus aureus	25.5	15.0
Diplococcus pneumoniae	23.5	21.0
Klebsiella pneumoniae	24.0	18.0
Salmonella schottmülleri	24.0	22.0
Salmonella typhi	—	—
Pseudomonas aeruginosa	—	—
Proteus vulgaris	—	—
E. coli W	24.0	22.0
E. coli/Streptomycin-resistant	22.0	21.0
E. coli/Cycloserin-resistant	26.0	23.0
E. coli/Pleocidin-resistant	35.0	30.0
E. coli/Chloramphenicol-resistant	35.0	28.0
E. coli/Chlortetracycline-resistant	35.0	31.0
E. coli/Oxytetracycline-resistant	35.0	26.0
E. coli/Neomycin-resistant	35.0	26.0
E. coli/Tetracycline-resistant	35.0	31.0
E. coli/Viomycin-resistant	—	—
E. coli/Grisein-resistant	—	—
E. coli/Albomycin-resistant	—	—

Spectrum of activity and minimum inhibitory concentration of sideromycins from groups 2 and 3 do not differ essentially in their antibiotic activity, and will be discussed together. HASKELL *et al.* (1963) refer to succinimycin as an antibiotic with a narrow spectrum of activity confined to Gram-positive bacteria, including staphylococci and streptococci. TSUKIURA *et al.* (1964) studied the antibacterial spectrum of danomycin in an agar dilution test and reported that the spectrum is restricted chiefly to Gram-positive bacteria. Exceptions within this Gram-positive group of bacteria are *Staphylococcus albus* and streptococci, which display a high degree of resistance. The spectrum of the related antibiotic A 22,765 does not differ significantly from that of danomycin (Table 3 and Fig. 8). SACKMANN *et al.* (1962) investigated the spectrum of ferrimycin, using the agar diffusion test and described ferrimycin as an antibiotic whose activity is mainly confined to Gram-positive bacteria such as micrococci, streptococci, corynebacteria, and bacilli (Table 4). *Bacillus megatherium* and *Streptococcus faecalis* are far more resistant than the other Gram-positive micro-organisms. As a general rule, ferrimycin is only active against Gram-negative organisms when employed in very high doses. Even in the high concentrations selected, ferrimycin proved inactive against anaerobic spore-forming micro-organisms as well as against *Candida albicans*. In the course of tests carried out with ferrimycin, SACKMANN *et al.* noted that the inhibitory effect exerted by this antibiotic depends to a high degree upon the media employed. They presume that there is a causal connection between this phenomenon and the inactivation of ferrimycin or, alternatively, its transformation into an antagonistic sideramine. As already mentioned, ferrimycin shows minimum pH-stability at physiological pH levels, and the elucidation of its constitution has also shown that it can be transformed into a sideramine. The results of our own studies indicate that microbial resistance to ferrimycin caused by nutritional fac-

Table 3. *Minimum growth-inhibiting concentrations (MIC) of antibiotic A 22,765 in a streak gradient plate test*

Organism	MIC mcg/ml
Staphylococcus aureus Z 2070	0.08
Staphylococcus aureus SG 511	0.07
Bacillus subtilis Z 2016	0.03
Bacillus megatherium	>0.1>1
Streptococcus faecalis	>1>50
Klebsiella pneumoniae	>50
Shigella dysenteriae	>50
Salmonella typhimurium	>50
Proteus vulgaris	>50
Pseudomonas aeruginosa	>50
Escherichia coli Z 2018	>50
Paecylomyces varioti	>50
Trichophyton interdigitale	>50
Candida albicans	>50

Table 4. *Inhibitory effect of ferrimycin A on various micro-organisms*[1] (SACKMANN *et al.*, 1962)

Strains	Inhibition zone[1] in mm
Staph. aureus ATCC 6538	30
Staph. aureus/Streptomycin-resistant	31
Streptococcus pyogenes A 1338	28
Streptococcus viridans 1326	21
Corynebacterium diphtheriae B 161	36
Bacillus subtilis Z 2016	30
Bacillus megatherium Z 2040	14
Escherichia coli Z 2018	12
Shigella sonnei E 355	13
Klebsiella pneumoniae AB 327	16
Pasteurella pestis B 343	27
Vibrio el Tor Irak 514	13
Streptococcus faecalis Z 2065	0
Salmonella typhi B 271	0
Salmonella schottmülleri B 272	0
Pseudomonas aeruginosa Z 2072	0
Clostridium perfringens B 443	0
Clostridium chauvoei B 444	0
Clostridium septicum B 442	0
Clostridium novyi B 441	0
Candida albicans Z 5897	0

[1] Disc agar diffusion test with 0.1% ferrimycin solution (20 mcg ferrimycin/disc).

tors, as postulated by BACHMANN and ZÄHNER (1961), can only be explained in terms of chemicophysical inactivation or transformation due to the nature of the substances employed as a medium.

Ferrimycin and antibiotic A 22,765 have a growth-inhibiting effect on the glutamic acid-producing bacteria *Micrococcus glutamicus* ATCC 13,058 and *Brevibacterium flavum* ATCC 14,067.

There are generally no differences between the antibacterial spectra and specific activities (minimum inhibitory concentration) of the sideromycins in groups 2 and 3. Against sensitive bacteria these antibiotics are active in very low concentrations. Their spectrum of activity is largely restricted to Gram-positive bacteria. Cross-resistance between the three groups of sideromycins is a consistent finding.

Antibiotic A 22,765 shows an interesting inhibitory effect on *Streptomyces griseoflavus*, strain A 9578, which is a producer of ferrimycin. Its inhibitory action on this strain of Streptomyces is very marked (Table 5). The ferrimycin-producing Streptomyces strain A 9578 reacted to the sideromycin A 22,765 like a highly sensitive bacterium. Ferrimycin itself had no effect. Neither ferrimycin nor antibiotic A 22,765 had any significant inhibitory effect on *Streptomyces aureofaciens*, from which antibiotic A 22,765 is produced.

ZÄHNER *et al.* (1960) have reported that ferrimycin inhibits growth of the ferrichrome-producing Basidiomycetes *Ustilago sphaerogena*. All the sideromycins appear to have a very high specific activity, as reflected in the clear-cut dividing

Table 5. *Effect of antibiotic A 22,765 on Streptomyces griseoflavus A 9578*[1]

Test substance	Concentration of test solution in mcg/ml	Halo of inhibition in mm 0.02 ml test solution per punched hole
Antibiotic A 22,765	1,000	42
	100	34
	10	24
Ferrimycin	1,000	0
	100	0
	10	0
Ferrioxamine	1,000	0
	100	0
	10	0
Desferrioxamine	1,000	0
	100	0
	10	0

[1] The strain *Streptomyces griseoflavus* A 9578 was incubated at 28°C for 40 hours in 100 ml of a complex nutrient solution (pure glucose 5.0 g, sucrose 10 g, bacto-trypton 5 g, Difco yeast extract 2.5 g, tap-water 1,000 ml; pH adjusted to 7.0 with $NaHCO_3$ prior to sterilisation; solution then autoclaved at 115°C/20 min) on a rotating shaking machine in 500 ml Erlenmeyer flasks. The mycelium was centrifuged off, washed with physiological NaCl, and, having been diluted with physiological NaCl 50 times in relation to the initial concentration, was re-suspended in the nutrient solution. Petri dishes containing yeast-extract agar were then surface-inoculated with 0.1 ml of the resultant suspension. Using an 8 mm ⌀ cork-drill, holes were punched in the agar and filled with 0.02 ml of the test solutions.

line between non-inhibitory and inhibitory concentrations (Fig. 9). Neither in the biophotometer nor in the Warburg apparatus was it possible to observe any concentration-dependent, smooth dose-effect pattern.

Toxicity, Pharmacology, and Chemotherapeutic Properties of the Sideromycins

The data contained in Table 6 show that, on the whole, the acute toxicity of the sideromycins is low. Thanks to their low ED_{50} (Table 7), these antibiotics have a very wide therapeutic margin. YAMADA and KAWAGUCHI (1964) carried out a detailed pharmacological analysis of danomycin. Not until they gave extremely high intravenous doses of 3—5 g/kg did they observe fatal poisoning in mice. Death was due to respiratory paralysis. These authors also studied the chronic toxicity of danomycin in rats receiving 100 mg/kg daily for 90 days. No significant effect on growth was observed, nor were any changes detected in the organs. The blood picture, as well as hepatic and renal function, were likewise investigated, and here again the findings were negative.

Sublethal doses of ferrimycin produced a similar, uncharacteristic syndrome of poisoning, with signs of general respiratory paralysis. In rats, ferrimycin — administered in daily subcutaneous doses of 100 mg/kg for 4 weeks — resulted in cessation of growth after one week. When the animals were sacrificed, the thymus, lymph nodes, and testes were found to be underdeveloped, but no other pathological changes attributable to the preparation could be demonstrated. Instilled into the rabbit's eye, solutions of ferrimycin containing concentrations as high as 10% were tolerated without signs of irritation. GAUSE (1955) also reported that albomycin is a pharmacologically inactive substance which is extremely well tolerated by laboratory animals.

GAUSE (1955) refers to studies on the behaviour of albomycin in the serum. Neither casein nor ovalbumin has any influence on the effect of this antibiotic, whereas its antibiotic activity is sharply reduced in the presence of a 10% solution of blood serum. It would appear that a portion of the albomycin is reversibly bound by blood serum. This reversible binding to protein accounts for the fact that, following a single subcutaneous injection, very little of the sideromycin is excreted through the kidneys.

The maximum concentration of albomycin in the rabbit's blood is attained 30 minutes after administration of a subcutaneous dose of 100,000 U/kg; 70—80% of the non-bound albomycin injected is excreted in the urine within 6—8 hours, whereas the portion bound to protein remains in the organism correspondingly longer than the free portion. The presence of albomycin could be demonstrated in the lymph and in various organs and tissues but not in the cerebrospinal fluid. SACKMANN *et al.* (1962) report that, 1 hour after subcutaneous administration of ferrimycin in a dose of 1—250 mg/kg, the antibiotic could be traced in the blood of mice in concentrations ranging from 0.1 to 8 mcg/ml.

YAMADA and KAWAGUCHI (1964) investigated the pharmacokinetic behaviour of danomycin in rabbits. In response to an intramuscular dose of 50 mg/kg, mean maximum blood levels of 20 mcg/ml were already attained 15 minutes after the injection. The levels subsequently showed a rapid decline; 12 hours after injection the antibiotic could no longer be traced in the serum. Oral doses failed to yield any demonstrable concentration in the blood. YAMADA and KAWAGUCHI also studied the distribution of danomycin in the organs of rats. Following an intraperitoneal dose of 10 mg/kg they were able to find the sideromycin only in the kidneys and small intestine.

Table 6. *Acute toxicity of the sideromycins*

Sideromycin	Animal experiment	LD_{50} mg/kg Intravenous	Subcutaneous	Per oral	Literature
Albomycin	Mouse, Rabbit, Cat, Guinea-pig	>5.10⁷ U (>70 mg)	>5.10⁷ U (>70 mg)		GAUSE (1955)
Grisein[1]	?	>500,000 U (>1.5 mg)			REYNOLDS and WAKSMAN (1948)
Succinimycin	Mouse	770			HASKELL *et al.* (1963)
Danomycin	Mouse	3,250			YAMADA and KAWAGUCHI (1964)
Ferrimycin	Mouse	100	300	3,000	SACKMANN *et al.* (1962)

[1] Species of animal used not stated.

Table 7. *Chemotherapeutic activity of the sideromycins*

Sideromycin	Animal species	Infection	Effective doses mg/kg Subcutaneous	Per oral	Literature
Albomycin	Mouse	*Pneumococci*	1.05 (ED_{100})		GAUSE (1955)
Albomycin	Mouse	*K. pneumoniae*	0.035 (ED_{100})		GAUSE (1955)
Grisein	Mouse	*S. aureus*	0.0024—0.0058 mg/mouse		REYNOLDS and WAKSMAN (1948)
Grisein	Mouse	*Salm. schottmülleri*	0.0024—0.0058 mg/mouse		REYNOLDS and WAKSMAN (1948)
Succinimycin	Mouse	*S. aureus*		0.33 (ED_{50})	HASKELL *et al.* (1963)
Danomycin	Mouse	*S. aureus* Smith strain	0.015 (ED_{50})	0.78 (ED_{50})	TSUKIURA *et al.* (1964)
Danomycin	Mouse	*S. aureus* pen.-resist.	0.075 (ED_{50})	0.95 (ED_{50})	TSUKIURA *et al.* (1964)
Ferrimycin	Mouse	*Staphylococci*	0.3 (ED_{50})	10.0 (ED_{50})	SACKMANN *et al.* (1962)
Ferrimycin	Mouse	*Streptococci*	10.0 (ED_{50})	10.0 (ED_{50})	SACKMANN *et al.* (1962)
Ferrimycin	Mouse	*Pneumococci*	10.0 (ED_{50})	33.0 (ED_{50})	SACKMANN *et al.* (1962)

In contrast to albomycin, neither danomycin nor ferrimycin appears to be bound to the blood serum (YAMADA and KAWAGUCHI, 1964; SACKMANN *et al.*, 1962).

Sideromycins are chemotherapeutic, even when given to animals in very small doses (Table 7). GAUSE (1955) states that experimental infections with various Gram-positive and Gram-negative bacteria have been successfully treated with albomycin. Albomycin exerted no effect, however, in animals infected with tubercle bacilli, Listeria, Salmonella, or Rickettsia. Comparative studies carried out by SACKMANN *et al.* (1962) showed that, in animals infected with *Staph. aureus* and *Strept. pyogenes*, ferrimycin, administered subcutaneously, was clearly superior to penicillin or erythromycin. On the other hand, ferrimycin proved completely ineffective against infections with Gram-negative micro-organisms such as *E. coli*, *K. pneumoniae*, and *Past. avicida*. Danomycin and succinimycin likewise were effective in the treatment of infections with Gram-positive bacteria.

SACKMANN *et al.* (1962) studied the effect of ferrimycin on a *Staph. aureus* population in the blood of infected animals. For this purpose, blood cultures were made at various intervals after infection and examined to determine to what extent the cultures were sterile or showed evidence of multiplication of bacteria which were either resistant or sensitive to ferrimycin.

Twenty-four hours after infection and simultaneous administration of the sideromycin, 19 out of 20 mice had ferrimycin-resistant staphylococci in their blood. On the following day, however, the bacteria in the new blood samples had become sensitive again. Between the 3rd and 7th day, the number of mice without staphylococci increased, and after the 8th day staphylococci could no longer be isolated from the blood of any of the animals. Animal experiments with pure, ferrimycin-resistant strains of staphylococci revealed that these micro-organisms displayed the same virulence as the ferrimycin-sensitive ones. This finding conflicts to some extent with the impressive therapeutic results obtained in animal experiments.

Biochemical Properties of the Sideromycins

Ferrimycin and antibiotic A 22,765 can be washed out of bacterial cells with the aid of physiological NaCl solution. *Bacillus subtilis* was incubated at 37° C for 3 hours in a physiological saline solution containing the sideromycin in a concentration of 100 mcg/ml. The bacteria were then centrifuged, washed or unwashed cells were suspended in glucose bouillon, and their oxygen uptake was studied in the Warburg apparatus. As shown in Fig. 12, bacterial respiration increases in direct proportion to the number of washings. The sideromycin, in contrast to penicillin, cephalosporin C, and the tetracyclines, can easy be removed from the bacterial cells. When the sideromycin has been washed out of the cells, their oxygen consumption rises appreciably, thereby testifing to the bacteriostatic activity of the antibiotic. The sideromycins appear to be only very loosely bound to the bacterial cell. Nothing is yet known about the sites at which they are attached.

Since the results of the antagonism test indicate that a competitive antagonism exists between the sideramines and the sideromycins, the two presumably compete for the sites of attachment, which may, for example be enzymes. When ferrimycin is added to a *Staphylococcus aureus* culture one hour before the addition of a sideramine (ferrioxamine) in a concentration sufficient to completely antagonise the action of the ferrimycin, the sideramine is no longer able to interfere with the antibiotic activity of the sideromycin. Conversely, prior addition of ferrioxamine affords the bacteria complete protection against the sideromycin. The two types of compounds thus seem to display a similar affinity for the sites of attachment at which they exert their effects — which, once again, suggests a competitive antagonism. ZÄHNER *et al.* (1960) report that, in the agar diffusion tests carried out which filter-discs, the ferrioxamine/ferrimycin concentration ratio at which the antibiotic effect on *B. subtilis* Z 2016 is completely neutralised remains constant over a concentration range of 0.01—100 mcg/ml in the case

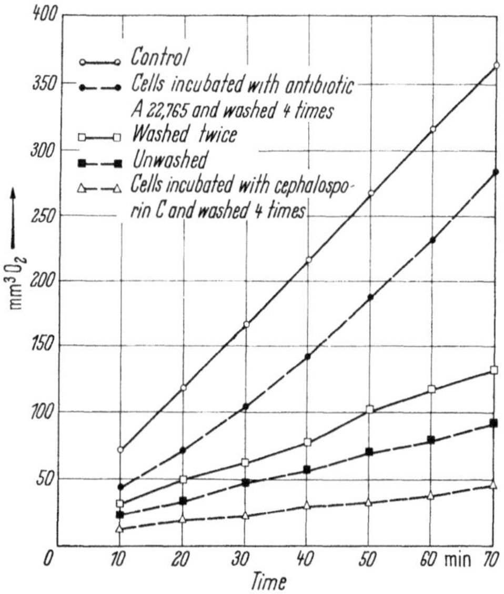

Fig. 12. Influence of washing upon bacterial cells after incubation with the antibiotic A 22,765 and cephalosporin C

of ferrimycin and 0.1—1,000 mcg/ml in the case of ferrioxamine. The quantitative ratio of ferrimycin to ferrioxamine is 1:10, and the molecular ratio 1:15.9, corresponding to the molecular weights, which are 977.26 and 613.10, respectively. In terms of both molecules and weights, much larger quantities of the sideramine than of the sideromycin are required to achieve a neutralising effect. This may be due to two factors: first, the postulated bivalent function of the sideramines may play a role and, second, the relative affinities for the binding sites may be important.

The relationships between desferrioxamine and antibiotic A 22,765 were investigated using a modified gradient-plate test. The experiments were carried out with *B. subtilis* strain W in a synthetic medium with separately sterilised glucose. Under these experimental conditions, growth of this strain occurs only in the presence of a chelating agent such as desferrioxamine B. In this instance, the weight ratio between antibiotic A 22,765 and desferrioxamine is 5:1.

One of the principal features of the sideromycins is the extraordinarily large number of individual cells within a sideromycin-sensitive bacterial population which are resistant. We have studied the resistance rates in *Bacillus subtilis* strain W, *Staphylococcus aureus* SG 511, and *Staphylococcus aureus* Z 2070 under the influence of the sideromycin A 22,765. The strains were cultivated in glucose bouillon at 37 C. After a cell density of approx. 10^9 cells/ml had been attained, the suspension was centrifuged and the bacteria resuspended in phosphate buffer (pH 7) in a concentration of 10^9 ml; 10^8 and 10^5 bacteria were then spread on to bouillon agar plates with antibiotic A 22,765 to produce a concentration of 50 mcg/ml. Corresponding control cultures were set up on plates to which no sideromycin was added. At the same time, the resistant colonies were transferred with the aid of the replica technique to agar plates to which the following enzyme-inhibitors were added: potassium cyanide, sodium arsenite, iodoacetate, and fluoroacetate. These inhibitors were employed in concentrations which were not sufficient to cause any growth inhibition in the initial populations. Besides the action of the inhibitors, the effects exerted by ferrioxamine and desferrioxamine, as well as catalase formation, were also investigated. Finally, the growth of normal populations and resistant populations were compared in B.B.L. anaerobic Petri dishes under conditions ranging from anaerobic to micro-aerophilic. The experiments were repeated three times and the results are summarised in Table 8. Five hundred to a thousand single colonies were examined. The values given in the Table, however, should not be regarded as statistically confirmed mean values. The resistance rates were in agreement with those quoted for the development of resistance to sideromycins in the literature. The two strains of staphylococci showed an extremely large number of resistant mutants, whereas the *B. subtilis* strain W tested displayed an appreciably lower resistance rate. In none of the strains studied were any changes in catalase formation observed. Under anaerobic to micro-aerophilic conditions, the capacity for growth is significantly reduced in resistant populations of *Staph. aureus* Z 2070 and *B. subtilis W*. Both resistant staphylococcal populations show larger numbers of desferrioxamine-sensitive colonies than the normal populations. The iron-containing form of the sideramine is devoid of activity. With the exception of the resistant colonies of *Staph. aureus* Z 2070, which are highly sensitive to sodium-arsenite, the two strains of staphylococci display no significant differences in their response to enzyme inhibitors. *B. subtilis W* differs fundamentally from the staphylococci; approx. 40—50% of the resistant colonies show enhanced sensitivity to the enzyme poisons tested. It is interesting to note that, in this autotrophic bacillus, both the iron-free and the iron-containing sideramine have an inhibitory effect on a large portion of the individual colonies from the normal strain, an effect which is considerably stronger than that exerted on the resistant population.

A comparison between the individual colonies of sideromycin-sensitive and sideromycin-resistant strains does not reveal any properties common to one or the other type. On the contrary, it would seem that the individual resistant colonies differ appreciably not only from one strain to another but also even within the same strain. For this reason it was impossible to find any general biochemical feature common to sideromycin-resistant clones.

The sensitivity of sideromycin-resistant staphylococci to iron-free forms of sideramines, to which reference has already been made, was studied in closer detail. Under the influence of albomycin and ferrimycin, as well as of antibiotic

Table 8. *Resistance rates for B. subtilis W, Staph. aureus Z 2070*, and *Staph. aureus SG 511, and comparison between resistant and sensitive populations*

Micro-organism	Resistance rate	Catalase formation	Growth of colonies as % of controls						
			Anaerobic	Desferri-oxamine 100 mcg/ml	Ferri-oxamine 100 mcg/ml	KCN	$NaAsO_2$	FCH_2COONa	$CH_2ICOONa$
Staph. aureus Z 2070 normal	6.10^{-3}	+	96	100	100	100	100	100	100
Staph. aureus Z 2070 resistant		+	42	63	100	100	15	100	100
Staph. aureus SG 511 normal	5.10^{-4}	+	74	92	91	100	100	100	100
Staph. aureus SG 511 resistant		+	74	69	95	95	100	100	100
B. subtilis W normal	3.10^{-6}	+	87	18	11	100	100	100	100
B. subtilis W resistant		+	52	91	54	41	37	40	55

A 22,765, sideromycin-resistant staphylococci, *E. coli*, and *B. subtilis* can be found which display a high degree of sensitivity to desferri-sideramines. In the dilution test, the ferrimycin-resistant mutant *Staph. aureus* SAR is completely inhibited by desferrioxamine B, in a concentration of 3—6 mcg/ml. Even in high concentrations, however, ferrioxamine B has no effect on *Staph. aureus* SAR. On the other hand, the growth of this bacterium is affected not only by iron-free sideramines, but also by iron-free ferrimycin (Fig. 13a, b). This strain is catalase-

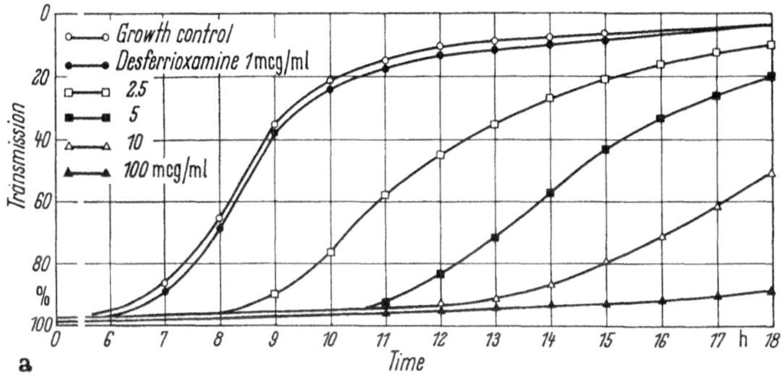

a

Fig. 13a. Influence of desferrioxamine on the growth of the ferrimycin-resistant mutant strain *Staph. aureus* SAR

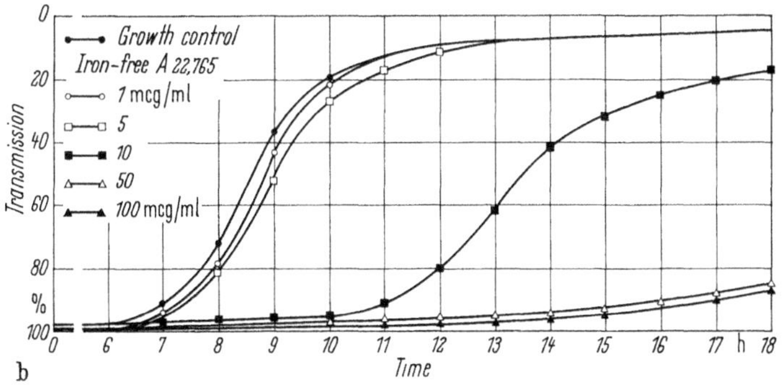

b

Fig. 13b. Influence of iron-free A 22,765 on the growth of the ferrimycin-resistant mutant strain *Staph. aureus* SAR

positive and its sensitivity to KCN is ten times higher than that of the ferrimycin-sensitive initial strain *Staph. aureus* Z 2070. In addition, *Staph. aureus* SAR is no longer capable of growing under strictly anaerobic conditions. These observations reveal that, despite their high binding constants for trivalent iron, the iron-free forms of sideramine are unable to bind this metal in a complex medium. The effect exerted by desferri-sideramines and desferri-sideromycins on the ferrimycin-resistant mutant *Staph. aureus* SAR can best be explained as an intracellular type of iron-complex formation similar to that observed with KCN. These findings suggest that, for its catabolic energy-yielding metabolism, the SAR mutant, has to confine itself to the central, aerobic tricarboxylic-acid cycle unlike the initial strain. *Staph. aureus* SAR can be employed for the quantitative estimation of desferrisideramines.

Despite their structural differences, all the siderochromes display one feature in common, their iron (III)-trihydroxamate complex. The three hydroxamate groups form an extremely stable complex with the ferri-atom. The iron-complexing capacity of the siderochromes for the trivalent iron is not only very high, but also extraordinarily specific.

The fact that the sideramines are so widely encountered and that, generally speaking, they are non-specifically interchangeable as growth factors for heterotrophic micro-organisms, would seem to suggest that the sideramines and their antagonists, the sideromycins, play some role in the iron metabolism of these micro-organisms. This supposition is further borne out by the general observation that larger quantities of sideramine are not produced by such micro-organisms except where there is an iron-deficiency.

To understand the action exerted by sideromycins it is necessary first of all to examine the effects which the sideramines are known to produce. According to NEILANDS (1957), the quantity of iron contained in the living cell is greater than that present in any of the known iron compounds. A portion of this remaining iron can be assigned to the respiratory enzymes discovered by GREEN and BEINERT (1955), which contain an iron component. Nothing is yet known, however, about the bulk of the remaining iron. The discovery of quite a large number of iron-containing growth factors and of corresponding heterotrophic micro-organisms provided the starting point for extensive studies on iron metabolism in micro-organisms.

NEILANDS (1957) refers to the smut fungus *Ustilago sphaerogena* as an organism with an "exaggerated" iron metabolism. WEISEL and ALLEN (1951) succeeded in demonstrating that this fungus produces large quantities of haemoproteins when cultured in a synthetic nutrient solution to which zinc has been added. These haemoproteins were C type cytochrome (NEILANDS, 1952). Even after all the cytochrome C had been removed, extracts of *Ustilago sphaerogena* still contained fairly large amounts of a coloured iron compound. This iron compound, which was subsequently prepared in crystalline form, was given the name "ferrichrome" by NEILANDS (1952). At the same time, PAGE (1952) reported that haemin served as a growth factor for the fungus *Pilobulus kleinii*. HESSELTINE *et al.* (1952) isolated from actinomycetes fermentation broths an iron-containing substance which proved 1,000 times more active than haemin as a growth factor for *Pilobulus kleinii;* they designated this substance as "coprogen". Ferrichrome was also discovered to be highly active as a growth factor for *Pilobulus kleinii* (PAGE, 1952).

LOCHHEAD *et al.* (1952) described an iron-containing substance which they had isolated from *Arthrobacter pascens* and which they found to be essential for the growth of *Arthrobacter terregens*. They gave this substance the name "terregens factor". Ferrichrome and coprogen also proved to be potent growth factors for *A. terregens*.

FRANCIS *et al.* (1953) isolated an iron-contaning factor, mycobactin P, from *Mycobacterium phlei* which promotes the *in vitro* growth of *Mycobacterium johnei*. SNOW (1965) has meanwhile elucidated the chemical structure of mycobactin. BURNHAM and NEILANDS (1961) have demonstrated that mycobactin is capable of replacing terregens factor in cultures of *Arthrobacter terregens*.

WOLIN and NAYLOR (1955) demonstrated that *Micrococcus lysodeikticus* could be grown on a simple synthetic medium only when all the components of the medium had been sterilised together. In a nutrient solution in which the ingredients had been sterilised separately and then mixed after allowing to cool, no growth took place. On the other hand, a good rate of growth was observed when traces of citric acid, 8-hydroxyquinoline, ferrichrome, or small quantities of an autoclaved solution of glucose and sodium glutamate were added to a medium consisting of separately sterilised ingredients.

When MORRISON *et al.* (1965) investigated the activity of synthetic metal-chelators as growth factor for *A. terregens*, they found that 8-hydroxyquinoline, salicylaldehyde, 8-hydroxyquinaldine, acetyl-acetone, and benzoyl-acetone were capable of replacing terregens factor. From this they concluded that two requirements have to be fulfilled by a synthetic metal-chelator if it is to prove satisfactory as a growth factor for *A. terregens:* first, it must be able to chelate ferric irons and, second, the metal chelate must be of lipophilic character.

Using *Microbacterium* sp. as a test organism, DEMAIN and HENDLIN (1959) showed that sideramines and other chelating agents exert a marked growth-promoting effect. ZÄHNER *et al.* (1962), however, describe ferrioxamine as an essential growth factor for *Microbact. lacticum.* In the experiments undertaken by DEMAIN and HENDLIN, ferrichrome shortened the lagphase but had no influence on the absolute extent of growth. A similar effect is displayed by heat-transformation products of an autoclaved glucose-phosphate solution (RAMSEY and LANKFORD, 1956). The glucose, which had been autoclaved in the presence of phosphate, stimulated growth initiation of various micro-organisms in chemically defined media, but did not exert any influence on the extent of growth or rate of growth in the exponential growth phase. When SERGEANT *et al.* (1957) investigated this effect in *Bacillus globigii*, they found that in a synthetic medium, these bacteria reacted in the same way to the transformation products. They then attempted to reproduce this effect of the autoclaved glucose-phosphate solution using various chemical compounds, and demonstrated that there were in fact several structurally differing types of substance which also displayed the desired growth-enhancing action. Most of the compounds which proved active in these experiments showed structural features characteristic of metal-chelating agents.

BICKEL *et al.* (1960), ZÄHNER *et al.* (1962), and KELLER-SCHIERLEIN *et al.* (1965) have reported a large number of iron-containing substances which have been isolated from micro-organisms of various groups and which act as sideromycin antagonists. These sideramines (ferrioxamine, ferrichrysin, ferricrocin, ferrirhodin, and ferrirubin) were also found to be growth factors for the heterotrophic strains described. GARIBALDI and NEILANDS (1956) demonstrated that, when cultured under conditions of iron-deficiency, *B. subtilis*, *B. megatherium*, and *A. niger* synthesise iron-binding compounds. Besides ferric iron-binding agents, *B. subtilis*, *Ustilago* species, and *A. niger* but not *B. megatherium* also secrete large quantities of porphyrin into the nutrient solution. The porphyrin produced by *B. subtilis* was identified by TOWNSLEY (1956) as coproporphyrin III.

According to NEILANDS (1957), ferrichrome possibly fulfils the function of a "co-enzyme" for the transport of iron in microbial cells. DEMAIN and HENDLIN

(1959) are basically in agreement with this hypothesis and refer to the sideramines as "iron-transport compounds".

The experimental data obtained with sideramines must now be examined in relation to studies on the mode of action of the sideromycins. GAUSE (1955) observed that albomycin is active only under aerobic but not under anaerobic conditions; in other words, it is capable of acting only when the necessary energy is obtained via the cytochrome system. GAUSE (1956) reports that an increase in the iron content of the nutrient agar causes the activity of albomycin against *Staph. aureus* to diminish by 30%.

BURNHAM and NEILANDS (1961) have succeeded in showing that, in the case of *Arthrobacter JG 9*, ferrichrome can be replaced by secondary hydroxamic acids or by a haemin compound in high doses. *Arthrobacter JG 9* is inhibited by ferrimycin A. According to the investigations of BURNHAM (1962a), this sideramine-heterotrophic strain is also able to take up free ferric-ions, but it cannot incorporate them into haemin. BURNHAM (1962b) employed *Arthrobacter JG 9* to study the antagonism between sideromycins and sideramines; catalase activity, rather than growth, was taken as a measure of antagonism of the sideramines.

The formation of catalase activity by *Arthrobacter JG 9* is dependent upon the addition of exogenous haemin, or the iron-containing growth factor ferrichrome. The iron-containing antibiotic ferrimycin A inhibited the synthesis of catalase in bacterial suspensions supplemented with ferrichrome but did not measurably alter catalase formation in suspensions supplemented with haemin. This suggests that ferrichrome is necessary for haemin (catalase) synthesis and that ferrimycin A acts by blocking this synthesis. Cell free extracts of *Rhodopseudomonas spheroides* were able to synthesise haemin when incubated with an oxidisable substrate, protoporphyrin IX, and iron supplied as ferrichrome.

In the light of these findings obtained with sideromycins and sideramines, ZÄHNER (1965) postulated a mode of action for the sideromycins as outlined in Fig. 14. Studies carried out by various research teams indicate that the incorporation of iron into protoporphyrin is an enzymatic process.

LOCHHEAD *et al.* (1963) use the term "iron-incorporating enzyme". PORRA and JONES (1963 a, b) have described the assay and the properties of ferrochelatase and have studied the role played by this enzyme in the biosynthesis of various haem prosthetic groups. There can be no doubt that iron-transport compounds or specific metal chelators do play a part in the transfer of iron to these iron-incorporating enzyme systems and, hence, also in the synthesis of haemin enzymes.

From what is at present known about the chemical structure of the sideramines, the process involved must certainly be a complicated one, since the strongly bound trivalent iron would first have to be reduced to bivalent iron before it could be incorporated by enzyme systems into the protoporphyrin molecule. It is certain that sideramines cannot function as electron-transfer catalysts.

If the sole function of the sideramines were to supply iron for enzymatic incorporation into the protoporphyrin molecule, and if the effect of the sideromycins consisted solely in inhibiting this process, then addition of exogenous haemin could be expected to counteract the inhibitory effect of the sideromycin. This deinhibitory effect would have to involve growth, and would not simply be confined to catalase formation, as demonstrated by BURNHAM (1962b) with *Arthrobacter*

JG 9. When exogenous haemin is added to cultures of *Arthrobacter JG 9* which have been inhibited by a sideromycin, catalase formation is resumed, but growth inhibition cannot be reversed. BURNHAM (1962b) postulated an additional mode of action which is still completely unexplained.

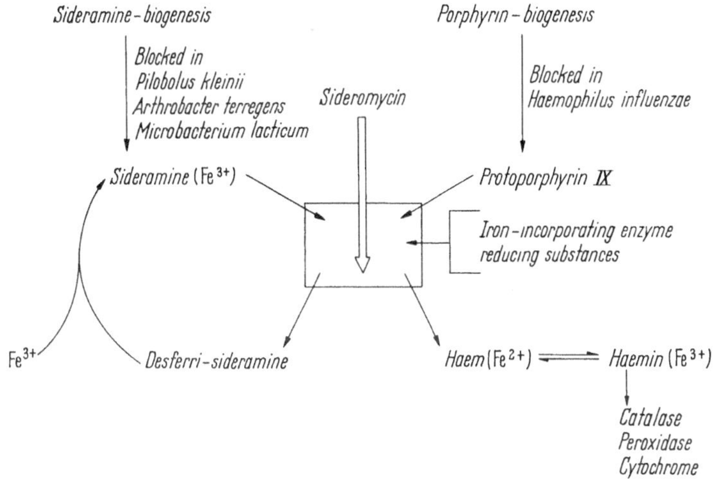

Fig. 14. Hypothesis of the mode of action of the siderochromes (ZÄHNER)

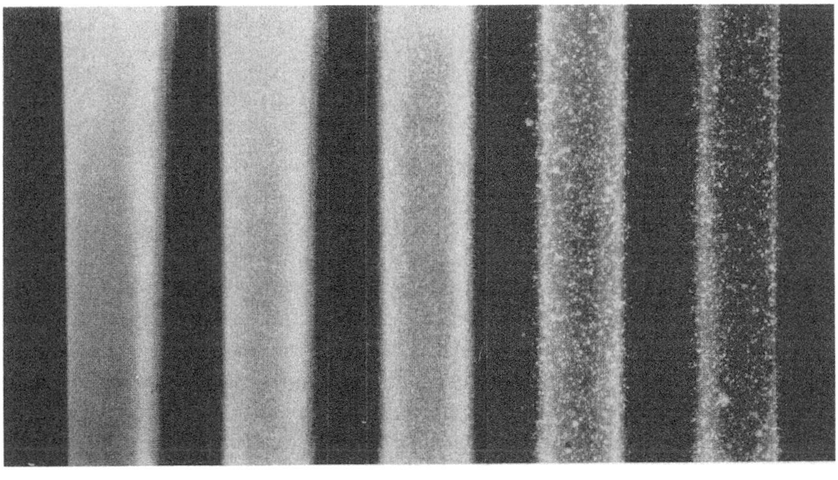

1 2 3 4 5

Fig. 15. Antibiotic activity of albomycin on *E. coli* under anaerobic conditions. 1 Growth control; 2 Albomycin 0.1 mcg/ml; 3 Albomycin 0.5 mcg/ml; 4 Albomycin 1 mcg/ml; 5 Albomycin 10 mcg/ml

It was the results reported by BURNHAM (1962b) which prompted us to re-examine more closely ZÄHNER's haemin-iron enzyme hypothesis. The following experimental findings soon led us to doubt this hypothesis (KNÜSEL and NÜESCH, 1965).

1. Sideromycins are also active under anaerobic conditions, the rate of resistance formation remaining equally high (Fig. 15). Biophotometric measurements

carried out with *Staph. aureus* and *E. coli* confirmed that ferrimycin and albomycin exert an inhibitory action under anaerobic conditions.

2. A ferrimycin-resistant strain of *Staph. aureus*, but not all of the ferrimycin-resistant micro-organisms, is inhibited by desferrioxamine and desferrimycin, but not by ferrioxamine (Fig. 13).

We were also able to isolate albomycin-resistant strains of *E. coli* which were inhibited by desferrioxamine, and it was only these resistant strains which grew only under aerobic conditions.

3. The iron-free form of antibiotic A 22,765, i.e. desferri-A 22,765, has just as strong an antibiotic effect as the ferri molecule (Table 9). Control experiments with the desferrioxamine-sensitive strain referred to above under point 2 showed that no iron is incorporated into the desferri molecule.

Table 9. *Comparison of the antibiotic activity between the iron-containing and the iron-free form of antibiotic A 22,765*

Addition to *Lascelles'* semisynthetic medium without glucose and with 2% of purified agar			Inhibition zone in mm 1% solutions		Catalase activity
			A 22,765	Desferri-22,765	
Glucose 0.5%			35	35	—
Glucose 0.5%	pyruvate	0.5%	30	30	—
Glucose 0.5%	oxalacetate	0.5%	28	25	—
Glucose 0.5%	acetate	0.5%	41	30	—
Glucose 0.5%	haemin	0.25 mcg/ml	30	30	+
	pyruvate	0.5%	37	36	—
	oxalacetate	0.5%	33	35	—
	acetate	0.5%	No growth	No growth	
	haemin	0.25 mcg/ml	29	30	+

All inhibition zones show the characteristic high numbers of resistant colonies.

4. Neither in *E. coli*, in *B. subtilis* nor *Staph. aureus* was it possible to reverse inhibition of growth or of oxygen consumption by administering exogenous haemin.

In none of the experiments with *E. coli*, *B. subtilis*, and *Staph. aureus*, in which attempts were made to counteract sideromycin inhibition by adding haemin, could any proof be obtained that these micro-organisms are capable of incorporating exogenous haemin into their own haemin enzymes.

In an excellent review by LASCELLES (1961) an account is given of the synthesis of tetrapyrroles by micro-organisms. She discusses the iron-binding factors and the fact that, in heterotrophic organisms, haemin is capable of replacing these factors, although it is far less active than they are. LASCELLES postulates that haemin serves the function of organically bound iron and that this iron then plays a role in the insertion of the metal into the tetrapyrrole nucleus. The haemin hypothesis advanced by ZÄHNER (1965) has been subjected to further critical analysis on the basis of two other facts obtained with bacteria. The first was the specificity of the haemin requirement of *Haemophilus influenzae;* protoporphyrin was just as active as haemin (GRANICK and GILDER, 1946). In this micro-organism it is therefore not the incorporation of iron into the protoporphyrin molecule which is disturbed, but a biochemical step in porphyrin synthesis. For this reason, *Haemophilus influenzae* is not suitable for studying the iron-incorporation hypothesis. The second fact that was examined is based on the synthetic capacities of a streptomycin-resistant strain of *Micrococcus pyogenes* var. *aureus* which was isolated by JENSEN and THOFERN (1953a, b). Under certain conditions of culture, this strain, *Staphylococcus aureus* JT 52, displays an absolute need for haemin. It possesses the ability to synthesize porphyrin via 8-δ-aminolaevulinic acid but cannot insert the iron into the protoporphyrin ring. According to THOFERN (1961) strain JT 52 utilizes exogenous sources of haemin for cytochrome synthesis. This microorganism is blocked at precisely the point where ZÄHNER (1965) presumes the site of action of the sideromycins to be located. It is able to incorporate exogenous haemin into its own haemin enzymes, and it therefore appeared to us to be the organism of choice with which to study the haemin hypothesis. The connection between streptomycin-resistance and haemin requirement, which has also been demonstrated in *E. coli* (BELJANSKI and BELJANSKI, 1957), is still unclear and calls for further investigation.

By culturing strain JT 52 in various nutrient solutions and under various conditions of culture, it is possible to influence the means by which proliferating cells of this mutant obtain their energy (KNÜSEL and NÜESCH, 1965; THOFERN, 1961; LASCELLES, 1956). The semi-synthetic nutrient solution used in our experiments has been described by LASCELLES (1956), who employed strain JT 52 for the determination of small quantities of iron-protoporphyrin produced by *Rhodopseudomonas sphaeroides*. These variations are summarized below.

1. When the mutant is cultured under aerobic conditions in a medium containing haemin, haemin enzymes are present; the population is catalase-positive. Atmospheric oxygen functions as a terminal H_2-acceptor and electron-transport takes place via the cytochrome system.

2. When the mutant is cultured under aerobic conditions in a nutrient solution containing no haemin, and with glucose and pyruvate serving as a source of carbon, no haemin enzymes can be detected; the population is catalase-negative. Some organic substance must therefore function as a terminal H_2-acceptor and there is no electron-transport via the cytochrome system.

3. When the mutant is cultured under anaerobic conditions in a nutrient solution containing haemin and sodium nitrate, the haemin enzymes needed for the activity of nitrate-reductase are present. Oxygen from the nitrate then functions as a terminal H_2-acceptor.

The influence exerted by potassium cyanide on the mutant JT 52 under these three conditions of culture offers additional proof that, when the organisms are cultured aerobically with glucose and pyruvate as a source of carbon, growth occurs without the participation of the cytochrome system (Fig. 16). JT 52, cultured under the three above-mentioned conditions, was employed to determine whether ferrimycin inhibition can be counteracted by the addition of exogenous haemin. The results obtained in studies with *Staph. aureus JT 52* can be summarised as follows:

Ferrimycin inhibits growth of this mutant under each of the three above mentioned conditions (Fig. 17). In other words, inhibition also occurs when the energy is obtained without recourse to the cytochrome system, i.e. even when haemin is not involved at all in the metabolism. When JT 52 is cultured on a solid nutrient medium with glucose and pyruvate as the carbon source, growth occurs without catalase formation, despite which it is still inhibited by sideromycins. An antagonism test with haemin showed that no reversal of inhibition occurs (Fig. 18). One striking feature in the case of this mutant is the large number of resistant organisms as compared with freshly isolated staphylococci.

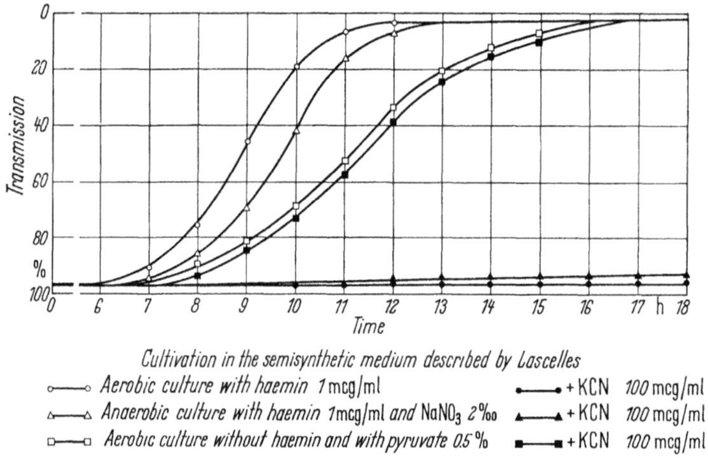

Fig. 16. Influence of KCN on the growth of *Staphylococcus aureus* JT 52 under various conditions of culture

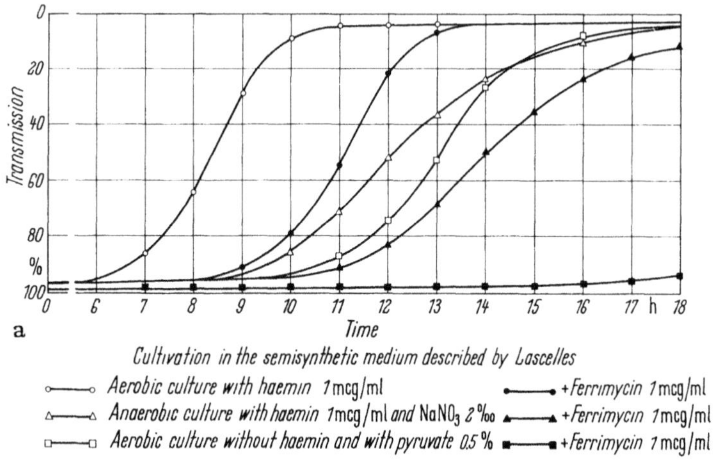

Fig. 17. Inhibitory effect of ferrimycin on *Staphylococcus aureus* JT 52 under various conditions of culture

From these experiments with *Staph. aureus JT 52*, it may be concluded that in the case of this bacterium the action exerted by the sideromycins can in all cases not be attributed to inhibition of haemin synthesis; moreover, there is certainly justification for assuming that the same applies to all other micro-organisms which are susceptible to sideromycin inhibition. If this is so, then the haemin hypothesis also becomes untenable.

The following conclusions can be drawn from the data that have thus far been discussed: sideramines and other metalchelators act as growth factors or growth stimulators on a small number of heterotrophic strains of bacteria from various systematic groups. Sideramines competitively reverse the antibiotic activity of the sideromycins. Intracellular haemin synthesis is not inhibited by the sideromycins.

To find out whether there is any connection between sideromycin inhibition and the activity of sideramines as growth factors, we studied the effect of autoclaved glucose-phosphate transformation products on *Bacillus subtilis* strain W (medium with glucose, NH_4Cl, inorganic salts, and trace elements) and *Brevibacterium flavum* ATCC 14,067 (medium: glucose 36 g, urea 10 g, KH_2PO_4 1 g,

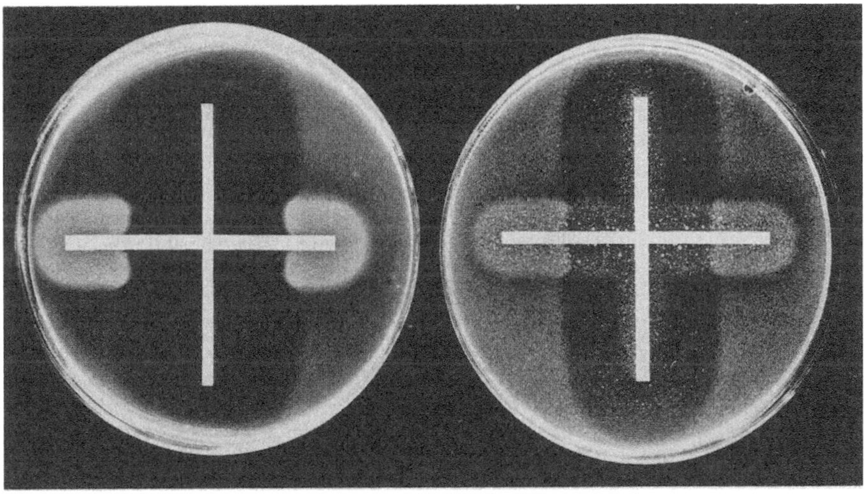

Fig. 18. Interaction between haemin and ferrimycin with the haemin-requiring *Staphylococcus aureus* JT 52 adapted and unadapted to neopyrithiamine. Cultivation on semisynthetic agar containing no haemin but 0.5% glucose and 0.5% pyruvate. Horizontal strip: Haemin 316 mcg/ml; Vertical strip: A 22,765 1,000 mcg/ml. Left: strain adapted to neopyrithiamine in a concentration of 100 mcg/ml. Right: untreated haemin-requiring mutant

$Na_2HPO_4 \cdot 2H_2O$ 1.6 g, $MgSO_4 \cdot 7H_2O$ 10 mg, $FeSO_4 \cdot 7H_2O$ 10 mg, $MnSO_4 \cdot 4H_2O$ 10 mg, casamino acids 100 mg, biotin 2 mcg, thiamine HCl 100 mcg, dist. water 1,000 cc).

If the glucose is separately sterilised using a membrane filter, neither of the two strains is capable of growing on the above-mentioned media when inoculated at a level of approx. 10^7 micro-organisms per Petri dish. In this experiment, the sideramines (e.g. desferrioxamine and ferrichrysin) exert a marked growth-enhancing action, and haemin and yeast extract also produce a slight stimulant effect on growth.

Under these conditions, ferrimycin has an equally marked growth-inhibiting action. The sideramines and sideromycins antagonise on another in the usual manner (Fig. 19). On the other hand, there is no antagonism between haemin or yeast extract and the sideromycins.

When cultured on the same media, but with autoclaved glucose-phosphate solution, the bacteria show an excellent rate of growth without the presence of a sideramine. Here too, however, ferrimycin has a strong growth-inhibiting effect, which can once again be competitively antagonised by a sideramine. It can thus be clearly demonstrated that the glucose-phosphate transformation products are capable of assuming one of the functions of the sideramines, i.e. their function as non-specific chelating agents. But there is no analogy between this and the effect exerted on the activity of ferrimycin, since the latter is not affected by these glucose-phosphate transformation products. The sideramines must therefore possess bifunctional properties; on the one hand, they show a specific mutual correlation *vis-à-vis* the sideromycins while, on the other hand, under certain conditions they act a snon-specific growth-promoting compounds. This is a property shared by many chelating agents of varying structure.

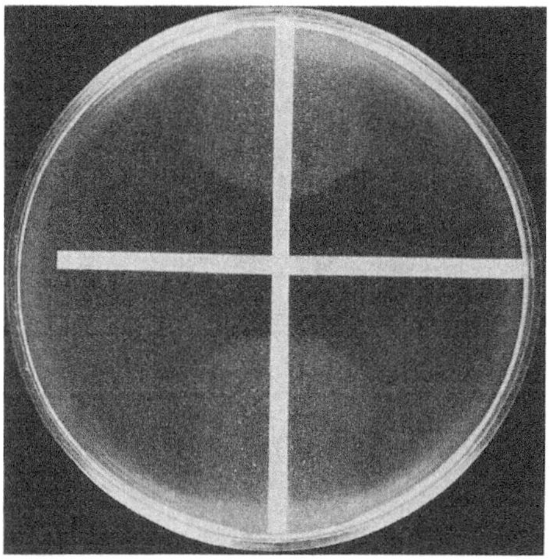

Fig. 19. Growth promoting effect of desferrioxamine B and the antibiotic activity of the sideromycin A 22,765 on *Brevibacterium flavum* on a chemically defined glucose medium. Horizontal: strip antibiotic A 22,765 100 mcg/ml; Vertical strip: Desferrioxamine B 50 mcg/ml

Carbohydrate Metabolism

The influence exerted by sideromycins on the degradation of glucose by resting cells was studied in two micro-organisms which are systematically quite different, i.e. *B. subtilis* ATCC 6633 and *Streptomyces griseoflavus* ETH 9578. We determined glucose degradation in the auto-analyser, and measured the oxygen uptake of cell masses suspended in a phosphate buffer containing glucose. Antibiotic A 22, 765 had no influence either on glucose degradation or on the oxygen uptake of resting *B. subtilis* ATCC 6633 cells, as indicated in Figs. 20 and 21, nor did it affect these two parameters when similar experiments were undertaken with *Streptomyces griseoflavus* ETH 9578.

The occurrence of large numbers of resistant organisms among all bacterial strains that are sensitive to the antibiotic action of sideromycins is a phenomenon of fundamental importance for an understanding of the mode of action of the sideromycins. Freshly isolated *Staph. aureus* strains, laboratory strains of the same species, and the haemin-requiring mutant JT 52 show very marked differences with regard to the number of resistant cells encountered. What is more, among these resistant cells, various types of resistance can be distinguished.

Another question of interest in this connection is whether the biochemical behaviour of a population of staphylococci repeatedly cultured *in vitro* can be compared with that of cells proliferating *in vivo*.

When cultured in a semi-synthetic nutrient solution with vitamin-free casamino acids as a source of nitrogen, staphylococci require the vitamins nicotinic acid and thiamine (HILLS, 1938). In our experience, thiamine acts only as a growth-enhancing substance. Accordingly, small doses of neopyrithiamine, which is a competitive antagonist of thiamine (ROBBINS, 1961; SCHOPFER, 1948), exerts a growth-inhibiting effect on staphylococci. Bacteria such as *E. coli* and *B. subtilis*, which are not thiamine-heterotrophic, are not inhibited by neopyrithiamine. With the aid of *Lactobacillus fermenti* ATCC 9338, for which the presence of thiamine

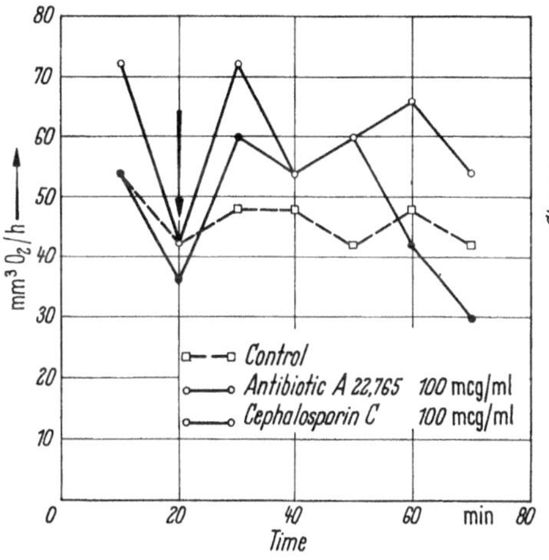

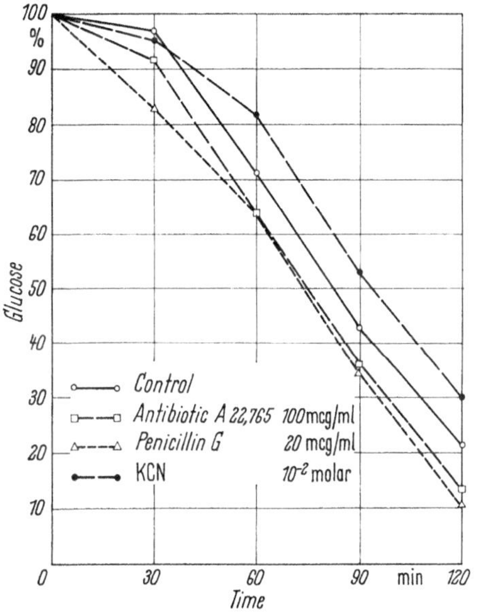

Fig. 20 Fig. 21

Fig. 20. Oxygen uptake of resting cells of *B. subtilis* ATCC 6633. *B. subtilis* ATCC 6633 was incubated in glucose broth at 37°C until a cell density of approx. 10^9 cells/ml was obtained. The mass of bacteria was then centrifuged off, washed twice with physiological saline solution, and resuspended at a concentration of 10^9 cells/ml in phosphate buffer (pH 7) with or without 1% glucose. Using these suspensions, the oxygen uptake was measured in the Warburg apparatus

Fig. 21. *B. subtilis* ATCC 6633 was cultured as already mentioned in Fig. 20. Having been washed with physiological saline, the moist sediment was resuspended in 200 ml. ERLENMEYER shaking flasks containing 60 ml phosphate buffer (pH 7) and the ingredients indicated in the Figure. The concentration of the bacterial mass amounted to 5% (w/v). The flasks were then incubated at 37°C on a shaking machine rotating at 120 r.p.m. After 0, 30, 60, 90, and 120 minutes, samples were removed, placed for 10 minutes in a water bath at 90°C, cooled, and centrifuged; the glucose content of the supernatant was then determined in the auto-analyser

is absolutely essential, the competitive antagonism between the vitamin and the antivitamin can be conclusively demonstrated. By continuously culturing *Staph. aureus* with increasing doses of neopyrithiamine, it is possible to adapt the bacteria to the antivitamin (DAS and CHATTERJEE, 1962). In our opinion, this adaptation is attributable to selection of those mutants in the population which are relatively insensitive to neopyrithiamine. The most striking biochemical changes occurring in the strain adapted to neopyrithiamine are an improvement in acetate utilisation coupled with a decrease in glucose consumption and high levels of isocitratase and malate synthetase (DAS and CHATTERJEE, 1963). These two enzymes are almost completely absent in the normal strain. Their presence indicates the existence of a glyoxalate by-pass in the adapted strain.

In a concentration of 10 mcg/ml, neopyrithiamine completely inhibits growth of the haemin-requiring mutant *Staphylococcus aureus* JT 52. When this strain was repeatedly cultured in nutrient solutions containing steadily increasing doses of the antivitamin, selection finally reached a point where the organisms continued to grow without thiamine in solutions in which the concentration of neopyrithiamine was as high as 100 mcg/ml.

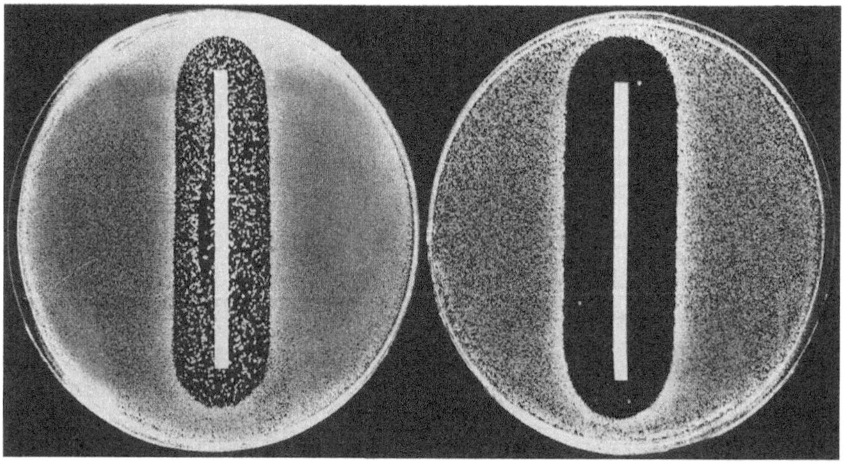

Fig. 22. Suppression of resistance formation by adaption of *Staphylococcus aureus* JT 52 to neopyrithiamine. Left: strain adapted to neopyrithiamine in a concentration of 100 mcg/ml. Rigth: untreated haemin-requiring mutant. Strips impregnated with a 1 mg/ml solution of antibiotic A 22,765

A study of the inhibitory effect exerted by a sideromycin on the adapted strain revealed the following interesting finding. In the adapted strain, the formation of sideromycin-resistant organisms was almost completely suppressed (KNÜSEL and NÜESCH, 1965) (Fig. 22). The resistance rate amounted to approx. 10^{-4} in the normal strain, whereas it was reduced to 10^{-8} as a result of selection. Since all sideromycin-sensitive bacterial populations contain an extremely large number of resistant organisms, it can be assumed that some mechanism common to all of them must underlie this phenomenon. The reduction in the number of resistant cells occurring as a result of adaptation to neopyrithiamine would therefore appear to be due to the loss of some step in metabolism which is responsible for the development of resistance.

Glutamic Acid Metabolism

The various experiments carried out with the sideromycins led us to postulate that the mechanism of action of these antibiotics might be linked with central, energy-yielding pathways of metabolism. For this reason, in our search for suitable biochemical tools, we attached great importance to those micro-organisms about which a great deal is already known and which accumulate measurable quantities of end-products connected with carbohydrate metabolism. Hence our particular interest in bacteria which produce glutamic acid. HUANG (1964) has published an excellent review summarising what is at present known about the biogenesis of glutamic acid. Glutamic-acid producers are to be found chiefly within a group of closely related bacteria which, as recent studies suggest (HUANG, 1964), probably belong to the genus *Arthrobacter*. This genus includes micro-organisms such as *Arthrobacter* JG 9, which is sensitive to ferrimycin and on which sideramines act as growth initiators. The organisms in question are non-sporulating, Gram-positive, catalase-forming, non-motile bacteria varying in morphology from coccoid to rod-shaped. They show an absolute need for biotin,

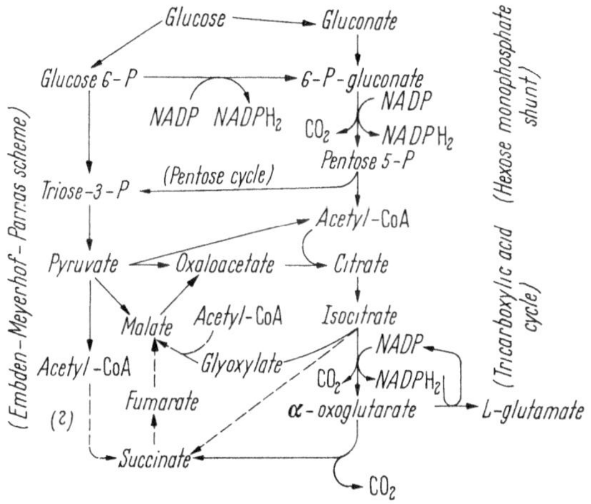

Fig. 23. Probable pathway of glutamate formation by *Micrococcus glutamicus* (KINOSHITA, 1963)

and when cultured in the presence of air they produce large quantities of L-glutamic acid from carbohydrates and ammonium. The mechanism of glutamic-acid biogenesis has been investigated in detail by Japanese workers, particularly as regards *Micrococcus glutamicus* and *Brevibacterium flavum*, and has also been reviewed by HUANG (1964).

The catabolic metabolism of carbohydrates by *Brevibacterium flavum* and *Micrococcus glutamicus* has now been largely elucidated. KINOSHITA (1963) has outlined in diagrammatic form the various intermediary and terminal metabolic pathways by which *Micrococcus glutamicus* breaks down carbohydrates (Fig. 23). Intermediary carbohydrate degradation seems to be possible via the glycolytic sequence as well as via the hexosemonophosphate shunt. According to HUANG (1964), the asymmetrical fixation of CO_2 to pyruvate plays an important role in L-glutamate synthesis. *Brevibacterium flavum* possesses all the enzymes of the tricarboxylic-acid cycle except α-oxoglutarate dehydrogenase. For this reason, it would also appear very unlikely that the Krebs cycle functions normally. Both *Brevibacterium* and *Micrococcus* display high isocitratase activity when cultured with acetate as their carbohydrate source. Since glutamic acid is also produced in the presence of acetate, an efficient glyoxylate cycle presumably operates side by side with an incomplete tricarboxylic-acid cycle. According to HUANG (1964), the following sequence of glucose oxidation leads to the synthesis of glutamic acid: glucose ⟶ pyruvate ⟶ citrate ⟶ α-oxoglutarate. The oxalacetate needed for citrate synthesis can also be obtained from acetate via the glyoxylate cycle. One major feature which distinguishes the glutamic-acid producing bacteria from other bacteria is the absence of an α-oxoglutarate dehydrogenase and the inability to oxidise L-glutamate to α-oxoglutarate. The biochemical problems which this poses have been discussed in detail by HUANG (1964). Finally, reference should also be made to the decisive role played by biotin in the biosynthesis of L-glutamic acid. It is the concentration of biotin which limits the production of glutamic acid; low biotin levels lead to maximal production, whereas an excess of biotin results in a rapid consumption of sugar and in marked cell growth, coupled with only a small accumulation of L-glutamic acid. In the studies described here, the microorganism generally employed was *Brevibacterium flavum* ATCC 14,067, *Micrococcus glutamicus* ATCC 13,058 being used only occasionally to provide confirmation of the results. Media[1] that were used in the experiments are given in the footnote. The results so far obtained must to some extent be regarded as merely preliminary, and will require confirmation and further study. As already described, when cultured on a semi-synthetic medium (medium A + 2% Bacto-agar) *Brevibacterium flavum* is inhibited by the sideromycin A 22,765. Optimal growth of the bacterium is observed only when the medium is sterilised at 120°C or when sterilisation is performed under mild conditions and a chelating agent such as desferrioxamine B is added. A good rate of growth also occurs in this liquid medium A when mild conditions of sterilisation are employed, provided that the medium is heavily inoculated. Fig. 24 indicates

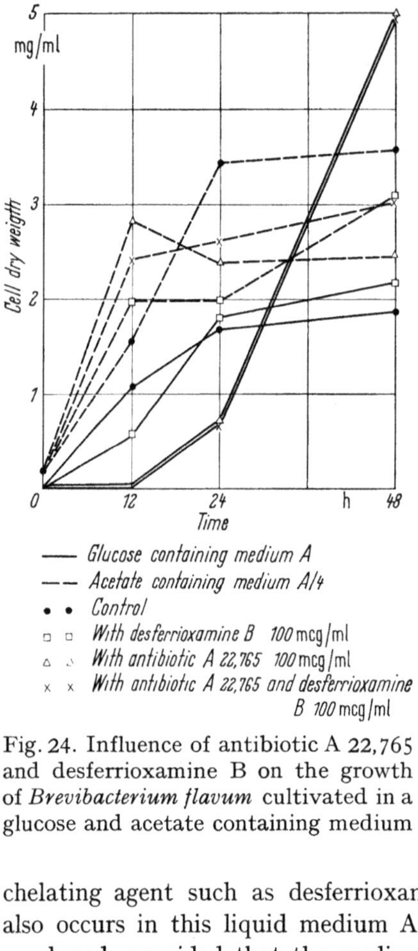

Fig. 24. Influence of antibiotic A 22,765 and desferrioxamine B on the growth of *Brevibacterium flavum* cultivated in a glucose and acetate containing medium

[1] Medium A-Glucose, 36 g; Urea, 10 g; KH_2PO_4, 1 g; $Na_2HPO_4 \cdot 2H_2O$, 1.6 g; $MgSO_4 \cdot 7H_2O$, 0.4 g; $FeSO_4 \cdot 7H_2O$, 10 mg; Casamino acids, 100 mg; $MnSO_4 \cdot 4H_2O$, 10 mg; Thiamine HCI, 100 mcg; Biotin, 2 mcg; Distilled H_2O to 1,000 ml; pH 7.0 after sterilization for 110°C, 20 minutes.

Medium A/4-Identical with Medium A, except that 25 g Na-acetate (as acetic acid) was substituted for the glucose.

Medium B-Glucose, 25 g; NH_4-acetate, 15 g; KH_2PO_4, 2 g; $Na_2HPO_4 \cdot 2H_2O$, 3.15 g; $MgSO_4 \cdot 7H_2O$, 0.4 g; $FeSO_4 \cdot 7H_2O$, 10 mg; $MnSO_4 \cdot 4H_2O$, 10 mg; Thiamine HCl, 100 mcg; Cornsteep liquor, 2 g; Tap water to 1,000 ml; pH 7.5 after sterilization for 110°C, 20 minutes.

the growth of *Brevibacterium flavum* under the influence of a sideramine (desferrioxamine B) and a sideromycin (antibiotic A 22,765) in the glucose-containing medium A and in the acetate- containing medium A/4.

The effect which the sideromycin exerts on growth is clearly dependent upon the carbohydrate source. In the medium containing glucose, the antibiotic inhibits multiplication of the cells for approx. 12 hours, after which very strong growth suddenly sets in. Both the rate of growth and the size of the cell mass formed are considerably greater under the influence of the sideromycin than in the control cultures. On the other hand, in comparison with the controls, far less L-glutamate is produced. Desferrioxamine B has no influence either on growth

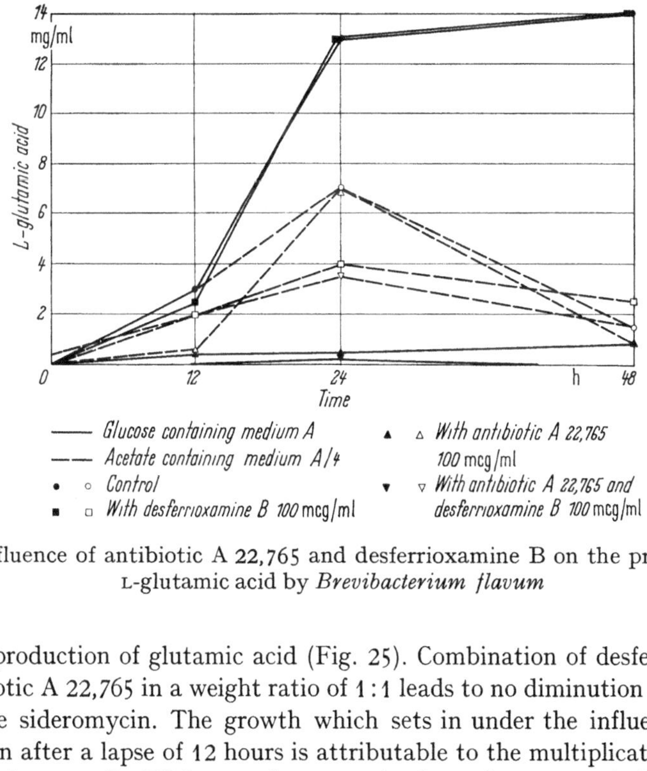

Fig. 25. Influence of antibiotic A 22,765 and desferrioxamine B on the production of L-glutamic acid by *Brevibacterium flavum*

or on the production of glutamic acid (Fig. 25). Combination of desferrioxamine and antibiotic A 22,765 in a weight ratio of 1:1 leads to no diminution in the activity of the sideromycin. The growth which sets in under the influence of the sideromycin after a lapse of 12 hours is attributable to the multiplication of sideromycin-resistant cells. With regard to growth, the resistant population behaves like the normal strain cultured in a medium containing an excess of biotin.

However, in the acetate-containing medium, and under the experimental conditions chosen, neither the sideromycin nor the iron-free sideramine was found to exert any clear-cut influence on growth or on glutamic-acid production (Fig. 24 and Fig. 25).

The siderochromes studied had the same type of effect on the degradation of glucose by growing cultures as on growth itself. The sideromycin-resistant population broke down the glucose in a much faster rate than did the normal strain. Desferrioxamine B, on the other hand, had no effect. The production of ammonia in the culture solutions is affected. In medium A, a high and uniform ammonia level is obtained after incubation for 24 hours (Fig. 26). This effect is far less pronounced in the presence of antibiotic A 22,765, while in the acetate-containing medium it is not observed at all, either with or without the sideromycin.

Determination of several carboxylic acids in the culture solutions of both media yielded the results presented in the following Figures. In medium A, containing glucose, maximal accumulation of lactate occurred after 12 hours under all experimented conditions. In the nutrient solution containing the sideromycin, the maximal lactate concentration after 12 hours was considerably higher than in the control solution; once multiplication of the resistant cells is well under way. On the other hand, the lactate concentration decreases to a lower level than in

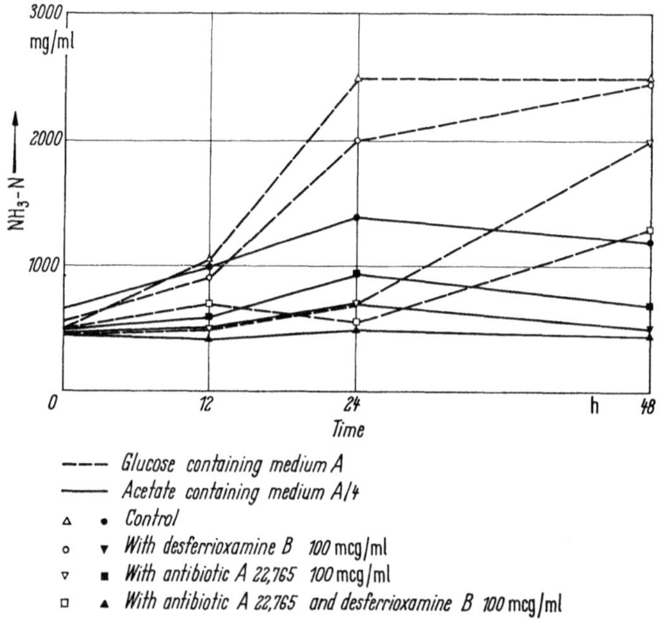

Fig. 26. Accumulation of ammonia by *Brevibacterium flavum* under the influence of antibiotic A 22,765 and desferrioxamine B

the cultures containing no sideromycin or in the cultures to which the sideramine has been added. In the case of the cultures grown in the acetate-containing nutrient solution A/4, no differences could be detected, as lactate production was invariably very small (Fig. 27).

As a general rule, pyruvate production in the culture filtrates from the glucose-containing medium did not rise to high levels. The pattern of pyruvate production, however, corresponded by and large to that of lactate production (Fig. 28).

In the glucose-containing medium, a brief accumulation of α-oxoglutaric acid also occurs, provided antibiotic A 22,765 is added to the solution; whereas in the acetate-containing medium only very small quantities of α-oxoglutaric acid could be found. In medium A/4 neither antibiotic A 22,765 nor desferrioxamine B has any effect (Fig. 29). In the glucose-containing medium, relatively large quantities of lactate, pyruvate, and α-oxoglutarate are secreted extracellularly over a brief period under the influence of the sideromycin. Once multiplication of the sideromycin-resistant population is in full swing, however, the carboxylic-acid level decreases again, the decrease being much more pronounced than in the control cultures. The sideramine exerts no measurable influence on the production of these carboxylic acids.

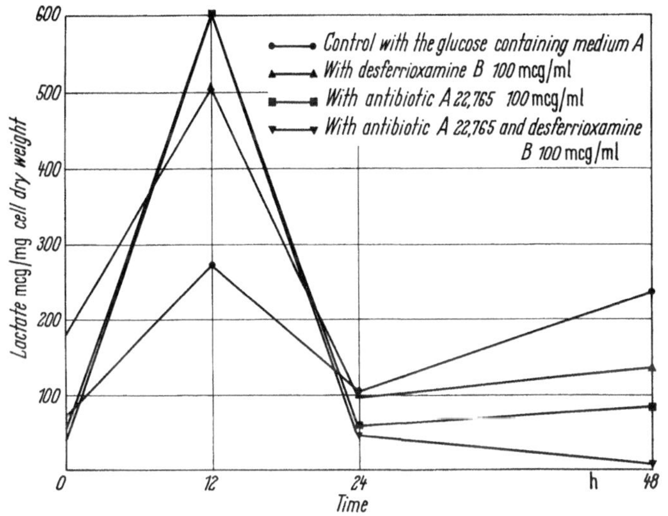

Fig. 27. Accumulation of lactate by *Brevibacterium flavum* under the influence of antibiotic A 22,765 and desferrioxamine B

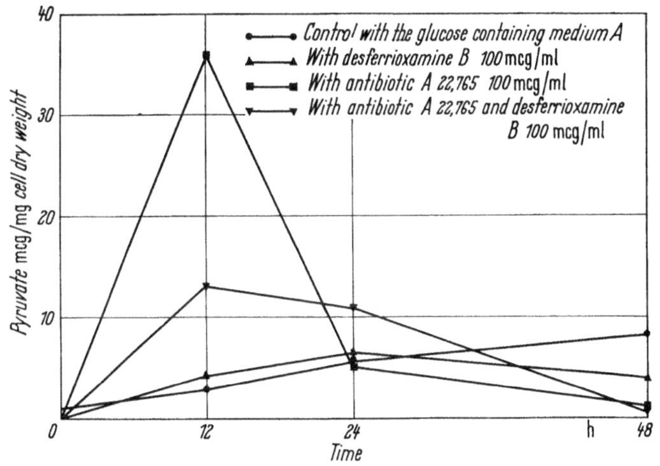

Fig. 28. Accumulation of pyruvate by *Brevibacterium flavum* under the influence of antibiotic A 22,765 and desferrioxamine B

No marked accumulation of carboxylic acid occurs in the acetate-containing medium. In medium A/4 neither antibiotic A 22,765 nor desferrioxamine B appears to have any influence on *Brevibacterium flavum*.

The situation is different on accumulation of glyoxylic acid, (Fig. 30). Whereas glyoxylic acid cannot be detected in significant quantities in the glucose-containing medium A, comparatively high extracellular concentrations of glyoxylic acid are built up in the same nutrient solution under the influence of the sideramine (desferrioxamine B) and, to a lesser extent, under the influence of the sideromycin (antibiotic A 22,765). In the acetate-containing medium and also in the control cultures, *Brevibacterium flavum* produces measurable amounts of glyoxylic

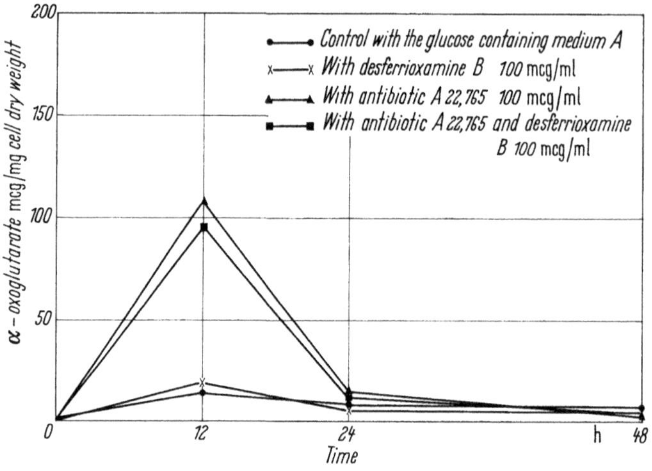

Fig. 29. Accumulation of α-oxoglutarate by *Brevibacterium flavum* under the influence of antibiotic A 22,765 and desferrioxamine B

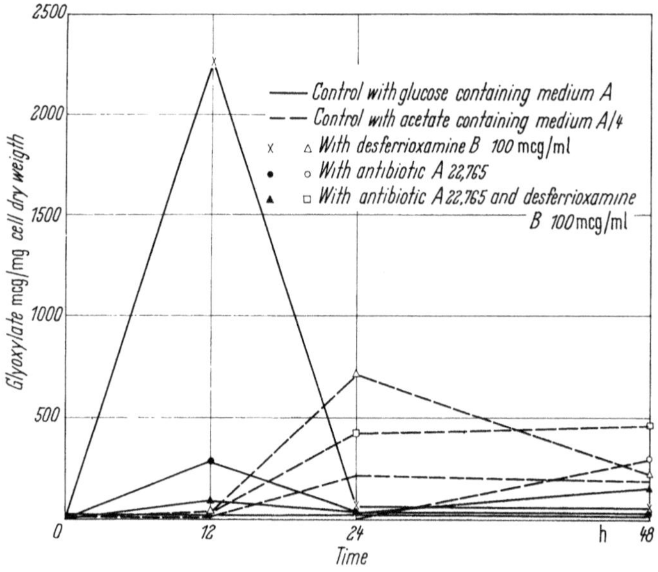

Fig. 30. Accumulation of glyoxylate by *Brevibacterium flavum* under the influence of antibiotic A 22,765 and desferrioxamine B

acid. Under our experimental conditions, this glyoxylic acid seems to be an integral part of acetate metabolism in *Brevibacterium flavum*. Though sideromycin has no significant influence on glyoxylic-acid formation, the sideramine appears to cause an earlier and stronger accumulation of this acid. The malate determinations yielded negative results under all experimental conditions. It was also impossible to detect any significant extracellular isocitrate dehydrogenase or glutamate-oxalacetate transaminase activity.

Conclusions

In view of the chemical properties displayed by the siderochromes, which are characteristic iron (III) trihydroxamate complexes, it has been postulated that these substances play a role in the iron metabolism of living cells. To the sideramines have been ascribed functions as co-factors for iron incorporation into enzymes of the haem type or for intracellular iron transport. The sideromycins have been assumed to inhibit such processes. The chemical structure of these compounds is such that the possibility of their exercising a function in an electron-transfer system could be excluded.

From experiments with the haemin-heterotrophic mutant *Staph. aureus* JT 52, whose haemin requirement is attributable to a defect in the incorporation of iron into protoporphyrin, it was clearly demonstrated that the sideromycins do not intervene in the biosynthesis of haemin. They also have no effect on haemin containing enzymes. Sideromycin-resistant micro-organisms obtain their energy chiefly via the respiratory chain which is catalysed by haemin enzymes and is linked to the tricarboxylic-acid cycle. Growth of *Staph. aureus JT 52* is also inhibited by sideromycins under conditions of culture which induce energy-yielding catabolism without the presence of haemin enzymes.

The data which appeared to support the iron-incorporation and iron-transport theories were based largely on the activity displayed by the sideramines as growth-factors — an activity which takes the form mainly of a growth-stimulating or growth-initiating effect. From a detailed study of the literature, as well as from our own experiments, it has been shown that the sideramines, in their capacity as organic iron compounds, do indeed play a role as iron donors. This property, however, is relatively unspecific and is shared by many different chelating agents, including, for example, heat-sterilised glucose-phosphate solutions. The sideromycins do not interfere in any way with this activity of the sideramines. The sideramines thus fulfil a dual function in the physiology of microbial cells: first, they act as non-specific iron donators and, second, they show a close specific relationship to the sideromycins. This, of course, does not preclude the possibility that the site of action of the sideromycins may not be related to an iron-containing enzyme system.

The precise mechanism of action of the sideromycins is still a matter of conjecture. The results of the studies discussed here suggest that the sideromycins effect carbohydrate metabolism. The fact that exposure to the action of neopyrithiamine — a competitive antagonist of thiamine — results in selection of a *Staph. aureus* population which is no longer able to develop a high degree of resistance to sideromycins, indicates, on the one hand, that the process of selection favours the emergence of a population whose metabolism is catalysed by thiamine-independent enzymes and, on the other hand, that the inhibitory mechanism of the sideromycins must be related to these thiamine-independent metabolic steps. Thiamine is known to function in the catabolism of carbohydrates.

Studies with the glutamic-acid producing *Brevibacterium flavum* reveal that there is an obvious connection between carbohydrate metabolism and the action of the sideromycins. A sideromycin-resistant population of this bacterium differs from a normal population in that it accumulates very little extracellular glutamic acid and that its pattern of growth and glucose degradation is indicative of a more rational utilisation of energy for carbohydrate metabolism. The activity of the sideromycins is dependent on the carbohydrate source and, consequently, on the enzyme systems responsible for catalysing carbohydrate metabolism. Micro-organisms have various pathways of carbohydrate metabolism, to serve the same end. The sideromycins appear to block one of these particular pathways. Sideromycin-resistant micro-organisms must therefore be capable of bypassing the metabolic step that has been blocked.

We propose to undertake further studies to investigate the metabolic steps which are sensitive or insensitive to the blocking action of the sideromycins. In particular, it will be necessary to examine the thiamine-dependent transketolases in the pentose-phosphate pathway, as well as the biosynthesis of leucine and valine. Since the biosynthesis of leucine and valine proceeds via acetolacetate, the suggestion made by HOGG *et al.* (1965) that an iron-containing enzyme system may be involved in the thiamine-dependent synthesis of acetoin, is especially interesting.

See Addendum

References

BACHMANN, E., u. H. ZÄHNER: Stoffwechselprodukte von Actinomyceten. 28. Mitt. Die „*in vitro*"-Resistenz gegen Ferrimycin. Arch. Mikrobiol. **38**, 326 (1961).

BELJANSKI, M., et M. BELJANSKI: Sur la formation d'enzymes respiratoires chez un mutant d'escherichia coli streptomycine-résistant et auxotrophe pour l'hémine. Ann. inst. Pasteur. **92**, 396 (1957).

BENZ, F., and H. BICKEL: Personal communication 1965.

BERGMEYER, H. U.: Methoden der enzymatischen Analyse (Glyoxalat, S. 300, Malat, S. 328, Pyruvat, S. 253). Weinheim: Verlag Chemie 1962.

BICKEL, H., E. GÄUMANN, W. KELLER-SCHIERLEIN, V. PRELOG, E. VISCHER, A. WETTSTEIN u. H. ZÄHNER: Über eisenhaltige Wachstumsfaktoren, die Sideramine und ihre Antagonisten, die eisenhaltigen Antibiotika Sideromycine. Experientia **16** (4), 129 (1960a).

BICKEL, H., E. GÄUMANN, G. NUSSBERGER, P. REUSSER, E. VISCHER, W. VOSER, A. WETTSTEIN u. H. ZÄHNER: Stoffwechselprodukte von Actinomyceten. 25. Mitt. Über die Isolierung und Charakterisierung der Ferrimycine A_1 und A_2, neuer Antibiotika der Sideromycin-Gruppe. Helv. Chim. Acta **43**, 2105 (1960b).

BICKEL, H., P. MERTENS, V. PRELOG, J. SEIBL, and A. WALSER: The constitution of Ferrimycin A_1. IVth Int. Congr. Chemother. 1965 (Abstracts) p. 15.

Boehringer: Glutamat-Oxalacetat-Transaminase „Boehringer". Biochemica Testcombination „Boehringer", C. F. Boehringer & Söhne GmbH Mannheim 1962.

Boehringer: Isocitronensäure-Dehydrogenase nach „Boehringer", Biochemica Informationen „Boehringer", C. F. Boehringer & Söhne GmbH Mannheim 1961.

Boehringer: Ketoglutarsäure-Test. Biochemica Testkombinationen „Boehringer", C. F. Boehringer & Söhne GmbH Mannheim 1962.

Boehringer: Lactat-Test. Biochemica Testkombination „Boehringer", C. F. Boehringer & Söhne GmbH Mannheim 1962.

BRINBERG, S. L., and T. I. GRINYUK: The physiological features of *Act. subtropicus* in connection with the biosynthesis of the antibiotic Albomycin. Antibiotics UdSSR **4**, 534 (1959).

BURNHAM, F. B.: Bacterial iron metabolism. Investigations on the mechanism of ferrichrome function Arch. Biochem. Biophys. **97**, 329 (1962a).

BURNHAM, F. B.: Personal communication 1962b.

BURNHAM, F. B., and J. B. NEILANDS: Studies on the metabolic function of the ferrichrome compounds. J. Biol. Chem. **236** (2), 554 (1961).

COULTAS, M. K., and D. I. HUTCHINSON: Metabolism of resistent mutants of streptococcus faecalis. IV. Use of a biophotometer in growth-curve studies. J. Bacteriol. **84**, 393 (1962).

DAS, S. K., and G. C. CHATTERJEE: Pyrithiamine adaptation of Staphylococcus aureus. I. Adaption and carbohydrate utilization. J. Bacteriol. **83**, 1251 (1962).

DAS, S. K., and G. C. CHATTERJEE: Pyrithiamine adaptation of Staphylococcus aureus. II. Tricarboxylic acid cycle and related enzymes. J. Bacteriol. **86**, 1157 (1963).

DEMAIN, A. L., and D. HENDLIN: "Iron transport" compounds as growth stimulators for *Microbacterium* sp. J. gen. Microbiol. **21**, 72 (1959).

FRANCIS, J., H. M. MACTURK, J. MADINAVEITIA, and G. A. SNOW: Mycobactin, a growth factor for *Mycobacterium johnei*. I. Isolation from *Mycobacterium phlei*. Biochem. J. **55**, 596 (1953).

GARIBALDI, J. A., and J. B. NEILANDS: Formation of iron binding compounds by micro-organisms. Nature **177**, 526 (1956).

GAUSE, G. F.: Recent studies on Albomycin, a new antibiotic. Brit. med. **1955**, 1177.

GAUSE, G. F., u. M. G. BRAZHNIKOVA: Die Wirkung von Albomycin gegen Bakterien [Russ.]. Novostin. Med., Akad. Med. Nauk S. S. S. R. **23**, 3 (1951).

GÄUMANN, E., E. VISCHER u. H. BICKEL: Verfahren zur Herstellung eines neuen Antibiotikums. Deutsche Auslegeschrift DAS 1129, 259 (1951).

GRANICK, S., and H. GILDER: The porphyrin requirements of *Haemophilus influenzae* and some functions of the vinyl and propionic acid side chains of heme. J. Gen. Physiol. **30**, 1 (1946).

GREEN, D. E., and H. BEINERT: Biological oxidations. Ann. Rev. Biochem. **24**, 1 (1955).

HASKELL, TH. H., R. H. BUNGE, J. C. FRENCH, and QU. R. BARTZ: Succinimycin, a new iron-containing antibiotic. J. Antibiotics (Japan), Serie A **16**, 67 (1963).

HESSELTINE, C. W., C. PIDACKS, A. R. WHITEHILL, N. BOHONOS, B. L. HUTCHINGS, and J. H. WILLIAMS: Coprogen, a new growth factor for coprophilic fungi. J. Am. Chem. Soc. **74**, 1362 (1952).

HILLS, G. M.: Aneurin (Vitamin B_1) and pyruvate metabolism by Staphylococcus aureus. Biochem. J. **32**, 383 (1938).

HOGG, R. W., CH. S. BISWAS, and H. P. BROQUIST: Interference with valine and isoleucine biosynthesis by cyclic hydroxamic acids. J. Bacteriol. **90**, 1265 (1965).

HUANG, H. T.: Microbial production of amino acids. Progr. Ind. Microbiol. **5**, 55 (1964).

HÜTTER, R.: Zur Systematik der Aktinomyceten. 10. Streptomyceten mit griseus Luftmycel. Giorn. microbiol. **11**, 191 (1963).

JENSEN, J., u. E. THOFERN: Chlorohämin (Ferriporphyrinchlorid) als Bakterienwuchsstoff. I. Z. Naturforsch. **8**, 595 (1953a).

JENSEN, J., u. E. THOFERN: Chlorohämin (Ferriporphyrinchlorid) als Bakterienwuchsstoff. II. Zur Synthese der Hämatinfermente. Z. Naturforsch. **8**b, 604 (1953b).

KELLER-SCHIERLEIN, W., V. PRELOG u. H. ZÄHNER: Siderochrome. Fortschr. Chem. org. Naturstoffe **22**, 279 (1964).

KELLER-SCHIERLEIN, W., P. MERTENS, V. PRELOG u. A. WALSER: Die Ferrioxamine A_1, A_2 und D_2. Helv. Chim. Acta **48**, 710 (1965).

KINOSHITA, SH.: Amino acids. From biochemistry of industrial micro-organisms, p. 206. London and New York: Academic Press 1963.

KNÜSEL, F., and J. NÜESCH: Mechanism of action of sideromycins. Nature **206**, 675 (1965).

KORNBERG, H. L.: Anaplerotic sequences in microbial metabolism (1). Angew. Chem. (internat. edit.) **4**, 558 (1965).

KRYSIN, E. P., u. N. A. PODDUBNAYA: Chemische Untersuchung der Struktur des Albomycin. IV. Bestimmung der Aminosäurezusammensetzung und Umwandlungen der Albomycin-Fraktionen. Zhurn. Obshchei Khim. **33**, 1370 (1963).

KUEHL, F. A., M. N. BISHOP, L. CHAIET, and K. FOLKERS: Isolation and some chemical properties of grisein. J. Am. Chem. Soc. **73**, 1770 (1951).

LASCELLES, J.: An assay of iron protoporphyrin based on the reduction of nitrate by a variant strain of Staphylococcus aureus; synthesis of iron protoporphyrin by suspension of *Rhodopseudomonas spheroides*. J. Gen. Microbiol. **15**, 404 (1956).

LASCELLES, J.: Synthesis of tetrapyrroles by micro-organisms. Phys. Rev. **41**, 417 (1961).

LOCHHEAD, A. G., M. O. BURTON, and R. H. THEXTON: A bacterial growth factor synthesized by a soil bacterium. Nature **170**, 282 (1952).

LOCHHEAD, A. G., S. KRAMER, and A. GOLDBERG: Quantitative measurement of the iron incorporating enzyme in relation to marrow cells and liver tissue in the rabbit. Brit. J. Haemat. **9**, 39 (1963).

MORRISON, N. E., A. D. ANTOINE, and E. E. DEWBREY: Synthetic metal chelators which replace the natural growth-factor requirements of *Arthrobacter terregens*. J. Bacteriol. **89**, 1630 (1965).

NEILANDS, J. B.: A crystalline organo iron compound from the fungus *Ustilago spaerogena*. J. Am. Chem. Soc. **74**, 4846 (1952).

NEILANDS, J. B.: Some aspects of microbial iron metabolism. Bacteriol. Rev. **21**, 101 (1957).

OKAMI, Y.: Studies on the characteristic of antibiotic Streptomyces. III. Characteristices of grisein producing strains. J. Antibiotics (Japan) **3**, 93 (1950).

PAGE, R. M.: The effect of nutrition on growth and sporulation of *Pilobolus*. Am. J. Bot. **39**, 731 (1952).

PORRA, R. J., and O. T. G. JONES: Studies on ferrochelatase 1. Assay and properties of ferrochelatase from a pig-liver mitochondrial extract. Biochem. J. **87**, 181 (1963a).

PORRA, R. J., and O. T. G. JONES: Studies on ferrochelatase 2. An investigation of the role of ferrochelatase in the biosynthesis of various haem prosthetic groups. Biochem. J. **87**, 186 (1963b).

PRELOG, V.: Iron-containing compounds in Micro-organisms Symposium Iron-Metabolism, Aix-en-Provence. Berlin-Göttingen-Heidelberg: Springer 1963.

RAMSEY, H. H., and C. E. LANKFORD: Stimulation of growth initiation by heat degradation products of glucose. J. Bacteriol. **72**, 511 (1956).

REYNOLDS, D. M., A. SCHATZ, and S. A. WAKSMAN: Grisein, a new antibiotic produced by a strain of *Streptomyces griseus*. Proc. Soc. Exptl. Biol. Med. **64**, 50 (1947).

REYNOLDS, D. M., and S. A. WAKSMAN: Grisein, an antibiotic produced by certain strains of *Streptomyces griseus*. J. Bacteriol. **55**, 739 (1948).

ROBBINSON, F. A.: The vitamin B complex. New York: John Wiley & Sons. Inc. 1951.

SACKMANN, W., P. REUSSER, L. NEIPP, F. KRADOLFER, and F. GROSS: Ferrimycin A, a new iron-containing antibiotic. Antibiotics & Chemotherapy **12**, 34 (1962).

SCHOPFER, W. H.: La pyrithiamine comme antivitamine B_1. Colloque internat. sur les Antivitamines, Lyon. Bull. soc. chim. biol. **30**, 940 (1948).

SEARGEANT, T. P., C. E. LANKFORD, and R. W. TRAXLER: Initiation of growth of Bacillus species in a chemically defined medium. J. Bacteriol. **74**, 728 (1957).

SENSI, P., and M. T. TIMBAL: Isolation of two antibiotics of the grisein and albomycin groups. Antibiot. & Chemotherapy **9**, 160 (1958).

SEVCIK, V.: Antibiotica aus Actinomyceten, 647 S. Jena: VEB Gustav Fischer 1963.

SNOW, G. A.: The structure of Mycobactin P, a growth factor for *Mycobacterium johnei*, and the significance of its iron complex. Biochem. J. **94**, 160 (1965).

STAPLEY, E. O., and R. E. ORMOND: Similarity of albomycin and grisein. Science **125**, 587 (1957).

STRASTERS, K. C., and K. C. WINKLER: Carbohydrate metabolism of Staphylococcus aureus. J. Gen. Microbiol. **33**, 213 (1963).

THOFERN, E.: Über Synthese, Struktur und Funktion bakterieller Haeminsysteme. Ergeb. Mikrobiol. **34**, 213 (1961).

THRUM, H.: Eine neue Methode zur Isolierung der Antibiotika vom Grisein-Typ. Naturwissenschaften **44**, 561 (1957).
TOWNSLEY, P. M.: The iron and porphyrin metabolism of *Micrococcus lysodeikticus*. Doctoral dissertation. Berkeley: University of California, 1956.
TSUKIURA, H., M. OKANISHI, T. OHMORI, H. KOSHIYAMA, T. MIYAKI, H. KITAZIMA, and H. KAWAGUCHI: Daunomycin, a new antibiotic. J. Antibiotics (Japan), Ser. A **17**, 39 (1964).
TURKOVA, J., O. MIKES, and F. SORM: Isolation of the biologically active component albomycin in pure form and its thermal degradation. Antibiotiki **7**, 878 (1962).
UMEZAWA, H., S. HAYANO, and Y. OGATA: Studies on an antibiotic substance of *Streptomyces griseus*, Grisein. J. Antibiotics (Japan), Ser. B **2**, 104 (1949).
WARREN, R. A. J., and J. B. NEILANDS: Mechanism of microbial catabolism of Ferrichrome A. J. Biol. Chem. **240**, 255 (1965).
WEISEL, P., and P. J. ALLEN: Abstr. Inst. Biol. Sci. Meeting. Minneapolis, September 1951.
WOLIN, H. L., and H. B. NAYLOR: Basic nutritional requirements of *Micrococcus lysodeikticus*. Bacteriol. Proc. 55th General Meeting 1955, 47.
YAMADA, SH., and H. KAWAGUCHI: Pharmacological studies on Danomycin, a new antibiotic. J. Antibiotics (Japan), Ser. A **17**, 48 (1964).
ZÄHNER, H., R. HÜTTER u. E. BACHMANN: Zur Kenntnis der Sideromycinwirkung. Arch. Mikrobiol. **36**, 325 (1960).
ZÄHNER, H., E. BACHMANN, R. HÜTTER u. J. NÜESCH: Sideramine, eisenhaltige Wachstumsfaktoren aus Mikroorganismen. Path. Mikrobiol. **25**, 708 (1962).
ZÄHNER, H.: Antibiotica in der Mikrobiologie. Naturw. Rundschau **17**, 391 (1964).

Antimycin A

John S. Rieske

Antimycin A is the name given to an antibiotic complex that consists of at least four components of closely related structure. Compounds of this family are produced by a number of species of microorganism of the genus *Streptomyces*. The antimycins first attracted considerable interest because of their toxicity toward a number of pathogenic fungi; however, scientific interest in these compounds has centered primarily on their action as potent inhibitors of aerobic respiration. Commercially, the most promising use of antimycin A appears to be as a fish poison for the removal of undesirable fish from lakes and ponds.

Possibly nine different organisms are known to produce antimycin A or antimycin A-like compounds (Table 1). Although crystalline preparations of antimycin A can be separated chromatographically into a number of components

Table 1. *Types and microbiological sources of antimycin A*

Organism	Culture designation	Name	Type of antimycin *	Reference
Streptomyces			mixture:	
(species not named)	isolate 35 **	antimycin A-35	A_1, A_2, A_3, A_4	LEBEN and KEITT (1948)
(species not named)	isolate 102	antimycin A-102	A_1, A_2, A_3, A_4	LOCKWOOD, LEBEN, and KEITT (1954)
(species not named)	X-41			—
(species not named)	X-4992			—
Streptomyces kitazawaensis	48 B 3	antipiricullin A	—	HARADA and TANAKA (1956)
Streptomyces kitazawaensis	21 A 2	antipiricullin A	—	HARADA and TANAKA (1956)
Resembles *Streptomyces olivochromogenus*		virosin	—	SAKAGAMI *et al.* (1956)
Streptomyces blastmyceticus	455 D_1	blastmycin	predominantly A_3	WATANABE *et al.* (1957)
Streptomyces umbrosus		phyllomycin	homologs of A-35 of lower R_f	SCHMIDT-KASTNER (1963)

* Designated according to the method of LOCKWOOD, LEBEN, and KEITT (1954).
** Culture NRRL 2288, Culture Collection Section, Fermentation Division, Northern Regional Research Laboratory, Peoria, Illinois (KEITT, LEBEN, and STRONG, 1953).

(LOCKWOOD, LEBEN, and KEITT, 1954; SCHMIDT-KASTNER, 1963) it is evident from their ability to co-crystallize that these components are closely related, if not identical, in basic structure.

As the result of chemical degradation studies conducted under the joint direction of VAN TAMELEN and STRONG (VAN TAMELEN *et al.*, 1960) the complete chemical structures of antimycin A_1 and A_3 have been determined. As illustrated in Fig. 1, the basic structure of the antimycins consist of an acyl and alkyl-substituted dilactone ring linked via an amide bond to 3-formamidosalicylic acid. Antimycins A_1 and A_3 differ only by two methylene carbons in the multicarbon, alkyl substituent of the dilactone ring. Although scarcity of purified antimycins other than A_1 and A_3 has precluded complete determination of the structures of these additional forms, it is probable that all of the antimycins differ only in the length or the degree of branching of the alkyl or acyl substituents of the dilactone portion of the molecule. All chemical species of antimycin A differ only quantitatively in biological and biochemical activity; therefore, unless noted otherwise this article will employ the general term antimycin A for either a single isolated species or for a co-crystallizable mixture of antimycins.

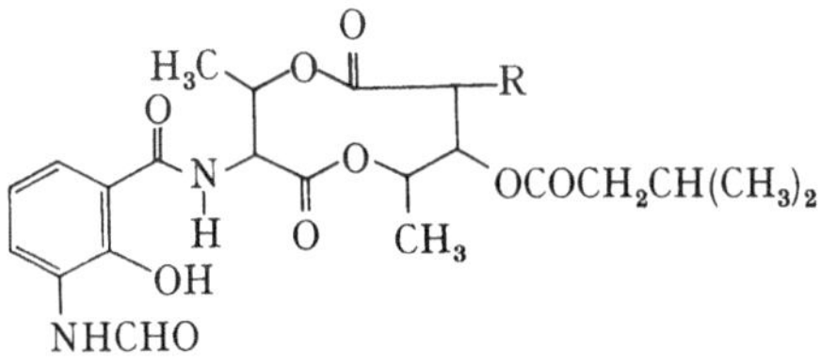

Antimycin A_1; R=n-hexyl
M.W.= 548

Antimycin A_3; R=n-butyl
M.W.= 520

Fig. 1. Chemical structures of antimycin A_1 and A_3

Toxicity of Antimycin A

The antibiotic properties of antimycin A were observed first as an inhibition of growth of a pathological mycotic organism (hence its name) (LEBEN and KEITT, 1948). Therefore, as would be expected, antimycin A was first tested extensively with regard to its antifungal properties. Of a large number of fungi tested about 31 types were found to be highly sensitive to the antibiotic when it was incorporated into the growth media. These fungi together with data of dosage of antimycin A and the type of antimycin A employed are listed in Table 2. It is apparent that a number of discrepancies exist in the response of a given organism to different preparations of antimycin A as well as in the response of different cultures of an organism to a single preparation of the antibiotic (LEBEN and KEITT, 1948). These discrepancies emphasize the complexity of the factors involved in the overall toxicity of the antibiotic. These factors probably include penetrability of the antibiotic through the cell wall and the degree of dependence of the organism on the function that is affected by the antibiotic. These possible

Table 2. *Pathogenic fungi inhibited strongly by the antimycins*

Organism	Antibiotic*	Conc. inhibitory to growth μg/ml	Reference**
Alternaria kikuchiana	antipiricullin	0.1	(4)
Alternaria kikuchiana	antipiricullin	>100	(1)
Alternaria kikuchiana	antimycin A	<1.0	(1)
Alternaria kikuchiana	virosin	10, >100	(1)
Alternaria kikuchiana	blastmycin	5.0	(6)
Candida albicans	antipiricullin	0.1	(4)
Candida albicans	blastmycin	>50	(6)
Candida krusei	antipiricullin	0.5	(4)
Candida lipolytica	antimycin A	<0.6	(3)
Candida parakrusei	antipiricullin	1.0	(4)
Ceratostomella fimbriata	antipiricullin	<1.0	(5)
Ceratostomella fimbriata	antipiricullin	52	(4)
Ceratostomella fimbriata	virosin	<1.0	(5)
Colletotrichum circinans	antimycin A	<1.6	(2)
Colletotrichum circinans	antimycin A	<0.6	(3)
Colletotrichum lindithialum	120 A	<1.0	(5)
Colletotrichum lindithialum	antipiricullin	<1.0	(5)
Colletotrichum lindithialum	virosin	<1.0	(5)
Colletotrichum phomoides	antimycin A	<0.8	(2)
Colletotrichum phomoides	blastmycin	>50	(6)
Colletotrichum pisi	antimycin A	<1.6	(2)
Corticium centrifugus	blastmycin	0.2	(6)
Elsinoe ampelina	120 A	<1.0	(5)
Elsinoe ampelina	antipiricullin	<1.0	(1), (5)
Elsinoe ampelina	virosin	<1.0	(1), (5)
Elsinoe ampelina	blastmycin	>50	(6)
Elsinoe ampelina	antimycin A	<1.0	(1)
Elsinoe fawcetti	720 A	<1.0	(5)
Elsinoe fawcetti	antipiricullin	<1.0	(1), (5)
Elsinoe fawcetti	virosin	<1.0	(1), (5)
Elsinoe fawcetti	blastmycin	>50	(6)
Elsinoe fawcetti	antimycin A	>1.0	(1)
Gibberella saubinetti	720 A	>1.0	(5)
Gibberella saubinetti	antipirucillin	>100	(1), (5)
Gibberella saubinetti	virosin	>100	(1), (5)
Gibberella saubinetti	antimycin A	>100	(1)
Gloesporium lacticola	blastmycin	0.01	(6)
Gloesporium kaki	720 A	<1.0	(1), (5)
Gloesporium kaki	antipirucillin	>100, <1.0	(1), (5)
Gloesporium kaki	virosin	>100, <1.0	(1), (5)
Gloesporium kaki	antimycin A	100, <1.0	(1)
Glomerella cingulata	720 A	<1.0	(5)
Glomerella cingulata	antipiricullin	>100, <1.0	(1), (5)
Glomerella cingulata	virosin	>100, 10	(1), (5)
Glomerella cingulata	blastmycin	0.2	(6)
Glomerella cingulata	antimycin A	0.8—62.5	(2)
Glomerella cingulata	antimycin A	>100, 0.6	(1), (3)
Helminthosporium sigmoideum	blastmycin	0.05	(6)
Nigrospora sphaerica	antimycin A	0.2	(2)
Ophiostoma fimbriata	blastmycin	0.2	(6)
Phoma lingam	antimycin A	0.4	(2)

Table 2. (Continued)

Organism	Antibiotic*	Conc. inhibitory to growth µg/ml	Reference**
Piricularia grisea	blastmycin	0.005	(6)
Piricularia oryzae	720 A	10—100	(5)
Piricularia oryzae	antipiricullin	0.025, <1.0	(4), (5)
Piricularia oryzae	virosin	<1.0	(5)
Piricularia oryzae	virosin	<1.0—>100	(1)
Piricularia oryzae	blastmycin	0.005	(6)
Piricularia oryzae	antimycin A	100	(1)
Sclerotinia arachidis	720 A	<1.0	(5)
Sclerotinia arachidis	antipiricullin	<1.0—>100	(1), (5)
Sclerotinia arachidis	virosin	>100	(1), (5)
Sclerotinia arachidis	blastmycin	>50	(6)
Sclerotinia arachidis	antimycin A	<1.0—100	(1), (5)
Sclerotinia fructicola	antimycin A	0.4, 1.6	(2)
Sclerotinia hydrophilium	blastmycin	0.05—0.2	(6)
Sclerotinia mali	blastmycin	0.05	(6)
Sclerotinia rolfsii	blastmycin	0.05—0.2	(6)
Stemphylium sarcinaeforme	antimycin A	1.6, 0.6	(2), (3)
Venturia inaequalis	antimycin A	0.8	(2)

* Cf. Table 1 for type of antimycin.
** (1) KOAZE *et al.* (1956); (2) LEBEN and KEITT (1948); (3) LOCKWOOD *et al.* (1954); (4) NAKAYAMA *et al.* (1956); (5) SAKAGAMI *et al.* (1956); (6) WATANABE *et al.* (1957).

factors will be examined in greater detail in the subsequent section on the toxicology of antimycin A.

In contrast to fungi, the toxicity of antimycin A to bacteria is of a very low level generally. Of the 14 species tested by LEBEN and KEITT only two: *Bacillus cereus* var. *mycoides* and *Eriwinia amylovora* were significantly inhibited in growth by antimycin A (LEBEN and KEITT, 1948). Later, LOCKWOOD, LEBEN, and KEITT (1954) tested the effect of antimycin A on ten types of bacteria. Inhibition of growth was noted only at high concentrations of the antibiotic (>80 µg/ml). NAKAYAMA, OKAMOTO, and HARADA (1956) also found that antimycin A inhibited the growth of *Mycobacterium* 607, *Bacillus subtilis* and *Escherichia coli* only at concentrations above 104 µg/ml. The growth of several pathogenic bacteria of plants, *Eriwinia arodeae, Pseudomonas solanacearum, Pseudomonas tabaci, Xanthomonas citri,* and *Xanthomonas pruni* was not inhibited at 100 µg/ml of antimycin A (KOAZE *et al.*, 1956).

Yeast was found to be highly sensitive to antimycin A. *Saccharomyces cerevisia* Y30 was inhibited completely by a concentration of 8 µg/l (1.5×10^{-8} M) of antimycin A. However, when yeast was grown on a natural medium containing peptone and yeast extract no effect of antimycin A was observed at a concentration of 40 µg/l (AHMAD, SCHNEIDER, and STRONG, 1950).

Toxicity measurements of antimycin A on higher forms of animal life have been somewhat fragmentary. Some representative results are listed in Table 3. Although considerable variability exists between different animal forms in the toxicity of antimycin A when ingested, it appears to be uniformly very toxic to animal life when administered by injection.

Table 3. *Toxicity of antimycin A toward higher forms of life*

Organism	Mode of administration	Dosage	Toxic action	Reference
Aphid (green peach)	Ingestion	200 ppm on leaves	86% mortality in 3 days	Harries and Mattson (1963)
Two spotted spider mite (*Tetranychus telarius*)	Ingestion	200 ppm in plant	99% mortality in 3 days	Harries (1963)
Housefly	Ingestion	10 ppm in food	38% mortality in 24 hrs	Kido and Spyhalski (1950)
Housefly	Applied to breast	20 μg/ml in soln.	87.5% mortality in 24 hrs	Sakagami *et al.* (1956)
Cockroach (German and American)	Ingestion Injection into body cavity	1.0 mg/g food >3.0 μg/g wt.	no mortality lethal within 24 hrs	Beck (1950) Beck (1950)
Fish	Water medium			Walker *et al.* (1964)
Trout (Rainbow and Brown)	Water medium (12°)	0.08 p.p.b.	100% mortality in 96 hrs	Walker *et al.* (1964)
Yellow perch	Water medium (12°)	0.20 p.p.b.	100% mortality in 96 hrs	Walker *et al.* (1964)
Yellow perch	Water medium (17°)	0.08 p.p.b.	100% mortality in 96 hrs	Walker *et al.* (1964)
Yellow perch	Water medium (22°)	0.06 p.p.b.	100% mortality in 96 hrs	Walker *et al.* (1964)
White sucker	Water medium (12°)	0.22 p.p.b.	100% mortality in 96 hrs	Walker *et al.* (1964)
Bigmouth buffalo	Water medium (12°)	0.40 p.p.b.	100% mortality in 96 hrs	Walker *et al.* (1964)
Green sunfish	Water medium (12°)	0.80 p.p.b.	100% mortality in 96 hrs	Walker *et al.* (1964)
Bluegill	Water medium (12°)	0.40 p.p.b.	100% mortality in 96 hrs	Walker *et al.* (1964)
Goldfish	Water medium (12°)	2.0 p.p.b.	Total lethality in 96 hrs	Walker *et al.* (1964)
Carp	Water medium (12°)	0.6 p.p.b.	Total lethality in 96 hrs	Walker *et al.* (1964)
Black and Yellow bullhead	Water medium (12°)	80.0 p.p.b.	Total lethality in 96 hrs	Walker *et al.* (1964)
Channel catfish	Water medium (12°)	20.0 p.p.b.	Total lethality in 96 hrs	Walker *et al.* (1964)
Mice	Intraperitoneal injection	1.8 mg/kg	LD_{50}	Watanabe *et al.* (1957)

Table 3. (Continued)

Organism	Mode of Administration	Dosage	Toxic action	Reference
Mice	Subcutaneous injection	1.6 mg/kg	LD_{50}	NAKAYAMA *et al.* (1956)
Mice (12—18 g)	Subcutaneous injection	21.25 mg/kg	LD_{50}	NAKAYAMA *et al.* (1956)
Mice	Intravenous injection	0.893 mg/kg	LD_{50}	NAKAYAMA *et al.* (1956)
Mice	Intraperitoneal injection	7.581 mg/kg	LD_{50}	REIF and POTTER (1953)
Rat, female (120—150 g)	Intraperitoneal injection	0.81 mg/kg	LD_{50}	REIF and POTTER (1953)
Rat, male and female (92—110 g)	Ingested with ration for 1 week	181.6 mg/kg	Weight loss, no deaths	AHMAD, SCHNEIDER, and STRONG (1950)
Rat (158 g)	Ingestion (stomach tube)	12 mg/kg	Non lethal	AHMAD, SCHNEIDER, and STRONG
		30 mg/kg	Lethal	AHMAD, SCHNEIDER, and STRONG
Guinea pig	Ingestion	1.8 ± 0.28 mg/kg	LD_{50}	Ayerst Res. Lab. (1965)
Rabbit	Ingestion	10 mg/kg	LD_{50}	Ayerst Res. Lab (1965)
Pigeon	Ingestion	2 mg/kg	LD_{50}	W.A.R.F. (1965a and b)
Chicken	Ingestion	>160 mg/kg	LD_{50}	W.A.R.F. (1965a and b)
Pheasant	Ingestion	5 mg/kg	LD_{50}	W.A.R.F. (1965a and b)
Duck (Mallard)	Ingestion	2.9 mg/kg	LD_{50}	Ayerst Res. Lab. (1965)
Quail	Ingestion	39 ± 11 mg/kg	LD_{50}	Ayerst Res. Lab. (1965)
Lamb	Ingestion	1—5 mg/kg	LD_{50}	Ayerst Res. Lab. (1965)
Dog	Ingestion	>5 mg/kg	LD_{50}	Ayerst Res. Lab. (1965)

Fish appear to be exceptionally sensitive to antimycin A when it is added to their water medium. With sensitive species, less than 0.1 part per billion of antimycin A is lethal. A striking characteristic of the action of antimycin A on fish is the extended length of time required for the lethal effect to appear at low concentrations of antimycin A. Also, the toxic effects of antimycin A appear to be accelerated as the temperature of the water is raised. Possibly, the sensitivity of fish to antimycin A may reflect a deficiency in the ability of fish to detoxify or excrete accumulated antimycin A. A puzzling result of the toxicity data on warm-blooded animals is the great difference in toxicity of ingested antimycin A towards chickens ($LD_{50} > 160$ mg/kg) and pheasants ($LD_{50} = 5$ mg/kg), respectively.

Data on the toxicity of antimycin A toward plants are sketchy. LEBEN and KEITT (1949) in conjunction with their studies of antimycin A as a protectant fungicide noted no phytotoxicity of an aqueous spray of the antibiotic when applied to young tomato, bean, cucumber, or cowpea plants. Later, they did note that if the antimycin A was applied as a solution in oil (0.3 μg per plant) it was injurious to the unfurled leaves of tomato plants (LEBEN and KEITT, 1956).

Toxicology of Antimycin

The high degree of toxicity of antimycin A toward susceptible organisms indicated that the antibiotic exerts its toxic action through a specific interaction with a vital function of the organisms. However, toxicity data alone are insufficient for a determination of how the antibiotic compound exerts its toxic action.

The first evidence of how antimycin A achieves its toxic effect was provided by the studies of AHMAD *et al.* (1949) and AHMAD, SCHNEIDER, and STRONG (1950). In their studies on the effects of antimycin A on the metabolism of yeast (*Saccharomyces cerevisia*) they found that the antibiotic stimulated fermentation and concomitantly inhibited respiration. Succinate oxidase activity was inhibited completely at a concentration of antimycin A of 3×10^{-6} M. The activity of succinic dehydrogenase was not affected under these conditions. The studies of BECK (1950) provided additional evidence that the toxicity of antimycin A is attributable to its action as a respiratory inhibitor; he found that the toxic action of antimycin A on the cockroach was paralleled by a depression of oxygen consumption.

Studies of the above nature were extended to mammals by POTTER, REIF, and associates. In studies with rats they determined that antimycin A was a potent inhibitor *in vitro* of succinate oxidation in all tissues examined, *i.e.* heart, kidney, brain, muscle, spleen, thymus, lung, and tumor. Also, the amount of antimycin A required to inhibit succinate oxidation in a given amount of tissue was proportional to the activity of the enzyme in the tissue (POTTER and REIF, 1952). Injection of lethal doses (1—3 mg/kg) of antimycin A into rats resulted in a strong inhibition *in vivo* of succinate oxidation in tissues of low succinate oxidase titer, i.e. spleen, lung, and thymus whereas tissues containing a high titer of the enzyme system, i.e. heart, brain, and muscle were barely affected. An exception to the above generalization was noted for liver, in which case the succinate oxidation was inhibited even though the activity of the enzyme system was high. Also, tumor tissues with relatively low succinate oxidation levels were not inhibited as much as expected. Succinate oxidation in brain tissue was unaffected even at doses of antimycin A up to 50 mg/kg. These discrepancies between the action of antimycin A *in vitro* and *in vivo* were attributed possibly to differences in rate of blood flow or capillary permeability in the various tissues. The relative insensitivity of brain tissue *in vivo* to the antibiotic was explained on the basis of the blood-brain barrier (REIF and POTTER, 1953a).

Another significant factor involved in the mammalian toxicology of antimycin A is the rate of detoxification. In their studies, REIF and POTTER discovered that the succinate oxidase activity of liver, lung, and spleen inhibited *in vivo* by sublethal doses of Antimycin A recovered completely 2—4 hours after injection of the antibiotic. Recovery of respiratory activity *in vitro* paralleled abatement of visible physiological symptoms. Also, reactivation of succinate oxidase activity in tissues from injected rats was obtained *in vitro* by the addition of serum or cell fractions from normal rats. Subsequent experiments implicated serum albumin as the factor responsible for this reactivation. This indicated that the reactivation *in vivo* of respiration was accomplished by transfer of the antimycin A from the inhibited site to serum albumin and then its subsequent excretion or inactivation after dissociation from the serum albumin. Experiments *in vitro* demonstrated that of nine tissues tested only the liver is capable of chemically inactivating antimycin A (REIF and POTTER, 1953a). The reactivating capability of serum albumin was supported further by subsequent experiments in which it was demonstrated that serum albumin can bind antimycin A and that reactivation of succinate oxidation by serum albumin is competitive with the inhibition of the enzyme system by antimycin A (REIF and POTTER, 1953a and b). Thus, REIF and POTTER described the biological action of antimycin A as a pseudo-irreversible inhibition of succinate oxidation. Although the antibiotic inhibits respiration in a stoichiometric manner, the inhibition can be reversed by appropriate reagents, in this case serum albumin.

The toxic effects of antimycin A on the development of embryo tissues have been studied by EBERT and his associates. Initially, DUFFY and EBERT (1957) found that antimycin A at very low concentrations (0.25—0.30 μg/ml) inhibited the developing heart in chick embryos. In an extension of these studies, the susceptibility of embryonic heart and somites to the antibiotic at different stages of development was tested. Although neither entodermal nor endodermal tissues were affected significantly by low concentrations of antimycin A, the development of heart and somites was inhibited (MCKENZIE and EBERT, 1960). REPORTER and EBERT (1965) made a detailed study of the effects of antimycin A on differentiation and morphogenesis in the chick embryo. The results of this study not only confirmed that only the mesodermal tissues were affected significantly by antimycin A but also that the toxic effects of antimycin A exhibits selectivity within this embryological layer. Thus, although the development of somite pairs was inhibited almost completely at 0.04 μg antimycin A per ml of medium, the formation of hemoglobin was unaffected. They also observed that the sensitivity of the embryo to antimycin A was affected by the oxygen tension in the growth medium. With normal oxygen tension (1.0 atmosphere of air) and an antimycin A concentration of 0.025 μg/ml of medium only heart and somite formation was inhibited; at higher oxygen tensions the antibiotic caused a pronounced general inhibition, the embryos developing only residual axial structure.

REPORTER and EBERT (1965) also tested the effects of antimycin A on the activities of several enzymes normally present in the chick embryo. Of the enzymes tested, i.e. lactic dehydrogenase (LDH-1, MARKERT, 1963), NADH oxidase, NADH-cytochrome *c* reductase, succinate-cytochrome *c* reductase and creatine kinase, only the activity of LDH displayed a consistent relationship to the concentration of antimycin A. The activity of LDH decreased with increasing concentrations of antimycin A. Apparently, the activity of LDH reflected the development of somite pairs since the enzyme activity appeared to be proportional to the number of somite pairs developed in the embryo. Other respiratory inhibitors (e.g. amytal) and inhibitors of mitochondrial oxidative phosphorylation (e.g. oligomycin) were found also to affect the chick embryo in a manner similar to the effects of antimycin A.

In a parallel study, REPORTER and EBERT (1965) in collaboration with, and in an extension of the original observations of KONIGSBERG (1964) observed selective effects of antimycin A on monolayer cultures of leg-muscle cells from chick embryos. Of the tissue elements present at the end of the growth period (5 days), fibroblasts, myoblasts, and syncytial (multinuclear) muscle, only the multinuclear muscle cells were affected at concentrations of antimycin A of 0.04—0.06 μg/ml of medium. At higher concentrations (0.1—0.3 μg/ml) the antibiotic began to affect fibroblasts. The effect of antimycin A on the multinuclear cells was characterized by a shriveling of the cells with a release of many of the cells into the medium. In absence of antimycin A the surviving mononuclear cells were capable of giving rise to multinucleated fibers. In contrast to the effects of antimycin A on enzymic activities during the development of somite pairs in the embryo, the antibiotic was found to inhibit either the synthesis of, or the activity of NADH oxidase and NADH-cytochrome *c* reductase of the embryo muscle cells whereas little or no effect of antimycin A on the activity of lactic dehydrogenase (LDH) was noted.

These studies of EBERT and his associates as decribed above reemphasize the complexity of effects of antimycin A on organisms *in vivo*. The differential responses of different types of tissues in the chick embryo are reminiscent of the selective responses to antimycin A of different tissues in the rat. Since other inhibitors of the mitochondrial respiratory chain and inhibitors of oxidative phosphorylation mimic, in certain respects, the toxic effects of antimycin A in the chick embryo, the concept of the primary toxic role of antimycin A as an inhibitor of respiration receives additional confirmation. Also, similar to the release of inhibition of succinate oxidase in rat tissue by serum albumin, the effects of antimycin A on the chick embryo were reversed or blocked by a specific protein, in this case, a protein isolated from chicken liver mitochondria (REPORTER and EBERT, 1965).

Antimycin A has been tested also on such diverse physiological processes as the renal tubular transport of p-amino hippurate (DOMINGUEZ and SHIDEMAN, 1955), release of histamine during the anaphylactic reaction (MOUSSATCHE and PROUVOST, 1962), influenza virus production by tissue cells (ACKERMANN, 1951), reticulocyte maturation and accumulation of hypoxanthine in reticulocytes

(HAYASHI and OCHI, 1965), and energy-yielding reactions in thymus nuclei (MCEWEN *et al.*, 1963). All of these processes were found to be inhibited by antimycin A. In support of the respiratory involvement of antimycin A, all of these processes also were inhibited by selected inhibitors of respiration (e.g. malonate, amytal, CN^-, or N_3^-) or uncouplers of oxidative phosphorylation (e.g. 2,4 dinitrophenol and dicoumarol).

Although all toxic effects of antimycin A in higher animals appear to be caused either directly or indirectly by an inhibition of terminal respiration; with the exception of yeast, the nature of the toxic effects of antimycin A on microorganisms is less well defined. However, in the case of fungi that are sensitive to antimycin A, selected data indicate that the antibiotic exerts its toxic effect in a manner that is similar, if not identical, to its effect on higher organisms.

MATSUNAKA (1961) examined the cytochromes and respiratory enzymes in *Piricularia oryzae*, the pathogen of blast disease of rice plants, and an organism that is particularly sensitive to antimycin A (cf. Table 1). This fungus was found to contain cytochromes of the types *a*, *b*, and *c* which correspond spectroscopically to the cytochromes that are present in the respiratory assemblies of higher organisms. In contrast, the pathogenic bacteria, *Xanthomonas oryzae*, which causes a leaf blight disease, was found to contain cytochromes of types a_1 and *b*, which are characteristic of bacterial respiratory chains of the *E. coli* type. Also in common with bacteria in general, this organism was found to be relatively insensitive to antimycin A. In keeping with their divergence in the cytochrome makeup, *Piricularia oryzae* and *Xanthomonas oryzae* displayed widely divergent characteristics with respect to respiratory enzymes. Subcellular particles of *Piricularia oryzae* contained enzymic activities corresponding to cytochrome *c* oxidase, succinate oxidase, and NADH oxidase. Both the succinate oxidase and the NADH oxidase required added cytochrome *c* for maximal activity; significantly, both activities were inhibited by antimycin A. The respiratory enzymes in subcellular particles of *Xanthomonas oryzae* consisted of NADH oxidase and NADPH oxidase. Neither enzyme was stimulated by cytochrome *c* nor inhibited by antimycin A. Succinate oxidase activity was absent.

In a similar study, RAMACHANDRAN and GOTTLIEB (1961) tested antimycin A on cell-free extracts of bacteria (*Escherichia coli* and *Pseudomonas fluorescens*) and fungi (*Sclerotinia fructicola*, *Gibberella Zeal*, *Phycomyces nitens*, and *Glomerella cingulata*). The antibiotic had no effect on the oxygen uptake of either the intact cells or cell-free extracts of the bacteria; however, it was a potent inhibitor of NADH-cytochrome *c* reductase in cell-free extracts of the fungi. Although the enzymic activities of the antimycin A-sensitive fungi resembled those present in the respiratory chain of higher organisms, a complete comparison is not possible since the nature of the cytochrome components was not determined.

From the above data, it would be tempting to make the generalization that all microorganisms which are sensitive to antimycin A contain cytochromes and enzyme activities similar to those found in mammalian mitochondria. However, a recent report by KURUP *et al.* (1966) appears to be an exception that disproves the rule. These investigators found that cell-free extracts of *Agrobacterium tumefaciens* contained a very active NADH-oxidase system which was inhibited strongly by antimycin A. Only one cytochrome was detectable in these extracts,

Table 4. *Enzyme systems inhibited by antimycin A*

Enzyme Activity and Source	Reaction	Concentration of Antimycin A*	Inhibition %	Reference
1. Succinate oxidases	Succinate + 1/2 O_2 → Fumarate + H_2O			
a) mitochondria				
beef heart		0.50 µmoles/g protein	89	BROWN *et al.* (1965)
rat liver		0.07—0.08 µmoles/g protein	90	ESTABROOK (1962)
Euglena gracilis		2.0 µM	80	BUETOW and BUCHANAN (1965)
Prototheca zopfii		1.0 µM	100	LLOYD (1966)
Saccharomyces carlsbergensis		2.3 µmoles/g protein	93.5	OHNISHI *et al.* (1966)
Neurospora crassa		0.4 µmoles/g protein	inhibited	HALL and GREENAWALT (1964)
Claviceps purpura (ergot fungus)		3.4 µM	100	ANDERSON *et al.* (1964)
Piricularia oryzae		—	inhibited	MATSUNAKA (1961)
lupine		3.0 µM	97	HUMPHREYS and CONN (1956)
b) mitochondrial fragments				
pig heart		0.34 µmoles/g protein	98	THORN (1956)
c) solubilized preparations				
"Succinic dehydrogenase" + S.C. Factor (pig heart)		0.2 µM	100	CLARK *et al.* (1954)
Reconstituted from solubilized complexes II, III, and IV		—	100	HATEFI *et al.* (1962)
2. NADH oxidases	NADH + H^+ + 1/2 O_2 → NAD^+ + H_2O			
a) mitochondria				
Saccharomyces carlsbergensis		2.3 µmoles/g protein	97	OHNISHI *et al.* (1966)
Claviceps purpura (ergot fungus)		3.4 µM	100	ANDERSON *et al.* (1964)

Prototheca zopfii		0.02 μM or 0.35 μmoles/g protein	82	Lloyd (1966)
Piricularia oryzae		2.0 μM	inhibited	Matsunaka (1961)
skunk cabbage		3.4 μM	80	Hackett (1957)
potato tuber		2.0 μM	88	Hackett (1956)
b) mitochondrial fragments				
ETP, beef heart		0.35 μmoles/g protein	94	Pumphrey (1962)
rat brain		3.5 μM	95	Strecker and DiPrisco (1963)
lupine, w/o cyt *c*		0.6 μM	100	Humphreys and Conn (1956)
lupine, cyt *c* added		0.6 μM	94	Humphreys and Conn (1956)
lupine		0.01 μM (7—8 μg protein/ml)	80	Humphreys and Conn (1956)
c) bacteria (subcellular particles)				
Bacillus subtilis		10—100 μM	inhibited	Szulmajster (1964)
Agrobacterium tumefaciens		0.34 μM or 2.5 μmoles/g protein	100	Kurup *et al.* (1966)
d) solubilized particles				
reconstituted form purified Complex I, III, and IV of beef heart mitochondria		—	100	Hatefi *et al.* (1962)
3. Succinate-cytochrome *c* reductases	Succinate + 2 (Fe^{+3}) cyt *c* → Fumarate + 2 (Fe^{+2}) cyt *c* + 2H^+			
isobutyl alcohol fraction of beef heart mitochondria		1.01 μmoles/g protein	100	Green *et al.* (1955)
purified from a t-amyl alcohol extract of beef heart mitochondria		2—10 μmoles/g protein	100	Green and Burkhard (1961)
purified from a heart muscle preparation		0.87 μmoles/g protein	97	Takemori and King (1964)
mitochondria (potato tuber)		2.0 μM	93	Hackett (1956)
particulate (tobacco root)		2.5 μmoles/g protein	>90	Sisler and Evans (1959)

Table 4. (Continued)

Enzyme Activity and Soure	Reaction	Concentration of Antimycin A*	Inhibition %	Reference
4. NADH-cytochrome *c* reductases	NADH + 2 (Fe^{+3}) cyt *c* → NAD^{+} + 2 (Fe^{+2}) cyt *c* + H^{+}			
purified from beef heart mitochondria		0.002 μM (preincubated with enzyme)	>90	HATEFI *et al.* (1961)
purified from beef heart mitochondria		0.016 μM (added to assay mixture)	100	HATEFI *et al.* (1961)
purified from beef heart mitochondria		0.16 μmoles/g protein	95	FOWLER and RICHARDSON (1961)
rat skeletal muscle (digitonin treated)		0.18 μmoles/g protein	100	NASON and LEHMAN (1956)
Sclerotinia fructicola (cell-free extract)		0.2 μM	ca. 65	RAMACHANDRAN and GOTTLIEB (1961)
Gibberella zeae (cell-free extract)		0.2 μM	76	RAMACHANDRAN and GOTTLIEB (1961)
Phycomyces nitens (cell-free extract)		0.2 μM	76	RAMACHANDRAN and GOTTLIEB (1961)
Glomerella cingulata (cell-free extract)		0.2 μM	75	RAMACHANDRAN and GOTTLIEB (1961)
potato mitochondria		2.0 μM	21, 33	HACKETT (1956)
wheat-root mitochondria		3.0 μmoles/mg protein N	30	MORTON and MORTON (1956)
corn-root mitochondria		0.2 μM	54	RAMACHANDRAN and GOTTLIEB (1961)
5. *Coenzyme Q oxidase*	$CoQH_2 + 1/2\ O_2 \rightarrow CoQ + H_2O$			
prepared from a deoxycholate extract of beef heart mitochondria		1.0 μmoles/g protein	>90	HATEFI (1959)

6. Reduced coenzyme Q-cytochrome *c* reductase	$CoQH_2 + 2\,(Fe^{+3})$ cyt *c* → $CoQ + 2\,(Fe^{+2})$ cyt *c* + $2\,H^+$			
purified from beef heart mitochondria		1.0 mole/mole cyt c_1	>90	RIESKE and ZAUGG (1962)
7. Light-induced phosphorylation	ADP + P_i + hν → ATP			
Rhodospirillum rubrum (cell-free extract)		3.0 μM	>95	BALTSCHEFFSKY and BALTSCHEFFSKY (1958)
Rhodospirillum rubrum (cell-free extract)	succinate as electron source	0.2 μM	83	GELLER and LIPMAN (1960)
+ phenazine methosulfate	succinate as electron source	2.0 μM	12	GELLER and LIPMAN (1960)
chloroplasts (spinach) + phenazine methosulfate	ascorbate as electron source	50.0 μM	81	BALTSCHEFFSKY (1960)
chloroplast fragments	no external electron source	10.0 μM	100	FEWSON *et al.* (1963)
(spinach) + PPNR**		1.0 μM	32	FEWSON *et al.* (1963)
8. *Photoreduction of NAD*	NAD^+ + 2e + H^+ + hν → NADH			
Rhodospirillum rubrum	succinate as electron source	—	inhibited	NAZAKI *et al.* (1961)
(cell-free extract)	succinate as electron source	—	inhibited	HINKSON (1965)
Rhodospirillum rubrum (cell-free extract)	ascorbate-dichloroindophenol as electron source	—	not inhibited	HINKSON (1965)
9. *Aldehyde oxidase*	RCHO + $1/2\,O_2$ → RCOOH			
(hog liver)		2.0 μM	62	RAJAGOPALAN *et al.* (1962)

* All concentrations of antimycin A originally listed on a weight basis have been converted to approximate molar dimensions.
** Photosynthetic pyridine nucleotide reductase (SAN PIETRO and LANG, 1958).

a cytochrome of type *b* (heme extractable with acidic acetone) with absorption maxima at 550, 520, and 420 mμ when in the reduced state.

Although antimycin A-sensitive organisms are limited generally to those containing respiratory chains with cytochromes of type *a*, *b*, and *c*, the converse argument, that organisms that contain these cytochromes will be sensitive to antimycin A may not be correct. In an examination by difference spectra of the cytochromes of thirteen varieties of bacteria by SMITH (1954), three types, *Bacillus subtilis*, *Micrococcus pyogenes var. albus*, and *Sarcina lutea* were found to contain cytochromes of types *a*, *b*, and *c*. Two of these bacteria (the only ones of this group tested), *Bacillus subtilis* and *Micrococcus pyogenes var. albus* were not affected by antimycin A with respect to either an alteration of oxidation state of cytochrome *b* or to an inhibition of respiration. It appears, therefore, that bacteria, even when possessing a respiratory chain, similar to that of mammalian mitochondria may be relatively insensitive *in vivo* to antimycin A. These bacteria may possess alternate pathways of electron transport that either by-pass the antimycin site or do not contain this site. Another case in point is provided by the study of RAMACHANDRAN and GOTTLIEB (1961) as referred to previously. Although respiratory activity of cell-free extracts of *Pseudomonas fluorescens* is unaffected by antimycin A; in other respects the respiratory chain resembles those present in mammalian mitochondria. The bacterium has a cytochrome-linked electron transport system that is sensitive to cyanide; also it contains enzymes that catalyze the reduction of cytochrome *c* by succinate, malate, glucose, and NADH, respectively. In the case of *Bacillus subtilis*, however, the insensitivity to antimycin A may not reflect a property of the respiratory chain. The impermeability of the cell wall to antimycin A, probably limits the effectiveness *in vivo* of the antibiotic. SZULMAJSTER (1964) reported that antimycin A at concentrations between 0.01 and 0.1 μmoles per ml inhibited electron transport in NADH-oxidizing particles derived from this bacterium. Also, the dihydrostreptomycin antagonist, 2-n-heptyl-4-hydroxyquinoline-N-oxide, which apparently acts at the same site as antimycin A, was observed to inhibit respiration *in vivo* of *Bacillus subtilis* (LIGHTBOWN and JACKSON, 1956). Apparently the cell wall of *Bacillus subtilis* is permeable to 2-n-heptyl-4-hydroxyquinoline-N-oxide but not to antimycin A.

In the case of at least one variety of bacteria, the antibiotic effect of antimycin A may not reflect its inhibitory action on respiration. Although the antibiotic is lethal for *Bacillus megaterium* at a concentration of 5 mμmoles per mg of bacterial cells, oxygen uptake of the cells is not inhibited at 30 mμmoles of antimycin A per mg of bacterial cells (MARQUIS, 1965). Upon further examination, MARQUIS found that the bactericidal action of antimycin A toward *Bacillus megaterium* could be correlated with its interference of plasma membrane function as measured by the concentrative uptake of α aminoisobutyrate and α methyl glucoside. At higher concentrations antimycin A induced extensive loss or inorganic phosphate and other substances from whole cells, inhibited aerobic respiration, and acted as a lytic agent of isolated protoplasts. The protoplasts concentrated antimycin A primarily on the plasma membrane.

Mitochondrial Electron Transport

A study of the toxic action of antimycin A provided valuable information on the effects of the antibiotic on living organisms. However, much of our understanding of details of the action of the antibiotic stems from measurements made with cell-free preparations of enzymes. About the time that antimycin A was recognized as a potent respiratory inhibitor (AHMAD *et al.*, 1949), it was determined that the terminal processes of respiration in most cells occurred in the mitochondria (SCHNEIDER and POTTER, 1949; LEHNINGER and KENNEDY, 1949). Since then a concerted effort has been made to elucidate the physiological and biochemical processes that occur within these organelles. Antimycin A proved to be an indispensable tool in the study of the mitochondrial processes, in return, the more complete dissection and characterization of the respiratory system that is found in mitochondria has led us to a more detailed knowledge of how antimycin A exerts its biological action. From the pioneering investigations of WARBURG (1927) and KEILEN and HARTREE (1939); and the more recent contributions principally from the laboratories of SLATER (1950), CHANCE (CHANCE and WILLIAMS, 1956), and GREEN (cf. GREEN and WHARTON, 1963), a picture of the components of the mitochondrial respiratory system and their reaction sequence has emerged (Fig. 2). The bracketed components appear to function as morphological and functional units and therefore are designated as electron-transfer complexes (HATEFI, 1963).

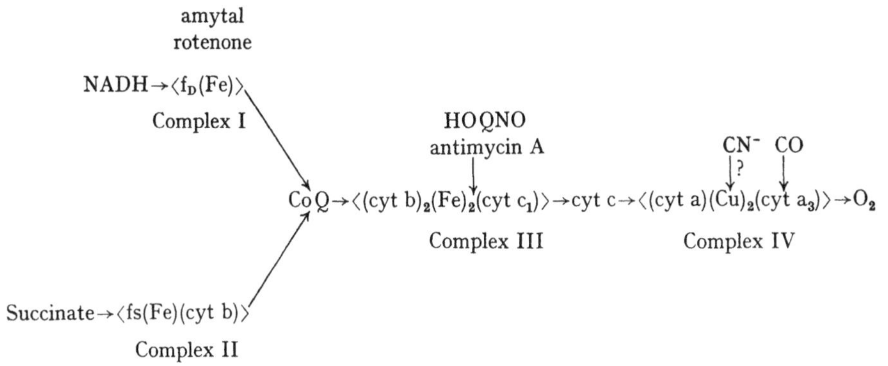

Fig. 2. Components and their sequence as proposed for the respiratory chain of mammalian mitochondria. Abbreviations: f_D, NADH-dehydrogenase flavoprotein; f_S, succinate-dehydrogenase flavoprotein; CoQ, coenzyme Q or ubiquinone; HOQNO, -2-n-heptyl-4-hydroxyquinoline-N-oxide

The early investigations of AHMAD *et al.* (1949) and AHMAD *et al.* (1950) established that antimycin A acts as a potent inhibitor of succinate oxidation. In an attempt to define more precisely the locus of action of antimycin A, AHMAD and his associates tested the inhibitory action of the antibiotic on the succinic dehydrogenase (reduction of methylene blue by succinate) and the cytochrome oxidase activities of the respiratory system. Antimycin A inhibited the succinic-dehydrogenase activity as measured but had no effect on the cytochrome-oxidase activity. These investigators concluded that antimycin A acts on the succinic-dehydrogenase portion of the respiratory chain. A clearer picture of the locus of

Table 5. *Inhibitory activity of derivatives and synthetic analogs of antimycin A*

Compound	Structure	Succinate → O_2* Conc. (µg/ml)	Succinate → O_2* Inhib (%)	Succinate → Cyt *c*** Conc. (µg/ml)	Succinate → Cyt *c*** Inhib (%)	QH_2 → Cyt *c**** Conc.	QH_2 → Cyt *c**** Inhib (%)
Antimycin A_1	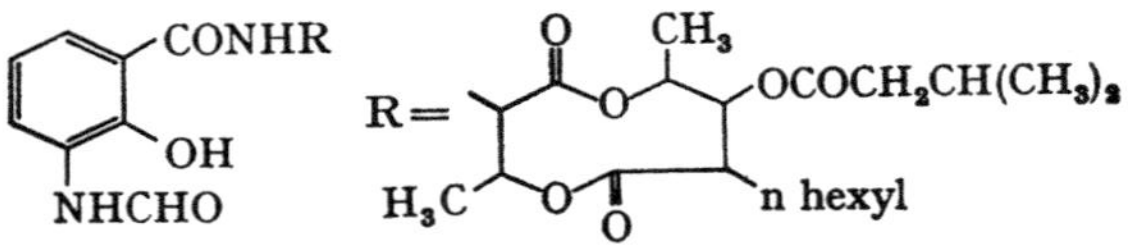			0.01 0.25 0.25 0.5	5 89 94 100	—	—
Antimycin A_3	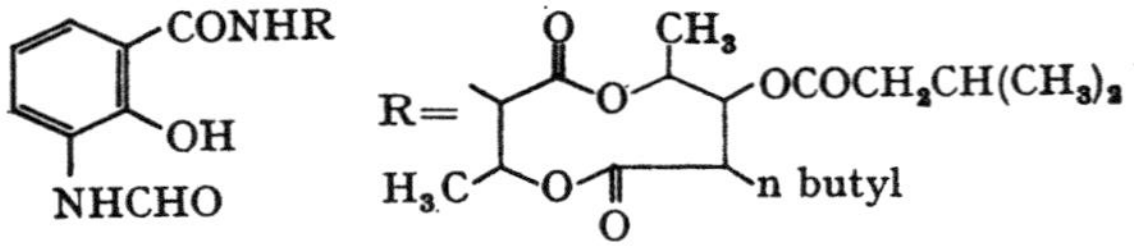	0.05	95	0.01	40	2 µg/mg protein	81
Deformyl Antimycin A_3 hydrochloride	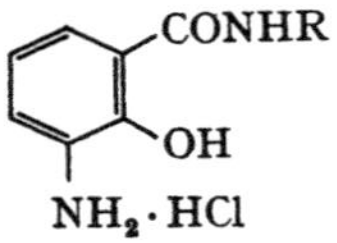 ,,	0.05	10	—	—	—	—
Antimycin A_3 diacetate	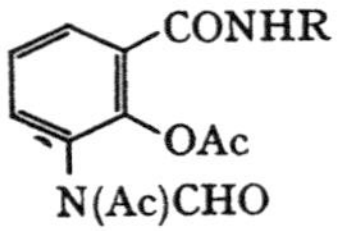 ,,	0.05	0	0.05 0.25 0.50	0 50 90	2 µg/mg protein	29 42
Deformyl Antimycin A_3 triacetate	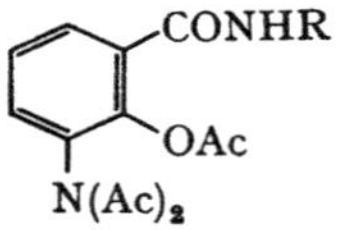 ,,	0.05	10	—	—	2 µg/mg protein	21

Antimycin A_3, O-methylether	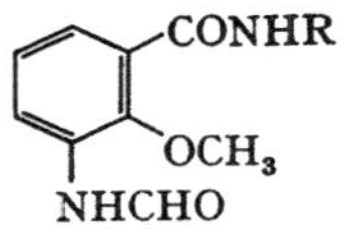	,,	0.05	0	0.5	0	2 µg/mg protein	0
Deformyl-N-acetylantimycin A_3	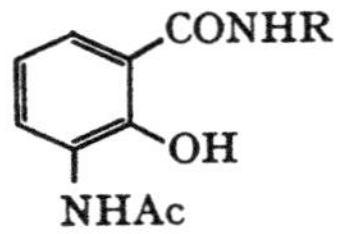	,,	0.05	85	—	—	2 µg/mg protein	63
Antimycin A_3 (reformylated deformyl antimycin A_3)	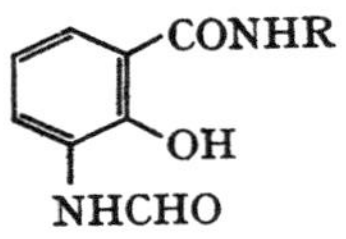	,,	0.05	95	—	—	—	—
Antimycic acid	,,	R=CH_3-CH(OH)-CH(-)-COOH	—	—	0.5	0	—	—
N-butyl-3-formamido salicylamide	,,	R=n butyl	—	—	—	—	5.0 µg/ml	11
N-octyl-3-formamido salicylamide	,,	R=n octyl	—	—	—	—	5.0 µg/ml	60
N-decyl-3-formamido salicylamide	,,	R=n decyl	—	—	—	—	5.0 µg/ml	85
N-dodecyl-3-formamido salicylamide	,,	R=n dodecyl	—	—	—	—	1.0 µg/ml	57
							2.0 µg/ml	73
N-hexadecyl-3-formamido salicylamide	,,	R=n hexadecyl	—	—	—	—	1.0 µg/ml	84
N-octadecyl-3-formamido salicylamide	,,	R=n octadecyl	—	—	—	—	1.0 µg/ml	50

* From VAN TAMELEN *et al.* (1961).
** From TAPPELL (1960).
*** From DICKIE *et al.* (1963) and RIESKE, previously unpublished data.

antimycin A inhibition emerged as a result of the investigations of POTTER and REIF (1952). They found that in addition to being an inhibitor of succinate oxidation, antimycin A also prevented completely the oxidation of α-ketoglutarate, fumarate, malate, pyruvate, citrate, and cis-aconitate in rat liver. Extending their studies to heart muscle, they observed that antimycin A inhibited the oxidation of reduced nicotinamide adenine dinucleotide (NADH) and the reduction of cytochrome *c* by NADH when both reactions were catalyzed by a KEILIN-HARTREE preparation of heart muscle. Furthermore, in collaboration with A. M. PAPPENHEIMER they found that antimycin A had no effect on the enzymic activity of a purified succinic dehydrogenase that was derived from *Corynebacterium diphtheriae* (PAPPENHEIMER and HENDEE, 1949). In retrospect, the validity of the results from their latter experiment is questionable, since bacteria, to begin with, are generally insensitive to antimycin A; however, subsequent experiments with purified succinic dehydrogenase derived from heart muscle have verified that the mitochondrial enzyme also is insensitive to antimycin A (SINGER, KEARNEY, and BERNATH, 1956). The deviant results of AHMAD *et al.* (1950) probably can be explained by a lack of specificity of methylene blue as an electron acceptor for succinic dehydrogenase when other components of the succinate-oxidase system are present. From the results of these early studies it became evident that antimycin A affects a respiratory component that is common to both the succinate-oxidase system and the NADH-oxidase system and that this component functions between succinic dehydrogenase and cytochrome *c* of the succinate-oxidase chain and between NADH and cytochrome *c* of the NADH-oxidase chain.

The first attempts at chemical dissection of the respiratory chain of heart muscle were attempted independently and almost simultaneously by CLARK *et al.* (1954) and GREEN *et al.* (1954). CLARK *et al.* obtained a solubilized fraction of pig-heart muscle by extraction of the muscle preparation with cholate (a bile salt with detergent properties). This extract catalyzed the reduction of cytochrome *c* by succinate. This preparation was designated the SC Factor because it was claimed that the protein linked the reduction of cytochrome *c* to succinic dehydrogenase. The factor was as sensitive to antimycin A as the succinate oxidase in extracts of heart muscle (i.e. mitochondria or mitochondrial fragments). Spectrally, the SC Factor in the reduced form displayed absorption peaks in the α region at 562 and 554 mμ. Reduction by ascorbate produced only the 554 mμ peak (WIDMER *et al.*, 1954). These spectra correspond to what are designated now as cytochromes *b* and c_1, respectively. The SC Factor probably is identical to a crude preparation of Complex III (cf. Fig. 2). GREEN *et al.* (1954) treated a purified NADH oxidase (prepared from beef-heart mitochondria) with deoxycholate. The NADH-oxidase activity was mostly lost, but concomitantly a NADH-cytochrome *c* reductase and a cytochrome *c* oxidase activity emerged. The untreated NADH-oxidase was inhibited completely by antimycin A. Also inhibited by antimycin A was the NADH-cytochrome *c* reductase of the deoxycholate-treated particle.

Knowledge of the location of the antimycin A-sensitive site of the respiratory chain in mitochondria was narrowed to a point between cytochromes *b* and c_1 by the studies of KEILEN and HARTREE, CHANCE and WILLIAMS, ESTABROOK and

DE BERNARD, RABINOWITZ and ESTABROOK. KEILEN and HARTREE (1955) observed that the reduction by either succinate or NADH of cytochrome c_1 in their heart muscle preparation was inhibited by antimycin A. CHANCE and WILLIAMS (1955, 1956) and ESTABROOK (1955) by the use of sensitive spectrophotometric techniques observed that when respiring mitochondria were treated with antimycin A, cytochromes c_1, c, a, and a_3 became completely oxidized whereas cytochrome b became completely reduced. This point of reversal of oxidation states of the electron carriers has been termed by CHANCE a crossover point or the point at which a block of electron flow occurs. DE BERNARD *et al.* (1956) found that in an extract of submitochondrial particles containing NADH-cytochrome c reductase, reduction of cytochrome b by succinate was stimulated by antimycin A, whereas the reduction of cytochromes c_1 and c was inhibited. ESTABROOK (1957), from kinetic measurements on a NADH-cytochrome c reductase preparation from heart muscle, found that antimycin A caused a blockage of the reaction between the reduced cytochrome b and cytochrome c_1 and c.

Table 6. *Properties of complex III of beef heart mitochondria*

Catalytic activity:	$CoQH_2$ — cyt c reductase
Molecular weight:	2.62—2.88 × 10^5 *
Composition:	
cytochrome b	7.4—8.2*, ** μmoles/g protein
cytochrome c_1	3.7—4.1** μmoles/g protein
nonheme iron	7.7 ± 0.6** μmoles/g protein
coenzyme Q_{10}	~1.0 μmoles/g protein
lipid	0.16* g/g protein
Inhibitors:	
antimycin A***	
2-n-heptyl (or nonyl)-4-hydroxyquinoline-N-oxide	
SN 5949 (a 3-alkyl-2-hydroxynaphthoquinone)	

* From TZAGOLOFF *et al.* (1965).
** Derived from data of HATEFI *et al.* (1962) and RIESKE *et al.* (1964).
*** Cf. Tables 4 and 5.

Isolation and purification of four electron-transfer complexes of the respiratory chain from heart mitochondria (cf. Fig. 2) allowed a direct test of the site of action of antimycin A. Of the four complexes, i.e. Complex I or NADH-coenzyme Q reductase (HATEFI, HAAVIK, and GRIFFITHS, 1962a), Complex II or succinate-coenzyme Q reductase (ZIEGLER and DOEG, 1959), Complex III or (reduced coenzyme Q) cytochrome c reductase (HATEFI *et al.*, 1962b), and Complex IV or cytochrome c oxidase (GRIFFITHS and WHARTON, 1961; FOWLER *et al.*, 1962), only Complex III is affected by antimycin A. An almost complete inhibition (>90%) of the reduced coenzyme Q-cytochrome c reductase activity is obtained after treatment of the enzyme with an amount of antimycin A equivalent in moles to the amount of cytochrome c_1 in the enzyme (RIESKE and ZAUGG, 1962). Since Complex III is the segment of the respiratory chain that contains cytochrome b and c_1 (cf. Table 6), the location of the antimycin A-sensitive site as determined in the intact respiratory chain has been substantiated by chemical isolation.

Most of the experimental work on mitochondria has involved the use of mammalian mitochondria. However, observations made on the respiratory system of mitochondria from plants and lower organisms give evidence that antimycin A acts on the respiratory chain of these mitochondria in a manner similar, if not identical, to its action on these systems in mammalian mitochondria. HUMPHREYS and CONN (1956) found that antimycin A strongly inhibited the oxidation of NADH as catalyzed by lupine mitochondria. MORTON and MORTON (1956) examined both microsomal and mitochondrial fractions of wheat roots. The mitochondrial fraction had active succinate- and NADH- cytochrome *c* reductase activities, both of which were partially inhibited by antimycin A. SISLER and EVANS (1959) reported that a succinate-cytochrome *c* reductase activity in particles from tobacco roots was inhibited by antimycin A. HACKETT (1957) observed that antimycin A partially inhibited the succinate oxidase and NADH oxidase in the mitochondria of skunk cabbage. Later, spectrophotometric measurements were made on the electron transfer system of these mitochondria. Although the overall respiration was relatively insensitive to antimycin A, the antibiotic did stimulate the reduction of a type *b* cytochrome. The effects of antimycin A on the respiration and phosphorylation of isolated yeast mitochondria (OHNISHI, KAWAGUCHI, and HAGIHARA, 1966), crab (*Carcinus maenas*) mitochondria (BURRIN and BEECHEY, 1964), and corn-root mitochondria (RAMACHANDRAN and GOTTLIEB, 1961; STONER and HANSON, 1966) were found to be very similar to its effects on these functions in mammalian mitochondria. BUETOW and BUCHANAN (1965) observed that antimycin A inhibited the oxidation of succinate and oxidative phosphorylation as catalyzed by isolated mitochondria of *Euglena gracilis*. In this case it is of interest that the mitochondria of this organism apparently contain a type *c* cytochrome with an α band at 556 mμ and a type *a* cytochrome, but no cytochromes of type *b* (PERINI *et al.*, 1964).

In a rather thorough investigation LUNDEGÅRDH (1962) found that the respiratory system of wheat-root mitochondria is very similar in cytochrome content to the respiratory systems of yeast and heart muscle mitochondria, being composed of cytochromes b, b_3, c_1, c, a, and a_3. Like the respiratory chain of mammalian mitochondria, electrons could be furnished to the cytochrome chain through either succinic dehydrogenase or pyridine nucleotide-linked dehydrogenases. However, in addition to the usual respiratory pathway involving cytochromes b, c, c_1, and a, wheat-root mitochondria also contain a cytochrome b_3 — oxygen shunt that is insensitive to cyanide. It is significant that only the cyanide-sensitive respiration was found to be sensitive to antimycin A.

Electron Transport and Phosphorylation of Photosynthesis

The ubiquity of the antimycin A-sensitive site in living organisms is emphasized by its presence in the photosynthetic apparatus of bacteria and plants as well as its presence in the aerobic respiratory systems of many of the forms of life that have been studied. GELLER and GREGORY (1956) first reported that light-induced phosphorylation (photophosphorylation) in cell-free extracts of the photosynthetic bacteria *Rhodospirillum rubrum* was inhibited by antimycin A. Almost simultaneously, SMITH and BALTSCHEFFSKY (1956) noted a similar inhibition of the same process by 2-n-heptyl-4-hydroxyquinoline-N-oxide (HOQNO), a compound that closely simulates the effects of antimycin A on mitochondrial respiration (LIGHTBOWN and JACKSON, 1956). These studies were extended by BALTSCHEFFSKY and BALTSCHEFFSKY (1958) and GELLER and LIPMANN (1960). Both groups confirmed that antimycin A at low concentrations strongly inhibited light-induced phosphorylation in cell-free extracts of *Rhodospirillum rubrum*. They also observed that in order to obtain this light-induced phosphorylation a suitable source of electrons was required (e.g. succinate, NADH, or lactate). When an electron-transfer mediator such as phenazine methosulfate (PMS) was present in the reaction mixture, the light-induced phosphorylation was found to be insensitive to antimycin A as well as to the other inhibitors, 2-n-heptyl-4-hydroxyquinoline-N-oxide and SN 5949 (a 3-alkyl-2-hydroxynaptho-quinone antimalarial). The inhibitory effects of antimycin A on bacterial photophosphorylation has been affirmed for *Chromatium* as well as for *Rhodospirillum rubrum*. NOZAKI *et al.* (1961) reported that cyclic photophosphorylation in *Chromatium* was suppressed by antimycin A.

Another reaction catalyzed by the photosynthetic system of photosynthetic bacteria is the photoreduction of NAD. This reaction has been observed in chromatophores of both *Chromatium* and *Rhodospirillum rubrum* and in both cases is strongly inhibited by antimycin A (NOZAKI *et al.*, 1961); HINKSON, 1965). However, the inhibitory effect of antimycin A (or HOQNO) appears to differ in the two organisms. HINKSON (1965) observed that the photoreduction of NAD catalyzed by chromatophores of both *Rhodospirillum rubrum* and *Chromatium* could be supported by succinate, ascorbate plus 2,6-dichloroindophenol, or reduced coenzyme Q_2. In the case of *Rhodospirillum rubrum* only the succinate-supported photoreduction was inhibited by HOQNO (and also by antimycin A). However, with chromatophores of *Chromatium*, HOQNO inhibited the reduction of NAD when supported by all three of the reductants.

Because both antimycin A and HOQNO were found to inhibit mitochondrial electron transfer between cytochromes *b* and c_1, BALTSCHEFFSKY and BALTSCHEFFSKY (1958) proposed that an electron transfer chain containing a type *b* cytochrome and a type *c* cytochrome is operative also in the photosynthetic apparatus of *Rhodospirillum rubrum*. This contention was supported by the observations of SMITH and BALTSCHEFFSKY (1959) and NISHIMURA (1963). In a spectroscopic examination of cell-free extracts of *Rhodospirillum rubrum* during the process of light-induced phosphorylation SMITH and BALTSCHEFFSKY observed an oxidation of the cytochromes including cytochrome c_2; however, after addition of HOQNO, difference spectra showed an increased reduction of a type *b* cytochrome having a Soret band at about 430 mμ. Simultaneously an increased oxidation of cytochrome c_2 was observed. NISHIMURA (1963) studied the effects of antimycin A and HOQNO on spectral changes in cell-suspensions of *Rhodopseudomonas sphaeroides* and *Rhodospirillum rubrum*. Introduction of the inhibitors to aerobic-cell suspensions in the dark caused changes in the steady-state oxidation level of cytochromes that correspond to a more reduced state of a *b*-type cytochrome and a more oxidized state of a *c*-type cytochrome. Upon depletion of the oxygen in the suspension of bacteria, normally both cytochromes became reduced; however, in bacteria treated with either antimycin A or HOQNO the reduction of the *c*-type cytochrome was blocked. With illuminated, aerobic suspensions the inhibitors induced a reduction of the *b*-type cytochrome and an oxidation of the *c*-type cytochrome. It was suggested that the site of inhibition of antimycin A is located in the photosynthetic and the respiratory electron transport chain between the *b*-type cytochrome and the *c*-type cytochrome. The *c*-type cytochrome is closer to the photochemical-oxidizing site, whereas the *b* type cytochrome is nearer to the photochemical-reducing site and to the dehydrogenases. Although the complete sequence of electron transfer in photosynthetic bacteria has yet to be elucidated, it is evident that the photosynthetic apparatus does contain a component analogous to Complex III of mitochondria with respect to both cytochrome content and to antimycin A sensitivity. Confirmation for the correctness of this hypothesis is provided by the observation of ZAUGG (1963) that chromatophores of *Rhodospirillum rubrum* contain a (reduced coenzyme Q) — cytochrome *c* reductase activity that is inhibited by antimycin A.

The antimycin A-sensitive component present in chromatophores of *Rhodospirillum rubrum* apparently is a part of the photosynthetic apparatus of this organism; however, it is likely that this component participates only in the nonphotochemical portion of the photosynthetic system. By the use of flashing-light techniques, NISHIMURA (1962a and b) found that the overall photochemical process in chromatophores of *R. rubrum* could be separated into a fast, photochemical process and a slower, light-independent, electron transfer. Only the slower electron-transfer process was inhibited by antimycin A.

The photosynthetic apparatus of plant chloroplasts appears also to contain an antimycin A-sensitive component or components. However, higher concentrations, generally, of antimycin A are required to inhibit photophosphorylation in spinach chloroplasts, than are required to inhibit photophosphorylation in photosynthetic bacteria. BALTSCHEFFSKY (1960) reported that in the presence of flavin mononucleotide (FMN), phenazine methosulfate (PMS) or menadione, and with ascorbate as a source of electrons, photophosphorylation as catalyzed by spinach chloroplasts was inhibited appreciably by antimycin A only at concentrations above 5×10^{-5} M. However, the conditions of the above reaction may have been unfavorable for maximal sensitivity to antimycin A, since PMS may have caused an electronic by pass of the antimycin A-sensitive component as is the case for bacterial photosynthesis. FEWSON *et al.* (1963) were able to demonstrate the photoreduction of NADP and a concomitant photophosphorylation by fragmented chloroplasts supplemented by PPNR (plant ferredoxin) (SAN PIETRO and LANG, 1958; TAGAWA and ARNON, 1962). Antimycin A at 10^{-5} M completely inhibited the reaction.

As a result of their own investigations, ARNON and his associates have proposed the existence of three overlapping pathways of electron transfer in the photochemical apparatus of chloroplasts (ARNON *et al.*, 1964). These are designated as 1. cyclic photophosphorylation, in which ATP is photochemically generated in the absence of oxygen evolution and in the absence of supplementary electron donors or acceptors (oxygen evolution can be suppressed by either p-chlorophenyl dimethyl urea (CMU) or by the employment of light of a wavelength longer than 700 mμ), 2. noncyclic photophosphorylation, in which ATP is generated concomitant to the reduction of a suitable electron acceptor (ferredoxin or NADP), and 3. pseudocyclic photophosphorylation, a form of noncyclic photophosphorylation in which the oxygen evolved during the reaction serves as an electron acceptor via reduced ferredoxin. Of the three types of photophosphorylation, only the cyclic type was inhibited significantly by antimycin A (0.44—1.25 $\times 10^{-5}$ M) (TAGAWA *et al.*, 1963 a and b; ARNON *et al.*, 1964). Based on ARNON's criterion of noncyclic photophosphorylation, the reaction studied by FEWSON *et al.* (1963) would be classified as noncyclic. In this case, it is difficult to understand why the FEWSON system displayed a sensitivity to antimycin A.

Although the presence of a specific antimycin A-sensitive site in spinach choroplasts has been established, an identification of this site with any specific component has not been made as yet. Cytochromes b_6 (α band at 562—563 mμ) and f (α band at 554—555 mμ) were identified as components of chloroplasts some time ago (HILL, 1954; DAVENPORT, 1952; DAVENPORT and HILL, 1952). Recently, LUNDEGÅRDH (1962, 1964) described a second cytochrome of type b that is present in chloroplasts of higher plants. This cytochrome was designated cytochrome b_3 (α band at 557—558 mμ). According to WITT *et al.* (1965) cytochrome f is sequential to a cytochrome b in the transfer of electrons from plastoquinone to chlorophyll a_1. Whether this cytochrome b is the b_3 species or the b_6 species is not clear. If the schemes presented by WITT *et al.* (1965) are correct, then with respect to electron donor (plastoquinone), type of cytochromes, and the span of oxidation potential, E_0' (—0.03 to +0.37 V) the cytochrome b — cytochrome f segment of the electron transfer system in chloroplasts is analogous to the cytochrome b — cytochrome c_1 segment of the mitochondrial respiratory chain. This similarity would make the cytochrome b — cytochrome f segment a likely candidate for the antimycin A-sensitive site in the chloroplasts.

Hepatic Aldehyde Oxidase

With but one known exception, the inhibitory action of antimycin A is confined to enzymes that participate in the electron transport chains of either cellular respiration or photosynthesis. This exception is hepatic aldehyde oxidase (RAJAGOPALAN *et al.*, 1961). This enzyme catalyzes the oxidation of a number of aldehydes including acetaldehyde, salicylaldehyde and principally N-methylnicotinamide. Suitable electron acceptors are oxygen, ferricyanide, certain dyes, silicomolybdate, and cytochrome *c*. Antimycin A is one of a number of compounds that inhibit the enzyme. The enzyme was reported to be inhibited 62% at 2×10^{-6}M antimycin A.

It might be argued that in the case of hepatic aldehyde oxidase, the inhibitory activity of antimycin A is unrelated by mechanism to its inhibitory activity toward respiratory systems. However, the reported presence in this enzyme of coenzyme Q_{10} (Ubiquinone 50) (RAJAGOPALAN *et al.*, 1961) and a nonheme-iron component that gives an electron paramagnetic resonance (EPR) signal at g = 1.94 (RAJAGOPALAN *et al.*, 1962) makes it probable that this enzyme contains a compound very similar to the antimycin A-sensitive component of the respiratory chain of mitochondria. Complex III, the segment of the respiratory chain of mitochondria that contains the antimycin A-site uses coenzyme Q_{10} as an electron donor and also contains a nonheme-iron component with an EPR signal of the g = 1.94 type (RIESKE, HANSEN, and ZAUGG, 1963).

Cleavage of Complex III of the Respiratory Chain

A novel effect displayed by antimycin A is its ability to block the chemical cleavage of Complex III into its individual, constituent cytochromes (RIESKE and ZAUGG, 1962). Incubation of Complex III in the presence of bile salts (>5%) and ammonium sulfate (0.20—0.30 saturation at 0 °C) results in the separation of cytochrome *b* as an insoluble protein; cytochrome c_1 remains in the supernatant solution. This reaction is blocked completely by antimycin A in an amount equivalent to the content of cytochrome c_1 of Complex III in the reaction mixture (cf. Fig. 3). It was postulated that antimycin A protects a reactive moiety connecting cytochrome *b* to cytochrome c_1 from hydrolytic cleavage. The detergent action of bile salts plus ammonium sulfate may allow free access of water into the interior of the complex. This reaction will be discussed in greater detail in later sections of this review.

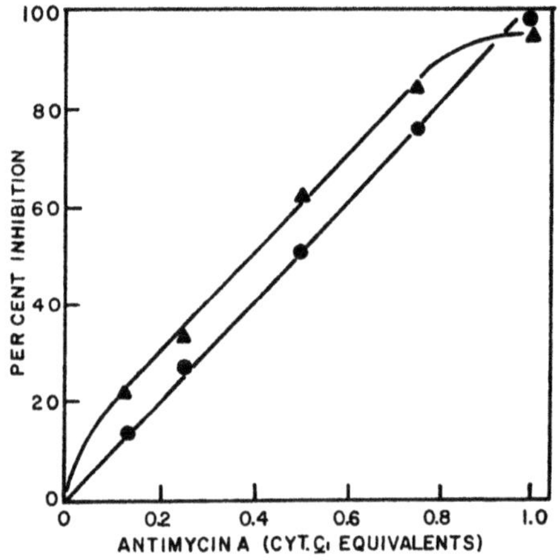

Fig. 3. Inhibitory effects of antimycin A on the Co QH_2-cytochrome *c* reductase activity and on the cleavage of Complex III. ●, Inhibition of Co QH_2-cytochrome *c* reductase ▲, Inhibition of cleavage of cytochrome *b* from Complex III

Mechanism of Inhibition of Respiration by Antimycin A

In recent years some effort has been expended in attempts to determine how antimycin A exerts its inhibitory effect on the respiratory chain. The enzymologist is motivated in this venture by the realization that a highly specific stoichiometric inhibitor such as antimycin A provides a useful tool for elucidation of the chemical nature of the component that interacts with the inhibitor. A knowledge of the nature of the site of inhibition and its role in the respiratory process goes hand-in-glove with a knowledge of the mechanism of inhibition. Chemical, kinetic, spectrophotometric, and isolation techniques have enabled us to gain a clearing but as yet indistinct image of the nature of interaction of antimycin A with its site of inhibition in the respiratory chain. In this section the accumulated data bearing on this problem will be discussed and evaluated in an effort to build a picture of the nature of the antimycin A-sensitive site and the mechanism by which antimycin A blocks electron flow at this site.

Chemical Characteristics of Antimycin A in Relationship to its Inhibitory Activity

With the determination of chemical structure of antimycin A (VAN TAMELEN *et al.*, 1961), the way was opened for an identification of the reactive groups of the molecule with respect to its inhibitory activity. In the classical manner, various derivatives of antimycin A_3 (blastmycin) were prepared and tested with regard to their inhibitory activity toward respiratory processes. The following derivatives, antimycin A_3 O-methyl ether, antimycin A_3 diacetate, deformylantimycin A_3 hydrochloride, deformylantimycin A_3 triacetate, reformylated deformylantimycin A_3 hydrochloride, and antimycic acid were tested with respect to their inhibitory activity toward succinate oxidase (VAN TAMELEN *et al.*, 1961), succinate-cytochrome *c* reductase (TAPPEL, 1960), and (reduced coenzyme Q)-cytochrome *c* reductase (RIESKE, unpublished experiments) (cf. Table 5). In all three assay systems, the inhibitory activity, respectively, of the o-methyl, the deformyl, and the deformyl-triacetate derivatives was almost absent when compared to the activity of the parent compound. Antimycic acid was found to have low inhibitory activity toward the succinate-cytochrome *c* reductase (TAPPEL, 1960). Although in the succinate oxidase system the diacetate derivative displayed little inhibitory activity, it did display a low, but significant, activity in the succinate-cytochrome *c* reductase and the (reduced coenzyme Q)-cytochrome *c* reductase systems. This residual activity may be a result of the unstable nature of the O-acetyl linkage in the aqueous system of the assay. Replacement of the N-formyl group with an acetyl group as in the deformyl-N-acetylantimycin A_3 resulted in little loss of inhibitory activity. From these results it is evident that the substituted dilactone ring, the phenolic hydroxyl group and an N-carbonyl group individually and collectively are indispensible for inhibitory activity of antimycin A.

In order to test the supposition that the dilactone-ring moiety of antimycin A merely provides a proper degree lipid solubility to the molecule, DICKIE *et al.* (1963) prepared and tested a series of synthetic analogs of antimycin A. These compounds were substituted amides of 3-formamidosalicylic acid and differed from antimycin A in having a straight-chain alkyl group substituting for the dilactone ring structure. All of the analogs from the n-butyl to the n-octadecyl-substituted compound were found to inhibit (reduced coenzyme Q) — cytochrome *c* reductase (Complex III); however, the effectiveness of inhibition and of binding of the analogs to the enzyme increased with increasing chain-length of the alkyl group. These data support the hypothesis that the dilactone portion of the antimycin A molecule merely confers the proper lipid solubility to the compound, and that the mechanism of inhibition is determined by the aromatic nucleus and its substituted groups. This generalization although probably correct in substance appears to be overly simplified. Even the most effective inhibitor of the analogs, the octadecyl homolog, reacts somewhat sluggishly with Complex III (30 minutes or longer for equilibration at 0 °C) in comparison to antimycin A (less than 5 minutes for equilibration at 0 °C) (RIESKE, unpublished data). In addition to conferring lipid solubility to antimycin A, the dilactone ring and its substituted alkyl groups may function in providing proper fit between the inhibitor and its binding site on the enzyme.

A property of antimycin A that has been considered with respect to its function as a respiratory inhibitor is its ability to form metal-chelates. TAPPEL (1960) proposed that antimycin A in common with other inhibitors of respiration (ie. 2-n-heptyl-4-hydroxyquinoline-N-oxide, 2-hydroxy-3-alkyl naphthoquinones, and 2-thenoyltrifluoroacetone) probably inhibits by reason of its capacity for chelation with metal ions. Nonheme-iron components in the lipid environment of the respiratory chain were proposed as probable targets for these inhibitors. The metal-complexing capabilities of antimycin A were verified by the finding of KOYAMA *et al.* (1960). They observed that complexes of antimycin A with cobalt, copper, nickel, zinc, lead, and mercury ions were less toxic than antimycin A alone. In a study of the complexes of antimycin A with ionic iron, FARLEY, STRONG, and BYDALEK (1965) deduced that at acid pH's Fe (III) formed with antimycin A a bidentate, six-membered ring involving the 1-carboxamide and the 2-hydroxyl of the aromatic moiety. The significance of this property of antimycin A with respect to the antimycin A-sensitive site will be discussed in a subsequent section.

Nature of the Antimycin Site

Despite rather extensive investigations the nature of the component inhibited by antimycin A remains obscure. Four measurable components of the mitochondrial respiratory chain may be considered as candidates for the locus of inhibition by antimycin A. These are: 1. cytochrome *b*, 2. nonheme iron-protein of Complex III, 3. the component involved in the cleavage of Complex III, and 4. the component involved in the coupling of energy-conserving reactions to respiration.

Cytochrome *b* has been an attractive candidate for the site of action of antimycin A because it is the only cytochrome of the respiratory chain that appears to be altered in its properties by antimycin A. CHANCE (1958) first reported that antimycin A modified the properties of cytochrome *b* with respect to both its kinetic behavior during oxidation and reduction and its absorption spectrum. Previously, CHANCE and WILLIAMS (1955) had demonstrated that in preparations of heart muscle (mitochondrial fragments) which had lost their capacity for oxidative phosphorylation cytochrome *b* was reduced by succinate at a much lower rate than the reduction of other electron-transfer components. However, after the preparation was treated with antimycin A, the rate of reduction of cytochrome *b* by succinate was increased 50-fold over the untreated preparation (CHANCE, 1958). Spectrally, after reduction by succinate or hydrosulfite, the preparation that had been treated with antimycin A displayed a cytochrome *b*-type component with an α band at 566 mμ and a Soret band at 432 mμ in contrast to analogous absorption bands at 562 mμ and 430 mμ for preparations untreated with antimycin A. CHANCE suggested that an inactive form of cytochrome *b* (α band at 566 mμ) was capable of being reduced only under conditions of rapid electron transfer to cytochrome *b* (α band at 562 mμ) as a result of treatment with antimycin A. SLATER and COLPA-BOONSTRA (1961) substantiated the observations of CHANCE (1958) regarding the effects of antimycin A on the reducibility and spectra of cytochrome *b* in heart muscle preparations. They suggested, however, that both forms of cytochrome *b* reacted with antimycin A leading to an increased oxidation-reduction potential with an increased reducibility of both forms of cytochrome *b* by succinate. PUMPHREY (1962) observed that upon graded additions of antimycin A to submitochondrial particles, spectral changes in cytochrome *b* occurred with much smaller amounts of antimycin A than the amounts required to inhibit NADH oxidase activity or to affect the reducibility of cytochrome *b* by NADH or reduced coenzyme Q_2 (cf. Fig. 4). In addition, treatment of the particles with high concentrations of bile salts (cholate) caused a blue-shift of the α band of cytochrome *b* from 563 mμ to 561 mμ and also resulted in a loss of reducibility of the cytochrome by menadiol. Addition of antimycin A prior to the addition of cholate protected cytochrome *b* from these effects of the bile salt.

Although the multiplicity of effects of antimycin A on cytochrome *b* indicate an intimate relationship at least between the antimycin A-sensitive site and the cytochrome, CHANCE (1958) dismissed cytochrome *b* itself as containing this site. This conclusion was based on the observation that the reduction of cytochrome *b* in mitochondrial preparations that had lost their phosphorylating capacity is much slower than the reduction of other electron-transfer components (eg. cytochrome c_1 or cytochrome *c*). Therefore, it was argued that in these nonphosphorylating particles cytochrome *b* does not function on the main pathway of respiration (CHANCE and WILLIAMS, 1955) and on this basis could not be the primary site of inhibition by antimycin A.

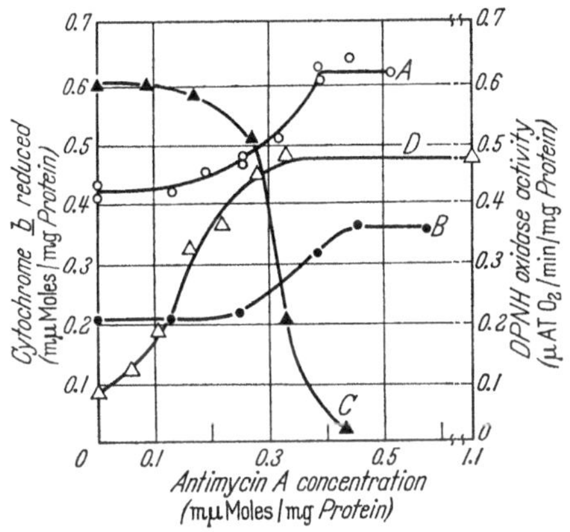

Fig. 4a

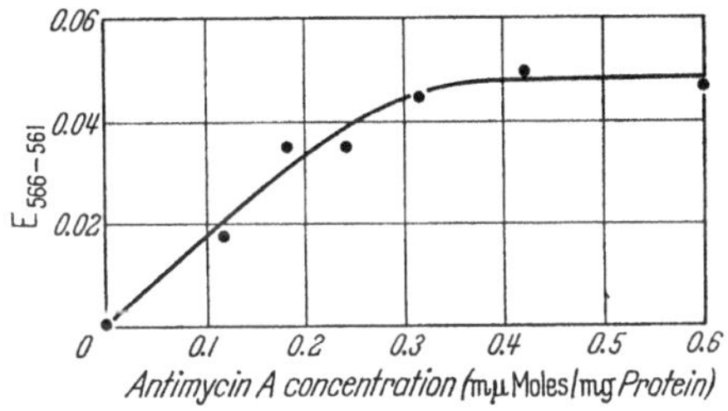

Fig. 4b

Fig. 4a. Relationships between antimycin A-titer and the degree of various effects of antimycin A on a respiratory particle (ETP) derived from beef heart mitochondria. *Curve A*, amount of cytochrome *b* reduced by NADH; *Curve B*, amount of cytochrome *b* reduced by CoQ_2H_2; *Curve C*, NADH oxidase activity; *Curve D*, amount of cytochrome *b* reduced by menadiol, in ETP treated with cholate (1.4 mg/mg of ETP protein). From PUMPHREY (1962)

Fig. 4b. Effect of antimycin A concentration on the magnitude of the red shift in the α band of reduced cytochrome *b* of ETP. From PUMPHREY (1962)

The possibility that a metal-containing compound is involved at the site of inhibition by antimycin A has been considered seriously ever since the chelating capabilities of antimycin A were first described (TAPPEL, 1960). This possibility was reinforced by the discovery that Complex III of the respiratory chain contained nonheme iron (HATEFI *et al.*, 1962). The discovery that nonheme iron of Complex III gives rise to a unique EPR (electron paramagnetic resonance) signal at $g = 1.90$ (RIESKE *et al.*, 1964a) and can be cleaved from the complex as an iron protein (RIESKE *et al.*, 1964b) provided means for testing the hypothesis that a nonheme iron compound is the locus of inhibition by antimycin A. The first intimation that nonheme iron could be involved only indirectly at most with the antimycin A-sensitive site was the observation that antimycin A inhibited the rate of formation of the EPR signal at $g = 1.90$ upon reduction with succinate but caused no alteration in the signal *per se* (RIESKE *et al.*, 1964a). Because the unique aspects of the EPR signal are caused by the ligand field in the vicinity of the iron, any new ligand formation between antimycin A and the iron of the $g = 1.90$ species would be expected to perturb the EPR signal.

Studies on the cleavage of Complex III provided further evidence that nonheme iron is not involved directly in the inhibitory effects of antimycin A. As mentioned previously, upon treatment with ammonium sulfate and high concentrations of bile salt Complex III separates into two principal subfractions, an insoluble protein that contains cytochrome *b* and a soluble protein that contains cytochrome c_1. In the presence of antimycin A this major cleavage does not occur (RIESKE and ZAUGG, 1962); however, a minor fraction of the protein of Complex III containing the nonheme iron is precipitated. Even after almost complete removal of the nonheme iron by this process the cleavage of Complex III into subfractions containing cytochrome *b* and cytochrome c_1, respectively, remains blocked by antimycin A (RIESKE *et al.*, 1964b). Unless antimycin A promotes a secondary bonding between cytochromes *b* and c_1 somewhat removed from the initial site of inhibition, it is evident that the component containing nonheme iron could not qualify as the factor inhibited by antimycin A.

The possible involvement of some metal other than iron at the antimycin A-sensitive site should be considered; however, analysis of Complex III has failed to detect any metals other than iron in sufficient amounts to qualify as a functional component of the complex (RIESKE, unpublished data).

A measurable function of the respiratory chain that probably is most intimately related to the antimycin A-sensitive site is the linkage connecting cytochromes *b* and c_1 that undergoes change in the presence of bile salts plus ammonium sulfate (RIESKE and ZAUGG, 1962). Unlike other functions of the respiratory chain that are affected by antimycin A, the cleavage of Complex III appears to be a chemical reaction that is non-enzymic in nature. Evidence to date support the contention that this cleavage actually occurs within the chemical structure of the antimycin A-sensitive site (RIESKE *et al.*, in preparation).

In the presence of ammonium sulfate and excess bile salt Complex III undergoes a cleavage into three principle fractions, containing cytochrome *b*, cytochrome c_1, and a nonheme-iron protein, respectively. An event preceding physical separation of cytochromes *b* and c_1 is a loss of the ability of antimycin A to block the cleavage process. The rate of this loss of sensitivity to antimycin A corresponds to a first order kinetic process and is increased at acidic and alkaline pH's. Concomitant with the loss of sensitivity to antimycin A, the effects of antimycin A on the properties of cytochrome *b* and the specific binding of the antibiotic to Complex III are lost (this latter observation will be discussed more fully in a subsequent section). These results support the contention that the antimycin A-sensitive site itself is a primary linkage between cytochromes *b* and c_1 and that this linkage undergoes a hydrolytic-type cleavage upon exposure of its lipid environment to the detergent action of salt plus bile acids. Furthermore, data indicate that this site of cleavage undergoes reversible oxidation-reduction during normal electron-transport in the complex. Reduction of Complex III with succinate, reduced coenzyme Q_2 and other, strictly chemical, reducing agents (i.e. borohydride and dithionite) protects Complex III from loss of antimycin A sensitivity and attendant with this loss of sensitivity the susceptibility of the complex to cleavage into separate cytochromes. Therefore, it appears that the antimycin A-sensitive site may be an electron-transfer component that is susceptible to cleavage only when in the oxidized state. In terms of potential, this electron-transfer component appears to be located between cytochromes *b* and c_1. Treatment of Complex III aerobically with ascorbate, which completely reduces cytochrome c_1 and leaves cytochrome *b* in the oxidized state, inhibited the cleavage reaction by 40%; therefore, the state of oxidation of the cleavage site apparently was intermediate between the states of oxidation of cytochromes *b* and c_1.

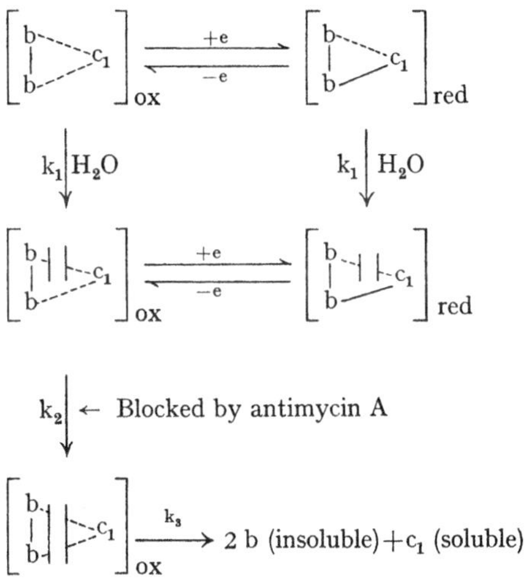

Fig. 5. Postulated scheme for the reactions involved in the cleavage of Complex III

Reduction of Complex III protects it from loss of sensitivity to antimycin A during exposure to cleavage conditions; however, the rate of loss of sensitivity to antimycin A upon reoxidation of the reduced complex after extended exposure to cleavage conditions is accentuated. Apparently, cleavage of the antimycin A-sensitive site is preceded by a slower reaction that is independent of the oxidation state of the site of cleavage. From pH studies of these individual reactions, it was found that only the slow reaction, that preceding the cleavage of the antimycin A-site, is highly dependent on pH. The slow reaction may reflect a cleavage of another bond between cytochromes *b* and c_1 that is parallel to the antimycin A-sensitive linkage. The possible reactions involved in the cleavage of Complex III are illustrated in Fig. 5.

Although antimycin A has been classified as strictly an inhibitor of electron transfer in the respiratory process, this classification may be an over-simplication. There are several striking similarities between the effects of antimycin A and the effects of energy-conserving intermediates on the reducibility and spectral properties of cytochrome *b*. These suggest a relationship between the site of inhibition by antimycin A and the primary site of energy coupling in the cytochrome *b* — cytochrome c_1 region of the respiratory chain. These similarities are summarized as follows: 1. The rate and extent of reduction of cytochrome by succinate in sub-mitochondrial preparations are decreased greatly upon loss of phosphorylative capacity; antimycin A causes a restoration of much of the rate and extent of reduction of cytochrome *b* observed in phosphorylating preparations (CHANCE, 1958, 1961). 2. CHANCE *et al.* (1965) have reported the detection of high energy forms of cytochrome *b* with α bands at 555 mμ and 565 mμ, respectively. These spectral forms of cytochrome *b* were detected at liquid nitrogen temperature in mitochondria and mitochondrial particles that had been inhibited with malonate and sulfide and then treated with glutamate and manganese (formation of a peak at 555 mμ), then inorganic phosphate (disappearance of the peak at 555 mμ and appearance of a peak at 565 mμ). These apparent shifts of absorption bands of cytochrome *b* are reminiscent of the shift of the α peak of cytochrome *b* to shorter wavelengths after cleavage of Complex III (PUMPHREY, 1962; RIESKE, unpublished observations) and to longer wavelengths (566 mμ) after treatment of mitochondrial preparations with antimycin A (CHANCE, 1958; PUMPHREY, 1962). 3. The cross-over point (point of reversal of oxidation state of adjacent components) of cytochrome reduction in the respiratory chain inhibited by antimycin A is the same as the crossover point between cytochromes *b* and c_1 observed during state-4 respiration (i.e. respiration in absence of a phosphate acceptor such as ADP) in mitochondria that are tightly coupled to oxidative phosphorylation (CHANCE, 1961). These similarities between energy-coupled respiration and antimycin A-inhibited respiration suggest the possibility that antimycin A inhibits respiration by stabilizing the initial compound involved in energy conservation in the coenzyme Q-cytochrome *c* segment of the respiratory chain. According to one concept of respiratory control, respiration can proceed only when the high-energy compound can turn-over by reacting with a suitable acceptor system. In a system coupled to phosphorylation the acceptor system transfers the available bond energy from the respiration-linked, high-energy compound to the ultimate high-energy bond of ATP. In an uncoupled system, it is believed that some side reaction (e.g. hydrolysis) decomposes the high-energy compound or compounds in preference to or in competition with the reactions that lead to phosphorylation. Therefore, on the basis of this argument, respiration as well as phosphorylation would be blocked by any reagent that interfers with the reaction of the high-energy compound with either phosphorylating acceptors or uncoupling compounds. Antimycin A may function as this type of reagent.

ESTABROOK (1962a) tested the possibility that antimycin A is an inhibitor of phosphorylation as well as of respiration. He observed that 2,4-dinitrophenol did not reverse the inhibition of respiration caused by antimycin A in contradistinction to its reversal of the inhibition of state-3 respiration (i.e. respiration in the presence of phosphate acceptor such as ADP) of mitochrondria by oligomycin. On the basis of this observation ESTABROOK concluded that antimycin A did not function as an inhibitor of phosphorylation in the same manner as did oligomycin. However, this observation of ESTABROOK can be explained on the basis that 2,4-dinitrophenol uncouples the energy-linked reactions somewhere between the antimycin A-inhibited site and the oligomycin-inhibited site. For purposes of illustration only, the relationships between respiration, the antimycin A-sensitive site, and respiration-linked phosphorylation as discussed in this section can be summarized by the following reactions. In this case A∼ designates an energized electron carrier and X designates the first acceptor of the high-energy moiety in the phosphorylation system.

$$b^{2+} + A \rightleftharpoons A^{\text{red.}} + b^{3+}$$
$$A^{\text{red.}} + c_1^{3+} \rightleftharpoons A{\sim} + c_1^{2+}$$
$$A{\sim} + X \underset{\text{Antimycin A}}{\overset{\uparrow}{\rightleftharpoons}} A + X{\sim}$$
$$X{\sim} \xrightarrow{(\text{Pi} + \text{ADP})} X + \text{ATP}$$
$$X{\sim} \xrightarrow[\text{H}_2\text{O}]{\text{2,4 DNP}} X + \text{heat}$$

Nature of Interaction of Antimycin A with its Site of Inhibition

As described in a preceding section the stoichiometric nature of the inhibition of respiration by antimycin A was first described by POTTER and REIF (1952). They found that in rat tissues, inhibition of succinate oxidation by antimycin A was dependent on the ratio of the amount of inhibitor to the amount of tissue rather than on the overall concentration of antimycin A. From these results they suggested that the respiratory system of rat tissues actually was titrated by antimycin A. The correctness of this suggestion was emphasized by CHANCE (1952) who reported that the respiratory chain of heart-muscle preparation was inhibited by antimycin A in amounts nearly stoichiometric to the content of cytochrome. The remaining problem was the establishment of the antimycin A titer of inhibition in terms of the concentration of respiratory chains or assemblies. Several values of antimycin A-titer in terms of various components of the respiratory chain of heart muscle have been reported. GREEN *et al.* (1955) determined that antimycin A inhibited succinate-cytochrome *c* reductase of a subfraction of beef-heart mitochondria in amounts stoichiometric with the content of flavin. THORN (1956) reported that the succinate oxidase of a heart-muscle preparation was inhibited completely by antimycin A in amounts of the same order of magnitude as the amount of a single component of the cytochrome system.

Although the above data suggest that antimycin A can titrate a single component per unit respiratory chain, the values given are based on rather vague analytical data. Also, in most of the preparations tested, the titration curves relating degree of inhibition to amount af antimycin A added to the preparation were sigmoid in shape rather than linear as would be expected for an uncomplicated titration. POTTER and REIF (1952) suggested two possible causes for this nonlinearity; either some component other that than inhibited by antimycin A was rate-limiting in the electron transfer process or antimycin A was bound in a noninhibitory manner to components other than the one specifically inhibited by antimycin A. In the first case, despite a nonlinear inactivation with respect to the amount of antimycin A added, the end point of the titration (amount of antimycin A required for complete inhibition) would be stoichiometric with the amount of inhibited components. In the second case, the endpoint would require amounts of antimycin A in excess of the amount of inhibited components.

In most cases, an evaluation of antimycin A-titration data on the basis of these criteria has been unsatisfactory; the principal reason being inadequate information on the concentration of the respiratory segment inhibited by antimycin A. However, the antimycin A-titration data of PUMPHREY (1962) provided good evidence that of the two mechanisms proposed by POTTER and REIF (1962), the first is the better explanation for the sigmoid shape of the titration curves, at least in the case of mitochondrial fragments (ETP) from beef heart. The curves relating antimycin A titer to the reducibility of cytochrome *b* by menadiol and to the changes in spectrum of cytochrome *b* are essentially linear and both curves extrapolate to completion at an antimycin A titer of approximately 0.27 mμ moles per mg of protein (cf. Fig. 5a). This titer corresponds precisely to the content of cytochrome c_1 (i.e. 0.27 mμ moles/mg of protein) in these particles (GREEN and WHARTON, 1963). In contrast, at this titer of antimycin A the NADH oxidation in this same system was inhibited about 10%. It is evident that the NADH oxidation was not inhibited appreciably until almost all of the antimycin A- sensitive sites were titrated by antimycin A.

Isolation and purification of Complex III from beef-heart mitochondria (HATEFI, HAAVIK, and GRIFFITHS, 1962) provided a more ideal system for titrations with antimycin A. Not only was the antimycin A-sensitive segment of the respiratory chain isolated from other portions of the chain but its purity allowed an accurate determination of its content of cytochromes *b* and c_1. RIESKE and ZAUGG (1962) titrated Complex III with antimycin A; the (reduced coenzyme Q) — cytochrome *c* reductase activity of the complex was inhibited completely by an amount of antimycin A equivalent to the content of cytochrome c_1 in the sample of enzyme (cf. Fig. 3). In confirmation of the suggestions of POTTER and REIF (1952) regarding the cause of the sigmoid form of the curve of inactivation of succinate oxidase by antimycin A, the inhibition of Complex III was a linear function of the amount of antimycin added. Agreement between the minimal molecular weight based on its content of cytochrome c_1 and the measured molecular weight (TZAGOLOFF *et al.*, 1965) indicate that each unit complex contains a single molecule of cytochrome c_1; therefore it is probable that each complex also contains a single site of inhibition by antimycin A.

Although it appears that each respiratory chain in heart mitochondria contains a single site of inhibition by antimycin A, ESTABROOK (1962a) presented evidence that in phosphorylating mitochondria from rat liver only one molecule of antimycin A is required to inhibit three respiratory chains. It must be pointed out, however, that ESTABROOK arrived at this conclusion on the assumption that each respiratory chain in rat-liver mitochondria contains one molecule of cytochrome *a*.

Although the stoichiometric nature of the reaction between antimycin A and its site of inhibition indicate a highly specific and irreversible interaction, there is evidence that under certain conditions the inhibitory effects of antimycin A can be reversed. In their studies on the toxic effects of antimycin A, POTTER and REIF (1952) observed a spontaneous recovery of succinate oxidase activity in the liver tissue of rats that had been treated with inhibitory amounts of antimycin A. Further investigations by these workers established that rat serum, specifically the albumin fraction, was responsible for this reactivation and was capable of reversing *in vitro* the inhibition of succinate oxidase by antimycin A of other tissues in the rat. Apparently, serum albumin competed with the respiratory chain for the binding of antimycin A. As the amount of antimycin A added to the tissue was increased the degree of reactivation obtained by addition of a given amount of serum albumin was decreased concomitantly. Also, serum albumin was found capable of binding antimycin A (REIF and POTTER, 1953; REIF, 1953). THORN (1956) tested the reversibility of the binding of antimycin A to the succinate oxidase system of a heart muscle preparation. He observed that the succinate oxidase activity of preparations that had been inactivated completely by antimycin A recovered most of the lost activity upon addition of an equal quantity of the preparation of heart muscle that had been inactivated irreversibly with respect to succinate oxidase by either p-aminophenylarsenoxide or BAL (2,3-dimercapto propanol). The arsenical was found to inactivate succinate dehydrogenase whereas BAL treatment apparently destroys an electron-transfer component located near cytochrome *b* of the respiratory chain (SLATER, 1949). Thorn interpreted these results as an indication that the binding of antimycin A to its specific site of inhibition was sufficiently reversible to permit a redistribution of antimycin A from the inhibited enzyme to its analogous binding site on the enzyme that had been inactivated by either BAL or the arsenical.

NASON and LEHMAN (1956) claimed that α-tocopherol was capable of partially reactivating a NADH-cytochrome *c* reductase preparation (from rat skeletal muscle) that had been treated with antimycin A; however, DEUL *et al.* (1958) failed to confirm this type of reversal. A similar reactivation of a particulate succinate cytochrome *c* reductase from heart muscle after inhibition by antimycin A was reported by TAKEMORI and KING (1964). They observed that the inhibition of the enzyme was reversed as much as 50% by 48 μM coenzyme Q_2. In the presence of 480 μM coenzyme Q_2 a prior addition of 0.9 mμmole of antimycin A per milligram of enzyme protein resulted in less than 5% inhibition. Antimycin A and coenzyme Q appeared to be competitive with regard to inhibition and reactivation, respectively. This observation would preclude a mechanism of reactivation involving an electronic bypass of an antimycin A-inhibited component. REPORTER and EBERT (1964) described the isolation and partial purification of a protein from chicken-liver mitochondria which prevented the inhibitory effects of antimycin A on early chick embryo and cultured muscle cells. This factor also alleviated the inhibition of respiration caused by antimycin A in phosphorylating mitochondrial preparations isolated from rat liver and from rat and embryonic chick hearts (REPORTER, 1965).

Although the pseudoirreversible nature of the interaction between antimycin A and its site of inhibition has been well documented for respiring particles using succinate as a reducing substrate, attempts to demonstrate a significant reactivation (>10%) of antimycin A-inhibited Complex III, (reduced coenzyme Q)-cytochrome *c* reductase, both purified and in mitochondrial fragments have failed uniformly (RIESKE, J. S., S. H. LIPTON, and H. BAUM; unpublished experiments). These attempts have employed reagents such as bovine serum albumin, excess coenzyme Q_2 and the reactivating factor isolated from chicken-liver mitochondria by REPORTER and EBERT. The discrepancy between these results and the reversals of inhibition of succinate oxidase or succinate-cytochrome c reductase may be a result of a low requirement of active Complex III to support a maximal rate of succinate oxidation. In this case, a relatively small reactivation of Complex III may be sufficient to support full succinate-oxidase activity. This suggestion is supported by the high turnover number of (reduced coenzyme Q)-cytochrome c reductase in comparison to the succinic dehydrogenase protein of the respiratory chain (HATEFI *et al.*, 1962). Also, ESTABROOK (1961a) found that during a titration of heart muscle particles with antimycin A the alteration by the antibiotic of the steady state reduction of cytochrome b was initiated at 40% of the titer required to initiate an inhibition of oxygen uptake.

The question of stoichiometry and reversibility of the interaction between antimycin A and Complex III has been studied recently with respect to the inhibition of cleavage of Complex III. Like the inhibition of electron transfer in Complex III, cleavage of Complex III into cytochrome b and cytochrome c_1 was inhibited completely by an amount of antimycin A equivalent to the amount of cytochrome c_1 in the sample (Fig. 3). However, at substoichiometric levels of antimycin A, the inhibitions of cleavage were greater than those expected on the basis of a simple titration of a single component of Complex III (RIESKE and ZAUGG, 1962). An investigation of the reversibility of this inhibition was conducted by RIESKE *et al.* (b) (manuscript in preparation). Complex III was treated with a stoichiometric amount of tritium-labelled antimycin A and then extracted several times with 10% taurocholate. Although this procedure removed 70% of the added antimycin A the complex was still incapable of cleavage. It was concluded that antimycin A either is capable of inhibiting the cleavage of Complex III at much less than stoichiometric quantities, or that antimycin A promotes the formation of a linkage between cytochromes b and c_1 that remains even after removal of the antimycin A. It is difficult to reconcile the apparent irreversibility of the inhibition of the cleavage reaction with the reactivations of succinate oxidase as described earlier in this section. Perhaps the interaction of antimycin A with its site of inhibition involves a transient, reversible inhibition followed by a slower formation of an irreversible linkage.

Although antimycin A is well characterized with respect to its chemical nature and to the chemical groups responsible for its inhibitory activity, nothing is known about the chemistry of its interaction with the respiratory chain. However, insight has been gained on some superficial aspects of this interaction. The possibility has been entertained that antimycin A undergoes a chemical alteration either before or during its interaction with its site of inhibition. ESTABROOK (1962a) observed that at an alkaline pH there was a pronounced lag in the onset of inhibition subsequent to addition to antimycin A to a succinate oxidase system of heart muscle. This lag was attributed by ESTABROOK to a conversion of antimycin A from a non-inhibitory form to an inhibitory form within the mitochondrial particle. Also, the requirement of the N-formyl group of the antimycin A molecule for inhibitory activity (cf. section on Chemical Characteristics of Antimycin A) suggested that antimycin A may inhibit respiration by a formylation of some chemical group required in the respiratory process. This hypothesis offered an attractive explanation for the inability to reverse the effects of antimycin A on the cleavage of Complex III by removal of most of the antimycin A.

However, the preceding hypothesis was discredited by experimental data that indicated an absence of any permanent loss of inhibitory activity of antimycin A after its interaction with Complex III of the respiratory chain. Acetone extraction of Complex III that had been pretreated with substoichiometric amounts of tritium-labeled antimycin A recovered 70% of the tritium that had been added to the enzyme. On the basis of specific radioactivity, antimycin A in these acetone extracts was fully inhibitory to the enzymic activity ($CoQH_2$ — cytochrome *c* reductase) of Complex III (RIESKE, J. S., S. H. LIPTON, H. BAUM, and I. SILMAN in preparation). Although these results argue against the possibility of a deformylation or any other permanent alteration leading to loss of inhibitory activity of antimycin A as a result of its interaction with the antimycin A-site, they do not disqualify the suggestion of ESTABROOK that antimycin A is converted from an inactive to an active form during its interaction with the respiratory chain.

Another question that has been clarified is the question regarding the oxidation state of the antimycin A blocked component. ESTABROOK (1958), on the basis of the effects of antimycin A on the steady-state reduction of the cytochromes concluded that antimycin A reacted with an oxidized component of the respiratory chain. This conclusion has been supported by the spectrophotometric observations of PUMPHREY (1962); SHORE and WAINIO (personal communication); and BAUM and RIESKE (1966). All of these investigators have observed independently an apparent paradox in which the addition of an oxidant to a respiratory particle pretreated with antimycin A triggers the further reduction of cytochrome *b*. PUMPHREY observed an increased reduction of cytochrome *b* upon admixture of air to an anaerobic preparation containing mitochondrial fragments (electron-transport particles), antimycin A, and menadiol. SHORE and WAINIO observed a similar effect upon admixture of air to mitochondrial preparations reduced by succinate and treated with antimycin A. The most striking effect of this type was the recent observation of BAUM and RIESKE. Treatment of Complex III with reduced coenzyme Q_2 reduced completely cytochrome c_1 and about 30% of the cytochrome *b*. Addition of antimycin A at this point resulted in no further reduction of cytochrome *b*; however, subsequent addition of a small amount of ferricyanide triggered an immediate but transient reduction of an additional 50% of the cytochrome *b* (cf. Fig. 6). Apparently, antimycin A although present in Complex III exerts no effect on the reducibility of cytochrome *b* until its site of interaction becomes oxidized temporarily. This interpetration supports the contention that antimycin A is reactive only toward the oxidized form of the antimycin A-sensitive component.

Recently, the relationship between the chemical integrity of the antimycin A-sensitive site and the capacity of this site to bind antimycin A has been investigated (RIESKE, J. S., S. H. LIPTON, H. BAUM, and I. SILMAN, in preparation). The capacity of Complex III after a selected treatment to bind antimycin A was assessed by a technique analogous to that described by THORN (1956). Under certain conditions (i.e. incubation at 40 C for 1 hour or short exposure to 10% sodium taurocholate) the enzymic activity ($CoQH_2$-cytochrome *c* reductase) of Complex III can be destroyed with little concomitant loss of sensitivity of the cleavage reaction to antimycin A. Admixture of the inactivated complex with active complex provided a system in which the relative affinity of antimycin A for the enzymically active and inactive components, respectively, could be measured. Therefore, any treatment that decreases the binding of antimycin A to the inactivated complex concomitantly will allow more antimycin A to react with, and to inhibit, the enzymically-competent complex. Experiments of this type confirmed that the chemical integrity of the antimycin A-sensitive site in Complex III is essential for a physical binding of antimycin A to this site. Conditions that resulted in loss of sensitivity of the cleavage reaction to antimycin A (e.g. prolonged exposure to high concentrations of bile salts) also destroyed the capacity of Complex III to bind antimycin A. A mild digestion of Complex III with trypsin also destroyed the capacity of the complex to bind the antibiotic; however, if antimycin A was added to Complex III prior to proteolysis the antimycin A remained bound. Analogous results were obtained when Complex III was exposed to 1.0 M guanidine.

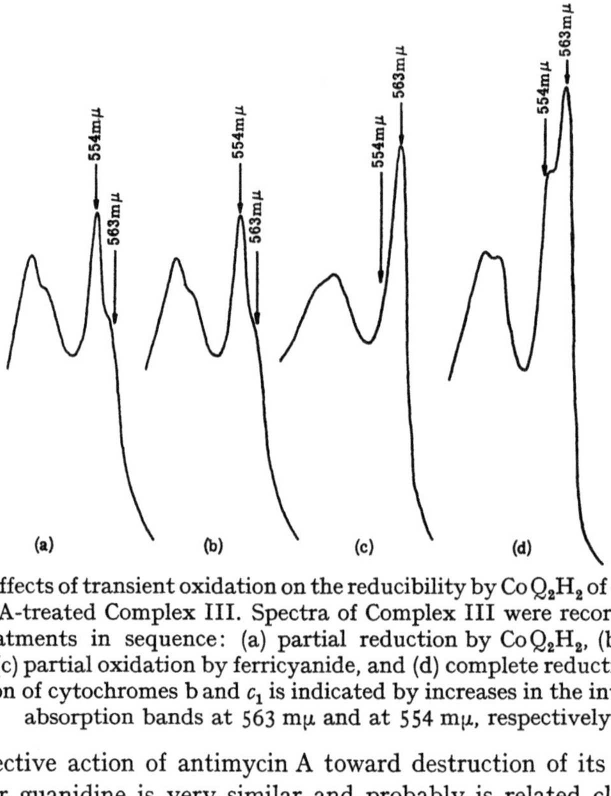

Fig. 6 a—d. Effects of transient oxidation on the reducibility by Co Q_2H_2 of cytochrome *b* in antimycin A-treated Complex III. Spectra of Complex III were recorded after the following treatments in sequence: (a) partial reduction by Co Q_2H_2, (b) addition of antimycin A, (c) partial oxidation by ferricyanide, and (d) complete reduction by dithionite. Reduction of cytochromes b and c_1 is indicated by increases in the intensity of the absorption bands at 563 mμ and at 554 mμ, respectively

The protective action of antimycin A toward destruction of its binding site by trypsin or guanidine is very similar and probably is related closely to the protective action of antimycin A toward cleavage of the complex. In either case it is not clear whether antimycin A exerts its protective effect directly on the chemical structure of the antimycin A-sensitive site or whether it promotes a conformation change in the entire complex that limits the accessibility of the antimycin A-sensitive site to destructive reagents.

Acknowledgements. The author appreciates the encouragement and advice of Professor D. E. GREEN during the research the results of which are reported in this article. Thanks are due also to Dr. H. BAUM for his constructive criticism of the manuscript.

See Addendum

References

ACKERMANN, W. W.: The relation of Krebs cycle to virus propagation. J. Biol. Chem. **189**, 421 (1951).

AHMAD, K., F. M. BUMPUS, B. R. DUNSHEE, and F. M. STRONG: Antimycin antibiotics. Federation Proc. **8**, 178 (1949).

AHMAD, K., H. G. SCHNEIDER, and F. M. STRONG: Studies on the biological action of antimycin A. Arch. Biochem. **28**, 281 (1950).

ANDERSON, J. A., F. KANG SUN, J. K. MCDONALD, and V. H. CHELDELIN: Oxidase activity and lipid composition of respiratory particles from *Claviceps purpura* (Ergot fungus). Arch. Biochem. Biophys. **107**, 37 (1964).

ARNON, D. I., H. Y. TSUJIMOTO, and B. H. MCSWAIN: Role of ferredoxin in photosynthetic production of oxygen and phosphorylation by chloroplasts. Proc. Natl. Acad. Sci. U.S. **51**, 1274 (1964).

ASH, O. K., W. S. ZAUGG, and L. P. VERNON: Photoreduction of methyl red and tetrazolium blue by spinach chloroplasts and chromatophores of *Rhodospirillum rubrum*. Acta Chem. Scand. **15**, 1629 (1961).

Ayerst Research Laboratories, New York, N.Y.: Toxicology study of antimycin. Unpublished Report, April 1965.

BALTSCHEFFSKY, H.: Inhibitor studies on light-induced phosphorylation in isolated spinach chloroplasts. Acta Chem. Scand. **14**, 264 (1960).

BALTSCHEFFSKY, H., and M. BALTSCHEFFSKY: On light-induced phosphorylation in *Rhodospirillum rubrum*. Acta Chem. Scand. **12**, 1333 (1958).

BAUM, H., and J. S. RIESKE: Involvement of water in electron transport in complexes III and IV if the mitochondrial electron transport chain. Biochem. Biophys. Research Commun. **24**, 1 (1966).

BECK, S. D.: Toxicology of antimycin A. J. Econ. Entomol. **43**, 105 (1950).

BROWN, C. B., J. R. RUSSEL, and J. L. HOWLAND: Antimycin-insensitive respiration in beef-heart mitochondria. Biochim. et Biophys. Acta **110**, 640 (1965).

BUETOW, D. E., and P. J. BUCHANAN: Oxidative phosphorylation in mitochondria isolated from *Euglena gracilis*. Biochim. et Biophys. Acta **96**, No. 1, 9 (1965).

BURRIN, D. H., and R. B. BEECHEY: The spectrophotometric dissection of the electron transfer system of mitochondria isolated from the hepatopancreas of *Carcinus maenas*. Comp. Biochem. Physiol. **12**, 245 (1964).

CHANCE, B.: The kinetics and inhibition of cytochrome components of the succinic oxidase system. III. Cytochrome *b*. J. Biol. Chem. **233**, 1223 (1958).

CHANCE, B.: Energy transfer and conservation in the respiratory chain. In: Haematin enzymes (ed. J. E. FALK, R. LEMBERG and R. K. MORTON), p. 597. Pergamon Press 1961.

CHANCE, B., and B. SCHOENER: High and low-energy states of cytochromes. III. In reactions with cations. J. Biol. Chem. **241**, 4577 (1966).

CHANCE, B., and G. R. WILLIAMS: Respiratory enzymes in oxidative phosphorylation. IV. The respiratory chain. J. Biol. Chem. **217**, 429 (1955).

CHANCE, B., and G. R. WILLIAMS: The respiratory chain and oxidative phosphorylation. In: Advances in enzymology (F. F. NORD, ed.), p. 65—137. New York: Interscience Publ., Inc. 1956.

CLARK, H. W., H. A. NEUFELD, C. WIDMER, and E. STOTZ: Purification of a factor linking succinic dehydrogenase with cytochrome *c*. J. Biol. Chem. **210**, 851 (1954).

DAVENPORT, H. E.: Cytochrome components in chloroplasts. Nature **170**, 1112 (1952).

DAVENPORT, H. E., and R. HILL: Preparation and some properties of cytochrome *f*. Proc. Roy. Soc. (London) B **39**, 327 (1952).

DE BERNARD, B., M. RABINOWITZ, and R. ESTABROOK: Preparation and enzymic properties of a succinate-reduced DPNH-cytochrome *c* reductase extract in particulate form from a hypomitochondrial respiratory fraction (ETP). Boll. soc. ital. biol. sper. **32**, 1096 (1956).

DEUL, D., E. C. SLATER, and L. VELDSTRA: The possible role of α-tocopherol in the respiratory chain II. Reactivation by α-tocopherol. Biochim. et Biophys. Acta **27**, 133 (1958).

DICKIE, J. P., M. E. LOOMANS, T. M. FARLEY, and F. M. STRONG: The chemistry of antimycin A. XI. N-substituted 3-formamidosalicylic amides. J. Med. Chem. **6** (4), 424 (1963).

DOMINQUEZ, A. M., and F. E. SHIDEMAN: Effect of malonate and antimycin A on renal tubular transport of p amino-hippurate. Proc. Soc. Exptl. Med. **90**, 329 (1955).

DUFFY, L. M., and J. D. EBERT: Metabolic characteristics of the heart-forming areas of the early chick embryo. J. Embryol. Exptl. Morphol. **5**, 324 (1957).

ESTABROOK, R. W.: Cytochromes of disrupted mitochondria. Federation Proc. **14**, 45 (1955).

ESTABROOK, R. W.: Kinetic properties of DPNH-cytochrome *c* reductase from heart muscle. J. Biol. Chem. **227**, 1093 (1957).

ESTABROOK, R. W.: Antimycin A inhibition of biological oxidations. I. Stoichiometry and pH effects. Biochim et Biophys. Acta **60**, 236 (1962a).

ESTABROOK, R. W.: Antimycin A inhibition of biological oxidations. II. Electronic analog computer studies. Biochim. et Biophys. Acta **60**, 249 (1962b).

FARLEY, T. M., F. M. STRONG, and T. J. BYDALEK: Chemistry of antimycin A. XII. Dissociation constants and iron (III) chelates of antimycin A_3 and some analogs. J. Am. Chem. Soc. **87**, 3501 (1965).

FEWSON, C. A., C. C. BLACK, and M. GIBBS: Photochemical production of TPNH and ATP by fragmented spinach chloroplasts. Plant Physiol. **38** (6), 680 (1963).

FOWLER, L. R., and S. H. RICHARDSON: Studies on the electron transfer system. L. On the mechanism of reconstitution of the mitochondrial electron transfer system. J. Biol. Chem. **238**, 456 (1963).

FOWLER, L. R., S. H. RICHARDSON, and Y. HATEFI: A rapid method for the preparation of highly purified cytochrome oxidase. Biochim. et Biophys. Acta **64**, 170 (1962).

GELLER, D. M., and J. D. GREGORY: Light-induced oxidation-reduction changes in *Rhodospirillum rubrum* extracts. Federation Proc. **15**, 260 (1956).

GELLER, D. M., and F. LIPMANN: Photophosphorylation in extracts of *Rhodospirillum rubrum*. J. Biol. Chem. **235**, 2478 (1960).

GREEN, D. E., and R. K. BURKHARD: Studies on the electron transport system. XXXII. Succinic-cytochrome *c* reductase. Arch. Biochem. Biophys. **92**, 312 (1961).

GREEN, D. E., B. MACKLER, R. REPASKE, and H. R. MAHLER: Oxidase of DPNH. Biochim. et Biophys. Acta **15**, 435 (1954).

GREEN, D. E., S. MII, P. M. KOHOUT, and H. TISDALE: The terminal electron transport system. I. Succinic dehydrogenase. J. Biol. Chem. **217**, 551 (1955).

GREEN, D. E., and D. C. WHARTON: Stoichiometry of the fixed oxidation-reduction components of the electron transfer chain of beef heart mitochondria. Biochem. Z. **338**, 335 (1963).

GRIFFITHS, D. E., and D. C. WHARTON: Studies of the electron transport system. XXXV. Purification and properties of cytochrome oxidase. J. Biol. Chem. **236**, 1850 (1961).

HACKETT, D. P.: Pathways of oxidation in cell-free potato fractions. Plant Physiol. **31**, 111 (1956).

HACKETT, D. P.: Pathways of oxidation in cell-free potato fractions. II. Properties of the soluble pyridine nucleotide oxidase system. Plant Physiol. **33**, 8 (1958).

HACKETT, D. P.: Respiratory mechanisms in *Aroid spadix*. J. Exptl. Botany **8**, 157 (1957).

HALL, D. O., and J. W. GREENAWALT: Oxidative phosphorylation by isolated mitochondria of *Neurospora Crassa*. Biochem. Biophys. Research Commun. **17**, 565 (1964).

HARADA, Y., K. KUMABE, T. KAGAWA, and T. SATO: Antifungal activity of antipiricullin for several growing stages of *Piricularia oryzae*. Nippon Shokubutsu Byori Gakkaiho **24**, 247 (1959).

HARADA, Y., and S. TANAKA: Studies on carzinocidin, antitumor substance produced by streptomyces Sp. III. On the taxonomic studies of the strain No. 48-B-3 identified as S. Kitazawaensis Nov. Sp. J. Antibiotics (Japan), Ser. A **14**, 113 (1956).

HARRIES, F. H.: Effects of some antibiotics and other compounds on fertility and mortality of orchard mites. J. Econ. Entomol. **56**, 438 (1963).

HARRIES, F. H., and V. J. MATTSON: Effects of some antibiotics on three aphid species. J. Econ. Entomol. **56** (3), 412 (1963).

HATEFI, Y.: Coenzyme Q oxidase. Biochim. et Biophys. Acta **34**, 183 (1959).

HATEFI, Y.: The pyridine nucleotide-cytochrome *c* reductase. In: The enzymes (ed. P. D. BOYER, H. LARDY and K. MYRBÄCK), vol. 7. New York: Academic Press 1963.

HATEFI, Y., A. G. HAAVIK, and D. E. GRIFFITHS: Studies on the electron transfer system. XLI. Reduced coenzyme Q (QH_2)-cytochrome *c* reductase. J. Biol. Chem. **237**, 1681 (1962b).

HATEFI, Y., A. G. HAAVIK, and P. JURTSHUK: Studies on the electron transport system. XXX. DPNH-cytochrome *c* reductase I. Biochim. et Biophys. Acta **52**, 106 (1961).

HAYASHI, K., and O. OCHI: Accumulation of hypoxanthine in reticulocytes affected by 2,4 DNP and antimycin A. Biochim. et Biophys. Acta **95** (4), 598 (1965).

HILL, R.: The cytochrome *b* component of chloroplasts. Nature **174**, 501 (1954).

HINKSON, J. W.: Nicotinamide adenine dinucleotide photoreduction with *Chromatium* and *Rhodospirillum rubrum* chromatophores. Arch. Biochem. Biophys. **112**, 478 (1965).

HUMPHREYS, T. E., and E. E. CONN: Oxidation of DPNH by lupine mitochondria. Arch. Biochem. Biophys. **60**, 226 (1956).

KEILIN, D., and E. F. HARTREE: Cytochrome and cytochrome oxidase. Proc. Roy. Soc. (London) B **127**, 167 (1939).

KEILIN, D., and E. F. HARTREE: Relation between certain components of the cytochrome system. Nature **176**, 200 (1955).

KIDO, G. S., and E. SPYHALSKI: Antimycin A, an antibiotic with insecticidal and mitocidal properties. Science **112**, 172 (1950).

KOAZE, Y., H. SAKAI, H. YONEHARA, M. ASAKAWA, and T. MISATO: Studies on the activities of antibiotics against plant pathogenic microorganisms. J. Antibiotics (JAPAN), Ser. A **9**, 89 (1956).

KONIGSBERG, I. R.: Clonal and biochemical studies of myogenesis. Carnegie Inst. Wash. Year Book **63**, 516—521.

KOYAMA, T., Y. HARADA, and K. KUMABE: Lowering of the toxicity of antimycin A. Kyowa Fermentation Industry Co. Ltd. Japan 3104 (1963). April 12 Appl. July 13, 1960 (1963).

KURUP, C. K., C. S. VAIDYANATHAN, and T. RAMASARMA: NADH oxidase system of *Agrobacterium Tumefaciens*. Arch. Biochem. Biophys. **113**, 548 (1966).

LEBEN, C., and G. W. KEITT: An antibiotic substance active against certain phytopathogens. Phytopathology **38**, 899 (1948).

LEBEN, C., and G. W. KEITT: Laboratory and greenhouse studies of antimycin preparations as protectant fungicides. Phytopathology **39**, 529 (1949).

LEBEN, C., and G. W. KEITT: Phytotoxicity of antimycin A. Antibiotics & Chemotherapy **6**, 191 (1956).

LEHMAN, I. R., and A. NASON: Role of lipides in electron transport. I. Properties of a DPN-cytochrome *c* reductase from rat skeletal muscle. J. Biol. Chem. **222**, 497 (1956).

LEHNINGER, A. L., and E. P. KENNEDY: Oxidation of fatty acids and tricarboxylic acid cycle intermediates by isolated rat liver mitochondria. J. Biol. Chem. **179**, 957 (1949).

LIGHTBOWN, J. W., and F. L. JACKSON: Inhibition of cytochrome systems of heart muscle and certain bacteria by antagonists of dehydrostreptomycin: 2-alkyl-4-hydroxyquinoline-N-oxides. Biochem. J. **63**, 130 (1956).

Lockwood, J. L., C. Leben, and G. W. Keitt: Production and properties of antimycin A from a new *Streptomyces* isolate. Phytopathology **44**, 438 (1954).

Lloyd, D.: Inhibition of electron transport in *Prototheca zopfii*. Phytochemistry **5**, 527 (1966).

Lundegårdh, H.: Quantitative relations between chlorophyll and cytochromes in chloroplasts. Physiol. Plantarum **15**, 390 (1962a).

Lundegårdh, H.: The respiratory system of wheat roots. Biochim. et Biophys. Acta **57**, 352 (1962b).

Lundegårdh, H.: The cytochromes of chloroplasts. Proc. Natl. Acad. Sci. U.S. **52**, 1587 (1964).

Markert, C. L.: Epigenetic control of specific protein synthesis in differentiating cells. In: Cytodifferentiation and macromolecular synthesis (M. Locke, ed.), p. 65—84. New York: Academic Press 1963.

Marquis, R. E.: Nature of the bactericidal action of antimycin A for *Bacillus megaterium*. J. Bacteriol. **89**, 1453 (1965).

Matsunaka, S.: Comparison of the electron transport systems in rice blast fungus and pathogenic bacterium of rice leaf blight. Koso Kagaku Shimpozium **15**, 229 (1961).

McEwen, B. S., V. G. Allfrey, and A. E. Mirsky: Energy yielding reactions in thymus nuclei. I. Comparison of nuclear and mitochondrial phosphorylation. J. Biol. Chem. **238**, 758 (1963).

McKenzie, J., and J. D. Ebert: Inhibitory action of antimycin A in early chick embryo. J. Embryol. Exptl. Morphol. **8**, 314 (1960).

Morton, E. M., and R. K. Morton: Enzymic and chemical properties of cytoplasmic particles from wheat roots. Biochem. J. **64**, 687 (1956).

Moussatche, H., and A. Prouvost-Danon: Influence of inhibitors of the respiratory chain on the release of histamine. Biochem. Pharmacol. **11**, 603 (1962).

Nakayama, K., F. Okamoto, and Y. Harada: Antimycin A: Isolation from *Streptomyces kitazawaensis* and its activity against rice plant blast fungi. J. Antibiotics (Japan), Ser. A 9, **63** (1956).

Nason, A., and I. R. Lehman: Tocopherol as an activator of cytochrome *c* reductase. Science **122**, 19 (1955).

Nishimura, M.: Studies on bacterial photophosphorylation. I. Kinetics of photophosphorylation in *Rhodospirillum rubrum* chromatophores by flashing light. Biochim. et Biophys. Acta **57**, 88 (1962a).

Nishimura, M.: Studies on bacterial photophosphorylation. II. Effects of reagents and temperature on light-induced and dark phases of photophosphorylation in *Rhodospirillum rubrum* chromatophores. Biochim. et Biophys. Acta **57**, 96 (1962b).

Nishimura, M.: Studies on the electron-transfer systems in photosynthetic bacteria. II. The effect of heptyl hydroxyquinoline-N-oxide and antimycin A on the photosynthetic and respiratory electron transfer system. Biochim. et Biophys. Acta **66**, 17 (1963).

Nozaki, M., K. Tagawa, and D. I. Arnon: Noncyclic photophosphorylation in photosynthetic bacteria. Proc. Natl. Acad. Sci. U.S. **97**, 1334 (1961).

Ohnishi, T., K. Kawaguchi, and B. Hagihara: Preparation and some properties of yeast mitochondria. J. Biol. Chem. **241**, 1797 (1966).

Pappenheimer, Jr., A. M., and E. D. Hendee: Diphtheria Toxin V. A comparison between the diphtherial succinoxidase system and that of beef heart muscle. J. Biol. Chem. **180**, 597 (1949).

Perini, F., J. A. Schiff, and M. D. Kamen: Iron-containing proteins in Euglena. II. Functional localization. Biochim. et Biophys. Acta **88**, 91 (1964).

Potter, V. R., and A. E. Reif: Inhibition of an electron-transport component by antimycin A. J. Biol. Chem. **194**, 287 (1952).

Pumphrey, A. M.: Studies on the electron transfer system. XLV. Some effects of antimycin on cytochrome *b*. J. Biol. Chem. **237**, 2384 (1962).

RAJAGOPALAN, K. V., V. ALEMAN, and P. HANDLER: Electron paramagnetic resonance studies of iron reduction and semi-quinone formation in metalloflavoproteins. Biochem. Biophys. Research Commun. **8**, 220 (1962).

RAJAGOPALAN, K. V., I. FRIDOVICH, and P. HANDLER: Hepatic aldehyde oxidase. J. Biol. Chem. **237**, 922 (1962).

RAMACHANDRAN, S., and D. GOTTLIEB: Mode of action of antibiotics. II. Specificity of action of antimycin A and ascosin. Biochim. et Biophys. Acta **53**, 396 (1961).

REIF, A. E.: Succinoxidase inhibition studies. II. Mechanism of the binding of a naphthoquinone and of antimycin A by serum albumin. Arch. Biochem. Biophys. **47**, 396 (1953).

REIF, A. E., and V. R. POTTER: *In vivo* inhibition of succinoxidase activity in normal and tumor tissues by antimycin A. Cancer Research **13**, 49 (1953a).

REIF, A. E., and V. R. POTTER: Succinoxidase inhibition. I. Pseudoirreversible inhibition by a naphthoquinone and antimycin A. J. Biol. Chem. **205**, 279 (1953b).

REIF, A. E., and V. R. POTTER: Oxidative pathways insensitive to antimycin A. Arch. Biochem. Biophys. **48**, 1 (1954).

REPORTER, M. C.: Interaction of antimycin A in biological system. J. Cell Biol. **27**, 83A (1965).

REPORTER, M. C., and J. D. EBERT: A mitochondrial factor that prevents the effects of antimycin A on myogenesis. Develop. Biol. **12**, 154 (1965).

RIESKE, J. S., R. E. HANSEN, and W. S. ZAUGG: Studies on the electron-transfer system. LVIII. Properties of a new oxidation-reduction component of the respiratory chain as studied by electron paramagnetic resonance spectroscopy. J. Biol. Chem. **239**, 3017 (1964).

RIESKE, J. S., H. BAUM, C. D. STONER, and S. LIPTON: In preparation (a).

RIESKE, J. S., S. LIPTON, H. BAUM, and I. SILMAN: In preparation (b).

RIESKE, J. S., and W. S. ZAUGG: The inhibition by antimycin A of the cleavage of one of the complexes of the respiratory chain. Biochem. Biophys. Research Commun. **8**, 421 (1962).

RIESKE, J. S., W. S. ZAUGG, and R. E. HANSEN: Studies on the electron-transfer system. LIX. Distribution of iron and of the component giving an electron paramagnetic resonance signal at $g = 1.90$ in subfractions of complex III. J. Biol. Chem. **239**, 3023 (1964).

SAKAGAMI, Y., S. TAKEUCHI, H. SAKAI, and M. TAKASHIMA: Antifungal substances No. 720A and No. 720B and the probable identity of No. 720A with antimycin A, virosin, and antipiricullin. J. Antibiotics (Japan), Ser. A **9**, 1 (1956).

SAN PIETRO, A., and H. M. LANG: Photosynthetic pyridine nucleotide reductase I. Partial purification and properties of the enzyme from spinach. J. Biol. Chem. **231**, 211 (1958).

SCHMIDT-KASTNER, G.: Phyllomycin, ein Antibiotikum aus *Actinomyceten*. Liebigs Ann. Chem. **668**, 122 (1963).

SCHNEIDER, W. C., and V. R. POTTER: Intracellular distribution of enzymes IV. The distribution of oxalacetic oxidase activity in rat liver and rat kidney fractions. J. Biol. Chem. **177**, 893 (1949).

SHORE, J. D., and W. W. WAINIO: Personal communication from Dr. WAINIO.

SINGER, T. P., E. B. KEARNEY, and P. BERNATH: Studies on succinc dehydrogenase. II. Isolation and properties of the dehydrogenase from beef heart. J. Biol. Chem. **223**, 599 (1956).

SISLER, E. C., and H. J. EVANS: Electron transport mechanisms in tobacco roots. I. Studies on the cytochrome and related systems. Plant Physiol. **34**, 81 (1959).

SLATER, E. C.: A respiratory catalyst required for the reduction of cytochrome *c* by cytochrome *b*. Biochem. J. **45**, 14 (1949).

SLATER, E. C.: The components of the dihydrocozymase oxidase system. Biochem. J. **46**, 484 (1950).

SLATER, E. C., and J. P. COLPA-BOONSTRA: Cytochrome *b* in the respiratory chain. In: Haematin enzymes (ed. J. E. FALK, R. LEMBERG and R. K. MORTON), p. 575. Pergamon Press 1961.

SMITH, L.: Bacterial cytochromes. Difference spectra. Arch. Biochem. Biophys. **50**, 299 (1954).
SMITH, L., and M. BALTSCHEFFSKY: Respiration and phosphorylation in extracts of *Rhodospirillum rubrum*. Federation Proc. **15**, 357 (1956).
STONER, C., and J. HANSON: Swelling and contraction of corn mitochondria. Plant Physiol. **41**, 255 (1966).
STRECKER, H. J., and G. DIPRISCO: Activation and inactivation of NADH (reduced nicotinamide adenine dinucleotide) oxidation by brain mitochondrial fragments. Acta Chem. Scand. **17**, Suppl. 1, S67—S73 (1963).
SZULMAJSTER, J.: Biochimie de la sporogenese chez *B. subtilis*. Bull. soc. chim. biol. **46**, 443 (1964).
TAGAWA, K., and D. I. ARNON: Ferredoxins as electron carriers in photosynthesis and in the biological production and consumption of hydrogen gas. Nature **195**, 537 (1962).
TAGAWA, K., H. Y. TSUJIMOTO, and D. I. ARNON: Role of chloroplast ferredoxin in the energy conversion process of photosynthesis. Proc. Natl. Acad. Sci. U.S. **49**, 567 (1963a).
TAGAWA, K., H. Y. TSUJIMOTO, and D. I. ARNON: Separation by monochromatic light of photosynthetic phosphorylation from oxygen evolution. Proc. Natl. Acad. Sci. U.S. **50**, 544 (1963b).
TAPPEL, A. L.: Inhibition of electron transport by antimycin A, alkylhydroxy naphthoquinones, and metal coordination compounds. Biochem. Pharmacol. **3**, 289 (1960).
TAKEMORI, S., and T. E. KING: Coenzyme Q: reversal of inhibition of succinate-cytochrome *c* reductase by lipophilic compounds. Science **144**, 852 (1964).
THORN, M. B.: Inhibition by antimycin A of succinic oxidase in heart muscle preparations. Biochem. J. **63**, 420 (1956).
TZAGOLOFF, A., P. C. YANG, D. C. WHARTON, and J. S. RIESKE: Studies on the electrontransfer system. LX. Molecular weights of some components of the electrontransfer chain in beef-heart mitochondria. Biochim. et Biophys. Acta **96**, 1 (1965).
VAN TAMELEN, E. E., J. P. DICKIE, M. E. LOOMANS, R. S. DEWEY, and F. M. STRONG: The chemistry of antimycin A. X. Structure of the antimycins. J. Am. Chem. Soc. **83**, 1639 (1961).
WALKER, C. R., R. E. LENNON, and B. L. BERGER: Investigations in fish control. II. Preliminary observations on toxicity of antimycin A to fish and other aquatic animals. U.S. Fish Wildlife Serv. Circ. No. 186 (1964).
WARBURG, O.: Über Kohlenoxydwirkung ohne Hämoglobin und einige Eigenschaften des Atmungsferments. Naturwissenschaften **15**, 546 (1927).
WIDMER, C., H. W. CLARK, H. A. NEWFELD, and E. STOTZ: Cytochrome components of the soluble SC factor preparation. J. Biol. Chem. **210**, 861 (1954).
Wisconsin Alumni Research Foundation, Madison, Wis. Unpublished report, March 29, 1965a.
Wisconsin Alumni Research Foundation, Madison, Wis.: Antimycin as a fish toxicant. Unpublished resumé, June 10, 1965b.
WITT, H. T., B. RUMBERG, P. SCHMIDT-MENDE, U. SIGGEL, B. SKERRA, J. VATER, and J. WEIKARD: On the analysis of photosynthesis by flashlight techniques. Angew. Chem. internat. ed. **4**, 799 (1965).
ZAUGG, W. S.: Coupled photoreduction of ubiquinone and photooxidation of ferrocytochrome *c* catalyzed by chromatophores of *Rhodospirillum rubrum*. Proc. Nat. Acad. Sci. U.S. **50**, 100 (1963).

Oligomycin Complex, Rutamycin and Aurovertin

Paul D. Shaw

The work described in this chapter resulted largely from the pioneering efforts of LARDY and his coworkers in their search for "toxic" antibiotics which inhibit respiration. The results of such studies have proved that this type of approach could be very fruitful, and much insight has been gained into the mechanism of oxidative phosphorylation and associated phenomena such as mitochondrial swelling and ion transport across membranes. In fact, the use of certain of the antibiotics has provided information which would have been difficult or perhaps impossible to obtain by any other means.

In general, all of the antibiotics have the same action, namely the inhibition of some phase of energy transformation associated with the terminal electron transport system; however, they do not act at the same site. Because of the complex nature of the processes occurring in mitochondria and because of the many mechanisms by which the energy derived from respiration is utilized, the precise mechanism of inhibition of the antibiotics is not known.

Oligomycin and Rutamycin

Oligomycin was isolated from cultures of an organism resembling *Streptomyces diastatochromogenes* by SMITH *et al.* (1954). MASAMUNE *et al.* (1958) and MARTY and McCOY (1959) separated the crude materials obtained from culture filtrates and mycelial extracts into three biologically active components which were designated oligomycins A, B, and C. The relative amounts of the three components varied with cultural conditions (LARSON and PETERSON, 1960). These components were very closely related chemically as indicated by their virtually identical ultraviolet spectra and the marked similarity of their infrared spectra (MASAMUNE *et al.*, 1958). A summary of their chemical and physical properties is given in Table 1.

An absorption maximum at 225 mμ for all three oligomycins indicates the presence of unsaturation, and the presence of bands at 1700 cm^{-1} in the infrared spectrum is indicative of a carbonyl group. Maxima at 3462 cm^{-1} show hydroxyl groups. The presence of weak hydroxyl absorption in the oligomycin diacetates suggests that one of the hydroxyl groups may be tertiary. The solubility properties of all three are similar in that they are generally soluble in organic solvents, except hydrocarbons, and are insoluble in water.

Rutamycin (A 272) was isolated by THOMPSON *et al.* (1961) from a strain of *Streptomyces rutgersensis* (NRRL B-1256). As can be seen in Table 1, rutamycin is very similar to the oligomycin complex in its physical and chemical properties.

In addition, ultraviolet and infrared spectra were very similar to the oligomycin spectra as were the solubility properties. Rutamycin could, however, be separated from oligomycin A, B, and C by paper chromatography.

The biological properties of the three oligomycins and rutamycin have many similarities. Neither the oligomycins (SMITH *et al.*, 1954; MARTY and McCOY, 1959) at 80 μg/ml nor rutamycin (THOMPSON *et al.*, 1961) at 100 μg/ml show any activity against Gram-positive bacteria, Gram-negative bacteria, or yeasts. All four antibiotics inhibit the growth of several fungi. However, the antifungal spectra of the four antibiotics are not identical. Table 2 gives the minimal inhibitory concentration of the antibiotics for several species of fungi.

Table 1. *Chemical and physical properties of the oligomycin complex and rutamycin*

	A[1]	B[1]	C[1]	Rutamycin[2]
Empirical formula	$C_{24}H_{70}O_6$	$C_{22}H_{36}O_6$	$C_{28}H_{46}O_6$	$C_{25}H_{42}O_6$
Molecular weight	424.56	396.51	478.64	438.59
Melting point	140—141 C	160—161 C	198—200 C	127—128 C
$[\alpha]^{23}$ (Dioxane)	—54.5	—46.4	—80.7	—40.5
Active hydrogen	4—5	4	—	6
C-Methyl	5	5	6	4
Double bonds	1.92—2.2	—	—	—

[1] From MASAMUNE *et al.* (1958).
[2] From TOMPSON *et al.* (1961).

Table 2. *Antifungal spectrum of the oligomycin complex and rutamycin*

Organism	Minimal inhibitory concentration (μg/ml)			
	A[1]	B[1]	C[1]	Rutamycin[2]
Alternaria solani	0.5	0.5	<1	3.13
Aspergillus niger	1	5	5	3.13
Blastomyces dermatitidis	0.01	0.1	0.1	—
Fusarium oxysporium	5	5	>50	6.25
Glomerella cingulata	0.1	0.5	0.5	1.56
Helminthosporium sativum	0.5	1	1	1.56
Verticillium albo-atrum	0.5	1	1	0.78
LD_{50} (mg/kg mouse, intraperitoneally)	1.5	2.9	8.3	18—74

[1] From MARTY and McCOY (1959).
[2] From THOMPSON *et al.* (1961).

Effects on Respiration

SMITH *et al.* (1954) reported that oligomycin inhibited only aerobic organisms. This prompted LARDY *et al.* (1958) to include the oligomycin complex in the large group of "toxic" antibiotics which were tested as potential inhibitors of mitochondrial respiration. In these studies, oligomycin A inhibited the oxidation of a variety of substrates by intact mitochondria. Subsequently LARDY *et al.* (1965) investigated the relative effectiveness of the three oligomycins and rutamycin as inhibitors of respiration. As can be seen from Table 3, the antibiotics vary in their affectiveness depending on the substrate used; the oxidation of succinate was affected least and β-hydroxybutyrate oxidation appeared to be most sensitive. LARDY *et al.* (1964) explained the relatively greater sensitivity of the NAD linked substrates by the fact that the oxidation of NADH is more tightly coupled with phosphorylation. There were also differences in the activities of the antibiotics among themselves. Oligomycin A was in general the most effective and oligomycin C the least effective. It is of interest that this same order (A > B > C) was reported by MARTY and McCOY (1959) for the effectiveness of the oligomycins in the inhibition of the growth of certain fungi.

Table 3. *Inhibition of mitochondrial oxidations by oligomycins and rutamycin*[1]

Substrate	Qo_2 (N)				
	Control	A	B	C	Rutamycin
L-Glutamate	330	21	80	130	40
α-Ketoglutarate	306	—	48	55	55
Succinate	410	150	130	150	125
DL-β-Hydroxybutyrate	260	15	20	50	60

Antibiotic concentrations were 0.67 μg/ml.
[1] From LARDY *et al.* (1965).

The inhibition of the oxidation of DPN linked substrates was not due to an inhibition of the dehydrogenases themselves but rather to the reoxidation of the reduced pyridine nucleotide (LARDY and McMURRAY, 1959). An important observation was that oligomycin inhibition was completely reversed by 2,4-dinitrophenol (DNP), an uncoupler of oxidative phosphorylation. This suggested that the antibiotic inhibited respiration by its action on some phase of energy transfer associated with the terminal electron transport system rather than the electron transfer itself. Since the final step in the energy transfer sequence is the incorporation of inorganic phosphate into ATP, and since DNP must uncouple at a site prior to the oligomycin sensitive site, it was concluded (LARDY and McMURRAY, 1959; HUIJING and SLATER, 1961) that DNP must act at a step before the introduction of inorganic phosphate into ATP. Oligomycin had no effect on anaerobic glycolysis (LARDY *et al.*, 1958).

In contrast to the above results with intact mitochondria oligomycin A was almost completely without effect on respiration in sub-mitochondrial particles obtained by sonic oscillation of rat liver mitochondria (LARDY *et al.*, 1958) or in digitonin treated mitochondria (WADKINS and LEHNINGER, 1963a, 1963b). β-Hydroxybutyrate and succinate were used as substrates in these latter experiments.

Levels of oligomycin A which gave maximum inhibition of respiration in intact rat liver mitochondria also, as would be expected, eliminated phosphorylation associated with the electron transport system (LARDY *et al.*, 1958). However, when oligomycin was used in levels which gave less than maximum inhibition of oxygen uptake, the synthesis of ATP and oxygen uptake were inhibited equally so that normal P/O ratios were obtained (LARDY *et al.*, 1964). The formation of GTP is unaffected by oligomycin in intact rat liver mitochondria (HELDT *et al.*, 1964), and the antibiotic does not inhibit the substrate phosphorylation associated with the oxidation of α-ketoglutarate (LARDY *et al.*, 1964; DANIELSON and ERNSTER, 1963b). Although the antibiotic had little effect on respiration in sub-mitochondrial particles, phosphorylation was completely inhibited (LARDY *et al.*, 1958; WADKINS and LEHNINGER, 1963a, 1963b). Light induced phosphorylation by extracts of *Rhodospirillum rubrum* is also inhibited by oligomycin (BALTSCHEFFSKY and BALTSCHEFFSKY, 1960).

The effects of oligomycin on respiration and associated phosphorylation were confirmed by HUIJING and SLATER (1961) and WADKINS and LEHNINGER (1963b). Phosphorylation coupled with the oxidation of ascorbate by cytochrome c in swollen rat heart sarcosomes is completely inhibited whereas oxygen uptake was not affected (HUIJING and SLATER, 1961). In addition, oligomycin had no effect on oxygen uptake in the absence of ADP in rat liver with either glutamate or succinate as the substrate or in rat heart sarcosomes in the absence of inorganic phosphate. Oxygen uptake by non-phosphorylating KEILEN and HARTREE heart-muscle preparations was not inhibited by 30 μg/ml of oligomycin. These results confirmed that oligomycin inhibition was associated with an energy coupled respiration rather than the electron transport system itself.

In the absence of inorganic phosphate, respiration by rat liver mitochondria is stimulated by arsenate, and this stimulation is inhibited by oligomycin (ESTABROOK, 1961; BRUNI *et al.*, 1964; HUIJING and SLATER, 1961). Even in the presence of inorganic phosphate, arsenate, in contrast to DNP, was unable to relieve oligomycin inhibition (HUIJING and SLATER, 1961). It was concluded that oligomycin, arsenate and DNP exert their inhibitory effects at different sites. The DNP presumably acts between the electron transport chain and the site of oligomycin inhibition, and the arsenate acts at the step which incorporates inorganic phosphate into the energy transfer sequence (ESTABROOK, 1961).

Inhibition of respiration in rat liver mitochondria by oligomycin is reversed by many agents which stimulate ATPase activity and uncouple oxidative phosphorylation. In addition to DNP, the following compounds were investigated by LARDY *et al.* (1964) using a variety of substrates[1]: O-methyl triac, usnic acid, dicoumarol, TCAP, valinomycin, SQ 15859, DNT, calcium chloride, selenite, and tellurite. Valinomycin, SQ 15859, DNT, and dicoumarol completely reversed oligomycin inhibition; DNP and TCAP were slightly less effective. Usnic acid and tellurite, which also partially inhibit respiration, restored that fraction of the activity observed with these compounds alone. O-Methyl triac, calcium and selenite were without effect on oligomycin inhibited respiration.

Oligomycin inhibition of respiration is not associated exclusively with rat liver mitochondria. LARDY *et al.* (1964) reported similar results with mitochondria from rat kidney, guinea pig liver and kidney, and bovine spermatazoa. Also, MINAKAMI and YOSHIKAWA (1963) found that as little as 0.25 μg/ml of rutamycin would inhibit respiration in ascites hepatoma cells, and this inhibition was reversed by DNP.

---

[1] The following abbreviations are used: O-methyl triac, O-methyl triiodothyroacetate; TCAP, 1,1,3-tricyano-2-amino-1-propene; DNT, 2,6-dinitrothymol. SQ15859 is an antibiotic.

The effect of oligomycin on whole tissues is in general different from that on intact mitochondria. DALLNER and ERNSTER (1962) reported that the antibiotic inhibited respiration only 70% in Ehrlich ascites tumor cells. This inhibition was reversed by DNP and also by vitamin K_3 if a substrate was present. Presumably K_3 provides a bypass from NAD to cytochrome b by way of a non-specific diaphorase. In rat kidney slices (WU, 1964), in frog muscle, and in rat diaphragm, brain and kidney (TOBIN and SLATER, 1965), oligomycin inhibited respiration only 30%. Lactate production was stimulated. The antibiotic completely inhibited the potassium stimulated respiration in rat brain. It was suggested that this inhibition is due to an inhibition of the utilization of the ADP which is formed by the sodium plus potassium induced ATPase in brain tissue. This same conclusion was reached by MINAKAMI *et al.* (1963) although previous results indicated that the sodium plus potassium activated ATPase in brain microsomes was not very sensitive to oligomycin. If these conclusions are valid, however, the primary site of action of oligomycin is on the respiratory chain, and there is no reason to introduce a second site on the mitochondrial membrane as suggested by WHITTAM *et al.* (1964) (c.f. the section in this chapter on ion transport). Furthermore, TOBIN and SLATER (1965) suggested that in whole tissues, the mitochondria are largely uncoupled; most of the energy is drained off by reactions which can utilize a high energy intermediate formed prior to ATP. Lactate production is stimulated because oligomycin prevents the accumulation of adenine nucleotides in the mitochondria so that they are available in the cytoplasm for glycolysis.

In contrast to the above results, CURRIE and GREGG (1965) found that respiration in the following tissues was nearly completely inhibited by low concentrations of oligomycin: Chinese Hamster Ovary, HeLa cells, L-51788, C13, and L forms. The response to the antibiotic was linear with no lag period as in intact mitochondria, and the inhibition was reversed by DNP.

In experiments with isolated heart cells, HARARY and SLATER (1965) found that beating was inhibited by DNP but not by oligomycin or iodoacetate. A combination of the latter two compounds, however, did inhibit beating. They concluded that in the presence of oligomycin, ATP formed by glycolysis was utilized for the beating and with iodoacetate, ATP from oxidative phosphorylation was used. When both inhibitors were present, no ATP was available. This indicated that the beating of the cells required ATP and that other high energy intermediates of oxidative phosphorylation could not be used.

The effect of oligomycin, arsenate and other uncouplers on mitochondrial energy transformations is summarized in Fig. 1. C is an electron carrier, either oxidized or reduced, and I and X are energy carriers. If oligomycin binds $I{\sim}X$ so that the transfer of inorganic phosphate cannot take place and no free I is available for the first reaction in the sequence, electron transport will be stopped. Uncoupling agents such as DNP, which cause the decomposition of a prior intermediate ($C{\sim}I$), would relieve the respiratory inhibition by regenerating I. It is possible that other uncouplers which are less effective in relieving oligomycin inhibition, act at a different site or are only less efficient than DNT, DNP, etc. in causing the decomposition of $C{\sim}I$. Arsenate for example may uncouple the third reaction, and because of the instability of the arsenic-containing intermediate, this ion acts as an uncoupler by cleaving the $I{\sim}X$ bond. In the presence of oligomycin, I~X is made unavailable to the arsenate, thereby preventing the cleavage from taking place. Inhibition of electron transport would, therefore, not be relieved by arsenate.

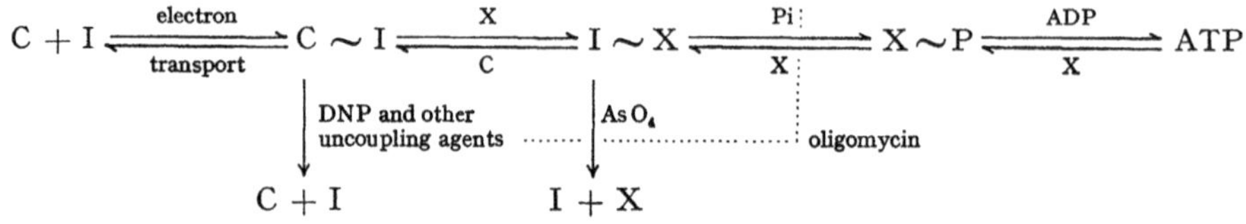

Fig. 1. Site of oligomycin inhibition in proposed scheme for mitochondrial energy transformations. From Ernster and Lee (1964)

Effects on ATPase Activity

In view of the results with agents which induce ATPase activity and which may also uncouple oxidative phosphorylation, the effect of the oligomycin complex on the mitochondrial ATPase induced by various of these compounds was investigated (Lardy *et al.*, 1958; Lardy and McMurray, 1959; Lardy *et al.*, 1964; Azzone and Ernster, 1961; Bruni *et al.*, 1965; Michel *et al.*, 1964). Oligomycin A caused an 80 to 100% inhibition of the induced ATPase activity with all of the compounds tested. These included compounds related to DNP, compounds related to the thyroid hormones, antibiotics, and the inorganic ions arsenate, selenite, and tellurite. A comparison of the effectiveness of the oligomycins and rutamycin on ATPase activity is given in Table 4.

Table 4. *Inhibition of mitochondrial ATPase by oligomycins and rutamycin*[1]

Inducer	Pi liberated per 0.2 mg N in control (μmoles)	Inhibition of Pi liberation (%)			
		A	B	C	Rutamycin
DNP (5×10^{-5} M)	4.42	90	87	74	87
DNT (1×10^{-6} M)	4.24	94	90	67	86
O-Methyl triac (4×10^{-5} M)	2.59	94	90	74	88
Aging 20 minutes at 37 C	0.58	82	78	62	73
Aging 20 minutes at 37 C + Mg^{++} (1.5×10^{-3} M)	1.52	86	85	70	81
Valinomycin	4.30			89	97
Gramicidin	4.85			93	98

Antibiotic concentrations were 1 μg/ml.

[1] From Lardy *et al.* (1965).

Oligomycin A and B and rutamycin have about the same activity with all the inducers; oligomycin C, however, shows somewhat less activity than the other three. The effects of oligomycin C on ATPase activity induced by valinomycin, gramicidin and aging was investigated to determine if that antibiotic was affecting only one phase of the ATPase activity[1]. The data in Table 4 show that oligomycin C is only quantitatively less effective than A, B, or rutamycin and does not

[1] Two catagories of mitochondrial ATPase activity have been postulated by Lardy *et al.* (1964) based on inhibition studies with the antibiotic, aurovertin.

act in the manner of aurovertin (c.f. the subsequent section of this chapter dealing with the mechanism of action of that antibiotic).

Oligomycin A also inhibits induced ATPase activity in sub-mitochondrial particles (LARDY *et al.*, 1958). In this case, however, the DNP induced ATPase activity is inhibited only about 50%, but magnesium induced activity is nearly completely inhibited. KAGAWA and RACKER (1965) reported that an oligomycin insensitive, soluble ATPase became oligomycin sensitive when added to sub-mitochondrial particles which had been treated with trypsin and urea. A colorless lipoprotein (colorless Fo) was obtained which could bind oligomycin and which conferred oligomycin sensitivity to the treated sub-mitochondrial particles. Treatment of colorless Fo with a phospholipase destroyed its ability to confer oligomycin sensitivity.

It is possible to explain the effect of oligomycin on mitochondrial ATPase activity by the same mechanism which has been postulated for its inhibition of respiration (Fig. 1). If the antibiotic binds I∼X, the transfer of phosphate from ATP to X, a reversal of the last step in the sequence, would be prevented; no free X would be available from the reversal of the second reaction in the sequence to act as an acceptor.

The action of oligomycin on the potassium and sodium ion activated, magnesium dependent ATPase of brain microsomes has been investigated by JÄRNEFELT (1962) who observed inhibition at antibiotic levels of 10 μg/ml but not at 1 μg/ml. JÖBSIS and VREMAN (1963) partially purified their ATPase from rabbit brain, and they found that the oligomycin concentration giving half-maximum inhibition was 0.9 μg/ml (12 μg/ml protein) for the crude preparation and 0.6 μg per ml (7 μg/ml protein) in the purified preparation. VAN GRONIGEN and SLATER (1963) compared the effect of oligomycin on the ATPase activities of brain mitochondria and microsomes. The mitochondrial ATPase activity was inhibited by the antibiotic. The addition of sodium and potassium slightly increased the ATPase activity, but this slight activation was apparently not affected by oligomycin. The microsomal ATPase was stimulated by sodium and potassium, and the activity was partially inhibited by oligomycin. Treatment of the microsomes and mitochondria with EDTA and deoxycholate stimulated ATPase activity in both cases. In mitochondria, the increased activity was not activated by sodium and potassium and was inhibited by oligomycin. In the microsomes the activity was activated by sodium and potassium and was partially inhibited by oligomycin. It was found that half maximal inhibition of the sodium and potassium activated ATPase required 100 times as much oligomycin as the mitochondrial ATPase. These results indicated that the mitochondrial and microsomal sodium plus potassium activated ATPase activities functioned by different mechanisms. GLYNN (1962) reported that the sodium and potassium stimulated, magnesium activated ATPase from the electric organ of the electric eel was inhibited 75% by oligomycin at a concentration of 1 μg/ml.

Effects on Exchange Reactions

Another phenomenon associated with oxidative phosphorylation is the exchange reaction involving ADP, ATP, inorganic phosphate and water. LARDY *et al.* (1958), LARDY and McMURRAY (1959) and COOPER and KULKA (1961), reported that the exchange of inorganic phosphate (^{32}P) into ATP by intact mitochondria was inhibited 94% by 0.5 μg/ml oligomycin. The loss of ^{18}O from ^{18}O-labeled phosphate was also inhibited by oligomycin. A comparison of the effectiveness of the oligomycins and rutamycin on inhibition of the ATP-Pi exchange in intact rat liver mitochondria is given in Table 5. The antibiotics are about equally inhibitory of the exchange of inorganic ^{32}P into ATP although oligomycin C and rutamycin are somewhat more effective at low concentrations.

Table 5. *Inhibition of ATP-Pi exchange reaction by oligomycins and rutamycin*[1]

Amount of Antibiotic	μmoles Pi → ATP				
		A	B	C	Rutamycin
None	2.23				
0.03 μg		2.16	1.97	1.71	1.67
0.3 μg		0.063	0.22	0.17	0.086
3 μg		0.078	0.055	0.056	0.062

Final volumes were 1 ml.
[1] From LARDY *et al.* (1965).

Initial reports (HUIJING and SLATER, 1961) indicated that the ADP-ATP exchange reaction was not inhibited by oligomycin. These results were not confirmed in subsequent work by COOPER and KULKA (1961) and KULKA and COOPER (1962) who found that the portion of the ADP-ATP exchange reaction sensitive to pentachlorophenol (presumably that activity not due to adenylate kinase) and the ATP-Pi exchange reaction were inhibited to an equal extent by oligomycin in digitonin treated particles. The antibiotic caused 50% inhibition at 0.11 to 0.14 μg per 0.3 mg particle protein per ml. WADKINS (1962) on the other hand found that oligomycin at 1 μg/ml inhibited the ADP-ATP exchange almost completely in fresh mitochondria and about 30% in mitochondria aged for 8 hr at 2 C. In mitochondria aged for 20 hr at 2 C or in phosphorylating sub-mitochondrial particles prepared by digitonin treatment, the exchange was inhibited only slightly or not at all. DNP was somewhat more inhibitory than oligomycin in aged mitochondria and in sub-mitochondrial particles. Arsenate was able to reverse oligomycin inhibition in intact mitochondria.

WADKINS and LEHNINGER (1963a, 1963b) and LEHNINGER (1963) found that the ADP-ATP exchange was inhibited 93% at 1 μg oligomycin per ml in the absence of magnesium. This reaction was also sensitive to DNP. These workers examined the ADP-ATP exchange reaction in nuclei, intact mitochondria, microsomes and a soluble fraction. Only the mitochondrial reaction was appreciably inhibited by either oligomycin (98%) or DNP (89%) in the absence of magnesium. With magnesium present, similar results were obtained except inhibition was reduced to 48% with oligomycin and 46% with DNP. It was also found that oligomycin at 1.0 μg/ml, while inhibiting the exchange reaction 95% in intact mitochondria, inhibited only 10% in digitonin treated particles. In fact, the inhibition of the exchange reaction by DNP in the digitonin particles is reversed by oligomycin.

A comparison of the effects of oligomycin on the oxygen uptake, P/O, ATP-ADP exchange reaction, ATPase and acceptor control was made by WADKINS and LEHNINGER (1963a, 1963b) and LEHNINGER (1963). Their results are given in Table 6. In the tightly coupled mitochondria, the effects of oligomycin on the various activities are similar. In the digitonin fragments, ATPase is completely inhibited and phosphorylation is uncoupled. Oxygen uptake is partially inhibited and the ADP-ATP exchange reaction is unaffected. Similar results were obtained with sonicated mitochondria except that oxygen uptake was completely unaffected. These results indicated that oligomycin sensitivity is best correlated with respiration and that some functional relationship exists between the exchange reaction and the tightness of respiratory control.

Table 6. *Effect of oligomycin on various functions of mitochondria and sub-mitochondrial particles*[1]

	Intact mitochondria		Digitonin fragments		Sonic fragments	
	—	+	—	+	—	+
O_2 Uptake	44	5	76	42	83	83
P:O	3.0	0.0	2.1	0.2	0.93	0.09
Respiratory control ratio	18	1.1	1.8	1.0	1.0	1.0
ATP-ADP exchange	69.0	3.1	72	72	28.3	28.0
ATPase	59	4.0	79	2.0	41	1.0

— and + indicate minus and plus oligomycin.

[1] From WADKINS and LEHNINGER (1963b).

WADKINS and LEHNINGER (1963b) modified the scheme shown in Fig. 1 to account for the differences between intact mitochondria and loosely coupled mitochondria. They suggested that the alterations in mitochondrial function resulting from the disruption of the mitochondria, might be caused by the dissociation of an enzyme complex. These theories are shown in Fig. 2. Oligomycin presumably binds the complexes containing M so that in the tightly coupled

1. Tightly coupled

$$\text{Ared} \xrightleftharpoons{\text{M}\cdot\text{E}} \text{Ared—M}\cdot\text{E} \xrightleftharpoons{-2\,\text{e}} \text{Aox} \sim \text{M}\cdot\text{E} \xrightleftharpoons[\text{Aox}]{\text{Pi}}$$

$$\text{P} \sim \text{M}\cdot\text{E} \rightleftharpoons \text{M}\cdot\text{E} \sim \text{P} \xrightleftharpoons{\text{ADP}} \text{ATP} + \text{M}\cdot\text{E}$$

Exchange reaction

$$\text{ATP} + \text{M}\cdot\text{E} \rightleftharpoons \text{M}\cdot\text{E} \sim \text{P} + \text{ADP}$$

2. Loosely coupled

$$\text{Ared} \xrightleftharpoons{\text{M}} \text{Ared—M} \xrightleftharpoons{-2\,\text{e}} \text{Aox} \sim \text{M} \xrightleftharpoons[\text{Aox}]{\text{Pi}}$$

$$\text{P} \sim \text{M} \xrightleftharpoons[\text{M}]{\text{E}} \text{P} \sim \text{E} \xrightleftharpoons{\text{ADP}} \text{ATP} + \text{E}$$

Exchange reaction

$$\text{ATP} + \text{E} \rightleftharpoons \text{E} \sim \text{P} + \text{ADP}$$

Fig. 2. Energy transformations and exchange reactions in tightly coupled and loosely coupled mitochondria. From WADKINS and LEHNINGER (1963b) mitochondria, the exchange reaction would be inhibited whereas in the loosely coupled system where M is not involved in the complex associated with the exchange, no inhibition would occur. DNP is thought to inhibit at a step before the oligomycin inhibition site.

Effects on Electron Transport Reversal

A postulated energy dependent reversal of the electron transport system was demonstrated by CHANCE (1961a), and oligomycin has proved useful in the study of this process. Oligomycin inhibited the ATP induced reduction of NAD and reduced cytochrome c oxidation by succinate in aerobic and sodium sulfide inhibited pigeon heart mitochondria (CHANCE, 1961b). Subsequently it was shown (DANIELSON and ERNSTER, 1963a; LEE *et al.*, 1964) that this antibiotic inhibited the ATP induced reduction of NADP by NADH in rat liver and beef heart mitochondria under anaerobic conditions. Under aerobic conditions ATP was not required and this reduction was inhibited by DNP but stimulated by oligomycin. This indicated that oligomycin could prevent the utilization of the energy from ATP in the transhydrogenase reaction but not the utilization of energy derived from the oxidation of NADH. These observations have also been made by ERNSTER (1963) who reported that in the presence of succinate and in the absence of a phosphate acceptor, acetoacetate could be reduced to β-hydroxybutyrate in the presence or absence of oligomycin. With a phosphate acceptor present, however, β-hydroxybutyrate was produced only if oligomycin was also present. It was concluded that oligomycin prevents ATP formation, and thereby stops the oxidation of succinate by succinic dehydrogenase. The succinate is available therefore for the reduction of NAD and the NADH in turn can reduce acetoacetate.

LEE and ERNSTER (1965), while working with nonphosphorylating sub-mitochondrial particles, reported similar effects of oligomycin on the transhydrogenase reaction, i.e. the antibiotic stimulated the NADH-NADP transhydrogenase reaction which was driven by aerobically generated high energy intermediates. They made the additional observations that the required concentration of oligomycin was much less (0.2 µg/mg protein) for this reaction and for the ATP supported reduction of NAD than that required to inhibit ATPase. It is of interest that in these sub-mitochondrial particles the ATP supported reduction of NADP was stimulated by low concentrations of oligomycin whereas in intact mitochondria oligomycin inhibited that process. They also demonstrated that the ATP-supported reduction of NAD by ascorbate plus tetramethyl-p-phenylenediamine was stimulated by oligomycin. Another interesting observation was that low concentrations (0.4 µg/mg protein) of oligomycin enhanced inorganic phosphate uptake with NADH or succinate as substrate. Oligomycin did not inhibit respiration under these conditions, but respiration was inhibited in the absence of magnesium, inorganic phosphate, or ADP. Respiration could be restored by the addition of these components or by DNP. These results were interpreted to mean that in the nonphosphorylating particles, some high energy intermediate before ATP (I$\sim$X in Fig. 1) was spontaneously broken down. In the presence of low concentrations of oligomycin this spontaneous decomposition was prevented, but ATP could still be formed. High concentrations of the antibiotic prevented not only the spontaneous decomposition of this high energy intermediate but also prevented the incorporation of inorganic phosphate and subsequent formation of ATP.

The energy dependent formation of glutamate from α-ketoglutarate and ammonia has been the subject of a series of papers from SLATER'S laboratory (TAGER and SLATER, 1963a; TAGER, 1963; TAGER *et al.*, 1963; SLATER and TAGER, 1963; SNOSWELL, 1961; SNOSWELL, 1962; SLATER *et al.*, 1962; TAGER and SLATER, 1963b). The synthesis of glutamate with succinate as the energy source was stimulated by ATP and by oligomycin (mixture of A and B) if a phosphate acceptor was present. Synthesis was inhibited by DNP. When ATP was used as the energy source, the reaction was inhibited by oligomycin. Antimycin on the other hand inhibited glutamate formation with succinate but not with ATP as the energy source. The explanation proposed for these observations is given in Fig. 3. Reaction (1) is stimulated by DNP, (2) is the normal

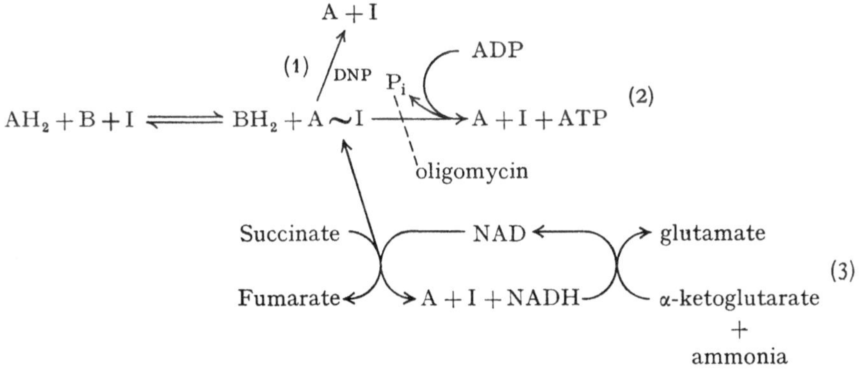

Fig. 3. Energy dependent synthesis of glutamate. From TAGER and SLATER (1963a)

oxidative phosphorylation pathway, and (3) requires α-ketoglutarate and ammonia. Oligomycin presumably stimulates the formation of glutamate by inhibiting (2) and thereby providing more A∼I which is the energy source for NADH formation. DNP inhibits glutamate formation by removing A∼I. Oligomycin inhibits synthesis with ATP as the energy source because the energy from ATP cannot be converted to A∼I, and the antibiotic fails to stimulate in the absence of a phosphate acceptor because under these conditions reaction (2) cannot proceed at the optimal rate. While this scheme describes only a mechanism for glutamate synthesis, it is also applicable to other reactions associated with electron transport reversal. A similar hypothesis was given by DANIELSON and ERNSTER (1963a) to explain the energy dependent reduction of NADP by NADH.

Effects on Ion Transport

An energy requirement for the transport of ions across cell membranes and the membranes of sub-cellular fragments has been well documented. One facet of the studies on the mechanism of action of oligomycin has been the effect of this antibiotic on the transport of ions across mitochondrial membranes. BRIERLY *et al.* (1962) showed that the uptake of inorganic phosphate and magnesium by beef-heart mitochondria was inhibited by DNP but not oligomycin. These experiments were conducted aerobically in the presence of oxidizable substrates and magnesium. Similar results were described by CHAPPELL *et al.* (1962) using rat liver mitochondria; in the presence of a substrate, the addition of manganese or magnesium and inorganic phosphate caused a burst of oxygen uptake with the concomitant uptake of the inorganic ions into the mitochondria and the production of hydrogen ions. This process was inhibited by DNP but not by oligomycin. These results indicate that the source of energy for the transport of magnesium, manganese and phosphate across the mitochondrial membrane is at a step prior to ATP synthesis, since oligomycin would be expected to inhibit a process which derives its energy from ATP. In similar experiments with rat kidney slices (WU, 1964), respiration was inhibited about 30% by DNP, oligomycin and azide. Only DNP inhibited inorganic phosphate uptake. He also suggested that a high energy intermediate located before the oligomycin sensitive site may be involved in phosphate transport. BRUNI *et al.* (1965) reported that intact rat liver mitochondria are capable of binding about four times as much oligomycin (mixture of A and B) as is required for complete inhibition of phosphate uptake. Damaged mitochondria can also bind the antibiotic. They conclude that there must be several oligomycin binding sites, but that the sites associated with oxidative phosphorylation must have a higher affinity for the antibiotic. They point out that small changes in protein concentrations could account for some of the discrepancies reported in the literature for oligomycin inhibition. Another explanation for this variability could be the instability of oligomycin A in aqueous ethanol (LARDY *et al.*, 1965). Oligomycins B and C and rutamycin were stable in aqueous solutions.

VAN ROSSUM (1962) reported that the transport of sodium and potassium through the cell membrane in slices of adult rat liver was inhibited a maximum of 50% by 10 μg/ml oligomycin. The remaining 50% was inhibited by DNP. Respiration was inhibited only 20% by 10 μg/ml of oligomycin, and this inhibition could be relieved by DNP. Respiration was, however, inhibited 90% by cyanide. Subsequently VAN ROSSUM (1964) found that respiration could be inhibited to the same extent as potassium ion uptake at a given oligomycin concentration. It was concluded that the oligomycin resistant uptake of potassium was dependent on the oligomycin resistant respiration.

In foetal rat liver slices, where a major fraction of the energy comes from the substrate phosphorylations which occur during anaerobic glycolysis, oligomycin at 10 μg/ml inhibited 50% of the cyanide resistant accumulation of potassium. At the oligomycin concentrations used, anaerobic glycolysis, as measured by lactic acid production, was not inhibited. The oligomycin insensitive potassium uptake of cyanide treated foetal livers was inhibited by DNP, and this inhibition was relieved by oligomycin. These observations were explained by the stimulatory action of DNP on the ATPase, which breaks down the ATP generated by anaerobic glycolysis. The oligomycin prevents this by inhibiting the ATPase.

Oligomycin had no effect on cation transport through erythrocyte membranes, since these cells presumably have no mitochondria and depend solely on anaerobic glycolysis for their energy. This observation is interesting in light of the report of VAN GRONIGEN and SLATER (1963) that oligomycin fails to inhibit the ATPase activity of erythrocytes except at high concentrations. In contrast to these results, WHITTAM *et al.* (1964) found that sodium and potassium transport in ethrocytes as well as lactate production were inhibited by oligomycin.

Two hypotheses were proposed (VAN ROSSUM, 1964) to explain the inhibition of sodium and potassium transport. The first was that oligomycin inhibited directly an ATPase associated with ion transport. The second hypothesis, which was favored by the author, was that the oligomycin sensitive ion uptake obtained its energy from an intermediate step in the energy transformation sequence (C∼I of Fig. 1), not directly from ATP. In addition to this pathway, a second transport sequence involving ATP as an energy source must also be operative, and this pathway is sensitive to oligomycin. The source of this ATP may be from respiration or from substrate level phosphorylation (VAN ROSSUM, 1964). A similar suggestion was made by JÖBSIS and VREMAN (1963) in their studies on oligomycin inhibition of the sodium and potassium ion stimulated ATPase from rabbit brain.

A possible mechanism for the action of oligomycin on sodium and potassium ion transport and on ATPase activity in rabbit-kidney cortex has been proposed by WHITTAM *et al.* (1964). In this tissue, oligomycin inhibited respiration, potassium uptake and a potassium plus sodium activated ATPase; however, high antibiotic concentrations (10 μg/ml) were required. When kidney slices were incubated with ATP-γ-^{32}P in the presence of both sodium and potassium, a trichloroacetic acid precipitable fraction was obtained which contained ^{32}P. Sodium promoted the formation of this labeled fraction and potassium stimulated the conversion to inorganic phosphate. Oligomycin had no effect on the sodium-activated reaction, but it inhibited the potassium-activated hydrolysis. These results lead to the postulated mechanism for potassium and sodium transport illustrated in the following scheme. The authors suggest that oligomycin has two mechanisms of action, one on the formation of ATP in mitochondria and the other on ATP utilization in membranes. TOBIN and SLATER (1965), however, feel that oligomycin has no effect on membranes.

$$\text{ATP} + \text{protein} \xrightarrow[\text{Na}^+]{\text{Internal}} \text{protein}-\text{PO}_4\text{H}_2 + \text{ADP}$$

$$\text{Protein} - \text{PO}_4\text{H}_2 \xrightarrow[\substack{\text{(inhibited by}\\ \text{oligomycin)}}]{\text{External K}^+} \text{protein} + \text{Pi}$$

$$\text{Sum: ATP} + \text{internal Na}^+ + \text{external K}^+ \rightarrow \text{ADP} + \text{internal K}^+ + \text{external Na}^+ + \text{P}$$

Oligomycin has also proved to be a useful tool in studies on the role of parathyroid hormone (PTH) on phosphate transport by mitochondria. Oligomycin B was used in all of the PTH experiments unless otherwise noted. FANG *et al.* (1963) reported that PTH caused a 20% increase in oxygen uptake in rat liver mitochondria and a decrease in P/O from 3 to 0.7 with glutamate or succinate as the substrate. In the presence of magnesium or manganese, oligomycin did not inhibit the hormone dependent, potassium stimulated respiration in isolated kidney or liver mitochondria (FANG and RASMUSSEN, 1964). When both oligomycin and PTH were added to the mitochondria, oxidation was restored but not phosphorylation. ATP, magnesium and inorganic phosphate were required for the restoration of oxygen uptake. Calcium ions could not replace magnesium. The effect of PTH on oligomycin inhibited mitochondria was prevented by cyanide, azide and antimycin A. DNP, like PTH, increased respiration in the oligomycin inhibited mitochondria. Unlike the hormone, however, it did not require inorganic phosphate.

In contrast to results with mitochondria, PTH did not stimulate respiration in rat renal tubules (ARNAUD and RASMUSSEN, 1964). In fact 7 μg/ml oligomycin inhibited respiration in this tissue. When PTH and oligomycin were used in combination, an increase in oxygen consumption of 33% over the control occurred; however, under these same conditions mitochondrial respiration may be stimulated as much as 500%.

In addition to its effects on respiration, oligomycin inhibits a PTH-dependent ATPase activity (SALLIS and DELUCA, 1964; SALLIS *et al.*, 1965) and a PTH-stimulated phosphate uptake in rat-liver mitochondria (SALLIS *et al.*, 1963a, 1963b). The inhibition of this latter reaction could be reversed by ATP, and in a later paper SALLIS *et al.* (1965) reported that ADP or AMP were also effective. In fact, AMP appeared to be the most effective. Oligomycin inhibition occurred with glutamate or α-ketoglutarate as the substrate but not with β-hydroxybutyrate, succinate, ascorbate or pyruvate plus malate. Oxygen consumption was also only inhibited with α-ketoglutarate or glutamate as substrate. These results were interpreted as follows: ATP, ADP and AMP relieve oligomycin inhibition by serving as phosphate acceptors for the substrate level phosphorylation associated with α-ketoglutarate oxidation. ATP is presumably partially hydrolyzed to ADP and/or AMP by the mitochondrial ATPase so that it can also serve as an acceptor, although not so readily as the mono- and dinucleotides. This role as inorganic phosphate acceptors for the adenine nucleotides was further substantiated by the findings that AMP could accept two equivalents of inorganic phosphate and ADP could accept one equivalent. These results provide an explanation for the lack of inhibition by oligomycin with other substrates since no phosphate acceptor is required for the oxidation of succinate, β-hydroxybutyrate etc. If oligomycin inhibits energy transformation at some step prior to the formation of ATP, a high energy intermediate located prior to the oligomycin sensitive site must be utilized for the PTH stimulated transport of inorganic phosphate. In the presence of the antibiotic, the energy for this process must come from the oxidation of substrate whereas in its absence, it can be derived from ATP.

Effects on Mitochondrial Swelling

The process of mitochondrial swelling is presumably closely associated with electron transport activity and associated energy transformations since inorganic phosphate can initiate the swelling process and ATP can reverse the effect of phosphate. CHAPPELL and GREVILLE (1959a, 1960) reported that oligomycin inhibited phosphate-induced mitochondrial swelling when β-hydroxybutyrate was present but not when it was absent. DNP reversed this inhibition. In aged mitochondria or in the presence of thyroxine as the inducer of swelling, oligomycin had no effect (CHAPPELL and GREVILLE, 1959b). However, neither oligomycin nor DNP inhibited mitochondrial swelling induced by an arginine rich histone fraction from calf thymus (UTSUMI and YAMAMOTO, 1965). Subsequently CHAPPELL and GREVILLE (1960) found that oxygen was not the obligatory terminal electron acceptor for this process but that, in cyanide inhibited mitochondria, ferricyanide could serve equally well as an electron acceptor.

When glutamate was used as substrate, respiration could not be maintained by liver mitochondria in the presence of oligomycin and DNP unless ADP was also present. In addition, DNP was unable to reverse the oligomycin inhibition of phosphate induced swelling unless ADP was present. The ADP was apparently serving as a phosphate acceptor for the obligatory substrate level phosphorylation during the oxidation of glutamate. These data provide further evidence that oligomycin does not inhibit substrate level phosphorylation, and furthermore that it is the electron transfer system not phosphorylation that is important in mitochondrial swelling (CHAPPELL and GREVILLE, 1961).

In another report, NEUBERT and LEHNINGER (1962) found that oligomycin inhibited the ATP (plus magnesium) reversal of glutathione induced mitochondrial swelling. Inhibition was 50% at 5×10^{-8} M and 100% at about 10^{-7} M; however, approximately 10^{-6} M is required for 50% inhibition of thyroxine induced swelling. Oligomycin inhibited contraction of the glutathione swollen mitochondria in a linear fashion dependent on antibiotic concentration. This led these workers to postulate a stoichiometric binding of the antibiotic to some structure in the mitochondria.

The phenomenon of mitochondrial swelling as related to energy transformation has also been studied by CONNELLY and LARDY (1964a, 1964b). These workers confirmed the inhibitory effect of oligomycin on ATP induced contraction of phosphate swollen mitochondria. In addition, they found that magnesium was able to depress the effectiveness of oligomycin. In contrast to the results of CHAPPELL and GREVILLE (1959b), CONNELLY and LARDY (1964b) found that oligomycin at 4 μg per 6 ml (1.54×10^{-6} M) also inhibited ATP reversal of thyroxine induced swelling. They point out that this apparent contradiction might be explained by differences in the medium used for the contraction studies. In sucrose, for example, the effect of oligomycin is the same as in potassium chloride although the inhibition is less pronounced.

In all of the previously described experiments on mitochondrial swelling, the pH was maintained at near neutrality. Under slightly acidic conditions (pH 6.1), ATP no longer stimulated the contraction of swollen mitochondria, but instead, it caused mitochondria to swell. Oligomycin inhibited this ATP-induced swelling, and DNP did not reverse the effect of the antibiotic (CONNELLY and LARDY, 1964a, 1964b). Inhibition occured either in the presence or absence of magnesium.

There is some disagreement as to the effect of substrate on the time of onset of phosphate induced swelling at pH 7.4. CHAPPELL and GREVILLE (1958) reported that substrate causes a decreased time of onset whereas CONNELLY and LARDY (1964b) found a slight increase with either succinate or glutamate. These latter workers also found that oligomycin alone causes a slight increase in the time of onset of swelling, but in combination with succinate, this time period is markedly increased. In neither case, however, is the rate or extent of swelling affected. At pH 6.1, succinate has about the same effect on phosphate treated mitochondria as does ATP. Oligomycin does not inhibit this reversal of swelling.

A rationalization for these observations on the effect of oligomycin on the mitochondrial swelling process has been discussed by CONNELLY and LARDY (1964b). They point out that oligomycin interferes with the utilization of ATP by mitochondrial ATPase and by the activities associated with membrane phenomena. It was assumed that these two means of ATP utilization involve a reversal of the ATP generating system of oxidative phosphorylation. This assumption becomes particularly important when attempting to rationalize the differences in behavior of oligomycin and aurovertin (c.f. the section on that antibiotic). A schematic representation that could explain the observations on the effect of oligomycin on mitochondrial swelling is shown in Fig. 4.

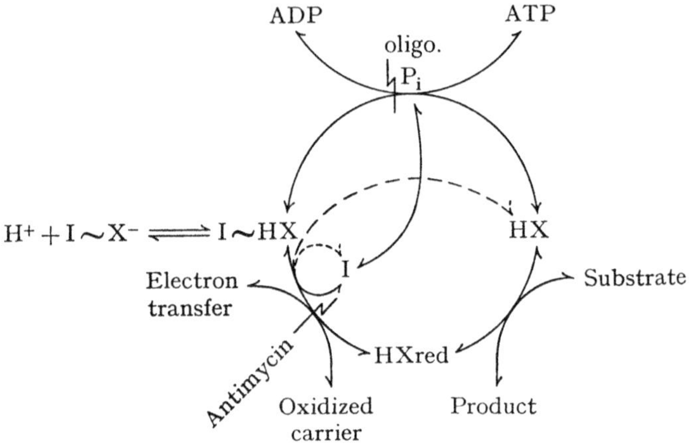

Fig. 4. Hypothetical scheme to explain the effect of oligomycin on mitochondrial swelling. From CONNELLY and LARDY (1964a)

It was theorized that the concentration of $I{\sim}X^-$ determines the extent of swelling. ATP and substrates would increase the $I{\sim}X^-$ concentration whereas hydrogen ions would reduce the concentration. Oligomycin in this scheme is an inhibitor of the utilization of I~HX for ATP formation; it would therefore enhance the effect of substrate. Utilization of ATP as an energy source for the formation of I~HX would, however, be inhibited. The relationship between mitochondrial swelling as visualized in this scheme and the other processes of mitochondrial energy transformation and utilization is given in Fig. 7 of the summary.

STONER and HANSON (1966) in their studies on the swelling phenomena in corn mitochondria reported that oligomycin, at 0.04 μg/ml, almost completely inhibited phosphorylation. At about this same level, respiration was inhibited about 50% and ATPase activity about 75%. Substrates such as succinate or NADH induced rapid contraction of corn mitochondria which had been swollen in potassium chloride. This contraction was inhibited by phosphate, and the inhibition was not reversed by oligomycin. The antibiotic does, however, inhibit ATP induced contraction. Inorganic phosphate was produced continuously during the time the mitochondria were maintained in the contracted state and phosphate inhibited the ATP induced contraction, presumably by mass action effects. The authors propose that a non-phosphorylated intermediate such as

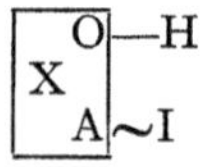

(Fig. 7) is required to maintain the mitochondria in a contracted state, and that the form ation of a phosphorylated intermediate such as

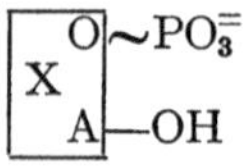

leads to mitochondrial swelling. Since oligomycin did not inhibit phosphate induced swelling of the substrate-contracted mitochondria, itmust not prevent the formation of the phosphorylated intermediate. These data therefore support the contention of LARDY *et al.* (1964) that the site of oligomycin inhibition is at the transfer of inorganic phosphate from the phosphorylated intermediate to ADP (reaction 5, Fig. 7).

Aurovertin

Aurovertin was isolated and purified from cultures of the fungus, *Calcarisporium arbuscula* PREUSS by BALDWIN *et al.* (1964). It is a yellow compound having an empirical formula $C_{26}H_{34}O_9$. It does not inhibit bacteria, yeasts or filamentous fungi even at a concentration of 10,000 μg/ml. It does inhibit *Trichomonas vaginalis* at 250 μg/ml. In spite of the lack of activity of aurovertin against microorganisms, it is very toxic to animals. The LD_{50} value (intravenously) is 1.65 mg/kg in mice and the LD_{100} is 1 mg/kg in rabbits and dogs.

Aurovertin is very similar to the oligomycin complex in its mechanism of action. In this discussion the similarities will be noted only in passing, and emphasis will be placed on the differences. Aurovertin has the following properties in common with oligomycin:

1. It causes inhibition of mitochondrial respiration by blocking associated energy transformations.
2. Inhibition of respiration is reversed by various uncouplers of oxidative phosphorylation.
3. It is ineffective as an uncoupler of oxidative phosphorylation in intact mitochondria. It does, however, inhibit phosphorylation but not oxidation in phosphorylating sub-mitochondrial particles with NADH, succinate or ascorbate plus phenazine methosulfate as substrates (LENAZ, 1965).
4. It does not inhibit substrate phosphorylation associated with α-ketoglutarate oxidation.
5. It inhibits the Pi-ATP and $HP^{18}O_4 - H_2O$ exchange reactions. In fact, equal mixtures of oligomycin and aurovertin give exactly the same level of inhibition as equivalent amounts of either antibiotic alone.

These results are from LARDY *et al.* (1964) and CONNELLY and LARDY (1964a, 1964b) unless otherwise noted. In other aspects, aurovertin does not act like oligomycin. For example, in Table 7 are shown some representative data on the effects of oligomycin and aurovertin on mitochondrial ATPase activity induced by various agents. These data show that, while oligomycin invariably inhibits this induced ATPase activity, aurovertin may inhibit, have no effect or actually enhance the activity. Only with arsenate as the inducer was ATPase activity markedly inhibited to approximately the same extent by both oligomycin and aurovertin. It should be pointed out that the four examples shown in Table 7 are from a total of 37 given by LARDY, and that these in turn represent about one-half of the compounds tested. In a further study of this phenomenon, it was demonstrated that the effects of aurovertin on ATPase activity induced by various compounds fell into six categories. These results, shown in Fig. 5, provide an explanation for the variable effects of aurovertin. As can be seen from the figure, one could observe stimulation, inhibition or no effect depending on which inducer is used and at what concentration. It was found that most of the inducers exhibited the pattern shown in B and C. In another report, Sallis and DeLuca (1964) state that aurovertin inhibited the PTH-dependent ATPase activity in rat-liver mitochondria.

Table 7. *Effects of oligomycin and aurovertin on mitochondrial ATPase activity*[1]

Uncoupler	Control	µmoles Pi liberated/0.2 mg N	
		Oligomycin, 2 µg	Aurovertin, 2 µg
None	0.23	0.17	0.24
DNP, 10^{-4} M	5.60	0.75	2.57
DBNP, 10^{-4} M	2.99	0.54	4.11
BDHB, 10^{-4} M	1.28	0.33	1.28
Arsenate, 10^{-2} M	0.72	0.20	0.14

Abbreviations used are DNP, 2,4-dinitrophenol; DBNP, 2,6-dibromo-4-nitrophenol; BDHB, N-butyl-3,5-diiodo-4-hydroxybenzoate.

[1] Data from Lardy *et al.* (1964).

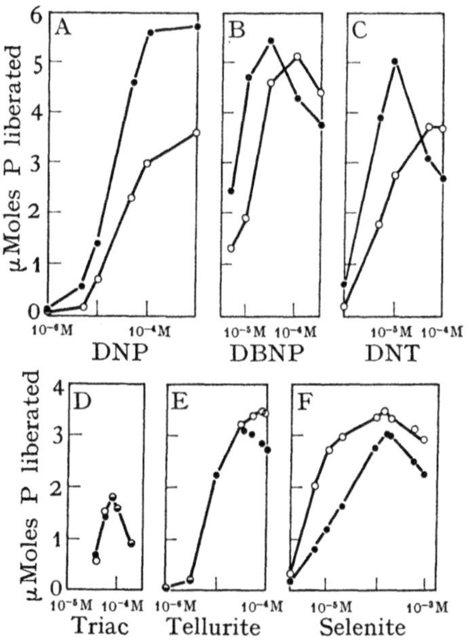

Fig. 5. The effect of aurovertin on ATPase activity induced by a variety of agents. From Lardy *et al.* (1964). Solid dots, without aurovertin; open circles, with 2 µg aurovertin per ml

One possible explanation for the observations that both oligomycin and aurovertin inhibit respiration in intact mitochondria while only oligomycin consistently inhibits ATPase activity is that in the respiration experiments, which contain glucose and hexokinase, the ATP level is lower than in the ATPase experiments. This possibility was tested by Lardy *et al.* (1964) by studying the oxidation of several substrates with a glucose-hexokinase acceptor system and a creatine-creatine kinase acceptor system. These two systems would be expected to maintain different ATP/ADP ratios. The inhibition of respiration by both rutamycin and aurovertin was the same with both acceptor systems, so it was concluded that the extent of aurovertin inhibition is probably not related to ATP concentration.

Aurovertin is also different from oligomycin in its effect on the various aspects of mitochondrial swelling (CONNELLY and LARDY, 1964a, 1964b). These differences are as follows: 1. it is less effective in inhibiting ATP reversal of phosphate induced swelling; 2. it has no effect on ATP reversal of thyroxine induced swelling; 3. it has only slight effect on ATP induced swelling at pH 6.1; 4. it shows no tendency to increase the time of onset of swelling. Aurovertin does, however, have essentially the same action as oligomycin in prolonging the time of onset of swelling induced by succinate.

From the results reported above, it is apparent that aurovertin and oligomycin have similar actions on the processes associated with ATP formation, but it is in the systems which utilize ATP where differences are observed. A comparison of some of these ATP requiring systems has been made by LENAZ (1965) using phosphorylating submitochondrial particles. Partial inhibition (43%) by aurovertin of the ATP mediated reduction of NAD by succinate was observed; however, the reduction by ascorbate plus tetramethyl-p-phenylenediamine was not inhibited. There was little inhibition of the NADH-NADP transhydrogenase activity, and the translocation of calcium ions across the mitochondrial membrane was inhibited partially when supported by ATP but only at high aurovertin concentrations. When this translocation was driven by the oxidation of succinate, no inhibition was observed. The relative sensitivity of these reactions to aurovertin was as follows: oxidative phosphorylation > reduction of NAD by succinate > translocation of calcium ions > NADH-NADP transhydrogenase.

Summary

CONNELLY and LARDY (1964a, 1964b) point out that previous attempts to explain energy transfer phenomena have probably been oversimplifications of the existing situation. In an attempt to incorporate the results obtained by the

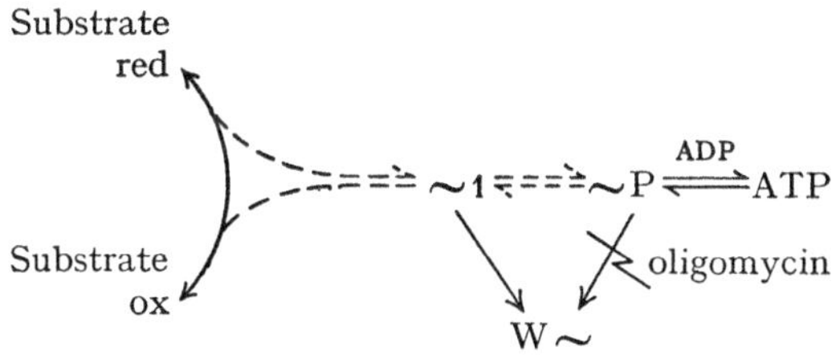

Fig. 6. The inhibition of ATP-utilizing systems by oligomycin. Dashed lines represent multiple steps in the reaction sequence. This scheme is a simplification of the one proposed by LARDY *et al.* (1964)

use of these antibiotics into a rational scheme which would provide a more adequate description of mitochondrial energy transfer, they proposed a scheme similar to that shown in Fig. 6. In this scheme ~I and ~P are high energy intermediates generated either by the oxidation of substrates or by reversal of ATP formation. Either of these intermediates can be utilized for the formation of W~ (work functions), another high energy intermediate not on the pathway for ATP synthesis. The hydrolysis of W~ could account for one type of uncoupling of oxidative phosphorylation and ATPase activity. W∼ may be utilized in the various energy requiring processes of the mitochondria. Oligomycin would inhibit the formation of W∼ from ATP but not from ∼I, but aurovertin would have little inhibitory effect from either direction. LENAZ (1965) suggested that each of the functions of W∼ may have a different energy acceptor and that the variable amounts of inhibition observed may reflect different sensitivities of the acceptors to the antibiotic.

The scheme in Fig. 7 represents a hypothetical mechanism for the energy transfer sequence coupled to respiration. It is essentially the scheme proposed by LARDY *et al.* (1964), but it has been modified by the addition of information from other sources.

The sequence of reactions (1) through (5) represents the pathway of ATP synthesis from a reduced component (AH_2) of the electron transport system. I and X are hypothetical energy carriers. Reaction (12) represents the reduction of the electron carrier, A, by either a substrate or a prior component of the electron transport system.

The exchange of ^{18}O and ^{32}P can be accomplished via reactions (4) and (5), assuming that the —OH group is dissociable from A. Two reactions are required for the exchange reaction in order to explain the observations that, although the rate of ^{18}O exchange is much more rapid than ^{32}P exchange, both reactions are inhibited equally on a percentage basis by oligomycin and aurovertin (LARDY *et al.*, 1964).

The reaction sequences (5) → (6) or (5) → (4) → (3) → (2) → (7) represent one type of ATPase activity. LARDY *et al.* (1964) has suggested that those agents, such as DNP, which induce ATPase activity and which are partially inhibited by aurovertin act at either the X∼P or the A∼I sites. Aurovertin blocks either reaction (3) or (4) and is therefore an inhibitor of the induced ATPase activity associated with electron transport.

A second type of ATPase activity is shown by reaction (11). This reaction represents a mechanism for the utilization of the energy from ATP for the formation of another high energy intermediate, W∼, which is not on the main pathway of oxidative phosphorylation. The energy from W∼ is used in such processes as ion transport, mitochondrial swelling, the energy-dependent reduction of NAD by succinate, or it may be lost by hydrolysis. These processes would in effect uncouple oxidative phosphorylation, and any compounds which promoted the processes would be uncoupling agents. Evidence has been presented that W∼ may be a multifunctional entity rather than a single factor (LENAZ, 1965). It was necessary to postulate an entity such as W∼ in order to account for the differences in susceptibility to oligomycin and aurovertin of certain reactions associated with ATP utilization processes. These differences are discussed in detail in the section of this chapter dealing with the mechanism of action of aurovertin. Reaction (11) is inhibited by oligomycin but not by aurovertin. It represents the ATPase activity induced by those agents which are weak uncouplers of oxidative phosphorylation and which are not inhibited by aurovertin. LARDY *et al.* (1964) suggested that both antibiotics act on X∼P but that they are bound at different sites.

The formation of W∼ must also occur from some intermediate before X is introduced into the sequence because the W∼ functions are not inhibited by

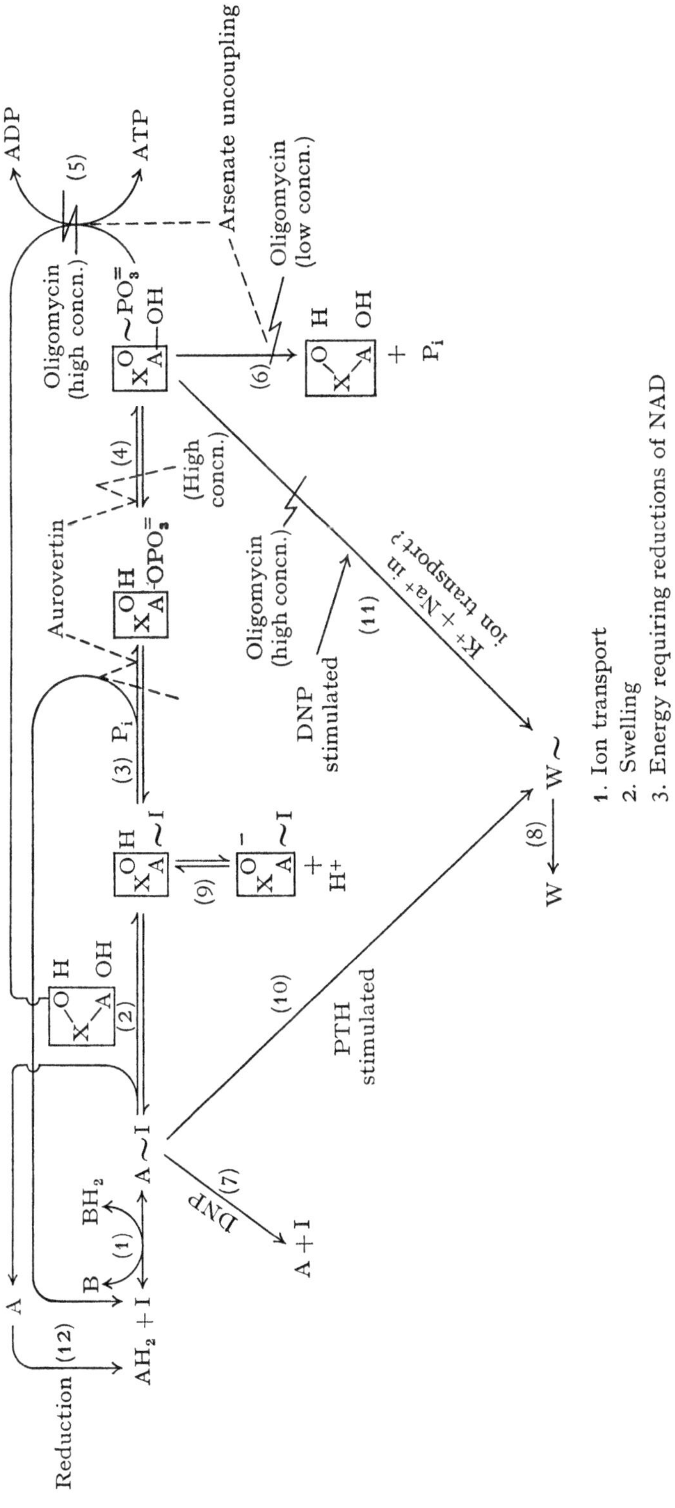

Fig. 7. A hypothetical scheme for the energy transformation reactions associated with the electron transport system. From Lardy *et al.* (1964)

oligomycin when the energy is derived from the oxidation of substrates. A second, oligomycin insensitive pathway reaction (10), was proposed to account for this observation. This reaction is stimulated by PTH, presumably because of the hormone-enhanced utilization of the energy from A∼I for ion transport. Apparently the ion transport induced by PTH cannot utilize energy from ATP via reaction (11), because that process is inhibited by aurovertin.

The site of arsenate uncoupling of oxidative phosphorylation was not definitely established by the use of oligomycin and aurovertin. Oxygen consumption is not restored by that ion in oligomycin or aurovertin inhibited mitochondria, nor is arsenate able to induce ATPase activity in the presence of these antibiotics. Arsenate may act at reaction (6), although LARDY *et al.* (1964) suggested that it may not uncouple until ADP-arsenate is formed.

Reaction (9) was included in this scheme in order to explain certain observations of CONNELLY and LARDY (1964a, 1964b) on mitochondrial swelling phenomena (c.f. Fig. 4). The hypotheses of WADKINS and LEHNINGER (1963b), described in Fig. 2, could also be incorporated into the scheme in Fig. 7 with little alteration. If an enzyme, E, is included in reaction (1) or (12), the sequence (1) through (5) becomes similar to WADKINS' and LEHNINGER'S tightly coupled system; if the following reaction is inserted into Fig. 7 between reactions (4) and (5) or if it is associated with reaction (11), the result is similar to their loosely coupled mitochondria. The enzyme bound phosphate would then presumably react with ADP to form ATP.

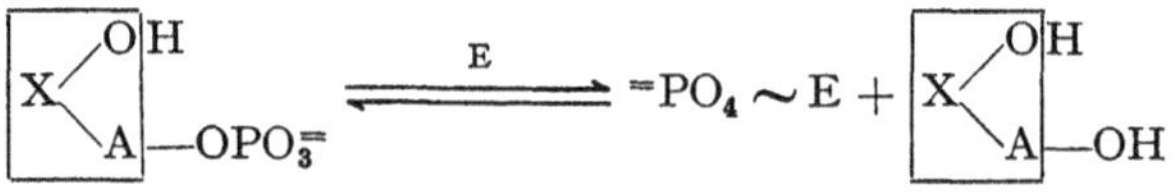

In addition to inhibiting reactions (4) and (11), oligomycin, at low concentrations, also inhibits reaction (6). This inhibition would explain the observations of LEE and ERNSTER (1965) who found that low concentrations of this antibiotic enhanced inorganic phosphate uptake by nonphosphorylating sub-mitochondrial particles.

The partial inhibition of sodium and potassium transport reported by several authors can also be explained by the scheme in Fig. 7. Presumably the energy required for this process can be derived partially from an intermediate such as A∼I and partially from ATP via X∼P. It is the utilization of energy from this latter intermediate that is inhibited by oligomycin, while the process of energy transformation from A∼I is not inhibited. Possibly reaction (11) has more than one step. One of the W∼ functions may be that of the protein moiety in the scheme of WHITTAM *et al.* (1964). They suggested that this protein was involved in the sodium plus potassium stimulated ATPase activity in rabbit-kidney cortex.

References

ARNAUD, C. D., and H. RASMUSSEN: Effect of purified parathyroid hormone added *in vitro* on the respiration of oligomycin-inhibited rat renal tubules. Endocrinology **75**, 277 (1964).

AZZONE, G. F., and L. ERNSTER: Compartmentation of mitochondrial phosphorylations as disclosed by studies with arsenate. J. Biol. Chem. **236**, 1510 (1961).

BALDWIN, C. L., L. C. WEAVER, R. M. BROOKER, T. N. JACOBSEN, C. OSBORNE, JR., and H. A. NASH: Biological and chemical properties of aurovertin, a metabolic product of *Calcarisporium arbuscula*. Lloydia **27**, 88 (1964).

BALTSCHEFFSKY, H., and M. BALTSCHEFFSKY: Inhibitor studies on light-induced phosphorylation in extracts of *Rhodospirillum rubrum*. Acta Chem. Scand. **14**, 257 (1960).

BRIERLY, G. P., E. BACHMANN, and D. E. GREEN: Active transport of inorganic phosphate and magnesium ions by beef heart mitochondria. Proc. Natl. Acad. Sci. U.S. **48**, 1928 (1962).

BRUNI, A., A. R. CONTESSA, and P. SCALLELA: The binding of atractyloside and oligomycin to liver mitochondria. Biochim. et biophys. Acta **100**, 1 (1965).

BRUNI, A., S. LUCIANI, A. R. CONTESSA, and D. F. AZZONE: Effects of atractyloside and oligomycin on energy-transfer reactions. Biochim. et Biophys. Acta **82**, 630 (1964).

CHANCE, B.: The interaction of energy and electron transfer reactions in mitochondria. V. The energy transfer pathway. J. Biol. Chem. **236**, 1569 (1961b).

CHANCE, B.: Energy-linked cytochrome oxidation in mitochondria. Nature **189**, 719 (1961a).

CHAPPELL, J. B., and G. D. GREVILLE: Dependence of mitochondrial swelling on oxidizable substrates. Nature **182**, 813 (1958).

CHAPPELL, J. B., and G. D. GREVILLE: Inhibition of electron transport and the swelling of isolated mitochondria. Nature **183**, 1525 (1959a).

CHAPPELL, J. B., and G. D. GREVILLE: Effects of 2,4-dinitrophenol and other agents on the swelling of isolated mitochondria. Nature **183**, 1737 (1959b).

CHAPPELL, J. B., and G. D. GREVILLE: Mitochondrial swelling and electron transport. I. Swelling supported by ferricyanide. Biochim. et Biophys. Acta **38**, 483 (1960).

CHAPPELL, J. B., and G. D. GREVILLE: Effects of oligomycin on respiration and swelling of isolated liver mitochondria. Nature **190**, 502 (1961).

CHAPPELL, J. B., G. D. GREVILLE, and K. C. BICKNELL: Stimulation of respiration of isolated mitochondria by manganese ions. Biochem. J. **84**, 61 P (1962).

CONNELLY, J. L., and H. A. LARDY: The effect of adenosine triphosphate and substrate on orthophosphate-induced mitochondrial swelling at acid pH. J. Biol. Chem. **239**, 3065 (1964a).

CONNELLY, J. L., and H. A. LARDY: Antibiotics as tools for metabolic studies. III. Effects of oligomycin and aurovertin on the swelling and contraction processes of mitochondria. Biochemistry **3**, 1969 (1964b).

COOPER, C., and R. G. KULKA: Properties of the inorganic orthophosphate-adenosine triphosphate and adenosine diphosphate-adenosine triphosphate exchange reactions of digitonin particles. J. Biol. Chem. **236**, 2351 (1961).

CURRIE, W. D., and C. T. GREGG: Inhibition of the respiration of cultured mammalian cells by oligomycin. Biochem. Biophys. Research Commun. **21**, 9 (1965).

DALLNER, G., and L. ERNSTER: Induction of a crabtree-like effect in Ehrlich ascites tumor cells by oligomycin. Exptl. Cell Research **27**, 372 (1962).

DANIELSON, L., and L. ERNSTER: Demonstration of a mitochondrial energy-dependent pyridine nucleotide transhydrogenase reaction. Biochem. Biophys. Research Commun. **10**, 91 (1963a).

DANIELSON, L., and L. ERNSTER: Energy dependence of pyridine nucleotide-linked dismutations in rat liver mitochondria. Biochem. Biophys. Research Commun. **10**, 85 (1963b).

ERNSTER, L.: The phosphorylation occurring in the flavoprotein region of the respiratory chain. Proc. Intern. Congr. Biochem., 5th, Moscow 1961, **5**, 115 (1963).

ERNSTER, L., and C. LEE: Biological oxidoreductions. Ann. Rev. Biochem. **33**, 729 (1964).

ESTABROOK, R. W.: Effect of oligomycin on the arsenate and 2,4-dinitrophenol (DNP) stimulation of mitochondrial oxidations. Biochem. Biophys. Research Commun. **4**, 89 (1961).

FANG, M., and H. RASMUSSEN: Parathyroid hormone and mitochondrial respiration. Endocrinology **75**, 434 (1964).
FANG, M., H. RASMUSSEN, H. F. DELUCA, and R. YOUNG: The influence of parathyroid hormone upon glutamate oxidation in isolated mitochondria. Biochem. Biophys. Research Commun. **10**, 260 (1963).
GLYNN, I. M.: An adenosine triphosphatase from electric organ activated by sodium and potassium and inhibited by ouabain or oligomycin. Biochem. J. **84**, 75 P (1962).
HARARY, I., and E. C. SLATER: Studies *in vitro* on single beating heart cells. VIII. The effect of oligomycin, dinitrophenol and ouabain on the beating rate. Biochim. et Biophys. Acta **99**, 227 (1965).
HELDT, H. W., H. JACOBS, and M. KLINGENBERG: Evidence for the participation of endogenous guanosine triphosphate in substrate level phosphate transfer in intact mitochondria. Biochem. Biophys. Research Commun. **17**, 130 (1964).
HUIJING, F., and E. C. SLATER: The use of oligomycin as an inhibitor of oxidative phosphorylation. J. Biochem. (Japan) **49**, 493 (1961).
JÄRNEFELT, J.: Properties and possible mechanism of the Na^+ and K^+-stimulated microsomal adenosinetriphosphatase. Biochim. et Biophys. Acta **59**, 643 (1962).
JÖBSIS, F. F., and H. VREMAN: Inhibition of sodium- and potassium-stimulated adenosinetriphosphatase by oligomycin. Biochim. et Biophys. Acta **73**, 346 (1963).
KAGAWA, Y., and E. RACKER: A factor conferring oligomycin sensitivity to mitochondrial ATPase. Federation Proc. **24**, 363 (1965).
KULKA, R. G., and C. COOPER: The action of oligomycin on the inorganic orthophosphate-adenosine triphosphate and adenosine diphosphate-adenosine triphosphate exchange reactions of digitonin particles. J. Biol. Chem. **237**, 936 (1962).
LARDY, H. A., J. L. CONNELLY, and D. JOHNSON: Antibiotics as tools for metabolic studies. II. Inhibition of phosphoryl transfer in mitochondria by oligomycin and aurovertin. Biochemistry **3**, 1961 (1964).
LARDY, H. A., D. JOHNSON, and W. C. MCMURRAY: Antibiotics as tools for metabolic studies. I. A survey of toxic antibiotics in respiratory, phosphorylative and glycolytic systems. Arch. Biochem. Biophys. **78**, 587 (1958).
LARDY, H. A., and W. C. MCMURRAY: The mode of action of oligomycin. Federation Proc. **18**, 269 (1959).
LARDY, H. A., P. WITONSKY, and D. JOHNSON: Antibiotics as tools for metabolic studies. IV. Comparative effectiveness of oligomycins A, B, C, and rutamycin as inhibitors of phosphoryl transfer reactions in mitochondria. Biochemistry **4**, 552 (1965).
LARSON, M. H., and W. H. PETERSON: Chromatographic study of the oligomycin complex produced under various conditions of fermentation. Appl. Microbiol. **8**, 182 (1960).
LEE, C. P., G. F. AZZONE, and L. ERNSTER: Evidence for energy coupling in nonphosphorylating electron transport particles from beef-heart mitochondria. Nature **201**, 152 (1964).
LEE, C., and L. ERNSTER: Restoration of oxidative phosphorylation in non-phosphorylating submitochondrial particles by oligomycin. Biochem. Biophys. Research Commun. **18**, 523 (1965).
LEHNINGER, A. L.: Intermediate enzymatic reactions in the coupling of phosphorylation to electron transport. Symp. Intracellular respiration: Phosphorylating and non-phosphorylating oxidation reduction. Proc. Intern. Congr. Biochem., 5th, Moscow 1961, **5**, 239 (1963).
LENAZ, G.: Effect of aurovertin on energy-linked processes related to oxidative phosphorylation. Biochem. Biophys. Research Commun. **21**, 170 (1965).
MARTY, E. W., JR., and E. MCCOY: The chromatographic separation and biological properties of the oligomycins. Antibiotics & Chemotherapy **9**, 286 (1959).
MASAMUNE, S., J. M. SEHGAL, E. E. VAN TAMELEN, F. M. STRONG, and W. H. PETERSON: Separation and preliminary characterization of oligomycins A, B, and C. J. Am. Chem. Soc. **80**, 6092 (1958).

MICHEL, R., P. HUET, and M. HUET: Action of rutamycin (A 272) on rat hepatic mitochondria adenosinetriphosphatases. Compt. rend. soc. biol. **158**, 994 (1964).

MINAKAMI, S., K. KAKINUMA, and H. YOSHIKAWA: The control of respiration in brain slices. Biochim. et Biophys. Acta **78**, 808 (1963).

MINAKAMI, S., and H. YOSHIKAWA: Effect of oligomycin on the phosphorylating respiration of ascites hepatoma cells. Biochim. et Biophys. Acta **74**, 793 (1963).

NEUBERT, D., and A. L. LEHNINGER: Effect of oligomycin, gramicidin and other antibiotics on reversal of mitochondrial swelling by adenosine triphosphate (ATP). Biochim. et Biophys. Acta **62**, 556 (1962).

SALLIS, J. D., and H. F. DELUCA: Parathyroid hormone interaction with the oxidative phosphorylation chain. Effect on adenosine-triphosphatase activity and the adenosine triphosphate-orthophosphate exchange reaction. J. Biol. Chem. **239**, 4303 (1964).

SALLIS, J. D., H. F. DELUCA, and D. L. MARTIN: Parathyroid hormone-dependent transport of inorganic phosphate by rat liver mitochondria. Effect of phosphorylation chain inhibitors. J. Biol. Chem. **240**, 2229 (1965).

SALLIS, J. D., H. F. DELUCA, and H. RASMUSSEN: Parathyroid hormone stimulation of phosphate uptake by rat liver mitochondria. Biochem. Biophys. Research Commun. **10**, 266 (1963a).

SALLIS, J. D., H. F. DELUCA, and H. RASMUSSEN: Parathyroid hormone-dependent uptake of inorganic phosphate by mitochondria. J. Biol. Chem. **238**, 4098 (1963b).

SLATER, E. C., and J. M. TAGER: Synthesis of glutamate from α-oxoglutarate and ammonia in rat-liver mitochondria. V. Energetics and mechanism. Biochim. et Biophys. Acta **77**, 276 (1963).

SLATER, E. C., J. M. TAGER, and A. M. SNOSWELL: The mechanism of the reduction of mitochondrial DPN^+ coupled with the oxidation of succinate. Biochim. et Biophys. Acta **56**, 177 (1962).

SMITH, R. M., W. H. PETERSON, and E. MCCOY: Oligomycin, a new antifungal antibiotic. Antibiotics & Chemotherapy **4**, 962 (1954).

SNOSWELL, A. M.: The mechanism of the reduction of mitochondrial diphosphopyridine nucleotide by succinate in rabbit-heart sarcosomes. Biochim. et Biophys. Acta **52**, 216 (1961).

SNOSWELL, A. M.: The reduction of diphosphopyridine nucleotide of rabbit-heart sarcosomes by succinate. Biochim. et Biophys. Acta **60**, 143 (1962).

STONER, C., and J. HANSON: Swelling and contraction of corn mitochondria. Plant Physiol. **41**, 255 (1966).

TAGER, J. M.: Synthesis of glutamate from α-oxoglutarate and ammonia in rat-liver mitochondria. III. Malate as hydrogen donor. Biochim. et Biophys. Acta **77**, 258 (1963).

TAGER, J. M., J. L. HOWLAND, E. C. SLATER, and A. M. SNOSWELL: Synthesis of glutamate from α-oxoglutarate and ammonia in rat-liver mitochondria. IV. Reduction of nicotinamide nucleotide coupled with the aerobic oxidation of tetramethyl-p-phenylenediamine. Biochim. et Biophys. Acta **77**, 266 (1963).

TAGER, J. M., and E. C. SLATER: Synthesis of glutamate from α-oxoglutarate and ammonia in rat-liver mitochondria. II. Succinate as hydrogen donor. Biochim. et Biophys. Acta **77**, 246 (1963a).

TAGER, J. M., and E. C. SLATER: Synthesis of glutamate from α-oxoglutarate and ammonia in rat-liver mitochondria. I. Comparison of different hydrogen donors. Biochim. et Biophys. Acta **77**, 227 (1963b).

THOMPSON, R. Q., M. M. HOEHN, and C. E. HIGGINS: Crystalline antifungal antibiotic isolated from a strain of *Streptomyces rutgersensis*. Antimicrobial Agents and Chemotherapy, p. 474 (1961).

TOBIN, R. B., and E. C. SLATER: The effect of oligomycin on the respiration of tissue slices. Biochim. et Biophys. Acta **105**, 214 (1965).

UTSUMI, K., and G. YAMAMOTO: Mitochondrial swelling and uncoupling of oxidative phosphorylation by arginine-rich histone extracted from calf thymus. Biochim. et Biophys. Acta **100**, 606 (1965).

VAN ROSSUM, G. D. V.: Effect of oligomycin on cation transport in slices of rat liver. Biochem. J. **84**, 35 P (1962).
VAN ROSSUM, G. D. V.: Effect of oligomycin on net movements of sodium and potassium in mammalian cells *in vitro*. Biochim. et Biophys. Acta **82**, 556 (1964).
VAN GRONIGEN, M. E. M., and E. C. SLATER: Effect of oligomycin on the ($Na^+ + K^+$)-activated Mg^{++} ATPase of brain microsomes and erythrocyte membranes. Biochim. et Biophys. Acta **73**, 527 (1963).
WADKINS, C. L.: Inhibition of the dinitrophenol-sensitive adenosine triphosphate (ATP)-adenosine diphosphate (ADP) exchange reaction by oligomycin. Biochem. Biophys. Research Commun. **7**, 70 (1962).
WADKINS, C. L., and A. L. LEHNINGER: Role of ATP-ADP exchange reaction in oxidative phosphorylation. Federation Proc. **22**, 1092 (1963a).
WADKINS, C. L., and A. L. LEHNINGER: Distribution of an oligomycin-sensitive adenosine triphosphate-adenosine diphosphate exchange reaction and its relationship to the respiratory chain. J. Biol. Chem. **238**, 2555 (1963b).
WHITTAM, R., K. P. WHEELER, and A. BLAKE: Oligomycin and active transport reactions in cell membranes. Nature **203**, 720 (1964).
WU, R.: Effect of azide and oligomycin on inorganic phosphate transport in slices of rat kidney. Biochim. et Biophys. Acta **82**, 212 (1964).

Usnic Acid

Paul D. Shaw

Usnic acid (usninic acid) is an antibiotic produced by many species of lichens (STOLL *et al.*, 1947). Its chemistry was studied by WIDMAN (1902), and the following structure was proposed by SCHOPF and ROSS (1938, 1947). Usnic acid was synthesized by BARTON *et al.* (1956).

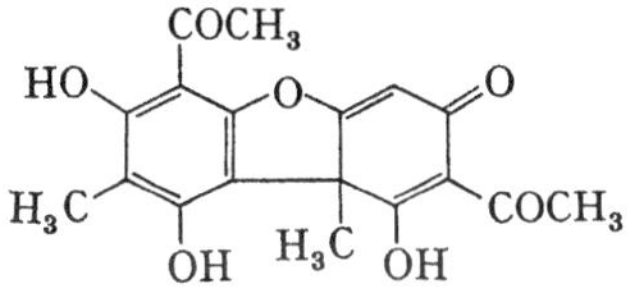

Usnic Acid

Usnic acid is somewhat unusual in that it has been isolated in both the d- and l-forms as well as a racemic mixture (STOLL *et al.*, 1947; SAVICH *et al.*, 1960). It has been obtained from cultures of the fungal portion of the lichen *Cladonia cristatella* (CASTLE and KUBSCH, 1949).

The biological activities of the usnic acid enantiomorphs are the same (STOLL *et al.*, 1947) so for this discussion, they will be regarded as a single compound. This antibiotic is active against Gram-positive bacteria such as *Bacillus subtilis*, *Sarcina lutea*, staphylococci, *Corynebacterium diphtheriae*, *Haemophilus pertussis* and *Mycobacterium tuberculosis* at about 1 part per million. Most Gram-negative bacteria, filamentous fungi and yeasts are not inhibited. The LD_{50} (intravenously) is 25 mg per kg in mice.

Usnic acid has had limited clinical use in the treatment of tuberculosis, and many derivatives have been prepared, such as complexes with other antibiotics (VIRTANEN, 1955) various hydrazones (NAITO *et al.*, 1957) and as the usnate of benzyldimethyl{2-{2-[p-(1,1,3,3-tetramethylbutyl)phenoxy]ethoxy}ethyl} ammonium hydroxide (TOMASELLI, 1957; VIRTANEN and KILPIO, 1957). Some of these derivatives have antibiotic properties different from the parent compound. For example, the last compound mentioned is less toxic than usnic acid, and it has activity against certain fungi that cause skin infections.

Although much work has been done on the isolation, chemistry and pharmacology of usnic acid, there has been very little work on its mechanism of action. One report (CREASER, 1955) stated that 30 μg/ml usnic acid inhibited the induction of *β*-galactosidase in *Staphylococcus aureus*. This line of investigations has apparently not been pursued.

JOHNSON *et al.* (1950) studied the effects of usnic acid on respiration in washed rat kidney particles. At 10^{-6} M, this antibiotic slightly inhibited oxygen uptake with succinate, fumarate and citrate. Respiration was increased or there was no effect with glutamate, α-ketoglutarate, malate, pyruvate plus fumarate or cis-aconitate as the substrate. At 10^{-4} M, the oxidation of all these substrates was inhibited from 55 to 89%. Hexokinase was not inhibited by usnic acid.

Usnic acid at 10^{-6} M caused a slight increase in inorganic phosphate uptake by liver homogenates with pyruvate as the substrate. Inhibition occurred at higher antibiotic concentrations and was nearly complete at 1.6×10^{-5} M. There was little effect on oxygen consumption at these concentrations. Similar results were obtained with α-ketoglutarate as substrate although slightly higher antibiotic concentrations were required.

Usnic acid, unlike the other antibiotics previously discussed, is an uncoupler of oxidative phosphorylation as well as a respiratory inhibitor (LARDY *et al.*, 1964). It can therefore restore oxygen consumption in mitochondria which have been inhibited by oligomycin or aurovertin to levels with usnic acid alone. Oxygen consumption with choline as substrate was more than doubled with 10^{-5} M usnic acid in place of a glucose-hexokinase, phosphate acceptor system.

The mechanism of action of usnic acid would appear to be at some site in the terminal electron transport system. It inhibits respiration and uncouples oxidation phosphorylation so inhibition may be associated with the energy transforming system in the terminal respiratory pathway.

References

BARTON, D. H. R., A. M. DEFLORIN, and O. E. EDWARDS: The synthesis of usnic acid. J. Chem. Soc. **1956**, 530.

CASTLE, H., and F. KUBSCH: The production of usnic, didymic and rhodocladonic acids by the fungal component of the lichen *Cladonia cristatella*. Arch. Biochem. **23**, 158 (1949).

CREASER, E. H.: The induced (adaptive) biosynthesis of β-galactosidase in *Staphylococcus aureus*. J. Gen. Microbiol. **12**, 288 (1955).

JOHNSON, R. B., G. FELDOTT, and H. A. LARDY: The mode of action of the antibiotic usnic acid. Arch. Biochem. (now Arch. Biochem. Biophys.) **28**, 317 (1950).

LARDY, H. A., J. L. CONNELLY, and D. JOHNSON: Antibiotics as tools for metabolic studies. II. Inhibition of phosphoryl transfer in mitochondria by oligomycin and aurovertin. Biochemistry **3**, 1961 (1964).

NAITO, M., R. WATANABE, R. KITAGAWA, K. IBA, S. IMAI, F. FUJIKAWA, S. NAKAZAWA, Y. YAGI, J. YAGI, and M. NISHIMOTO: Effect of some compounds on tubercle bacilli in vitro. VIII. Antibacterial activity of several hydrazone compounds *in vitro*. Yakugaku Zasshi **77**, 1251 (1957) [Chem. Abstr. **52**, 4016a (1958)].

SAVICH, V. P., M. A. LITVINOV, and E. N. MOISEEVA: An antibiotic from lichens as a medicinal product. Planta Med. **8**, 191 (1960).

SCHOPF, C., and F. ROSS: Die Konstitution der Usninsäure. Naturwissenschaften **26**, 772 (1938).

SCHOPF, C., and F. ROSS: Die Konstitution der Usninsäure. II. Justus Liebigs Ann. Chem. **1** (1941).

STOLL, A., A. BRACK and J. RENG: Die antibakterielle Wirkung der Usninsäure auf Mykobakterien und andere Mikroorganismen. Experientia **3**, 115 (1947).

TOMASELLI, R.: New usnic acid derivative used therapeutically. Farmaco (Pavia), Ed. pract. Ed. sci. **12**, 137 (1957) [Chem. Abstr. **51**, 9091c (1957)].

VIRTANEN, O. E., and O. E. KILPIO: Fungistatic activity of an usnic acid preparation with the trade name USNO. Suomen Kemistilehti **30**, 8 (1957) [Chem. Abstr. **51**, 10743e(1957)].

VIRTANEN, O. E.: Derivatives of usnic acid with the most important tuberculostatic agents. Suomen Kemistilehti B **28**, 125 (1955).

WIDMAN, D.: Zur Kenntnis Usninsäure. Justus Liebigs Ann. Chem. **324**, 139 (1902).

Nigericin

Paul D. Shaw

Nigericin was isolated from an unidentified streptomycete by HARNED *et al.* (1951). Subsequently the producing organism was reported to be *Streptomyces* "Nig-1" (BENEDICT, 1953). The antibiotic has the empirical formula $C_{39}H_{69}O_{11}$. It forms a monosodium salt and has one —OCH_3 group. Nigericin inhibits gram-positive bacteria at levels below 0.5 μg/ml, but levels above 60 μg/ml are required to inhibit gram- negative bacteria such as *Escherichia coli* (HARNED *et al.*, 1951). *Mycobacterium smegmatis* and *Candida albicans* are inhibited at 2 μg/ml, and fungi are inhibited at somewhat higher concentrations. The antibiotic is not active against bacteriophages at 500 μg/ml (HALL *et al.*, 1951). The LD_{50} (intraperitoneally) is 2.5 mg/kg in mice.

The inhibition of respiration by nigericin in intact mitochondria is dependent in the substrate used. Table 1 summarizes the available information on the inhibition by this antibiotic of the oxidation of a variety of substrates. The oxidation of glutamate, pyruvate and caprylate is nearly completely inhibited. Succinate, α-ketoglutarate, proline and choline oxidations are partially inhibited. There is only slight inhibition of oxidation of either the cytochrome c-ascorbate or cytochrome c-adrenaline systems. The effect of the antibiotic on β-hydroxybutyrate oxidation is variable; although the maximum reported inhibition is only 33%.

P/O values for most of the substrates used were not altered by nigericin except where oxidation was completely inhibited. However, phosphorylation associated with the oxidation of choline was completely inhibited, and that associated with

Table 1. *The effect of nigericin on the oxidation of a variety of substrates*

	Percent inhibition of oxygen uptake	
Succinate	71[1]	50 (1 μg antibiotic)
β-Hydroxybutyrate	28[1]	0
Glutamate	93[1]	88
α-Ketoglutarate		74
Proline		64
Pyruvate		100
Caprylate		93
Cyt. c-Ascorbate		9 (5 μg antibiotic)
Cyt. c-Adrenaline		2
Choline		16 (57 at 100 μg antibiotic)

[1] These data are from LARDY *et al.* (1958). All other data are from CHA (1962). In all cases, except where noted, the antibiotic concentrations were 10 μg per 3.0 ml.

the cytochrome c-ascorbate and cytochrome c-adrenaline systems was partially inhibited (CHA, 1962). Respiration was not inhibited by nigericin in sub-mitochondrial particles with β-hydroxybutyrate or succinate as substrate (LARDY *et al.*, 1958). Phosphorylation is partially inhibited (28 to 58%) with β-hydroxybutyrate as substrate and markedly inhibited (82%) with succinate as substrate (CHA, 1962). These results are somewhat different than those reported by LARDY *et al.* (1958) who found a similar decrease in P/O value with β-hydroxybutyrate but only a 20% decrease with succinate.

2,4-Dinitrophenol (DNP) is an uncoupler of oxidative phosphorylation, and it reverses oligomycin inhibition of the oxydation of most substrates. When this agent was added with nigericin, no reversal of succinate oxidation was observed. DNP did however restore a small protion of the activity with α-ketoglutarate, glutamate, proline and pyruvate as substrates (CHA, 1962).

The effect of nigericin on respiration in the absence of a phosphate acceptor was investigated by CHA (1962). With the exception of β-hydroxybutyrate, the oxidation of all the substrates was inhibited by the antibiotic. With that substrate, a stimulation in respiration was observed. This indicated that a partial uncoupling of oxidative phosphorylation had occurred. Respiration with all the substrates but succinate was stimulated by DNP, and this stimulated oxygen uptake was inhibited by the antibiotic except when β-hydroxybutyrate was the substrate. It was concluded that if the nigericin inhibited coupled phosphorylation, the site of action must be before the site of DNP uncoupling.

High concentrations of nigericin stimulated mitochondrial ATPase slightly (LARDY *et al.*, 1958; CHA, 1962). ATPase activity was inhibited about 24% by low levels of the antibiotic when DNP was the inducer, 29% when deoxycholate was the inducer, but the activity was not inhibited when Triac[1] was the inducer (LARDY *et al.*, 1958). Neither calcium nor magnesium induced activity was inhibited, but the ATPase activity induced by magnesium plus calcium was inhibited. SALLIS and DE LUCA (1964) reported that nigericin did not inhibit the parathyroid hormone-dependent ATPase activity in rat-liver mitochondria. The hormone-dependent transport of inorganic phosphate was however inhibited when pyruvate plus malate or α-ketoglutarate was the energy source (SALLIS *et al.*, 1965). The inhibition was not relieved by addition of adenine nucleotides. This indicates that the mechanism of action of nigericin is different from oligomycin because inhibition of phosphate transport by this last antibiotic is prevented by adenine nucleotides.

The conversion of proline or glutamic acid to α-ketoglutarate was studied by incubating these amino acids with mitochondria in the absence of a phosphate acceptor system (CHA, 1962). In the presence of nigericin, α-ketoglutarate accumulated; this indicated that α-ketoglutarate dehydrogenase was inhibited by the antibiotics. This conclusion was supported by the lack of disappearance of α-ketoglutarate when this acid was used in place of the amino acids. Pyruvate, when used as substrate in place of α-ketoglutarate, gave identical results. However, when α-ketoglutarate dehydrogenase was assayed in the presence of the antibiotic, no inhibition of enzyme activity was found. In addition, the activities of the following enzyme systems were not inhibited by the antibiotic: succinic dehydrogenase, NADH-cytochrome c reductase, NADH-coenzyme Q reductase,

[1] Triac is 3,3',5-triiodothyroacetate.

succinic-coenzyme Q reductase, reduced coenzyme Q-cytochrome c reductase, cytochrome oxidase, isocitric dehydrogenase, malic dehydrogenase and succinic thiokinase. Substrate phosphorylation with α-ketoglutarate as substrate was not inhibited.

The only enzyme of the Krebs cycle that was inhibited by nigericin was fumarase (CHA, 1962). This reaction was inhibited by low concentrations of the antibiotic with either fumarate or malate as the substrate. At high antibiotic concentrations (ca. 2 μg/ml) however, enzyme activity was restored to the level of the controls. The mechanism of inhibition of fumarase is unknown. The antibiotic did not act as a substrate for the enzyme, but rather it behaved in the manner of a polyanion (CHA, 1962). It was suggested by this author that the primary mechanism of action of nigericin might be an inhibition of fumarase activity; this would interrupt the Krebs cycle, prevent NADH formation and cause a buildup of fumarate. This conclusion fails to consider that at the levels of antibiotic required for maximal inhibition of fumarase (0.02 to 0.4 μg/ml), mitochondrial respiration is only partially inhibited. Fumarase activity was restored at approximately 2 μg/ml, whereas, at about this same concentration, inhibition of the nigericin sensitive oxidation of glutamate or α-ketoglutarate is maximal. The inhibition of fumarase therefore may not be related to the inhibition of respiration. However, since these studies on fumarase utilized a purified enzyme preparation in place of the mitochondria used in the respiratory studies, the results may only reflect the ability of the antibiotic to penetrate the mitochondrial membrane.

In addition to inhibition of respiration, nigericin at 2 μg/ml nearly completely inhibited the ATP-^{32}Pi exchange reaction in intact mitochondria (LARDY *et al.*, 1958). This reaction was not inhibited however in sub-mitochondrial particles. Similarly, the $H_2{}^{18}O$-Pi exchange is also inhibited to varying degrees (CHA, 1962). The extent of inhibition depended on the antibiotic concentration, pH, and the presence or absence of ATP and EDTA.

The failure of nigericin to inhibit β-hydroxybutyrate oxidation was explained by the incomplete oxidation of that substrate. The acetoacetate produced by the oxidation was not further oxidized by the mitochondria. These results support the hypothesis that nigericin inhibits some step in the Krebs cycle but does not effect the terminal electron transport system.

Another material seems to act similarly to nigericin. The name dianemycin was used for this agent by investigators studying the effect of various poisons on the respiratory systems (LARDY *et al.*, 1958; CHA, 1962; SALLIS and DE LUCA, 1964; SALLIS *et al.*, 1965). No publications exist on the organism that synthesizes such a material nor on its antibiotic spectrum. There is no information available in the literature on its isolation, chemistry, or its purity.

References

BENEDICT, R. G.: Antibiotics produced by actinomycetes. Bot. Rev. **19**, 271 (1953).

CHA, C. M.: Inactivation of oxidative and phosphorylative systems in mitochondria by dianemycin and nigericin. Ph. D. Thesis, University of Wisconsin 1962.

HALL, E. A., F. KAVANAGH, and I. N. ASHESHOV: Action of forty-five antibacterial substances on bacterial viruses. Antibiotics & Chemotherapy **1**, 369 (1951).

HARNED, R. L., P. H. HIDY, C. J. CORUM, and K. L. JONES: Nigericin, a new crystalline antibiotic from an unidentified *Streptomyces*. Antibiotics & Chemotherapy **1**, 594 (1951).
LARDY, H. A., D. JOHNSON, and W. C. MCMURRAY: Antibiotics as tools for metabolic studies. I. A survey of toxic antibiotics in respiratory, phosphorylative and glycolytic systems. Arch. Biochem. Biophys. **78**, 587 (1958).
SALLIS, J. D., and H. F. DE LUCA: Parathyroid hormone interaction with the oxidative phosphorylation chain. Effect on adenosine-triphosphatase activity and the adenosine triphosphate-orthophosphate exchange reaction. J. Biol. Chem. **239**, 4303 (1964).
SALLIS, J. D., H. F. DE LUCA, and D. L. MARTIN: Parathyroid hormone-dependent transport of inorganic phosphate by rat liver mitochondria. Effect of phosphorylation chain inhibitors. J. Biol. Chem. **240**, 2229 (1965).

Flavensomycin

David Gottlieb

Flavensomycin was first isolated from a culture of *Streptomyces tanaschiensis* by CRAVERI and GIOLITTI (1957) and later from a culture of *S. griseus* (CHACKO and GOTTLIEB, 1965). A culture, *S. cavourensis*, has also been denoted by Dr. R. CRAVERI as a flavensomycin producer. A literature survey failed to reveal whether *S. cavourensis* was originally *S. tanaschiensis* or is a different organism. Recent studies indicate the possibility that *S. cavourensis* belongs to the species *S. griseus.*

Flavensomycin is deleterious in various degrees to the growth of a wide variety of organisms. Fungi are generally sensitive between 5 and 100 μg per ml of antibiotic (CHACKO and GOTTLIEB, 1965) though some are inhibited as low as 0.05 μg (CRAVERI and GIOLITTI, 1957; CRAVERI *et al.*, 1958) and others required more than 100 μg. Gram positive bacteria were inhibited between 32 and 125 μg per ml but Gram negative bacteria were generally not readily inhibited (CHACKO and GOTTLIEB, 1965). The antibiotic did not inactivate viruses per se but did prevent infection of tobacco by the tobacco mosaic virus (CHACKO and GOTTLIEB, 1965). Flavensomycin was also insecticidal at very low concentrations (CRAVERI and GIOLITTI, 1957). It is very toxic and mice are killed on interperitoneal injections at 1 mg per kilogram body weight (CRAVERI and GIOLITTI, 1957).

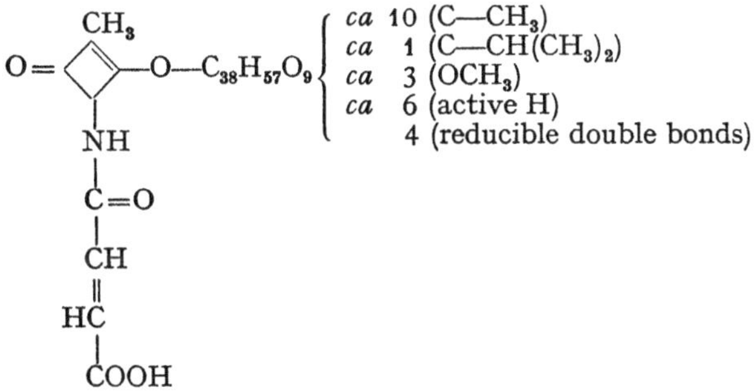

Flavensomycinic acid

Fig. 1. Flavensomycin

The antibiotic has been obtained as pale yellow crystals which melt at about 152° C; a partial structure was determined by CANONICA *et al.* (1961 a). Their data indicate a molecular formula $C_{38}H_{58}N_2O_{10}$. Methanolysis resulted in the formation of a new crystalline compound, flavensomycinic acid. The structure of flavensomycinic acid was subsequently determined (Fig. 1) (CANONICA *et al.*, 1961 a, 1961 b, 1961 c). Most recent data by mass spectrograph analysis indicate a molecular weight of 870 and an empirical formula, $C_{47}H_{67}NO_{14}$ (DYER, 1965). The structure and composition of that part of the molecule which is known at present is indicated in Fig. 1 (DYER, 1965). Data on the mechanism of action of flavensomycin are from recent studies of INOUE and GOTTLIEB (1966). *Penicillium oxalicum* was used for all experiments. Its growth in liquid or agar culture was inhibited by low levels of the antibiotic, 5 μg per ml solution. At this concentration, exogenous respiration of the fungus was inhibited, but endogenous respiration was unaffected. The oxidation of some mono or disaccharides was inhibited 70% ; the oxidation of some amino acids was prevented and succinate oxidation was completely inhibited.

Detailed studies on the mechanism of action of the antibiotic have been almost entirely confined to the nature of the inhibition of the oxidation of succinic acid and related compounds. The oxidations of succinate and NADH are via the usual type of terminal electron transport mechanism associated with animal and fungal cells (Fig. 2). With mitochondria, oxygen consumption is inhibited by sodium azide, indicating the presence of cytochrome c oxidase. The operation of a normal cytochrome system was also indicated by the sensitivity of succinic and NADH cytochrome c reductases to antimycin A, and amytal. Thenoyltrifluoroacetone and diethylstilbesterol prevented the reduction of cytochrome c to various degrees, again pointing to a mammalian type electron transport system. The addition of exogenous cytochrome c and phenazine methosulfate increased mitochondrial oxidation.

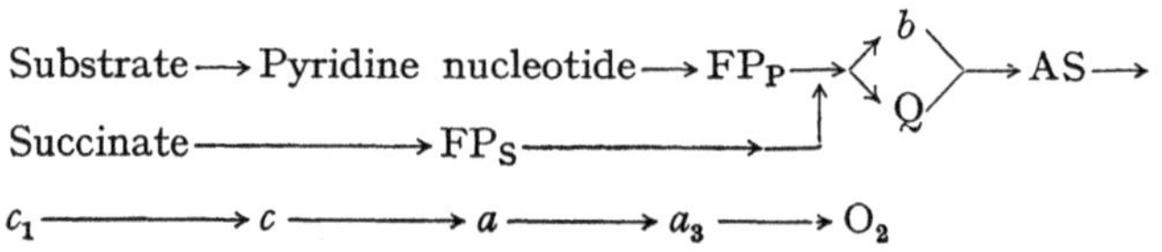

Fig. 2. Terminal electron transport system in Penicillium oxalicum

Cell-free preparations of *P. oxalicum* which normally oxidase succinate and NADH cannot carry out this process in the presence of flavensomycin. The antibiotic also inhibits the oxidation of succinate and NADH by washed mitochondria from the fungus. Flavensomycin reduced substrate oxidation progressively as the concentration of the antibiotic increased. At 10 and 100 μg per ml, succinate oxidation was inhibited 38 and 100%, respectively. NADH oxidation responded similarly and was inhibited 98% at the higher concentration. These results are at variance with those reported for liver mitochondria by LARDY *et al.* (1958). The difference is probably caused by the difference in the concentrations tested. Much higher concentrations than 10 μg per ml of flavensomycin are needed to inhibit these reactions, and the inhibition would not have been detected at the low concentrations that were used by LARDY.

The site of action of flavensomycin in inhibiting succinate or NADH oxidation is not far from the removal of hydrogen from the substrate. Action on cytochrome oxidase was ruled out because only 18% inhibition of the oxidation of reduced cytochrome c occurred with the antibiotic compared 97% with sodium azide. Furthermore, succinate and NADH cytochrome c reductases were inhibited by flavensomycin and by antimycin A, indicating an action was prior to cytochrome oxidase. As concentration of the antibiotic increased, there was an increasing inhibition of formazan formation from various tetrazolium dyes when phenazine methosulfate was present. With succinate as the substrate, two of them, INT[1] and NBT[2], accept hydrogen between *b* and the antimycin sensitive site or CoQ and the antimycin sensitive site. The other, TTC[3], accepts hydrogen at cytochrome oxidase (NACHLAS *et al.*, 1960). The reduction of 2,6-dichlorphenolindophenol was also inhibited when phenazine methosulfate was present and the same trend occurred when NADH was the substrate except that the NADH system was less sensitive.

A further narrowing of potential sites of action was possible when experiments revealed that even in the presence of antimycin A, flavensomycin inhibited the reduction of the dyes. The antimycin prevents the reduction of dye from that portion of the cytochrome system at or beyond the antimycin sensitive site. Under such conditions, any reduction of dyes had to occur before this point, and the inhibition of the transfer of hydrogen must then have been somewhere between the substrate and CoQ. CoQ_6 and CoQ_{10} were not reduced by succinate of NADH probably because they did not enter the mitochondria. CoQ_1, however, was reduced by succinate and NADH; this reduction was inhibited by flavensomycin at concentrations similar to those that inhibited the entire oxidase systems.

The site of action on the electron transfer is thus between the substrate and CoQ_1. That CoQ_1 itself is not altered by flavensomycin is indicated by the absence of any change in its ultra violet absorption spectrum. The mitochondrial dehydrogenases for the respective substrates are probably the site of action. Indirect evidence supporting this concept was obtained from studies with 1-amino acid oxidase. This enzyme and succinic dehydrogenase are flavoproteins. Since flavensomycin inhibited these oxidases as well, it is reasonable to assume for the moment that succinic and NADH dehydrogenases are also inactivated by the antibiotic.

Though it is evident that flavensomycin acts on the succinic dehydrogenase to interrupt electron transfer, the question remains whether or not this is the primary means for its growth inhibiting activity. The concentrations of antibiotic that are needed to inhibit the electron flow are 20 times that required to inhibit growth. Even though the protein concentration used in the studies of the terminal electron transport system is much greater than that in the inoculum for growth studies, one would feel in firmer ground if there were less needed to inhibit growth and to inhibit respiration disparity in concentrations, that are large.

References

CANONICA, L., G. JOMMI, F. PELLIZONI e G. GIOLITTI: Antibiotici de streptomyces. Nota I. Sulla flavensomycin. Gazz. chim. ital. **91**, 1306 (1961a).

CANONICA, L., G. JOMMI, and P. PELIZZONI: Structure of flavensomycinic acid. Tetrahedron Letters 537 (1961b).

CANONICA, L., G. JOMMI e F. PELIZZONI: Antibiotici de streptomyce. Nota II. Sulla struttura dell'acido flavensomicinico. Gazz. chim. ital. **91**, 1315 (1961c).

CHACKO, C. I., and DAVID GOTTLIEB: The isolation of flavensomycin and humidin from the same strain of *Streptomyces griseus* and their antimicrobial properties. Phytopathology **55**, 587 (1965).

[1] INT = 2-p-iodophenyl-3-p-nitrophenyl-5-phenyl-tetrazolium chloride.

[2] NBT = 2,2'-di-p-nitrophenyl-(3,3'-dimethoxy-4,4'-biphenylene)-5,5'-diphenylditetrazolium.

[3] TTC = 2,3,5-triphenyltetrazolium chloride.

CRAVERI, R., and G. GIOLITTI: An antibiotic with fungicidal and insecticidal activity produced by streptomyces. Nature **179**, 1307 (1957).
CRAVERI, R., A. M. LUGULI e G. GIOLITTI: Attivita antifungina della flavensomicina nuovo antibiotica da *Streptomyces sp.* Nuovi ann. igiene e microbiol. **9**, 185 (1958).
DYER, J. R.: Personal communication 1965.
INOUE, Y., and DAVID GOTTLIEB: The mechanism of antifungal action of flavensomycin. (Paper in preparation 1966.)
LARDY, H. A., D. JOHNSON, and W. E. MCMURRAY: Antibiotics as tools for metabolic studies. I. A survey of toxic antibiotics in respiratory phosphorylative and glycolytic systems. Arch. Biochem. Biophys. **78**, 587 (1958).
NACHLAS, M. M., S. I. MARGULIES, and A. M. SELIGMAN: Sites of electron transfer to tetrazolium salts in the succinoxidase system. J. Biol. Chem. **235**, 2739 (1960).

Patulin*

Jaswant Singh

Patulin, 4-hydroxy-4H-furo [3,2c] pyran-2 (6H)-one, has an empirical formula $C_7H_6O_4$ and molecular weight 154. It has been isolated as colorless crystals, melting at 110.5°C, and is optically inactive. The ultraviolet absorption spectrum of the antibiotic has a single peak at 276 mμ. Patulin is unstable in alkali and loses biological activity (CHAIN *et al.*, 1942; ATKINSON, 1942; HOOPER *et al.*, 1944; and KAROW and FOSTER, 1944), but it is stable in acid (CHAIN *et al.*, 1942). The antibiotic was isolated from several species of *Penicillium* and *Aspergillus*, and a species of *Gymnoascus*. Details of the history of discovery of patulin and the various names given to it can be found in the reviews by FLOREY *et al.* (1949) and SINGH (1966). WOODWARD and SINGH (1949, 1950) elucidated its chemical structure (Fig. 1).

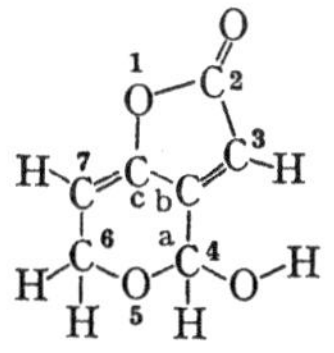

Fig. 1

Patulin has been found toxic to all kinds of microorganisms (Table 1). It inhibits the growth of Gram positive and Gram negative bacteria. Of the more than 70 species which were tested, none was completely resistant to the inhibitory effect of patulin. Most bacteria were inhibited at less than 20 μg patulin/ml but some required as much as 500 μg/ml. *Actinomyces scabies* was inhibited at about 6 μg/ml. Not all fungi are sensitive to patulin, and there is a considerable variation in the sensitivity of different species. Some species were inhibited at 5 μg patulin/ml whereas others, such as *Aspergillus clavatus*, were not affected even at 1000 μg/ml. Patulin is toxic to all protozoa that have been tested. The sensitivity of different species is dependent on the concentration of the antibiotic and the period of incubation. *Glaucoma piriformis*, for instance, required 24 hours for complete kill at 2 μg/ml, and only one hour at 200 μg/ml (JIROVEC, 1949). Some species, such as those of *Strigomonas* are more resistant and required 24 hours' exposure to 200 μg/ml for complete killing. Patulin also inhibited the growth of various individual cells and tissue cultures. VOLLMAR (1947) reported that mouse leucocytes and the normal epithelium cultures from rabbit cornea were stimulated at lower concentrations, 20 to 40 μg patulin/ml, and inhibited at higher concentrations, 100 to 200 μg/ml.

* Synonyms — clavacin, clavatin, claviformin, expansin, leucopin, mycoin c, penicidin, and tercinin.

Patulin proved ineffective in checking the multiplication of influenza virus in mice inoculated with that virus (RUBIN and GIARMAN, 1947). Effect of *in vitro* incubation of bacterial viruses with patulin varied with the concentrations of the antibiotic. High concentrations of patulin inactivated *Escherichia coli* phages (JONES, 1945) and 11 other bacterial viruses (HALL *et al.*, 1951). Low concentrations of the antibiotic, on the other hand, did not inactivate the phages of *Pseudomonas pyocyanea* (DICKINSON, 1948).

Table 1. *Toxicity of patulin to microorganisms*

Microorganism	Growth inhibitory concentration µg/ml	Reference
Bacteria		
Gram negative		
Agrobacterium tumefaciens	2 to 3	KLEMMER *et al.* (1955)
Eberthella typhi	20	OOSTERHUIS (1945/1947)
Escherichia coli	6 to 10	DE ROSNAY *et al.* (1952)
Gram positive		
Bacillus subtilis	4	KAVANAGH (1947)
	12.5 to 100	LEMBKE and FRAHM (1947)
Micrococcus pyogenes	12.5 to 100	LEMBKE *et al.* (1950)
Staphylococcus aureus	8	KAVANAGH (1947)
	12.5 to 30	RAISTRICK *et al.* (1943)
Actinomycetes		
Actinomyces scabies	6.25	GILLIVER (1946)
Fungi		
Aspergillus clavatus	1000 (Not inhibited)	KATZMAN *et al.* (1944)
Bodinia violacea	6.25	SANDERS (1946)
Candida albicans	300	REILLY *et al.* (1945)
Penicillium nigricans	62.5	WRIGHT (1955)
Pythium debaryanum	3.3	ANSLOW *et al.* (1943)
Ustilago tritici	10	TIMONIN (1946)
Protozoa		
Euglaena gracilis	100	JIROVEC (1949)
Glaucoma piriformis	2	JIROVEC (1949)
Paramecium aurelia	10	AUSTIN *et al.* (1956)
Strigomonas oncopelti	200	JIROVEC (1949)
Trypanosoma equiperdon	0.10	RUBIN (1947/1948)
Cells and tissue cultures		
Mouse leucocytes and the normal rabbit corneal epithelium cultures	100 to 200	VOLLMAR (1947)
Ehrlich carcinoma	20 to 40	VOLLMAR (1947)
Leucocytes	1.25	CHAIN *et al.* (1942)
L-cells in suspension culture	1.00	PERLMAN (1959)
Chick fibroblast cultures and ciliary movement in frog's buccal cavity	100	BROOM *et al.* (1944)
Chick heart and fibroblast cultures	10	KEILOVA-RODOVA (1949, 1951)
Mouse ascites tumor cells	60	LETTRE *et al.* (1954)

Patulin is highly toxic to plants. It inhibited the germination of seeds (GATTANI, 1957; TIMONIN, 1946; WALLEN and SKOLKO, 1951) and the growth of all plant parts, and also caused wilting (GÄUMANN and JAAG, 1947; IYENGAR and STARKEY, 1953; KLEMMER *et al.*, 1955; NICKELL and FINLAY, 1954; WANG, 1948; WRIGHT, 1951; VAN DER LAAN, 1947). The antibiotic inhibited the plasma streaming in *Elodea canadensis* (GAUMANN *et al.*, 1947), and the release of scopoletin from oat roots (MARTIN, 1958). It arrested the motility of *Chlamydomonas* and prevented the plasmolysis of *Spirogyra* (GAUMANN and v. ARX, 1947; MEYER *et al.*, 1952).

Patulin is highly toxic to animals (BROOM *et al.*, 1944; CHAIN *et al.*, 1942; FREERKSEN and BONICKE, 1951; KATZMAN *et al.*, 1944; and SCHWEITZER, 1946). However, OOSTERHUIS (1945/1947) showed that the application of the antibiotic as an ointment was useful for curing clinical dermatomycosis. The data of VOLLMAR (1947) suggested a possible use of patulin in the healing of corneal wounds. BOLLAG (1949) reported that the lymphocyte count decreased markedly in the blood of mice injected with 100 μg patulin/day but the granulocyte count was unaffected. After the injections were stopped, the lymphocyte count increased again and was sometimes accompanied by an increase in the granulocytes. The general consensus of all the pharmacological studies is that patulin increases vascular permeability causing strong edema. A rise, followed by a fall in the blood pressure occurred in animals injected with the antibiotic. KATZMAN *et al.* (1944) reported that the antibiotic suppressed the formation of urine and caused a rise in the blood sugar. The LD_{100} i.v. for mice is about 25 mg/kg body weight (BROOM *et al.*, 1944; RAISTRICK *et al.*, 1943).

Cytological Effects

Patulin inhibits the cell and/or nuclear division but the observations regarding the precise nature of its action are quite conflicting. BABUDIERI (1948) reported that patulin inhibited the reproductive function of bacteria causing the appearance of giant forms among them. WANG (1948) found that the antibiotic caused the appearance of binucleate cells in corn and onion roots. He did not find any alteration in the chromosome behaviour and, therefore, thought that patulin probably inhibited the cell wall formation. KEILOVA-RODOVA (1949, 1951) reported on the mitostatic action of patulin in the fibroblast and osteoblast cultures of chick embryo. She found that the chromosomes were in pathological condition at all stages of mitosis especially at the metaphase. She reported that there was a reduction in the number of prophases, an increase in the number of reconstruction phases, and a frequent formation of binucleate cells. SENTEIN (1955) revealed that patulin caused total or partial fragmentation of chromosomes during mitosis in avian eggs. A deleterious action of patulin on the nucleus and chromosomes of *Allium cepa* and *Lepidium sativum* was reported by STEINEGER and LEUPI (1956) who believed that spindle mechanism was not affected. On the other hand, RONDANELLI *et al.* (1957) found that sulfhydryl compounds such as glutathione, cysteine and dimercaptopropanol could prevent the mitostatic effect of patulin and concluded that the spindle mechanism was the site of patulin action; they thought that the antibiotic might have reacted with the sulfhydryl groups of the contractile fibers and thereby rendered them inelastic.

Sulfhydryl compounds such as cysteine, glutathione, thioglycollate, and dimercaptopropanol, prevent the toxic action of patulin (ATKINSON, 1943a, b; BUSTINZA and LOPEZ, 1949; DANIEL *et al.*, 1955; DELAUNAY *et al.*, 1955; DE ROSNAY *et al.*, 1952; GEIGER and CONN, 1945; MIESCHER, 1950; RINDERKNECHT *et al.*, 1947; RONDANELLI *et al.*, 1957). CAVALLITO and BAILEY (1944) found the inactivation of patulin only with cysteine and not with glutathione or thioglycollate. On the other hand, AFRIDI (1962) reported that cysteine, glutathione, and tryptophan augment the inhibitory effect of patulin on the formation of induced nitrate reductase in higher plants. Although cysteine reacts with patulin resulting in decrease in the ultraviolet absorption of the antibiotic, the reaction requires very high concentrations of cysteine to patulin and is very slow even at the favorably high concentrations of cysteine (SINGH, 1966).

The antibiotic activity of patulin is also decreased by other compounds such as peptone, glycine, methionine, asparagine, p-aminobenzoic acid (DE ROSNAY *et al.*, 1952; WAKSMAN and BUGIE, 1943); by wheat flour (TIMONIN, 1946); and by sodium sulfite, sodium thiosulfate, and sodium pyrosulfite (MIESCHER, 1950). On the other hand, tryptophan, urea, and thiourea increased the toxicity of patulin (DE ROSNAY *et al.*, 1952).

Biochemical Effects

Patulin inhibits the aerobic respiration of bacteria (CHAIN *et al.*, 1942, 1944; LEMBKE and FRAHM, 1947; LEMBKE and HAHN, 1954), fungi (GOTTLIEB and SINGH, 1964), phagocytic cells (DELAUNAY *et al.*, 1955), and guinea pig kidney slices and brain homogenates (ANDRAUD *et al.*, 1963). Oxygen consumption by the cell-free extracts of *Claviceps purpurea* was inhibited at the growth inhibitory concentrations (GOTTLIEB and SINGH, 1964). Mycelial respiration was inhibited to a progressively increasing extent with incubation time and complete suppression occurred in about 3 to 6 hours. On the other hand, the inhibition of the oxygen consumption by the cell-free extracts was very rapid and completely suppressed within 40 minutes. ANDRAUD *et al.* (1963) had found that inhibition of the oxygen consumption by the guinea pig brain homogenates was much stronger than that by the kidney slices. The disparity in the time required to completely inhibit the respiration of the mycelia and their cell-free extracts might be due to the presence of a membrane barrier to patulin in whole mycelia and its absence in cell-free extracts.

There have been reports that patulin affects the semipermeability of cell membranes. GÄUMANN *et al.* (1947) found that the antibiotic caused leakage of anthocyanins from beet root slices. Patulin inhibited the absorption of potassium ions by erythrocytes (KAHN, 1957). Recent experiments have shown that concomitant with the inhibition of respiration of fungal mycelium, there is an inhibition of the uptake of glucose by the mycelium (SINGH, 1966). However, patulin did not cause leakage of metabolites (inorganic phosphate, sugars, amino acids, etc.) from *C. purpurea* mycelium, or of hemoglobin from bovine erythrocytes (GOTTLIEB and SINGH, 1964). LETTRÉ *et al.* (1954a, b) reported that the antibiotic did not affect the permeability of mouse ascites tumor cells to ^{32}P.

Patulin probably does not interfere directly in any of the synthetic processes. The antibiotic did not inhibit the multiplication of influenza virus in mice (RUBIN and GIARMAN, 1947), and therefore, should not inhibit the synthesis of the protein and RNA of which this virus is composed. Recent studies on *C. purpurea* have shown that patulin does not change the gross chemical composition of fungal mycelium grown in the presence of lethal or sublethal concentrations of the antibiotic (SINGH, 1966). These mycelia were analyzed for total lipids, soluble carbohydrates, total carbohydrates, ribonucleic acid, desoxyribonucleic acid, protein, chitin, and residue. In the presence of sublethal concentrations of patulin, a partial respiratory inhibition resulted in a reduced supply of energy for all the synthetic processes, and therefore, the growth proceeded at slower rate without any effect on the gross chemical composition.

Patulin partially inhibited co-carboxylase at 5.2×10^{-2} M (KARRER and VISCONTINI, 1947). The general dehydrogenase activity of mouse ascites tumor cells measured with tetrazolium salts using glucose, phenylalanine, succinate, and hypoxanthine as substrates was inhibited at 20 μg patulin/ml (HOLSCHER, 1950, 1951). However, SCHMITZ (1950) did not find any inhibition of the dehydrogenase activity of mouse ascites cells measured with the Thunberg technique at 30 to 120 μg patulin/ml.

GOTTLIEB and SINGH (1964) investigated the effect of patulin on the terminal electron transport system of *C. purpurea* cell-free extracts. Succinate oxidase and succinate dehydrogenase activities were strongly inhibited (90% and about 60 to 80% respectively) at 5×10^{-2} M (1,155 μg patulin/mg protein). NADH oxidase, succinate cytochrome c reductase, and cytochrome oxidase activities were inhibited 40, 30, and 30% respectively at 5×10^{-2} M (7,000 μg/mg protein). Inhibition of the succinate-cytochrome c reductase increased from 30% when the antibiotic was added at the time of measurement of the activity, to over 80% if the cell-free extract was preincubated with patulin for about 30 minutes before the activity was measured.

Incubation of patulin with the cell free extract caused some changes in the antibiotic which made it more toxic. Similar changes occurred in aqueous solutions of patulin on standing at 26 C. Inhibition of the NADH oxidase of mitochondria by patulin from freshly made solutions, 5-day old solutions, and from 9-day old solutions was 40, 60, and 90%, respectively. Crystalline glucose oxidase and glyceraldehyde-3-phosphate dehydrogenase were not inhibited by patulin (SINGH, 1966).

Inhibition of respiration by patulin can cause suppression of the growth of microorganisms. But the growth and respiration of an organism may also be inhibited indirectly by the effect of an antibiotic on the permeability of cellular membranes. The membrane permeability can be affected in two ways. First, the cell membrane may be so damaged by an antibiotic action that it can no longer hold vital metabolites inside the cell; compounds such as inorganic phosphate, sugars, amino acids, nucleotides, and cofactors, etc. may leak out of the cell resulting in the cessation of all cellular functions. Second, although the general integrity of the membrane may remain unaltered, some nutrient transport mechanism on or in the cell membrane may be altered by the antibiotic thus impeding the nutrient absorption, and therefore, arresting respiration and growth. Patulin does not completely change membrane permeability in fungi and erythrocytes since no leakage occurred (GOTTLIEB and SINGH, 1964); but it inhibits the uptake of potassium ions in the case of erythrocytes (KAHN, 1957), and of glucose in the case of fungal mycelium (SINGH, 1966). This indicates that patulin may disturb some nutrient transport mechanism(s). However, the inhibition by patulin of the oxygen consumption of cell-free systems, in which the respiration does not depend upon substrate permeability, shows that the antibiotic has a direct effect on the respiration. Since glucose and potassium uptake require energy which is produced by respiration, the inhibition of the nutrient absorption may be the result rather than the cause of respiratory inhibition.

Cytological effects of patulin can also be interpreted on the basis of respiratory inhibition. It is known that powerful inhibitors of respiration such as cyanide, azide, malonate, iodoacetate, fluoride, dinitrophenol, etc. strongly inhibit mitosis (BULLOUGH and JOHNSON, 1951). The importance of the respiratory inhibition as the mode of patulin action is further strengthened by the insensitivity of anabolic systems such as nucleic acid synthesis and protein synthesis *in vivo*.

The exact site of patulin action on respiration is not yet very clear. The inhibition of the terminal electron transport from NADH and succinate by fungal cell-free extracts required patulin in concentrations much higher than those required for the inhibition of growth, and the respiration of the whole mycelia or the cell-free extracts. Because the relative insensitivity of the terminal electron transport system contrasts sharply with the sensitivity of oxygen consumption by the whole mycelia or their cell-free extracts, it is possible that a vulnerable site may occur in the respiratory reactions prior to the terminal electron transport chain. Inhibition of the growth of anaerobic bacteria (DE ROSNAY *et al.*, 1952) also suggests that patulin has a site of action other than that in the terminal part of aerobic respiration. Nevertheless, one cannot entirely rule out the terminal electron transport as one area of patulin action because of its relative insensitivity to the antibiotic, since the preincubation of patulin with fungal cell-free extracts markedly increased the inhibition of succinate-cytochrome c reductase and an increased inhibition of mitochondrial NADH oxidase occurred with aged (changed) solutions of patulin.

The earliest hypothesis regarding the mechanism of action of patulin was based on the inactivation of patulin by sulfhydryl compounds. Patulin would thus interfere with cell metabolism by complexing with vital sulfhydryl groups of certain enzymes or metabolites (CAVALLITO and BAILEY, 1944; CAVALLITO and HASKELL, 1945; CAVALLITO *et al.*, 1945; GEIGER and CONN, 1945; and RINDERKNECHT *et al.*, 1947). Investigations by SINGH (1966) do not support this concept. The reaction of patulin with cysteine was extremely slow even with very high concentrations of cysteine. In addition, patulin did not inhibit glyceraldehyde-3-phosphate dehydrogenase, an enzyme having sulfhydryl groups in its active center.

The available evidence shows that patulin acts on respiration, and that a modified form of patulin may be the real toxic agent. The exact site and mechanism is not known at present, although terminal electron transport is one segment vulnerable to the antibiotic. Some step(s) prior to the terminal electron transport may also be sensitive to the action of patulin or its changed product.

References

AFRIDI, M. M. R. K.: Effect of some antibiotics on the induced formation of nitrate reductase in higher plants. Hindustan Antibiot. Bull. **5**, 51—54 (1962).

ANDRAUD, G., A. M. AUBLET-CUVELIER, J. COUQUELET, R. CUVELIER et P. TRONCHE: Activité comparée sur la respiration cellulaire de la patuline naturelle et d'un isomere synthese. Compt. rend. Soc. biol. (Paris) **157** (7), 144—146 (1963).

ANSLOW, W. K., H. RAISTRICK, and G. SMITH: Antifungal substances from molds. Part 1. Patulin, (anhydro-3-hydroxymethylene-tetrahydro-1:4-pyrone-2-carboxylic acid), a metabolic product of *Penicillium patulum* BAINIER and *Penicillium expansum* (LINK) THOM. Chem. & Ind. (London) **62**, 236—238 (1943).

ATKINSON, N.: Antibacterial substances produced by molds. I. Penicidin a product of the growth of *Penicillium*. Australian J. Exptl. Biol. Med. Sci. **20**, 287—288 (1942).

ATKINSON, N., and N. F. STANLEY: Antibacterial substances produced by molds. 4. The detection and occurrence of suppressors of penicidin activity. Australian J. Exptl. Biol. Med. Sci. **21**, 249—253 (1943).

ATKINSON, N., and N. F. STANLEY: Antibacterial substances produced by molds. 5. The mechanism of action of some penicidin suppressors. Australian J. Exptl. Biol. Med. Sci. **21**, 255—257 (1943).

AUSTIN, M. L., D. WIDMAYER, and L. M. WALKER: Antigenic transformation as an adaptive response of *Paramoecium aurelia* to patulin; relation to cell division. Physiol. Zool. **29**, 261—287 (1956).

BABUDIERI, B.: L'azione antibatterica di alcuni antibiotici, studiata col microscopio elettronico. Rend. ist. super. sanità (Rome). **11**, 577—598 (1948). Abstract World Med. **5**, 662—663 (1949). Chem. Abstract **46**, 7178b (1952).

BOLLAG, W.: Die Wirkung von Patulin auf das myclo- und lymphopoetische System der Maus. Experientia **5**, 447—448 (1949).

BROOM, W. A., E. BULBRING, C. J. CHAPMAN, J. W. F. HAMPTON, A. M. THOMSON, J. UNGAR, R. WIEN, and G. WOOLFE: The pharmacology of patulin. Brit. J. Exptl. Pathol. **25**, 195—207 (1944).

BULLOUGH, W. S., and M. JOHNSON: Energy relations of mitotic activity in adult mouse epidermis. Proc. Roy. Soc. (London) B **138**, 562—575 (1951).

BUSTINZA, L. F., and A. C. LOPEZ: Preliminary tests in the study of influence of antibiotics on the germination of seeds. Rept. Proc. 4th Intern. Congr. Microbiol., 1947, 160—161 (1949).

CAVALLITO, C. J., and J. H. BAILEY: Preliminary note on the inactivation of antibiotics. Science **100**, 390 (1944).

CAVALLITO, C. J., and T. H. HASKELL: The mechanism of action of antibiotics. J. Am. Chem. Soc. **67**, 1991 (1945).

CAVALLITO, C. J., J. H. BAILEY, T. H. HASKELL, J. R. MCCORMICK, and W. F. WARNER: The inactivation of antibacterial agents and their mechanism of action. J. Bacteriol. **50**, 61 (1945).

CHAIN, E., H. W. FLOREY, and M. A. JENNINGS: An antibacterial substance produced by *Penicillium claviforme*. Brit. J. Exptl. Pathol. **23**, 202—205 (1942).

CHAIN, E., H. W. FLOREY, and M. A. JENNINGS: Identity of patulin and claviformin. Lancet **246**, 112—114 (1944).

DANIEL, P., E. LASFARGUES, and A. DELAUNAY: Sur la dissociation possible du pouvoir antibiotique et du pouvoir antimitotique de la patuline. Compt. rend. Soc. Biol. (Paris) **149**, 18—19 (1955).

DELAUNAY, A., P. DANIEL, C. DE ROQUEFEUIL, and M. HENON: Effets exercés par la patuline et des mélanges patuline-cystéine sur les propriétés physiologiques des cellules phagocytaires. Ann. inst. Pasteur **88**, 699—712 (1955).

DE ROSNAY, C. D., MARTIN-DUPONT, and R. JENSEN: An antibiotic, mycoin c. J. méd. Bordeaux et Sud-Ouest **129**, 189—199 (1952).

DICKINSON, L.: Bacteriophages of *Pseudomonas pyocyanea*. I. The effect of various substances upon their development. J. Gen. Microbiol. **2**, 154—161 (1948).

FLOREY, H. W., E. CHAIN, N. G. HEATLEY, M. JENNINGS, A. G. SANDERS, E. P. ABRAHAM, and M. E. FLOREY: Antibiotics, 2 vols., 1774 p. London-New York-Toronto: Oxford University Press 1949.

FREERKSEN, E., u. R. BONICKE: Die Inaktivierung des Patulins in vivo (Modellversuche zur Bestimmung des Wertes antibakterieller Substanzen für therapeutische Zwecke). Z. Hyg. Infektionskrankh. **132**, 274—291 (1951).

GATTANI, M. L.: Control of damping off of safflower with antibiotics. Plant Disease Reptr. **41**, 160—164 (1957).

GÄUMANN, E., u. A. v. ARX: Antibiotika als pflanzliche Plasmagifte. II. Ber. schweiz. botan. Ges. **57**, 174—183 (1947).

GÄUMANN, E., u. O. JAAG: Die physiologischen Grundlagen des parasitogenen Welkens. II. Ber. schweiz. botan. Ges. **57**, 132—148 (1947).

GÄUMANN, E., O. JAAG u. R. BRAUN: Antibiotika als pflanzliche Plasmagifte. Experientia **3**, 70—71 (1947).

GEIGER, W. B., and J. E. CONN: The mechanism of antibiotic action of clavacin and penicillic acid. J. Am. Chem. Soc. **67**, 112—116 (1945).

GILLIVER, K.: Inhibitory action of antibiotics on plant pathogenic bacteria and fungi. Ann. Botany (London) **10**, 271—282 (1946).

GOTTLIEB, D., and J. SINGH: The mechanism of patulin inhibition of fungi. Riv. patol. vegetale, Ser. III **4** (4), 455—479 (1964).

HALL, E. A., F. KAVANAGH, and I. N. ASHESHOV: Action of forty-five antibacterial substances on bacterial viruses. Antibiotics & Chemotherapy **1**, 369—378 (1951).

HOLSCHER, H. A.: Über den Nachweis von Dehydrasen der Tumorzelle mittels Tetrazoliumsalzen. Z. Krebsforsch. **56**, 587—595 (1950).

HOLSCHER, H. A.: Einige Beobachtungen an Tumorzellen und den darin enthaltenen Granula. Z. Krebsforsch. **57**, 634—636 (1951).

HOOPER, J. R., H. W. ANDERSON, P. SKELL, and H. E. CARTER: The identity of clavacin with patulin. Science **99**, 16 (1944).

IYENGAR, M. R. S., and R. L. STARKEY: Synergism and antagonism of auxin by antibiotics. Science **118**, 357—358 (1953).

JIROVEC, O.: Der Einfluß des Streptomycins und Patulins auf einige Protozoen. Experientia **5**, 74—77 (1949).

JONES, D.: The effect of antibiotic substances upon bacteriophages. J. Bacteriol. **50**, 341—348 (1945).

KAHN, JR., J. B.: Effects of various lactones and related compounds on cation transfer in incubated cold stored human erythrocytes. J. Pharmacol. Exptl. Therap. **121**, 234—251 (1957).

KAROW, E. O., and J. W. FOSTER: An antibiotic substance from species of *Gymnoascus* and *Penicillium*. Science **99**, 265—266 (1944).

KARRER, P., u. M. VISCONTINI: Einfluß verschiedener Zusätze auf die Wirksamkeit der Cocarboxylase. Helv. Chim. Acta **30**, 268—271 (1947).

KATZMAN, P. A., E. E. HAYS, C. K. CAIN, J. J. VAN WYK, F. J. REITHEL, S. A. THAYER, and E. A. DOISY: Clavacin, an antibiotic substance from *Aspergillus clavatus*. J. Biol. Chem. **154**, 475 (1944).

KAVANAGH, F.: Activities of 22 antibacterial substances against 9 species of bacteria. J. Bacteriol. **54**, 761—766 (1947).

KEILOVA-RODOVA, H.: Effect of patulin on tissue cultures. Experientia **5**, 242 (1949).

KEILOVA-RODOVA, H.: Effect of antibiotics on tissue cultures. Časopis lékáru českých **90**, 38—42 (1951).

KLEMMER, H. W., A. J. RIKER, and O. N. ALLEN: Inhibition of crown gall by selected antibiotics. Phytopathology **45**, 618—625 (1955).

LEMBKE, A., u. H. FRAHM: Untersuchungen über Mycoine. II. Zentr. Bakteriol. Parasitenk., Abt. I. Orig. **152**, 221—230 (1947).

LEMBKE, A., and B. HAHN: The action of metabolic products of *Penicillium claviforme* on cells and tissues varying in their stage of development. Kiel. Milchwirtsch. Forschungsber. **6**, 41—58, 219—241 (1954).

LEMBKE, A., M. KORNLEIN u. H. FRAHM: Beiträge zum Brucellose-Problem. I. Mitteilung. Zentr. Bakteriol. Parasitenk., Abt. I. Orig. **155**, 16—31 (1950).

LETTRÉ, H., E. SEIDLER u. H. WRBA: Untersuchung der Hemmstoffe in Wirkung auf Verdopplungsgeschwindigkeit und Phosphataufnahme von Tumoren mit Hilfe von ^{32}P. Z. Krebsforsch. **60**, 86—90 (1954).

LETTRÉ, H., H. WRBA u. E. SEIDLER: Charakterisierung von Tumorhemmstoffen mit Hilfe markierter Tumorzellen. Naturwissenschaften **41**, 122—123 (1954).

MARTIN, P.: Einfluß der Kulturfiltrate von Mikroorganismen auf die Abgabe von Scopoletin aus den Keimwurzeln des Hafers (*Avena sativa* L.). Arch. Mikrobiol. **29**, 154—168 (1958).

MEYER, J., R. SARTORY, J. MALGRAS, and J. TOUILLIER: Animal and plant control tests for antibiotics. Bull. Assoc. Diplomes Microbiol Fac. Pharm. Nancy **46**, 30—42 (1952).

MIESCHER, G.: Über die Wirkungsweise von Patulin auf höhere Pflanzen, insbesondere auf *Solanum lycopersicum* L. Chem. Zentr. 1950 II, **121**, 546. Phytopathol. Z. **16**, 369—397 (1950).

NICKELL, L. G., and A. C. FINLAY: Antibiotics and their effects on plant growth. J. Agr. Food Chem. **2**, 178—182 (1954).

OOSTERHUIS, H. K.: Antibiotica uit Schimmels. Mededel. Lab. Physiol. Chem. Univ. Amsterdam **10**, (3) 116 pp. (1945/47).

PERLMAN, D., N. A. GIRFFRE, P. N. JACKSON, and F. E. GIARDINELLO: Effects of antibiotics on multiplication of L-cells in suspension culture. Proc. Soc. Exptl. Biol. Med. **102**, 290—292 (1959).

RAISTRICK, H., J. H. BIRKINSHAW, S. E. MICHAEL, ARTHUR BRACKEN, W. E. GYE, W. A. HOPKINS, and MAJOR GREENWOOD: Patulin in the common cold. Collaborative research on a derivative of *Penicillium patulum* BAINIER. Lancet **245**, 625—635 (1943).

REILLY, H. C., A. SCHATZ, and S. A. WAKSMAN: Antifungal properties of antibiotic substances. J. Bacteriol. **49**, 585—594 (1945).

RINDERKNECHT, H., J. L. WARD, F. BERGEL, and A. L. MORRISON: Studies on antibiotics. Biochem. J. **41**, 463—469 (1947).

RONDANELLI, E. G., P. GORINI, E. STROSSELTI, and D. PICORARI: Inhibition of the metaphase effect of patulin by thiols. Experimental research *in vivo* and *in vitro*. Haematologia (Pavia) **42**, 1427—1440 (1957).

RUBIN, B. A.: The trypanocidal effect of antibiotic lactones and of their analogs. Yale J. Biol. and Med. **20**, 233—271 (1947/48).

RUBIN, B. A., and N. J. GIARMAN: The therapy of experimental influenza in mice with antibiotic lactones and related compounds. Yale J. Biol. and Med. **19**, 1017—1022 (1947).

SANDERS, A. G.: Effect of some antibiotics on pathogenic fungi. Lancet **250**, 44—46 (1946).

SCHMITZ, H.: Über den Nachweis von Dehydrasen am Ascitestumor der Maus mit der Thunberg-Methode. Z. Krebsforsch. **56**, 596—600 (1950).

SCHWEITZER, A.: Pharmacological studies on the effects of clavatin. Exptl. Med. Surg. **4**, 289—305 (1946).

SENTEIN, P.: Alterations du fuseau mitotique et fragmentation des chromosomes par l'action de la patuline sur l'oeuf d'Urodeles en segmentation. Compt. rend. Soc. Biol. (Paris) **149**, 1621—1622 (1955).

SINGH, J.: Mechanism of antifungal action of patulin. Ph. D. Thesis, University of Illinois, Urbana, Illinois, U.S.A. 1966.

STEINEGGER, E., and H. LEUPI: Influence of plant substances on root growth of *Allium cepa* and germination of *Lepidium sativum*. Pharm. Acta Helv. **31**, 45—51 (1956).

TIMONIN, M. I.: Activity of patulin against *Ustilago tritici* (PERS.) JEN. Can. J. Agr Sci. **26**, 358—368 (1946).

VAN DER LAAN, P. A.: Emploi de substances antibiotiques comme fongicides dans la lutte centre *Cercospora nicotianae* attaquant le tabac. Tijdschr. Plantenziekten **53**, 180—187 (1945). Chim. & ind. (Paris) **61**, 61 (1949).
VOLLMAR, H.: Versuche über die Beeinflussung des Wachstums von Gewebe durch Patulin. Z. Hyg. Infektionskrankh. **127**, 316—321 (1947).
WAKSMAN, S. A., and E. BUGIE: Action of antibiotic substances upon *Ceratostomella ulmi*. Proc. Soc. Exptl. Biol. Med. **54**, 79—82 (1943).
WALLEN, V. R., and A. J. SKOLKO: Activity of antibiotics against *Ascochyta pisi*. Can. J. Botany **29**, 316—323 (1951).
WANG, F. H.: The effects of clavacin on root growth. Botan. Bull. Acad. Sinica **2**, 265—269 (1948).
WOODWARD, R. B., and G. SINGH: The structure of patulin. J. Am. Chem. Soc. **71**, 758—759 (1949).
WOODWARD, R. B., and G. SINGH: The synthesis of patulin. J. Am. Chem. Soc. **72**, 1428 (1950).
WRIGHT, J. M.: Phytotoxic effects of some antibiotics. Ann. Botany (London) **15**, 493—499 (1951).
WRIGHT, J. M.: The production of antibiotics in soil. II. Production of griseofulvin by *Penicillium nigricans*. Ann. Appl. Biol. **43**, 288—296 (1955).

Valinomycin

F. Edmund Hunter, Jr. and Lois S. Schwartz

The isolation of and chemical studies on valinomycin from *Streptomyces fulvissimus* were first reported by BROCKMANN and SCHMIDT-KASTNER (1955). SHEMYAKIN *et al.* (1965) reported its structure to be a cyclododecadepsipeptide consisting of three repetitions of the sequence, D-valine, L-lactic acid, L-valine, and D-α-hydroxyvaleric acid. The empirical formula is $C_{54}H_{90}O_{18}N_6$ with a molecular weight of 1110. The structural formula is indicated in Fig. 1.

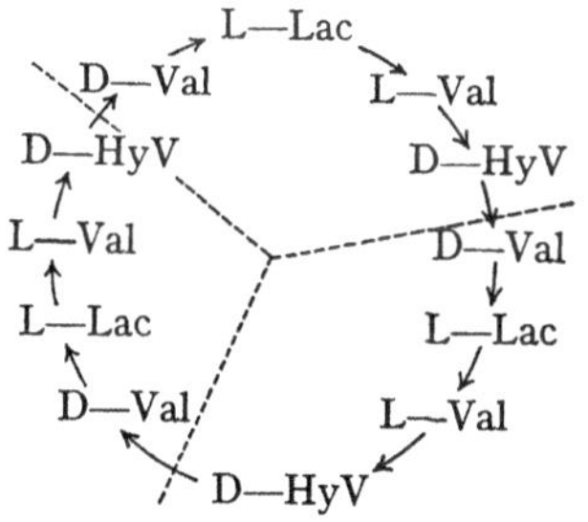

Fig. 1. Structure of valinomycin

The minimal growth inhibiting concentration of valinomycin for *Mycobacterium tuberculosis* or *phlei*, many fungi, and some strains of *Staphylococcus* aureus is 1—2μg/ml, or 10^{-6} M. *Bacillus subtilis*, *E. coli*, *B. mycoides*, and some strains of staphylococcus require 50μg/ml and more for inhibition (BROCKMANN and SCHMIDT-KASTNER, 1955; SHEMYAKIN *et al.*, 1965). Structure activity relationships have been studied in detail by SHEMYAKIN *et al.* (1965). The cyclic structure is absolutely essential, with the 36 atom ring being optimal. The presence of both D- and L-amino acids is also essential, although some variations are possible.

In vivo subcutaneous doses protected mice against *Trypanosoma brucei* infection (BROCKMANN and SCHMIDT-KASTNER, 1955).

Many cyclopeptides are not toxic on oral administration, probably because the ring is opened by digestive enzymes or they are not absorbed. Valinomycin, however, is reported to have an LD_{50} for mice of 2.5 mg/kg orally (SHEMYAKIN *et al.*, 1965) and 1.0 mg/kg subcutaneously or intraperitoneally (BROWN *et al.*, 1962; MCMURRAY and BEGG, 1959). These amounts of valinomycin, if evenly distributed, would give concentrations of 10^{-6} M, about the same as effective against the more sensitive microorganisms and ten-fold higher than the concentrations (10^{-7} M) which uncouple phosphorylation or affect ion transport in isolated mitochondria. Therefore, the type of effect observed on mitochondria could be the principal mode of action of valinomycin on microorganisms and on higher animals.

No specific effects of valinomycin on carbohydrate, fat, protein, or nucleic acid metabolism have been reported. However, if valinomycin uncouples oxidative phosphorylation, indirect effects on many systems must be expected.

McMURRAY and BEGG (1959) found that concentrations of valinomycin as low as 0.1 μg/ml (10^{-7} M) would completely uncouple oxidative phosphorylation in rat liver mitochondria with essentially no effect on the oxygen uptake when ADP, hexokinase, and glucose were present. In the absence of a phosphate acceptor system respiration was stimulated five fold. ATPase was stimulated to a degree very similar to that with 2,4-dinitrophenol. PRESSMAN (1963) confirmed these observations and showed that there was an instantaneous stimulation of respiration in phosphate-acceptor limited systems when valinomycin was added. The exact site of uncoupling could not be pinpointed. Valinomycin also disrupts oxidative phophorylation in mitochondria from pigeon heart, rabbit kidney, and potato tuber.

BALTSCHEFFSKY (1961, 1962) tested valinomycin on photophosphorylation in chromatophores of *Rhodospirillum rubrum* and in spinach chloroplasts. The antibiotic inhibited 40—50% in *R. rubrum*, but had no effect on photophosphorylation in the chloroplasts. This was interpreted to mean that there were two phosphorylation sites in *R. rubrum*, with only one being sensitive to valinomycin. The valinomycin insensitive phosphorylation was the one still present when the dye phenazine methosulfate was used. The absence of the valinomycin-sensitive photophosphorylation step in chloroplasts may be an artifact from preparation rather than inherent differences in mechanism.

PRESSMAN (1963) noted that valinomycin was quite different from 2,4-dinitrophenol as an uncoupler of phosphorylation. There was ejection of H^+ ion from the mitochondria during electron transport in the presence of valinomycin. Further studies by MOORE and PRESSMAN (1964, 1965a, 1965c) indicated that the ability of valinomycin to uncouple phosphorylation was dependent on the presence of K^+. Measurements with cationic electrodes demonstrated K^+ uptake in large amounts. MOORE and PRESSMAN postulated that valinomycin stimulated energy dependent accumulation of K^+, with the apparent uncoupling of phosphorylation being due to the fact that all of the energy supply was being used for ion transport. Further studies (HARRIS, COCKRELL and PRESSMAN, 1966; CHAPPELL and CROFTS, 1965; OGATA and RASMUSSEN, 1966; AZZI and AZZONE, 1965) have confirmed that there is an energy dependent uptake of K^+ in the presence of valinomycin, but the mechanism responsible for this is a matter of debate. The high energy intermediate used is non-phosphorylated and is formed prior to the site of oligomycin action. It can be formed with ATP, and in this case the reaction is inhibited by oligomycin. Whether there is any direct uncoupling effect of valinomycin at higher concentrations is uncertain.

SHEMYAKIN (1965), in collaboration with PRESSMAN, carried out a most important study showing (a) highly specific structural requirements in valinomycin analogs and (b) both qualitative and quantitative correlation between antimicrobial activity and the ability of valinomycin analogs to induce K^+ uptake by mitochondria. PRESSMAN (1966) has reported that valinomycin also accelerates K^+ uptake by azotobacter, so there are strong indications that the mechanism of action on microorganisms and on mitochondria are the same. If correct, this means that the antibiotic action arises from diversion of cellular energy into an unprofitable cyclic flux of ions. Werner, Harris and Pressman (1966) have shown that valinomycin does affect mitochondria inside ascites tumor cells, and Hofer, Crockrell and Pressman (1966) have suggested that K^+ concentrations may have a regulatory role in energy metabolism.

The effects of valinomycin on mitochondria have been studied in detail by several workers (Harris *et al.*, 1966; Ogata and Rasmussen, 1966; Azzi and Azzone, 1965; Chappell and Crofts, 1965). The cation uptake is fairly selective for K^+ as against Na^+. The apparent requirement for phosphate was due to phosphate acting as a permeant anion to enter with the K^+. It can be replaced by arsenate, acetate, and others. Chloride penetrates very poorly. The amount of substrate that will be required, the degree to which respiration will be stimulated, the extent of mitochondrial swelling, and the degree of uncoupling (failure to phosphorylate ADP) are determined by the K^+ concentration and by the permeant anions present. This is because without a permeant anion the process is limited. However, with a permeant anion the uptake of K^+ is large and the secondary effects of swelling as well the direct effects of valinomycin set the stage for an energy requiring but cyclic and futile flux of ions.

That valinomycin acts on mitochondrial membranes to increase permeability to K^+ and K^+ uptake is generally accepted, but different conclusions have been drawn with respect to mechanisms. Chappell and Crofts (1965), Ogata and Rasmussen (1966), Mitchell and Moyle (1965), and Lynn and Brown (1965a) have concluded that the primary effect of valinomycin is increased permeability to K^+. Chappell and Crofts (1965) and Mitchell (1965) consider the uptake of K^+ to be a secondary electrochemical response to a metabolically driven extrusion of H^+. Ogata and Rasmussen do not favor the simple H^+ pump explanation, but do believe that swelling is due to osmotic forces. Lynn and Brown (1965b) suggest that exchanges are responsible for ejection of H^+. In the view of Mitchell and Chappell the H^+ pump is always ready to work, but the net operation in normal mitochondria is limited by ions available and the pH gradient which can be created. Pressman (1965a, 1965c) and Harris, Crockrell and Pressman (1966) have reported that H^+ extrusion and K^+ uptake are not at all equivalent under some conditions and that swelling changes cannot be explained completely on osmotic grounds. They believe that passive permeability to K^+ is increased, as indicated by outward flux, but that a major effect of valinomycin is stimulation of an energy driven pump for uptake of K^+. Inherent in this pump mechanism are mechanochemical changes that cause alterations in light scattering (Pressman, 1965b). Harris *et al.* (1966) point out that increased permeability to K^+ induced by valinomycin could not alone explain experimentally observed shifts from K^+ loss to K^+ uptake.

There is general agreement that if the mitochondria have not undergone too much alteration, interruption of the energy supply by anaerobiosis, electron transport inhibition, or true uncoupling by dinitrophenol results in reversal of the changes as the accumulated K^+ moves out of the mitochondria (Harris, Crockrell and Pressman, 1966; Chappell and Crofts, 1965; Ogata and Rasmussen, 1966). Remarkable is the immediate disappearance of the H^+ gradient, first observed with dinitrophenol by Mitchell and Moyle (1965).

The mechanism by which valinomycin produces the selective increase in apparent pore size is not known. Direct reaction with changes in lipid-protein relationships have been proposed. In preliminary experiments CHAPPELL, CROFTS and BANGHAM (1965) have observed increased cation permeability in phospholipid micelles viewed as model membranes. However, valinomycin did not increase the permeability of the erythrocyte membrane. Energy dependent changes in mitochondrial membrane permeability may explain some of the complexity (AZZI and AZZONE, 1965; HUNTER, 1963). Yet to be explained are the effects of sucrose and the inhibition of phosphate-induced swelling and ATP-induced contraction by valinomycin under some circumstances.

See Addendum

References

AZZI, A., and G. F. AZZONE: Potassium-transport-linked swelling induced by valinomycin in liver mitochondria. Biochem. J. **96**, 1C (1965).

BALTSCHEFFSKY, H.: Electron transport and phosphorylation in light induced phosphorylation. In: Biological structure and function (T. W. GOODWIN and O. LINDBERG, eds.). IUBS/IUB International Symposium, Stockholm 1960, vol. II, p. 431. New York: Academic Press 1961.

BALTSCHEFFSKY, H., and B. ARWIDSSON: Evidence for two phosphorylation sites in bacterial cyclic photphosphorylation. Biochim. et Biophys. Acta **65**, 425 (1962).

BROCKMANN, H., and G. SCHMIDT-KASTNER: Valinomycin-Mitteilungen über Antibiotica aus Actinomyceten. Chem. Ber. **88**, 57 (1955).

BROWN, K., J. BRENNAN, and C. KELLEY: An antifungal agent identical with valinomycin. Antibiotics & Chemotherapy **12**, 482 (1962).

CHAPPELL, J. B., and A. R. CROFTS: Ion transport and reversible volume changes of isolated mitochondria. Symposium on the Regulation of Metabolic Processes in Mitochondria, Bari, Italy, April 1965. (In press, 1966).

HARRIS, E. J., R. COCKRELL, and B. C. PRESSMAN: Induced and spontaneous movements of potassium into mitochondria. Biochem. J. (in press, 1966).

HOFER, M., R. COCKRELL, and B. C. PRESSMAN: Effect of induced mitochondrial K^+ transport on ATP synthesis. Federation Proc. Abstract, March (1966).

HUNTER, JR. F. E.: The role of electron transfer and phosphorylation in various parts of the electron transport chain in control of mitochondrial swelling. Symposium V. Fifth Internat. Congr. of Biochemistry, Moscow, 1961, p. 287. Oxford: Pergamon Press 1963.

LYNN, W. S., and R. H. BROWN: Role of anions in mitochondrial swelling and contraction. Biochim. et Biophys. Acta **110**, 445 (1965a).

LYNN, W. S., and R. H. BROWN: Cation exchange and oxidative phosphorylation in mitochondria. Biochim. et Biophys. Acta **110**, 459 (1965b).

MCMURRAY, W., and R. W. BEGG: Effect of valinomycin on oxidative phosphorylation. Arch. Biochem. Biophys. **84**, 546 (1959).

MITCHELL, P., and J. MOYLE: Stoichiometry of proton translocation through the respiratory chain and adenosinetriphosphatase systems of rat liver mitochondria. Nature **208**, 147 (1965).

MOORE, C., and B. C. PRESSMAN: Mechanism of action of valinomycin on mitochondria. Biochem. Biophys. Research Commun. **15**, 562 (1964).

OGATA, E., and H. RASMUSSEN: Valinomycin and mitochondrial ion transport. Biochemistry **5**, 57 (1966).

PRESSMAN, B. C.: Specific inhibitors of energy transfer. In: Energy-linked functions of mitochondria (B. CHANCE, ed.), p. 181. New York: Academic Press 1963.

PRESSMAN, B. C.: Induced active transport of ions in mitochondria. Proc. Natl. Acad. Sci. U. S. **53**, 1076 (1965a).

PRESSMAN, B. C.: Mechanochemical oscillations of mitochondria. Abstract, Division of Biological Chemistry, American Chemical Society Meeting, September 1965b.

PRESSMAN, B. C.: Mitochondrial light scattering changes associated with induced ion transport. J. Cell. Biol. **27**, 79A (1965c).
PRESSMAN, B. C.: Ion transport induction by valinomycin and related antibiotics. Abstract, Symposium on Mechanism of Fungicides and Antibiotics, Reinhardsbrun, East Germany, 1966.
SHEMYAKIN, M. M., E. I. VINOGRADOVA, M. Y. FEIGNIA, N. A. ALDANOVA, N. F. LOGINOVA, I. D. RYABOVIA, and I. A. PAVLENKO: The structure-antimicrobial relation for valinomycin depsipeptides. Experientia **21**, 548 (1965).
WERNER, C. E., E. J. HARRIS, and B. C. PRESSMAN: Relationship of the light scattering properties of mitochondria to the metabolic state in ascites tumor cells. Abstract, Biophysics Society Meeting, Boston, Feb. 1966.

Tyrocidines and Gramicidin S (J_1, J_2)

F. Edmund Hunter, Jr. and Lois S. Schwartz

Tyrocidine

Tyrocidine is produced by *Bacillus brevis* (Hotchkiss, 1944). Since its separation from tyrothricin, a mixture of about 60% tyrocidine and 20—25% gramicidin, by Hotchkiss and Dubos in 1940—1941, it has been considered one of the foremost examples of an antibiotic which causes direct damage to microorganisms and erythrocytes by a surfactant property.

The amino acid sequences were established for tyrocidine A (Battersby and Craig, 1952; Paladini and Craig, 1954) and for tyrocidine B (King and Craig, 1955) some years ago. Recently the structure for tyrocidine C was also established (Ruttenberg, King and Craig, 1965). These substances are cyclic decapeptides. Although there are some variations in part of the ring, all contain the sequence L-Val-L-Orn-L-Leu-D-Phe-L-Pro. The structures are indicated below.

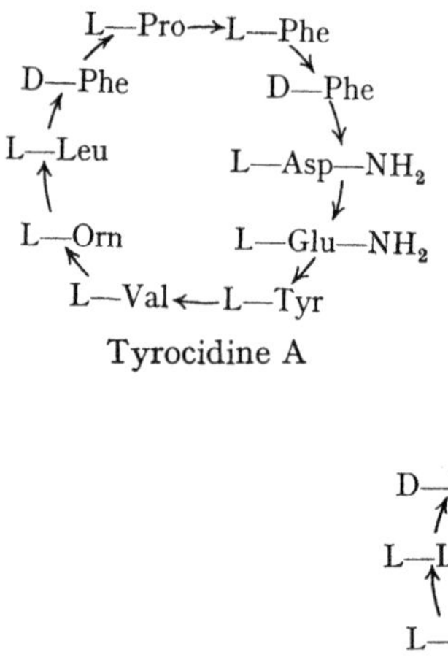

Tyrocidine A

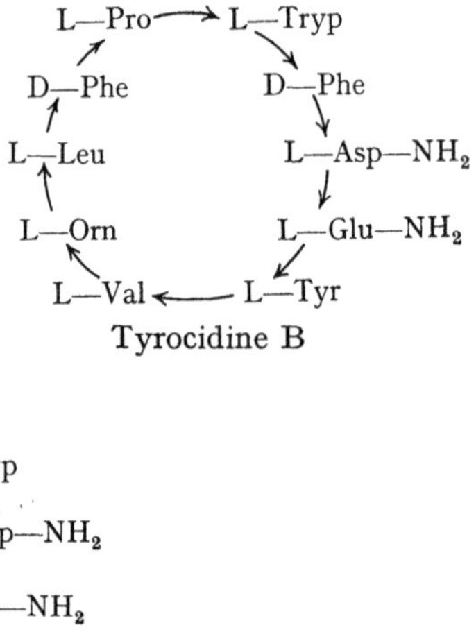

Tyrocidine B

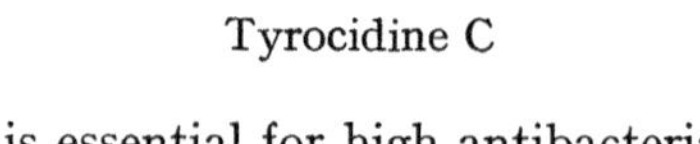

Tyrocidine C

The cyclic structure is essential for high antibacterial activity in these decapeptides. They have several basic groups and a number of non-polar side chains. This combination appears to give them properties of cationic detergents. The tyrocidines show a strong tendency to associate with each other (Ruttenberg, King, and Craig, 1965), and similar forces undoubtedly come into play when the tyrocidines combine with membrane structures. Several models of tyrocidine-like structures indicate that the mixture of D- and L-amino acids may be important for having the lipophilic groups lie in one orientation and the lipophobic in another.

The tyrocidines are bactericidal for many Gram-positive and for some Gram-negative organisms. The Gram-negative organisms are much less sensitive than the Gram-positive. The range between bacteriostatic and bactericidal concentrations is extremely narrow, being only two-fold (HOTCHKISS, 1944; FLOREY *et al.*, 1949). One to 100μg/ml will kill *Pneumococcus*, *Staphylococcus aureus*, *Cl. welchii*, and *B. subtilis*. The sensitivity of Streptococci varies enormously. Some strains of *E. coli* and *Aerobacter aerogenes* are not killed by 1000μg/ml. These differences indicate specificity of interaction between antibiotic and organism, with some organisms being very resistant to cationic detergents. Bactericidal action is sometimes accompanied by bacteriolysis, but since this is characteristic primarily of the organisms capable of rapid autolysis (pneumococcus and staphylococcus, for example), the surfactant action of the antibiotic would appear not to be directly responsible for lysis of bacteria. Several cationic and anionic detergents give the same effect as tyrocidine in about the same concentrations, so HOTCHKISS (1944) concluded that tyrocidine was a bactericidal detergent, unique only in its origin and complexity of chemical structure. Basic tyrocidine is rendered inactive by interaction with acidic groups in proteins, peptones, and phospholipids. Interference by phospholipids is reduced by addition of protamines, which precipitate the cephalins.

The early studies on toxicity to animals and indications for limited local use have been thoroughly summarized by FLOREY *et al.* (1949). Because the prospects for systemic use were so poor, there have been few additional studies. Oral doses of 1000 mg/kg are tolerated, presumably because the substance is not absorbed or the ring is split by digestive enzymes. The LD_{50} for mice is 15 mg/kg i.v. and 40 mg/kg for i.p. Even distribution of these amounts in body water would yield the concentrations (50μg/ml) which cause rapid lysis of washed erythrocytes. However, in the presence of serum a much higher concentration of tyrocidine is required, presumably because the basic polypeptide interacts with acidic groups in the proteins. HOTCHKISS (1944) reported that a few μg of tyrocidine per ml caused immediate and complete inhibition of the respiration of leucocyctes, with subsequent disintegration. Others (RAMMELKAMP and WEINSTEIN, 1942; HEILMAN and HERRELL, 1941) found that much higher concentrations were needed to produce effects. The amount of serum present may account for some of these differences. Despite some interference by serum protein, hemolysis is probably a significant toxic mechanism. Petechial hemorrhages and necroses in liver, spleen, heart, and lungs have been reported (FLOREY *et al.*, 1949). Tyrocidine has been reported to inhibit the developing frog egg but to have little effect on spermatozoa, while the reverse is true for gramicidin (HOTCHKISS, 1944; FLOREY *et al.*, 1949).

Evidence for a direct effect of tyrocidine is available from a number of observations. The age, point on the growth curve, and metabolic state of the organisms seem to make no difference. HEILMAN and HERRELL (1941) reported that tyrocidine had an instantaneous effect on surface tension. The probable relationship of this property to the cationic group and the hydrophobic groups, and its possible role in antibacterial action has been discussed in detail by FLOREY *et al.* (1949). Acetylation of tyrocidine eliminates its cationic nature and destroys its antibacterial action.

Other experiments indicate a direct and immediate attack on the permeability barrier provied by the plasma membrane. There is an immediate and rapid leakage from the cell of nitrogenous and phosphorus containing substances known to exist in a free and sometimes concentrated state in the cell (HOTCHKISS, 1944; GALE, 1963). The cationic detergent cetyl trimethyl ammonium bromide has very similar effects. The loss of amino acids, purines, pyrimidines, phosphate esters, etc. results in dilution of essential metabolites to the point where cell respiration and metabolism virtually stop (HOTCHKISS, 1946). Disintegration of the cell wall of several organisms in the presence of tyrocidine has been reported (FLOREY *et al.*, 1949), but the cell membrane seems to be the real target. Complete disintegration may occur only when autolytic enzymes are active (HOTCHKISS, 1944; GALE, 1963; DUBOS, 1939).

In low concentrations (10^{-6} M or about 1 µg/ml) tyrocidine uncouples oxidative phosphorylation without inhibiting oxygen uptake, activates ATPase, causes mitochondrial swelling, and inhibits ATP induced contraction of mitochondria (NEUBERT and LEHNINGER, 1962). These actions could all result from relatively mild surface action effects. Although the results are essentially identical in description to effects seen with gramicidin, there is evidence that they are not due to identical mechanisms. For example, gramicidin S, which is really a tyrocidine, does not induce ion transport into mitochondria like the true gramicidins do (PRESSMAN, 1965).

The detergent type of action could result in tyrocidines, in sufficient concentration, having either stimulating or inhibiting properties (even denaturation) on enzymes which are lipoproteins. Inhibition of metabolism by such direct action on enzymes seems not to be a major factor in the antibacterial action of tyrocidine.

Gramicidin S (J_1, J_2)

Gramicidin S (Soviet), produced by an organism very similar to *Bacillus brevis*, was isolated and named by GAUSE and BRAYHNIKOVA in 1944. However, on further investigation the biological and chemical properties of gramicidin S indicated that it was more closely related to the tyrocidines than to the gramicidins. These characteristics included the smaller molecular weight, the presence of free amino groups, the amino acid composition, bactericidal effects, and action against certain Gram-negative organisms as well as Gram-positive organisms. These properties distinguish gramicidin S from the true gramicidins, which are neutral polypeptides of higher molecular weight and active against certain Gram-positive bacteria, neisseriae, and mycobacteria (FLOREY *et al.*, 1949).

Recent work on the structure of gramicidin J_1 and gramicidin J_2 (Japan) has demonstrated that these antibiotics are identical with gramicidin S (OTANI and SAITO, 1964; KURAHASHI, 1964), so they are all tyrocidines. All reports on their actions must be reviewed with this new information in mind.

The early work on the structure of gramicidin S has been discussed by FLOREY *et al.* (1949). The amino acid composition and cyclopeptide nature were established, but there was uncertainty as to whether it was a pentapeptide or a decapeptide. ERLANGER and GOODE (1954) presented evidence favoring the decapeptide, and the structure has now been thoroughly established as a cyclic decapeptide closely related to the tyrocidines. In fact, it is a dimer of the one half the ring which never seems to vary in the tyrocidine structures (RUTTENBERG, KING, CRAIG, 1965). The formula of gramicidin S is shown below.

Like other antibacterial peptides, gramicidin S contains some D-amino acids. The proline can be replaced by glycine without loss of activity (AOYAGI *et al.*, 1964) but ornithine with a free amino group is essential. The cyclic structure has always been considered essential in tyrocidines, but KATCHALSKI *et al.* (1955) reported some activity in linear decapeptides related to gramicidin S. The probable orientation of the hydrophobic and hydrophilic groups in the gramicidin S structure, which is important for surfactant properties, has been discussed by WARNER (1961).

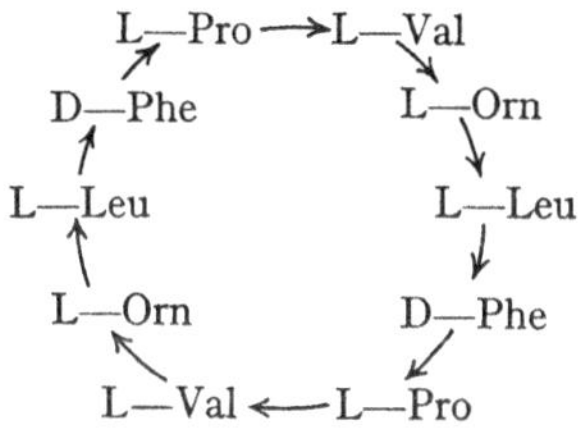

Gramicidin S

Gramicidin S inhibits organisms like *Staph. aureus.*, *B. subtilis*, *Salmonella paratyphi*, *M. tuberculosis*, and *Candida albicans*, with 10—100μg/ml being effective. The antibiotic does bind to cell membranes, but this occurs in resistant as well as sensitive strains. Morphological, biochemical, virulence and antigenic changes have been reported. Relatively high concentrations (100μg/ml) inhibit the respiration of staphylococci. HIRAMATSU (1961) has demonstrated that 10μg/ml causes the lysis of protoplasts from sensitive cells like *Micrococcus lysodeikticus* but has very little effect on protoplasts from insensitive *E. coli* or *B. brevis*. When low concentrations of gramicidin S inhibit hemolytic microorganisms it appears to protect against hemolysis, but slightly higher concentrations have a direct hemolytic action.

The mechanism of action of gramicidin S on bacteria, erythrocytes, and mitochondria, as well as the toxicity for mammals (LD_{50} for rats, 17 mg/kg i.p.) is very similar to that for tyrocidine [SPECTOR (1957), FLOREY *et al.* (1949)]. It has direct action which disturbs the organization of lipoprotein systems and destroys the permeability barrier of membranes. The degree of alteration is dependent on the amount of drug present.

OKUDA *et al.* (1960) have studied in detail the effects of gramicidin S (J) on rat liver mitochondria. Graded effects, presumably all due to the detergent type of action, could be obtained by selecting the concentration of gramicidin S. At 10^{-6} M there was rapid swelling. With 10^{-5} M there was loss of NAD linked oxidations due to release and splitting of NAD. There was no direct effect on any dehydrogenase or on the electron transport chain. At 2.5×10^{-5} M there was loss of other adenine nucleotides and most of the phosphorylating capacity. ATPase activity was increased. The changes are identical with those seen with other treatments which alter the mitochondrial membrane and produce swelling (for example, procedures as simple as incubation with phosphate buffer). They occur with concentrations of gramicidin S which act on microorganisms. Upon exposure to high concentrations of gramicidin S for one hour at 0^0 (2×10^{-4} M or 200μg/ml) mitochondrial structure is considerably disrupted with release of some β-hydroxybutyrate dehydrogenase and NADH oxidase, but no release of succinoxidase. In fact succinoxidase activity is increased as permeability barriers are decreased. HAGIHARA *et al.* (1962) and ZVYAGILSKAYA and KOTELNIKOVA (1962) have also studied uncoupling by gramicidin S. The latter workers found that extremely high concentrations (6×10^{-3} M) would disrupt the succinoxidase system.

Inhibition of mitochondrial ATPase by high concentrations of gramicidin S has been reported by several workers (KOTELNIKOVA and ZVYAGILSKAYA, 1964). This result is entirely consistent with surfactant disruption of lipoprotein systems. MIZUNO (1960) has shown that the loss of intramitochondrial Mg^{++} is a significant factor.

Gramicidin S has no effect on phosphorylase, aldolase, or other enzymes of carbohydrate metabolism (YUDELOVICH, 1950), but it has been reported to inhibit invertase and photosynthesis. However, the concentration reported to cause 80% inhibition of photosynthesis was 10^{-2} M.

References

AOYAGI, H., T. KATO, M. OHNO, M. KONDO, and N. IZUMIYA: Cyclo-(L-valyl-L-ornithyl-L-leucyl-D-phenylalanylglycyl)$_2$, an active analog of gramicidin S. J. Am. Chem. Soc. **86**, 5700 (1964).

BATTERSBY, A. R., and L. C. CRAIG: The chemistry of tyrocidine. I. Isolation and characterization of a single peptide. II. Molecular weight studies. J. Am. Chem. Soc. **74**, 4019, 4023 (1952).

DUBOS, R. J.: Studies on a bactericidal agent extracted from a soil bacillus. I. Preparation of the agent. Its activity *in vitro*. J. Exptl. Med. **70**, 1 (1939).

ERLANGER, B. F., and L. GOODE: Gramicidin S: Relationship of cyclic structure to antibiotic activity. Nature **174**, 840 (1954).

FLOREY, H. W., E. CHAIN, N. G. HEATLEY, M. A. JENNINGS, A. G. SANDERS, E. P. ABRAHAM, and M. E. FLOREY: Antibiotics, vols. I and II. London: Oxford University Press 1949.

GALE, E. F.: Mechanisms of antibiotic action. Pharmacol. Revs. **15**, 481 (1963).

GAUSE, G. F., and M. G. BRAYHNIKOVA: Gramicidin S and its use in the treatment of infected wounds. Nature **154**, 703 (1944).

HAGIHARA, B., J. L. CONELLY, K. SHIKAMA, R. OSHINO, and K. OKUNUKI: Effects of antibiotics on respiration and phosphorylative systems of mitochondria. Koso Kagaku Shimposiumu **17**, 58 (1962). Chem. Abstr. **59**, 6859d.

HEILMAN, D. H., and W. E. HERRELL: Mode of action of gramicidin. Proc. Soc. Exptl. Biol. Med. **47**, 480 (1941).

HIRAMATSU, T.: Action of gramicidin J on protoplasts. Osaka Shiritsu Daigaku Igaku Zasshi **10**, 267 (1961). Chem. Abstr. **56**, 14720h.

HOTCHKISS, R. D.: Gramicidin, tyrocidine, and tyrothricin. Advances in Enzymol. **4**, 153 (1944).

HOTCHKISS, R. D.: The nature of bactericidal action of surface active agents. Ann. N.Y. Acad. Sci. **46**, 479 (1946).

KATCHALSKI, E., A. BERGER, L. BICHOWSKY-SOLMNITZKI, and J. KURTZ: Antibiotically active amino acid copolymers related to gramicidin S. Nature **176**, 118 (1955).

KING, T. P., and L. C. CRAIG: The chemistry of tyrocidine. IV. Purification and characterization of tyrocidine B. J. Am. Chem. Soc. **77**, 6624, 6627 (1955).

KOTEL'NIKOVA, A. V., and R. A. ZVYAGILSKAYA: Adenosinetriphosphatase activity of mitochondria from *Endomyces magnusii*. Biokhimiya **29**, 662 (1964). (Chem. Abstr. **61**, 14921c).

KURAHASHI, K.: Identity of gramicidin S, J_1, and J_2. J. Biochem. (Japan) **56**, 101 (1964).

MIZUNO, A.: Effects of gramicidin J_1 on the adenosinetriphosphatase of rat liver mitochondria. Osaka Shiritsu Daigaku Igaku Zasshi **9**, 1957 (1960). Chem. Abstr. **54**, 17516b.

NEUBERT, D., and A. L. LEHNINGER: The effect of oligomycin, gramicidin and other antibiotics on reversal of mitochondrial swelling by adenosinetriphosphate. Biochim. et Biophys. Acta **62**, 556 (1962).

OKUDA, K., Y. AKIYAMA, Y. MIKI, and I. UEMURA: Effects of gramicidin J_1 on rat liver mitochondria. I. Respiratory enzyme activities. II. Acid soluble nucleotides and oxidative phosphorylation. III. Morphology and enzyme activities. Osaka Shiritsu Daigaku Igaku Zasshi **9**, 2767, 2901, 3373 (1960). Chem. Abstr. **55**, 9519i.

OTANI, S., and Y. SAITO: Reinvestigation of the chemical structure of gramicidin J_1. J. Biochem. (Japan) **56**, 103 (1964).

PALADINI, A., and L. C. CRAIG: The chemistry of tyrocidine. III. The structure of tyrocidine A. J. Am. Chem. Soc. **76**, 688 (1954).

PRESSMAN, B. C.: Induced active transport of ions in mitochondria. Proc. Natl. Acad. Sci. U. S. **53**, 1076 (1965).

RAMMELKAMP, C. H., and L. WEINSTEIN: Toxic effects of tyrothricin, gramicidin, and tyrocidine. J. Infectious Diseases **71**, 166 (1942).

RUTTENBERG, M. A., T. P. KING, and L. C. CRAIG: The chemistry of tyrocidine. VI. The amino acid sequence of tyrocidine C. Biochemistry **4**, 11 (1965).

SPECTOR, W. S. (ed.): Handbook of toxicology, vol. II. Antibiotics, p. 88. Philadelphia: W. B. Saunders Co. 1957.

WARNER, D. T.: Proposed molecular models of gramicidin S and other polypeptides. Nature **190**, 120 (1961).

YUDELOVICH, R. Y.: The mechanism of action of gramicidin S on oxidative phosphorylation. Doklady Akad. Nauk. S. S. S. R. **74**, 111 (1950). Chem. Abstr. **45**, 2098d.

ZVYAGILSKAYA, R. A., and A. V. KOTEL'NIKOVA: Effect of gramicidin S upon oxidative phosphorylation and respiration in rat liver mitochondria. Biokhimiya **27**, 849 (1962). Chem. Abstr. **58**. 7259a.

Gramicidins

F. Edmund Hunter, Jr. and Lois S. Schwartz

Gramicidin, produced by *Bacillus brevis*, was isolated along with tyrocidine in 1941 (Hotchkiss, 1944) from the crude material described by Dubos (1939). Early preparations were called gramicidin D (Dubos). Later, countercurrent distribution techniques resolved gramicidin into four groups of polypeptides now specifically designated as gramicidins A, B, C, D. Many commercial preparations are mixtures of the Dubos type.

Hotchiss (1944) and Florey *et al.* (1949) have reviewed the early work on structure. The absence of free amino and carboxyl groups suggested a neutral cyclopolypeptide. James and Synge (1951) established that there was one ethanolamine for each glycine. Okuda, Lin and Winnick (1962) presented additional information on the amino acid composition differences in gramicidins A, B, and C, suggesting a structure of 30 amino acids and 2 ethanolamines with a molecular weight of about 3725. In 1963 Ramachandran reported that further countercurrent distribution studies indicated heterogeneity in the A, B, C peaks. He named one new component gramicidin D, but favored the molecular weights near 1800—2000, as reported by Ishii and Witkop (1963).

Recently Sarges and Witkop (1965a, 1965b) concluded that gramicidins A, B, and C probably are not cyclic in structure, but more likely consist of chains containing 15 amino acids (D- and L-forms), one ethanolamine, and one formyl group. Their commercial sample of gramicidin contained 85% A, 9% B, 6% C, and a trace of D. The only difference between the first three gramicidins is at position No. 11, A having L-tryptophan; B, L-phenylalanine; and C, L-tyrosine. The D component may have 5 or 6 additional amino acids. Gramicidins A, B, and C each consist of two chains differing only in the amino acid in the No. 1 position. The chain which comprises 80—95% of each gramicidin has valine in the amino terminal (No. 1) position, and the other chain has isoleucine. The molecule is neutral because the amino end-group is covered by the formyl group, and the other end is the hydroxy group of ethanolamine. Sarges and Witkop presented evidence that these chains associate to dimers in head to tail arrangements with strong hydrogen bonding between amino acids along the chain. These properties may explain the finding of molecular weights related to the 1850 and 3700 range, depending on methods and solvents.

The chain of gramicidin A with L-valine at position No. 1 has the following structure: HCO-L-Val-Gly-L-Ala-D-Leu-L-Ala-D-Val-L-Val-D-Val-L-Try-D-Leu-L-Try-D-Leu-L-Try-D-Leu-L-Try-NH-CH_2CH_2OH. Note the alternating D- and L-configurations.

Gramicidin acts on many but not all gram-positive organisms with a primarily bacteriostatic rather than bactericidal action, as it does not lyse the bacteria

(HOTCHIKSS, 1944; FLOREY *et al.*, 1949). Concentrations of 1 to 30μg/ml (10^{-6} to 10^{-5} M) are effective in many cases. A very few gram-negative cocci are inhibited. The action of gramicidin is little affected by peptones, proteins, carbohydrates, sterols, and fatty acids. However, the action is inhibited by phospholipids of the ethanolamine and serine type. Gramicidin appears to interact directly with the cephalin phospholipids. Carbohydrates have been reported not to affect the action of gramicidin on bacteria, but sucrose certainly does alter its effect on mammalian mitochondria (NEUBERT and LEHNINGER, 1962a; GUERRA and HUNTER, 1965a). Under specific conditions gramicidin can protect animals against some experimental infections (FLOREY *et al.* (1949).

Gramicidin causes hemolysis of red blood cells at concentrations (0.5—1 μg/ml) lower than those which inhibit many bacteria, and much lower than required for hemolysis with tyrocidine. However, the hemolysis is not rapid, as with tyrocidine and saponin, but is delayed and takes many hours (HOTCHKISS, 1944). The hemolytic action is partially inhibited by 5% glucose and considerably inhibited by 1% horse serum (FLOREY *et al.*, 1949). Cholesterol also reduces the hemolytic action. The inhibitory action of glucose on hemolysis may be similar to the effect of sucrose in the case of mitochondria.

RAMMELKAMP and WEINSTEIN (1942) reported that 1000—3000μg/ml of gramicidin had no effect on numbers or activity of leucocytes. HOWEVER, HERRELL and HEILMAN (1943) found that 10μg/ml affected macrophages and 100μg/ml decreased migration of lymphocytes. Motility of spermatozoa is eliminated by 10μg/ml (HENLE and ZITTLE, 1941). Frog embryos and tissue culture cells are quite resistant, being unaffected by 100μg/ml (HERRELL and HEILMAN, 1941 and 1943; POMERAT, 1942).

The pharmacology and toxicity of gramicidin to higher animals has been reviewed by HOTCHKISS (1944) and by FLOREY *et al.* (1949). There is virtually no effect orally; gramicidin must be given parenterally to have any systemic effect. However, its systemic toxicity is so high that clinical use is limited to local application. Miscellaneous pharmacological and degenerative changes have been reported. For mice the lethal dose is about 3 mg/kg i.v. and 30 mg/kg i.p. The toxic doses would produce tissue concentrations equal to or higher than those which affect sensitive microorganisms. Uncoupling of phosphorylation and increased permeability of membranes may be the basis for action in both cases. Slow hemolysis is probably also an important factor, since it occurs at very low concentrations and is only partially inhibited by serum.

High concentration of gramicidin do not cause lysis or dissolution of the bacterial cell, and ordinarily autolysis does not set in. However, long exposure to relatively high concentrations of gramicidin may cause death due to disturbances in energy metabolism.

HEILMAN and HERRELL (1941, 1943) found that gramicidin did lower surface tension, but the effect was much slower and more complicated than the instantaneous effects seen with tyrocidine and detergents. This property may underlie the action of gramicidin on all membranes, but the effect is not great enough to cause dissolution of the permeability barrier in staphylococci, for GALE (1963) found that gramicidin did not lead to loss of cell constituents, as does tyrocidine. Many organisms are not sensitive to gramicidin, so either it does not bind or it does not alter the surface tension in some cases. Interference by cephalins has been proposed as a possible explanation for differences in sensitivity.

DUBOS, HOTCHKISS, and COBURN (1942) showed that 1—30μg/ml of gramicidin could greatly stimulate the oxygen consumption of *Staphylococcus aureus*. Inhibition of respiration and death of the cells occurred only with high concentrations and after several hours of increased respiration. Death may have resulted from disorganization in the respiratory system or from long term effects of uncoupling (see next section). HOTCHKISS (1944) analyzed these observations and pointed out that stimulation of respiration was not correlated with antibacterial action. For example, it did not occur with gramicidin insensitive *E. coli*, but did occur with some gramicidin-resistant strains of staphylococci. Moreover, it occurred only when K^+ ions were present and NH^{4+} ions absent.

HOTCHKISS (1944) observed that gramicidin prevented uptake of phosphate by staphylococci, and this has been confirmed for other cells. Inhibition of phosphate uptake was correlated with antibacterial action. Noting that 2,4-dinitrophenol produced some effects like gramicidin, HOTCHKISS (1944) postulated that gramicidin had an uncoupling action potentially capable of affecting phosphate uptake in all cells. Differences in permeability and the presence of inhibitors like cephalins may explain why gramicidin does not affect all cells. If gramicidin acts like 2,4-dinitrophenol, only electron transport chain phosphorylations would be eliminated. ATP derived from glycolysis and numerous dismutations would be unaffected. Years later BRODIE and GRAY (1956) reported that gramicidin inhibited esterification of phosphate without affecting O_2 consumption in bacterial extracts. This direct study of uncoupling was important because bacterial electron transport and phosphorylation mechanisms are not identical with mammalian systems.

If gramicidin is an uncoupling agent, its presence would be expected to (a) decrease the uptake of any substance whose uptake requires energy, and (b) to decrease the ability of the cell to concentrate substances from the medium. Interference with energy supply by uncoupling could decrease the syntheses of polysaccharides, lipids, nucleic acids and proteins. Syntheses dependent on organized membranous structures might also be affected in a more direct way. Inhibition of protein synthesis is clearly indicated by blocking of the formation of the inducible enzyme, β-galactosidase (CREASER, 1955), and in blocking of M-protein synthesis (BROCK, 1963). The synthesis of bacteriophage in bacteria (PRICE, 1947) and tobacco mosaic virus in tobacco leaves is also decreased (BOBYR, 1963). The observed inhibition of bacteriophage formation does not prove direct inhibition of protein or nucleic acid synthesis, as it is known that phosphate must be taken up from the external medium in order to make bacteriophage.

Glycolytic enzymes are not affected directly by gramicidin, but glycolysis could increase if there were an uncoupling effect or increased metabolic demand. There are a few reports of inhibition of enzymes in the citric acid cycle (MIURA, 1961). The high concentrations of gramicidin used may cause partial disorganization by surface action. Uncoupling effects or abnormal burdens of ion pumping would increase oxidative activity; extensive disorganization in lipoproteins of membrane systems might inhibit oxidations. Hyaluronidase activity of several strains of staphylococcus is suppressed by gramicidin at 100μg/ml according to

SHIRYAEVA (1954). These are rather high concentrations of gramicidin and the action may be a detergent-like one. Hydrolysis of poly-β-hydroxybutyrate — MERRICK (1965) has demonstrated that gramicidin at 4×10^{-6} M causes 50% inhibition of both synthesis and depolymerization of poly-β-hydroxybutyrate in the storage granule system found in many bacteria. This is believed to be due to changes in the structure of the membrane, which is intimately involved in the metabolism of the granules.

BALTSCHEFFSKY and BALTSCHEFFSKY (1960) noted that gramicidin was a strong inhibitor of photophosphorylation in extracts of *Rhodospirillum rubrum*. Similar observations have been made for chloroplasts.

Uncoupling of phosphorylation in mammalian mitochondria by gramicidin was first reported by CROSS *et al.* (1949). The effective concentrations were similar to those inhibiting sensitive microorganisms. The action appeared to be similar to that of DNP. Further studies have been summarized by NEUBERT and LEHNINGER (1962a). As would be predicted, gramicidin stimulates oxygen O_2 consumption in the absence of phosphate acceptor systems (HUNTER, 1956; SANTI, 1962). The recent work suggesting that gramicidin should be classed as an apparent uncoupler rather than a true uncoupler will be discussed under ion uptake.

HUNTER (1956) showed that gramicidin, like DNP, could stimulate mitochondrial ATPase at low concentrations. At high concentrations gramicidin inhibited the gramicidin-activated and the DNP-activated ATPase. COOPER and LEHNINGER (1957) observed stimulation of ATPase by gramicidin in digitonin fragments of mitochondria. NEUBERT and LEHNINGER (1962a) obtained near maximal uncoupling and stimulation of ATPase by the same concentration (10^{-8} M).

The inhibitory action on ATPase probably occurs at a different site from that which produces stimulation (HUNTER, 1956). NEUBERT and LEHNINGER (1962a, 1962b) demonstrated that extremely low concentrations of gramicidin (10^{-10} M) can interfere with ATP induced contraction of GSH swollen mitochondria. Also, WEINBACH *et al.* (1963) observed that gramicidin inhibits ATP-induced contraction of mitochondria after swelling produced by 50μM pentachlorophenol. Since the mitochondria have already been fully uncoupled by the pentachlorophenol, gramicidin inhibits contraction by a mechanism other than uncouplingor ATPase activation.

NEUBERT and LEHNINGER (1962a) and WEINSTEIN, SCOTT and HUNTER (1964) observed that extremely low concentrations of gramicidin would induce swelling of liver mitochondria in potassium chloride medium but not in sucrose medium. The inhibitory effect of sucrose was studied further by GUERRA and HUNTER (1965a). The induction of swelling by gramicidin in potassium chloride medium does not seem to be due to simple surfactant effects, nor is it like the direct swelling-inducing action of pentachlorophenol (WEINSTEIN, SCOTT and HUNTER, 1964). It is produced by the same concentrations which cause uncoupling, activate ATPase, and inhibit bacteria. NEUBERT and LEHNINGER (1962a) postulated that discharge of some high energy intermediate was the common basis for these effects. However, WEINSTEIN, SCOTT and HUNTER (1964) demonstrated that dinitrophenol as well as certain electron transport inhibitors could partially block gramicidin-induced swelling. GUERRA and HUNTER (1965b) presented considerable additional evidence that much of gramicidin induced swelling in high potassium chloride medium is dependent on electron transport and intermediates of oxidative phosphorylation.

In sucrose medium, gramicidin behaves like a typical uncoupler, accelerating swelling at low concentrations and completely blocking phosphate-induced swelling at uncoupling concentrations. These higher concentrations cause very rapid swelling instead of blocking swelling in potassium chloride medium. The ability of gramicidin to prevent swelling in sucrose medium under certain circumstances may be due to a true uncoupling effect, but there is little indication of such an action under other conditions.

CHAPPELL and CROFTS (1965a) and PRESSMAN (1965) observed that mitochondria in a sucrose medium respond in very specific ways to the addition of gramicidin if monovalent cations are present. Without added substrate or phosphate, gramicidin causes the ejection of H^+ ions and the uptake of some K^+, Na^+, Li^+, etc. Unlike valinomycin, gramicidin does not produce an effect selective for K^+. Gramicidins are required in concentrations 20—25 times greater than valinomycin to induce ion uptake (PRESSMAN, 1965).

If phosphate, arsenate, acetate, or some other anion more permeant than Cl^- is present, the uptake of cations is greatly increased, they are accompanied by anions, and swelling of the mitochondria takes place. The energy demands for these changes cause a large increase in oyxgen consumption and endogenous substrate no longer suffices, so that substrate must be added. Anaerobiosis, electron transport inhibitors, and true uncoupling agents not only prevent these changes, but the swelling and the pH changes actually reverse as accumulated ions diffuse out and H^+ ion moves back in. The process is dependent on generation of a high energy intermediate by electron transport. Apparent uncoupling of phosphorylation by low concentrations of gramicidin is due to diversion of the energy supply to ion transport work.

PRESSMAN (1965) has suggested that gramicidin stimulates energy requiring transport of K^+ as well as producing some increase in passive permeability. However, CHAPPELL and CROFTS (1965b) have postulated that the mitochondrial membrane possesses an energy dependent H^+ pump for ejecting protons, and that the entry of K^+ and other ions is a passive electrochemical response to the H^+ pumping when gramicidin makes the membrane more permeable to K^+. They have shown that gramicidin increases the permeability of erythrocyte membranes and phospholipid micelles to monovalent cations. They have also presented interesting experiments with ammonia and carbon dioxide which support the key role for H^+ pumping. The mechanisms for cation shifts with gramicidin appear to be identical with those for valinomycin, except that the lack of selectivity for K^+ with gramicidin indicates a greater effect on membrane structure with a larger apparent pore size.

Whether the induced movement of monovalent cations as seen in isolated mitochondria has any relationship to the antibacterial action of gramicidin is a largely unanswered question. Further work on the monovalent cation dependence of gramicidin action on bacteria is needed. HOTCHKISS (1944) did note that the presence of K^+ and the absence of NH_4^+ were essential for gramicidin to stimulate

O_2 uptake by staphylococci. On the other hand, uncoupling effects have been reported in "extracts", where something besides alteration of permeability to K^+ would have to occur unless vesicular structures still exist.

References

Baltscheffsky, H., and M. Baltscheffsky: Inhibitor studies on light induced phosphorylation in extracts of *Rhodospirillum rubrum*. Acta Chem. Scand. **14**, 257 (1960).

Bobyr, A. D.: Antiviral activity of some antibiotics and other substances depending on the period of infection development. Mikrobiol. Zhur., Akad. Nauk Ukr. R.S.R., **23**, 27 (1961). Chem. Abstr. **57**, 3822b.

Brock, T. D.: Effect of antibiotics and inhibitors on M protein synthesis. J. Bacteriol. **85**, 527 (1963).

Brodie, A. F., and C. T. Gray: Phosphorylation coupled to oxidation in bacterial extracts. J. Biol. Chem. **219**, 853 (1956).

Chappell, J. B., and A. R. Crofts: Gramicidin and ion transport in isolated liver mitochondria. Biochem. J. **95**, 393 (1965a).

Chappell, J. B., and A. R. Crofts: Ion transport and reversible volume changes of isolated mitochondria. Symposium on the Regulation of Metabolic Processes in Mitochondria, Bari, Italy. April 1965 (1965b).

Cooper, C., and A. L. Lehninger: Oxidative phosphorylation by an enzyme complex from extracts of mitochondria. IV. Adenosinetriphosphatase activity. J. Biol. Chem. **224**, 547 (1957).

Creaser, E. H.: The induced (adaptive) biosynthesis of β-galactosidase in *Staphylococcus aureus*. J. Gen. Microbiol. **12**, 288 (1955).

Cross, R. J., J. Taggert, G. Covo, and D. E. Green: Studies on the cyclophorase system. VI. The coupling of oxidation and phosphorylation. J. Biol. Chem. **177**, 655 (1949).

Dubos, R. J.: Studies on a bactericidal agent extracted from a soil bacillus. I. Preparation of the agent. Its activity *in vitro*. J. Exptl. Med. **70**, 1 (1939).

Dubos, R. J., R. D. Hotchkiss, and A. F. Coburn: Effect of gramicidin and tyrocidine on bacterial metabolism. J. Biol. Chem. **146**, 421 (1942).

Florey, H. W., E. Chain, N. G. Heatley, M. A. Jennings, A. G. Sanders, E. P. Abraham, and M. E. Florey: Antibiotics, vols. I and II. London: Oxford University Press 1949.

Gale, E. F.: Mechanisms of antibiotic action. Pharmacol. Rev. **15**, 481 (1963).

Guerra, L., and F. E. Hunter Jr.: Sucrose inhibition of gramicidin induced swelling of isolated rat liver mitochondria. Broteria, Serie de Ciencias Naturais XXXIV (LXI), 227. Lisbon 1965a.

Guerra, L., and F. E. Hunter Jr.: Relationship of gramicidin induced swelling of liver mitochondria to electron transport and high energy intermediates. Federation Proc. **24**, No. 2, March—April (1965b).

Henle, G., and C. A. Zittle: Effect of gramicidin on metabolism of bovine spermatozoa. Proc. Soc. Exptl. Biol. Med. **47**, 193 (1941).

Herrell, W. E., and D. Heilman: Experimental and clinical studies on gramicidin. J. Clin. Invest. **20**, 583 (1941).

Herrell, W. E., and D. Heilman: Tissue culture studies on cytotoxicity of bactericidal agents. III. Cytotoxicity and antibacterial activity of gramicidin and penicillin, comparison with other germicides. Am. J. Med. Sci. **206**, 221 (1943).

Hotchkiss, R. D.: Gramicidin, tyrocidine, and tyrothricin. Advances in Enzymology **4**, 153 (1944). New York: Interscience Publ. 1944.

Hunter, Jr., F. E.: The relationship of dinitrophenol activated adenosinetriphosphatase to uncoupling mechanisms and possible phosphorylation of electron transfer catalysts. Proceedings of the Third Internat. Congr. of Biochemistry, Brussels 1955 (C. Liebecq, ed.), p. 298. New York: Academic Press 1956.

ISHII, S. I., and B. WITKOP: Gramicidin A. I. Determination of composition and amino acid configuration by enzymatic and gas chromatographic methods. J. Am. Chem. Soc. **85**, 1832 (1963).

JAMES, A. T., and R. L. M. SYNGE: Non-peptide linkages in gramicidin. Biochem. J. **50**, 109 (1951).

MERRICK, J. M.: Effect of polymixin B, tyrocidine, gramicidin D, and other antibiotics on the enzymatic hydrolysis of poly-β-hydroxybutyrate. J. Bacteriology **90**, 965 (1965).

MIURA, Y.: Metabolism of rat ascites tumors with nitrogen mustard sensitive and resistant strains. VII. Effect of ubiquinone and vitamin K_3 on succinate and α-glycerophosphate-neotetrazolium reductases. J. Biochem. (Japan) **52**, 43 (1962).

NEUBERT, D., and A. L. LEHNINGER: The effect of oligomycin, gramicidin, and other antibiotics on reversal of mitochondrial swelling by adenosinetriphosphate. Biochim. et Biophys. Acta **62**, 556 (1962a).

NEUBERT, D., and A. L. LEHNINGER: Role of C-factor in water uptake and extrusion by mitochondria and interference by various drugs. Biochem. Pharmacol. **9**, 127 (1962b).

OKUDA, K., C. S. LIN, and T. WINNICK: Amino acid composition of gramicidin. Nature **195**, 1067 (1962).

POMERAT, C. M.: Effect of direct applications of tyrothricin and allantoin to cells *in vitro*. Proc. Soc. Exptl. Biol. Med. **51**, 345 (1942).

PRESSMAN, B. C.: Induced active transport of ions in mitochondria. Proc. Natl. Acad. Sci. (U.S.) **53**, 1076 (1965).

PRICE, W. H.: Bacteriophage formation without bacterial growth. III. Effect of iodoacetate, fluoride, gramicidin, and azide on the formation of bacteriophage. J. Gen. Physiol. **31**, 135 (1947).

RAMACHANDRAN, L. K.: On the heterogeneity of gramicidin. Biochemistry **2**, 1138 (1963).

RAMMELKAMP, C. H., and L. WEINSTEIN: Toxic effects of tyrothricin, gramicidin, and tyrocidine. J. Infectious Diseases **71**, 166 (1942).

SANTI, R.: Drugs with selective action on oxidative phosphorylation. Arch. ital. sci. farmacol. **12**, 5 (1962). Chem. Abstr. **58**, 7258e.

SARGES, R., and B. WITKOP: Gramicidin. V and VII. The structure of valine and isoleucine gramicidin A and B. J. Am. Chem. Soc. **87**, 2011, 2027 (1965a).

SARGES, R., and B. WITKOP: Gramicidin. VIII. The structure of valine and isoleucine gramicidin C. Biochemistry **4**, 2491 (1965b).

SHIRYAEVA, V. L.: Influence of penicillin and gramicidin on certain properties of staphylococcus. Zhur. Mikrobiol., Epidemiol. Immunobiol. No. 6, 64 (1954). Chem. Abstr. **49**, 7059e.

WEINBACH, E. C., H. SHEFFIELD, and J. GARBUS: Restoration of oxidative phosphorylation and morphological integrity to swollen, uncoupled rat liver mitochondria. Proc. Natl. Acad. Sci. U.S. **50**, 561 (1963).

WEINSTEIN, J., A. SCOTT, and F. E. HUNTER JR.: The action of gramicidin D on isolated liver mitochondria. J. Biol. Chem. **239**, 3031 (1964).

Nonactin and Related Antibiotics

Paul D. Shaw

Nonactin, monactin, dinactin and trinactin (Fig. 1) are related antibiotics whose structures and sterochemistry have been elucidated by GERLACH and PRELOG (1963). They were isolated from a *Streptomyces* sp. which also produced cycloheximide (DOMINGUEZ *et al.*, 1962). The nonactins have little or no antimicrobial activity.

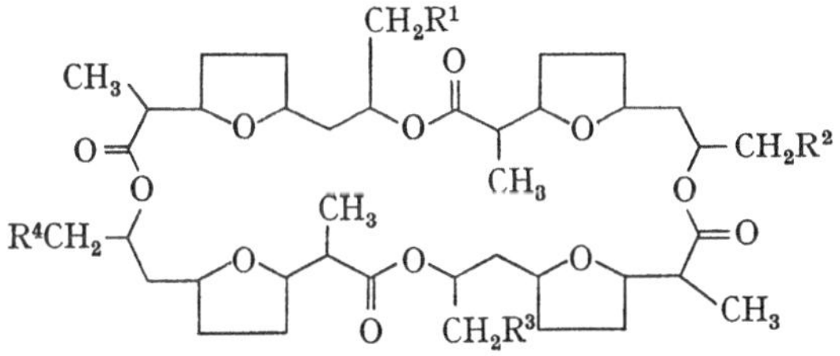

Fig. 1. Nonactin $R^1, R^2, R^3, R^4 = H$; Monactin $R^1, R^2, R^3 = H$, $R^4 = CH_3$; Dinactin $R^1, R^2 = H$; $R^3, R^4 = CH_3$; Trinactin $R^1 = H$; $R^2, R^3, R^4 = CH_3$. The configuration about the four carbon atoms bearing R^1—R^4 differ in the four antibiotics

GRAVEN *et al.* (1966a) reported that $1 \times 10^{-7}\,M$ monactin, dinactin and trinactin completely uncoupled oxidative phosphorylation in rat liver mitochrondria with glutamate, succinate or ascorbate plus tetramethylphenylenediamine as the substrate. Nonactin was somewhat less active. In addition, these antibiotics stimulated respiration with either glutamate or pyruvate as substrate. This stimulation was optimal at the lowest antibiotic concentration which uncoupled oxidative phosphorylation. Stimulation occurred in the presence or absence of inorganic phosphate, although it was greater in the presence of phosphate. The observation, that acetate could replace phosphate with no loss of respiratory stimulation, led the authors to conclude that the stimulation in the presence of phosphate was due to its role as an anion and not related to any phosphorylated intermediate or phosphorylation process.

Nonaction and its homologs induce ATPase activity in the presence of sodium or potassium ions (GRAVEN *et al.*, 1966a). Nonactin is the least active. At $10^{-7}\,M$ trinactin, ATP hydrolysis was induced by cesium, rubidium, potassium or sodium ions. Lithium and ammonium ions did not induce hydrolysis. The antibiotics oligomycin D and peliomycin nearly completely inhibited the induction of ATPase activity by all of the nonactin homologs in the presence of sodium or potassium ions. Aurovertin inhibited ATPase activity 50 to 70% under the same conditions.

The authors concluded that the nonactin homologs function in a manner similar to the gramicidins, valinomycin and tyrocidine. All of these antibiotics act by some mechanism associated with cation movement across the mitochondrial membrane. The cation specificities are different however, and the authors suggest that these differences are associated with the molecular configurations of the antibiotics.

The nonactin antibiotics induce swelling in mitochondria (GRAVEN *et al.*, 1966b). This swelling requires a monovalent, alkali metal cation, a source of energy and an anion. All of the alkali metal cations are effective except lithium, and the energy source may be either ATP or a substrate such as β-hydroxybutyrate or succinate. The anion may be either phosphate or acetate. ATP induced swelling is blocked by oligomycin, but substrate induced swelling is not. It was suggested that the antibiotics act on a non-phosphorylated, high energy intermediate involved in ATP synthesis but not necessarily on the same pathway (c. f. LARDY *et al.*, 1964 and the chapter on oligomycin in this book).

All four antibiotics induce a damped oscillatory swelling of mitochondria in the presence of all alkali metal cations except lithium. An energy source and either phosphate or acetate are also required (GRAVEN *et al.*, 1966b). Oscillations induced by ATP were prevented by respiratory inhibitors. The amplitude and period of the oscillations were dependent on the amount of energy available, the concentration of the monovalent cation, the concentration and type of anion, the concentration of antibiotic, temperature, and the age or condition of the mitochondria. It was suggested that the oscillations induced by the nonactin antibiotics were caused by the cyclic interruptions in the energy available to sustain the mitochondria in a swollen state.

A relationship apparently exists between cation movement, ATP hydrolysis (or substrate oxidation) and mitochondrial swelling. ATP hydrolysis induced by the antibiotics requires an alkali metal cation while mitochondrial swelling requires both an alkali metal cation and an anion. Thus ATP hydrolysis is associated with mitochondrial swelling, but such ATP hydrolysis or substrate oxidation does not necessarily cause mitochondria to swell. The nature of the relationships between these three phenomena are still unclear.

See Addendum

References

DOMINGUEZ, J., J. D. DUNITZ, H. GERLACH, and V. PRELOG: Stoffwechselprodukte von Actinomyceten. Über die Konstitution von Nonactin. Helv. Chim. Acta **45**, 129 (1962).

GERLACH, H., and V. PRELOG: Über die Konfiguration der Nonactinsäure. Liebigs Ann. Chem. **669**, 121 (1963).

GRAVEN, S. N., H. A. LARDY, D. JOHNSON, and A. RUTTER: Antibiotics as tools for metabolic studies. V. Effect of nonactin, monactin, dinactin, and trinactin on oxidative phosphorylation and adenosine triphosphatase induction. Biochemistry **5**, 1729 (1966a).

GRAVEN, S. N., H. A. LARDY, and A. RUTTER: Antibiotics as tools for metabolic studies. VI. Oscillatory swelling of mitochondria induced by nonactin, monactin, dinactin and trinactin. Biochemistry **5**, 1735 (1966b).

LARDY, H. A., J. L. CONNELLY, and D. JOHNSON: Antibiotics as tools for metabolic studies. II. Inhibition of phosphoryl transfer in mitochondria by oligomycin and aurovertin. Biochemistry **3**, 1961 (1964).

Novobiocin*

Thomas D. Brock

The recent review by MACEY and SPOONER (1964) provides an excellent compliation for novobiocin on the chemistry, antimicrobial spectrum *in vitro*, assay and chromatographic procedures, development of resistance, *in vivo* activity, pharmacology, and toxicity in animals and humans, and the use of the antibiotic in non-medical situations. The present article will thus concentrate on a discussion of the mode of action of the antibiotic.

Although the activity of novobiocin is best against gram-positive bacteria, it does act on certain gram-negative bacteria as well, especially certain *Klebsiella* and *Proteus* strains. It has only weak or negligible activity against fungi and is less active against mycobacteria and corynebacteria than against other gram-positive bacteria. Two early observations related to its mode of action were that the antibiotic causes filamentation of gram-negative rods (SMITH *et al.*, 1956) and that its growth inhibiting activity especially for gram-negative bacteria is reversed readily by magnesium ions, and to a lesser extent by other alkaline earth metals (BROCK, 1956). A little later it was shown that novobiocin induced the accumulation of uridine nucleotide mucopeptides in *Staphylococcus aureus* (STROMINGER and THRENN, 1959). Because penicillin also induced accumulation of the uridine nucleotides, it was natural to assume that novobiocin inhibited cell wall formation. However, attempts to demonstrate specific inhibition of cell wall synthesis were unsuccessful (BROCK, 1960, 1962a). It was also found that growth of wall-less protoplasts (L-forms) was very sensitive to the antibiotic under conditions in which penicillin was not active (BROCK and BROCK, 1959; SHOCKMAN and LAMPEN, 1962). It thus seemed unlikely that the primary mode of action of novobiocin was in the inhibition of cell wall synthesis, and the original workers have now withdrawn this hypothesis (WISHNOW et al., 1965), although this idea has persisted in a number of textbooks and review articles.

In the integrated cell, the inhibition of one process may lead to the inhibition (or stimulation) of other processes indirectly, through the alteration of feedback systems or other control mechanisms, so that it is not possible to draw firm conclusions from the study of the effect of an antibiotic on a single process. It is necessary to study the temporal changes in a wide variety of processes from the moment of antibiotic addition, and attempt to identify the earliest processes which are affected. The target of an antibiotic is that element or elements within the cell with which the antibiotic combines and so affects that it alters the functioning of the cell. The target may be a specific substance such as a protein, enzyme or nucleic acid, but it may also be some less specific element such as a phospholipid or a divalent cation.

* Novobiocin has also been known by the names streptonivicin, Cathomycin, Albamycin and Cardelmycin.

The thesis of the present article is that novobiocin inhibits growth by combining with magnesium ions. A wide variety of enzyme and cell functions require magnesium ions for activity. Most enzymes which catalyze reactions involving phosphate groups require magnesium ions, such as nucleic acid synthetases, amino acid activating enzymes, teichoic acid synthesizing enzymes, glycolytic enzymes, phospholipases, etc. In addition, magnesium ions play a structural role in the cell membrane, probably by linking phospholipid molecules together, and magnesium ions also play a role in stabilizing the double-stranded form of DNA and in keeping the 30 S and 50 S ribosomal subunits together in the normal 70 S configuration. Clearly, a magnesium deficiency can have profound influences on the functioning of a cell. However, not all magnesium-related processes require equivalent amounts of the cation, so that some reactions may be more readily affected by a magnesium deficiency than others. Furthermore, some reactions can be measured more precisely or more sensitively than others, because of methodological factors, and thus it will be more likely that the early inhibition of these reactions will be detected. Finally, some organisms have a greater requirement for magnesium ions that others (WEBB, 1953), so that the growth of these organisms may be more readily affected. All of the above factors can contribute an element of specificity to the effects of an antibiotic which binds magnesium ions, making it seem that the antibiotic really inhibits in a specific manner a single reaction, even though it may inhibit many reactions. It is possible that novobiocin does have specific effects on certain organisms under certain conditions, perhaps related to the activity of the coumarin portion of the molecule (WEBER and ROSO, 1963), but there is no present evidence that these effects are in any way directly related to the growth inhibitory properties of the antibiotic.

Chemistry of Novobiocin and its Cation-Binding Properties

The structure of novobiocin is shown in Fig. 1. The antibiotic has two acidic groups, a weakly acidic phenol, and a more strongly acidic enol on the coumarin ring. The solubility of novobiocin is markedly affected by pH, and the free acid is insoluble in water, whereas the sodium salt is highly water soluble. Novobiocin forms insoluble salts with a variety of divalent and trivalent cations, including the alkaline earth metals, zinc, aluminium, manganese, and iron.

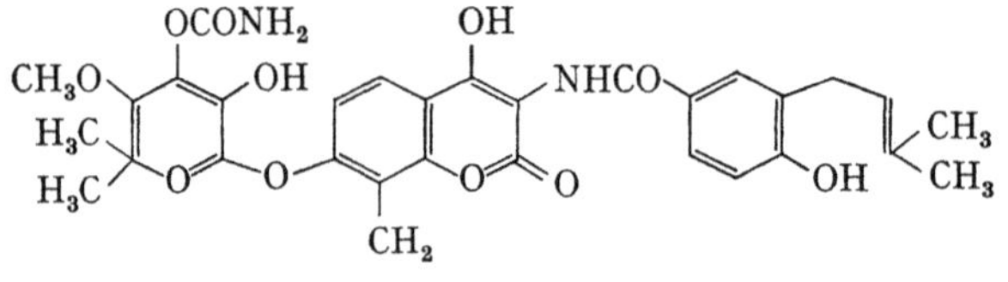

Fig. 1. Structure of novobiocin

The double bond of the 3-methyl-2-butenyl group can be reduced by catalytic hydrogenation, yielding dihydronovobiocin, with no loss in biological activity. However, the existence and position of the O-carbamyl group on the noviose sugar are essential for activity. Thus both descarbamyl novobiocin and isonovobiocin have greatly reduced biological activity.

Formation of a Novobiocin-Magnesium Ion Complex

When a variety of biological and biochemical data suggested that novobiocin might be inducing a magnesium deficiency (BROCK, 1962a), attempts were made to see if novobiocin could interact with magnesium ions in any additional way other than by forming an insoluble salt. No evidence of typical chelating properties for novobiocin could be found, but the following evidence (BROCK, 1962a) suggests that a charge-transfer complex (SZENT-GYÖRGI, 1960) might form between novobiocin and magnesium ions:

1. An aqueous mixture of 0.01 M novobiocin and 0.01 M $MgCl_2$ fluoresces under ultraviolet light when frozen or when dried on filter paper but not in the liquid state. A similar fluorescent complex is not formed with calcium ions. The novobiocin-magnesium complex occurs at pH 7.5 or 10.0. At pH less than 7.0 the free acid of novobiocin is formed which fluoresces in the solid state even in the absence of added cations.

2. Mixtures of 0.01 M novobiocin and 0.01 M $MgCl_2$ are more yellow than solutions of the antibiotic alone. The difference spectrum between novobiocin and novobiocin-magnesium chloride mixtures shows a peak at 390 mμ, as shown in Fig. 2. When the height of this peak is plotted versus magnesium ion concentration, a straight line is obtained. No peak is obtained when calcium chloride is substituted for magnesium chloride and no peak is obtained when descarbamyl novobiocin is used instead of novobiocin (Fig. 2). The lack of evidence for a charge transfer complex for descarbamyl novobiocin is interesting, and suggests that the carbamyl group may interact with the enolic or other electron donating group of the antibiotic molecule. It would be desirable to ascertain by modern chemical techniques the precise conformation of the antibiotic molecule.

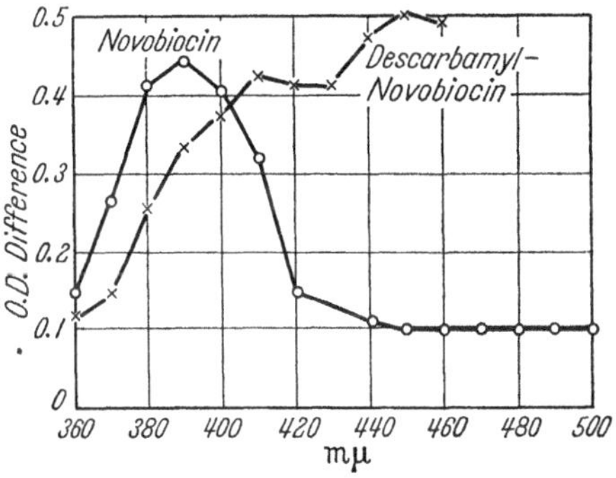

Fig. 2. Difference spectra of novobiocin and descarbamyl novobiocin in magnesium ions. 0.01 M antibiotic plus 0.01 M $MgCl_2$, pH 10.0. Absorption spectrum in Beckman DU spectrophotometer, 1 cm light path. Difference spectrum calculated as follows:

$$\frac{(\text{O.D. Nov.} + \text{Mg}) - (\text{O.D. Nov.})}{(\text{O.D. Nov.} + \text{Mg})}$$

3. Potentiometric titrations of 0.01 M solutions of novobiocin in the presence and absence of 0.02 M magnesium chloride revealed a small but definite and reproducible alteration in the titration curve brought about by magnesium ions.

4. If, instead of concentrated solutions, dilute solutions of novobiocin (1.6×10^{-5} M) are used, there is no spectral evidence of chelate formation when magnesium ion-novobiocin ratios of 1:1, 10:1, 100:1 and 1000:1 are used, at neutral, acid or alkaline pH, in water or ethanol. The existence of a magnesium ion novobiocin interaction in concentrated solutions and in the solid state, and its absence in dilute solutions, is evidence of a weak interaction of the charge transfer type.

5. Novobiocin has good electron donating properties as evidenced by its ability to form a dark brown complex with iodine on filter paper (SZENT-GYÖRGI,

1960), and other common antibiotics (e.g. penicillin, chloramphenicol) do not form such a complex.

6. Novobiocin is able to form insoluble salts with a variety of divalent and trivalent cations including calcium although no evidence of a charge transfer complex with calcium could be found. This indicates that novobiocin is able to interact with cations in at least two ways, by salt formation and by charge transfer complex.

Although high concentrations of antibiotic must be used before the magnesium-novobiocin complex is seen, the data below on binding of the antibiotic reveal that such concentrations may exist in the cell.

Adsorption of Novobiocin to Cells

In any study of drug action, it is essential to know the actual antibiotic concentration at the site of action. Unpublished work of C. G. SMITH (quoted in BROCK and BROCK, 1959) had shown that novobiocin was bound to bacteria, but the thick suspension technique used by him was not amenable to use with cells growing under physiological conditions or for short incubation times. Since novobiocin has attached to the aromatic ring an unsaturated side chain which can be catalytically hydrogenated (HINMAN *et al.*, 1957), and the resulting dihydronovobiocin retains full biological activity, it is possible to obtain tritium-labeled novobiocin of high specific radioactivity.

The tritiation was carried out by the New England Nuclear Corp. Twenty mg of novobiocin free acid and 25 mg of Adams catalyst in 4 ml ethyl acetate were treated with 3 curies of tritium gas. The catalyst was filtered and the residue was exchanged twice with 10 ml methanol. The specific activity of the resulting material was 82 mc/mg. Fifty µl of a 50 µc/ml solution was chromatographed on Whatman No. 1 filter paper in 96 water: 4 n-butanol. The strips were counted on a Vanguard windowless gas flow strip counter. One radioactive peak was obtained which had the correct R_f value for dihydronovobiocin. To make the sodium salt, nonradioactive dihydronovobiocin was added to a methanolic solution of radioactive antibiotic to produce a final specific activity of 10 mc/mg. The methanol was carefully evaporated to dryness on a steam bath and the material dissolved in the calculated amount of sodium hydroxide solution. This material was then used in the binding experiments.

Streptococcus faecium strain X3 was used in all binding experiments. In preliminary experiments, attempts were made to remove the cells from the radioactive medium on membrane filters (Millipore, Type HA). Unfortunately, the radioactive antibiotic itself was strongly bound to the filters. Therefore, the cells were centrifuged in the cold at 5000 rpm and washed three times with cold medium. In some experiments the cells were then resuspended in cold medium, aliquots filtered, and the filters glued directly to planchets and counted. In other experiments the washed cell pellet was extracted with ethyl acetate to remove the antibiotic and the extract plated and counted.

The radioactive ditritionovobiocin was as active in inhibiting growth as the non-radioactive parent substance, showing that the preparation of the radioactive material did not affect its antibiotic properties. The data in Table 1 show the time course of binding at 0° C and 37° C. At 0° C binding occurs quickly, and little additional binding occurs if the incubation is extended. The results at 37° C are anomalous, since more radioactivity seems to be retained in short incubations than in longer incubations. It is possible that at 37° C some metabolism of the radioactive compound takes place, with release of radioactivity. This might be either due to a breakdown of the molecule or to an exchange of the tritium atoms. Because of this, further binding studies were carried out at 0° C. The results in Table 2 show that the concentration of antibiotic bound to the cells was generally proportional to the concentration in the external medium, and the concentration of antibiotic on the cells was 7—60 times the external concentration. Another experiment using filtered cells instead of ethyl acetate extracts had given similar results.

These results show that novobiocin is quickly bound to cells, even at 0° C, and that the amount bound is roughly proportional to the external concentration. When 100 μg/ml of antibiotic was used, the concentration achieved per ml of wet cells was 2500 μg/ml, or 0.004 M, assuming that the drug is uniformly distributed throughout the cell fluid. If there were any localization in a structure of the cell such as the cell membrane, the local concentration might be much higher. Since novobiocin at 0.01 M forms a complex with magnesium ions these calculations show that concentrations in this range are achieved in cells, and this lends more credence to the theory that novobiocin inhibits growth by inducing a magnesium deficiency.

Table 1. *Effect of time and temperature on binding of 10 μg/ml radioactive ditritionovobiocin to growing cells of S. faecium*

Time of uptake	cpm/ml cells 0° C	cpm/ml cells 37° C
1 min	220	482
10 min	306	236
30 min	280	300
60 min	246	276

Radioactive novobiocin — 10 μg/ml (specific activity, 10 mc/mg). Antibiotic added to growing cells when cell O.D. reached 0.160. Cells centrifuged and washed in the cold. Volume of cells filtered, 0.5 ml. Cells counted directly on filters.

Table 2. *Quantitation of ditritionovobiocin binding to S. faecium*

Concentration of radioactive novobiocin	cpm/ml extract	μg antibiotic / ml wet cells	Concentration factor
1 μg/ml	35	60	60 ×
10 μg/ml	630	108	11 ×
50 μg/ml	2130	368	7 ×
100 μg/ml	14500	2500	25 ×

Cell concentration — O.D. 0.150 (400 μg wet weight cells/ml). Binding — 1 minute, 0° C. Extraction — 5 ml washed cells with 5 ml ethyl acetate. Radioactive standard — 0.1 μg/ml, 145 cpm/0.01 μg.

Novobiocin has a marked capacity to bind to proteins (Ritzenfeld, 1958; Tennent et al., 1957; Lubash *et al.*, 1956), and novobiocin solvates can bind to cellulose filter paper (Sokolski *et al.*, 1956). In a quantitative study using the ultracentrifuge, Grostic, Sokolski, Johnson and Colovos (unpublished), showed that binding to plasma proteins was proportional to external concentration, and that the concentration of antibiotic per mass of plasma protein was greater than 50 times the external concentration. In equilibrium dialysis experiments (LUBASH *et al.*, 1956) up to 94% of the added antibiotic was bound to serum proteins or to crystalline serum albumin. C. G. SMITH (unpublished) has shown that microorganisms sensitive and resistant to novobiocin bound similar amounts of the drug. Since novobiocin also binds readily to membrane filters, it seems unlikely that there is any specificity in the binding.

The main contribution of the work with labeled novobiocin is to show the rapidity with which binding takes place, the lack of temperature coefficient, and the concentration achieved on the bacterial cells. In all respects, binding of novobiocin to *S. faecium* is quite analogous to binding to serum albumin.

As discussed below, sensitive cells undergo several divisions in the presence of the antibiotic before inhibition is established. From the present results it is unlikely that this requirement is caused by a delay in binding of the antibiotic to the cells.

Biological and Biochemical Aspects of Novobiocin Action

Many studies have been made on the mechanism of novobiocin activity against microbes which have aerobic respiration, such as *Escherichia coli* (BROCK and BROCK, 1959; D. H. SMITH and DAVIS, 1965), *Staphylococcus aureus* (WISHNOW *et al.*, 1965) and *Micrococcus lysodeikticus* (BROCK, 1960). It was also desirable to investigate a sensitive organism which lacked both an aerobic metabolism and oxidative phosphorylation, but yet had a simple gram-positive cell wall and a reasonable sensitivity to the antibiotic. A strain of *Streptococcus faecium* was selected because it had no ability to take up oxygen in Warburg experiments, and thus its sensitivity to novobiocin was not likely to be related to a specific inhibition of oxydative phosphorylation (WEBER and ROSSO, 1963). The minimum inhibitory concentration of novobiocin for this strain of *S. faecium* was: 1 μg/ml in a complex medium and 25 μg/ml in a synthetic medium. This strain therefore showed a sensitivity to novobiocin of the same order as reported by earlier workers (SMITH *et al.*, 1956; WILKINS *et al.*, 1956). The marked difference in activity between the complex and the synthetic medium is similar to that reported earlier for gram-negative bacteria (BROCK, 1956). However, although antibiotic sensitivity appeared high, when various concentrations of novobiocin were added during the early logarithmic phase of growth in a complex medium, complete growth inhibition occurred immediately only after 1000 μg/ml of antibiotic was added. When growth was determined by turbidity measurements, it was apparent that only three or four divisions could take place before growth ceased due to nutrient exhaustion. Since novobiocin did not bring about complete inhibition of growth even at concentrations 100 times the minimum inhibitory concentration, it seemed possible that the organism might undergo a number of divisions in the presence of the antibiotic before it became completely inhibited. Consequently, an experiment was set up in which cells were kept continually growing by periodic 2-fold dilutions into fresh medium, always maintaining the same antibiotic concentration. The number of cell divisions necessary before growth inhibition was complete was determined for different novobiocin concentrations: at 100 μg/ml, inhibition became complete after 1 division; at 10 μg/ml, after 3 divisions; and 1 μg/ml, after 5 divisions.

The requirement of cell division for development of inhibition was further confirmed by experiments in which the growth rate of cells was reduced either by lowering the temperature or by using a synthetic medium at 37° C. When novobiocin was added to these slower growing cells, the cells went through the same number of divisions before inhibition was complete as when growing faster. The requirement for cell division to achieve complete inhibition at low concentrations of novobiocin complicates biochemical studies where non-growing cells are used in short term experiments. As noted above, cell division is not required for the binding of novobiocin to the cells, since binding is almost instantaneous, even at 0° C.

Table 3. *Effect of novobiocin on incorporation of labeled compounds into the intracellular pool of S. faecium*

^{14}C labelled compound	% of change over control			
	Polymyxin 1000 µg/ml	Nov. 1000 µg/ml	Nov. 100 µg/ml	Nov. 10 µg/ml
Lysine	—65	—99	0	—24
Glycine	—70	—66	—30	+7
Uracil	—47	+349	+285	+144
Na Acetate	—	—76	+17	—

Control values — lysine, 1265 cpm/ml; glycine, 263 cpm/ml; uracil, 1785 cpm/ml; acetate, 491 cpm/ml. Incubation—glycine, 13 minutes, 37° C; others, 60 minutes, 37° C.

Direct microscopic counts revealed that when novobiocin was added to growing cultures of *S. faecium*, chain formation occurred. Chaining began almost immediately upon addition of novobiocin and was more marked at 1 µg/ml than at higher concentrations. Growth was probably necessary for chaining to occur, and higher concentrations of antibiotic probably inhibited growth quicker. ROCHFORD and MANDLE (1953) have shown that magnesium deficiency induces chain formation in *Diplococcus pneumoniae*. Their method was used to prepare a magnesium-deficient complex medium to determine whether *S. faecium* also formed chains under these conditions, and it was found that magnesium deficiency does induce chain formation in this organism. Although exogenous magnesium ions only weakly reverse the action of novobiocin against *S. faecalis*, this does not rule out the magnesium deficiency hypothesis since exogenous magnesium ions may not be available to the magnesium-deficient site within the cell in this organism.

Isotope methods have been used in short-term experiments to measure the effects of novobiocin on macromolecular and cell synthesis in *S. faecium*. Since the cells must undergo several divisions in the presence of the antibiotic before inhibition is complete, 1000 µg/ml of antibiotic was used to achieve growth inhibition immediately, since this concentration correlates with that needed to inhibit growth in short term experiments.

The effect of novobiocin on uptake of several labeled compounds into the intracellular pool is shown in Table 3. The pool is defined as that fraction of the radioactivity not removed by a buffer wash, but removed by treatment with cold 5% trichloroacetic acid. The pool may thus contain both free material as well as low molecular weight derivatives of the compound supplied. Novobiocin inhibits the uptake of lysine, glycine and acetate, but strongly stimulates uptake of uracil. The uracil effect, to be discussed further below, reveals that novobiocin is not acting as a general cytotoxic agent, and is not non-specifically disrupting the semi-permeable membrane. For comparison, polymyxin, known to act directly on the physical structure of the membrane (Newton, 1956), inhibits transport of both uracil and the amino acids.

The glycine transport system in *S. faecium* has been studied in detail (Brock and Moo-Penn, 1962; Brock and Wooley, 1964), and has been shown to be a stereospecific, energy-requiring, exchange-diffusion process. Although novobiocin strongly inhibits the uptake of radioactive glycine, it has little effect on the exit of radioactive glycine from preloaded cells. This is a further indication that novobiocin is not a general cytotoxic agent.

Table 4. *Effect of antibiotics on incorporation of ^{14}C labeled lysine into the cell wall and other macromolecules of S. faecium*

Antibiotic	% change over control			
	Pool	Wall	Soluble RNA	Protein
Penicillin, 1000 µg/ml	+1	—65	+8	+73
Bacitracin, 1000 µg/ml	+30	—80	—63	—57
Chloramphenicol, 50 µg/ml	+35	—13	—58	—51
Novobiocin, 1000 µg/ml	—99	—69	—92	—89
Novobiocin, 100 µg/ml	0	—8	—89	—85
Novobiocin, 10 µg/ml	—24	—7	—39	—36

Control values — pool, 1265 cpm/ml; wall, 258 cpm/ml; soluble RNA, 715 cpm/ml; protein, 847 cpm/ml. Incubation — 1 hr., 37° C.

For the purposes of this discussion the incorporation of radioactive lysine into soluble RNA is evaluated by incubating the cells with radioactive lysine and determining the radioactivity resistant to treatment with cold 5% trichloracetic acid but extracted by 5% trichloracetic acid in 10 minutes at 100° C; incorporation of radioactive lysine into protein is evaluated by determining the radioactivity not extracted by the above procedure but extracted by 1 N NaOH in 20 minutes at 100° C; cell wall synthesis is evaluated by determining the residual incorporated radioactivity after further treatment with 1 N NaOH at 100° C for 1 hour.

The data in Table 4 show the marked differences between novobiocin and several other common antibiotics in inhibiting macromolecular syntheses. As expected, chloramphenicol inhibits incorporation into protein but not into cell wall. Novobiocin, on the other hand, inhibits incorporation into cell wall the least. By a comparison of the soluble RNA and protein figures, it seems possible that novobiocin inhibits incorporation into protein because of inhibition of incorporation into soluble RNA.

Novobiocin only partially inhibits the induced synthesis of β-galactosidase in *Escherichia coli* K-12 (Brock and Brock, 1959), and does not inhibit M protein synthesis in group A streptococcus at concentrations of 100 µg/ml or less, although this same process is inhibited at 0.1 µg/ml by erythromycin, and at 10 µg/ml by chloramphenicol (Brock, 1963). These results agree with the suggestions made above that novobiocin inhibits protein synthesis only indirectly through an effect on incorporation of amino acids into soluble RNA.

Table 5. *Effect of antibiotics on incorporation of radioactive uracil into pool and nucleic acids of S. faecium*

Antibiotic	% of change over controls	
	Pool	RNA
Novobiocin, 1000 μg/ml	+349	—93
Novobiocin, 100 μg/ml	+285	—81
Novobiocin, 10 μg/ml	+144	+163
Penicillin, 1000 μg/ml	—29	—9
Chloramphenicol, 50 μg/ml	+117	+217
Bacitracin, 1000 μg/ml	+297	—63
Streptomycin, 1000 μg/ml	—19	+135
Polymyxin, 100 μg/ml	—44	—47
Erythromycin, 1000 μg/ml	—16	+141
Cycloserine, 1000 μg/ml	—8	+188

Control values — pool, 1785 cpm/ml; nucleic acids, 2425 cpm/ml.

All of the radioactive uracil incorporated in *S. faecium* is found either in the pool or in the RNA fraction under the conditions used. Table 5 shows the results obtained for a number of antibiotics. The stimulation of RNA synthesis by chloramphenicol, streptomycin, and erythromycin is not surprising and has been reported earlier (Brock and Brock, 1959a; Hahn and Ciak, 1959). Novobiocin inhibits RNA synthesis strongly at 100 and 1000 μg/ml, while strongly stimulating incorporation into the pool. It is possible that the stimulation of incorporation into the pool, also seen with bacitracin, is due to inhibition of synthesis of nucleic acids and any other subsequent reactions involving uracil or uridine nucleotides, without the inhibition of the incorporation of uracil. The formation of an excess of a variety of uridine nucleotides, including the cell wall nucleotides, might thus occur in the presence of novobiocin. This would reconcile the observation (Strominger and Threnn, 1959) that novobiocin promotes accumulation of cell wall nucleotides with the observation made here that incorporation of lysine into the cell wall is less affected than other reactions. Lysine incorporation is a more direct measure of inhibition of cell wall synthesis than accumulation of uridine nucleotides. This hypothesis would also explain the data in *S. aureus* of Wishnow *et al.* (1965). Novobiocin is also an effective inhibitor of nucleic acid synthesis in *E. coli* (Smith, D. H., and Davis, 1965).

Incorporation of radioactive glucose into the polysaccharide (cell wall) is unaffected by novobiocin even at 1000 μg/ml. This concentration has only a minimal effect on incorporation of radioactive acetate into lipid. Incorporation of leucine and glycine into soluble RNA and protein are inhibited in a manner similar to that of lysine (Table 4).

Frei *et al.* (1958) have reported the inhibition by novobiocin of respiration and oxidative phosphorylation in rat liver homogenates and Weber and Rosso (1963) reported a similar inhibition in *Mycobacterium phlei*. Brock and Brock

(1959) reported the inhibition by the antibiotic of the nitrate reductase of *E. coli*. Novobiocin at 1000 µg/ml also inhibits oxygen uptake by cells of *Micrococcus lysodeikticus* with ethanol, succinate or glucose as substrates. It inhibits reduction of 2,3,5-triphenyltetrazolium chloride and potassium ferricyanide by whole cells and cell extracts of *M. lysodeikticus* with succinate or ethanol as electron donors. With ethanol as electron donor, diphosphopyridine nucleotide was used as an intermediate electron carrier. Reduction of tetrazolium chloride by whole cells of *S. faecium* is also inhibited. The production of lactic acid from glucose by *S. faecium* is inhibited by novobiocin as measured by CO_2 release from bicarbonate buffer in the Warburg apparatus in an atmosphere of 95% N_2-5% CO_2 or as measured by color change of brom cresol purple indicator.

Luminescence of *Photobacterium phosphorium* is inhibited by 1000 µg/ml novobiocin, and this luminescence cannot be reactivated by extensive washing of the cells in fresh medium.

However, motility of *Salmonella typhimurium* and of a motile strain of *S. faecium* are not inhibited by 5 mg/ml novobiocin. It is interesting that motility is also not inhibited by 0.01 M sodium azide.

Novobiocin at 1 mg/ml causes 25% inhibition of the ATPase activity of sonic extracts of *S. faecium* using the system of ABRAMS *et al.* (1960). KESSLER and RICKENBERG (personal communication) have found that novobiocin at 0.01 M completely inhibits the ATPase of *E. coli*. They also found sodium azide to be an effective inhibitor although not as active as novobiocin. It is interesting that sodium azide potentiates novobiocin action in *E. coli*.

Discussion of the Mode of Action of Novobiocin

The present paper and previous reports (BROCK, 1956; BROCK and BROCK, 1959; BROCK, 1962a) reveal a wide variety of effects that are induced by novobiocin. There is an induction of filament formation in gram-negative rods, chain formation in *S. faecium*, and permeability effects in *E. coli* ML 35. Novobiocin inhibits respiration, electron transfer, ATPase activity, amino acid and acetate transport, the incorporation of amino acids into soluble RNA and of radioactive uracil into RNA. The antibiotic also inhibits luminescence, and the activity of DNA and RNA polymerases (SMITH, D. H., and DAVIS, 1965).

Also significant are the processes less affected or unaffected by novobiocin such as incorporation of lysine into cell wall, motility, protein synthesis, and the efflux of radioactive amino acids from preloaded cells. One process that was markedly stimulated was the uptake of radioactive uracil into the cell. These latter results show that novobiocin is not a general cytotoxic agent but affects a wide variety of specific processes in the cell.

Each process affected by novobiocin is related to magnesium requirements of cells as indicated below:

1. Filamentation is induced by magnesium deficiency (WEBB, 1953).
2. Chain formation is induced by magnesium deficiency (ROCHFORD and MANDLE, 1953; BROCK, unpublished).
3. Permeability effects in *E. coli* ML 35 are induced by magnesium deficiency (BROCK, 1962b).

4. Respiration, fermentation, electron transport and oxidative phosphorylation all show absolute requirements for magnesium ions, at least for certain key enzymes (FRUTON and SIMMONDS, 1958).

5. ATPase activity requires magnesium ions (ABRAMS *et al.*, 1960; DIXON and WEBB, 1958).

6. Amino acid transport requires magnesium ions (GALE, 1953; PAL and CHRISTENSEN, 1959).

7. The incorporation of amino acids into soluble RNA has an absolute requirement for magnesium ions (HECHT *et al.*, 1959; ROBERTS *et al.*, 1959).

8. The synthesis of RNA and DNA have absolute requirements for magnesium ions (ROBERTS *et al.*, 1959).

9. Although there is no apparent metal requirement for the luminescence process itself, electron transport is necessary for luminescence and luminescence is inhibited by agents that inhibit electron transport (MCELROY, 1961).

10. DNA and RNA polymerases have absolute requirements for magnesium ions (DAVIDSON, 1960).

The processes that are unaffected or little affected by novobiocin have not been shown to require magnesium ions.

An interesting parallelism exists between magnesium and the bactericidal effects of the antibiotic. Cells of *S. faecium* die only slowly during growth in magnesium deficient medium (MACLEOD, 1951), and novobiocin is only slowly bactericidal to this organism. On the contrary, *E. coli* ML 35 is killed much more quickly in magnesium deficient medium (BROCK, 1962b), and novobiocin is more bactericidal to this organism (BROCK and BROCK, 1959).

Effects of magnesium deficiency are potentiated by zinc (WEBB, 1953), and novobiocin inhibition is potentiated by zinc (BROCK, 1962a). Antagonisms between zinc and magnesium ions have also been noted by ABELSON and ALDOUS (1950) and MILSTEIN (1961).

The inhibition of cell wall synthesis is not a primary effect of the antibiotic. This concept is confirmed by data showing that growth of L forms (BROCK and BROCK, 1959) protoplasts (SHOCKMAN and LAMPEN, 1962) and pleuropneumonia-like organisms (PPLO) (CARSKI and SHEPARD, 1961) are strongly inhibited by novobiocin. Since magnesium ions are essential for the stability of the cell membrane (WEIBULL, 1956; HERSHKO *et al.*, 1961) and since the cell membrane is of crucial importance for the cellular integrity of both L forms and PPLO, this effect of novobiocin is understandable.

Magnesium deficiency has been shown to induce a variety of morphological effects on bacteria. In rod-shaped bacteria the predominant effect is the formation of filaments (WEBB, 1953; NICKERSON and SHERMAN, 1952; BROWN and GIBBONS, 1955; BLAKENSHIP and DOETSCH, 1961). In cocci chain formation is the predominant effect (ROCHFORD and MANDLE, 1953). Novobiocin also induces both filament formation in rods and chain formation in cocci, and this striking similarity in action of antibiotic and magnesium deficiency in quite unrelated bacteria hardly seems accidental. The degradation and excretion of RNA has also been shown to be induced by magnesium ion deficiency (HOLDEN, 1958). These results are all consistent with the effect of novobiocin on morphology and RNA stability.

At least 58 different enzymes are known to require magnesium ions for activity (HASTINGS, 1961). Magnesium ions also stabilize the cell membrane (WEIBULL, 1956) and ribosomes (TISSIÈRES *et al.*, 1959). This wide variety of roles is consistent with the wide variety of effects inducible by novobiocin.

Recent observations on chlorpromazine (NATHAN, 1961; BOURDON, 1961) and aminosidine (BARDI *et al.*, 1961) are consistent with hypothesis that these agents also affect magnesium related processes. It has also been shown recently that the effect of phenol is reversed by various divalent ions (HARVIS and RICHARDS, 1961). This observation is especially interesting, since novobiocin is a phenolic compound.

The evidence for the present hypothesis, although extensive, is indirect. It can always be argued that the effects observed are only secondary results of some still unknown primary reaction. However, it is hard to design an experiment which will provide direct evidence. Cells growing in the presence of novobiocin might retain all the magnesium ions they have, or continue to take up more magnesium ions, but in the presence of novobiocin, these ions, although measurable in a chemical assay, might be non-functional, as far as the cell is concerned. Thus a direct demonstration of induction of a magnesium deficiency might not be possible. The absence of a good radioactive isotope of magnesium makes experimentation in this field difficult.

Chemical studies described above have revealed that novobiocin is able to form specific complexes with magnesium ions. There is no need, however, to postulate that novobiocin affects only magnesium ions. The antibiotic forms insoluble salts with a variety of group IIA, IIB, IIIA and VIII metals. Magnesium, however, is quantitatively the most important metal in the cell, since it plays a large number of functional and structural roles. WEINBERG (1961) has reviewed the importance of metal coordination and the action of antimicrobial drugs. It is readily understandable that a magnesium deficiency might be an early manifestation of novobiocin inhibition.

The relationship between sodium azide and novobiocin is of some interest. Azide at subinhibitory concentrations strongly potentiates novobiocin activity. A number of cell functions are inhibited both by azide and novobiocin: respiration, electron transport, oxidative phosphorylation, ATPase, and amino acid transport. Significantly, azide and novobiocin both have no effect on motility. The inhibition by azide of a wide variety of metal-containing enzymes is well known (DIXON and WEBB, 1958, p. 374—375), and this may be further suggestive evidence that novobiocin acts by binding metals. On a molar basis, novobiocin is more active than azide and cyanide in inhibiting electron transport.

If novobiocin does inhibit growth because it induces a magnesium deficiency, it is of interest to consider the reason for its selective toxicity. As WEBB (1953) has shown, gram-positive organisms have a ten-fold higher requirement for magnesium than gram-negative organisms. Novobiocin is more active against gram-positive than gram-negative organisms although certain gram-negative bacteria, i.e. *Proteus* and *Klebsiella* (WILKINS *et al.*, 1956) are fairly sensitive. Since all organisms presumably require magnesium, and since there seems to be no selective binding of novobiocin to antibiotic-sensitive cells, it seems likely that novobiocin would inhibit growth of all organisms to degrees parallel with their magnesium requirements. Novobiocin also inhibits the growth of a gram-negative marine organism *Leucothrix mucor* (BROCK, unpublished), and the high magnesium requirement of marine organisms is well known.

Novobiocin action is not restricted to bacteria. The antibiotic can inhibit the fungi, *Blastomyces* and *Monospermum*, and the protozoan, *Trichomonas*, at relatively low concentrations (SPECTOR, 1957). It is also interesting that the antibiotic inhibits the growth of *S. niveus*, the organism that produces novobiocin (HOEKSEMA and SMITH, 1961). NORMAN (1960) has shown that novobiocin inhibits primary root elongation in cucumbers at 50—250 μg/ml, and induces a leakage of materials absorbing at 270 mμ in barley roots. This latter effect is reversed by calcium ions.

Cells must undergo several divisions in the presence of the antibiotic before growth inhibition becomes complete. This may be because a dilution of the magnesium existing at sensitive cell sites must occur to achieve growth inhibition. In infected animals, the parasite usually divides much more rapidly than the host cells and so would be inhibited more quickly. Because of this difference in rate of cellular multiplication, novobiocin could be used in the therapy of acute diseases even if it acted on host cells. Dosage of the antibiotic could be so regulated that novobiocin would not be in the tissues long enough to induce effects on the host. In extended usage of the antibiotic, however, toxicity might occur.

Acknowledgements. Unpublished data of the author are based on work supported by a research grant from U.S. Public Health Service, E-3722. The author is a Research Career Development Awardee of the U.S.P.H.S. The technical assistance of M. L. BROCK is gratefully acknowledged.

See Addendum

References

ABELSON, P. H., and E. ALDOUS: Ion antagonisms in microorganisms: interference of normal magnesium metabolism by nickel, cobalt, cadium, zinc, and manganese. J. Bacteriol. **60**, 401 (1950).

ABRAMS, A., P. MCNAMARA, and F. B. JOHNSON: Adenosine triphosphatase in isolated bacterial cell membranes. J. Biol. Chem. **235**, 3659 (1960).

BARDI, U., G. BORETTI, and A. DIMARCO: Inhibition of oxidative phosphorylation by aminosidine and other antibiotics in rat liver mitochondria. Biochem. Pharmacol. **1**, 165 (1961).

BLANKENSHIP, L. C., and R. N. DOETSCH: Influence of a bacterial cell extract upon the morphogenesis of *Arthrobacter ureafaciens*. J. Bacteriol. **82**, 882 (1961).

BOURDON, J. L.: Contribution a l'étude des proprietés antibiotiques de la chlorpromazine ou 4560 RP. Ann. inst. Pasteur **101**, 876 (1961).

BROCK, T. D.: Studies on the mode of action of novobiocin. J. Bacteriol. **72**, 320 (1956).

BROCK, T. D.: Permeability and the mode of action of antibiotics. Antimicrobial Agents Ann., p. 297 (1960).

BROCK, T. D.: Magnesium binding as an explanation of the mode of action of novobiocin. Science **136**, 316 (1962a).

BROCK, T. D.: Effects of magnesium ion deficiency on *Escherichia coli* and possible relation to the mode of action of novobiocin. J. Bacteriol. **84**, 679 (1962b).

BROCK, T. D.: Effect of antibiotics and inhibitors on M protein synthesis. J. Bacteriol. **85**, 527 (1963).

BROCK, T. D., and M. L. BROCK: Effect of novobiocin on permeability of *Escherichia coli*. Arch. Biochem. Biophys. **85**, 176 (1959).

BROCK, T. D., and M. L. BROCK: Similarity in mode of action of chloramphenicol and erythromycin. Biochim. et Biophys. Acta **33**, 274 (1959a).

Brock, T. D., and G. Moo-Penn: An amino acid transport system in *Streptococcus faecium*. Arch. Biochem. Biophys. **98**, 183 (1962).
Brock, T. D., and S. O. Wooley: Glycylglycine uptake in streptococci and a possible role of peptides in amino acid transport. Arch. Biochem. Biophys. **105**, 51 (1964).
Brown, H. J., and N. E. Gibbons: The effect of magnesium, potassium and iron on the growth and morphology of red halophilic bacteria. Can. J. Microbiol. **1**, 486 (1955).
Carski, T. R., and C. C. Shepard: Pleuropneumonia-like (Mycoplasma) infections of tissue culture. J. Bacteriol. **81**, 626 (1961).
Davidson, J. N.: The biochemistry of the nucleic acids. London: Methuen & Co. 1960.
Dixon, M., and E. C. Webb: Enzymes. NewYork: Academic Press 1958.
Frei, J., N. Canal, and E. Gori: Novobiocin as uncoupling agent. Experientia **14**, 377 (1958).
Fruton, J. S., and S. Simmonds: General biochemistry. New York: John Wiley & sons 1958.
Gale, E. F.: Assimilation of amino acids by gram-positive bacteria and some actions of antibiotics thereon. Advances in Protein Chem. **8**, 287 (1953).
Hahn, F. E., and J. Ciak: Studies on the mode of action of streptomycin, I. Inhibition of bacterial protein synthesis by streptomycin. Bacteriol. Proc. (Soc. Am. Bacteriologists) **1959**, 131 (1959).
Harvis, N. D., and J. P. Richards: Influence of adding salts to the medium on counts of phenol-treated *Escherichia coli* on membrane filters. Nature **192**, 87 (1961).
Hastings, A. B.: Discussion of paper by L. A. Johnson, and M. J. Seven, Biological aspects of metal-binding. Federation Proc. **20**, Suppl. **10**, 226 (1961).
Hecht, L. I., M. L. Stephenson, and P. C. Zamecnik: Binding of amino acids to the end group of a soluble ribonucleic acid. Proc. Natl. Acad. Sci. U.S. **45**, 505 (1959).
Hershko, A., S. Amos, and J. Mager: Effect of polyamines and divalent metals on *in vitro* incorporation of amino acids into ribonucleoprotein particles. Biochim. et Biophys. Acta **5**, 46 (1961).
Hinman, J. W., E. L. Caron, and H. Hoeksema: The structure of novobiocin. J. Am. Chem. Soc. **79**, 3789 (1957).
Hoeksema, H., and C. G. Smith: Novobiocin. Prog. Industrial Microbiol. **3**, 91 (1961).
Holden, J. T.: Degradation of intracellular nucleic acid and leakage of fragments by *Lactobacillus arabinosus*. Biochim. et Biophys. Acta **29**, 667 (1958).
Lubash, G., J. van der Meulen, C. Berntsen, and R. Tompsett: Novobiocin: a laboratory investigation. Antibiotic Med. **2**, 233 (1956).
Macey, P. E., and D. F. Spooner: Experimental chemotherapy, vol. III. Chemotherapy of bacterial infections, part II. New York: Academic Press 1964.
MacLeod, R. A.: Further mineral requirements of *Streptococcus faecalis*. J. Bacteriol. **62**, 337 (1951).
McElroy, W. D.: Bacterial luminescence. In: The bacteria, vol. II, p. 479. NewYork: Academic Press 1961.
Milstein, C.: Inhibition of phosphoglucomutase by trace metals. Biochem. J. **79**, 591 (1961).
Nathan, H. A.: Alteration of permeability of *Lactobacillus plantarum* caused by chlorpromazine. Nature **1961**, 471.
Newton, B. A.: The properties and mode of action of the polymyxins. Bacteriol. Rev. **20**, 14 (1956).
Nickerson, W. J., and F. G. Sherman: Metabolic aspects of bacterial growth in the absence of division. II. Respiration of normal and filamentous cells of *Bacillus cereus*. J. Bacteriol. **64**, 667 (1952).
Norman, A. G.: Microbial products affecting root development. Seventh Intern. Congr. Soil Sci., vol. II; Commission III, 531 (1960).
Pal, P. R., and H. W. Christensen: Interrelationships in the cellular uptake of amino acids and metals. J. Biol. Chem. **234**, 613 (1959).

ROBERTS, R. B., K. McQUILLEN, and I. Z. ROBERTS: Biosynthetic aspects of metabolism. Ann. Rev. Microbiol. **13**, 1 (1959).
ROCHFORD, E. J., and R. J. MANDLE: The production of chains by *Diplococcus pneumoniae* in magnesium deficient media J. Bacteriol. **66**, 554 (1953).
SHOCKMAN, G. D., and J. D. LAMPEN: Inhibition by antibiotics of the growth of bacterial and yeast protoplasts. J. Bacteriol. **84**, 508 (1962).
SMITH, C. G., A. DIETZ, W. T. SOKOLSKI, and G. M. SAVAGE: Streptonivicin, a new antibiotic. Antibiotics & Chemotherapy **6**, 135 (1956).
SMITH, D. H., and B. D. DAVIS: Inhibition of nucleic acid synthesis by novobiocin. Biochem. Biophys. Research Commun. **18**, 796 (1965).
SOLKOLSKI, W., N. J. EILERS, and J. W. SHELL: Adsorption of novobiocin solvates on paper during development in paper chromatography. Antibiotics Ann. **1956/57**, 1031 (1957).
SPECTOR, W. S.: Handbook of toxicology, vol. II. Antibiotics. Philadelphia: W. B. Saunders Co. 1957.
STROMINGER, J. L., and R. H. THRENN: The optical configuration of the alanine residues in a uridine nucleotide and in the cell wall of *Staphylococcus aureus*. Biochim. et Biophys. Acta **33**, 280 (1959).
SZENT-GYÖRGYI, A.: Introduction to a submolecular biology. New York: Academic Press 1960.
TISSIÈRES, A., J. D. WATSON, D. SCHLESSINGER, and B. R. HOLLINGWORTH: Ribonucleoprotein particles from *Escherichia coli*.. J. Mol. Biol. **1**, 221 (1959).
WEBB, M.: Effects of magnesium on cellular division in bacteria. Science **118**, 607 (1953).
WEBER, M. M., and G. ROSO: Novobiocin inhibition of electron transport in *Mycobacterium phlei*. Bacteriol. Proc. (Soc. Am. Bacteriologists), p. 95 (1963).
WEIBULL, C.: Bacterial protoplasts; their formation and characteristics. In: Bacterial anatomy, p. 111. Cambridge University Press 1956.
WEINBERG, E. D.: Known and suspected role of metal coordination in actions of antimicrobial drugs. Federation Proc. **20**, Suppl. **10**, 132 (1961).
WILKINS, J. R., C. LEWIS, and A. R. BARBIERS: Streptonivicin, a new antibiotic. III. *In vitro* and *in vivo* evaluation. Antibiotics & Chemotherapy **6**, 149 (1956).
WISHNOW, R. M., J. L. STROMINGER, C. H. BIRGE, and R. H. THRENN: Biochemical effects of novobiocin on *Staphylococcus aureus*. J. Bacteriol. **89**, 1117 (1965).

Actithiazic Acid

Paul G. Caltrider

Actithiazic acid was discovered and isolated concurrently in four different laboratories. Names proposed for the organisms producing the antibiotic were *Streptomyces virginiae* (GRUNDY *et al.*, 1952), *S. acidomyceticus* (MIYAKE *et al.*, 1953a), *S. lavendulae* (TEJERA *et al.*, 1952), and *S. cinnamonensis* (MAEDA *et al.*, 1953). Synonyms for actithiazic acid are acidomycin, cinnamonin and mycobacidin.

Actithiazic acid is (—)2-(5 carboxypentyl)-4-thiazolidone. Its molecular structure is given below (MCLAMORE *et al.*, 1952; SCHENCK and DEROSE, 1952; MCLAMORE *et al.*, 1953; MIYAKE *et al.*, 1953b; and GRUNDY *et al.*, 1954).

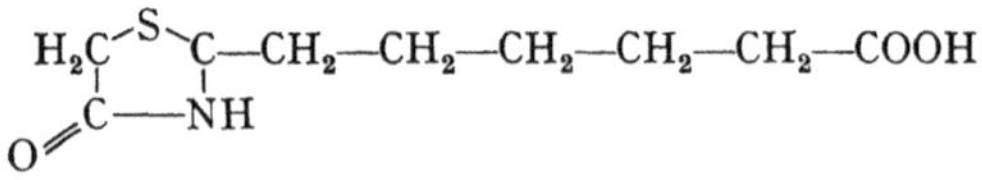

Several derivatives and analogs of the antibiotic have been synthesized in efforts to study the relationship between chemical structure and antibacterial activity (CLARK and SCHENCK, 1952; MIYAKE, 1953a; and KAWASHIMA *et al.*, 1956). The amide and lower alkyl esters were active against *Mycobacterium* spp. *in vitro*, and a side chain containing five methylene groups was optimal for antibiotic activity. Both the carbonyl group at ring position four and the bivalent sulfur atom were essential for biological activity.

The antibiotic activity of actithiazic acid is limited to species of mycobacteria. Generally, concentrations of 1 to 10 μg/ml are required to inhibit growth of mycobacteria *in vitro*. Under the same assay conditions, concentrations of the antibiotic up to 1 mg/ml do not inhibit growth of Gram-positive and Gram-negative bacteria and fungi (GRUNDY *et al.*, 1953; TEJERA *et al.*, 1952). Slight antibiotic activity was found at high concentrations of the antibiotic with the latter organisms in a chemically defined medium.

In vivo tests showed that actithiazic acid or its derivatives were practically non-toxic, but they also showed no activity against *M. tuberculosis* infection in animals (HWANG, 1952; SOBIN, 1952). The LD_{50} in mice was 3.5 g/kg intravenously and 2 g/kg subcutaneously (MIYAKE *et al.*, 1953a). Data of HWANG (1952) showed that actithiazic acid was inactivated very rapidly after injection into mice.

Because of the structural similarity of actithiazic acid to biotin, the antagonism between biotin and this antibiotic was investigated. *In vitro* tests showed that biotin reversed the growth inhibition of mycobacteria (GRUNDY *et al.*, 1952; HAMADA *et al.*, 1953; KAWASHIMA and FUJII, 1953; UMEZAWA *et al.*, 1953a, b). The addition of 0.01 μg per ml of biotin to KIRCHNER'S medium could eliminate the antitubercular effect of less than 20 μg per ml of the antibiotic. Further evidence for actithiazic acid acting as a biotin antagonist was reported by STIM *et al.* (1959). Known biotin antagonists, such as isonicotinic hydrazide, in conjunction with actithiazic acid gave a synergistic effect in the inhibition of growth of *Bacillus subtilis* var. *niger*, and this selective synergism was completely counteracted by biotin. The mechanism of biotin-antagonism by actithiazic acid is not known. Mycobacteria do not require exogenous biotin; therefore, the antibiotic must interfere with the synthesis of the vitamin. PITTILLO and FOSTER (1954) reported that actithiazic acid reduced the biosynthesis of biotin in *Aerobacter aerogenes*.

It is believed that actithiazic acid is inactive *in vivo* because sufficient quantities of biotin to reverse its inhibitory effects are present in tissues of the host. When the antibiotic was administered to rabbits, the biotin level in the urine markedly increased (HAMADA *et al.*, 1953; KAWASHIMA and FUJII, 1953). The biotin present in this urine antagonized the activity of the antibiotic *in vitro*. No antagonism was found between the antibiotic and its degradation products in a biotin-deficient medium (KAWASHIMA *et al.*, 1953).

References

CLARK, JR., R. K., and J. R. SCHENCK: Actithiazic acid. III. The synthesis of DL-actithiazic acid, derivatives of homologs. Arch. Biochem. **40**, 270 (1952).

GRUNDY, W. E., A. L. WHITMAN, E. G. RDZOK, E. J. RDZOK, M. E. HANES, and J. C. SYLVESTER: Actithiazic acid. I. Microbiological studies. Antibiotics & Chemotherapy **2**, 399 (1952).

GRUNDY, W. E., A. L. WHITMAN, J. C. SYLVESTER, J. R. SCHENCK, and A. F. DEROSE: 4-thiazolidone-2-n-caproic acid and salts and methods of preparing. U.S. Patent Office 2,678,929 (1954).

HAMADA, Y., M. KAWASHIMA, A. MILAKE, and K. OKAMOTA: Antiacidomycin factor in rabbits urine oberved by cylinder plate method. J. Antibiotics (Japan), Ser. A **6**, 158 (1953).

HWANG, K.: Actithiazic acid. IV. Pharmacological studies. Antibiotics & Chemotherapy **2**, 453 (1952).

KAWASHIMA, M., and S. FUJII: Acidomycin. II. Increase of urinary biotin excretion of acidomycin-tested rabbits. Pharm. Bull. (Tokyo) **1**, 328 (1953).

KAWASHIMA, M., Y. HAMADA, and S. FUJII: Acidomycin. VI. Metabolic antagonism with biotin. Pharm. Bull. (Tokyo) **1**, 94 (1953).

KAWASHIMA, M., A. MIYAKE, T. HEMMI, and S. FUJII: Acidomycin. III. Antibiotin activity of acidomycin and its related compounds. Pharm. Bull. (Tokyo) **4**, 53 (1956).

MAEDA, K.: Chemical studies on antibiotic substances. III. An antimycobacterial antibiotic produced by *Streptomyces cinnamonensis*. Japan J. Med. Sci. & Biol. **6**, 143 (1953).

MCLAMORE, W. M., W. D. CELMER, V. V. BOGERT, F. C. PENNINGTON, B. A. SOBIN, and I. A. SOLOMONS: Structure and synthesis of a new, thiazolidone antibiotic. J. Am. Chem. Soc. **75**, 105 (1953).

MIYAKE, A.: Antibiotic. II. Acidomycin. Antitubercular activity of compounds related to acidomycin. Pharm. Bull. (Tokyo) **1**, 89 (1953).

MIYAKE, A., A. MORIMATO, and T. KINOSHITA: Antibiotics. I. Acidomycin. Isolation and chemical structure. Pharm. Bull. (Tokyo) **1**, 84 (1953).

PITTILLO, R. F., and J. W. FOSTER: Potentiation of inhibitor action through determination of reversing metabolites. J. Bacteriol. **67**, 53 (1954).

SCHENCK, J. R., and A. F. DEROSE: Actithiazic acid. II. Isolation and characterization. Arch. Biochem. Biophys. **40**, 263 (1952).

SOBIN, B. A.: A new streptomyces antibiotic. J. Am. Chem. Soc. **74**, 2947 (1952).

STIM, T. B., B. C. ARNWINE, and J. W. FOSTER: Further studies on potentiation of inhibitor action through determination of reversing metabolites. J. Bacteriol. **77**, 566 (1959).

TEJERA, E., E. J. BACKUS, M. DANN, C. D. ERVIN, A. J. SHAKOFSKI, S. O. THOMAS, N. BOHONOS, and J. H. WILLIAMS: Mycobacidin: An antibiotic active against acid-fast organism. Antibiotics & Chemotherapy **2**, 333 (1952).

UMEZAWA, H., K. OIKAWA, K. MAEDA, and Y. OKAMI: Antibiotin activity of thiazolidone antibiotic. Japan J. Med. Sci. & Biol. **6**, 395 (1953).

UMEZAWA, H., K. OIKAWA, Y. OKAMI, and K. MAEDA: Thiazolidone antibiotic as an antimetabolite to biotin. J. Bacteriol. **66**, 118 (1953).

Minomycin

Paul G. Caltrider

Minomycin is an orange-pigmented antibiotic produced by *Streptomyas minoensis* n. sp. (NISHIMURA *et al.*, 1960; NISHIMURA, 1964). The molecular structure has not been elucidated but analytical data show that the antibiotic contains C-61.17%, H-6.52%, O-30.77% and OCH_3-3.76% (NISHIMURA *et al.*, 1960).

In vitro, minomycin is highly active against a wide variety of Gram-positive bacteria, but it shows little or no activity against Gram-negative bacteria (Table 1). It does not possess antifungal activity (NISHIMURA *et al.*, 1960). Minomycin showed appreciable activity against Ehrlich mouse ascites tumor and mouse Crocker sarcoma *in vitro*, but no carcinostatic activity was observed *in vivo*

Table 1. *Antimicrobial spectrum of minomycin* (NISHIMURA *et al.*, 1960)

Test organism	Minimal inhibitory concentration μg/ml
Staphylococcus, 209P	0.50
Bacillus subtilis, PCI-219	0.05
Sarcina lutea	0.20
Bacillus anthracis	0.02
Diplococcus pneumoniae, type I	0.01
Streptococcus hemolyticus, D	0.05
Klebsiella pneumoniae	> 50
Escherichia coli	> 50
Salmonella typhosa	> 50
Shigella dysenteriae	> 50
Aspergillus niger	> 50
Candida albicans	> 50
Torula sp.	> 50

(NISHIMURA *et al.*, 1960; NISHIYAMA and KATAGIRI, 1964). However, a prophylactic effect on poliomylitis in mice has been reported (NISHIYAMA and KATAGIRI, 1964). *In vivo*, minomycin exhibited marked activity against experimental pneumococcal infection in mice when administered intraperitoneally, slight activity when administered subcutaneously, and no therapeutic effect by the oral route (NISHIMURA *et al.*, 1960).

The intraperitoneal acute LD_{50} of minomycin in mice was 15 mg/kg (NISHIMURA *et al.*, 1960). Single oral doses of the drug (600 mg/kg) were well tolerated apparently, due to poor absorption.

NISHIMURA and SHIMOHIRA (1963) found more absorption of minomycin by a sensitive organism (*S. aureus*) than by less sensitive organisms (*E. coli* and *C. albicans*). Respiration of *S. aureus* was inhibited markedly by the antibiotic. SHINOHIRA (1960) reported that minomycin showed a marked bactericidal action on multiplying cells of *S. aureus*, but none on resting cells. The synthesis of an adaptive enzyme which mediates the oxidation of arabinose by *B. subtilis* was also inhibited by minomycin. SHIMOHIRA (1962) showed that minomycin activity was bound mainly in the RNA fraction in cells of *S. aureus*. Although critical data are lacking, these studies suggest that protein or nucleic acid synthesis may be the primary site of action of minomycin.

References

NISHIMURA, H.: Method of producing the antibiotic minomycin. U.S. Patent Office 3,146,174 (1964).

NISHIYAMA, S., and K. KATAGIRI: Antiviral action of minomycin against poliomyelitis in mice. Ann. Rep. Shionogi Res. Lab. 210 (1964).

NISHIMURA, H., K. SASAKI, M. MAYAMA, N. SHIMAOKA, K. TAWARA, S. OKAMOTO, and K. NAKAJIMA: Minomycin, a new antibiotic pigment from a *Streptomyces sp.* J. Antibiotics (Japan), Ser. A **13**, 327 (1960).

NISHIMURA, H., and M. SHIMOHIRA: Inhibition de la respiration bactérienne par la minomycine, un nouvel antibiotique. Compt. rend. Soc. Biol. **157**, 441 (1963).

SHIMOHIRA, M.: Some observations on the in vitro action of a new antibiotic, minomycin. Ann. Rep. Shionogi Res. Lab. 241 (1960).

SHIMOHIRA, M.: Electrophoretic distribution of minomycin in minomycin-fixed bacterial cells. Ann. Rep. Shionogi Res. Lab. 222 (1962).

Protoanemonin

Paul G. Caltrider

Protoanemonin is an antibiotic substance produced mainly by species of *Ranunculaceae*. Reports of its presence are in the following references: BOAS (1934), ZECHNER and WOHLMUTH (1954), KIPPING (1935), SHEARER (1938), BAER *et al.* (1946), HERZ *et al.* (1951), BERNARD and METZGER (1960) and TASHKOV *et al.* (1961).

In the intact plant, protoanemonin exists as a glucoside (ranunculin). On maceration of the plant tissues, it is released by an enzymatic process (HILL and VAN HEYNINGEN, 1951). Protoanemonin is the lactone of α-hydroxyvinyl-acrylic acid with the following molecular structure (ASAHINA and FUJITA, 1920; KIPPING, 1935; MORIARTY *et al.*, 1965):

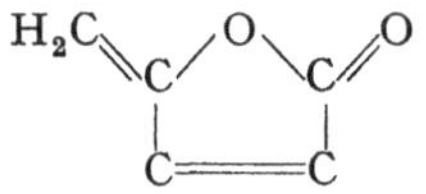

In purified form, the antibiotic substance is an oil which polymerizes to form the insoluble crystalline product anemonin.

Biological activity. A wide spectrum of microorganisms are sensitive to protoanemonin. HOLDEN *et al.* (1947) investigated the activity of a synthetically prepared protoanemonin against a number of bacteria and fungi *in vitro*. Data representative of these experiments are shown in Table 1.

Protoanemonin inhibited growth of Gram-positive and Gram-negative bacteria, and of fungi, but the degree of inhibition varied widely. Growth of two protozoa was inhibited in dilutions of protoanemonin ranging from $^1/_{200,000}$ to $^1/_{600,000}$. No inhibition of bacteriophage or influenza virus was demonstrated. The polymer of protoanemonin (anemonin) exhibited little antibiotic activity toward *E. coli*, *C. albicans*, and *S. aureus* and other microorganisms (BAER *et al.*, 1946; BRODERSON and KJAER, 1946).

Toxicity experiments with guinea pigs and mice showed that the antibiotic was lethal if doses were administered to give titers required to inhibit bacterial growth (ROTTER *et al.*, 1949). A dilution of 10^{-6} of the antibiotic was toxic to chicken epithelial and fibroblastic cells in tissue culture (HOLDEN *et al.*, 1947). Mitochondria of root tip cells of *Zea mays* exposed to protoanemonin disintegrated and mitotic division of meristematic tissue was affected (ERICKSON, 1948; ERICKSON and ROSEN, 1949). TOSHKOV *et al.* (1961) reported a cytopathogenic effect on both normal and tumor tissue cultures.

Protoanemonin was reported to be a potent vesicant, sternutator, and lacrymator by MCCAWLEY *et al.* (1946). ZECHNER and WOHLMUTH (1954) found that

Table 1. *The inhibition of microorganisms by protoanemonin* (HOLDEN *et al.*, 1947)

Test organism	Dilution of protoanemonin x1000
Staphylococcus aureus	66
Micrococcus lysodeikticus	44
Mycobacterium tuberculosis var. *hominis*	100—300
Bacillus subtilis	20—50
Klebsiella pneumonia	40
Pseudomonas aerugenosa	30—100
Proteus vulgaris	80
Shigella dysenteriae	250
Saccharomyces cerevisiae	50—166
Candida albicans	100—200
Trichophyton purpureum	83

anemonin caused a steady contraction of ganglion-free leach muscle and strong rhythmic contraction of a nerve-muscle preparation.

There have been no systematic studies on the mode of action of protoanemonin. The generally wide spectrum of biological activity, however, suggest that the site of action is common among biological systems. There is some evidence that protoanemonin inhibits growth by reacting with sulfhydryl enzymes. Cysteine caused a reduction in bacteriostatic properties of anemonin (CAVALLITO and BAILEY, 1944). Elongation of *Avena* coleoptiles was inhibited by protoanemonin but the inhibition was reversed by dimercaptopropanol (THIMANN and BONNER, 1949). ROTTER and GRUBER (1949) found that the inhibition of pyruvic acid oxidase by protoanemonin was comparable to that of monoiodoacetate. The inactivating effect against bacterial enzyme systems occurred in some cases at much lower concentration of protoanemonin than was effective for the inhibition of bacterial cells. Therefore, reactions with cellular components other than SH groups must be involved.

References

ASAHINA, Y., and A. FUJITA: Synthesis and constitution of anemonin. J. Pharm. Soc. Japan **455**, 1 (1920). Chem. Abstr. **14**, 1384 (1920).

BAER, H., M. HOLDEN, and B. C. SEEGAL: The nature of the antibacterial agent from *Anemone pulsatilla*. J. Biol. Chem. **162**, 65 (1946).

BERNARD, M., and M. J. METZGER: Antibiotic substances from Ranunculaceae. Proc. Indiana Acad. Sci. **70**, 83 (1960).

BOAS, F.: Contributions to the operating physiology of native plants. I. Ber. deut. botan. Ges. **52**, 126 (1934). Chem. Abstr. **28**, 3443 (1934).

BOAS, F., and R. STEUBE: Über die Wirkung von Anemonin auf Mikroorganismen. Biochem. Z. **279**, 417 (1935).

BRODERSEN, R., and A. KJAER: The antibacterial action and toxicity of some unsaturated lactones. Acta Pharmacol. Toxicol. **2**, 109 (1946).

CAVALLITO, C. J., and J. H. BAILEY: Preliminary note on the inactivation of antibiotics. Science **100**, 390 (1944).

ERICKSON, R. O.: Protoanemonin as a mitotic inhibitor. Science **108**, 533 (1948).

ERICKSON, R. O., and G. U. ROSEN: Cytological effects of protoanemonin on the root tip of *Zea mays*. Ann. J. Bot. **36**, 317 (1949).

HERZ, W., A. L. PATES, and G. C. MADSEN: The antimicrobial principle of *Clematis dioscoreifolia*. Science **114**, 206 (1951).
HILL, R., and R. VAN HEYNINGEN: Ranunculin: The precursor of the vesicant substance of the buttercup. J. Chem. Soc. **49**, 332 (1951).
HOLDEN, M., B. C. SEEGAL, and H. BAER: Range of antibiotic activity of protoanemonin. Proc. Soc. Exptl. Biol. Med. **66**, 54 (1947).
KIPPING, F. B.: Lactone of γ-hydroxyvinylacrylic acid, protoanemonin. J. Chem. Soc. **1935**, 1145.
McCAWLEY, E. L., B. A. RUBIN, and N. J. Giacomino: A preliminary survey of certain lactone antibiotics. Federation Proc. **5**, 191 (1946).
MORIARTY, R. M., C. R. ROMAIN, I. L. KARLE, and J. KARLE: The structure of anemonin. J. Am. Chem. Soc. **87**, 3251 (1965).
ROTTER, K., and W. GRUBER: Antibiotic activity and toxicity of protoanemonin. Mikrobiol. Hochschule Bodenkult. **3**, 108 (1949). Chem. Abstr. **47**, 7094e (1953).
SHEARER, G. D.: Some observations on the poisonous properties of buttercups. Vet. J. **94**, 22 (1938).
THIMANN, K. V., and W. D. BONNER: Inhibition of plant growth by protoanemonin and coumarin and its prevention by BAL. Proc. Natl. Acad. Sci. U.S. **35**, 272 (1949).
TOSHKOV, AS., V. IVANOV, U. SOBEVA, T. GANCHEVA, S. PANGELOVA, and V. TONEVA: Antibacterial, antiviral, antitoxic, and cytopathogenic properties of protoanemonin and anemonin. Antibiotiki **6**, 918 (1961). Chem. Abstr. **56**, 15612b (1962).
ZECHNER, L., and H. WOHLMUTH: Anemonin and protoanemonin. I. New method of isolation of anemonin from *Ranunculus acer* L. Sci. Pharm. **22**, 74 (1954a). Chem. Abstr. **48**, 13169c (1954).
ZECHNER, L., and H. WOHLMUTH: Anemonin and protoanemonin. II. Vermicidal action. Sci. Pharm. **22**, 90 (1954b). Chem. Abstr. **48**, 13169d (1954).

Trichothecin

Paul G. Caltrider

Antibiotic activity of culture filtrates of *Trichothecium roseum* against fungi was reported first by BRIAN and HEMMING (1947). The antibiotic substance, trichothecin, was isolated and its chemical properties described by FREEMAN and MORRISON (1949a), FREEMAN *et al.* (1949c), FREEMAN and GILL (1950), and FREEMAN *et al.* (1959). It was shown to be the isocrotyl ester ($C_{19}H_{25}O_5$) of the ketonic alcohol, trichothecolone ($C_{15}H_{20}O_4$) with the structure:

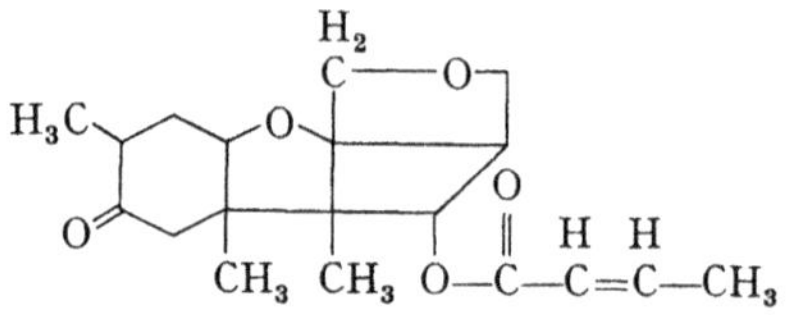

A modified structure was proposed recently by GUTZWILLER *et al.* (1964):

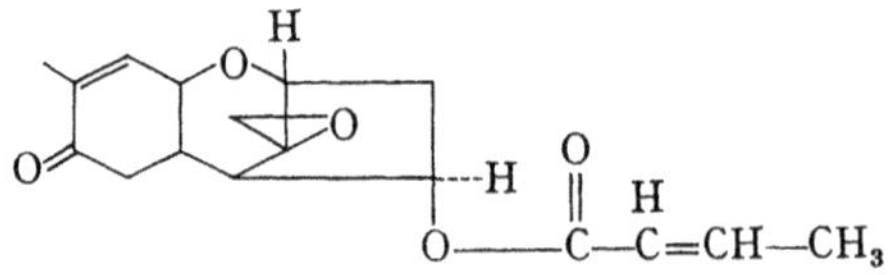

Trichothecin is active against fungi. FREEMAN and MORRISON (1949b) tested the antibiotic *in vitro* against 27 species of fungi from the *Fungi Imperfecti*, *Ascomycetes* and *Zygomycetes*. Various degrees of growth inhibition occurred with the concentrations of trichothecin tested (1.3 to 80 μg/ml). Of the fungi tested, *Penicillium digatatum* was the most sensitive to the antibiotic. Growth of this organism was completely inhibited by 0.64 μg/ml of the antibiotic.

In vitro tests showed that growth of several fungi pathogenic to man were inhibited by trichothecin (FREEMAN, 1955). The pathogenic fungi tested were *Actinomyces asteroides*, *Coccidioides immitis*, *Blastomyces dermatitidis*, *Torulopsis neoformans*, *Candida albicans*, *Hormodendron langeroni*, *Sporotrichum tropicalis*, *S. schencki*, *S. beurmanni*, *Geotrichum cutaneum*, *Histoplasma capsulatum*, *Epidermophyton floccosum*, *Trichophyton rubrum*, *T. interdigitale*, *T. sulphureum*, *T. mentagrophytes*, and *Microsporium canis*. These fungal pathogens generally were inhibited at trichothecin concentrations of 16 μg/ml or less, and the addition of blood serum did not influence their antifungal activity. *A. asteroides* and *C. immitis* were not inhibited by concentrations of trichothecin of 80 μg/ml. Trichothecin also inhibits growth of several plant pathogenic fungi *in vitro* and *in vivo* (YOSHII, 1949, 1950; DARPAUX and FAIVRE-AMOIT, 1952; VOROS, 1955; BELIMOVA and LAPATIN, 1963).

YASUE (1948, 1949) reported that a culture filtrate of *Cephalothecium roseum* (*T. roseum*) inhibited the growth of *Staphalococcus aureus*. However, the antibiotic substance isolated and characterized by FREEMAN *et al.* (1949a) had no antibacterial activity at 400 µg/ml. The active substance reported by YASUE may have been rosein II, a weakly antibacterial substance from mycelia and culture filtrates (FREEMAN *et al.*, 1949c).

Infection by mechanically transmitted plant viruses was prevented if trichothecin was applied to the leaves of the host plant (GUPTA and PRICE, 1950; SINHA, 1960). Systemic infection by aphid-transmitted viruses also was reduced markedly by the antibiotic (BRADLEY and MACKINNON, 1958). BAWDEN and FREEMAN (1952) found that the extent to which viral infection was inhibited by trichothecin depended on the species of the host plant and not on the specific virus. They suggested that the antibiotic acted indirectly by altering the metabolism of the host plant cells.

Trichothecin is of no therapeutic value in animals because of its extreme toxicity. FREEMAN (1955) found that in mice and rats, dosages as low as 12.5 to 50 mg/kg, when administered intravenously or subcutaneously, caused almost instant paralysis of the legs. Larger doses (500 mg/kg) caused mice to die within 30 sec after administration. Application of trichothecin to the skin of guinea pigs caused severe irritation.

Very little is known about the mode of action of trichethecin. The few studies which have been reported deal with general effects of the antibiotic and not with specific metabolic systems.

Growth of *Fusarium oxysporium* var. *cubense in vitro* was stimulated by low levels of trichothecin. At fungicidal levels (10 units/ml), swelling and bursting of hyphal tips were observed (HESSAYON, 1951). YOSHII (1953) reported that carbohydrase activity in *Piricularia oryzae* increased at certain dilutions of crude broths containing cephalothecin (trichothecin). Ammonia nitrogen was lower in leaf blades of rice plants treated with cephalothecin (trichothecin) than in nontreated plants (YOSHII, 1954). That the mechanism of action of the antibiotic does not involve sulfhydryl groups directly is suggested by the inability of cysteine to inactivate trichothecin (CAVALLITO and BAILEY, 1944).

References

BAWDEN, F. C., and G. G. FREEMAN: The nature and behavior of inhibitors of plant viruses produced by *Trichothecium roseum* LINK. J. Gen. Microbiol. **7**, 154 (1952).

BELIMOVA, A. V., and M. I. LOPATIN: Use of the antibiotic trichocetin in control of lodging or fusarial wilt of common pine seedlings. Sb. Nauchn. Rabot. Kurgansk. Sel'skokhoz. Inst. **8**, 85 (1963). Chem. Abstr. **62**, 16899c (1965).

BRADLEY, R. H. E., and J. P. MACKINNON: Effects of trichothecin on some viruses transmitted by aphids. Can. J. Microbiol. **4**, 555 (1958).

BRIAN, P. W., and H. G. HEMMING: Production of antifungal and antibacterial substances by fungi; preliminary examination of 166 strains of Fungi Imperfecti. J. Gen. Microbiol. **1**, 158 (1947).

CAVALLITO, C. J., and J. H. BAILEY: Inactivation of antibiotics. Science **100**, 390 (1944).

DARPOUX, H., et A. FAIVRE-AMIOT: Action de produits du metabolism du *Trichothecium roseum* LK sur l'oidium de l'arge (*Erysyphe graminis*). Phytiat.-Phytopharm. **1**, 21 (1952). Rev. Appl. Mycol. **33**, 532 (1954).

FREEMAN, G. G.: Further biological properties of trichothecin, an antifungal substance from *Trichothecium roseum* LINK, and its derivatives. J. Gen. Microbiol. **12**, 213 (1955).
FREEMAN, G. G., and J. E. GILL: Alkaline hydrolysis of trichothecin. Nature **166**, 698 (1950).
FREEMAN, G. G., J. E. GILL, and W. S. WARING: The structure of trichothecin and its hydrolysis products. J. Chem. Soc. 1105 (1959).
FREEMAN, G. G., and R. I. MORRISON: The isolation and chemical properties of trichothecin, an antifungal substance from *Trichothecium roseum* LINK. Biochem. J. **44**, 1 (1949a).
FREEMAN, G. G., and R. I. MORRISON: Some biological properties of trichothecium, an antifungal substance form *Trichothecium roseum* LINK. J. Gen. Microbiol. **3**, 60 (1949b).
FREEMAN, G. G., R. I. MORRISON, and S. E. MICHAEL: Metabolic products of *Trichothecium roseum* LINK. Biochem. J. **45**, 191 (1949c).
GUPTA, B. M., and W. E. PRICE: Production of plant virus inhibitors by fungi. Phytopathology **40**, 642 (1950).
GUTZWILLER, J., R. MAULI, H. P. SIGG, and C. TAMM: Die Konstitution von Verrucarol und roridin C. verrucarine und roridine. 4. Mitt. (1). Helv. Chim. Acta **47**, 2234 (1964). Chem. Abstr. **62**, 5301f. (1965).
HESSAYON, D. G.: Double action of trichothecin and its production in soil. Nature **168**, 998 (1951).
SINHA, R. C.: Effects of temperature and of virus inhibitors on infection of French-bean leaves by red clover mottle virus. Ann. Appl. Biol. **48**, 749 (1960).
VOROS, J.: A trichothecin antibiotikum alkalmazasa novenyi korokozok illen. Novenytermelis **4**, 233 (1955). Rev. Appl. Mycol. **35**, 476 (1956).
YASUE, Y.: Antibacterial activity of culture filtrate of *Cephalothecium roseum* I. Science (Japan) **18**, 565 (1948). Chem. Abstr. **45**, 6243c (1951).
YASUE, Y.: Studies on the antibacterial activity of the culture filtrate of *Cephalothecium roseum*. J. Japan Chem. **19**, 92 (1949).
YOSHII, H.: Studies on *Cephalothecium* as a means of the artificial immunization of agricultural crops. Ann. Phytopath. Soc. Jap. **13**, 37 (1949). Rev. Appl. Mycol. **29**, 475 (1950).
YOSHII, H.: On the germination of the conidia of *Piricularia oryzae* in the water drops on the leaves of rice seedlings treated with cephalothecin. Ann. Phytopath. Soc. Jap. **15**, 13 (1950). Rev. Appl. Mycol. **31**, 82 (1952).
YOSHII, H.: The influence of cephalothecin upon the secretion of carbohydrases by the blast fungus. Ann. Phytopath. Soc. Jap. **17**, 124 (1953). Chem. Abstr. **48**, 4053h (1954).
YOSHII, H.: Influence of cephalothecin upon the development of blast fungus in the cell of the ear-neck of rice plant. Ann. Phytopath. Soc. Jap. **18**, 17 (1954). Chem. Abstr. **48**, 8886b (1954).

Viomycin

Paul G. Caltrider

Viomycin is produced by *Streptomyces floridae* (EHRLICH *et al.*, 1951; BARTZ *et al.*, 1951), *S. paniceus* (FINLAY *et al.*, 1951), and *S. vinaceus* (MARSH *et al.*, 1953; MAYER *et al.*, 1954). The antibiotic also has been referred to as vinactane, viocin and vinactin.

Data on the chemistry of viomycin show that it is a strongly basic polypeptide with an empirical formula for the free base of $C_{23}H_{38}N_{12}O_9$. The structure of the antibiotic has not been elucidated completely, but the structure shown below is consistent with much of the physical and chemical data obtained for viomycin (HASKELL *et al.*, 1952; DYER *et al.*, 1965).

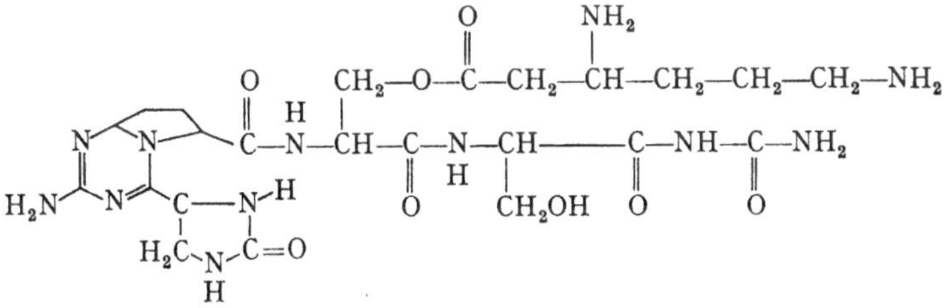

Viomycin differs from most antibiotics in that it is more active against mycobacteria than other groups of bacteria (EHRLICH *et al.*, 1951; MARSH *et al.*, 1953; FINLAY *et al.*, 1951; MAYER *et al.*, 1954). The antimicrobial activity of viomycin

Table 1. *Antimicrobial activity of viomycin sulfate in vitro* (EHRLICH *et al.*, 1951)

Test organism	Concentration for complete inhibition of growth (μg/ml)
Actinomyces bovis	25
Aerobacter aerogenes	25
Bacillus subtilis	25
Brucella abortus	50
Diplococcus pneumonia, Type I	50
Escherichia coli (ST-R)	>100
Klebsiella pneumonia, Type A	10
Mycobacterium tuberculosis	0.78
M. tuberculosis var. homimis (H37RV)	2.5—7.8
Neisseria catarrhalis	10
Proteus vulgaris	>100
Pseudomonas aerugenosa	>100
Salmonella typhosa	10

sulfate *in vitro* is shown in Table 1. These data show that viomycin is most active against mycobacteria, moderately active against Gram-positive bacteria and least active against Gram-negative bacteria.

In vitro, viomycin is inactive against human and plant pathogenic fungi at concentrations as high as 250 μg/ml (EHRLICH *et al.*, 1951; HOBBY *et al.*, 1951; KOAZE *et al.*, 1956). EHRLICH *et al.* (1951) reported that the antibiotic showed no activity against two protozoans (at 2 mg/ml) and several small viruses. Antiphage activity of viomycin, however, was reported for inordinately high concentrations (5 mg/ml) by HALL *et al.* (1951).

NITTA (1957) reported that HeLa cells were not affected by viomycin *in vitro*. Growth of embryonic cells in tissue culture was reduced by 300 μg/ml of the antibiotic (METZGER *et al.*, 1952). SATO (1959) found that chlorophyll formation was reduced in *Pheum pratense* by 200 μg/ml of viomycin.

Viomycin produces beneficial effects in the treatment of human tuberculosis provided it is given in high enough dosage (FINLAY *et al.*, 1951; STIENKEN and WOLINSKY, 1950). Mycobacteria develop resistance to viomycin more slowly than to streptomycin (EHRLICH *et al.*, 1951). STEENKEN and WOLINSKY (1951) reported that strains highly resistant to the action of viomycin *in vitro* were produced after eight transfers in a liquid medium containing increasing or graded concentrations of the drug.

Viomycin is an antibiotic of relatively low toxicity when given over short periods. Long-term treatment of tuberculosis, however, has given rather serious side effects. In mice, the intravenous and subcutaneous LD_{50} of viomycin sulfate was 240 and 1380 mg/kg, respectively (FINLAY *et al.*, 1951; P'AN *et al.*, 1951). Oral administration of the drug equivalent to 7500 mg/kg was tolerated by mice. Renal damage was not observed in rats receiving daily doses of 50 to 200 mg of viomycin hydrochloride or sulfate per kg of body weight subcutaneously for periods of five days (FINLAY *et al.*, 1951). Toxic symptoms for i.v. injection of a lethal dose of viomycin into mice were those of the central nervous system, such as irritability, tremors of extremities, chronic convulsions, followed by flaccid paralysis (P'AN *et al.*, 1951). No ill effects were demonstrated in rats given daily subcutaneous injections of 50 to 100 mg/kg over a period of six weeks. Daily i.m. injections of 50 to 100 mg/kg were tolerated by dogs for a period of more than 150 days (P'AN *et al.*, 1951). KELLER *et al.* (1955, 1956) found that toxicity of viomycin was reduced substantially if the pantothenic acid salts were used instead of the sulfate.

The mode of action of viomycin on bacteria has received minor consideration. Most of the observations are not the result of intensive systematic studies and thus appear to be unrelated. GUPTA and VISWANATHAN (1956) and GRIEDER *et al.* (1960) studied changes of tubercle bacilli upon exposure to the antibiotic. After 24 hr treatment with the drug, they observed bacilli which were dense to the electron beam. After 48 and 72 hr, the majority of the elongated bacilli developed swelling at one or both ends. No abnormal differentiation of the internal structure could be detected.

According to TSUKAMURA (1960), viomycin (5 μg/ml) inhibited incorporation of ^{32}P into the protein and nucleic acid fractions of *My. avium*. Incorporation of ^{35}S into the protein fraction was also inhibited. Viomycin forms aggregates with RNA and DNA at pH values lower than 5.5—6.0 (TSUKAMURA and TSUKAMURA, 1959).

MICHALSKA (1962) reported, however, that the precipitate reaction between viomycin and nucleic acids was non-spezific and that bacteriostasis cannot be explained on this basis.

Oxygen uptake by *Azotobacter chroococcum* on different substrates was reduced by viomycin (1 mg/ml) (FEDOROV and SEGI, 1961). An inhibition of dehydrogenase activity was suggested. Concentrations of the antibiotic $^1/_{10}$ to $^1/_{1000}$ those inhibiting respiration were sufficient for the suppression of growth and multiplication. Thus, the respiratory system appears not to be the primary site of viomycin activity. At a concentration of 10 μg/ml, viomycin was bacteriostatic, but growth of the bacteria occurred when transferred to an antibiotic-free medium.

SKULA and NIGAM (1962) reported that viomycin caused a decrease in catalase activity in *E. coli* unless the cells were previously adapted to the antibiotic. A bacteriostatic effect resulting from the accumulation of hydrogen peroxide was suggested. An inhibition of pyruvic decarboxylase activity by viomycin has been reported by HERNANDEZ *et al.* (1956).

SERVELL and NICOL (1958) attempted to determine if viomycin *in vivo* stimulated phagocytes, but they found little or no effect on phagocytic activity.

See Addendum

References

BARTZ, A. R., J. EHRLICH, J. D. MOLD, M. A. PENNER, and R. M. SMITH: Viomycin, a new tuberculostatic antibiotic. Am. Rev. Tuberc. **63**, 4 (1951).

DYER, J. R., C. K. KELLOGG, R. F. NASSAR, and N. E. STREETMAN: Viomycin: II. The structure of viomycin. Tetrahedron Letters 585 (1965).

EHRLICH, J., R. M. SMITH, M. A. PENNER, L. E. ANDERSON, and A. C. BRATTON, JR.: Antimicrobial activity of *Streptomyces floridae* and of viomycin. Am. Rev. Tuberc. **63**, 7 (1951).

FEDOROV, M. V., and I. SEGI: Effect of certain antibiotics on the physiological activity of *Azotobacter chroococcum*. Microbiology **30**, 247 (1961). Transl. of Mikrobiologiya **30**, 275 (1961).

FINLAY, A. C., G. L. HOBBY, F. HOCHSTEIN, T. M. LAS, T. F. LENERT, J. A. MEANS, S. Y. P'AN, P. P. REGNA, J. B. ROUTIEN, B. A. SOBIN, I. B. TATE, and J. H. KANE: Viomycin, a new antibiotic active against mycobacteria. Am. Rev. Tuberc. **63**, 1 (1951).

GRIEDER, FR., L. NEIPP, and R. MEIER: Characterization of the type of action of antibiotics by observation of their morphological effect and their influence on oxygen consumption during the logarithmic growth phase. Helv. Physiol. et Pharmacol. Acta **18**, 274 (1960). Chem. Abstr. **54**, 23022f (1960).

GUPTA, R. C., and R. VISWANATHAN: Electromicroscopic and phase-contrast studies of effects of p-aminosalicylic acid, isonazid, and viomycin on tubercle bacilli. Am. Rev. Tuberc. **73**, 291 (1956).

HALL, E. A., F. KAVANAGH, and IGOR ASBESHOV: Action of forty-five antibacterial substances on bacterial viruses. Antibiotics & Chemotherapy **1**, 369 (1951).

HASKELL, T. H., S. A. FUSARI, R. P. FROHARDT, and Q. R. BARTZ: The chemistry of viomycin. J. Am. Chem. Soc. **74**, 599 (1952).

HOBBY, G. L., T. F. LENERT, M. DONKIAN, and D. PIKULA: The activity of viomycin against *Mycobacterium tuberculosis* and other microorganisms in vitro and in vivo. Am. Rev. Tuberc. **63**, 17 (1951).

KELLER, H., W. KRUPE, H. SOUS, and H. MÜCKTER: Reduction of the toxicity of basic streptomyces antibiotics. II. Further observations. Arzneimittel-Forsch. **6**, 61 (1956). Chem. Abstr. **50**, 8913c (1956).

KELLER, H., W. KRUPE, H. SOUS, and H. MÜCKTER: The pathothenates of streptomycin, viomycin and neomycin, new and less toxic salts. Antibiotics Ann. **1955/56**, 35.

KOAZE, Y., H. SAKAI, H. YONEHARA, M. OSAKAWA, and T. MISATO: Studies on the activities of antibiotics against plant pathogenic microorganisms. J. Antibiotics (Japan), Ser. A **9**, 89 (1956).

MARSH, W. S., R. L. MAYER, R. P. MULL, C. R. SCHOLZ, and R. W. TOWSLEY: Antibiotics and method of preparing same. U.S. Patent Office 2,633,445 (1953).

MARTIN-HERNANDEZ, D., G. DE AL FUENTE SANCHEZ, and A. SANTOS-RUIZ: Carboxylases. X. Enzymic inhibition of pyruvic carboxylase by antibiotics of protein nature. Rev. españ. fisiol. **12**, 143 (1956). Chem. Abstr. **51**, 5878d (1957).

MAYER, R. L., P. C. EISMAN, and E. A. KONOPKA: Antituberculosis activity of vinactane. Experimentis **10**, 335 (1954).

METZGER, J. F., M. H. FUSILLO, and D. M. KUHNS: Effect of polymyxin and viomycin on embryonic cells in tissue cultures. Antibiotics & Chemotherapy **2**, 227 (1952).

MICHALSKA, K.: Action of antituberculous antibiotics on nucleic acid and related compounds. Gruzbica **30**, 13 (1962). Chem. Abstr. **57**, 8884d (1962).

NITTA, K.: Studies on the effects of actinomycetes products on the culture of human carcinoma cells (strain hela) I. The effect of known antibiotics having no or slight tumor-inhibitory activity on hela cells. Japan. J. Med. Sci. & Biol. **10**, 277 (1957).

P'AN, S. Y., T. V. HALLEY, J. C. REILLY, and A. M. PEKICH: Viomycin: acute and chronic toxicity in experimental animals. Am. Rev. Tuberc. **63**, 44 (1951).

SATO, Y.: Effect of streptomycin on chlorophyll formation in timothy. I. Morphological observation. Keijo J. Med. **8**, 187 (1959). Chem. Abstr. **54**, 16559h (1960).

SEWELL, I. A., and T. NICOL: Effect of antibiotics on the phagocytic activity of the reticulo-endothelial system. Nature **181**, 1662 (1958).

SKULA, J. P., and R. K. NIGAM: Effect of viomycin adaptation on catalase activity of Escherichia coli. Naturwissenschaften **49**, 135 (1962).

STEENKEN, JR., W., and E. WOLINSKY: Effects of antimicrobial agents on the tubercle bacilli and on experimental tuberculosis. Am. J. Med. **9**, 633 (1950).

STEENKEN, W., and E. WOLINSKY: Viomycin in experimental tuberculosis. Am. Rev. Tuberc. **63**, 30 (1951).

TSUKAMURA, M.: Mechanism of action of viomycin. J. Biochem. (Tokyo) **47**, 685 (1960).

TSUKAMURA, M., and S. TSUKAMURA: Precipitation of nucleic acid by kanamycin and viomycin. J. Biochem. (Tokyo) **46**, 1193 (1959).

WERNER, C. A., R. TOMPSETT, C. MUSCHENHEIM, and W. MCDERMOTT: The toxicity of viomycin in humans. Am. Rev. Tuberc. **63**, 49 (1951).

Actinomycetin

P. G. Caltrider

The bacteriolytic cell-free fluid of culture filtrates of actinomycetes was designated as actinomycetin (WELSCH, 1937c). Although the production of actinomycetin has been studied most intensively in *Streptomyces albus*, it is produced by most species of Streptomyces (WELSCH, 1942; TAI and VAN HEYNINGEN, 1951; SALTON, 1955; SLADE and SLAMP, 1960). Actinomycetin-like activity also has been reported for species of *Proactinomyces* and *Micromonospora* (WELSCH, 1942).

Most of the studies on the antibiotic activity of actinomycetin were carried out with crude broths acting on dead bacterial cells. Therefore, it is difficult to describe actinomycetin as an antibiotic with properties characteristic of most antibiotics. Under specific conditions, however, actinomycetin does cause rapid lysis of a few bacterial strains in the living state. Thus, it can be stated that actinomycetin contains antibiotic activity. WELSCH (1962) has reviewed the bacteriolytic enzymes from streptomycetes with special reference to actinomycetin. Only those factors of the actinomycetin "complex" which have been characterized will be included in this paper.

Killed bacteria have been used for most of the investigations on the activity of actinomycetin. Bacteriolytic activity of actinomycetin has been reported for live cells of *Streptococcus pyogenes, Diplococcus pneumonia, Staphylococcus aureus, Corynebacterium diphtheriae, Bacillus megaterium, Candida pulcherrima, Sarcina lutea, Micrococcus lysodeikticus*, and *B. subtilis* (WELSCH, 1947, 1959; SALTON, 1955; GHUYSEN, 1954, 1957). Live Gram-negative bacteria are generally not susceptible to lysis by actinomycetin (WELSCH, 1959). SMOLIAR (1952), however, reported lysis of *E. coli* by actinomycetin in the presence of high concentrations of glycine.

There is some evidence that actinomycetin is inhibitory to viruses. Purified preparations of the antibiotic prevented or reduced hemagglutination of red blood cells by strains of influenze virus but not by Newcastle disease virus (MALCHAIR, 1958). Influenza virus became non-infective for chick embryos. VYASELEVA (1949) reported that actinomycetin does not possess anti-spirochete activity.

The bacteriolytic activity of the actinomycetin „complex" is the consequence of an enzymatic destruction of the bacterial cell wall. Lysis of cell walls of *S. faecalis* has been used as a technique for the detection of actinomycetin-producing organisms (SALTON, 1955). A biochemical and electron microscopic study of the lytic action of actinomycetin showed a release of carbohydrate from the cell wall and release of nucleic acid from the protoplast (SLADE and SLAMP, 1960). After the cells were lysed, there remained fragments of the cell wall which contained approlimately half the carbohydrate of the original cell wall.

Several factors in actinomycetin contribute to its lytic action. GHUYSEN (1953, 1957) isolated two bacteriolytic fractions, designated F_1 and F_2, from actinomycetin. Both F_1 and F_2 fractions were peptidases, but the F_1 fraction was the primary lytic enzyme. F_2 fraction was a crude mixture of enzymes which potentiated the lysis of staphylococci by F_1. Solubilization of bacterial cell walls by F_1 or F_2 was accompanied by a release of dialyzable and non-dialyzable products (GHUYSEN, 1957; SALTON and GHUYSEN, 1957). Glycine and alanine were among the compounds detected. On the basis of these data, peptidases were proposed as the active enzymes. Further investigations with walls of *M. lysodeickticus* showed that the F_1 enzyme released N-acetylamino sugar compounds and N-acetylamino sugar peptide complexes (SALTON and GHUYSEN, 1959). These compounds were identified as di- and tetra-saccharides, and β(1—4)N-acetylhexosaminidase activity was suggested (SALTON and GHUYSEN, 1960). Although the same products were produced from lysozyme and the F_1 enzyme, they were shown to be two distinct enzymes (GHUYSEN, 1960). A second enzyme which released teichoic acid from the cell wall of *B. megaterium* has been isolated from the F_1 enzyme (GHUYSEN, 1961 b).

The F_2 fraction from actinomycetin was separated further into F_2A and F_2B. The latter fraction contained an enzyme which split the amidic acetylmuraminyl-alanine linkage in the cell wall (GHUYSEN, 1960, 1961 a).

MCCARTY (1952a and b) showed evidence that the lysis of streptococci by crude broths of *Streptomyces albus* was due to a carbohydrase. Thus it appears that the antibiotic activity of actinomycetin is caused by several different exoenzymes.

References

GHUYSEN, J. M.: Purification of actinomycetin (to Societe Belge de l'azote et des produits chimiques du S. H. MARLY). Belg. 517, 191 (1953). Chem. Abstr. **53**, 5600e (1959).

GHUYSEN, J. M.: Activite pneumolytique de l'actinomycetine. Compt. rend. soc. biol. **148**, 729 (1954).

GHUYSEN, J. M.: Bacteriolytic activities of the actinomycetin of Streptomyces albus. Arch. intern. physiol. et biochem. **65**, 173 (1957).

GHUYSEN, J. M.: Acetylhexosamine compounds enzymatically released from *Micrococcus lysodeikticus* cell walls. Biochim. et Biophys. Acta **40**, 473 (1960).

GHUYSEN, J. M.: Precisions sur la structure des complexes disaccharidepeptide liberes des parois de *Micrococcus lysodeikticus*. Biochim. et Biophys. Acta **47**, 561-(1961 a).

GHUYSEN, J. M.: Complexe acide teichoique-mucopeptide des parois cellulaires de *Bacillus megaterium* KM. Biochim. et Biophys. Acta **50**, 413 (1961 b).

MALCHAIR, R.: Effects de l'actinomycetin sur the virus grippal. Giorn. microbiol. **5**, 137 (1958). Biol. Abstr. **35**, 56723 (1960).

MCCARTY, M.: The lysis of group A hemolytic streptococci by extracellular enzymes of *Streptomyces albus*. I. Production and fractionation of the lytic enzymes. J. Exptl. Med. **96**, 555 (1952).

SALTON, M. R. J.: Isolation of *Streptomyces* spp. capable of decomposing preparations of cell walls from various microorganisms and a comparison of their lytic activities with those of certain *Actinomycetes* and *Mycobacteria*. J. Gen. Microbiol. **12**, 25 (1955).

SALTON, M. R. J., et J. M. GHUYSEN: Action de l'actinomycetine sur les parois cellulaires bacteriennes. Biochim. et Biophys. Acta **24**, 160 (1957).

SALTON, M. R. J., and J. M. GHUYSEN: The structure of di- and tetra-saccharides released from cell walls by lysozyme and *Streptomyces* F_1 enzyme and the β1—4)N-acetylhexosaminidase activity of these enzymes. Biochim. et Biophys. Acta **36**, 552 (1959).

SALTON, M. R. J., and J. M. GHUYSEN: Acetylhexosamine compounds enzymatically released from *Micrococcus lysodeikticus* cell walls. III. The structure of di- and tetra-saccharides released from cell walls by lysozyme and *Streptomyces* F_1 enzyme. Biochim. et Biophys. **45**, 355 (1960).

SLADE, H. D., and W. C. SLAMP: Studies on *Streptococcus pyogenes* V. Biochemical and microscopic aspects of cell lysis and digestion by enzymes from *Streptomyces albus*. J. Bacteriol. **79**, 103 (1960).

SMOLIAR, V.: Synergic bacteriolytique de l'actinomycetine et de la glycine. Compt. rend. soc. biol. **146**, 1620 (1952).

TAI, T. Y., and W. E. VAN HEYNINGEN: Bacteriolysis by a species of *Streptomyces*. J. Gen. Microbiol. **5**, 110 (1951).

VYASELEVA, S. M.: The action of some antibiotics on cultures of the spirochete. Vestnik Venerol. i Dermatol. No. 1, 4 (1949). Chem. Abstr. **43**, 54451 (1949).

WELSCH, M.: Influence de la nature du milieu de culture sur la production de lysines par les *Actinomyces*. Compt. rend. soc. biol. **126**, 244 (1932).

WELSCH, M.: Bacteriostatic and bacteriolytic properties of actinomycetes. J. Bacteriol. **44**, 571 (1942).

WELSCH, M.: Actinomycetin. J. Bacteriol. **53**, 101 (1947).

WELSCH, M.: Transformation in spheroplastes et lyse d'*Escherichia coli* par l'actinomycetine. Compt. rend. soc. biol. **153**, 370 (1959).

WELSCH, M.: Bacteriolytis enzymes from *Streptomyces*. A review. J. Gen. Physiol. **45**, 115 (1962).

Bacteriocins

I. B. Holland

The simple definition of bacteriocins proposed by JACOB, LWOFF, SIMINOVITCH and WOLLMAN in 1953 is still applicable and defines a bacteriocin as a highly specific anti-bacterial protein, produced by certain strains of bacteria, and active against some other strains of the same species. The restricted activity spectra of bacteriocins usually precludes their consideration as "classical" antibiotics. Nevertheless they are highly effective anti-bacterial agents and although no direct chemotherapeutic value of these compounds is evident at this time, their curiously abundant distribution amongst bacterial species and their seemingly specific effects upon bacterial regulatory processes are attracting increasing attention. HÁMON (1964) has reviewed the present reported incidence of bacteriocinogenic (bacteriocin producing or B^+) bacteria and whilst 27 families of B^+ bacteria are noted by this author, the more striking fact is that in many cases 30—100% of individual strains of each species tested are found to produce one or other bacteriocins. Bacteriocinogeny is therefore at least as prevalent in nature as is lysogeny. In fact these two phenomena have several other features in common and these will be very briefly considered later.

The preliminary identification of possible bacteriocinogenic strains is readily achieved by mixed plating of a small number of the suspected B^+ bacteria with an excess of a suitable (sensitive) indicator strain or by simply overlaying B^+ colonies on plates with the indicator. In both cases after overnight incubation, clear inhibition zones may be seen surrounding the B^+ colonies. When material is removed from such inhibition zones and again mixed and plated with indicator, no new "plaques" appear. Bacteriocins therefore unlike phage cannot multiply in sensitive strains. They do not contain any nucleic acid and in fact current evidence suggests that they are simple proteins. Although precise chemical information is still restricted to a small number of examples a large number of general observations note the sensitivity of bacteriocins to proteolytic enzymes and their large molecular weights (30,000—100,000). HINSDELL and GOEBEL (1964) in a recent review noted that of the 7 bacteriocins that have been purified, all appear to be protein although only in one case (megacin A) is it clearly established that the bacteriocin is a simple unconjugated protein (HOLLAND, 1961). Probably in all other cases, perhaps significantly in all produced by gram negative organisms, the protein bacteriocin is found to be in chemical combination with lipo-polysaccharide of cell wall origin. Nevertheless it is the protein moiety of this complex which contains the bacteriocin activity (GOEBEL and BARRY, 1958). Some interesting exceptions to these general statements are recent findings that bacteriocins are also found as components of or in association with incomplete phage particles and an example of this will be mentioned later. The significance of the apparent specific association of bacteriocin proteins with cell surface components or with phage particles of the producing bacteria has not yet been determined but may have profound implications for an understanding of the mode of action of these compounds. Similarly, these associations may have some relevance to the as yet un-understood immunity of a B^+ strain to its own bacteriocin.

The activity spectrum of each bacteriocin is extremely narrow, often restricted to a few particular strains of the same species. In addition to this, the prolific variety of different types produced makes classification and precise recognition extremely difficult. Furthermore, one strain may produce several distinct bacteriocins and reciprocal antagonisms between different producing strains are a common phenomena. Thus, when newly isolated strains are tested, they are invariably found to produce one or other bacteriocin and/or to be sensitive to a variety of others. Despite these complexities, the work concerned with the most extensively studied group, colicins formed by *Escherichia coli* and related species, has fortunately been greatly facillitated by the work of PIERRE FREDERICQ. By carrying out cross resistance tests with bacterial mutants resistant to specific colicins FREDERICQ was able to characterize 17 distinct groups of colicin (FREDERICQ, 1948). Several additional types have subsequently been discovered and currently the number is about 23 (HÁMON and PERON, 1963). As will be described in later articles, bacteriocins act through the intermediacy of specific receptor sites in the cell walls of sensitive bacteria and the specificity of this process determines the basis of FREDERICQ's classification. With further study on the specific action and chemical constitution of colicins, additional types will undoubtedly appear but this classification for the moment is a perfectly acceptable one. To utilize this system maximally, several workers have suggested that when reference to various colicins is made, both class (e.g. E or I) and strain of origin should be noted and this is being increasingly adopted (see REEVES, 1965).

Some mention should be made of the methods of titrating bacteriocin solutions. Two procedures are in common use; 1. the more sensitive method entails the direct measurement of the surviving cell fraction after treatment with bacteriocin under standard conditions of time and temperature; 2. a less sensitive but convenient routine method consists simply of spotting serial dilutions of bacteriocin on to a previously sown lawn of indicator and determining the end point of inhibition after appropriate incubation of the plates. Units of activity of bacteriocin may then be determined in terms of actual numbers of cells killed/ml or from the serial dilution assay from the reciprocal of the final dilution at the end point which is arbitarily designated as the activity in units/ml of the particular solution.

The abundance and variety of different bacteriocin types amongst many species has been referred to above, nevertheless the actual mode of action of bacteriocins of different types is in fact remarkably similar in that they act via a common basic mechanism. Thus all bacteriocins appear to be particulate killing agents, and one particle (or molecule) can be sufficient to kill one cell (JACOB, SIMINOVITCH and WOLLMAN, 1952) after fixation to a specific cell wall receptor (see FREDERICQ, 1957). These cell wall receptors are completely analogous to phage receptors and loss of a receptor confers resistance upon the bacteria to the corresponding bacteriocin. Two possible, alternative hypotheses for the mechanism of action of probably most or all bacteriocins arise out of these findings; 1. although specific cell-wall fixation is the first step this must be followed by penetration of the bacteriocin to the sensitive loci; 2. the less likely possibility that after fixation the bacteriocin is able to induce its effect directly from the extracellular position. In fact, evidence in support of the latter mechanism rather than the former has now been provided (NOMURA and NAKAMURA, 1962; REYNOLDS and REEVES, 1962). Detailed studies on the actual intra-cellular effects induced by the external bacteriocin are still relatively few but several interesting results have been reported, including specific inhibition of DNA and protein synthesis; uncoupling of energy metabolism or damage to the osmotic membrane. It may be tentatively postulated that in contrast to "antibiotics" which appear to block or inhibit stochiometrically a particular metabolic raction, often the action of a single enzyme, a single bacteriocin molecule may interact with what might be called the regulatory circuits of a bacterial cell (see JACOB and MONOD, 1962), thereby affecting many individual metabolic functions simultaneously. These regulatory centres presumably are a part of or are associated with the cytoplasmic membrane of sensitive bacteria and therefore accessible to interaction with the surface bound bacteriocin.

As pointed out by LURIA (1964) what is particularly needed now is much more information about the physical and biochemical nature of the cytoplasmic membrane itself. This would facillitate a better understanding of bacteriocin action which in turn might illuminate the role of the membrane in cellular organisation.

Lysogeny and Bacteriocinogeny

FREDERICQ (1957) and REEVES (1965) have outlined some of the undoubted similarities between these two natural phenomena. I will briefly point out here only the similarities between bacteriocins and bacteriophage rather than between their genetic determinants.

Following the fixation of a single particle of either a phage or a bacteriocin to its specific cell wall receptor a sensitive cell may be killed. In some cases one receptor may be common to both a bacteriocin and a phage (see FREDERICQ, 1957). It has been suggested in fact that a bacteriocin may be related to a similar protein component of a phage tail and this is supported by the findings that T phage ghosts (lacking DNA) can still kill sensitive cells (FREDERICQ, 1952, 1957). Furthermore some strains provisionally classified as bacteriocinogenic have subsequently been shown to be defective lysogens producing phage "tail units" only but which presumably contain the bacteriocin protein (ISHII, NISHI, IKEDA and EGAMI; cited by KAZIRO and TANAKA, 1965). There is therefore some evidence for some formal relationship between at least some bacteriocins and some phage components. It should be added however that as yet no one has succeeded in either isolating a bacteriocin-like protein from a phage tail, defective or otherwise, or elucidating the function of this hypothetical protein.

References

FREDERICQ, P.: Actions antibiotiques réciproques chez les enterobacteriaceae. Rev. belge pathol. et med. exptl. **29** (Suppl. **4**), 1—107 (1948).

FREDERICQ, P.: Action bactériocide de la colicine K. Compt. rend. **146**, 1295—1297 (1952).

FREDERICQ, P.: Colicins. Ann. Rev. Microbiol. **11**, 7—22 (1957).
GOEBEL, W. F., and G. T. BARRY: Colicine K. II. The preparation and properties of a substance having colicine K activity. J. Exptl. Med. **107**, 185—209 (1958).
HÁMON, Y., et Y. PÉRON: Individualisation de quelques nouvelles familles d'entérobacteriocines. Compt. rend. **257**, 309—311 (1963).
HÁMON, Y.: Les bactériocines. Ann. Inst. Pasteur **107** (Suppl.), 18—53 (1964).
HINSDELL, R. D., and W. F. GOEBEL: The chemical nature of bacteriocins. Ann. Inst. Pasteur **107** (Suppl.), 54—66 (1964).
HOLLAND, I. B.: The purification and properties of megacin, a bacteriocin from *Bacillus megaterium*. Biochem. J. **78**, 641—648 (1961).
JACOB, F., L. SIMINOVITCH et E. WOLLMAN: Sur la biosynthèse d'une colicine et sur son mode d'action. Ann. Inst. Pasteur **83**, 295—315 (1952).
JACOB, F., A. LWOFF, L. SIMINOVITCH et E. WOLLMAN: Définition de quelques termes relatifs à la lysogénie. Ann. Inst. Pasteur **84**, 222—224 (1953).
JACOB, F., and J. MONOD: Elements of regulatory circuits in bacteria. Unesco Symp. on Biological Organization 1962.
KAZIRO, Y., and M. TANAKA: Studies on the mode of action of pyocin. I. Inhibition of macromolecular synthesis in sensitive cells. J. Biochem. **57**, 689—695 (1965).
LURIA, S. E.: On the mechanisms of action of colicins. Ann. Inst. Pasteur **107** (Suppl.), 67—73 (1964).
NOMURA, M., and M. NAKAMURA: Reversibility of inhibition of nucleic acids and protein synthesis by colicin K. Biochem. Biophys. Research Commun. **7**, 306—309 (1962).
REYNOLDS, B. L., and P. R. REEVES: Some observations on the mode of action of colicin F. Biochem. Biophys. Research Commun. **11**, 140—145 (1962).
REEVES, P. R.: The bacteriocins. Bacteriol. Rev. **29**, 24—45 (1965).

Megacins

I. B. Holland

IVÁNOVICS and ALFÖLDI (1954) were the first to observe bacteriocin formation in *Bacillus megaterium*. Later IVÁNOVICS and NAGY (1958) using a phage resistant indicator strain to detect megacinogenic (M^+) strains, found that almost half of 200 strains tested were indeed M^+ and a similar frequency of M^+ strains was also found by HOLLAND and ROBERTS (1964). The megacins, like other bacteriocins, behave like proteins and have extremely narrow antibacterial spectra, being virtually restricted to other strains of *B. megaterium*. HOLLAND and ROBERTS (1964) proposed the classification of megacins into 3 types, A, B, C. The formulation of their classification drew heavily upon the work of IVÁNOVICS and coworkers and was based upon the known general properties and mode of production of megacins. Megacin resistant mutants have so far proved impossible to isolate and hence a Fredericq-type classification was not possible. Nevertheless the groups which emerged showed remarkably consistant group properties when antibacterial activity tests on stab plates were carried out against a wide range of indicator organisms. The C megacins constitute the most homogeneous group displaying identical activity spectra with no reciprocal activity between different C-producers. In fact 14 of 15 non-megacinogenic strains were found to be sensitive to megacin C whereas all the M^+ strains were resistant. With 51 strains tested HOLLAND and ROBERTS found that all strains, including other A producers, were inhibited by the A megacins. The universal antibacterial effect of megacin A on *B. megaterium* strains was also noted by IVÁNOVICS and co-workers. The activity spectra of the B megacins was much narrower with certain strains showing marked sensitivity to all the B group but of 51 strains tested, 18, including all the A producing strains were completely resistant. With B producers as with A^+ strains, there was considerable reciprocal activity between producers and presumably reflected different chemical types of the A and B megacins. It should be noted that in all these investigations M^+ strains have been isolated initially with the aid of only one indicator strain. The use of other selective indicators will undoubtedly reveal other types.

Examples from only 2 groups of megacin, A and C, have so far been studied and the mode of action of each of these will now be considered in turn.

Megacin A

Megacin A corresponds to the first megacin observed by IVÁNOVICS and ALFÖLDI and is the only megacin whose production has been shown to be inducible by ultra-violet light. The most studied member of this group is the megacin produced by *B. megaterium* 216, and the following information will therefore refer almost exclusively to this strain.

As described above, megacin A is active against all strains of *B. megaterium* even including its own producing strain although in this case sensitivity is only slight. Incomplete immunity to the homologous bacteriocin is, however, often found amongst bacteriocinogenic bacteria.

Although one particle of colicin, after fixation to a specific receptor in the cell surface of sensitive bacteria, may be sufficient to kill one cell (JACOB, SIMINOVITCH and WOLLMAN, 1952) sensitive cells nevertheless carry some thousands of receptor sites (HELINSKI, D. R., personal communication). The adsorption of colicin by sensitive bacteria may therefore be measured simply by mixing sensitive bacteria with a bacteriocin preparation, and then by assaying the residual supernatant activity after centrifuging down the cells. In the case of megacin A however the number of receptor sites appears to be relatively few and only a very sensitive assay and with dilute solutions of megacin can be used. The assay measures the actual decrease in viable cell number of a suspension of sensitive cells treated with megacin A. With *B. megaterium* special care must also be taken in assays of this kind to ensure that the bacteria are in fact unicellular and have a high plating efficiency (> 70%). Using such an assay the adsorption of mμg amounts of megacin A by sensitive bacteria can be determined. Thus different amounts of bacteriocin and bacteria were first mixed, kept at 37° for 20 minutes and then centrifuged. A second suspension of cells was then treated with the supernatants and the percent kill determined. The results showed that megacin sensitive cells readily adsorbed the bacteriocin, whereas resistant cells adsorbed only poorly (HOLLAND, 1962). Since purified megacin A was used in these experiments and the molecular weight was known it was possible to calculate the molecular multiplicity per cell of the added bacteriocin. Thus under conditions where a 50% kill of initial cells was obtained, between 100—150 molecules of megacin/cell were adsorbed. Although no strict proportionality was established from the limited data obtained, when the saturation levels for adsorption were determined they were indeed found to be close to the bacteriocidal levels under these conditions. It appears therefore that sensitive cells may on the average adsorb up to about 100 molecules of megacin before a lethal hit occurs. This was a somewhat unexpected result since killing in cell suspensions by this bacteriocin as with other bacteriocins shows single hit kinetics.

This apparent paradox has been discussed by several workers (LURIA, 1964; NOMURA, 1964; REEVES, 1965) and in the main, three alternative hypotheses are possible.

1. B^+ strains produce heterogeneus populations of bacteriocin, so that only a relatively small fraction, 1/x, are capable both of fixation to receptor and of inducing killing after that fixation.

2. All bacteriocin molecules after fixation do have an equal, but low, 1/x, probability of inducing killing.

3. All bacteriocin molecules have an equal probability of 1, of inducing killing but only 1/x of the cell receptors is capable, after fixation, of transmitting the lethal effect to the killing target[1]. The first hypothesis is the least likely and may be discounted. From the currently available evidence however we are unable to distinguish between the latter two possibilities.

[1] For further models of mechanism of action of bacteriocins see NOMURA (1964).

In the case of megacin A it is possible to say that fixation of the bacteriocin by sensitive cells is a specific process necessary to its lethal action and since the receptor sites appear to be close to saturation before killing takes place it may be argued that perhaps the second hypothesis is the more likely. The nature and location of the actual receptor sites involved in this process is unknown although by analogy with other bacteriocins the receptors may be supposed to reside in the cell surface.

Since bacteriocin fixation by sensitive bacteria is reminiscent of phage adsorption it might be anticipated that bacteriocin action like phage infection is also a step-wise process leading to a final and irreversible phase. No study has been made of the physio-chemical factors influencing the actual process of adsorption but evidence is available of a reversible phase of megacin A action following fixation (HOLLAND, 1962). Thus, when sensitive cells were treated with megacin for 20 minutes at 37°, diluted at room temperature, plated in several series and then incubated at different temperatures, it was found that the amount of killing was a direct function of temperature. Whilst at 37°, the kill was 70%, at 15° 80% of the cells survived and produced colonies. Over the range 25—35° killing was inversely proportional to temperature with a Q^{10} almost 2. Despite the adsorption of a potentially lethal dose of megacin therefore the cells survived when grown at low temperature. Killing and fixation are not therefore co-incident processes. Following adsorption a second step, presumably involving an enzyme and/or the synthesis of some protein, is necessary before the presence of megacin is converted into a lethal event. Nomura has suggested that colicin action is also a stepwise process, and that following adsorption the effect of the bacteriocin is transmitted somehow through the cytoplasmic membrane to the biochemical target, the hitting of which may ultimately lead to the death of the cell. Assuming that megacin A is acting in the same way, some step in the transmission process would appear to be temperature dependent and thus at low growth temperatures the effect of adsorbed bacteriocin is never converted into a successful hit on the biochemical target. The nature of this step however remains obscure. Much more information is now needed to establish which *cell* functions are necessary in order to convert megacin fixation into a lethal event.

IVÁNOVICS, ALFÖLDI and NAGY (1959) reported that megacin A killing in cell suspensions was also temperature dependent. In their studies, sensitive bacteria were treated with megacin for different times at different temperatures, diluted into ice cold broth and then plated for viable colonies at 37°. In essentially similar experiments, but using bacteriophage Tl, GAREN and PUCK (1951) showed that phage adsorbed at 4° could in fact be largely eluted on dilution into cold broth, but that the phage adsorbed at 37° could not, i.e. there is a very low temperature coefficient for reversible adsorption. A similar reversible change in the case of bacteriocin would also give rise to the results obtained by IVÁNOVICS *et al.* who were perhaps therefore simply measuring the effect of temperature on reversible adsorption and not upon killing. Unfortunately their data cannot exclude this possibility.

No studies have so far been carried out on the effects of megacin A on cellular metabolism, however from the work of IVÁNOVICS and collaborators it appears clear that treatment of sensitive bacteria with the bacteriocin induces drastic changes in the permeability properties of protoplasts and of whole cells. IVÁNOVICS *et al.* (1959) found that cultures treated with megacin A underwent characteristic cytological changes. The homogeneity and density of the cell cytoplasm gradually decreased until finally, only almost empty envelopes remained. These changes although accompanied by marked decrease in turbidity did not affect the total count of bacteria and furthermore a specific test for lysozyme, the addition of megacin to chloroform or heat-killed bacteria, was negative. The authors concluded therefore that megacin action leaves the cell wall intact although the cellular contents leak out. Effect of megacin on cell permeability was checked directly by determining the release of UV absorbing material and the increased permeability of cells to substrates of β-galactosidase. Thus megacin was added to a suspension of sensitive bacteria and after a lag of about 15 minutes, release of 260 mμ absorbing material took place. In a further experiment exponentially growing cells (on lactose) were treated with megacin, samples taken at intervals and the β-galactosidase activity of the suspension determined in the presence of O-nitrophenyl-β-γ-galactoside. The results showed that after a lag of about 8 minutes the megacin treated cells became permeable to the substrate and thereafter availability of the enzyme increased linearly with time for 30 minutes.

IVÁNOVICS *et al.* also measured the effect of megacin upon protoplast preparations of sensitive and resistant organisms (non-*B. megaterium* strains). Protoplasts of sensitive cells were rapidly lysed and transformed into ghosts whilst protoplasts of resistant strains were unaffected. The identification of megacin as the lytic agent was confirmed by the demonstration that extracts of producer cells not making megacin were inactive whilst the lytic activity of extracts from cells actively engaged in megacin production showed an increase in lytic action parallel with the increase in megacin. Control experiments showed that the protoplasts used in these experiments were not affected by trypsin or ribonuclease (100 μg/ml) or by the addition of a megaterium phage preparation. It was concluded from these results therefore that megacin acts at the level of the cytoplasmic membrane and kills by directly or indirectly destroying the permeability properties of this membrane. With a preparation of purified megacin A, HOLLAND (1962) also showed that protoplasts could be lysed but that when actual bacteriocidal levels of bacteriocin were used, lysis was delayed for up to 90 minutes before the protoplasts abruptly burst. It was also noted that lysis of protoplasts in fact left the macrostructure of the protoplast intact although the cytoplasmic contents were largely discharged. Furthermore isolated cytoplasmic membranes of sensitive cells were not detectably hydrolysed by added megacin. Thus although megacin A action is accompanied by characteristic permeability changes involving the cytoplasmic membrane we cannot be sure that this is the primary action of the protein. In any event, it seems unlikely that megacin is acting like a lipase with a direct hydrolytic effect. Alternatively and perhaps more likely, the primary action of megacin may be the introduction of a series of subtle local weakenings and changes in structure of the membrane leading eventually to the abrupt loss of the osmotic properties of the whole membrane. A study of the effect of megacin A on the energy metabolism of sensitive cells and upon the synthesis of structural components of the membrane might be a very fruitful approach to the problem at this stage.

A few other examples of A megacins have been examined by IVÁNOVICS and co-workers (NAGY, ALFÖLDI, and IVÁNOVICS, 1959). All were found to be produced in a similar manner by different producing strains and to induce lysis of protoplasts. Nevertheless no cross interactions were obtained with anti-serum obtained with different megacins and so they are chemically distinguishable.

Megacin C

The bacteriocin produced by *B. megaterium* C4MA$^-$ is the only group C megacin so far studied. This strain was derived from a parent producing both A and C megacins but a segregant was obtained producing megacin C alone (HOLLAND and ROBERTS, 1964). Although the studies of the mode of action of megacin C so far are limited, some interesting results have nevertheless been obtained.

As in the case of colicin, fixation of megacin C by bacteria can easily be demonstrated by mixing cells and bacteriocin and determining the decrease in supernatant activity by simple serial dilution assay. Presumably therefore megacin C receptors like those of colicin but unlike A receptors are present in relatively large numbers. In addition to fixation by whole cells preliminary experiments have also shown that purified cell wall preparations were equally effective in removing megacin C from solution. Isolated cytoplasmic membranes, however, did not adsorb megacin. Fixation by both cells and cell walls appeared to be a temperature independent process (HOLLAND, all unpublished results). It is therefore reasonable to assume that megacin C like other bacteriocins acts via the intermediacy of specific cell wall receptors. Nevertheless, the nature of these receptors, the mechanism of fixation or the number of molecules of bacteriocin per cell necessary to achieve the single hit kill are all unknown.

In preliminary purification studies megacin C was found to behave as would be expected of a protein although it is possible that this bacteriocin protein is also part of a lipo-polysaccharide complex. Unfortunately the inherent instability of the protein has so far precluded a successful purification (HOLLAND, unpublished). For this reason also, mode of action studies have been carried out so far simply using sterile culture supernatants from exponentially growing cultures of the producing strain, which contains considerable amounts of soluble bacteriocin (HOLLAND, 1963). Such supernatants do not contain any contaminating phage particles and moreover the supernatants from megacin C$^-$ strains derived from the parent strain have no detectable effects upon megacin C sensitive bacteria.

Killing curves with megacin C are the usual bacteriocin, one hit type and so one particle is sufficient to kill one cell. Megacin C does not affect the turbidity of growing cultures or cell suspensions of protoplasts of sensitive bacteria. This bacteriocin clearly does not therefore act in the same way as megacin A.

The study of megacin C action on sensitive bacteria has been restricted to an investigation of its effect upon protein and nucleic acid synthesis and evidence has been presented that megacin C specifically affects DNA synthesis of the treated bacteria (HOLLAND, 1965). Thus when exponentially growing cultures of sensitive strains were treated with bacteriocidal concentrations (5—200 units/ml) of megacin C it was found that the extent of inhibition of DNA synthesis was proportional to the amount of megacin added. In contrast, protein and RNA syntheses were completely unaffected at low concentrations (5—75 units/ml) and only partially inhibited at higher concentrations. At these higher concentrations megacin actually induced the rapid breakdown of acid precipitable DNA of the cells. With the destruction of the template for DNA dependent RNA synthesis, it is not surprising that RNA and protein syntheses were also inhibited. The rapid loss of DNA observed on addition of megacin C could not be induced when the cells were treated in a variety of other ways, e.g. with actinomycin D, puromycin, chloramphenicol, streptomycin, phenethyl alcohol, sodium azide or by oxygen starvation. It should be noted that under all these conditions DNA synthesis in *B. megaterium* is inhibited, specifically or otherwise, nevertheless there is no degradation of DNA. A primary effect of megacin C therefore is the specific induction of the inhibition of synthesis and the breakdown of DNA and the action of this bacteriocin is therefore similar to that of colicin E2 (NOMURA, 1963). As further evidence of their effect on DNA synthesis both of these agents have been shown to induce phage production in lysogenic organisms (ENDO, KAMIYA and ISHIZAWA, 1963; HOLLAND, 1963) a process which appears to be exclusive to compounds or radiations which specifically act upon DNA. It has not been possible as yet to determine whether degradation of DNA is the primary cause or the effect of megacin-induced inhibition of DNA synthesis. From the evidence available at the moment the simplest interpretation would be that inhibition of DNA synthesis results from the breakdown of DNA at a faster rate than the rate of synthesis.

Some attempt has been made to elucidate the mechanism of action of the bacteriocin and in particular the effect of inhibition of protein or DNA synthesis or energy metabolism in treated bacteria has been studied (HOLLAND, 1965). When DNA synthesis is inhibited (by mitomycin C) prior to the addition of megacin the degradation of DNA is unaffected and hence DNA in the process of active duplication is not an essential pre-requisite for its destruction on addition of the bacteriocin. It would nevertheless be of interest to determine what effect megacin had upon cells at different stages in their growth cycle, i.e. after synchronisation, and in particular whether chromosomal DNA on completion of a complete duplication cycle but before the initiation of a second, is still sensitive to megacin action.

The inhibition of both protein synthesis or energy metabolism does markedly reduce the degradative effects of the bacteriocin. Moreover, at least in the case of energy metabolism, restoration of normal aeration immediately initiates DNA degradation. In these experiments, inhibition of energy metabolism was achieved merely by cessation of shaking of the experimental cultures. Under such conditions, protein and nucleic acid metabolism of growing *B. megaterium* is immediately halted. Megacin C (400 units/ml) was then added to such a static culture, but no breakdown of DNA was observed. The cells were next washed, resuspended in fresh media, and aerated, whereupon DNA breakdown immediately commenced. Energy metabolism is therefore needed for the completion of some step in the action of megacin C following its adsorption. That this requirement is probably a requirement for protein synthesis was demonstrated by experiments in which protein synthesis was inhibited during treatment with megacin. Exponentially growing bacteria were first treated with concentrations of chloromycetin or streptomycin sufficient to cause an apparent 100% inhibition of protein synthesis. After 10 minutes megacin C was added and the effect on degradation of DNA was examined. Under such conditions breakdown of DNA was markedly reduced. At the same time, the slight inhibition of RNA synthesis usually observed at these concentrations of megacin C was completely abolished confirming the previous supposition that the effects of megacin on RNA synthesis (and perhaps therefore on protein synthesis) are only secondary and dependent upon the destruction of the DNA template.

These results pose several interesting questions concerning the mode of action of megacin C. Degradation of DNA must presumably involve the action of a DNase which must be synthesised or "activated" in some way in response to the presence of megacin. Since inhibition of protein synthesis suppresses breakdown of DNA it might be postulated that megacin action directly or indirectly induces the synthesis of a previously repressed DNase which then degrades the DNA. Alternatively, and more especially if the actual degradation of DNA does prove to be secondary to the primary effect of megacin, inhibition of protein synthesis may rather block in some way the *transmission* of the effect of megacin to its biochemical target whatever that may be. Both these alternative hypotheses are open to experimental test. Finally it should be pointed out that although a direct hydrolytic effect of megacin C upon DNA itself seems unlikely in view of these results, it has not been completely excluded. It should be noted however that the very similar colicin E2 has no detectable DNase activity (NOMURA and MAEDA, 1964). How the postulated "transmission" or "induction" processes could be actually achieved is of course obscure but this is a problem basic to an understanding of the mode of action of all bacteriocins. How do fixed extra-cellular proteins transmit their specific lethal effects across the cytoplasmic membrane to the appropriate targets within the cell or at least within the membrane? It is tempting to invoke the concept of allosteric protein interactions as a possible explanation and basis for future experimental approach to these problems.

Another type of bacteriocin in *B. megaterium* was previously reported by MARJAI and IVÁNOVICS (1962). This bacteriocin, named KP (killer principle) is clearly distinct from megacin A and was thought to be a part of a defective phage particle. The conditions for the formation and liberation of this bacteriocin are however very reminiscent of megacin C, and IVÁNOVICS (1965) suggested that KP might indeed be a megacin of the C group. This was supported by the finding that KP could also induce phage liberation from a lysogenic culture. IVÁNOVICS also reported the isolation of an interesting mutant form of the KP producing strain which illustrates another important future approach to the question of bacteriocin immunity and the mode of action of bacteriocins. The mutant, designated KP^1, was isolated as a streptomycin resistant mutant of the original strain but was found to produce a new KP^1 bacteriocin showing a different host range. Moreover the original strain was now sensitive to KP^1 and *vice versa*. A single mutation resulting in a mutant form of bacteriocin simultaneously therefore led to a change in the corresponding immunity mechanism. Elucidation of the way in which this is achieved and the isolation of more mutants of this type should be fruitful indeed.

References

ENDO, H., T. KAMIYA, and M. ISHIZAWA: λ phage induction by colicin E2. Biochem' Biophys. Research Commun. **11**, 477—482 (1963).

GAREN, A., and T. T. PUCK: The first two steps of the invasion of host cells by bacterial viruses. J. Exptl. Med. **94**, 177 (1951).

HOLLAND, I. B.: Further observations on the properties of megacin, a bacteriocin formed by *Bacillus megaterium*. J. Gen. Microbiol. **29**, 603—614 (1962).

HOLLAND, I. B.: Effect on DNA synthesis of preparations of a bacteriocin formed by *Bacillus megaterium*. Symp. Bacterial Transformation and Bacteriocinogeny, Budapest 1963 (in press) (1963).

HOLLAND, I. B., and C. F. ROBERTS: Some properties of a new bacteriocin formed by *Bacillus megaterium*. J. Gen. Microbiol. **35**, 271—285 (1964).

HOLLAND, I. B.: A bacteriocin specifically affecting DNA synthesis in *Bacillus megaterium*. J. Mol. Biol. **12**, 429—438 (1965).

IVÁNOVICS, G., and L. ALFÖLDI: A new antibacterial principle: megacin. Nature **174**, 465 (1954).

IVÁNOVICS, G., and E. NAGY: Heriditary aberrancy in growth of some *Bacillus megaterium* strains. J. Gen. Microbiol. **19**, 407—418 (1958).

IVÁNOVICS, G., L. ALFÖLDI, and E. NAGY: Mode of action of megacin. J. Gen. Microbiol. **21**, 51—60 (1959).

IVÁNOVICS, G.: Megacin and megacin-like substances. Zentr. Bakteriol. Parasitenk., Abt. I **196**, 318—329 (1965).

JACOB, F., L. SIMINOVITCH et E. WOLLMAN: Sur la biosynthèse d'une colicine et sur son mode d'action. Ann. Inst. Pasteur **83**, 295—315 (1952).

LURIA, S. E.: On the mechanisms of action of colicins. Ann. Inst. Pasteur **107** (Suppl.), 67—73 (1964).

MARJAI, E. H., and G. IVÁNOVICS: A second bacteriocin-like principle of *Bacillus megaterium*. I. The characteristics of the bacteriocidal principle. Acta Microbiol. Acad. Sci. Hung. **9**, 285—295 (1962).

NAGY, E., L. ALFÖLDI, and G. IVÁNOVICS: Megacins. Acta Microbiol. Acad. Sci. Hung. **6**, 327—336 (1959).

NOMURA, M.: Mode of action of colicines. Cold Spring Harbor Symposia Quant. Biol. **28**, 315—324 (1963).

NOMURA, M.: Mechanism of action of colicines. Proc. Natl. Acad. Sci. U.S. **52**, 1514—1521 (1964).

NOMURA, M., and A. MAEDA: Mechanism of action of colicines. Zentr. Bakteriol. Parasitenk., Abt. I **196**, 216—239 (1965).

Colicins

Masayasu Nomura

Colicins are bactericidal substances, protein in nature, which are synthesized by certain strains of Enterobacteriaceae and kill bacteria of the same or related species.

Colicins can not reproduce themselves and thus are distinct from bacteriophages. However, there are striking similarities between colicins and bacteriophages: 1. The killing action of colicins resembles that of virulent phage as will be described below. Most striking is the fact that it requires the presence of specific receptors which are sometimes common for a colicin and a bacteriophage (FREDERICQ, 1958). 2. The capacity to synthesize colicins is determined by a genetic factor, called a colicin factor (or colicinogenic factor), which has many similarities to prophage in lysogenic cells. Various agents which are known to induce prophage development are also effective in inducing the synthesis of colicin in colicinogenic cells. Both prophage development and colicin synthesis are lethal biosyntheses (JACOB, SIMINOVITCH and WOLLMAN, 1952; LWOFF, 1953). Finally, the presence in a cell of prophage or colicin factor renders that cell immune to homologous phage or to the killing action of "external" homologous colicin (FREDERICQ, 1958). Thus, colicins are distinct from ordinary antibiotics. Bactericidal substances similar to colicins are also produced by other bacterial species and the general name bacteriocin has been given to these bactericidal proteins (JACOB, LWOFF, SIMINOVITCH, and WOLLMAN, 1953).

Studies on the mode of action of colicins may be of interest for several reasons; first, because of their resemblances to bacteriophages, and second, because of their usefulness in the study of the functional importance of the cellular membrane as well as regulatory mechanisms controlling macromolecular syntheses in general. In this article, the mode of action of colicins will be described. Information about other aspects of colicins and colicinogeny can be obtained in several other review articles (FREDERICQ, 1957a, 1958, 1963; IVÁNOVICS, 1952; CLOWES, 1964; HAMON, 1964; REEVES, 1965a). The mode of action of another bacteriocin, megacin, is described by Holland elsewhere in this volume.

Colicins are usually classified according to the specificity of their receptors, and are further divided into subgroups according to the specificity of their immunity (FREDERICQ, 1948, 1965). For example, colicins E1, E2 and E3 differ from each other in their immunity pattern but are classified as E group, because all of them adsorb to the same receptor. This receptor is also shared by a bacteriophage, BF23 (FREDERICQ, 1949). Similarly, Ia and Ib share a common receptor, but can be distinguished from each other by their immunity specificity (STOCKER, 1965). About 20 different colicins are known. Only a few of them, which have been studied with respect to their mode of action, will be discussed in this article.

Colicins are produced by colicinogenic strains, either original "wild" strains isolated from natural sources or strains obtained by transfer of the colicin factor into noncolicinogenic strains. The colicin factor, a cytoplasmic genetic factor, can be transferred by cell to cell contact (FREDERICQ, 1954; OZEKI, STOCKER and SMITH, 1962; STOCKER, SMITH and OZEKI, 1963). Some of the colicinogenic strains pertinent to the colicins to be discussed here are described in Table 1. Since the properties of colicins are sometimes different depending on their origin, even though they are classified in the same group according to receptor and immunity specificity as described in the previous section. It has been suggested that one should refer to colicins by the name of the original producer strain (REEVES, 1965; LEWIS and STOCKER, 1965; cf. Table 1).

Table 1. *Some colicinogenic strains*

	Colicins	Colicinogenic strains	Colicin factors in the strain	Description or references[1]
K	K-K235	*E. coli* K235	K-K235	FREDERICQ's original strain
	K-K49	*E. coli* K49	K-K49	FREDERICQ's original strain
		S. typhimurium cys C-7 (K-49)		col K-K49 factor transferred to *S. typhimurium* CysC-7 by OZEKI *et al.* (1962)
E1	E1-ML	*E. coli* ML	E1-ML	JACOB *et al.* (1952)
	E1-K30	*E. coli* K12-30	E1-K30	FREDERICQ's original strain
	E1-a	*S. typhimurium* SL1015	E1-a	LEWIS and STOCKER (1965)
	E1-b	*S. typhimurium* SL1051	E1-b	LEWIS and STOCKER (1965)
E2	E2-P9	*Shigella sonnei* P9	E2-P9, Ib-P9	FREDERICQ's original strain
		*S. typhimurium cys*D-36 (E2-P9)	E2-P9	OZEKI *et al.* (1962)
		E. coli W3110 (E2-P9)	E2-P9	NOMURA (1964)
	E2-CA42	*E. coli* CA42	E2-CA42	Isolated by FREDERICQ
	E2-317	*E. coli* K12-317	E2-317	Isolated by FREDERICQ
	E2-W	*S. typhimurium* SL1057	E2-W	LEWIS and STOCKER (1965)
E3	E3-CA38	*E. coli* CA38	E3-CA38, I	FREDERICQ's original strain
Ia	Ia-CA53	*E. coli* CA53	Ia-CA53	FREDERICQ's original strain
Ib	Ib-P9	*Shigella sonnei* P9	Ib-P9, E2-P9	FREDERICQ's original strain
		S. typhimurium cysD-36 (Ib-P9)	Ib-P9	OZEKI *et al.* (1962)

[1] Concerning FREDERICQ's original strains, see FREDERICQ (1948), and FREDERICQ (1965).

Colicin preparations can be obtained either from old cultures of colicinogenic bacteria (GOEBEL, BARRY and SHEDLOVSKY, 1956) or from the cultures of exponentially growing colicinogenic bacteria by induction with various inducing agents (JACOB *et al.*, 1952; FREDERICQ, 1963). Mitomycin C at a concentration of 0.2 to 2μg/ml is a convenient inducing agent to be used in the laboratory.

Colicins can be purified by several methods (GOEBEL and BARRY, 1958; GOEBEL, 1962; REEVES, 1963; HELSINKI, 1966). GOEBEL's group purified colicin K produced by *E. coli* K235 as a lipocarbohydrate protein complex (GOEBEL and BARRY, 1958; GOEBEL, 1962). However, upon dissociation, the colicin activity was associated with the protein moiety (GOEBEL and BARRY, 1958). Colicin E2 (E2-P9) was purified recently to the extent that the preparation is pure as judged by ordinary chemical and physicochemical criteria (HELINSKI, 1966). Purified E2 does not contain any carbohydrate and is a simple protein. Another colicin E2 (E2-42) was purified by REEVES (1963). Although only a few colicins have been purified and characterized, it is reasonable to make a general conclusion that colicins are protein in nature. The fact that most of the colicins are inactivated by proteolytic enzymes such as trypsin (FREDERICQ, 1958) also agrees with this conclusion.

In contrast to all ordinary antibiotics, colicins act only on *E. coli* strains or closely related bacteria (such as *Shigella*) which have the necessary specific receptors on their cell surface. Even among *E. coli* strains, there are several strains which are resistant to a given colicin. Sensitive strains can mutate to the resistant state, either by a loss of specific receptor (FREDERICQ, 1957b) or by a change in some other mechanism (NOMURA, 1964; CLOWES, 1965). The former type of resistant mutant, which is more common, does not adsorb that colicin, while the latter type does. A sensitive strain also becomes resistant to a colicin after acquisition of the colicin factor (FREDERICQ, 1957b). This resistance property is called immunity. FREDERICQ (1957b) suggested that immune cells retain the receptor and adsorb colicins. This has recently been demonstrated by using a purified radioactive colicin, also by using a defective colicinogenic strain (MAEDA and NOMURA, 1966).

The requirement for the presence of specific receptors for colicin action was mentioned above. If a low concentration of a colicin solution is treated with sensitive cells, colicin activity disappears from the solution. As mentioned in the previous section, the most common type of resistant mutant does not remove colicin from the solution (HAMON and PERON, 1960). Actual adsorption of colicin to bacterial surface structure has recently been demonstrated using purified radioactive colicins (MAEDA and NOMURA, 1966).

As first shown by JACOB, SIMINOVITCH, and WOLLMAN (1952), the killing action of most colicins is a single hit process as is the killing of bacteria by bacteriophage particles (NOMURA, 1963; REEVES, 1965b). Thus, colicins behave like particles and their killing titer can be assayed in terms of the number of "killing particles" (or "killing units") (NOMURA, 1963; MAEDA and NOMURA, 1965). This is done by measuring the fraction of survivors after incubation of sensitive cells with various concentrations of colicin. The number of "killing particles", thus enumerated, is not necessarily equal to the actual number of active colicin molecules. Using a purified E2 preparation and taking the molecular weight for E2 as 60,000 (Helinski, personal communication), it has been calculated that one killing unit corresponds to about 100 molecules (MAEDA and NOMURA, 1966). The deviation from the value one is either due to inactive particles in the preparation and/or to the low probability (1%) of a successful killing action per adsorbed particle. The second explanation includes the possibility of heterogeneity of receptors. Since changes in assay conditions (e.g., temperature, the physiological state of sensitive cells) affect the estimation of the number of killing units, the second explanation accounts for at least a part of the deviation from one. However, the problem remains to be solved by future studies.

Colicin K and El

In their pioneer studies, JACOB, SIMINOVITCH, and WOLLMAN (1952) showed that colicin E1 (E1-ML) inhibits DNA and RNA synthesis and cell growth, but not respiration. Similarly, colicin K (K-235 or K-49) does not inhibit respiration even at high multiplicity [input ratio of colicin (number of killing units) to bacteria] (NOMURA, unpublished experiments), but inhibits DNA, RNA, and protein synthesis. In fact, a slight stimulation of respiration is usually observed. At low multiplicity, the degree of inhibition of the macromolecular synthesis corresponds approximately to the fraction of killed cells (NOMURA, 1963). Apparently the inhibition takes place in a relatively short time in every killed cell. Colicin K does not cause leakage of ^{32}P-substances from ^{32}P-labeled cells or of β-galactosidase from fully induced cells (NOMURA, 1963). However, it inhibits the functioning of certain permeases (permeases for β-D-galactosides, isoleucine and potassium) as does colicin E1 (LURIA, 1964). Inhibition of active transport of potassium has been confirmed also by NOMURA and MAEDA (1965).

It is known that the active transport, or permease function, depends on a supply of energy. Any agent which inhibits the energy supply inhibits the active transport of the metabolites. LEVINTHAL and LEVINTHAL (cited by LURIA, 1964) discovered that colicin E1 inhibited oxidative phosphorylation. This inhibition could explain the inhibition by E1 of active transport as well as the inhibition of macromolecular synthesis. Colicin K was also shown to inhibit the accumulation of ^{32}P-ATP in sensitive cells incubated in the presence of glucose and radioactive inorganic phosphate. About 70% inhibition was observed at a multiplicity of about 10 (NOMURA, unpublished experiments: also, cf. NOMURA and MAEDA, 1965). Thus, colicin K interferes with energy supply either by inhibiting ATP formation or by inducing ATP breakdown. However, interference with the energy supply system is not complete: at a high multiplicity where incorporation of ^{32}P into DNA and RNA is more than 98% inhibited, ^{32}P-inorganic phosphate is still esterified to the β-, and γ-position of ATP to an extent as much as 30% of the control, is incorporated into the phospholipid fraction to the same extent (about 20 to 40% of the control), and is incorporated into the non-nucleotide organic phosphate fraction without noticeable inhibition (NOMURA and MAEDA, 1965). Thus, specificity of inhibition of colicin K is distinct from other inhibitors such as 2, 4-dinitrophenol, a known uncoupler of oxidative phosphorylation. At 2×10^{-4} M concentration, 2, 4-dinitrophenol inhibits the incorporation of ^{32}P-inorganic phosphate into all the fractions, i.e., nucleotides, non-nucleotide organic phosphate, phospholipid, RNA and DNA fractions, more or less to the same extent (NOMURA, unpublished experiments). Two possibilities could be conceived: 1. There are at least two distinct energy supplying mechanisms. Colicin K (and E1) inhibits specifically one of them (probably, oxidative phosphorylation at the bacterial membrane), but not some other mechanisms (for example, glycolysis in the cytoplasm). Nucleic acid synthesis under the conditions studied depends primarily on the former system, while the latter system is responsible for the assimilation of ^{32}P into non-nucleotide organic phosphates or some of the phospholipids. Thus, colicin K inhibits macromolecular syntheses rather specifically by inhibiting the former energy supplying mechanism. 2. Alternatively, the inhibition of macromolecular synthesis by colicin K may not be the result of the inhibition of energy supply. Some unknown alteration of the bacterial membrane induced by the colicin may cause both the inhibition of the energy supplying system and the inhibition of macromolecular synthesis. Although some experiments with E1 performed by LEVINTHAL and LEVINTHAL (cited by LURIA, 1964) favors the first alternative, further experiments are desirable to make a more definite conclusion.

One striking feature of the action of colicin K is its reversibility (NOMURA and NAKAMURA, 1962). The inhibition of macromolecular synthesis, phage growth, and colony formation in colicin K-treated cells can be reversed to a great extent by treatment with trypsin. The degree of reversal with trypsin is greater when the colicin acts on resting cells than when it acts on growing cells (NOMURA and NAKAMURA, 1962). The reversal of the action of colicins does not seem to be due to the destruction of a pre-existing trypsin-sensitive structure necessary for colicin action, since pretreatment of cells with trypsin does not significantly change the sensitivity of the cells to colicin after washing to remove trypsin NOMURA, 1964). Therefore, the reversal seems to be due to the digestion of the adsorbed colicin particle itself. If, as suggested, the reversal of colicin action by treatment with trypsin is due to digestion of the colicin particle, the colicin must remain at the receptor site on the bacterial surface. The significance of this conclusion will be discussed later.

Reversibility by trypsin can also be demonstrated with several other colicins, if irreversible damages caused as a terminal step of colicin action (for example, DNA breakdown in the case of E2, see below) are prevented by some means (REYNOLDS and REEVES, 1963; NOMURA, 1963).

Colicin E2

Colicin E2 (E2-P9) at relatively high multiplicities does not inhibit respiration (less than 10% inhibition at multiplicities up to about 20), but does affect macromolecular synthesis (NOMURA, 1963, and unpublished experiments). However, by using a very high multiplicity, PERSIEL (1965) could observe a significant inhibition of respiration in growing cells after a certain time lag. Since both DNA degradation and inhibition of macromolecular synthesis (see below) can be observed under conditions where no inhibition of respiration is observed, the observed inhibition is certainly not a major biochemical effect. As was suggested (PERSIEL, 1965), the inhibition might be due to an alteration of the cell membrane structure caused by a very high multiplicity of the colicin.

Colicin E2 at high multiplicity inhibits the synthesis of DNA, RNA and protein in sensitive *E. coli* cells. At low adsorbed multiplicities (1 to 2), no inhibition of ^{35}S sulfate incorporation into total protein was observed for at least one hour. Synthesis of DNA and RNA also continued for at least 30 to 60 minutes under these conditions (NOMURA, 1963; NOMURA and MAEDA, 1965). The inhibition of macromolecular synthesis could be explained by the damage in DNA caused by E2; it was demonstrated that E2 induces the degradation of DNA and the rate of degradation depends strongly on the multiplicity of E2 (NOMURA, 1963). No degradation of RNA was observed. Since infection of E2-inhibited cells with T4 phage can cause the resumption of macromolecular synthesis in such cells (NOMURA, 1963), the extrachromosomal synthetic machinery including the oxidative phosphorylation system seems to be intact. In fact, when incorporation of ^{32}P-inorganic phosphate into the nucleotide fraction was followed, a significant stimulation rather than an inhibition, was observed (NOMURA, unpublished experiments). The observed stimulation could be due to a residual incorporation of ^{32}P into DNA followed by degradation of the radioactive DNA. Inhibition of the incorporation of ^{32}P-inorganic phosphate into the phospholipid fraction is also much less than the inhibition of ^{32}P incorporation into RNA and DNA (NOMURA, unpublished experiments). In contrast to E1 or K, colicin E2 does not inhibit the active transport of potassium and the functioning of some other permeases (LURIA, 1964; NOMURA and MAEDA, 1965).

Colicin E2, but not E3 or K, induces the development of phage λ in lysogenic *E. coli* cells (ENDO, KAMIYA and ISHIZAWA, 1963; NOMURA, 1963). A single event caused by E2, presumably a certain specific change in the state of DNA may be responsible for both the induction of λ and the degradation of DNA (NOMURA, 1963).

The observation that colicin E2 increases the frequency of genetic recombination between two mutants of bacteriophage T4 (NOMURA, unpublished experiments) could also be explained by a slow breakdown of phage DNA molecules induced by E2.

It seems that the damage to DNA is the main observable biochemical effect of colicin E2, and possibly the primary cause of the killing of sensitive strains. Another colicin E2, E2-CA42, also induces DNA degradation, and seems to be very similar to E2-P9 in its mode of action (REEVES, 1965). Interaction of colicin E2 with bacterial cells was studied using radioactive colicin (MAEDA and NOMURA, 1966).

Colicin E3

Colicin E3 (E3-CA38) at high multiplicity does not inhibit respiration (NOMURA, unpublished experiments), DNA or RNA synthesis, but inhibits protein synthesis (NOMURA, 1963; NOMURA and MAEDA, 1965). At lower multiplicity, no immediate inhibitory effect is observed on protein, DNA or RNA synthesis. The time lag before the complete inhibition of protein synthesis is strongly dependent on the multiplicity of E3.

Colicin E3 does not cause DNA degradation or induction of λ in lysogenic cells even at a high multiplicity. In contrast to colicin K, E3 has no effect on active transport of potassium (NOMURA and MAEDA, 1965). E3 does not significantly inhibit the assimilation of ^{32}P-inorganic phosphate into any of several organic phosphate fractions (nucleotide, non-nucleotide organic phosphate, lipid, RNA and DNA fractions) at the high multiplicities which cause the nearly complete inhibtion of protein synthesis (NOMURA and MAEDA, 1965). The inhibition of protein synthesis does not seem to be due to the inhibition of messenger RNA synthesis as shown by experiments using phage T4 infected cells (NOMURA and MAEDA, 1965).

In several respects, apparent effects of E3 on sensitive cells resemble those of chloramphenicol. Owing to the continuous RNA synthesis in the absence of protein synthesis, sensitive cells treated with E3 in complex growth medium gradually accumulate incomplete ribosomes which are similar to chloramphenicol particles (KONISKY and NOMURA, unpublished experiments; concerning chloramphenicol particles, see NOMURA and WATSON, 1959, and KURLAND, NOMURA and WATSON, 1962). It seems that the inhibition of protein synthesis is the major observable biochemical effect of colicin E3 on sensitive cells.

Recent experiments have shown that ribosomes obtained from E3 inhibited cells are physically intact, but inactive when the activity is assayed using a poly U-directed phenylalanine incorporation system (KONISKY and NOMURA, 1966). "Hybridization" with control ribosomes showed that the 30S ribosome is inactive, but that the 50S ribosome from E3 inhibited cells is active. However, about 10 to 20% residual activity is usually, observed even when ribosomes are taken from cells in which more than 95% of protein synthesis is inhibited by E3 *in vivo*. Thus, it is still not clear whether or not the observed inactivation of the 30S ribosomes is the cause of the inhibition of protein synthesis *in vivo*.

Other Colicins

Both colicin Ia (Ia-CA53) and Ib (Ib-P9) do not inhibit respiration, but inhibit RNA, DNA and protein synthesis. At low multiplicity, the degree of inhibition is approximate to the fraction of killed cells. They do not cause DNA degradation in sensitive cells. Thus, the apparent biochemical effects of colicin Ia and Ib resemble those of colicin K and E1 (LEVISOHN and NOMURA, manuscript in preparation).

As already described, colicin E2 induces the development of phage λ in lysogenic *E. coli* strains. HAMON and PERON (1965) examined the possible induction of λ with colicins B, D, E1, K, L, N and P (origins were not described) and compared them with E2. Only colicin P induced λ development as does colicin E2. However, they noted that colicin P does not cause DNA degradation, and thus seems to be distinct from E2 and from the other colicins studied so far.

It appears that further studies with other colicins may reveal a still greater diversity in their apparent mode of action. However, it is important for such studies to use a purified material in order to eliminate any possible effect due to contaminating substances.

Possible Mechanism of Action

Two major features of colicin action should be emphasized: first, a single colicin particle apparently is enough to kill a sensitive *E. coli* cell, and the colicin particle stays at the receptor site and acts from there. Second, although all the colicins have fundamental common features (see Introduction), different colicins exert different biochemical effects on sensitive cells: for example, as described in detail in the previous section, colicin E2 causes DNA degradation, colicin E3 inhibits only protein synthesis and inactivates ribosomes, and colicin K and E1 inhibit all the macromolecular synthesis presumably through inhibition of oxidative phosphorylation. It should be noted that colicin E1, E2, and E3 share a common receptor and yet their mode of action is entirely different.

The conclusion that the colicin stays at the receptor site and affects the biochemical targets from there was first obtained indirectly from the results on the reversibility of colicin K action by treatment with trypsin as described in the previous section. Recent experiments using purified radioactive colicin E2 have confirmed this conclusion (MAEDA and NOMURA, 1966): Sensitive cells of *E. coli* K12 treated with the radioactive E2 were disrupted by a French Pressure Cell, and fractionated by differential centrifugation. Most of the radioactivity stayed with the cell envelope fraction. Trypsin removed a major part of radioactivity from cells treated with radioactive E2. Furthermore, it was shown that the trypsin treatment causes a recovery of the capacity of E2-pretreated cells to adsorb further colicin E2. Thus, it appears that colicins stay at the receptor site and acts from there. This implies that the primary action of colicin is on the cytoplasmic membrane. The specificity of the biochemical action of different colicins suggests that bacterial cytoplasmic membrane is a mosaic, consisting of several specific parts, each of which has an important function, and that these functions can be inhibited individually by specific chemical stimuli initiated by specific colicins at the receptor site. It has been suggested that immunity is due to an alteration in the mechanism responsible for the initiation and/or the transmission of such a specific stimulus (NOMURA, 1964). The nature of this stimulus as well as the mechanism of its possible transmission through the membrane is still a matter of speculation, but presents a challenging subject for future studies. The significance and further discussion of these problems are described in the published papers (LURIA, 1964; NOMURA, 1964; NOMURA and MAEDA, 1965).

See Addendum

References

CLOWES, R. C.: Transfer génétique des facteurs colicinogènes. Ann. inst. Pasteur **107**, 74 (1964).

CLOWES, R. C.: Transmission and elimination of colicin factors and some aspects of immunity to colicin E1 in *Escherichia coli*. Zentr. Bakteriol. Parasitenk. Abt. I **196**, 152 (1965).

ENDO, H., T. KAMIYA, and M. ISHIZAWA: λ phage induction by colicine E2. Biochem. Biophys. Research Commun. **11**, 477 (1963).

FREDERICQ, P.: Actions antibiotiques réciproques chez les Enterobacteriaceae. Rev. belge pathol. et méd. exptl. **29** (Suppl. 4), 1 (1948).

FREDERICQ, P.: Sur la résistance croisée entre colicine E et bacteriophage II. Compt. rend. soc. biol. **143**, 1011 (1949).

FREDERICQ, P.: Transduction genetique des propriétés colicinogènes chez *Escherichia coli* et Shigella sonnei. Compt. rend. soc. biol. **148**, 399 (1954).

FREDERICQ, P.: Colicins. Ann. Rev. Microbiol. **11**, 7 (1957a).

FREDERICQ, P.: Genetics of two different mechanisms of resistance to colicins: Resistance by loss of specific receptors and immunity by transfer of colicinogenic factors. Ciba Foundation Symposium on Drug Resistance to Microorganism 1957b, p. 323.

FREDERICQ, P.: Colicins and colicinogenic factors. Symposia Soc. Exp. Biol. **12**, 104 (1958).

FREDERICQ, P.: On the nature of colicinogenic factors: a review. J. Theoret. Biol. **4**, 159 (1963).

FREDERICQ, P.: A note on the classification of colicines. Zentr. Bakteriol., Parasitenk. Abt. I **196**, 140 (1965).

GOEBEL, W. F.: The chromatographic fractionation of colicine K. Proc. Natl. Acad. Sci. U. S. **48**, 214 (1962).
GOEBEL, W. F., and G. T. BARRY: Colicine K. II. The preparation and properties of a substance having colicine K activity. J. Exptl. Med. **107**, 185 (1958).
GOEBEL, W. F., G. T. BARRY, and T. SHEDLOVSKY: Colicine K. I. The production of colicine K in media maintained at constant pH. J. Exptl. Med. **102**, 577 (1956).
HAMON, Y.: Les Bactériocines. Ann. inst. Pasteur **107**, 18 (1964).
HAMON, Y., and Y. PÉRON: Étude du mode de fixation des colicines et des pyocines sur les bactéries sensibles. Compt. rend. **251**, 1840 (1960).
HAMON, Y., and Y. PÉRON: Etude des propriétés inductrices de certaines colicines. Compt. rend. **260**, 5948 (1965).
HELINSKI, D.: Manuscript in preparation.
IVÁNOVICS, G.: Bacteriocins and bacteriocin-like substances. Bacteriol. Rev. **26**, 108 (1962).
JACOB, F., A. LWOFF, L. SIMINOVITCH, and E. L. WOLLMAN: Définition de quelques termes relatifs à la lysogénie. Ann. inst. Pasteur **84**, 222 (1953).
JACOB, F., L. SIMINOVITCH, and E. WOLLMAN: Sur la biosynthèse d'une colicine et sur son mode d'action. Ann. inst. Pasteur **83**, 295 (1952).
KONISKY, J., and M. NOMURA: Specific alteration of *Escherichia coli* ribosomes induced by colicin E3 *in vivo*. J. Mol. Biol. (1967 in press).
KURLAND, C., M. NOMURA, and J. D. WATSON: The physical properties of the chloromycetin particles. J. Mol. Biol. **4**, 388 (1962).
LURIA, S. E.: On the mechanisms of action of colicins. Ann. inst. Pasteur **107**, 67 (1964).
LEWIS, M. J., and B. A. D. STOCKER: Properties of some group E colicine factors. Zentr. Bakteriol., Parasitenk. **196**, 173 (1965).
LWOFF, A.: Lysogeny. Bacteriol. Rev. **17**, 269 (1953).
MAEDA, A., and M. NOMURA: Interaction of colicins with bacterial cells. I. Studies with radioactive colicins. J. Bacteriol. **91**, 685 (1966).
NOMURA, M.: Mode of action of colicines. Cold Spring Harbor Symposium Quant. Biol. **28**, 315 (1963).
NOMURA, M.: Mechanism of action of colicines. Proc. Natl. Acad. Sci. U. S. **52**, 1514 (1964).
NOMURA, M., and J. D. WATSON: Ribonucleoprotein particles within chloromycetin-inhibited Escherichia coli. J. Mol. Biol. **1**, 204 (1959).
NOMURA, M., and M. NAKAMURA: Reversibility of inhibition of nucleic acids and protein synthesis by colicin K. Biochem. Biophys. Research Commun. **7**, 306 (1962).
NOMURA, M., and A. MAEDA: Mechanism of action of colicines. Zentr. Bakteriol. Parasitenk. Abt. I **196**, 216 (1965).
OZEKI, H., B. A. D. STOCKER, and S. M. SMITH: Transmission of colicinogeny between strains of *Salmonella typhimurium* grown together. J. Gen. Microbiol. **28**, 671 (1962).
PERSIEL, I.: Beitrag zur Wirkungsweise des Colicins S3. Zentr. Bakteriol. Parasitenk. Abt. I **196**, 275 (1965).
REEVES, P. R.: Preparation of a substance having colicin F activity from *Escherichia coli* CA 42. Australian J. Exptl. Biol. Med. Sci. **41**, 153 (1963).
REEVES, P.: The bacteriocins. Bacteriol. Rev. **29**, 24 (1965a).
REEVES, P.: The adsorption and kinetics of killing by colicin CA 42-E2. Australian J. Exptl. Biol. Med. Sci. **43**, 191 (1965b).
REYNOLDS, B. L., and P. R. REEVES: Some observations on the mode of action of colicin F. Biochem. Biophys. Research Commun. **11**, 140 (1963).
STOCKER, B. A. D.: Heterogeneity of I colicines and of Col I factors. Microbial Genetics Bull. **23**, 11 (1965).
STOCKER, B. A. D., S. M. SMITH, and H. OZEKI: High infectivity of Salmonella typhimurium newly infected by the Col I factor. J. Gen. Microbiol. **30**, 201 (1963).

Enzymatic Reactions in Bacterial Cell Wall Synthesis Sensitive to Penicillins, Cephalosporins, and Other Antibacterial Agents*

Jack L. Strominger

The purpose of the present account of enzymatic reactions sensitive to penicillins, cephalosporins and other antibacterial agents is to complement the preceding chapter by providing an account of recent discoveries of the precise reactions inhibited by these agents. Bacterial cell walls are synthesized in three distinct stages which occur at three different sites in the bacterial cell. Antibiotics are known which specifically inhibit the activity of enzymes at each of these sites.

The uridine nucleotide precursors of the bacterial cell wall, UDP-acetylmuramyl-pentapeptide and UDP-acetylglucosamine, are synthesized in the cytoplasmic fraction of the cell (Fig. 1). The antibiotic, D-cycloserine, inhibits the

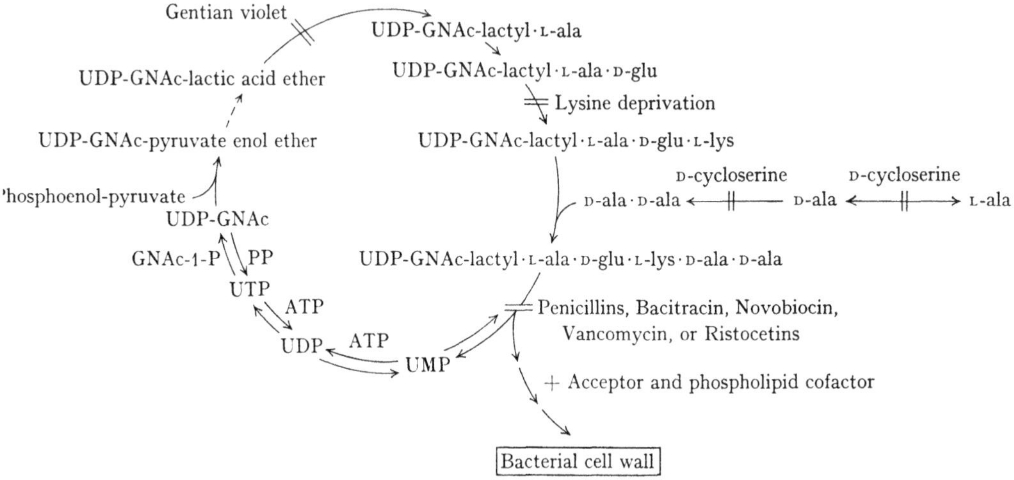

Fig. 1. Biosynthesis of the uridine nucleotide precursors of the cell wall (Strominger *et al.*, 1967). This sequence occurs in the cytoplasmic fraction of the cell and is inhibited by D-cycloserine

biosynthesis of UDP-acetylmuramyl-pentapeptide by inhibiting two sequential reactions catalyzed by alanine racemase and D-alanyl-D-alanine synthetase (fully described elsewhere in this volume) which are essential for synthesis of this nucleotide (Strominger *et al.*, 1960).

* Supported by research grants from the U.S. Public Health Service (AI-06247) and the National Science Foundation (GB-4552).

The second stage of cell wall synthesis is the utilization of these uridine nucleotide precursors and other substrates for the introduction of new disaccharide-pentapeptide units into a growing peptidoglycan in the cell wall. In this complex sequence, the sugar fragments of the nucleotides are first transferred to a membrane-bound phospholipid carrier with the formation of disaccharide-pentapeptide-P-P-phospholipid. The disaccharide-pentapeptide moiety may then be modified in a manner which depends on the particular bacterial species (e.g. by the addition of a pentaglycine chain to the ε-amino group of lysine and an amide to the α-carboxyl group of glutamic acid in *S. aureus*, or by the addition of a single glycine residue to the α-carboxyl group of glutamic acid in *M. lysodeikticus*), so that eventually a complete subunit of the peptidoglycan is synthesized (Fig. 2). Then this modified disaccharide-penta-

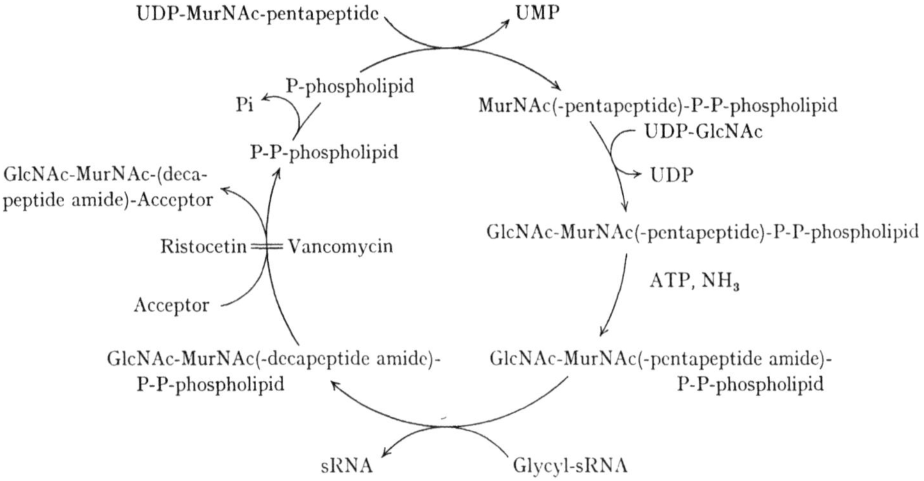

Fig. 2. Utilization of uridine nucleotides for the biosynthesis of a linear peptidoglycan in *S. aureus* (STROMINGER *et al.*, 1967). This reaction sequence occurs in the cell membrane and is inhibited by vancomycin and ristocetin at the locus indicated. Bacitracin has recently been found to be an inhibitor of the dephosphorylation of P-P-phospholipid

peptide moiety is transferred to the growing peptidoglycan with the release of P-P-phospholipid. The latter compound is then dephosphorylated to form P-phospholipid and inorganic phosphate. The phospholipid carrier then reenters the cycle. Presumably, the attachment of the sugar fragments to the phospholipid carrier serves as a means of rendering these polar compounds lipid soluble so that they can be transported through the cell membrane to the site of synthesis of the cell wall at the outside of the membrane. Vancomycin and ristocetin are specific inhibitors of the utilization of the lipid intermediates for peptidoglycan synthesis (ANDERSON *et al.*, 1965 and ANDERSON *et al.*, 1966). They inhibit the terminal reaction in the cycle in which the modified disaccharide-pentapeptide moiety is transferred to peptidoglycan. Bacitracin, on the other hand, is a specific inhibitor of the dephosphorylation of P-P-phospholipid (SIEWERT and STROMINGER, 1967).

The third stage in bacterial cell wall synthesis is the cross-linking of the linear peptidoglycan strands which are formed by the mechanism just described. This cross-linking reaction is a transpeptidation in which two linear peptidoglycan strands interact with each other with the formation of an interpeptide cross-bridge and the elimination of D-alanine (Fig. 3). This reaction occurs at the outside of the cell membrane. This site is extracellular in the sense that it is outside of the cell membrane, the permeability barrier of the cell, as is the cell wall to which new units have been attached. At this site, little or no ATP is available for catalyzing synthetic reactions and it is presumably for this reason that a mechanism of transpeptidation, which requires no additional energy source, has been evolved as the terminal step in bacterial cell wall synthesis. It is this

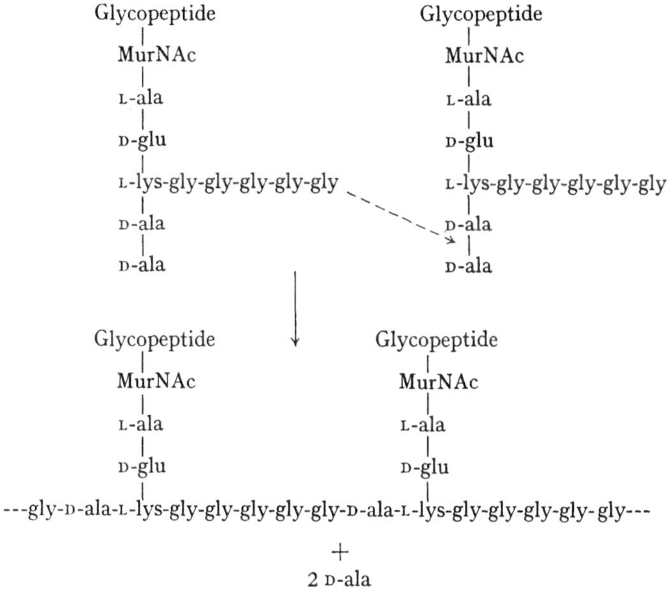

Fig. 3. Closure of glycine bridges in *S. aureus* by transpeptidation

last step in cell wall synthesis which is specifically inhibited by penicillins and cephalosporins. This hypothesis was arrived at independently by MARTIN from studies of the structure of rod-shaped cell walls of *Proteus mirabilis* and of the sphere shaped cell walls which are obtained when this organism is grown in the presence of penicillin (MARTIN, 1964a und b) and by WISE and PARK (1965) and TIPPER and STROMINGER (1965) who studied the biosynthesis of the cell wall in whole cells of *S. aureus* in the presence of penicillin. In thinking about what penicillins might do to this reaction it was recalled that, although a free carboxyl group in penicillins is not absolutely essential for their activity, this group greatly enhances their activity. The only free carboxyl group in the substrate is the carboxyl group of the terminal D-alanine residue and it seemed possible that penicillins might be structural analogs of the end of the pentapeptide chain. Molecular models of the D-alanyl-D-alanine end of the chain and of penicillin were built (Fig. 4) (TIPPER and STROMINGER, 1965). The model of penicillin was built from its crystallographic structure. The β-lactam ring of penicillin (the highly reactive four membered ring) and the thiazolidine ring (the sulfur containing ring) are almost at right angles to each other. The edge of the penicillin

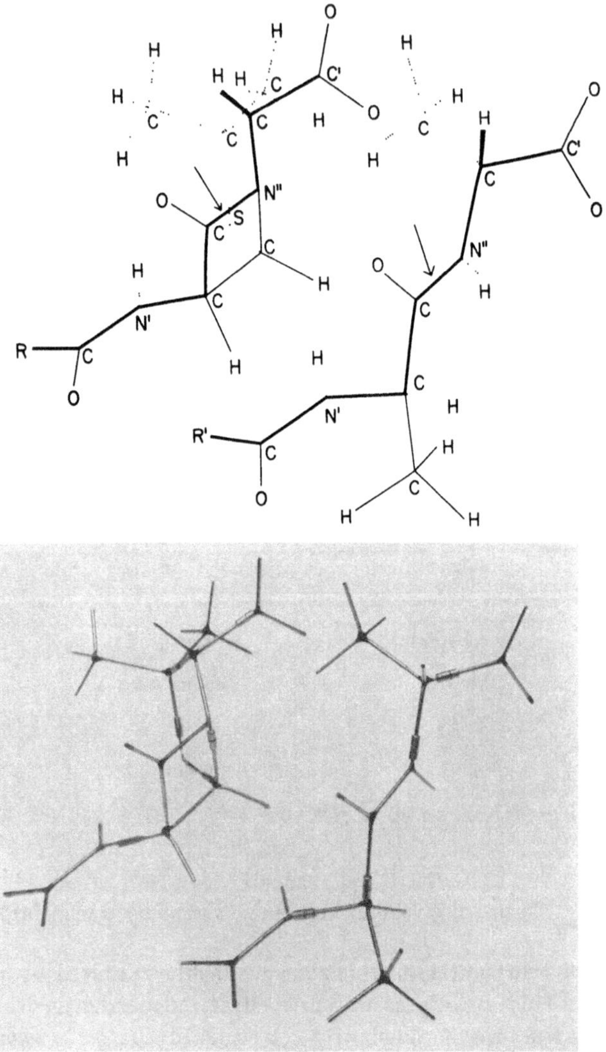

Fig. 4. Dreiding stereomodels of penicillin (left) and of the D-alanyl-D-alanine end of the peptidoglycan (right) (Tipper and Strominger, 1965)

molecule as photographed has nearly the same conformation as does the backbone of D-alanyl-D-alanine at the end of the peptide chain. The highly reactive CO-N bond in the β-lactam ring of penicillin occupies the same position as does the CO-N bond in D-alanyl-D-alanine. A mechanism for inhibition of the reaction by penicillins was therefore postulated (Fig. 5). By analogy with other reactions of this type, it was proposed that first a transpeptidase which catalyzed the cross-linking reaction would react with the end of the pentapeptide to form an acyl-enzyme intermediate with the elimination of D-alanine. This acyl-enzyme intermediate would then react with the free amino end of a pentaglycine chain in another peptidoglycan strand to form the cross-bridge. If penicillins were analogs of the end of the peptide, they might then also interact with transpeptidase. Since the CO-N bond of the β-lactam ring lies in the same position as the bond involved in transpeptidation, it might then acylate the enzyme and thereby inactivate it. A number of types of experiments with whole cells led to the conclusion that this was in fact the site of penicillin action. Similar structural and biosynthetic considerations also apply to the mechanism of action of cephalosporins.

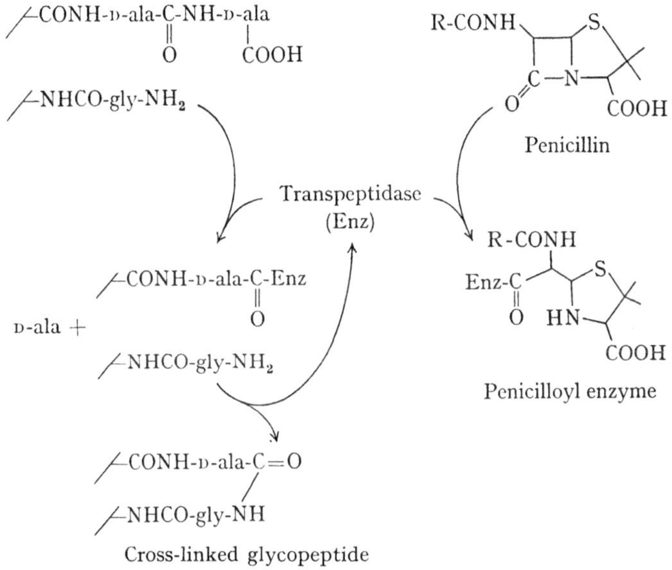

Fig. 5. Proposed mechanism of inhibition of transpeptidase by penicillins (TIPPER and STROMINGER, 1965)

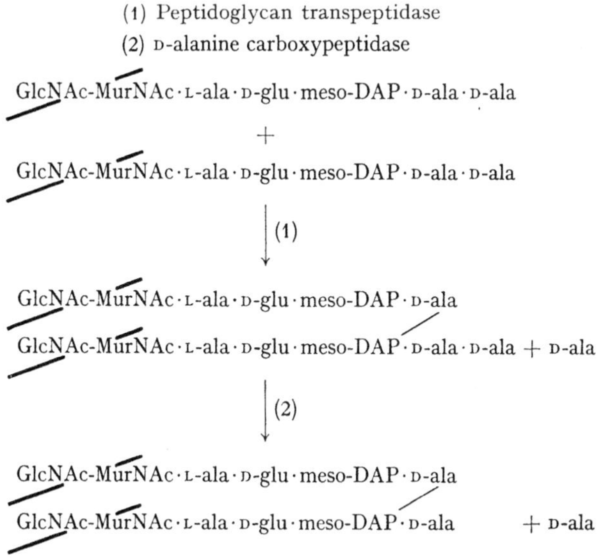

Fig. 6. Reactions catalyzed by peptidoglycan transpeptidase and D-alanine carboxypeptidase in *E. coli*

The next step was to find a cell-free preparation which catalyzed the transpeptidation. It was found, not in *Staphylococcus aureus*, the organism in which cell wall synthesis had been studied for many years, but in *Escherichia coli* (IZAKI, *et al.*, 1966; ARAKI *et al.*, 1966). For experiments with this organism labeled UDP-Mur-NAc-pentapeptide containing meso-diaminopimelic acid (rather than L-lysine) was employed, since the peptidoglycan of this organism contains this dibasic amino acid as the third residue in the peptide. There are in fact two terminal reactions in peptidoglycan synthesis in *E. coli* (Fig. 6). One of them is the transpeptidation and the other is catlayzed by a D-alanine carboxypeptidase which removes the D-alanine residue from the second strand. Presumably, the action of the carboxypeptidase limits the size of the peptide-linked oligomers in the cell wall of *E. coli* to dimers, a structural fact which has been demonstrated earlier in WEIDEL'S laboratory (WEIDEL and PELZER, 1964). In *S. aureus* no carboxypeptidase has been found and the peptide-linked oligomers may be as large as decamers. Both the transpeptidase and the carboxypeptidase are inhibited by penicillins and cephalosporins.

Table 1. *Effects of penicillins on peptidoglycan synthesis in Escherichia coli strain Y-10*

Amount added µg/ml	Penicillin G		Ampicillin	
	Peptidoglycan	Ala	Peptidoglycan	Ala
0	4100	3730	—	—
1	4900	2740	4250	2610
10	7000	890	4220	1650
100	8600	235	4780	680
1000	7300	150	5710	255

[1] Similar data were obtained with methicillin and cephalothin.

With the uridine nucleotide substrate labeled in both of the terminal D-alanine residues, during the course of the reaction one of the ^{14}C-D-alanines was liberated as free alanine while the other was incorporated into the polymer (Fig. 7). In the presence of penicillin, the release of free alanine was eliminated and both alanine residues appeared in the polymer. A physical difference in the products formed in the absence or presence of penicillin was also evident. The cross-linked product formed in the control system was a highly water insoluble polymer which remained exactly to its point of application to the filter paper while the water soluble polymer formed in the presence of penicillin spread on the paper so that it had a disc-like appearance (Fig. 7). With increasing amounts of penicillin, increasing amounts of alanine were found in the polymer until finally the amount found was doubled (Table 1). In parallel, the liberation of alanine was progressively decreased and finally eliminated. All the penicillins and cephalosporins which have been examined had the same effects on this system, and all similarly inhibited the carboxypeptidase (Table 2). The sensitivity data are summarized in Table 3. The growth inhibitory concentration for the organism studied is shown for four penicillin or cephalosporin preparations. The carboxypeptidase was exquisitely sensitive to these substances and, since it was completely inhibited at concentrations far below those required to inhibit growth, the inhibition of this enzyme is obviously not lethal. However, the sensitivity of the transpeptidase to these substances, with one exception, exactly paralleled the growth inhibitory concentrations. The important exception was penicillin G which inhibited the enzyme at a far lower concentration than it inhibited growth of this organism. This fact may provide an explanation of FLEMING's original observation that gram-negative organisms are relatively insensitive to penicillins. This insensitivity is probably not due to any lack of the sensitive enzyme but due to the fact that the antibiotic can not penetrate to the site of this enzyme in the bacterial cell.

Table 2. *Inhibition by penicillins of* D-*alanine carboxypeptidase in Escherichia coli strain B*

Amount added µg/ml	c.p.m. of D-ala released in the presence of	
	Penicillin G	Ampicillin
0	2230	—
0.04	527	338
0.4	319	242
4.0	87	164
40.0	37	58

This fact is even more strikingly illustrated by the example of three other antibiotics, ristocetin, vancomycin and bacitracin, which inhibit the preceding steps catalyzed by earlier enzymes. The intact cells of *E. coli* were virtually insensitive to these antibiotics but the enzymes obtained from these cells was just as sensitive to them as the same enzymes in *S. aureus* (Table 3). These antibiotics also must be unable to penetrate to the site of the sensitive components in the intact cell.

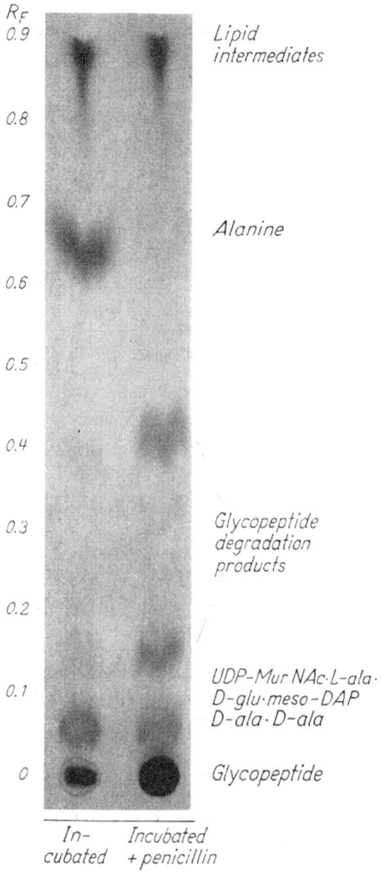

Fig. 7. Utilization of UDP-MurNAc-L-ala · D-glu · Meso-DAP · ^{14}C-D-ala-^{14}C-D-ala for peptidoglycan synthesis with *E. coli* enzyme in the absence and in the presence of penicillin G (IZAKI *et al.*, 1966)

The transpeptidase was irreversibly inactivated by penicillin (IZAKI *et al.*, 1966). After inhibition, activity could not be recovered by treatment of the enzyme preparation with penicillinase or by washing out the penicillin. Another interesting property of the transpeptidase is that the reaction it catalyzes can be reversed to some extent by addition of D-alanine or of other D-amino acids, or by high concentrations of glycine, but it cannot be reversed by the addition of L-amino acids. D-Amino acids and glycine are also known to induce formation of protoplasts and spheroplasts. This induction of spheroplasts is presumably due to reversal of the terminal cross-linking reaction in cell wall synthesis. Unlike the transpeptidase, the carboxypeptidase is reversibly inhibited by penicillins and activity can be recovered by treatment of inhibited enzyme with penicillinase (IZAKI, 1967). This enzyme has been purified to some extent and its substrate specificity is being studied.

Table 3. *Inhibition of growth and enzymes by antibiotics*

Antibiotic	Growth	Concentrations required for 50% inhibition, μg/ml		
		Peptidoglycan synthetase	Peptidoglycan trans-peptidase	D-alanine carboxy-peptidase
Ampicillin	3	—[1]	3	0.04
Penicillin G	30	—	3	0.02
Cephalothin	50	—	50	1
Methicillin	1000	—	1000	1
Ristocetin	1000	3	—	—
Vancomycin	100	10	—	—
Bacitracin	1000	40	—	—

[1] — Not inhibited.

Fibrous strands have been seen at the growing site in penicillin-inhibited bacteria by electron microscopy (FITZ-JAMES and HANCOCK, 1965). These fibrous strands are undoubtedly the uncross-linked peptidoglycan which is formed in the presence of penicillin. Similarly, fibrous material produced in the presence of D-amino acids has been visualized by electron microscopy (LARK *et al.*, 1963). Again, this fibrous material presumably represents the uncross-linked peptidoglycan strands which, in the presence of the D-amino acids, cannot be efficiently cross-linked.

Thus, the precise sites of inhibition of cell wall synthesis by penicillins, cephalosporins and a number of other substances are now known. Purification of the transpeptidase and a description of its precise mode of interaction with penicillins and cephalosporins remains an important problem for the future. According to the present hypothesis penicillins should acylate the active site of this enzyme and may thus provide another tool for studying the mechanism of enzyme action. It seems likely also that the transpeptidase is the component of bacterial cells which irreversibly binds penicillins and has been studied for many years.

References[1]

ANDERSON, J. S., M. MATSUHASHI, M. A. HASKIN, and J. L. STROMINGER: Lipid-phosphoacetylmuramyl-pentapeptide and lipid-phosphodisaccharide-pentapeptide: Presumed membrane transport intermediates in bacterial cell wall synthesis. Proc. Natl. Acad. Sci. U.S. **53**, 881 (1965).

ANDERSON, J. S., P. M. MEDDOW, M. A. HASKIN, and J. L. STROMINGER: Biosynthesis of the peptidoglycan of bacterial cell walls. 1. Utilization of uridine diphosphate acetylmuramyl pentapeptide and uridine diphosphate acetylglucosamine for peptidoglycan synthesis by particulate enzymes from *Staphylococcus aureus* and *Micrococcus lysodeikticus*. Arch. Biochem. Biophys. **116**, 487 (1966).

[1] Only a few key references have been provided. Interested readers are referred to a recent review for further references and details of the work described (STROMINGER *et al.*, 1967).

ARAKI, Y., A. SHIMADA, and E. ITO: Effect of penicillin on cell wall mucopeptide synthesis in a *Escherichia coli* particulate system. Biochem. Biophys. Res. Commun. **23**, 518 (1966).

FITZ-JAMES, P., and R. HANCOCK: The initial structural lesion of penicillin action in *Bacillus megaterium*. J. Cell Biol. **26**, 657 (1965).

IZAKI, K.: Purification and properties of the penicillin sensitive D-alanine carboxypeptidase. Federation Proc. (Abstr.) **26**, 388 1967.

IZAKI, K., M. MATSUHASHI, and J. L. STROMINGER: Glycopeptide transpeptidase and D-alanine carboxypeptidase: Penicillin-sensitive enzymatic reactions. Proc. Natl. Acad. Sci. U.S. **55**, 656 (1966).

LARK, C., D. BRADLEY, and K. G. LARK: Further studies on the incorporation of D-methionine into the bacterial cell wall. Its incorporation into the R-layer and the structural consequences. Biochim. et Biophys. Acta **78**, 278 (1963).

MARTIN, H. H.: Composition of the mucopolymer in cell walls of the unstable and stable form of *Proteus mirabilis*. J. Gen. Microbiol. **36**, 441 (1964a).

MARTIN, H. H.: Chemical composition of cell wall mucopolymer from penicillin spheroplasts and normal cells of *Proteus mirabilis*. Abstracts, Sixth Internat. Congr. of Biochem., New York 1964b, p. 518.

SIEWERT, G., and J. L. STROMINGER: Bacitracin: An inhibitor of the dephosphorylation of lipid pyrophosphate, an intermediate in biosynthesis of the peptidoglycan of bacterial cell walls. Proc. Natl. Acad. Sci. U.S. **57** 161 (1967).

STROMINGER, J. L., E. ITO, and R. H. THREN: Competitive inhibition of enzymatic reactions by oxamycin. J. Am. Chem. Soc. **82**, 998 (1960).

STROMINGER, J. L., K. IZAKI, M. MATSUHASHI, and D. J. TIPPER: Peptidoglycan transpeptidase and D-alanine carboxypeptidase: Penicillin sensitive enzymatic reactions. Federation Proc. (Symposium) **26**, 9 1967.

TIPPER, D. J., and J. L. STROMINGER: Mechanism of action of penicillins: A proposal based on their structural similarity to acyl-D-alanyl-D-alanine. Proc. Natl. Acad. Sci. U.S. **54**, 1133 (1965).

WEIDEL, W., and H. PELZER: Bagshaped macromolecules — a new outlook on bacterial cell walls. Advances in Enzymol. **26**, 193 (1964).

WISE, E. M., and J. T. PARK: Penicillin: Its basic site of action as an inhibitor of a peptide cross-linking reaction in cell wall mucopeptide synthesis. Proc. Natl. Acad. Sci. U.S. **54**, 75 (1965).

Actinomycin

E. Reich, A. Cerami and D. C. Ward

Actinomycins (AM)[1] are bright-red, highly toxic polypeptide antibiotics (Fig. 1). The actinomycins form complexes with DNA *in vivo* and *in vitro*, and there seems little reason to doubt that the interaction with DNA, and the associated effects on nucleic acid function account for most, if not all of the biological properties of these antibiotics.

The chemistry (BROCKMANN, 1960a and b) and the mechanism of action of actinomycins have been the subject of several recent reviews (REICH, 1963; GOLDBERG and REICH, 1964; REICH and GOLDBERG, 1964; REICH, 1966) which contain references and a discussion of previous experimental work. Consequently, only a brief summary of the earlier experiments and a consideration of more recent findings will be presented in this article.

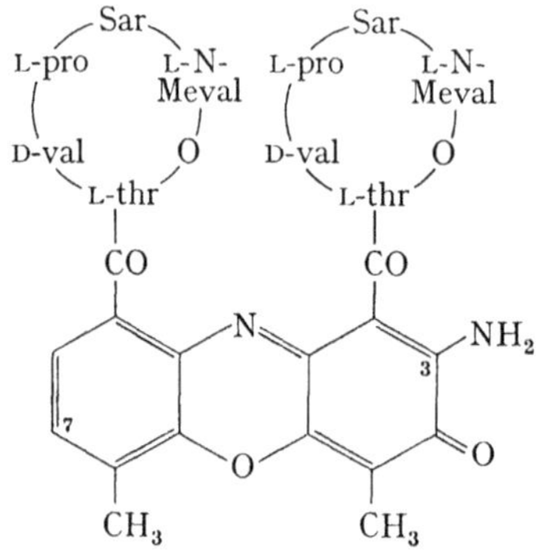

Actinomycin C_1 (D)

Fig. 1. Structure of actinomycin D; L-thr is L-threonine; D-val is D-valine; L-pro is L-proline; sar is sarcosine; and L-N-meval is L-N-methylvaline

Formation of Complexes between Actinomycins and DNA

The formation of complexes between AM and DNA, first reported by KIRK (1960), is the result of a highly specific interaction which occurs in intact cells and under controlled experimental conditions *in vitro*.

[1] The following abbreviations are used: AM — actinomycin; A, G, T, C, I, DAP, 2-AP — adenine, guanine, thymine, cytosine, hypoxanthine, 2,6-diaminopurine, 2-aminopurine, respectively; DNA, RNA — deoxyribonucleic and ribonucleic acid, respectively; dDAP-MP, dDAP-TP — 5′-monophosphate and triphosphate, respectively of 2,6-diaminopurine deoxynucleoside; AMP, UMP — adenylic acid and uridylic acid; dDAP-T — deoxynucleotide polymer, in which 90% of the residues are arranged in alternating sequence of DAP + T, the remaining 10% consisting of alternating A + T residues; dAT, alternating deoxynucleotide copolymer of A + T; dAT (A/DAP = 10) — dAT copolymer in which 10% of the purine residues are occupied by DAP, 90% by A.

1. AM forms complexes with DNA, but not with other cellular constituents. Despite its solubility in organic solvents AM accumulates in lipid membranes only after saturation of binding sites in DNA (SHATKIN, personal communication). A study of the cellular distribution of radioactive AM has shown that AM is selectively concentrated in the nucleus where it is found in association with DNA (DINGMAN and SPORN, 1965).

2. The cellular processes which require direct participation of DNA molecules in some way appear to be most sensitive to inhibition by AM. For example, the life cycles of numerous RNA viruses in mammalian cells are unaffected by AM; this indicates that the many cellular functions on which virus growth depends are unimpaired by the antibiotic. Conversely, cell division, chromosome morphology, bacteriophage maturation and non-viral RNA synthesis, all of which depend on direct physical involvement of DNA, are very sensitive to AM. Because the redox potential of the actinomycin chromophore could permit its reduction under biological conditions, and since the reduced chromophore is readily autoxidisable in air, the possibility exists that AM might function as an unnatural electron carrier under certain conditions. However, no data supporting such a possibility have been reported.

3. AM interacts specifically only with helical deoxypolynucleotides which contain guanine. Polyribonucleotides and deoxynucleotide polymers (such as apurinic acid, dAT, dAdT, or dIdC) which are free of guanine, do not form complexes with AM, and function as templates for nucleic acid polymerases with complete immunity to AM.

The helical conformation of DNA is another important determinant of the AM-DNA interaction as shown by the following facts:

a) Apyrimidinic DNA, which is devoid of ordered structure, shows much lower affinity for AM than does native DNA.

b) Denaturation of DNA, by heat or acid, is always associated with dissociation of AM-DNA complexes (REICH, 1964; GELLERT *et al.*, 1965; FROMAGEOT, personal communication).

c) Single-stranded DNAs show a lower AM-binding capacity than native DNA of equivalent base composition.

4. The functional groups of the AM molecule which are required for DNA-binding and for the characteristic biological properties of the antibiotic have been identified by studying the correlation of activity and structure with a variety of biosynthetic and chemically modified derivatives; most of these actinomycins have been produced by BROCKMANN'S laboratory in Göttingen.

The results of such experiments show that very similar structure-activity series are defined by assaying actinomycin action at the level of the tumour-bearing animal, the mammalian cell in culture, the bacterial cell, the enzyme reaction and the isolated polydeoxynucleotide. These findings strongly support the idea that the biological properties of AM are the product of a single, primary molecular event — namely, the formation of complexes between AM and DNA, with consequent impairment of DNA function (BROCKMANN, 1960b; REICH *et al.*, 1962; MÜLLER, 1962; BURCHENAL *et al.*, 1960; HARTMANN *et al.*, 1962).

The functional groups of AM which are indispensable for biological activity and for complex formation with DNA are the chromophore amino group, an unreduced quinoidal oxygen, and the intact, cyclic pentapeptide lactones. The requirement for the amino group and the quinoidal oxygen are shown by the disappearance of biological activity which accompanies modification of these structures.

The peptide chains with intact lactones are also indispensable for biological activity, and for binding to DNA. Although certain variations in amino acid sequence may cause only minor changes in AM activity, recent observations suggest that the conformational properties of the pentapeptides are a basic determinant of AM activity.

The chemical synthesis of AM derivatives by Wade and Mauger (personal communication) at the Chester Beatty Institute in London is now providing the opportunity for probing further the role of the peptides in the AM-DNA interaction. Compounds containing the following modifications of AM, generously provided by them, have been tested for complex formation with DNA and inhibition of RNA polymerase function *in vitro* (A. Cerami and D. C. Ward, unpublished results):

a) Replacement of the two cyclic pentapeptides of AM by a single, neutral, cyclic decapeptide[1].

b) Replacement of the pentapeptide sequences by either of the following hexapeptide sequences:

L-ser → D-val → L-pro → sar → L-pro → L-leu
|______________O______________|

L-thr → D-val → L-pro → sar → L-pro → L-leu
|______________O______________|

c) Replacement of C-terminal L-N-methylvaline by L-valine.

All of the above modifications totally abolish the characteristic properties of AM, although the spectra and solubility properties of the derivatives closely resemble those of the parent compound. These results are consistent with the idea that certain functional groups of the peptides interact in some way with specific counterparts on the surface of the DNA helix, and that the stereochemically reactive configuration is determined by the structure of the peptide lactones.

The above summary indicates the AM-DNA complex is an unusual and highly specific molecular interaction based on unique combination of stereochemical properties of the antibiotic and DNA. This interaction can be viewed as a model for a variety of biologically interesting phenomena such as antigen-antibody, enzyme-substrate and other drug-receptor associations; and the detailed study of any of these interactions may be expected to contribute useful insights for the understanding of some of the others.

A Model for the Structure of Actinomycin-DNA Complexes

A model for the structure of actinomycin-DNA complexes (Fig. 2), based on X-ray and model-building studies, has been proposed recently (Hamilton *et al.*,

[1] Such a molecule has been synthesized (Mauger and Wade, 1966) by coupling the chromophore of actinomycin, through its carboxyl groups, to the δ-NH_2 groups of the ornithine residues in Gramicidin S.

1963). According to this model, actinomycin is considered to be located in the minor groove of helical DNA, with which it can form up to seven hydrogen bonds. The geometry of three of these H-bonds has been studied in detail and has been found to be stereochemically satisfactory (Fig. 2). The properties of the complex deduced from this model fit most of the known facts concerning the reaction of actinomycin with DNA and the associated inhibition of DNA-dependent RNA synthesis.

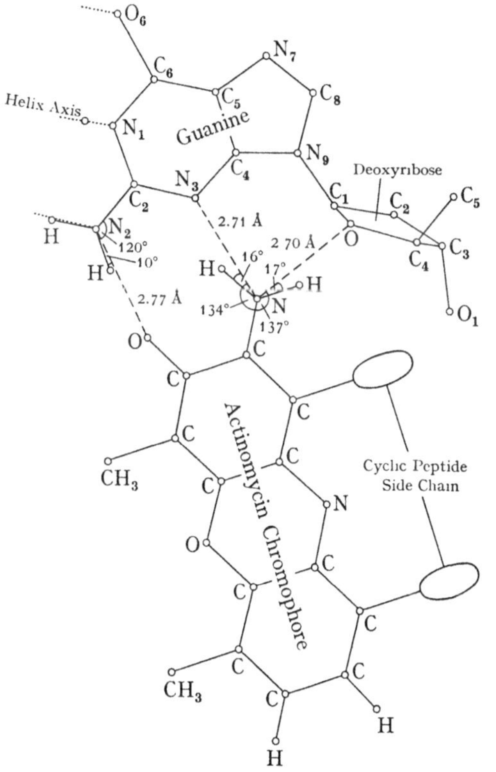

Fig. 2. Proposed model of AM binding to deoxyguanosine of DNA in the B conformation. Hydrogen bond lengths and angles calculated from coordinates measured on skeletal wire models. Hydrogen bonds between AM and DNA indicated by --- Hydrogen bonds between guanine and cytosine in DNA indicated by .... Rep. from HAMILTON *et al.*, Nature **198**, 538 (1963)

1. The model accounts for the role of the structures of actinomycin known to be required for biological activity. Thus, reduction of the quinoidal oxygen would restrict the ability of the oxygen atom to function as an H-bond acceptor. Alterations involving the amino group would eliminate one or both of the hydrogen bonds formed, or in the case of large alkyl substituents, actually prevent interaction of the quinoidal portion of the chromophore with the DNA constituents. The lactones can be visualized as stabilizing the peptide chains in a conformation permitting the formation of four additional H-bonds between the four peptide-NH groups and the phosphodiester oxygens of the DNA strand opposite to that containing the guanine interacting with the chromophore. It is of interest that the

model predicts the non-involvement in complex formation of position 7 of the chromophore which is seen to project away from the DNA helix. It is therefore of interest that the presence at this position of even rather bulky substituent groups does not interfere with binding of actinomycin to DNA (MÜLLER, 1962 and personal communication).

2. The model accounts for the structures in DNA on which complex formation is known to depend. Thus, only guanine can furnish the H in the DNA minor groove for which the quinoidal oxygen of actinomycin can serve as acceptor. The model depends critically on the relative positions of the DNA constituents as they are disposed in helical DNA in the B conformation, and thus is in accord with the fact that actinomycin binds poorly, if at all, to single-stranded DNA, and does not bind to RNA's such as Reovirus RNA and s-RNA, which are thought to exist in the A conformation (SHATKIN, 1966).

The model proposed for the actinomycin-DNA interaction concerns only those structural elements which appear to determine the specificity of complex formation; it does not cover a potentially wide variety of non-specific intermolecular forces, which could participate in the formation and stabilization of complexes. With this reservation, the model permits some specific predictions to be made. Many of these can be tested, and such experiments are the subject of current investigation.

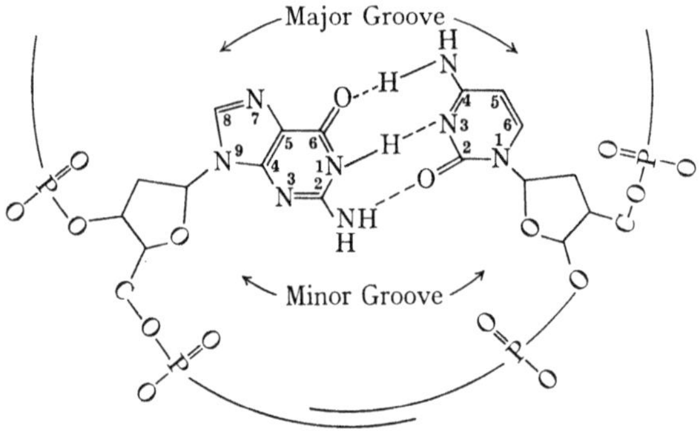

Fig. 3. Structure of guanine-cytosine base pair in DNA

In helical DNA only the edges of the base pairs are accessible. These are located in the DNA grooves, and since bound actinomycin interacts with guanine, the antibiotic must be located in one of the grooves, and not along the sugar-phosphate backbone. In a G-C base pair, the exposed atoms are as follows (Fig. 3): 1. for the purine, C_8, N_7, and O_6 in the major groove, N_3 and the 2-amino group in the minor groove; 2. for the pyrimidine, C_5, C_6, and the 4-amino group in the major groove, and O_2 in the minor groove. All available evidence supports the assumption that the helical structure of DNA is retained in actinomycin-DNA complexes. If this is so, and if actinomycin does not intercalate between adjacent base pairs, the only constituents of guanine and cytosine which could participate in complex formation are those located in the grooves. With this in mind, some of the predictions derived from the model can be examined.

1. The model predicts that alkylation of N-7 of guanine should not interfere with binding of actinomycin, and conversely that actinomycin should not interfere

with alkylation of DNA. DNA heavily alkylated with mustard gas (REICH, 1964), β-propiolactone (W. TROLL, personal communication) or methyl groups (MICHELSON, personal communication) forms complexes with AM as effectively as the control-starting material; and, in preliminary experiments, actinomycin did not inhibit the rate of alkylation of DNA (REICH, 1964).

2. A second prediction from the model is that the removal of the amino group of guanine from the minor groove should abolish complex formation. This can be accomplished by substituting hypoxanthine for guanine in DNA, as in the case of the synthetic DNA polymer dIdC. This polymer does not form complexes with actinomycin (REICH, 1964).

3. The model predicts that constituents in the major groove of DNA should not affect complex formation. When the AM-binding capacity of the DNAs of bacteriophages T_2, T_4 and T_6 was compared with that of the corresponding non-glycosylated DNAs, no difference was observed (C. C. RICHARDSON, personal communication).

4. Although subject to uncertainties discussed by the authors, the measured dichroism of actinomycin-DNA complexes provided a calculated orientation of the chromophore almost precisely that predicted by the model (GELLERT *et al.*, 1965).

5. The above findings are fully in accord with the predictions drawn from the model. The principle of a further experimental test of the model (CERAMI *et al.*, 1967a) is outlined in Fig. 4. As noted above, the removal of the 2-amino group of guanine from the AM-sensitive G-C base pair yields the AM-resistant I-C pair. The A-T base pair is known not to interact with AM; however, the structure of this base pair permits the insertion of an amino group at the position in the helix normally occupied by the amino group of guanine. Such an insertion can be accomplished by substituting 2,6-diaminopurine or 2-aminopurine for adenine, since it has been found that the corresponding deoxynucleotides serve as substrates for DNA polymerase. This finding has made it possible to produce and isolate a

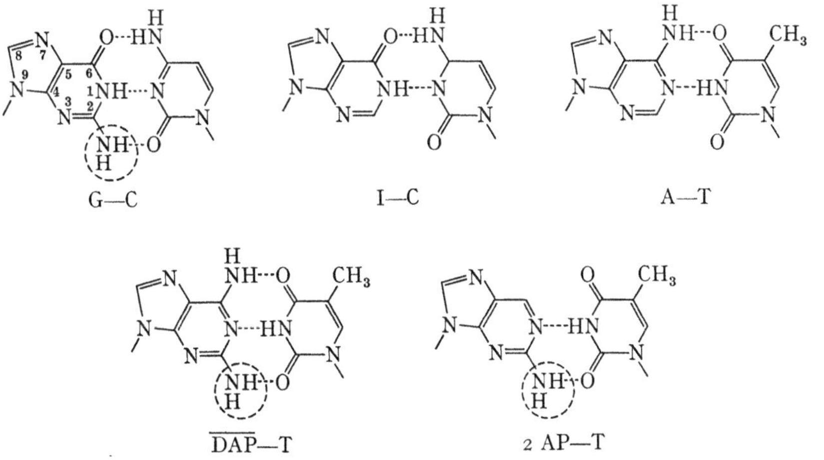

Fig. 4. Structure of hydrogen-bonded purine-pyrimidine base pairs; G-C, guanine-cytosine; I-C, hypoxanthine-cytosine; A-T, adenine-thymine; DAP-T, 2,6-diaminopurine-thymine; 2 AP-T, 2-aminopurine-thymine. The 2-amino group of the purine components is encircled

deoxynucleotide copolymer (d$\overline{\mathrm{DAP}}$-T) with an alternating sequence of diaminopurine and thymine residues. If the specificity of AM-binding is determined simply by a purine amino group suitably located in the minor groove, this polymer should interact with AM. As predicted by the model, the formation of complexes between d$\overline{\mathrm{DAP}}$-T and AM may be demonstrated in various ways.

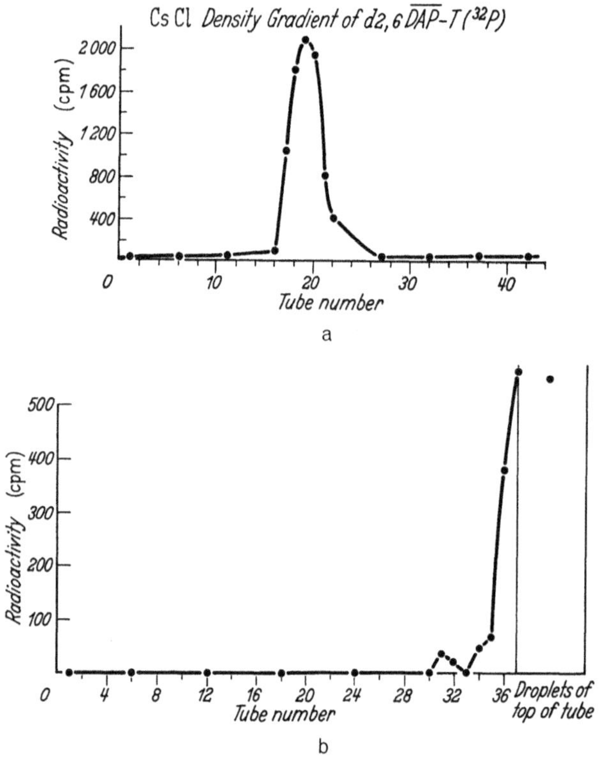

Fig. 5. Preparative equilibrium centrifugation in CsCl density gradients. Each tube contained 5 ml. CsCl ($\varrho = 1.710$), and 0.14 O.D. units (260 mμ) of radioactive d$\overline{\mathrm{DAP}}$-T, a total of 20 mμmoles of polymer nucleotide. A. Control. B. As in A, but containing a total of 20 mμmoles of actinomycin D. The specific radioactivity of the polymer in A was twice that in B. Following 120 hrs. of centrifugation (Spinco SW-39 rotor, 33,000 rpm, 25°) the tubes were punctured, 2-drop fractions were collected, and the acid insoluble radioactivity of the indicated samples was determined. The density of fraction 19 (Fig. A) corresponded to $\varrho = 1.715$

a) AM alters the distribution of DNA in CsCl density gradients (KERSTEN *et al.*, 1966). Figs. 5a and 5b show the results of an experiment undertaken to characterize the interaction of AM and d$\overline{\mathrm{DAP}}$-T by preparative ultracentrifugation in CsCl density gradients. In the absence of AM, the radioactivity of the polymer, which was due to incorporated d$\overline{\mathrm{DAP}}$-MP^{32}, was distributed in a single symmetrical band with a density corresponding to $\varrho = 1.715$. The addition of AM caused a remarkable alteration in the sedimentation of the polymer; one-half the radioactivity was located at the very top of the gradient, where AM normally forms a micelle; the other half was found in small yellow droplets which adhered to the centrifuge tube at the level of the meniscus. An analogous experiment was performed in the analytical ultracentrifuge with a dAT-like polymer in which DAP accounts for 10% of the purines; as seen in Fig. 6, the buoyant density of this polymer is indistinguishable from that of dAT. The addition of AM to the centrifuge cell leads to the appearance of a new, symmetrical band at a density $\varrho = 1.661$ which differs significantly from that of the control specimen. This is additional evidence for the interaction of AM with DAP incorporated in a polydeoxynucleotide.

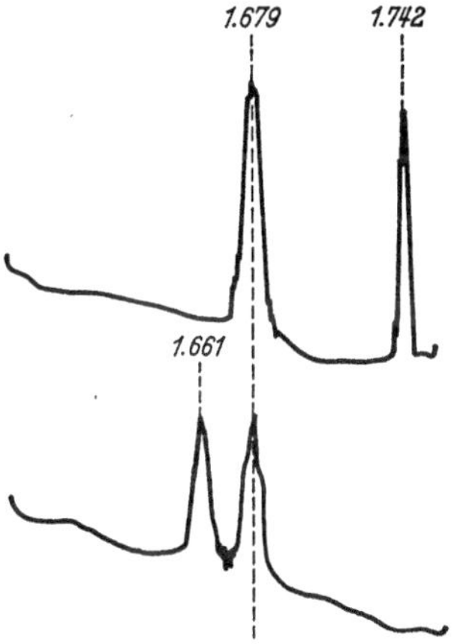

Fig. 6. Analytical equilibrium centrifugation of dAT (A/DAP = 10) in CsCl density gradient. The analytic cell corresponding to the upper densitometer tracing contained dAT (A/DAP=10) 0.01 O.D. unit (260 mμ); pure dAT and bacteriophage SP-8 DNA were present as reference standards. The buoyant density of dAT (A/DAP = 10) $\varrho = 1.679$ is not detectably different from that of pure dAT. The cell corresponding to the lower tracing contained dAT (A/DAP = 10) and pure dAT as above, with added actinomycin (4 mμmoles/ml); a new band is seen at $\varrho = 1.661$. This band is considered to represent dAT (A/DAP= 10) with bound actinomycin. Actinomycin is known not to affect the buoyant density of dAT.

b) Effect of AM on thermal denaturation of d$\overline{\text{DAP}}$-T: It has been shown that bound AM significantly stabilizes DNA to denaturation by heat (HASELKORN, 1964; REICH, 1964b); elevations of the transition temperature (Tm) due to AM of up to 12—15° have been observed with naturally occurring native DNAs. The data in Figs. 7 and 8 show a substantial increase in Tm of dAT (A/DAP = 10) on addition of AM; the corresponding increase for d$\overline{\text{DAP}}$-T is almost 40° — a change far greater than that previously recorded for any DNA.

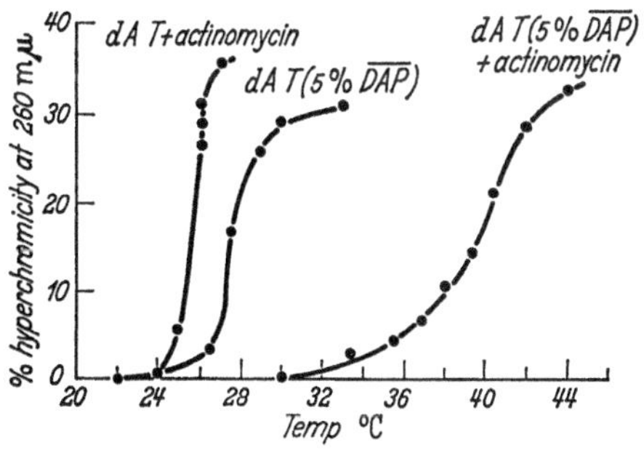

Fig. 7. Thermal denaturation of dAT (A/DAP = 10): Effect of actinomycin. dAT (A/DAP = 10) 36 mμmoles/ml was dissolved in 0.001 M Na^+. AM, where present, was added to a final concentration of 6.1 mμmoles/ml; this concentration of AM did not alter the Tm of pure dAT

c) Spectral changes in actinomycin solutions produced by d$\overline{\text{DAP}}$-T: The change in the spectrum of AM solutions on addition of guanine-containing DNAs is a characteristic parameter of the AM-DNA interaction. The difference spectrum shown in Fig. 9 demonstrates that dDAP-T, like DNA, produces alterations in the spectrum of AM. This difference spectrum resembles that produced by DNA at wavelengths below 470 mμ, but differs somewhat at higher wavelengths.

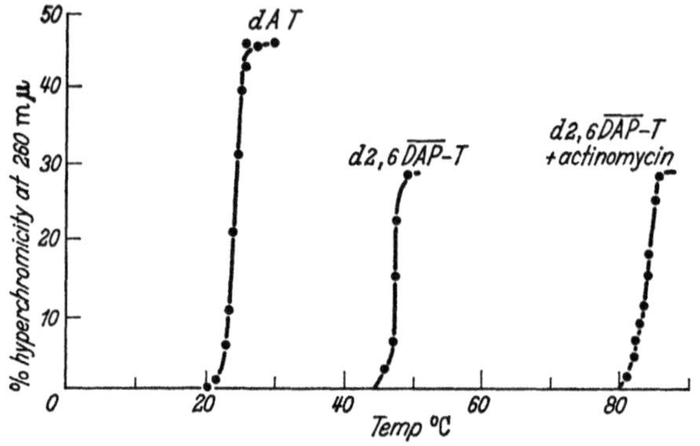

Fig. 8. Thermal denaturation of dDAP-T: Effect of actinomycin. dDAP-T, 54 mμ moles/ml, was dissolved in 0.001 M Na^+. Where present, AM was added to a final concentration of 10.5 mμmoles/ml

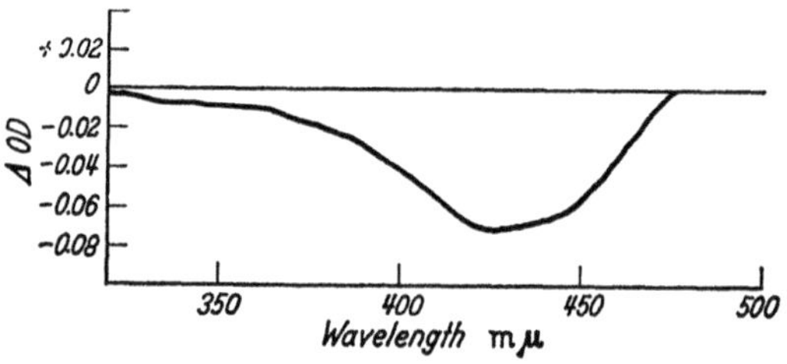

Fig. 9. Difference spectrum of AM in the presence of dDAP-T. A solution of AM (0.85 O.D./ml at 440 mμ) containing dDAP-T (24 mμmoles/ml) was read against a control solution of AM in Cary Model 14 spectrophotometer

d) Template function of dDAP-T with RNA polymerase: effect of AM: The results of experiments which will be described in detail elsewhere (CERAMI *et al.*, 1967b) show that dDAP-T possesses an alternating sequence of DAP and T residues, and functions as a template for RNA synthesis catalysed by *E. coli* RNA polymerase. Although a much less effective template than dAT, dDAP-T directs the formation of RNA containing only A + U in perfectly alternating sequence. The synthesis of RNA is linear for several hours; the concentration of polymer selected for the experiment reported here was on the linear portion of the velocity/template relationship.

The effect of AM on RNA synthesis directed by dDAP-T and by dAT (A/DAP = 10) is shown in Fig. 10. The template function of both polymers is progressively inhibited by increasing concentrations of AM. The ratio AM/DNA nucleotide which provides 50% inhibition of synthesis is 1:100 for dDAP-T, 1:100 for dAT (A/DAP = 10) as compared with 1:800 for native calf thymus DNA. Two points concerning the effect of AM on dDAP-T may be noted. The first is that a small fraction of RNA synthesized appears absolutely resistant to AM; this is considered to reflect the template activity of the residual dAT which had been used to prime d$\overline{\text{DAP}}$-T formation. Secondly, the inhibition curve shows a single, very steep slope as the concentration of AM is increased. With naturally occurring native DNAs the effect of AM is usually biphasic — an initial steep decline is seen at low concentration, followed by a more gradual inhibition. It is suggested that this difference may be due to the greater heterogeneity of the structure, sequences and configuration of calf thymus DNA as compared with the perfectly regular structure of d$\overline{\text{DAP}}$-T.

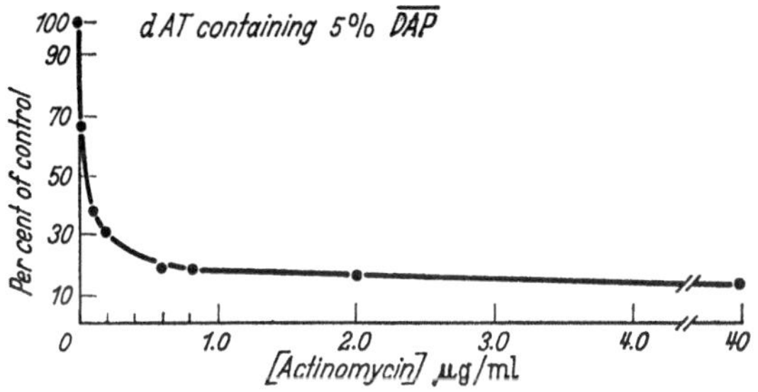

a

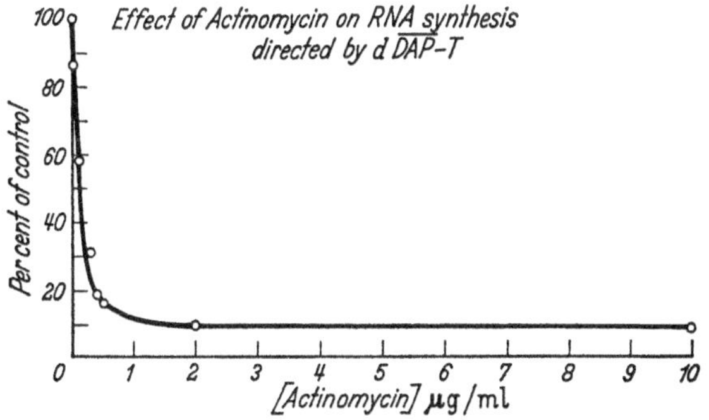

b

Fig. 10a and b. Effect of AM on RNA synthesis directed by (A) d$\overline{\text{DAP}}$-T and (B) dAT (A/DAP = 10). Enzyme incubations were performed at 37° for 30′, in a final volume of 0.125 ml, containing 9mμmoles/ml of the respective polymer templates. 100% incorporation corresponds in (A) to 11.6 mμmoles/ml of ^{3}H-UMP and in (B) to 39.2 mμmoles/ml ^{3}H-AMP

Due to the location of its two amino groups, DAP is structurally similar in some respects to both adenine and guanine. However, its chemical and biochemical properties make DAP an analogue of adenine, not of guanine. Thus, in its pK values (ADRIEN and BROWN, 1954), base pairing pattern, and substrate behavior for enzymes[1] DAP closely resembles only adenine, not guanine. Moreover, the 2-amino group of DAP differs significantly from that of guanine in its susceptibility to chemical deamination. These facts lead to the conclusion that the $\overline{\text{DAP}}$-T base pair is analogous to the A-T base pair chemically, as well as in the

[1] DAP ribonucleoside is a substrate for yeast (KORNBERG, 1950) and rabbit liver (ACS, personal communication) adenosine kinases, and for adenosine deaminase (WOLFENDEN personal communication); DAP nucleotides can substitute for adenine nucleotides with adenylic kinase and RNA polymerase (unpublished observations).

distribution of its functional groups; the outstanding property which $\overline{DAP}$-T and G-C pairs have in common is a purine 2-amino group and its location in the minor groove of helical DNA.

When AM forms complexes with native DNA the spectrum of the antibiotic changes, and the buoyant density, thermal stability and template function of the DNA are markedly affected. The interaction of AM with d$\overline{DAP}$-T faithfully reproduces (and in some respects exaggerates) each of these qualities of AM-DNA complexes. dAT does not interact with AM, and d$\overline{DAP}$-T differs from dAT in its possession of the additional purine 2-amino groups. Thus, the introduction of a purine 2-amino group into the minor groove of helical DNA is sufficient, and perhaps the sole requirement, for converting a base pair from AM-resistance to AM-sensitivity. Preliminary results obtained with a dAT-like polymer containing a proportion of 2-aminopurine residues are entirely analogous to those shown above for d$\overline{DAP}$-T.

The findings summarized above suggest that the 2-amino group of purines in helical DNA provides an indispensable component in the attachment site for AM in helical DNA. Therefore, disregarding the particular stereochemical details of the model, it appears likely that AM is indeed located in the minor groove of the DNA helix.

Even if it is assumed that the model accurately reflects some of the structural properties of the AM-DNA complex, the proposed interaction between deoxyguanosine in DNA and the AM chromophore could not account for the binding energy corresponding to the observed dissociation constant of the complex (GELLERT *et al.*, 1965). It is reasonable to postulate that the interaction of the AM-peptides with DNA makes a major contribution to the stability of the complex, and the detailed elucidation of this component of the AM-DNA complex is a challenging target for future investigations.

References

ADRIEN, A., and P. S. BROWN: Purine studies. Part I. Stability to acid and alkali. Solubility. Ionization. Comparison with pteridines. J. Chem. Soc. **1954**, 2060.

BROCKMANN, H.: Structural differences of the actinomycins and their derivatives. Ann. N.Y. Acad. Sci. **89**, 323 (1960a).

BROCKMANN, H.: Die Actinomycine. Fortschr. Chem. org. Naturstoffe **18**, 1 (1960b).

BURCHENAL, J. H., H. F. OETTGEN, J. A. REPPERT, and V. COLEY: The effect of actinomycins and their derivatives on a spectrum of transplanted mouse leukemia. Ann. N.Y. Acad. Sci. **89**, 399 (1960).

CERAMI, A., E. REICH, D. C. WARD, and I. H. GOLDBERG: The interaction of actinomycin with DNA; requirement for the 2-amino group of purines. Proc. Nat. Acad. Sci. Washington (in press) (1967a).

CERAMI, A., D. C. WARD, E. REICH, and I. H. GOLDBERG: The utilization of purine analogue nucleotides by nucleic acid polymerases. In preparation (1967b).

DINGMAN, W., and M. SPORN: Actinomycin D and hydrocortisone: intracellular binding in rat liver. Science **149**, 1251 (1965).

GELLERT, M., C. E. SMITH, D. NEVILLE, and G. FELSENFELD: Actinomycin binding to DNA; mechanism and specificity. J. Mol. Biol. **11**, 445 (1965).

GOLDBERG, I. H., and E. REICH: Actinomycin inhibition of RNA synthesis directed by DNA. Federation Proc. **23**, 958 (1964).

HAMILTON, L., W. FULLER, and E. REICH: X-ray diffraction and molecular model building studies of the interaction of actinomycin with nucleic acids. Nature **198**, 538 (1963).

HARTMANN, G., U. COY u. G. KNIESE: Zum biologischen Wirkungsmechanismus der Actinomycine. Z. Physiol. Chem. Hoppe Seyler's **330**, 227 (1962).
HASELKORN, R.: Actinomycin D as a probe for nucleic acid secondary structure. Science **143**, 682 (1964).
KERSTEN, W., H. KERSTEN, and W. SZYBALSKI: Physico-chemical properties of complexes between deoxyribonucleic acid and antibiotics which affect ribonucleic acid synthesis. Biochemistry **5**, 236 (1966).
KIRK, J. M.: The mode of action of actinomycin D. Biochim. et Biophys. Acta **42**, 167 (1960).
KORNBERG, A.: Enzymatic phosphorylation of adenosine and 2,6-diamino-purine riboside. J. Biol. Chem. **193**, 481 (1950).
MAUGER, A. B., and R. WADE: The synthesis of actinomycin analogues. Part II. Actinocylgramicidin S. J. Chem. Soc. **1966**, 1406.
MÜLLER, W.: Bindung von Actinomycenen und Actinomycin-Derivaten an Deoxyribonucleinsäure. Naturwissenschaften **49**, 156 (1962).
REICH, E.: Biochemistry of actinomycin. Cancer Research **23**, 1428 (1963).
REICH, E.: Actinomycin: Correlation of structure and function of its complexes with purines and DNA. Science **143**, 684 (1964a).
REICH, E.: Binding of actinomycin as a model for the complex-forming capacity of DNA. In: The role of chromosomes in heredity, p. 73 (ed. by M. LOCKE). New York: Academic Press 1964b.
REICH, E.: Binding to DNA and inhibition of DNA functions by actinomycins. In: Symposia of the Society for General Microbiology, vol. XVII, p. 266 (1966).
REICH, E., and I. H. GOLDBERG: Actinomycin and nucleic acid function (a review). In: Progress in nucleic acid research and molecular biology, vol. III, p. 184 (ed. by J. N. DAVIDSON and WALDO E. COHN). New York: Academic Press 1964.
REICH, E., I. H. GOLDBERG, and M. RABINOWITZ: Structure activity correlations of actinomycin and their derivatives. Nature **196**, 743 (1962).

The Effect of Streptomycin and Other Aminoglycoside Antibiotics on Protein Synthesis

G. A. Jacoby and L. Gorini

Streptomycin (Sm), the first nontoxic broad spectrum antibiotic also effective against the tubercle bacillus, was isolated from *Streptomyces griseus* by Schatz, Bugie, and Waksman in 1944. The structures of Sm and several of its active derivatives are shown in Fig. 1. It is composed of streptidine, an inositol substituted with two guanido groups, and streptobiosamine, a disaccharide containing a methylamino group. Streptidine can also be considered a substituted streptamine, which emphasizes a chemical moiety found in other aminoglycoside antibiotics, Fig. 3 and 4. Antibacterial activity is destroyed by cleavage of the glycosidic bond between streptidine and streptobiosamine, by replacing the guanido groups with amino groups, or by carbobenzyloxylation of the secondary amine (Polglase, 1965).

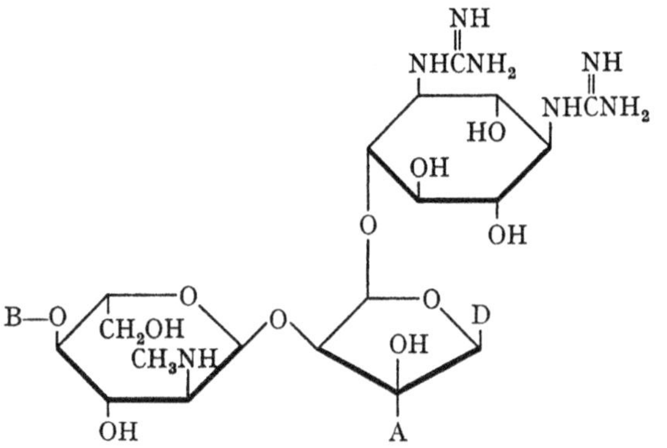

	A	B	D
Streptomycin	CHO	H	CH_3
Dihydrostreptomycin	CH_2OH	H	CH_3
Mannosidostreptomycin	CHO	See below	CH_2
Hydroxystreptomycin	CHO	H	CH_2OH

For mannosidostreptomycin, B =

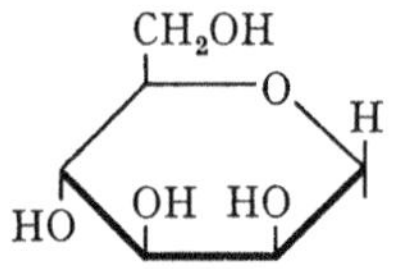

Fig. 1. The structure of streptomycin and some analogues

Sm is bactericidal for a wide variety of bacterial species, both gram-positive and gram-negative. Representative inhibitory concentrations for selected organisms appear in Table 1. An extensive tabulation of *in vitro* Sm sensitivity is given by YOUMANS and FISHER (1949). The amount of drug required for inhibition may vary over a considerable range within the same species and is influenced by a number of factors including the absence of oxygen and the pH and ionic strength of the medium. Fungi, rickettsiae, protozoa, and animal viruses are insensitive to Sm. The penetration of some bacterial viruses, however, is inhibited by Sm (REITER, 1963; BROCK *et al.*, 1965; SCHINDLER, 1965). Animal cells are relatively insensitive to Sm (MOSKOWITZ and KELKER, 1963, 1965), although in clinical use ototoxicity, nephrotoxicity, and hypersensitivity reactions have been recognized.

Table 1. *Streptomycin sensitivity of various organisms*[1]

Organism	Minimum inhibiting concentration μg/ml
Aerobacter aerogenes	2.7
Brucella abortus	0.8
Escherichia coli	6.0
Hemophilis influenzae	2.3
Klebsiella pneumoniae	1.8
Mycobacterium tuberculosis, var. *hominis*	0.5
Salmonella typhosa	12.2
Shigella sonnei	7.4
Staphylococcus aureus	0.8
Streptococcus pyogenes	11.7

[1] Modified from RAKE, PANSY, JAMBOR, and DONOVICK (1948).

The mechanism of Sm action has been intensively studied since its discovery, and a wide variety of biochemical effects have been reported. The reader is referred to the original papers and to several recent reviews (DAVIS and FEINGOLD, 1963; GALE, 1963; HURWITZ, 1963; BROCK, 1964, 1966) for further details.

From its cationic structure Sm would be expected to interact electrostatically with many cellular anionic components, and it has, indeed, been reported to precipitate DNA (COHEN, 1949) and RNA (COHEN and LICHTENSTEIN, 1960; MOSKOWITZ, 1963). The drug impairs the oxidation of a variety of substrates biy treated cells (OGINSKY, 1953), causes damage to the cell membrane in certa n strains producing leakage of essential metabolites (ANAND and DAVIS, 1960; ROTH *et al.*, 1960; DUBIN and DAVIS, 1961; TZAGOLOFF and UMBREIT, 1963), interferes with protein synthesis (see below), alters RNA metabolism (DUBIN, 1964; STERN *et al.*, 1966), and produces depolymerization of ribosomes (DUBIN and DAVIS, 1962).

A major problem has thus been to distinguish the primary site of the lethal action of Sm from secondary consequences of this lethal event. A major aid in determining this site has been the identification of the 30 S subunit of the bacterial ribosome as the altered component in a cell which has acquired single-step, high level Sm resistance. Sm resistant (Sm^R) mutants are thus ribosomal mutants and can be studied as such to elucidate ribosomal structure and function. Furthermore, since it has been shown both *in vivo* and *in vitro* that Sm, by interacting with the ribosome, causes misreading of the genetic code, the antibiotic itself has become a tool for understanding the control of the fidelity of translation of genetic information. This review will be largely restricted to these recent developments.

Streptomycin Inhibition of Protein Synthesis

An early indication that Sm affects protein synthesis was the observation by FITZGERALD *et al.* (1948) that the antibiotic inhibits adaptive enzyme formation in *Mycobacteria*. Later work showed that net formation of protein ceases five to fifteen minutes after addition of Sm to sensitive cells, while RNA and DNA synthesis continue for a longer period of time (ANAND and DAVIS, 1960; HAHN *et al.*, 1962; WHITE and FLAKS, 1962). A specific effect on protein synthesis was also suggested by SPOTTS and STANIER (1961) who observed that growth of a Sm dependent (Sm^D) mutant of *Escherichia coli* in suboptimal concentrations of Sm results in a decreased concentration of protein and an increased concentration of RNA. Since genetic studies (e.g., HASHIMOTO, 1960) had shown that Sm sensitivity, resistance, and dependence are very closely linked or possibly allelic, SPOTTS and STANIER postulated that the same cellular unit must be involved in each case and further that this unit is the ribosome. They therefore suggested that in sensitive cells Sm interacts with ribosomes so as to prevent messenger RNA (mRNA) attachment, in resistant cells this interaction does not occur, and in dependent cells Sm is necessary for proper mRNA attachment and function.

Direct demonstration of Sm impairment of amino acid incorporation in cell-free systems from *E. coli* soon followed (FLAKS *et al.*, 1962a and b; SPEYER *et al.*, 1962). Although the antibiotic does not interfere with the function of already attached native messenger, polyuridylic acid (poly U) directed phenylalanine incorporation is inhibited by a Sm concentration as low as 10^{-7} M, and the inhibition becomes complete as the ratio of Sm molecules to ribosomes approaches one. Furthermore, as observed earlier by ERDÖS and ULLMAN (1959) in another system, a cell-free system derived from a Sm^R organism requires a much higher antibiotic concentration to show a corresponding inhibition. As predicted by SPOTTS and STANIER, the resistance is determined by the ribosomes rather than by a factor in the supernatant from Sm^R cells. Similar results have been obtained using a cell-free system from *Diplococcus pneumoniae* (SAWADA and SUZUKI, 1964).

Further studies using labelled messenger have shown that mRNA binding is not inhibited by the antibiotic (DAVIES, 1964; COX *et al.*, 1964), but that Sm does inhibit the binding of certain transfer RNA (sRNA) molecules to the mRNA-ribosome complex. For example, Sm decreases the binding of phenylalanyl-sRNA directed by UpUpU or UpUpC to 70 S ribosomes from Sm sensitive (Sm^S) but not Sm^R cells (PESTKA *et al.*, 1965) and also depresses the binding of phenylalanyl-sRNA to 30 S subunits in the presence of poly U (KAJI *et al.*, 1966).

There are some indications that mRNA bound to ribosomes protects against Sm inhibition. For example, Sm killing is enhanced by puromycin (WHITE and WHITE, 1964). Puromycin inhibition of protein synthesis produces stripping of unfinished polypeptide chains and mRNA from ribosomes. WHITE and WHITE (1964) propose that puromycin synergizes Sm action by thus exposing Sm sensitive sites. However, most workers agree that *in vitro* Sm inhibition of poly U directed phenylalanine incorporation is the same whether Sm is added before or after the synthetic messenger (DAVIES, GORINI, and DAVIS, 1965; KNIPPENBERG *et al.*, 1965a).

When 70S ribosomes from Sm^S and Sm^R cells are dissociated into 30S and 50S subunits by lowering the magnesium concentration and hybrid ribosomes reconstructed from the subunits, the determinant of Sm sensitivity proved to be on the 30S subunit, which is also the site of messenger attachment (DAVIES, 1964; COX *et al.*, 1964). Further dissociation of the 30S subunit in cesium chloride produces 23S ribonucleoprotein cores and free protein at the meniscus. Sm sensitivity resides in the core (STAEHELIN and MESELSON, 1966), while mRNA binding requires the meniscus fraction as well (RASKAS and STAEHELIN, 1967).

No structural differences between ribosomes of Sm^S, Sm^R, and Sm^D cells have been unequivocally demonstrated as yet by polyacrylamide gel electrophoresis (LEBOY *et al.*, 1964). However, by other criteria physical differences between Sm^S and Sm^R ribosomes have been found: if Sm^S cells are treated briefly with Sm before harvesting, the ribosomes dissociate to a lesser extent into 30S and 50S subunits on lowering the magnesium concentration than ribosomes prepared from untreated or Sm^R cells (HERZOG, 1964). HERZOG (1964) was unable to reproduce this "sticking" effect of Sm by comparable amounts of the antibiotic added *in vitro* to protect against dissociation. However, LEON and BROCK (1967) recently reported that Sm at a concentration of 100 μg/ml added *in vitro* does protect against ribosomal dissociation on lowering the magnesium concentration and that the protective effect is greater with Sm^S than Sm^R ribosomes. In addition, Sm^R ribosomes dissociate more readily than Sm^S ribosomes in the absence of the antibiotic. Sm also protects Sm^S 70S ribosomes against thermal denaturation, but has no effect on the thermal dissociation of Sm^R ribosomes (LEON and BROCK, 1967). These results suggest that Sm can directly alter certain physical properties of the ribosome, but whether these changes are related to the effect of the antibiotic on protein synthesis is not known.

Streptomycin Induced Misreading

A major advance in the understanding of Sm action has been the discovery that the antibiotic produces not only inhibition of protein synthesis but also misreading of the genetic code. In 1961, GORINI, GUNDERSEN and BURGER reported that an arginine auxotroph of *E. coli* B, lacking ornithine transcarbamylase (OTC) in minimal medium, produces a low level of this enzyme in the presence of Sm. This observation was pursued by GORINI and KATAJA (1964a) who found that 1% of all auxotrophic mutants obtained after nitrosoguanidine mutagenesis of Sm^R *E. coli* are able to grow in the absence of their specific growth factors providing that Sm is present in the medium. Such mutants were termed "conditionally streptomycin dependent (CSD)" since Sm is required for growth only in minimal medium and not in medium supplemented with the growth factor required by the mutant.

In every case, the growth rate in the presence of Sm alone is slower than with the specific requirement, and in the original OTC CSD-mutant the OTC activity after growth in Sm is only about one thousandth of that produced by a corresponding OTC^+ strain. For a given CSD defect certain Sm^R alleles allow Sm correction while others do not. In strains which permit Sm correction, Sm mimics the action of a suppressor (a mutation at a second distinct site which reverses the mutant phenotype produced by a previous mutation), but unlike genetic suppression, the correction produced by Sm is phenotypic and not heritable.

GORINI and KATAJA (1964a) proposed that either mutation to certain types of Sm resistance allows Sm to suppress CSD mutations directly, or that there is a genetic suppressor present gratuitously in the parent of the CSD strains which requires Sm and certain Sm^R alleles to function. Since Sm resistance affects the ribosome, they further proposed that Sm affects the translation of mutant mRNA, and that the ribosome, rather than acting as a passive framework on which protein synthesis takes place, can influence the reading of the genetic code.

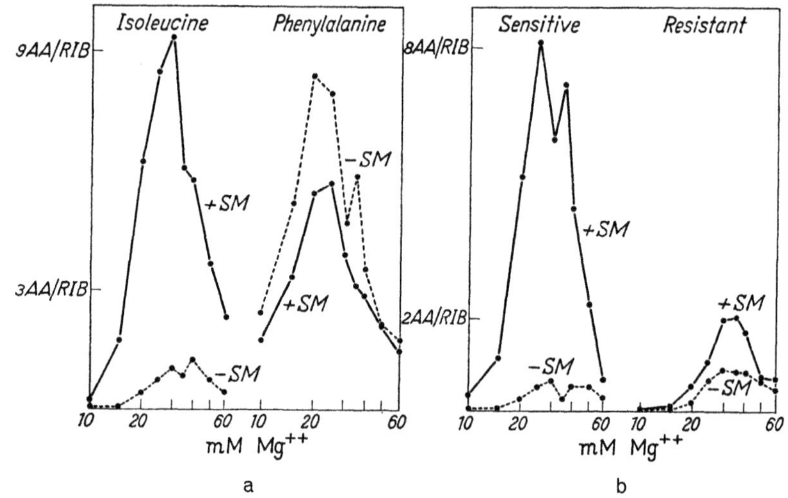

Fig. 2, a and b. (a) The magnesium dependence of the streptomycin stimulation of isoleucine incorporation and inhibition of phenylalanine incorporation on sensitive ribosomes primed with poly U. (b) Comparison of the stimulation of isoleucine incorporation on Sm^S and Sm^R ribosomes. [From DAVIES, GILBERT, and GORINI (1964)]

This hypothesis was confirmed by examining the ability of Sm to cause misreading in an *in vitro* amino acid incorporating system (DAVIES, GILBERT, and GORINI, 1964). Using extracts from Sm^S cells and poly U as primer, it was found that Sm and other aminoglycoside antibiotics inhibit phenylalanine incorporation as expected but at the same time stimulate the incorporation of isoleucine, serine, tyrosine, and leucine: amino acids not normally coded for by this synthetic messenger. Fig. 2 shows this effect as a function of the magnesium concentration and demonstrates that Sm-induced misreading is virtually absent when Sm^R ribosomes are used.

It is the recognition of codon by anticodon on the ribosome which Sm affects. In the absence of the antibiotic, poly U stimulates some binding of isoleucyl-sRNA to ribosomes at magnesium concentrations of 0.015 M or greater, but in the presence of 10^{-6} M Sm, this binding is markedly enhanced. The binding of leucyl-sRNA and seryl-sRNA is stimulated by Sm as well, but to a lesser extent (PESTKA *et al.*, 1965; KAJI and KAJI, 1965). Presumably, Sm introduces recognition ambiguity by changing the conformation of the ribosomes, but this has not been directly demonstrated.

The extent and spectrum of misreading varies with the antibiotic used and with the sRNA concentration. With polycytidylic acid (poly C) as messenger, incorporation of the "correct" amino acid, proline, is stimulated by Sm and misreading is observed for histidine, serine, threonine, leucine, and alanine. With polyadenylic acid (poly A), Sm stimulates lysine incorporation. With polyinosinic acid (poly I), glycine incorporation is stimulated by the drug and misreading occurs for arginine, tyrosine, valine, and lysine (DAVIES *et al.*, 1965). Table 2 shows the codon assignments for the amino acids affected when poly U and poly C are used as messengers. In general, only one base of a triplet is misread for poly U or poly C but all three bases may be misread in poly A or poly I. Both transition misreadings (purine to purine or pyrimidine to pyrimidine) and transversion misreadings (purine to pyrimidine or vice versa) are seen with these homopolynucleotides.

Table 2. *Misreading of poly U and poly C expressed in terms of amino acid codons*[1]

Input codon	Amino acid incorporated	Codons	
UUU	Phenylalanine	UU U/C	
	Isoleucine	AU U/C	
	Serine	UC U/C	UC A/G
	Tyrosine	UA U/C	
	Leucine	CU U/C	CU A/G
CCC	Proline	CC U/C	CC A/G
	Histidine	CA U/C	
	Serine	UC U/C	UC A/G
	Threonine	AC U/C	AC A/G
	Leucine	CU U/C	CU A/G
	Alanine	GC U/C	GC A/G

[1] From DAVIES (1965).

With messengers containing repeating dinucleotide sequences the specificity of Sm misreading is more restricted: 1. only pyrimidine bases are misread, 2. pyrimidine bases in the 5'-terminal position of a codon are misread as pyrimidines, 3. internal pyrimidines can be misread as either pyrimidines or purines, 4. 3'-terminal bases are not misread, and 5. misreading of a base in influenced by the nature of neighboring bases (DAVIES, JONES and KHORANA, 1966). Thus a substantial number of the 64 triplets should be refractory to Sm-induced misreading.

It might be supposed that the inhibition of "correct" amino acid incorporation would exactly parallel the stimulation of "misread" amino acids. In fact, with poly U as messenger the misincorporation of isoleucine alone exceeds the inhibition of phenylalanine incorporation: there is a net stimulation of amino acid synthesis (DAVIES *et al.*, 1964; OLD and GORINI, 1965). For other messengers either stimulation or inhibition of amino acid incorporation can be produced by Sm depending on the magnesium and sRNA concentrations and apparently independently of Sm-induced misreading (KNIPPENBERG *et al.*, 1965a, 1965b; DAVIES *et al.*, 1965). In general, with increasing sRNA concentration Sm inhibition of the "correct" reading becomes more prominent and the relative degree of misreading less prominent.

The manner in which the ribosomes are prepared for the *in vitro* system also differentially affects the inhibition and misreading observed. For example, with poly U as messenger Sm inhibits phenylalanyl-sRNA binding to ribosomes, which have been dissociated by lowering the magnesium concentration and then reassociated, much more than to nondissociated ribosomes; but Sm stimulates isoleucyl-sRNA binding to nondissociated ribosomes while inhibiting binding to reassociated ribosomes (PESTKA, 1966).

It is pertinent to recall that very low concentrations of Sm actually may stimulate bacterial growth (CURRAN and EVANS, 1947). While the explanation for Sm stimulation of protein synthesis remains unknown, Sm-induced misreading and inhibition of protein synthesis appear to involve different mechanisms.

In vivo, both nonsense and missense mutations respond to Sm-induced misreading. The original OTC CSD-mutation, for example, is now known to be an amber (UAG) nonsense mutation (GORINI, JACOBY, and BRECKENRIDGE, 1966); moreover, amber and ochre (UAA) mutants of phages T4 and T7 (ORIAS and GARTNER, 1966) and f2 (VALENTINE and ZINDER, 1964) are Sm-suppressible. In the *C* gene of the histidine operon of *Salmonella typhimurium*, while Sm suppressed 22 of 22 amber mutants and 5 of 6 ochre mutants, only 5 of 21 presumed missense mutations were suppressed, and none of 16 frameshift mutations were suppressed (WHITFIELD *et al.*, 1966).

According to the *in vitro* data of DAVIES *et al.*, (1966), Sm suppression of amber or ochre triplets should give CAG and CAA, respectively, codons for glutamine. Analysis of the protein products produced after Sm-induced misreading *in vivo* has not yet been accomplished due to the low level of suppression. There are, nonetheless, several indications that Sm suppression involves misreading of natural messengers. For example, in the presence of Sm, induced *E. coli* produces an altered β-galactosidase which has lost enzymatic activity but still cross-reacts with antiserum to the normal protein (BISSELL, 1965). *In vitro*, when amino acid incorporation is directed by f2 phage RNA under conditions in which a lack of asparagine in the incubation mixture limits incorporation, addition of either asparagine or Sm allows incorporation to proceed (SCHWARTZ, 1965). Presumably Sm allows the substitution of some other amino acid, perhaps lysine (SCHWARTZ, 1967), for the missing asparagine. Also, analysis of the polypeptide product made by poly U when Sm is present has shown it to be a random copolymer of phenylalanine and the misread amino acids leucine and isoleucine (OLD and GORINI, 1965; BODLEY and DAVIE, 1966).

Streptomycin Resistance

Mutants able to grow in the presence of Sm have arisen in many bacterial species. In a given species single step Sm^R mutants can be characterized by distinct levels of resistance to the antibiotic. In pneumococci and streptococci such mutants constitute a single locus but are genetically separable (RAVIN and MISHRA, 1965). In *E. coli* Sm resistance maps between *Mal A* and spectinomycin resistance (SCHWARTZ, 1966; DAVIES, ANDERSON, and DAVIS, 1965), and again appears to be a single locus (NEWCOMBE and NYHOLM, 1950; HASHIMOTO, 1960). Sm^R mutants differing in the degree of Sm resistance have also been reported in *E. coli* and they have been found to differ in growth rate and stability on subculture (MITCHISON, 1953); however, their genetic basis has not been analyzed. As a matter of fact, recombination between different Sm^R alleles of *E. coli* has been extremely difficult to detect, although recombination at a very low frequency is seen between Sm^R and Sm^D mutants, suggesting that they map in a single complex locus or in two closely linked sites (HASHIMOTO, 1960). Diploids containing both Sm^S and Sm^R alleles are sensitive to the antibiotic (LEDERBERG, 1951), a result currently interpreted by the participation of polyribosomes, containing a mixture of Sm^R and Sm^S components, in protein synthesis (LEDERBERG *et al.*, 1964), or by the fact that an equal mixture of good and bad ribosomes would produce bad protein because of the multimeric forms of many proteins (DAVIES *et al.*, 1964).

Further studies on CSD mutants have revealed differences between Sm^R alleles in their ability to allow Sm suppression and Sm-induced misreading. In the first place, a Sm^R allele is not necessary for Sm suppression. Providing that a low concentration of Sm is used, CSD mutants can be isolated at low frequency from Sm^S cells (GORINI and KATAJA, 1965). In a strain carrying a given Sm-suppressible defect, certain Sm^R alleles are competent for Sm suppression while the majority are not (GORINI and KATAJA, 1964a). From either type of strain it is generally possible to isolate CSD mutants for a second marker, and it is conceivable that no Sm^R allele is absolutely incompetent for Sm suppression of some defect (ANDERSON, GORINI, and BRECKENRIDGE, 1965). Although Sm-induced misreading using ribosomes from Sm^R strains was not at first demonstrated, by increasing the sensitivity of the *in vitro* system, it is possible to show that there is misreading by Sm^R ribosomes, even in the absence of the antibiotic, but at a ten-fold lower level than with Sm^S ribosomes. Furthermore, ribosomes from Sm^R competent and incompetent strains differ in the pattern of Sm-induced misreading (ANDERSON *et al.*, 1965).

These *in vitro* results did not distinguish between quantitative or qualitative differences in the misreading permitted by competent and incompetent Sm^R strains. By introducing different Sm^R alleles into a strain carrying two potentially Sm-suppressible defects, one an amber and the other presumably a missense mutation, it can be shown, Table 3, that either one defect or both or neither is corrected by Sm depending on the Sm allele present (GORINI *et al.*, 1966). Thus the nature of the ribosomal mutation seems to determine qualitatively the spectrum of misreading permitted, a powerful demonstration of the active role played by the ribosome in determining the specificity of protein synthesis.

Table 3. *Effect of different Sm alleles on the phenotype of two CSD mutations*[1]

Strain	Derivation	Arginine phenotype		Leucine phenotype	
		without Sm	with Sm	without Sm	with Sm
T 19—32	Sm^S parent	±	+	—	—
T 25—11	Sm^R transductant	—	+	—	+
T 23—11	Sm^R transductant	—	—	—	—
T 22—11	Sm^R transductant	—	—	—	+
T 23—61	Sm^R transductant	±	+	±	+

[1] From GORINI, JACOBY, and BRECKENRIDGE (1966).

There are other mechanisms by which Sm resistance may arise in bacteria. It has been observed that strains may become resistant to high levels of the antibiotic in multiple rather than single steps. In *S. typhimurium* multiple-step resistance is determined by multiple loci none of which are linked genetically to high level resistance (WATANABE and WATANABE, 1959a, 1959b). Furthermore, Sm resistance can be carried by an extrachromosomal R factor (RTF) conferring resistance to several antibiotics at once (WATANABE, 1963). The mechanism of Sm resistance due to R factors is quite different, however, from that due to mutation at the classical chromosomal Sm locus. Ribosomes from such a Sm^R strain are still sensitive to Sm *in vitro* (ROSENKRANZ, 1964). In one strain carrying an R factor conferring Sm resistance a soluble enzyme inactivating the antibiotic has been demonstrated (OKAMOTO and SUZUKI, 1965); in others altered permeability to the antibiotic is inferred. Finally, Sm resistance in *E. coli* can also be produced by an episome-like mutator factor (GUNDERSEN, 1963).

Streptomycin and Genetic Suppression

Since mutation to Sm resistance alters the interaction between messenger codons and sRNA anticodons on the ribosome, it would be expected that the interaction of a specific sRNA molecule responsible for genetic suppression might be altered by Sm resistance as well. The first example was found by LEDERBERG *et al.* (1964) who observed that when a strain which had reverted from Gal^- to Gal^+ by a suppressor mutation (Gal^- Su^+ Sm^S) became Sm^R the action of the suppressor disappeared unless Sm was present. The Sm^R derivative appeared like a CSD mutant in its response to Sm because mutation to Sm resistance had restricted the action of the genetic suppressor. A similar restriction of suppressor activity by mutation to Sm^R has been noted for suppressor-sensitive mutants of λ, T4, and T7 phages (COUTURIER *et al.*, 1964; GARTNER and ORIAS, 1966).

GARTNER and ORIAS (1966) distinguished at least four classes of Sm^R mutations on the basis of their ability to restrict the translation of amber and ochre codons by an ochre suppressor. Sm suppression of T4 nonsense mutants was evident in a Sm^S Su^- host, and Sm addition not only relieved restriction in some Sm^R Su^+ hosts but also allowed suppression in certain cases to approach 100% (ORIAS and GARTNER, 1966), i.e., the combined effects of phenotypic and genetic suppression can be more than additive. The mechanism by which Sm improves the conditions for genetic suppression and the specificity of this effect is not yet known.

Also, the relationship between competence to correct a bacterial CSD mutation and restriction of suppressor function remains to be systematically explored. Those incompetent Sm^R alleles examined to date are more restrictive than competent alleles (GORINI *et al.*, 1966), but the interaction of genetic suppression and Sm^R alleles can vary depending on the mutation examined, the nature of the genetic suppressor, and the presence of Sm. Furthermore, the efficiency of one suppressor is actually enhanced rather than restricted when a Sm^R allele is introduced (STRIGINI and GORINI, unpublished).

The interdependence between ribosomal structure and sRNA function is also illustrated by the difficulty of excluding the presence of a suppressor gene in a CSD strain. The original OTC amber CSD-mutant of GORINI, GUNDERSEN, and BURGER (1961) was obtained in a Sm^S strain in which no Sm suppression was evident because the potential to make the enzyme was low due to a peculiarity in the regulation of the arginine pathway in *E. coli* B (JACOBY and GORINI, 1967). When the potential to make OTC is raised by a mutation producing derepression of the arginine pathway, this OTC mutant appears CSD since enzyme formation is stimulated by Sm; however, it grows slowly even without Sm or arginine. When a Sm^R allele competent for correction is introduced in such a derepressed OTC mutant, then the strain becomes strictly arg^- CSD (Table 3). Although no suppressor for a variety of T4 phage amber or ochre mutants can be detected in any of these OTC CSD-derivatives by conventional techniques (GORINI *et al.*, 1966), it can be argued that some sRNA (suppressor) molecule capable of translating the amber codon in the OTC message must be present in the parent strain when it is Sm^S but that the less ambiguous Sm^R ribosome "restricts" this suppressor rendering it silent. Apparently, the degree of nonsense suppression must be too low to be detected using phage mutants yet high enough to allow cell growth by restoring a low level of OTC activity. For this reason it is operationally difficult to define a Su^- cell and important to consider both ribosomal and sRNA specificity in studies on suppression.

Ribosomal Ambiguity

Since the ribosome appears to play an active role in determining the specificity of messenger translation it would be expected that alterations in ribosomal structure may be brought about not only by an external agent like Sm, but also by mutations occurring in the genes determining ribosomal RNA or protein, i.e., some suppressor mutations may be ribosomal mutations producing a change in ribosomal specificity.

In the system in which the most extensive work has been done, namely nonsense suppression, two of the known amber suppressors, Su_I and Su_{III}, result from an alteration, probably in the anticodon, of an sRNA molecule. Thus Su_I is an altered serine sRNA (CAPECCHI and GUSSIN, 1965; ENGELHARDT *et al.*, 1965), while Su_{III} is a tyrosine sRNA (SMITH *et al.*, 1966); the result of suppression by Su_I or Su_{III} is the insertion of serine or tyrosine, respectively, at the site in a polypeptide chain corresponding to the UAG triplet. As yet there is no convincing evidence that Su_{II} also corresponds to a mutated sRNA although it is known to result in the insertion of glutamine. On the contrary, there is suggestive evidence that Su_{II} involves the ribosome, since ribosomes from an Su_{II}^+ strain differ from the Su_{II}^{-} parent in their dissociation as a function of the magnesium concentration and in the pattern of protein bands on polyacrylamide gel electrophoresis (BOLLEN and HERZOG, 1966; BOLLEN *et al.*, 1966). Ribosomal protein differences have also been reported in a strain carrying a less well characterized ochre suppressor (REID *et al.*, 1965). In either case, however, it can be argued that the observed ribosomal change is not the cause but a result of the suppressor mutation.

Furthermore, because of the interdependence of ribosomal specificity and sRNA suppression, a ribosomal mutation appears as a suppressor only in relation to the sRNA complement present in the cell. If this sRNA complement includes a minor component potentially able to translate a mutant codon, a mutation allowing more ribosomal ambiguity would appear as a ribosomal suppressor. In another genetic environment, with a different set of sRNA molecules, such a ribosomal mutation could be silent or lethal. Conversely, as seen above, an sRNA mutation appears a suppressor in the presence only of a given type of ribosome. Both sRNA and ribosomal specificity, therefore, must be taken into account.

Sm^R mutations are frequently pleiotropic (see review by GORINI and BECKWITH, 1966). They may simultaneously confer auxotrophy, alter control of inducible or repressible enzymes (ROSENKRANZ *et al.*, 1964), change host-prophage relationships or host-controlled modification of infecting bacteriophage, and alter patterns of genetic suppression. These pleiotropic effects of Sm mutations may have more than one basis, but it is reasonable that a different level of ribosomal ambiguity is at least one cause.

As previously noted, the amount of misreading observed in a cell-free system made up of mutant Sm^R ribosomes is ten-fold less than with wild type Sm^S ribosomes, even in the absence of antibiotics. Is a certain degree of ambiguity in translation advantageous to the naturally selected bacterial cell? In a haploid cell ambiguity may be selectively advantageous since certain mutations may thus remain unexpressed but available for future evolutionary trial. On the other hand, in higher organisms diploidy provides a genetic storehouse of unexpressed recessive mutations and ribosomal ambiguity may not be necessary. For whatever reason, it has in fact been found that with ribosomes from mammalian sources there is less *in vitro* misreading than with bacterial ribosomes and no Sm enhancement (WEINSTEIN *et al.*, 1966a, 1966b). In bacterial cells, with a short life span and rapid cellular renewal, a low level of errors would not be expected to produce cumulative effects.

One prediction of this hypothesis is that the apparent mutation rate for a given marker may be greater in Sm^R than Sm^S cells because the Sm^S ribosome by its ambiguity may permit certain mutations, including CSD mutations, to remain silent. In agreement with this prediction, GORINI and KATAJA (1965) found that the frequency of CSD mutants among auxotrophs from Sm^S strains is about seven times lower than from Sm^R strains.

Streptomycin Dependence

It is well known that an appreciable fraction of the survivors isolated from a plate containing high levels of streptomycin are Sm^D; i.e., they require streptomycin for growth even in a rich medium. They arise in one step from wild type Sm^S prototrophic strains and their phenotype is determined by a mutation allelic with (or very close to) the Sm^R locus. This genetic situation is quite different from that determining the conditionally streptomycin dependent (CSD) phenotype which results from the interaction of two independent genes: a structural gene harboring a Sm-suppressible mutation and a Sm gene harboring a competent allele.

The phenomenon of streptomycin dependence has intrigued microbiologists ever since its discovery. Different Sm^D mutants of *E. coli* vary remarkably in their properties, for example, in the incidence of reversion to Sm sensitivity or resistance, growth rate, UV sensitivity, requirement for Sm, and ability to grow on compounds related or unrelated to Sm (DEMEREC, 1950; SZYBALSKI and COCITO-VANDERMEULEN, 1958). It has not yet been possible to confirm the hypothesis of SPOTTS and STANIER (1961) that Sm is necessary for ribosomal function in Sm^D strains because *in vitro* protein synthesis using ribosomes from Sm^D mutants shows no Sm requirement (FLAKS *et al.*, 1962b). This failure may be due to the difficulty of removing bound Sm, but the discovery of CSD mutants and of the misreading effect of Sm offers another possibility (GORINI and KATAJA, 1964a). In both *E. coli* and *S. typhimurium* it has been frequently observed that mutation to Sm resistance and especially to Sm dependence also produces definable auxotrophic requirements (NEWCOMBE and NYHOLM, 1950; DEMEREC *et al.*, 1960; GOLDSCHMIDT *et al.*, 1962). This phenomenon has often been attributed to a multisite mutation affecting the Sm locus and neighboring genes. However, an attractive alternative is that Sm^D mutants represent a special class of Sm^R mutants in which ribosomal specificity has been restricted to such an extent that certain codons in the cell's mRNA can no longer be read efficiently, and specific requirements, not all replaceable by defined metabolites, become apparent unless Sm or some other agent producing misreading is present. The dependence on Sm, according to this interpretation, represents a requirement for an agent able to overcome ribosomal restriction by reintroducing selective translational ambiguity.

This explanation accounts for the observations that deficiencies in control mechanisms as well as nutritional deficiencies may appear with mutation to Sm dependence (ROSENKRANZ, 1963; BRAGG and POLGLASE, 1965), that upon Sm withdrawal from dependent cells a variety of metabolically unrelated enzyme activities decrease (SPOTTS and STANIER, 1961; SPOTTS, 1962), and that organic solvents like ethanol and methanol, known to introduce misreading in cell free systems (SO and DAVIE, 1964), may in certain Sm^D strains replace the Sm requirement (GADÓ and HORVÁTH, 1963). If this analysis is true, then protein synthesis *in vitro* employing Sm^D ribosomes might show no Sm requirement for the translation of specific synthetic messengers but would be expected to require Sm for the translation of natural mRNA.

Sm independent mutants can be easily selected by plating Sm^D strains on media lacking Sm. HASHIMOTO (1960) found that "revertants" to Sm independence in *E. coli* are actually due to suppressor mutations at a second site near the Sm locus and that the original Sm^D mutation remains unchanged. In *S. typhimurium* there are several sites for such suppressor mutations, unlinked to the Sm locus, but able to modify or remove a Sm requirement. Furthermore, "true" revertants from dependence to wild type Sm sensitivity can be found by using an unstable strain carrying a mutator gene (GOLDSCHMIDT *et al.*, 1962). True revertants from Sm dependence to wild type sensitivity as well as suppressed revertants have also been found in pneumococcus (MISHRA and RAVIN, 1966) and *B. subtilis* (FRASER and McDONALD, 1966).

In one such "revertant" of a Sm^D *E. coli* it has been shown that a 43 S ribosomal precursor accumulates in abnormal amounts during exponential growth (LEWANDOWSKI and BROWNSTEIN, 1966). This same revertant appears sensitive to Sm, although like the "oversuppressed" mutants of GORINI and KATAJA (1964b), Sm is not bactericidal. *In vitro*, the ribosomes from this strain show Sm inhibition of poly U directed phenylalanine incorporation and misincorporation of leucine and isoleucine like Sm^S ribosomes; i.e., the suppressor restores these Sm effects although the strain retains the Sm^D allele (BROWNSTEIN and LEWANDOWSKI, personal communication). If such a presumed suppressor mutation relieves the Sm requirement of a Sm^D strain by reintroducing misreading and the combined effects of genetic and phenotypic suppression produce apparent Sm sensitivity, then the same suppressor should also cause a classical Sm^R cell to appear relatively Sm^S. Such an effect was found by HASHIMOTO (1960).

Other Aminoglycoside Antibiotics

Bluensomycin, kanamycin (Km), neomycin (Nm), and paromomycin (Pm) (catenulin) are other chemically related aminoglycoside antibiotics produced by *Streptomyces* which have been shown to cause misreading *in vivo* (GORINI and

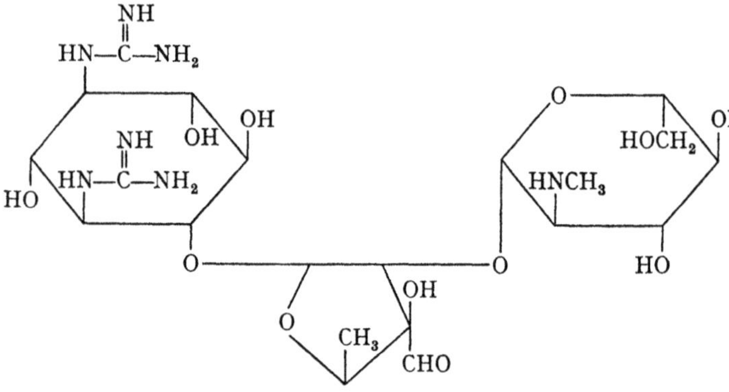

Streptomycin

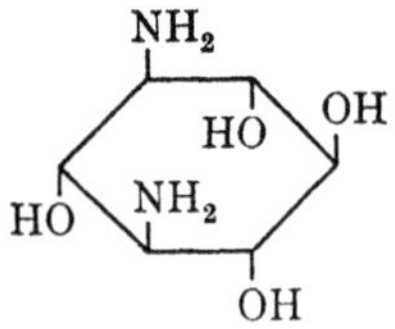

The streptamine nucleus of streptomycin and bluensomycin

Fig. 3. A comparison of streptomycin and bluensomycin. Bluensomycin posseses a structure similar to streptomycin with but two differences: 1. one of the guanido groups in the streptamine nucleus is substituted by $—OCONH_2$ in bluensomycin; 2. the —CHO group in streptomycin is substituted by $—CH_2OH$ in bluensomycin

KATAJA, 1965) and *in vitro* (DAVIES *et al.*, 1965). The evidence for their chemical structures given in Fig. 3 and 4 has been summarized by RINEHART (1964). Gentamicin and hygromycin B are other aminoglycoside antibiotics which have been shown to produce misreading *in vitro* (DAVIES *et al.*, 1965). Their chemical structure is, however, not completely known.

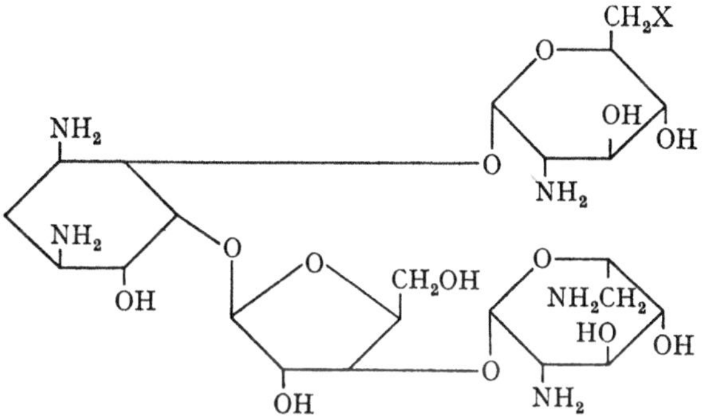

Neomycin B ($X = NH_2$) and Paromomycin I ($X = OH$)

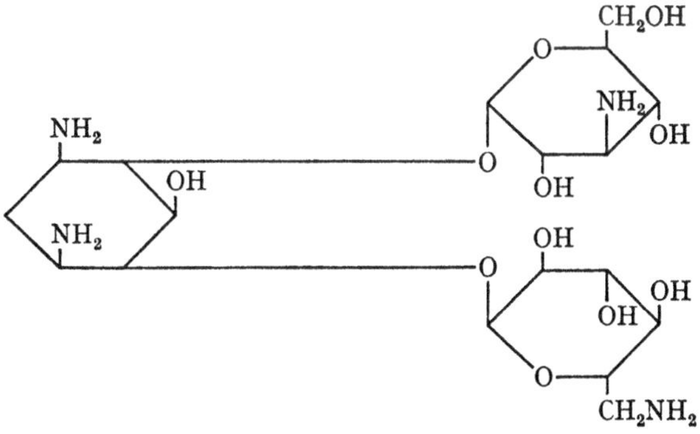

Kanamycin

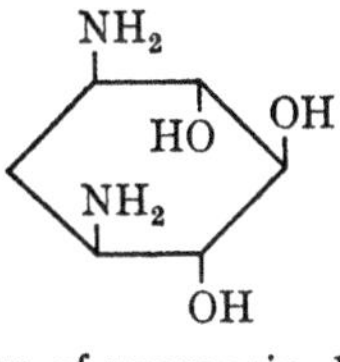

The 2-deoxystreptamine nucleus of neomycin, kanamycin, and paromomycin

Fig. 4. Structure of kanamycin A, neomycin B, and paromomycin I

There is evidence that different aminoglycoside antibiotics induce different, specific types of ambiguity. For instance, certain auxotrophic mutants of *E. coli* correctable by Sm are suppressed, at sub-lethal drug concentrations, by Nm but not Km and others by Km but not Nm (GORINI and KATAJA, 1965). Specificity is also seen *in vitro* where the different aminoglycoside antibiotics show different patterns of misreading. For example, Nm-induced misreading is more extensive and nonspecific than that produced by Sm and may involve two bases in a triplet as well as the 3′-terminal base (Davies *et al.*, 1966). Even denatured DNA functions as an effective template for amino acid incorporation in the presence of Nm or Km (McCarthy and Holland, 1965).

Aminoglycoside antibiotics were originally classified on the basis of their chemical structure. Subsequent studies, however, have shown that the class also possesses a functional unity. All those aminoglycosides which have been thoroughly studied appear to act on protein synthesis at the level of the 30S ribosomal subunit. Most of them produce ambiguity in translation, but there are exceptions. Spectinomycin (actinospectacin), for instance, inhibits protein synthesis at the level of messenger-ribosome interaction without causing misreading, although the genetic determinant for spectinomycin resistance has been shown to be associated with the 30S ribosomal subunit and to map near the Sm locus (Davies, Anderson and Davis, 1965).

As yet the chemical structure responsible for misreading is not understood, but suggestive hypotheses are on hand. According to Tanaka *et al.* (1967), the chemical moiety responsible for misreading is streptamine or deoxystreptamine which is present in the molecules of Sm, Km, Nm, Pm, bluensomycin, gentamicin, and hygromycin B (Fig. 3 and 4). Although the streptamines lack antibacterial activity, it can be shown that deoxystreptamine produces stimulation and misreading of synthetic messengers *in vitro* (Tanaka *et al.*, 1967). By contrast, in spectinomycin the streptamine nucleus is replaced by a stereoisomer, actinamine (Fig. 5), and the misreading property is lost. Kasugamycin is another aminoglycoside antibiotic lacking streptamine which inhibits protein synthesis but does not cause misreading (Tanaka *et al.*, 1966a, 1966b). Kasugamycin and spectinomycin appear to differ in the stage of protein synthesis inhibited since kasugamycin inhibits the binding of sRNA to ribosomes while spectinomycin does not.

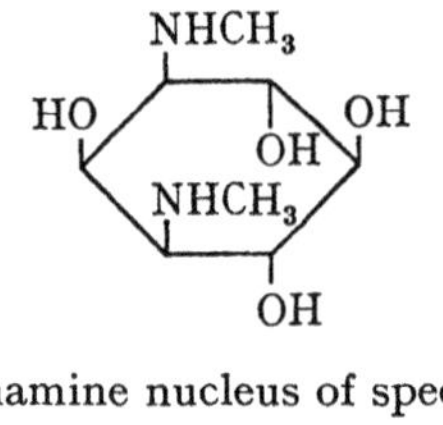

The actinamine nucleus of spectinomycin

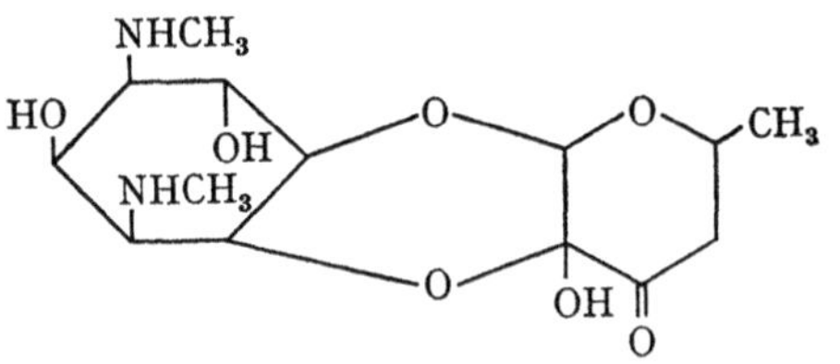

Spectinomycin

Fig. 5. Structure of spectinomycin. Only the actinamine nucleus is indicated in stereochemical form

If resistance to each aminoglycoside antibiotic is due to a different alteration in the 30S ribosomal subunit, some degree of cross resistance might be expected between the different drugs. Complete cross resistance has been found in *E. coli* between streptomycin, dihydrostreptomycin and bluensomycin, which are closely related chemically. A low level of cross resistance between Nm, Km, and Sm resistant mutants of *E. coli* has been reported (SZYBALSKY and BRYSON, 1952), and Nm^R mutants of *S. aureus* have been found resistant also to Sm, Km and Pm (SOKOLSKI *et al.*, 1962). Among the survivors to high concentrations of Pm or Sm is a class of one-step mutants resistant to both drugs when tested separately, but sensitive to the two drugs in combination. In contrast, two-step Sm^R Pm^R mutants are also resistant to a mixture of the two drugs (GORINI, unpublished). It should be anticipated that the study of these different drug resistances will clarify ribosomal structure. However, genetic studies have been hampered by the instability of aminoglycoside resistant mutants with the exception of the classical Sm^R mutants. Indeed, since ribosomal mutations affecting ambiguity would be expected to produce profound alterations in cell physiology, it may be fortunate for the experimenter that stable resistant mutants exist even for Sm.

Streptomycin Lethality

Consideration of the number of different hypotheses which have been advanced to explain Sm action suggests caution in assuming that the mechanism of Sm lethality is now known. Biochemical studies suggest the following sequence of events when Sm is added to growing cells. There is an almost immediate uptake of the drug, followed by an accelerated efflux of potassium and a transient stimulation of RNA synthesis. Next protein synthesis is inhibited, and viability declines. Still later more Sm is bound to the cells, respiration is impaired, RNA and DNA synthesis is inhibited, RNA breakdown occurs, and nucleotides are excreted (DUBIN, HANCOCK and DAVIS, 1963).

It is tempting to believe that these effects, and Sm lethality in particular, are related fundamentally to Sm-induced misreading. However, it is not clear why the accumulation of faulty protein alone should be rapidly bactericidal. In fact, GORINI and KATAJA (1964b) showed that a genotypically Sm^R cell containing a certain genetic suppressor appeared unable to grow in the presence of Sm due to the high level of misreading produced by the combined action of genetic and phenotypic suppression, but that despite the amount of faulty protein being produced, Sm was only bacteriostatic. Similarly the revertants from Sm dependence studied by BROWNSTEIN and LEWANDOWSKI are unable to grow in the presence of Sm, but in this case also Sm is not bactericidal despite *in vitro* evidence of misreading. Perhaps a special kind of misreading, such as that affecting membrane formation, is required for Sm lethality.

Nonetheless, there is good evidence for a close relationship between Sm killing and misreading. Firstly, bactericidal resistance *in vivo* and misreading resistance *in vitro* parallel each other. Wild type *E. coli* is sensitive to both Sm and Nm and its ribosomes are induced to misread with either drug, whereas ribosomes from Sm^R Nm^S mutants show appreciable misreading only with Nm, and conversely ribosomes from Sm^S Nm^R mutants show misreading only with Sm. Secondly, when certain chemical derivatives of Sm are compared for their bactericidal action and for their ability to cause misreading, the dose effect relationship is the same (GORINI, 1967). Thirdly, aminoglycoside antibiotics like spectinomycin which do not cause misreading are not bactericidal (DAVIES, ANDERSON and DAVIS, 1965). Finally, as predicted by the misreading hypothesis, if protein synthesis is prevented by chloramphenicol or starvation for a required amino acid, Sm killing ceases (ANAND and DAVIS, 1960; JAWETZ *et al.*, 1951).

However, the requirement of protein synthesis for Sm lethality has been challenged by COHEN and coworkers who obtained Sm killing, although at a slower rate, when a multiply auxotrophic strain of *E. coli* was starved for a required amino acid. Under these conditions Sm alters the distribution of the polyamines putrescine and spermidine in cells and produces a marked stimulation of RNA synthesis, which these authors believe to be closely related to the lethal event (STERN *et al.*, 1966; RAINA and COHEN, 1966).

Undoubtedly continued study of Sm action will reveal further surprises. However, any theory of how the drug acts as a bactericidal agent must encompass the genetic evidence thus far accumulated.

References

ANAND, N., and B. D. DAVIS: Damage by streptomycin to the cell membrane of *Escherichia coli*. Nature **185**, 22 (1960).

ANDERSON, W. F., L. GORINI, and L. BRECKENRIDGE: Role of ribosomes in streptomycin-activated suppression. Proc. Natl Acad. Sci. U.S. **54**, 1076 (1965).

BISSELL, D. M.: Formation of an altered enzyme by *Escherichia coli* in the presence of neomycin. J. Mol. Biol. **14**, 619 (1965).

BODLEY, J. W., and E. W. DAVIE: A study of the mechanism of ambiguous amino acid coding by poly U: the nature of the products. J. Mol. Biol. **18**, 344 (1966).

BOLLEN, A., et A. HERZOG: Altération du comportement des ribosomes à la suite d'une mutation "supersuppresseur". Arch. intern. physiol. et biochem. **73**, 139 (1965).

BOLLEN, A., A. HERZOG et R. THOMAS: Altération du comportement des ribosomes à la suite d'une mutation "superpresseur". III. Etude électrophorétique des proteines ribosomiales. Arch. intern. physiol. et biochem. **73**, 557 (1965).

BRAGG, P. D., and W. J. POLGLASE: Biosynthesis of valine in streptomycin-dependent *Escherichia coli*. J. Bacteriol. **89**, 1158 (1965).

BROCK, T. D.: Action of streptomycin and related antibiotics. Federation Proc. **23**, 965 (1964).

BROCK, T. D.: Streptomycin. In: Biochemical studies of antimicrobial drugs. Sixteenth symposium of the society for general microbiology. Cambridge: University Press 1966.

BROCK, T. D., R. M. JOHNSON, and W. B. DEVILLE: Physical and chemical properties of a bacterial virus as related to its inhibition by streptomycin. Virology **35**, 439 (1965).

CAPECCHI, M. R., and G. N. GUSSIN: Suppression in vitro: identification of a serine-sRNA as a "nonsense" suppressor. Science **149**, 417 (1965).

COHEN, S. S.: Streptomycin and desoxyribonuclease in the study of variations in the properties of a bacterial virus. J. Biol. Chem. **168**, 511 (1947).

COHEN, S. S., and J. LICHTENSTEIN: The isolation of deoxyribonucleic acid from bacterial extracts by precipitation with streptomycin. J. Biol. Chem. **235**, PC55 (1960).

COUTURIER, M., L. DESMET, and R. THOMAS: High pleiotropy of streptomycin mutations in *Escherichia coli*. Biochem. Biophys. Res. Commun. **16**, 244 (1964).

COX, E. C., J. R. WHITE, and J. G. FLAKS: Streptomycin action and the ribosome. Proc. Natl Acad. Sci. U.S. **51**, 703 (1964).

CURRAN, H. R., and F. R. EVANS: Stimulation of sporogenic and nonsporogenic bacteria by traces of penicillin or streptomycin. Proc. Soc. Exptl Biol. Med. **64**, 231 (1947).

DAVIES, J.: Studies on the ribosomes of streptomycin-sensitive and resistant strains of *Escherichia coli*. Proc. Natl Acad. Sci. U.S. **51**, 659 (1964).

DAVIES, J.: Effects of streptomycin and related antibiotics on protein synthesis. Antimicrobial Agents Chemotherapy 1965, p. 1001.

DAVIES, J., P. ANDERSON, and B. D. DAVIS: Inhibition of protein synthesis by spectinomycin. Science **149**, 1096 (1965).

DAVIES, J., W. GILBERT, and L. GORINI: Streptomycin, suppression, and the code. Proc. Natl Acad. Sci. U.S. **51**, 883 (1964).

DAVIES, J., L. GORINI, and B. D. DAVIS: Misreading of RNA codewords induced by aminoglycoside antibiotics. Mol. Pharmacol. **1**, 93 (1965).

DAVIES, J., D. S. JONES, and H. G. KHORANA: A further study of misreading of condons induced by streptomycin and neomycin using ribopolynucleotides containing two nucleotides in alternating sequence as templates. J. Mol. Biol. **18**, 48 (1966).

DAVIS, B. D., and D. S. FEINGOLD: Antimicrobial agents: mechanism of action and use in metabolic studies. In: The bacteria: a treatise on structure and function (I. C. GUNSALUS and R. Y. STANIER, eds.). New York: Academic Press 1963.

DEMEREC, M.: Reaction of populations of unicellular organisms to extreme changes in environment. Am. Naturalist **84**, 5 (1950).

DEMEREC, M., E. L. LAHR, E. BALBINDER, T. MIYAKE, J. ISHIDSU, K. MIZOBUCHI, and B. MAHLER: Bacterial genetics. Carnegie Inst. Wash. Yearbook **59**, 426 (1960).

DUBIN, D. T.: Some effects of streptomycin on RNA metabolism in *Escherichia coli*. J. Mol. Biol. **8**, 749 (1964).

DUBIN, D. T., and B. D. DAVIS: The effect of streptomycin on potassium flux in *Escherichia coli*. Biochim. et Biophys. Acta **52**, 400 (1961).

DUBIN, D. T., and B. D. DAVIS: The streptomycin-triggered depolymerization of ribonucleic acid in *Escherichia coli*. Biochim. et Biophys. Acta **55**, 793 (1962).

DUBIN, D. T., R. HANCOCK, and B. D. DAVIS: The sequence of some effects of streptomycin in *Escherichia coli*. Biochim. et Biophys. Acta **74**, 476 (1963).

ENGELHARDT, D. L., R. E. WEBSTER, R. C. WILHELM, and N. D. ZINDER: *In vitro* studies on the mechanism of suppression of a nonsense mutation. Proc. Natl Acad. Sci. U.S. **54**, 1791 (1965).

ERDÖS, T., and A. ULLMANN: Effect of streptomycin on the incorporation of aminoacids labelled with carbon-14 into ribonucleic acid and protein in a cell-free system of *Mycobacterium*. Nature **183**, 618 (1959).

FITZGERALD, R. J., F. BERNHEIM, and D. B. FITZGERALD: The inhibition by streptomycin of adaptive enzyme formation in *Mycobacteria*. J. Biol. Chem. **175**, 195 (1948).

FLAKS, J. G., E. C. COX, and J. R. WHITE: Inhibition of polypeptide synthesis by streptomycin. Biochem. Biophys. Res. Commun. **7**, 385 (1962a).

FLAKS, J. G., E. C. COX, M. L. WITTING, and J. R. WHITE: Polypeptide synthesis with ribosomes from streptomycin-resistant and dependent *E. coli*. Biochem. Biophys. Res. Commun. **7**, 390 (1962b).

FRASER, S. J., and W. C. MCDONALD: Analysis of mutations from streptomycin dependence to nondependence in *Bacillus subtilis* by transformation. J. Bacteriol. **92**, 1582 (1966).

GADÓ, I., and I. HORVÁTH: The effect of methanol on the growth of a streptomycin-dependent strain of *Escherichia coli* in streptomycin-free media. Life Sci. **10**, 741 (1963).

GALE, E. F.: Mechanism of antibiotic action. Pharmacol. Revs **15**, 481 (1963).

GARTNER, T. K., and E. ORIAS: Effects of mutations to streptomycin resistance on the rate of translation of mutant genetic information. J. Bacteriol. **91**, 1021 (1966).

GOLDSCHMIDT, E. P., T. S. MATNEY, and H. T. BAUSUM: Genetic analysis of mutations from streptomycin dependence to independence in *Salmonella typhimurium*. Genetics **47**, 1475 (1962).

GORINI, L.: Induction of code ambiguity by aminoglycoside antibiotics. Federation Proc. **26**, 5 (1967).

GORINI, L., and J. R. BECKWITH: Suppression. Ann. Rev. Microbiol. **20**, 401 (1966).

GORINI, L., W. GUNDERSEN, and M. BURGER: Genetics of regulation of enzyme synthesis in the arginine biosynthetic pathway of *Escherichia coli*. Cold Spring Harbor Symposia Quant. Biol. **26**, 173 (1961).

GORINI, L., G. JACOBY, and L. BRECKENRIDGE: Ribosomal ambiguity. Cold Spring Harbor Symposia Quant. Biol. **31** (in press) (1966).

GORINI, L., and E. KATAJA: Phenotypic repair by streptomycin of defective genotypes in *E. coli*. Proc. Natl Acad. Sci. U.S. **51**, 487 (1964a).

GORINI, L., and E. KATAJA: Streptomycin-induced oversuppression in *E. coli*. Proc. Natl Acad. Sci. U.S. **51**, 995 (1964b).

GORINI, L., and E. KATAJA: Suppression activated by streptomycin and related antibiotics in drug sensitive strains. Biochem. Biophys. Res. Commun. **18**, 656 (1965).

GUNDERSEN, W. B.: New type of streptomycin resistance resulting from action of the episomelike mutator factor in *Escherichia coli*. J. Bacteriol. **86**, 510 (1963).

HAHN, F. E., J. CIAK, A. D. WOLFE, R. E. HARTMAN, J. L. ALLISON, and R. S. HARTMAN: Studies on the mode of action of streptomycin. II. Effects of streptomycin on the synthesis of proteins and nucleic acids and on cellular multiplication in *Escherichia coli*. Biochim. et Biophys. Acta **61**, 741 (1962).

HASHIMOTO, K.: Streptomycin resistance in *Escherichia coli* analyzed by transduction. Genetics **45**, 49 (1960).

HERZOG, A.: An effect of streptomycin on the dissociation of *Escherichia coli* 70 S ribosomes. Biochem. Biophys. Res. Commun. **15**, 172 (1964).

HURWITZ, C.: Mechanism of action of streptomycin. Antimicrobial Agents Chemotherapy 1963, p. 371.

JACOBY, G. A., and L. GORINI: Genetics of control of the arginine pathway in *Escherichia coli* B and K. J. Mol. Biol. **24**, 41 (1967).

JAWETZ, E., J. B. GUNNISON, and R. S. SPECK: Studies on antibiotic synergism and antagonism; the interference of aureomycin, chloramphenicol, and terramycin with the action of streptomycin. Am. J. Med. Sci. **222**, 404 (1951).

KAJI, H., and A. KAJI: Specific binding of sRNA to ribosomes: effect of streptomycin. Proc. Natl Acad. Sci. U.S. **54**, 213 (1965).

KAJI, H., I. SUZUKA, and A. KAJI: Binding of specific soluble ribonucleic acid to ribosomes. Binding of soluble ribonucleic acid to the template-30 S subunits complex. J. Biol. Chem. **241**, 1251 (1966).

KNIPPENBERG, P. H. VAN, J. C. VAN RAVENSWAAY CLAASEN, M. GRIJM-VOS, H. VELDSTRA, and L. BOSCH: Stimulation and inhibition of polypeptide synthesis by streptomycin in ribosomal systems of *Escherichia coli*, programmed with various messengers. Biochim. et Biophys. Acta **95**, 461 (1965a).

KNIPPENBERG, P. H. VAN, M. GRIJM-VOS, H. VELDSTRA, and L. BOSCH: Effects of streptomycin on the translation of turnip yellow mosaic virus RNA *in vitro*. Biochem. Biophys. Res. Commun. **20**, 4 (1965b).

LEBOY, P. S., E. C. COX, J. G. FLAKS: The chromosomal site specifying a ribosomal protein in *Escherichia coli*. Proc. Natl Acad. Sci. U.S. **52**, 1367 (1964).

LEDERBERG, E. M., L. CAVALLI-SFORZA, and J. LEDERBERG: Interaction of streptomycin and a suppressor for galactose fermentation in *E. coli* K-12. Proc. Natl Acad. Sci. U.S. **51**, 678 (1964).

LEDERBERG, J.: Streptomycin resistance: a genetically recessive mutation. J. Bacteriol. **61**, 549 (1951).

LEON, S. A., and T. D. BROCK: Effect of streptomycin and neomycin on physical properties of the ribosome. J. Mol. Biol. **24**, 391 (1967).

LEWANDOWSKI, L. J., and B. L. BROWNSTEIN: An altered pattern of ribosome synthesis in a mutant of *E. coli*. Biochem. Biophys. Res. Commun. **25**, 554 (1966).

McCARTHY, B. J., and J. J. HOLLAND: Denatured DNA as a direct template for *in vitro* protein synthesis. Proc. Natl Acad. Sci. U.S. **54**, 880 (1965).

MISHRA, A. K., and A. W. RAVIN: Genetic linkage of streptomycin-dependence and resistance in pneumococcus. Genetics **53**, 1197 (1966).

MITCHISON, D. A.: The occurrence of independent mutations to different types of streptomycin resistance in *Bacterium coli*. J. Gen. Microbiol. **8**, 168 (1953).

MOSKOWITZ, M.: Differences in precipitability of nucleic acids with streptomycin and dihydrostreptomycin. Nature **200**, 335 (1963).

MOSKOWITZ, M., and N. E. KELKER: Sensitivity of cultured mammalian cells to streptomycin and dihydrostreptomycin. Science **141**, 647 (1963).

MOSKOWITZ, M., and N. KELKER: Amino-acid control of streptomycin action on mammalian cells. Nature **205**, 476 (1965).

NEWCOMBE, H. B., and M. H. NYHOLM: The inheritance of streptomycin resistance and dependence in crosses of *Escherichia coli*. Genetics **35**, 603 (1950).

OGINSKY, E. L.: Mode of action of streptomycin. Part III of Symposium on the mode of action of antibiotics. Bacteriol. Rev. **17**, 17 (1953).

OKAMOTO, S., and Y. SUZUKI: Chloramphenicol-, dihydrostreptomycin-, and kanamycin-inactivating enzymes from multiple drug-resistant *Escherichia coli* carrying episome 'R'. Nature **208**, 1301 (1965).

OLD, D., and L. GORINI: Amino acid changes provoked by streptomycin in a polypeptide synthesized *in vitro*. Science **150**, 1290 (1965).

ORIAS, E., and T. K. GARTNER: Suppression of *amber* and *ochre* RII mutants of bacteriophage T4 by streptomycin. J. Bacteriol. **91**, 2210 (1966).

PESTKA, S.: Studies on the formation of transfer ribonucleic acid-ribosome complexes. I. The effect of streptomycin and ribosomal dissociation on ^{14}C-aminoacyl transfer ribonucleic acid binding to ribosomes. J. Biol. Chem. **241**, 367 (1966).

PESTKA, S., R. MARHALL, and M. NIRENBERG: RNA codewords and protein synthesis. V. Effects of streptomycin on the formation of ribosome-sRNA complexes. Proc. Natl Acad. Sci. U.S. **53**, 639 (1965).

POLGLASE, W. J.: Contribution of the cationic groups of dihydrostreptomycin to biological activity. Nature **206**, 298 (1965).

RAINA, A., and S. S. COHEN: Polyamines and RNA synthesis in a polyauxotrophic strain of *E. coli*. Proc. Natl Acad. Sci. U.S. **55**, 1587 (1966).

RAKE, G., F. E. PANSY, W. P. JAMBOR, and R. DONOVICK: Further studies on the dihydrostreptomycins. Am. Rev. Tuber. **58**, 479 (1948).

RASKAS, H. J., and T. STAEHELIN: Messenger and s-RNA binding by ribosomal subunits and reconstituted ribosomes. J. Mol. Biol. **23**, 89 (1967).

RAVIN, A. W., and A. K. MISHRA: Relative frequencies of different kinds of spontaneous and induced mutants of pneumococci and streptococci capable of growth in the presence of streptomycin. J. Bacteriol. **90**, 1161 (1965).

REID, P. J., E. ORIAS, and T. K. GARTNER: Ribosomal protein differences in a strain of *E. coli* carrying a suppressor of an ochre mutation. Biochem. Biophys. Res. Commun. **21**, 66 (1965).

REITER, H.: The location of the inhibitory action of KCN and several polyamines on bacteriophage replication. Virology **21**, 636 (1963).

RINEHART, jr., K. L.: The neomycins and related antibiotics. New York: John Wiley & Sons 1964.

ROSENKRANZ, H. S.: Unusual alkaline phosphatase levels in streptomycin-dependent strains of *E. coli*. Biochemistry **2**, 122 (1963).

ROSENKRANZ, H. S.: Basis of streptomycin resistance in *Escherichia coli* with a "multiple drug resistance" episome. Biochim. et Biophys. Acta **80**, 342 (1964).

ROSENKRANZ, H. S., A. J. BENDICH, and H. S. CARR: The isolation of two streptomycin-resistant mutants of *Escherichia coli* ML 35 differing in constitutive enzymes. Biochim. et Biophys. Acta **82**, 110 (1964).

ROTH, H., H. AMOS, and B. D. DAVIS: Purine nucleotide excretion by *Escherichia coli* in the presence of streptomycin. Biochim. et Biophys. Acta **37**, 398 (1960).
SAWADA, F., and K. SUZUKI: Streptomycin-sensitive and resistant ribosomes of *Diplococcus pneumoniae*. Biochim. et Biophys. Acta **80**, 160 (1964).
SCHATZ, A., E. BUGIE, and S. A. WAKSMAN: Streptomycin, a substance exhibiting antibiotic activity against gram-positive and gram-negative bacteria. Proc. Soc. Exptl Biol. Med. **55**, 66 (1944).
SCHINDLER, J.: Interaction of basic antibiotics with phage f2 particles. Biochim. Biophys. Res. Commun. **18**, 119 (1965).
SCHWARTZ, J. H.: An effect of streptomycin on the biosynthesis of the coat protein of coliphage f2 by extracts of *E. coli*. Proc. Natl Acad. Sci. U.S. **53**, 1133 (1965).
SCHWARTZ, J. H.: Modification of the coat protein of coliphage f2 synthesized in cell-free extracts of *E. coli* in the presence of streptomycin. Federation Proc. **26**, 865 (1967).
SCHWARTZ, M.: Location of the maltose A and B loci on the genetic map of *Escherichia coli*. J. Bacteriol. **92**, 1083 (1966).
SMITH, J. D., J. N. ABELSON, B. F. C. CLARK, H. M. GOODMAN, and S. BRENNER: Studies on amber suppressor sRNA. Cold Spring Harbor Symposia Quant. Biol. **31** (in press) (1966).
So, A., and E. W. DAVIE: The effect of organic solvents on protein biosynthesis and their influence on the amino acid code. Biochemistry **3**, 1165 (1964).
SOKOLSKI, W. T., R. L. YEAGER, and J. K. MCCOY: Cross-resistance studies with neomycin antibiotics. Nature **195**, 623 (1962).
SPEYER, J. F., P. LENGYEL, and C. BASILIO: Ribosomal localization of streptomycin sensitivity. Proc. Natl Acad. Sci. U.S. **48**, 684 (1962).
SPOTTS, C. R.: Physiological and biochemical studies on streptomycin dependence in *Escherichia coli*. J. Gen. Microbiol. **28**, 347 (1962).
SPOTTS, C. R., and R. Y. STANIER: Mechanism of streptomycin action on bacteria: a unitary hypothesis. Nature **192**, 633 (1961).
STAEHELIN, T., and M. MESELSON: Determination of streptomycin sensitivity by a subunit of the 30 S ribosome of *Escherichia coli*. J. Mol. Biol. **19**, 207 (1966).
STERN, J. L., H. D. BARNER, and S. S. COHEN: The lethality of streptomycin and the stimulation of RNA synthesis in the absence of protein synthesis. J. Mol. Biol. **17**, 188 (1966).
SZYBALSKI, W., and V. BRYSON: Genetic studies on microbial cross resistance to toxic agents. I. Cross resistance of *Escherichia coli* to fifteen antibiotics. J. Bacteriol. **64**, 489 (1952).
SZYBALSKI, W., and J. COCITO-VANDERMEULEN: Neamine and streptomycin dependence in *Escherichia coli*. Bacteriol. Proc. 37 (1958).
TANAKA, N., H. MASUKAWA, and H. UMEZAWA: Structural basis of kanamycin for miscoding activity. Biochem. Biophys. Res. Commun. **26**, 544 (1967).
TANAKA, N., K. SASHIKATA, T. NISHIMURA, and H. UMEZAWA: Activity of ribosomes from kanamycin-resistant *E. coli*. Biochem. Biophys. Res. Commun. **16**, 216 (1964).
TANAKA, N., H. YAMAGUCHI, and H. UMEZAWA: Mechanism of kasugamycin action on polypeptide synthesis. J. Biochem. (Tokyo) **60**, 429 (1966a).
TANAKA, N., Y. YOSHIDA, K. SASHIKATA, H. YAMAGUCHI, and H. UMEZAWA: Inhibition of polypeptide synthesis by kasugamycin, an aminoglycoside antibiotic. J. Antibiotics (Japan) **19**A, 65 (1966b).
TZAGOLOFF, H., and W. W. UMBREIT: Influence of streptomycin on nucleotide excretion in *Escherichia coli*. J. Bacteriol. **85**, 49 (1963).
VALENTINE, R. C., and N. D. ZINDER: Phenotypic repair of RNA-bacteriophage mutants by streptomycin. Science **144**, 1458 (1964).
WATANABE, T.: Transductional studies of thiamine and nicotinic acid requiring streptomycin resistant mutants of *Salmonella typhimurium*. J. Gen. Microbiol. **22**, 102 (1960).
WATANABE, T.: Infective heredity of multiple drug resistance in bacteria. Bacteriol. Rev. **27**, 87 (1963).

WATANABE, T., and M. WATANABE: Transduction of streptomycin resistance in *Salmonella typhimurium*. J. Gen. Microbiol. **21**, 16 (1959a).
WATANABE, T., and M. WATANABE: Transduction of streptomycin sensitivity into resistant mutants of *Salmonella typhimurium*. J. Gen. Microbiol. **21**, 30 (1959b).
WEINSTEIN, I. B., S. M. FRIEDMAN, and M. OCHOA jr.: Fidelity during translation of the genetic code. Cold Spring Harbor Symposia Quant. Biol. **31** (in press) (1966).
WEINSTEIN, I. B., M. OCHOA jr., and S. M. FRIEDMAN: Fidelity of the translation of messenger ribonucleic acid in mammalian subcellular systems. Biochemistry **5**, 3332 (1966).
WHITE, J. R., and J. G. FLAKS: Inhibition of protein synthesis and other effects of streptomycin on *E. coli*. Federation Proc. **21**, 412a (1962).
WHITE, J. R., and H. L. WHITE: Streptomycinoid antibiotics: synergism by puromycin. Science **146**, 772 (1964).
WHITFIELD jr., H., R. MARTIN, and B. AMES: Classification of aminotransferase (*C* gene) mutants in the histidine operon. J. Mol. Biol. **21**, 335 (1966).
YOUMANS, G. P., and M. W. FISHER: Action of streptomycin on microorganisms *in vitro*. In: Streptomycin, nature and practical applications (S. A. WAKSMAN, ed.). Baltimore: Williams & Wilkins Co. 1949.

Addenda

Penicillin-Cephalosporin

Although we don't see how the recent data on multiple drug resistance is related to the mechanism of action of the penicillin-cephalosporin drugs, we feel that certain aspects of resistance development should be noted at this time. OCHIAI *et al.* (1959) and AKIBA (1959) independently reported the hereditary character of multiple drug resistance in strains of *Enterobacteriaceae.* The medical importance of the extrachromosomal episomal infective drug resistance transfer factors has only recently been emphasized (WALTON, 1966; KABINS and COHEN, 1966). Penicillinase synthesis has been adequately demonstrated to be mediated via R-factor episomes in *E. coli* by DATTA and RICHMOND (1966). How these infective transfer factors (R-factors) relate to the plasmids described in staphylococci is not clear but there are similarities in the conceptual status of these factors (POSTON, 1966; ASHESHOV, 1966). The character of infectious drug resistance transfer in complex environments and during chemotherapeutic regimens between various bacterial species and their morphological variants appears to be a most vital area for intensive future research. For further consideration of these "current events" we refer the reader to PETROVSKAYA *et al.* (1964), ANDERSON (1965), ANDERSON and LEWIS (1965), and DE COURCY and SEVAG (1966).

An interesting and perhaps related, sidelight also is discussed in HUGO and STRETTON's (1966) intriguing paper concerned with the effect of cellular lipids on bacterial sensitivity to the penicillin group of drugs.

Evidence supporting a β-1,4 linkage of the N-acetylglucosamine residues in the cell wall polysaccharide of *S. aureus* has been reported by TIPPER and STROMINGER (1966).

ROLINSON (1965) has described studies which he interprets as showing that the variations in antibacterial activity of penicillins may be ascribed to different "affinities" for the bacterial cell rather than to differences in mode of action.

References

AKIBA, T.: Mechanism of development of resistance in Shigella. Medicine of Japan in 1959. [In Japanese.] Proc. 15th Gen. Meeting of the Japan Med. Assoc. **5**, 299 (1959).

ANDERSON, E. S.: Origin of transferable drug-resistance factors in the Enterobacteriaceae. Brit. Med. J. **1965 II**, 1289.

ANDERSON, E. S., and M. J. LEWIS: Drug resistance and its transfer in *S. typhimurium*. Nature **206**, 579 (1965).

ASHESHOV, E. H.: Chromosomal location of the genetic elements controlling penicillinase production in a strain of *S. aureus*. Nature **210**, 804 (1966).

DATTA, N., and M. H. RICHMOND: The purification and properties of a penicillinase whose synthesis is mediated by an R-factor in *Escherichia coli*. Biochem. J. **98**, 204 (1966).

De Courcy, S. J., and M. G. Sevag: Specificity and prevention of antibiotic resistance in *S. aureus*. Nature **209**, 373 (1966).
Hugo, W. B., and R. J. Stretton: The role of cellular lipid in the resistance of gram-positive bacteria to penicillins. J. Gen. Microbiol. **42**, 133 (1966).
Kabins, S. A., and S. Cohen: Resistance-transfer factor in Enterobacteriaceae. New Engl. J. Med. **275**, 248 (1966).
Ochiai, K., T. Yamanaka, K. Kimura, and O. Sawada: Studies on inheritance of drug resistance between Shigella strains and *Escherichia coli* strains. [In Japanese.] Nippon Iji Shimpo **1861**, 34 (1959).
Petrovskaya, V. G., V. S. Levashev, and H. V. Davydova: Loss of the ability to transmit the colicinogenic factor I by penicillin spheroplasts and L-forms. [In Russian.] Zhur. Mikrobiol. Epidemiol. Immunol. (3) March, 22 (1966).
Poston, S. M.: Cellular location of the genes controlling penicillinase production and resistance to streptomycin and tetracycline in a strain of *S. aureus*. Nature **210**, 802 (1966).
Rolinson, G. N.: Antibacterial activity of penicillin. I. The nature of the activity of different acyl derivatives of 6-aminopenicillanic acid. Proc. Roy. Soc. (London), Ser. XIII **163**, 417 (1965).
Tipper, D. J., and J. L. Strominger: Isolation of 4-O-β-N-acetylmuramyl-N-acetylglucosamine and 4-O-β-N,6-O-diacetylmuramyl-N-acetylglucosamine and the structure of the cell wall polysaccharide of *Staphylococcus aureus*. Biochem. Biophys. Res. Commun. **22**, 48 (1966).
Walton, J. R.: *In vivo* transfer of infectious drug resistance. Nature **211**, 312 (1966).

Edwin H. Flynn and Carl W. Godzeski

Polyenes

Since the completion of the review of polyenes in November, 1965, several additional articles on these antibiotics have appeared. These papers deal with: an indirect effect of nystatin on the nucleus of *Candida* (Fujino *et al.*, 1962); the effect of nystatin on germination of *Aspergillus* spores (Stanley and English, 1965); the effect of amphotericin B on toad bladder permeability (Lichtenstein and Leaf, 1965); the action of filipin on *Pythium* species of fungi (Schlösser and Gottlieb, 1966a) and bovine erythrocytes (Schlösser and Gottlieb, 1966b); the effect of these antibiotics on lysosomes (Weissmann *et al.*, 1966), liposomes (Sessa, 1966), and artificial bilayer membranes (Zutphen, van Deenen, and Kinsky, 1966).

The experiments discussed in Section VIII of the review suggest that the polyene antibiotics may act by inducing a rearrangement of lipids within the cell membrane. Further evidence has now been obtained by electron microscopic examination of natural and artificial membranes which had been negatively stained with phosphotungstate (Kinsky, Luse, and van Deenen, 1966). "Pits" were apparent in erythrocyte membranes prepared by lysis with filipin, amphotericin B, or nystatin; they were not present in ghosts obtained by dilution with water. Similar pits were found in polyene treated membrane systems prepared from equimolar quantities of lecithin and cholesterol; they were not found after antibiotic treatment of membranes containing lecithin only. It seems particularly significant that the pits obtained with the polyenes were markedly different from those which saponin produced in the same membrane preparations. Whereas the latter are hexagonal in shape and appear in regular array, those produced by the antibiotics are more nearly circular and are distributed randomly. Thus, it appears likely the detailed mode of action of the polyenes and saponins is not identical although both classes of compounds interact with sterols. The pits obtained with the polyenes are, in fact, remarkably similar to those found in erythrocyte membranes after immune lysis in the presence of complement (BORSOS, DOURMASHKIN, and HUMPHREY, 1964).

References

BORSOS, T., R. R. DOURMASHKIN, and J. H. HUMPHREY: Lesions in erythrocyte membranes caused by immune hemolysis. Nature **202**, 251 (1964).

FUJINO, T., T. KAMIKI, Y. AKITA, and M. AKAGI: Morphological studies on the mode of action of nystatin on *Candida albicans*. Biken J. **5**, 233 (1962).

KINSKY, S. C., S. A. LUSE, and L. L. M. VAN DEENEN: Interaction of polyene antibiotics with natural and artificial membrane systems. In: Symposium on Lipid-Protein Interactions. Federation Proc. **25**, 1503 (1966).

LICHTENSTEIN, N. S., and A. LEAF: Effect of amphotericin B on permeability of the toad bladder. J. Clin. Invest. **8**, 1328 (1965).

SCHLÖSSER, E., and D. GOTTLIEB: Sterols and the sensitivity of Pythium species to filipin. J. Bacteriol. **91**, 1080 (1966a).

SCHLÖSSER, E., and D. GOTTLIEB: Mode of hemolytic action of antifungal polyene antibiotic filipin. Z. Naturforsch. **21**b, 74 (1966b).

SESSA, G.: Effect of polyene antibiotics on artificial liposomes. Federation Proc. **25**, 358 (1966).

STANLEY, V. C., and M. P. ENGLISH: Some effects of nystatin on the growth of four Aspergillus species. J. Gen. Microbiol. **40**, 107 (1965).

WEISSMANN, G., R. HIRSCHHORN, M. PRAS, and V. BEVANS: Effect of polyene antibiotics on lysosomes. Federation Proc. **25**, 358 (1966).

ZUTPHEN, H. VAN, L. L. M. VAN DEENEN, and S. C. KINSKY: The action of polyene antibiotics on bilayer lipid membranes. Biochem. Biophys. Res. Commun. **22** (1966).

STEPHEN C. KINSKY

Polymyxins and Circulin

B. colistinus was reported to elaborate a colistin-inactivating enzyme (colistinase) which was partially purified. Preliminary data indicated that the material also inactivated polymyxin sulfate and casein. The protein was immunologically indistinguishable from Nagarse, a proteinase elaborated by *B. subtilis*.

Reference

ITO, M., T. AIDA, and Y. KOYAMA: Studies on the bacterial formation of a peptide antibiotic, colistin. I. On the enzymatic inactivation of colistin by *Bacillus colistinus*. Agr. Biol. Chem. **30**, 1112 (1966).

OLDRICH. K. SEBEK

Sarkomycin

DNase from Ehrlich ascites tumor cells is inhibited by sarkomycin and the inhibition can be prevented by the addition of 2-mercaptoethanol [Proc. Canad. Fed. Biol. Soc. **9**, 10 (1966)]. The DNase activity when native DNA is the substrate is more resistant to sarkomycin than when heat denatured DNA is used as substrate.

SHAN-CHING SUNG

Chloramphenicol

The idea that susceptibility to chloramphenicol resides in ribosomes and that ribosomes are the site of action of the antibiotic has been further advanced by studies of ANDERSON and SMILLIE (1966) which show that cytoplasmic ribosomes of green plants bind less chloramphenicol than do chloroplast ribosomes from the same plant cells. Cytoplasmic protein synthesis in plants is insensitive to the antibiotic while the synthesis of chloroplast proteins is inhibited by chloramphenicol.

WEBER and DE MOSS (1966) have shown that the binding of messenger RNA to ribosomes *in vivo* as indicated by polysome formation is not inhibited in *E. coli* by chloramphenicol and that the release of finished protein molecules from the ribosome-messenger RNA assemblage is also not influenced by the antibiotic. However, chloramphenicol inhibits the process of peptide chain growth, i.e. steps that are common to the formation of all peptide bonds of a protein.

References

ANDERSON, L. A., and R. M. SMILLIE: Binding of chloramphenicol by ribosomes from chloroplasts. Biochem. Biophys. Res. Commun. **23**, 535 (1966).

WEBER, M. J., and J. A. DE MOSS: The inhibition by chloramphenicol of nascent protein formation in *E. coli*. Proc. Natl. Acad. Sci. U.S. **55**, 1223 (1966).

FRED E. HAHN

Chloramphenicol

A series of structural analogues of chloramphenicol have been prepared by COUTSOGEORGOPOULOS (1966) and were tested as inhibitors of protein synthesis in an *Escherichia coli* cell-free system. In all cases, the chloramphenicol was modified by replacement of the dichloroacetyl group with an α-aminoacyl group and/or reduction of the nitro group to an amino group.

The author reported that, of the twelve compounds tested, only the following three were as effective as chloramphenicol in the inhibition of poly-U directed incorporation of L-phenylalanine-^{14}C: 1. the L-leucyl analogue, 2. the L-p-methoxyphenylalanyl analogue and 3. the reduced L-leucyl analogue. None of the derivatives were as effective as chloramphenicol in the inhibition of poly-(U, C) directed incorporation of L-phenylalanine-^{14}C; however, the following compounds were about 60—80% as effective: 1. the glycyl analogue, 2. the L-leucyl analogue, 3. the L-phenylalanyl analogue, and 4. the L-p-methoxyphenylalanyl analogue. The structure of the N-acyl group and the presence of a nitro group are therefore important in determining the effectiveness of the chloramphenicol derivatives as inhibitors of protein synthesis. The nature of the messenger-RNA is apparently critical in determining the effectiveness of the analogues.

The author points out that chloramphenicol may exist in a conformation in which the three carbon side chain in part of a cyclic structure which results from hydrogen bond formation between the primary and secondary hydroxyl groups. In this conformation, chloramphenicol resembles uridylic acid as well as the antibiotics blasticidin S and gougerotin. It thus may act as a conformational analogue of peptidyl-sRNA or aminoacyl-sRNA and thereby inhibit either the formation of the peptide bond or the growth of the polypeptide chain.

Reference

COUTSOGEORGOPOULOS, C.: On the mechanism of action of chloramphenicol in protein synthesis. Biochim. et Biophys. Acta **129**, 214 (1966).

PAUL D. SHAW

Tetracyclines

In a review article on the mode of action of the tetracyclines, FRANKLIN (1966) discussed the various effects of the tetracyclines and concluded that the specific inhibition of protein biosynthesis at some late stage in the synthetic sequence appeared to be their most important effect at bacteriostatic concentrations. CARTER and MCCARTY (1966), in a general review of molecular mechanisms of antibiotic action, suggested that the specific step inhibited is the aminoacyl-sRNA binding reaction.

Based on the kinetics of inhibition of growth by subinhibitory concentrations of tetracycline and chloramphenicol, GARRETT *et al.* (1966) proposed a quantitative model for the inhibition, which is consistent with a binding of the antibiotics to receptor sites on the ribosomes, resulting in lowered protein synthesis.

DAY (1966a and b) reported on his detailed studies on binding of tetracycline to the components of the *E. coli* cell-free system for protein synthesis. He observed binding to both the 30 S and 50 S subunits of the 70 S ribosomes as well as to polyuridylic acid (poly U) and polyadenylic acid (poly A). Only when bound to ribosomes, however, was the antibiotic inhibitory to the cell-free assay (DAY, 1966b). When isolated 50S ribosomal subunits were treated with tetracycline, recombined with 30S subunits to form 70S ribosomes, and then again dissociated, tetracycline was found to be bound to both subunits (DAY, 1966b). It was not possible, therefore, to resolve the location of the precise site of inhibition on the ribosome by these techniques.

SUZUKA *et al.* (1966) determined that the 30S subunits of *E. coli* ribosomes bound phenylalanyl-sRNA in the presence of polyuridylic acid, and that this binding was inhibited by the tetracyclines. When 50S subunits were added, twice as much phenylalanyl-sRNA was bound; the 50S subunits alone did not bind aminoacyl-sRNA. They postulated that there is a tetracycline-sensitive sRNA binding site on the 30S subunit and that a second sRNA binding site is generated by the formation of 70S ribosomes when the 50S subunits are added.

IZAKI *et al.* (1966) demonstrated that the decreased uptake of tetracycline by resistant *E. coli* cells (IZAKI and ARIMA, 1963; FRANKLIN and GODFREY, 1965) occurred simultaneously with an increased level of resistance, and that these effects occurred only when the cells were grown in the presence of antibiotics of the tetracycline group. Other antibiotics, such as chloramphenicol or streptomycin did not cause such a decrease in the uptake of tetracycline, despite the fact that the organism carried the multiple resistance factor and was also resistant to these drugs. Resistance in these cells, therefore, was attributed to a specific decrease in the ability of the cells to take up the tetracyclines.

HOLMES and WILD (1966) extended their earlier studies (HOLMES and WILD, 1965) on inhibition of protein synthesis and stimulation of RNA synthesis by tetracyclines to include results with 6-methylene-5-hydroxy-tetracycline and demethylchlortetracycline. All tetracyclines tested with *E. coli* caused the formation of RNA-containing particles similar to those previously reported with chlortetracycline.

FUWA and OKUDA (1966) reported that tetracyclines (0.5 mM) could inhibit purified polynucleotide phosphorylase from *Micrococcus lysodeikticus* by competing either with substrate, with Mg^{++} or with K^{+}. Binding of Mg^{++} by tetracycline in the reaction mixture was demonstrated.

The arginine desimidase of *Streptococcus lactis* was found by MIKOLAJCIK (1966) to be markedly sensitive to a wide variety of antibiotics, including oxytetracycline and chlortetracycline, but the mechanism of the inhibition has not been elucidated.

YEH and SHILS (1966) attempted to clarify the situation with respect to the effect of tetracyclines on mammalian tissues. They found that tetracycline decreased incorporation of labeled amino acids into the proteins of a number of organs when given intragastrically, intramuscularly or intravenously to intact rats. The authors concluded that tetracycline can inhibit protein synthesis in mammalian species as well as in bacteria, and that such effects as negative nitrogen balance, azotemia and other uremic changes in certain patients are attributable to this inhibition.

NIKOLOV *et al.* (1966) reported that the tetracyclines inhibited antibody formation in spleen cells. Chlortetracycline was more inhibitory than either oxytetracycline or tetracycline.

References

CARTER, W., and K. S. MCCARTY: Molecular mechanisms of antibiotic action. Ann. Internal Med. **64**, 1087 (1966).
DAY, L. E.: Tetracycline inhibition of cell-free protein synthesis. I. Binding of tetracycline to components of the system. J. Bacteriol. **91**, 1917 (1966a).
DAY, L. E.: Tetracycline inhibition of cell-free protein synthesis. II. Effect of the binding of tetracycline to the components of the system. J. Bacteriol. **92**, 197 (1966b).
FRANKLIN, T. J.: Mode of action of the tetracyclines. Biochemical studies of antimicrobial drugs (B. A. NEWTON and P. E. REYNOLDS, eds.). Sixteenth Symposium, Soc. Gen. Microbiol. Cambridge: Cambridge University Press 1966, p. 192.
FUWA, I., and J. OKUDA: Inhibitory action of tetracyclines of polynucleotide phosphorylase. J. Biochem. **59**, 95 (1966) [Japan.].
GARRETT, E. R., G. H. MILLER, and M. R. W. BROWN: Kinetics and mechanisms of action of antibiotics on microorganisms. V. Chloramphenicol and tetracycline affected *Escherichia coli* generation rates. J. Pharm. Sci. **55**, 593 (1966).
HOLMES, I. A., and D. G. WILD: Consequences of inhibition of *Escherichia coli* by tetracycline antibiotics. Nature **210**, 1047 (1966).
IZAKI, K., K. KIUCHI, and K. ARIMA: Specificity and mechanism of tetracycline resistance in a multiple drug resistant strain of *Escherichia coli*. J. Bacteriol. **91**, 628 (1966).
MIKOLAJCIK, E. M.: Antibiotic influence on arginine desimidase activity by *Streptococcus lactis*. J. Dairy Sci. **48**, 1445 (1966).
NIKOLOV, T. K., B. D. STANTCHEV et S. I. BOYADJIEV: Influence des antibiotiques sur la formation des anticorps *in vitro*. I. Etude comparee de l'influence inhibitrice des tétracyclines et du chloamphénicol. Ann. inst. Pasteur **110**, Suppl. 3, 181 (1966).
SUZUKA, I., H. KAJI, and A. KAJI: Binding of specific SRNA to 30S ribosomal subunits: Effect of 50S ribosomal subunits. Proc. Natl. Acad. Sci. U.S. **55**, 1483 (1966).
YEH, S. D. J., and M. E. SHILS: Tetracycline and incorporation amino acids into proteins of rat tissues. Proc. Exptl. Biol. Med. **121**, 729 (1966).

ALLEN I. LASKIN

Streptogramin and Macrolide Antibiotics

VAZQUEZ and MONRO (1966) found that streptogramin A and the macrolide antibiotics do not affect binding of prolyl- and lysyl-s-RNA to bacterial ribosomes. Streptogramin A and a number of the macrolide antibiotics (spiramycin and derivatives, erythromycin, oleandomycin, carbomycin, and angolamycin) cause some inhibition of the binding of phenylalanyl-s-RNA to ribosomes. This inhibition is not enough to explain the inhibitory effect of the antibiotics on protein synthesis; this action is on the 50S subunit of the ribosome. On the other hand, streptogramin B and viridogrisein stimulate the binding of phenylalanyl-, prolyl- and lysyl-s-RNA to ribosomes; this effect is located on the 30S subunit of the bacterial ribosome. VAZQUEZ (1966) has shown that streptogramin A and spiramycin III act specifically on the 50S ribosomal subunit of 70S bacterial ribosomes Ammonium ions are required for this binding.

EBRINGER (1965) has shown that the macrolide antibiotics do not affect growth of *Euglena gracilis* but cause complete bleaching of the same algae; this is not surprising as it is known that cytoplasmic ribosomes of green plants (80 S ribosomes) are different than chloroplast ribosomes (70 S). G. A. M. CROSS (personal communication) found that streptogramin A and antibiotics of the streptogramin B and macrolide groups do not inhibit protein synthesis in a cell-free system from the protozoa *Crithidia oncopelti* (ribosomes 80 S). From these reports and from the evidence included in previous chapters in this book, it can be concluded that antibiotics of the streptogramin A, streptogramin B and macrolide groups act on 70 S but not on 80 S ribosomes. Antibiotics of the streptogramin A and the macrolide groups act specifically on the 50 S subunit of 70 S ribosomes at some step after the binding of aminoacyl-s-RNA to ribosomes. Antibiotics of the streptogramin B group act on the 30 S subunit of the 70 S ribosomes.

References

EBRINGER, L.: Macrolide antibiotics as bleaching factors for *Euglena gracilis*. Naturwissenschaften **52**, 666 (1965).

VAZQUEZ, D.: Inhibitors of protein synthesis at the ribosome level. Studies on their site of action. Biochem. Biophys. Res. Commun. (submitted) (1966).

VAZQUEZ, D., and R. E. MONRO: Effects of some inhibitors of protein synthesis on the binding of aminoacyl-s-RNA to ribosomes. Science (submitted) (1966).

D. VAZQUEZ

Erythromycin

In a recent personal communication, TAUBMAN *et al.* have reported that H^3-erythromycin binds to the 50 S ribosomal subunits of sensitive *Bacillus subtilis* but fails to bind to the same subunits of an erythromycin-resistant mutant of *B. subtilis*. The ribosomal binding of erythromycin was not reversed by chloramphenicol. TAUBMAN *et al.* relate the binding of erythromycin to ribosomes of susceptible bacteria to the effects of the antibiotic on bacterial growth and protein synthesis.

WOLFE and HAHN (in preparation) have recently found that erythromycin inhibits the polymerization of phenylalanine in a poly U-ribosome system of *E. coli* origin twice as strongly as the poly U-directed binding of transfer RNA in the analogous dynamic system. In time course experiments on the poly U-directed binding of phenylalanyl-transfer RNA to ribosomes, erythromycin decreased significantly the rate of binding.

FRED E. HAHN

Sparsomycin

More recent studies on the action of sparsomycin have confirmed the studies of Slechta that its action is indeed on protein synthesis with RNA synthesis continuing in the presence of the antibiotic, and that polypeptide synthesis is also inhibited in cell free preparations of *Escherichia coli*. In their current paper, GOLDBERG and MITSUGI (1967a) showed that with either synthetic or natural messenger, polypeptide synthesis was inhibited. The poly C, poly A, and poly U directed syntheses with proline, lysine, and phenyl alanine, respectively, were most sensitive to sparsomycin in that order. The order was similar with free amino acids or aminoacyl RNA. The synthesis directed with copolymers of uridylate was more sensitive than that directed by uridylate alone. No significant miscoding resulted from the action of sparsomycin when compared to that of streptomycin. The site action of sparsomycin is after the formation of the aminoacyl-sRNA-ribosome complex for it did not interfere with the formation of the complex. There appeared to be no antagonism between chloramphenicol and sparsomycin for the binding site, unlike the action of erythromycin in which the binding of chloramphenicol was decreased 94%. A sparsomycin resistant amino acid incorporating system was also present when endogenous messenger was used. Sparsomycin probably acts differently from chloramphenicol and gougerotin in inhibiting protein synthesis.

Sparsomycin also hinders the release by puromycin of polyphenylalanine containing polypeptides from prelabeled ribosomes. The antibiotic is a competitive inhibitor or puromycin. Its main action appears to be on the peptide bond forming step (GOLDBERG and MITSUGI, 1967b).

References

GOLDBERG, I. H., and K. MITSUGI; Sparsomycin inhibition of polypeptide synthesis promoted by synthetic and natural polynucleotides. Biochemistry **6**, 372 (1967a).

GOLDBERG, I. H., and K. MITSUGI: Inhibition by sparsomycin and other antibiotics of the puromycin induced relase of polypeptide from ribosomes. Biochemistry **6**, 383 (1967b).

DAVID GOTTLIEB

Cordycepin

Recently WILLIAMSON [WILLIAMSON, J.: Cordycepin, an antitumor antibiotic with trypanocidal properties. Trans. Roy. Soc. of Trop. Med. Hyg. **60**, 8 (1966)], has shown that cordycepin is trypanocidal. *In vitro*, it inhibits the infectivity, respiration, and glycolysis of *Trypanosoma rhodesiense* at concentrations of 10^{-6} to 10^{-7} M. A curative dose for *T. rhodesiense in vivo* has not yet been achieved. It is not curative at 400 mg/kg although it is therapeutically active at 12.5 mg/kg. It has also been tested *in vivo* against *T. cruzi* and *T. congolense*. On the former there appears to be little effect; on the latter it appears to be curative at 25 mg/kg and therapeutic as low as 6.25 mg/kg. Therapeutic doses of cordycepin produce abnormal division forms of *T. rhodesiense* and *T. congolense*. It appears to produce aberrant multinuclear forms. This would seem to imply in these organisms that a direct effect on nucleic acids is involved.

ARMAND J. GUARINO

Sideromycins

The DNA dependent DNA synthesis does not seem to be inhibited by sideromycins (these tests were carried out by Dr. G. HARTMANN, Institut für organische Chemie, Universität Würzburg, Würzburg, Germany). There is also evidence that the DNA dependent RNA synthesis is also not influenced by sideromycins. Our data show that protein synthesis is influenced by sideromycins. There was a strong inhibition of leucine-^{14}C incorporation into proteins by low doses of sideromycins.

It has been possible to demonstrate with a cell-free system that the formation of glutamic acid from citrate is not inhibited by sideromycins. In a resting cell system with the capacity to synthesize high amounts of glutamic acid, we could demonstrate that the inhibition of the formation of glutamic acid by sideromycins must primarily be due to an inhibition of growth. Secondarily, there is a selection of a sideromycin resistant population which no longer excretes high amounts of glutamic acid. This population does not seem to be genetically very stable, since there is a remarkable tendency to back mutation.

J. NÜESCH and F. KNÜSEL

Antimycin A

An antimycin A-sensitive function has been implicated in the mechanism of blood clotting. MÜRER (1966) has observed that antimycin A is a potent inhibitor of clot retraction as promoted by blood platelets under conditions of restricted glycolysis (low glucose).

REPORTER (1966) reported further investigations on the reversal of inhibition of respiration caused by antimycin A. A soluble protein (CAAF), obtained from chicken liver mitochondria, was found to mitigate inhibition of respiration in antimycin A-treated mitochondria. This reversal of inhibition was only obtained in mitochondria that were tightly coupled with respect to oxidative phosphorylation. Bovine serum albumin (BSA) was observed to enhance the fluorescence of antimycin A at 421 mμ when excited at 348 mμ. The BSA-bound antimycin A also exhibited a characteristic fluorescence on excitation of the protein at 278 mμ. Both types of fluorescence were quenched by CAAF. It was postulated that antimycin A is capable of forming a ternary complex with BSA and CAAF, and that this type of complex formation is a possible cause of the effects of antimycin A on mitochondrial respiration. It also was suggested that antimycin A may react at two sites in the respiratory chain, the site and tenacity of binding being different for coupled and noncoupled respiratory systems, respectively.

Recent studies conducted in the laboratory of the author (RIESKE *et al.*, 1966a and b) have added significant information on the nature of the binding of antimycin A to Complex III of the respiratory chain. Antimycin A bound to Complex III that had been inactivated by heating or by bile salts does not equilibrate significantly in its binding after addition of enzymically active Complex III. Under certain conditions guanidinium salts and organic mercurials can cause the cytochrome *b*-cytochrome c_1 cleavage even after treatment of the complex with antimycin A. Under these circumstances the binding of antimycin A to the treated complex is destroyed concomitant to cleavage as indicated by release of antimycin A in a fully inhibitory form. These results emphasize the necessity of an intact protein conformation in Complex III for the binding of antimycin A at its specific site of inhibition.

Recent studies in this laboratory indicate that the three-step cleavage of Complex III by taurocholate plus ammonium sulfate (cf. Fig. 4 in the review) may not be applicable to a general mechanism of cleavage. Guanidinium salts were found to be more potent reagents for the cleavage of Complex III than bile salts. However, with these reagents, steps of cleavage corresponding to K_2 and K_3 only are observed. Also, because of the well-known action of guanidinium salts in protein denaturation, the proposed mechanism of cleavage involving hydrolysis as the principal feature may require modification.

References

MÜRER, E. H.: Role of energy metabolism of platelets in clot retraction. *Information Exchange Group No. 2*, Scientific Memo No. 123 (1966).

REPORTER, M.: Interaction of antimycin A with biological systems. Biochemistry **5**, 2416 (1966).

RIESKE, J. S., S. LIPTON, and H. BAUM: In preparation.

RIESKE, J. S., C. D. STONER, and H. BAUM: In preparation.

JOHN S. RIESKE

Valinomycin

A recent report by HÖFER and PRESSMAN (1966) provides additional evidence that valinomycin acts by altering the permeability of mitochondrial membranes. This antibiotic is known to be an uncoupler of oxidative phosphorylation. These workers have observed, however, that not only respiration but also phosphorylation is stimulated in the presence of valinomycin plus appropriate levels of potassium ions. Oxygen consumption is increased to about the levels observed with uncouplers such as 2,4-dinitrophenol, but P/O ratios are not altered. It was suggested that the antibiotic acts by inducing the transport of potassium ions into the mitochondria. When the potassium transport reaches a certain rate, the concentration of potassium rises to a level sufficiently high to activate the transfer of energy from a high-energy intermediate into ATP.

The authors point out that the induction of potassium transport is not sufficient in itself to cause an increase in ATP formation. Gramicidin, for example, which induces both potassium and sodium ion transport, does not stimulate phosphorylation in the presence of either ion. The actin antibiotics on the other hand, resemble valinomycin; they also induce both potassium and sodium transport but stimulate phosphorylation only in the presence of potassium.

Reference

Höfer, M., and B. C. Pressman: Stimulation of oxidative phosphorylation in mitochondria by potassium in the presence of valinomycin. Biochemistry 5, 3919 (1966).

Paul D. Shaw

Nonactin

Graven *et al.* (1967) have reported that the nonactin antibiotics at concentrations as low as $10^{-9}\,M$ induced the energy dependent uptake of potassium by mitochondria. This uptake was observed at potassium concentrations as low as 1 mM. At high concentrations of potassium (>100 mM), the nonactin antibiotics stimulated respiration and induced mitochondrial swelling. Since these processes all require an anion such as phosphate or acetate, it was suggested that potassium and the anion move into the mitochondria together. The nonactin-stimulated ion uptake was inhibited by nigericin; however, this inhibition was reversed by pretreatment of the mitochondria with higher concentrations of potassium and phosphate.

In mitochondria that were disrupted by sonic oscillation, monactin no longer was able to cause an accumulation of potassium. Under these conditions, respiration was stimulated and an alteration of the light scattering behavior was observed. Nigericin, which inhibited the oxidation of glutamate in intact mitochondria, did not inhibit oxidation of that substrate in the sonic disrupted mitochondria. From these observations the authors concluded that the monactin stimulated respiration was related to an increased energy requirement which was necessary to maintain an ion concentration gradient within the intact mitochondria. Under these conditions, nigericin inhibited the uptake of potassium and phosphate into inner compartments which contain potassium and phosphate requiring dehydrogenases. In sonic oscillated mitochondria, on the other hand, the compartments were disrupted, and the inhibition of respiration by nigericin was prevented.

Reference

GRAVEN, S. N., H. A. LARDY, and S. ESTRADA-O.: Antibiotics as tools for metabolic studies. VIII. Effect of nonactin homologs on alkali metal cation transport and rate of respiration in mitochondria. Biochemistry **6**, 365 (1967).

PAUL D. SHAW

Novobiocin

In *Escherichia coli* strain 15 T⁻Arg⁻, growth is inhibited by novobiocin. After 60 minutes the net synthesis of DNA and RNA were 19 and 48% of the control respectively, but protein synthesis and permeability were only affected later. Removal of the drug allowed synthesis of nucleic acids to proceed. *In vitro* studies indicated that the antibiotic probably interfered with the polymerization of DNA. Moreover, novobiocin inhibited the replication of RNA phage, MS-2 and the DNA phages, T_2 and T_3. No DNA bound antibiotic was found (SMITH and DAVIS, 1965).

Further studies with *E. coli* confirm that the primary effect of novobiocin is on DNA synthesis. RNA synthesis decreased later, then protein and cell wall synthesis. The inhibition of nucleic acid synthesis by the antibiotic is on the template-polymerase complexes (SMITH and DAVIS, 1967).

Reference

SMITH, D. H., and B. D. DAVIS: Mode of action of novobiocin in *Escherichia coli*. J. Bacteriol. **93**, 71 (1967).
SMITH, D. H., and B. D. DAVIS: Inhibition on nucleic acid synthesis by novobiocin. Biochem. Res. Commun. **18**, 796 (1965).

DAVID GOTTLIEB

Viomycin

Viomycin apparently inhibits protein synthesis. The studies of DAVIES *et al.* (1965) showed the reduction of amino acid incorporation into polypeptides using the following synthetic polynucleotides: poly U for phenylalanine, poly C for proline and poly A for lysine. The antibiotic did not increase the incorporation of other amino acids and did not cause a misreading of the code.

Reference

DAVIES, J., L. GORINI, and B. D. DAVIS: Misreading of RNA code words induced by aminoglycoside antibiotics. Mol. Pharmacol. **1**, 93 (1965).

PAUL D. SHAW

Colicin

BEPPU and ARIMA (1967) have shown that in media of high osmotic pressure the lethal effects of Colicin E_2 and K were reduced. They suggest that the reason for this is a structural change in the cell membrane so that the colicin is not as readily transported into the cell. Thus one mechanism of action of the antibiotic is on a membrane transport system.

Reference

BEPPU, T., and K. ARIMA: Protection of *Escherichia coli* from lethal effect of colicin by high osmotic pressure. J. Bacteriol. **93**, 80 (1967).

DAVID GOTTLIEB

Antibiotic U-20,661

U-20,661 is a new antibiotic isolated from the culture broth of *Streptomyces steffisburgensis var. steffisburgensis sp. n.* The agent inhibits gram-positive but not gram-negative bacteria *in vitro*. It is extremely cytotoxic in mammalian cell cultures and remarkably non-toxic in mice.

The agent inhibits DNA-directed RNA synthesis specifically by binding to the double-stranded DNA template. Specific binding to DNA was verified by difference spectroscopy, reversal of the RNA polymerase inhibitory effect by increasing concentrations of DNA template and by increasing the melting temperature (Tm) of double-stranded DNA in the presence of the antibiotic. The RNA polymerase reaction primed with synthetic poly dAT was inhibited considerably but not completely despite high concentrations of antibiotic. Thus, the agent might bind to adenine or thymidine or both bases in the double-stranded DNA-helix.

F. REUSSER

Antibiotic 6270 (Echinomycin-like)

Antibiotic 6270 suppressed RNA synthesis selectively in both *Bacillus subtilis* and Ehrlich ascites carcinoma cells. In acellular systems from *Escherichia coli* it also inhibited the RNA dependent synthesis of RNA. The effect is caused by the inhibition of the RNA polymerase reaction.

Reference

GAUZE, G. G., V. DUDNIK, N. B. LOSHGAREVA, and I. B. ZBARSKY: Inhibition of RNA synthesis by antibiotic 6270 from Echinomycin group in bacterial and tissue cells. Antibiotics [Russian] **11**, 423 (1966).

DAVID GOTTLIEB

Amicetin

Amicetin is produced by *Streptomyces vinaceus, S. fasciculatus* and *S. plicatus.* Allomycin and sacromycin are identical with amicetin. The antibiotic inhibits many Gram positive bacteria at low concentrations, between 1 and 23 μg/ml, but other bacteria such as *Corynebacterium xeros* and *Sarcina lutea* were not inhibited by 100 μg. Growth of Gram negative bacteria and fungi were not readily prevented. The structure of amicetin is that of a substituted cytosine as given below:

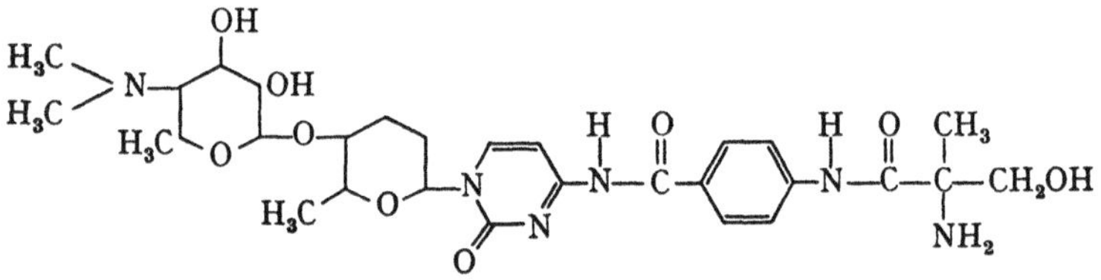

BROCK (1963) first pointed to its possible role in protein synthesis. Recent studies by BLOCH and COUTSOGEORGOPOULOS (1966) showed that amicetin inhibited protein synthesis in growing *Escherichia coli* cells, then reduced RNA and DNA synthesis, thus implicating protein synthesis as the prime site of action. This synthesis was also inhibited in a cell-free system. Amicetin did not prevent the formation of phenylalanyl-RNA, nor did the antibiotic prevent the binding of L-[^{14}C]-phenylalanine-RNA to the ribosomes. There is some speculation that the presence of an aminoacyl group on one end of the molecule and a second center at the other end is responsible for the binding to ribosomes of amicetin as well as other similar antibiotics.

References

BLOCH, T. D., and C. COUTSOGEORGOPOULOS: Inhibition of protein synthesis by amicetin, a nucleoside antibiotic. Biochem. **5**, 3345 (1966).

BROCK, T. D: Effect of antibiotics and inhibitors on M protein synthesis. J. Bacteriol. **85**, 527 (1963).

DAVID GOTTLIEB

Bruneomycin

Bruneomycin is produced by *Streptomyces albus var bruneomycini* and is structurally related to streptonigrin. Bruneomycin selectively inhibits the synthesis of DNA in whole cells of *Escherichia coli*. The antibiotic caused degradation of DNA in these cells even when the reduplication of DNA was not occurring or when protein synthesis had been blocked by chloramphenicol. The antibiotic did not depress DNA synthesis in *E. coli* acellular systems. Decreasing the temperature down to 2 C terminated the degradation of DNA which had been induced by bruneomycin. It strongly inhibited the growth of transplantable tumors in laboratory animals when administered orally. Bruneomycin was clinically effective when given orally in the treatment of leukemia reticulosis and lymphogranulomatosis. The antibiotic induced phage production in lysogenic bacteria.

References

DUDNIK, Y. V.: Induction of lysogenic Micrococcus lysodecticus by antibiotics with the ability to affect DNA synthesis. Antibiotiki **10**, 112 (1965).

DUDNIK, Y. V., and G. G. GAUSE: Studies of the mechanism of action of bruneomycin. Antibiotiki **10**, 880 (1965).

GAUSE, G. F.: Aspects of antibiotic research. Chem. & Ind. (London) **1966**, 1506.

DAVID GOTTLIEB

Phytoactin

Phytoactin is a non-cyclic polypeptide that inhibits the growth of some fungi and bacteria. It does not affect the permeability of *Saccharomyces pastorianus* to phosphorus containing compounds nor to the uptake of inorganic phosphorus. Respiration is inhibited to only a small degree. With glucose-^{14}C as substrate, the synthesis of small molecules and polysaccharides was not inhibited. Protein synthesis was retarded somewhat, but the greatest effect was on the formation of RNA. Relatively long exposures of the yeast to phytoactin reduced RNA synthesis 80 to 90%.

Reference

LYNCH, J. P., and H. D. SISLER: Mechanism of action of phytoactin in *Saccharomyces pastorianus*. Phytopathology **57**, 367 (1967).

DAVID GOTTLIEB

List of Antibiotics According to their Sites of Action

The antibiotics are arranged in various inhibition categories on the basis of the available information on their primary sites of action. Occasionally, the same antibiotic is listed under two headings because two sites of action might be possible. The action of some of the antibiotics are exactly known whereas, information on others is less exact and their position in the table will have to be changed as more information becomes available.

Cell Wall Synthesis

Bacitracin
Cephalosporin
D-Cycloserine
O-Carbamyl-D-serine
Penicillin
Ristocetin
Vancomycin

Membrane Function

Albomycin
Amphotericins
Antimycoin
Ascosin
Bacitracin
Candicidin
Candidin
Circulin
Colicin E 1, K
Colistin
Endomycin
Etruscomycin
Filipin
Flavicid
Fungichromin
Gramicidin S, J 1, J 2, A
Gramicidin B, C, D
Hamycin
Lagosin
Nystatin
Pentamycin
Perimycin
Pimaricin
Polyenes
Polymyxins
Rimocidin
Streptomycin
Trichomycin
Tyrocidines
Valinomycin

Ribonucleic Acid Metabolism

Aurantin
Chromomycin
Cinerubin
Colicin E 1, K, E 2, 1 a, 1 b
Daunomycin
Griseofulvin
Kanamycin
Minomycin
Mithramycin
Neomycin
Nogalamycin
Novobiocin
Olivomycin
Phytoactin
Pluramycin
Streptomycin
Streptonigrin

Deoxyribonucleic Acid Metabolism

Actidione
Actinomycin
Bruneomycin
Cinerubin
Colicin E 1, K, E 2, 1 a, 1 b, E 2, CA-42
Cycloheximides
Daunomycin
Edeine
Griseofulvin
Mitomycin A, B, C
Novobiocin
Phleomycin
Pluramycin
Porfiromycin
Sarkomycin
Streptonigrin
Xanthomycin

Purine and Pyrimidine Synthesis

Angustmycin A
Azaserine
Cordycepin
Decoyinine
DON (6-diazo-5-oxo-L-norleucine)
Hadacidin
Psicofuranine
Sangivamycin
Sarkomycin
Toyocamycin
Tubercidin

Protein Synthesis

Acetoxycycloheximide
Actinospectacin

Actiphenol
Amicetin
Angolamycin
Bacitracin
Blasticidin S
Bluensomycin
Carbomycin
Catenulin
Chalcomycin
Chloramphenicol
Chlortetracycline
Colicin E2, E3, 1a, 1b
Cycloheximide
Demethylchlortetracycline
Dihydrostreptomycin
Edeine
Erythromycin
Fermicidin
Framycetin
Fusidic Acid
Fusidin
Gentamycin
Glutarimides
Gougerotin
Hygromycin B
Hydroxystreptomycin
Inactone
Kanamycin
Kasugamycin
Lancamycin
Lincomycin
Mannosidostreptomycin
Methymycin
Mikamycin
Minomycin
Naramycin B
Neomycin
Niromycin
Nucleocidin
Ostreogrycins
Oxytetracycline
Pactomycin
Paromomycin
Protomycin
Pristinamycins
Puromycin
Rifamycin
Sarkomycin
Sparsomycin
Spectinomycin
Spiramycin
Staphylomycins
Streptimidone
Streptogramins A, B
Streptomycin
Streptonigrin
Streptoviticins
Synergistins
Tenuazonic Acid
Tetracycline
Vernamycins
Viomycin
Viridogrisein

Respiration

Antimycin A1, A2, A3, A4, A-35, A-102
Aurovertin
Flavensomycin
Nigericin
Oligomycins
Patulin
Pyocyanine
Rutamycin
Usnic Acid

Oxidative Phosphorylation

Aurovertin
Colicin E1, K
Dinactin
Gramicidin S, J1, J2, A, B, C, D
Monactin
Nonactin
Oligomycin
Rutamycin
Trinactin
Tyrocidine
Usnic Acid
Valinomycin

Other Sites

Bacitracin
Novobiocin
Sideromycin

Subject Index

Page numbers in *italics* refer to formulae and tables

Index of Organisms

GPSR Compliance

The European Union's (EU) General Product Safety Regulation (GPSR) is a set of rules that requires consumer products to be safe and our obligations to ensure this.

If you have any concerns about our products, you can contact us on ProductSafety@springernature.com

In case Publisher is established outside the EU, the EU authorized representative is:

Springer Nature Customer Service Center GmbH
Europaplatz 3
69115 Heidelberg, Germany

Batch number: 10844817

Printed by Printforce, the Netherlands